Nanoparticles for Biomedica

Nanoparticles for Biomedical Applications

Fundamental Concepts, Biological Interactions and Clinical Applications

Edited by

Eun Ji Chung
Department of Biomedical Engineering, University of Southern California
Los Angeles, CA, United States

Lorraine Leon
Department of Materials Science and Engineering, NanoScience and Technology Center
University of Central Florida Orlando, FL, United States

Carlos Rinaldi
Department of Chemical Engineering, Department of Biomedical Engineering,
University of Florida, Gainesville, FL, United States

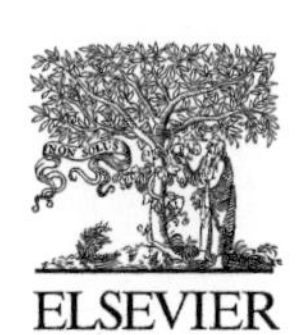

ELSEVIER

Elsevier
Radarweg 29, PO Box 211, 1000 AE Amsterdam, Netherlands
The Boulevard, Langford Lane, Kidlington, Oxford OX5 1GB, United Kingdom
50 Hampshire Street, 5th Floor, Cambridge, MA 02139, United States

Library of Congress Cataloging-in-Publication Data
A catalog record for this book is available from the Library of Congress

British Library Cataloguing-in-Publication Data
A catalogue record for this book is available from the British Library

ISBN: 978-0-12-816662-8

For information on all Elsevier publications visit our website at
https://www.elsevier.com/books-and-journals

Publisher: Matthew Deans
Acquisition Editor: Simon Holt
Editorial Project Manager: Isabella C. Silva
Production Project Manager: Anitha Sivaraj
Cover Designer: Greg Harris

Typeset by TNQ Technologies

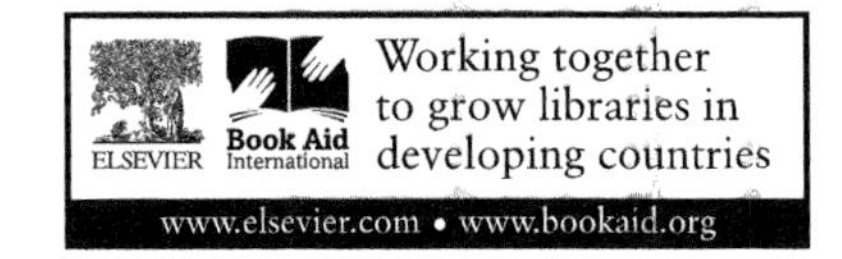

Contents

Contributors

Nicholas J. Abuid, J. Crayton Pruitt Family Department of Biomedical Engineering, University of Florida, Gainesville, FL, United States

Aitor Álvarez, Centro Singular de Investigación en Química Biolóxica e Materiais Moleculares (CiQUS), Departamento de Física de Partículas, Universidade de Santiago de Compostela, Santiago de Compostela, Spain

Candace Benjamin, Department of Chemistry and Biochemistry, University of Texas at Dallas, Richardson, Texas, United States

Agata Blasiak, N.1 Institute for Health (N.1); Department of Biomedical Engineering, NUS Engineering, National University of Singapore, Singapore

Olivia Brohlin, Department of Chemistry and Biochemistry, University of Texas at Dallas, Richardson, Texas, United States

Sean Burkitt, Department of Biomedical Engineering; Michelson Center for Convergent Biosciences, Los Angeles, CA, United States

Jos Campbell, Department of Biomedical Engineering; Michelson Center for Convergent Biosciences, Los Angeles, CA, United States

Carolina Carrillo-Carrión, Centro Singular de Investigación en Química Biolóxica e Materiais Moleculares (CiQUS), Departamento de Física de Partículas, Universidade de Santiago de Compostela, Santiago de Compostela, Spain

Yahya Cheema, Fischell Department of Bioengineering, University of Maryland, College Park, MD, United States

Andreina Chiu-Lam, Department of Chemical Engineering, University of Florida, Gainesville, FL, United States

Eun Ji Chung, Department of Biomedical Engineering; Department of Chemical Engineering and Materials Science; Eli and Edythe Broad Center for Regenerative Medicine and Stem Cell Research; Norris Comprehensive Cancer Center; Department of Surgery, Division of Vascular Surgery and Endovascular Therapy; Department of Medicine, Division of Nephrology and Hypertension, Keck School of Medicine, University of Southern California, Los Angeles, CA, United States

Nathan D. Donahue, Stephenson School of Biomedical Engineering, University of Oklahoma, Norman, OK, United States

Natalie Dong, Department of Biomedical Engineering; Michelson Center for Convergent Biosciences, Los Angeles, CA, United States

Mitsushita Doomra, NanoScience Technology Center; Burnett School of Biomedical Science, University of Central Florida, Orlando, FL, United States

Marco A. Downing, Department of Chemical Engineering, Herbert Wertheim College of Engineering, University of Florida

Omolola Eniola-Adefeso, Department of Chemical Engineering; Department of Biomedical Engineering; Macromolecular Science and Engineering Program, University of Michigan, Ann Arbor, MI, United States

Allen Eyler, Department of Materials Science and Engineering, University of Central Florida, Orlando, FL, United States

Catherine A. Fromen, Department of Chemical and Biomolecular Engineering, University of Delaware, Newark, DE, United States

Eric Fuller, J. Crayton Pruitt Family Department of Biomedical Engineering, University of Florida, Gainesville, FL, United States

Tiffany RX. Gan, N.1 Institute for Health (N.1); Department of Biomedical Engineering, NUS Engineering, National University of Singapore; Department of Surgery, National University Health System, Singapore

Jeremiah J. Gassensmith, Department of Chemistry and Biochemistry, University of Texas at Dallas, Richardson, Texas, United States

Kerim M. Gattás-Asfura, J. Crayton Pruitt Family Department of Biomedical Engineering, University of Florida, Gainesville, FL, United States

Mengjie Gu, Department of Pharmacology, National University of Singapore, Singapore; Cancer Science Institute of Singapore, National University of Singapore, Singapore, Singapore

Hao Guo, Department of Pharmacology and Pharmaceutical Sciences, School of Pharmacy, University of Southern California, Los Angeles, CA, United States

Ankur Gupta, Department of Mechanical and Aerospace Engineering; Princeton University, Princeton, NJ, United States

Dean Ho, N.1 Institute for Health (N.1); Department of Biomedical Engineering, NUS Engineering; Department of Pharmacology, Yong Loo Lin School of Medicine, National University of Singapore, Singapore

Leaf Huang, Division of Pharmacoengineering and Molecular Pharmaceutics and Center for Nanotechnology in Drug Delivery, Eshelman School of Pharmacy, University of North Carolina at Chapel Hill, Chapel Hill, NC, United States

Huang-Chiao Huang, Fischell Department of Bioengineering, University of Maryland, College Park, MD; Marlene and Stewart Greenebaum Cancer Center, University of Maryland School of Medicine, Baltimore, MD, United States

Collin T. Inglut, Fischell Department of Bioengineering, University of Maryland, College Park, MD, United States

Aaron J. Sorrin, Fischell Department of Bioengineering, University of Maryland, College Park, MD, United States

Piyush K. Jain, Department of Chemical Engineering, Herbert Wertheim College of Engineering, University of Florida

Bader M. Jarai, Department of Chemical and Biomolecular Engineering, University of Delaware, Newark, DE, United States

Edward Kai-Hua Chow, Department of Pharmacology; Cancer Science Institute of Singapore, National University of Singapore, Singapore, Singapore

Theodore Kee, N.1 Institute for Health (N.1); Department of Biomedical Engineering, NUS Engineering, National University of Singapore, Singapore

Jeffrey Khong, N.1 Institute for Health (N.1); Department of Biomedical Engineering, NUS Engineering, National University of Singapore, Singapore

Forrest M. Kievit, University of Nebraska, Department of Biological Systems Engineering, Lincoln, NE, United States

Jonathan Kin-Hun Lee, Department of Chemical Engineering, University of Michigan, Ann Arbor, MI, United States

Emily L. Kolewe, Department of Chemical and Biomolecular Engineering, University of Delaware, Newark, DE, United States

Truong Thanh Lan Anh, N.1 Institute for Health (N.1); Department of Biomedical Engineering, NUS Engineering, National University of Singapore, Singapore

Daniel J. LaShoto, J. Crayton Pruitt Family Department of Biomedical Engineering, University of Florida, Gainesville, FL, United States

Tram Le, Stephenson School of Biomedical Engineering, University of Oklahoma, Norman, OK, United States

Dao P. Le, Stephenson School of Biomedical Engineering, University of Oklahoma, Norman, OK, United States

Joanne C. Lee, Stephenson School of Biomedical Engineering, University of Oklahoma, Norman, OK, United States

Lorraine Leon, Department of Materials Science and Engineering; NanoScience and Technology Center, University of Central Florida, Orlando, FL, United States

Barry J. Liang, Fischell Department of Bioengineering, University of Maryland, College Park, MD, United States

John Andrew MacKay, Department of Pharmacology and Pharmaceutical Sciences, School of Pharmacy; Department of Biomedical Engineering, Viterbi School of Engineering; Department of Ophthalmology, Roski Eye Institute, Keck School of Medicine, University of Southern California, Los Angeles, CA, United States

Raquel Martínez, Centro Singular de Investigación en Química Biolóxica e Materiais Moleculares (CiQUS), Departamento de Física de Partículas, Universidade de Santiago de Compostela, Santiago de Compostela, Spain

Tyler Maxwell, Department of Chemistry; NanoScience Technology Center, University of Central Florida, Orlando, FL, United States

Michael McKenna, Department of Chemical Engineering, University of Washington, Seattle, WA, United States

Samantha A. Meenach, Department of Biomedical and Pharmaceutical Sciences, College of Pharmacy; Department of Chemical Engineering, College of

Engineering, University of Rhode Island, Kingston, RI, United States

Michael Mellas, Pritzker School of Molecular Engineering, University of Chicago, Chicago, IL, United States

Martina Migliavacca, Centro Singular de Investigación en Química Biolóxica e Materiais Moleculares (CiQUS), Departamento de Física de Partículas, Universidade de Santiago de Compostela, Santiago de Compostela, Spain

Daniel Najafali, Fischell Department of Bioengineering, University of Maryland, College Park, MD, United States

Elizabeth Nance, Department of Chemical Engineering; Department of Radiology; Center on Human Development and Disability; Molecular Engineering and Sciences Institute, University of Washington, Seattle, WA, United States

Steven M. Narum, Stephenson School of Biomedical Engineering, University of Oklahoma, Norman, OK, United States

María F. Navarro Poupard, Centro Singular de Investigación en Química Biolóxica e Materiais Moleculares (CiQUS), Departamento de Física de Partículas, Universidade de Santiago de Compostela, Santiago de Compostela, Spain

Jiansheng Ng, N.1 Institute for Health (N.1); Department of Biomedical Engineering, NUS Engineering, National University of Singapore, Singapore

Maria Gabriela Nogueira Campos, NanoScience Technology Center, University of Central Florida, Orlando, FL, United States; Institute of Science and Technology, Federal University of Alfenas, Poços de Caldas, Minas Gerais, Brazil

Beatriz Pelaz, Centro Singular de Investigación en Química Biolóxica e Materiais Moleculares (CiQUS), Departamento de Física de Partículas; Centro Singular de Investigación en Química Biolóxica e Materiais Moleculares (CiQUS), Departamento de Química Inorgánica, Universidade de Santiago de Compostela Santiago de Compostela, Spain

Pablo del Pino, Centro Singular de Investigación en Química Biolóxica e Materiais Moleculares (CiQUS), Departamento de Física de Partículas, Universidade de Santiago de Compostela, Santiago de Compostela, Spain

Ester Polo, Centro Singular de Investigación en Química Biolóxica e Materiais Moleculares (CiQUS), Departamento de Física de Partículas, Universidade de Santiago de Compostela, Santiago de Compostela, Spain

Alexia M. Poulos, J. Crayton Pruitt Family Department of Biomedical Engineering, University of Florida, Gainesville, FL, United States

Nisha Raman, Department of Chemical and Biomolecular Engineering, University of Delaware, Newark, DE, United States

Carlos Rinaldi, Department of Chemical Engineering; J. Crayton Pruitt Family Department of Biomedical Engineering, University of Florida, Gainesville, FL, United States

Angelie Rivera-Rodriguez, J. Crayton Pruitt Family Department of Biomedical Engineering, University of Florida, Gainesville, FL, United States

Hanieh Safari, Department of Chemical Engineering, University of Michigan, Ann Arbor, MI, United States

Swadeshmukul Santra, Department of Chemistry, University of Central Florida, Orlando, FL, United States; NanoScience Technology Center, University of Central Florida, Orlando, FL, United States; Burnett School of Biomedical Science, University of Central Florida, Orlando, FL, United States; Department of Materials Science and Engineering, University of Central Florida, Orlando, FL, United States

Shehaab Savliwala, Department of Chemical Engineering, University of Florida, Gainesville, FL, United States

Kacoli Sen, Department of Chemical Engineering, University of Florida, Gainesville, FL, United States

Nishan K. Shah, Department of Biomedical and Pharmaceutical Sciences, College of Pharmacy, University of Rhode Island, Kingston, RI, United States

Sachit Shah, Department of Materials Science and Engineering, University of Central Florida, Orlando, FL, United States

Arezoo Shahrivarkevishahi, Department of Chemistry and Biochemistry, University of Texas at Dallas, Richardson, Texas, United States

Stephen Smith, Department of Chemistry, University of Central Florida, Orlando, FL, United States; NanoScience Technology Center, University of Central Florida, Orlando, FL, United States

Enrica Soprano, Centro Singular de Investigación en Química Biolóxica e Materiais Moleculares (CiQUS), Departamento de Física de Partículas, Universidade de Santiago de Compostela, Santiago de Compostela, Spain

Jillian Stabile, Fischell Department of Bioengineering, University of Maryland, College Park, MD, United States

Cherie L. Stabler, J. Crayton Pruitt Family Department of Biomedical Engineering, University of Florida, Gainesville, FL, United States; University of Florida Diabetes Institute, Gainesville, FL, United States

Zachary S. Stillman, Department of Chemical and Biomolecular Engineering, University of Delaware, Newark, DE, United States

Sara Tabandeh, Department of Materials Science and Engineering, University of Central Florida, Orlando, FL, United States

Aria W. Tarudji, University of Nebraska, Department of Biological Systems Engineering, Lincoln, NE, United States

Marcus Threadcraft, College of Medicine, University of Florida, Gainesville, FL, United States

Zon Thwin, Department of Chemistry, University of Central Florida, Orlando, FL, United States; NanoScience Technology Center, University of Central Florida, Orlando, FL, United States

Matthew Tirrell, Pritzker School of Molecular Engineering, University of Chicago, Chicago, IL, United States

Elisa A. Torrico Guzmán, Department of Chemical Engineering, College of Engineering, University of Rhode Island, Kingston, RI, United States

Mythreyi Unni, Department of Chemical Engineering, University of Florida, Gainesville, FL, United States

Swapna Vaja, Fischell Department of Bioengineering, University of Maryland, College Park, MD, United States

Jonathan Wang, Biomedical Engineering, University of Southern California, Los Angeles, CA, United States

Peter Wang, N.1 Institute for Health (N.1), National University of Singapore, Singapore; Department of Biomedical Engineering, NUS Engineering, National University of Singapore, Singapore

Zimeng Wang, Phosphorex Inc., Hopkinton, MA, United States

Stefan Wilhelm, Stephenson School of Biomedical Engineering, University of Oklahoma, Norman, OK, United States; Stephenson Cancer Center, Oklahoma City, OK, United States

Jingru Xu, Department of Pharmacology, National University of Singapore, Singapore; Cancer Science Institute of Singapore, National University of Singapore, Singapore, Singapore

Wen Yang, Stephenson School of Biomedical Engineering, University of Oklahoma, Norman, OK, United States

Cristina Zavaleta, Department of Biomedical Engineering, University of Southern California, Los Angeles, CA, United States; Michelson Center for Convergent Biosciences, Los Angeles, CA, United States

Yuan Zhang, Department of Biomedical and Pharmaceutical Sciences, College of Pharmacy, University of Rhode Island, Kingston, RI, United States

Chapter 1

A brief history of nanotechnology and introduction to nanoparticles for biomedical applications

Lorraine Leon[1,2], Eun Ji Chung[3] and Carlos Rinaldi[4,5]

[1]Department of Materials Science and Engineering, University of Central Florida, Orlando, FL, United States; [2]NanoScience and Technology Center, University of Central Florida, Orlando, FL, United States; [3]Department of Biomedical Engineering, University of Southern California, Los Angeles, CA, United States; [4]Department of Chemical Engineering, University of Florida, Gainesville, FL, United States; [5]Department of Biomedical Engineering, University of Florida, Gainesville, FL, United States

According to the United States National Nanotechnology Initiative, nanotechnology is the understanding and control of matter at dimensions approximately between 1 and 100 nm that enable unique size-dependant properties.[1] However, slight variations of this definition exist depending on the governing body, such as the European Commission or the International Organization for Standardization (ISO) Technical Committee 229, and sometimes sizes in the 1000 nm range are considered nanomaterials. As this is an evolving field, the nomenclature is being constantly updated, most recently via the creation of an international working group establishing a uniform descriptor system for materials on the nanoscale.[2] This 1−100 nm size range can correspond to individual molecules for polymers or other macromolecules but can also include higher-order assemblies into nanoparticles. For smaller, angstrom-sized atoms and molecules, this size range consists of small clusters or nanoparticles. Material properties at the nanoscale are different compared with that of bulk materials, generally stemming from the characteristics that are pertinent to the larger surface area to volume ratio leading to changes in chemical reactivity and quantum confinement effects. For biological systems, the nanometer size range can be ideal for circulating in the blood stream, traversing tissues, and entering cells. This book surveys a variety of nanoparticles and their applications in the biomedical arena paying close attention to fundamental concepts in nanoparticle design and synthesis, the interactions and transport of nanoparticles within biological systems, and ultimately the use of nanoparticles in a clinical setting.

Examples of nanomaterials are abundant in nature, ranging from magnetotactic bacteria that use iron oxide nanoparticles to sense magnetic fields[3] to the unique colors of butterfly wings which originate from the interactions of light with complex nanoarchitectures and not absorption due to dyes or pigments.[4] Evidence of use of nanomaterials in human history can be found dating back to the fourth century AD in the form of the "Lycurgus Cup," which has unusual optical properties arising from metallic nanoparticles that make the cup appear either red or green in transmitted or reflected light, respectively.[5] These unique properties of metallic nanoparticles were analyzed by Michael Faraday in 1857, who concluded that gold at small size scales produces unusual colors.[6] A related observation that the optical properties of gold at small length scales would differ from bulk properties was made by Gustav Mie in 1908.[7] However, purposefully manipulating matter at the nanoscale is a relatively recent concept, famously conceptualized by Richard Feynman in a lecture given at the American Physical Society in 1959 titled "There is Plenty of Room at the Bottom: An Invitation to Enter a New Field of Physics".[8] This speech outlined a vision for manipulating and observing things on a small scale and how this would revolutionize many industries as well as provide answers to many fundamental questions, particularly in the context of understanding biology. The forward vision for the medical field was attributed to Albert Hibbs and his concept of "swallowing the surgeon" such that diagnosis could be made by tiny robots that access the interior of the body to identify the problem and repair it.[8] Following this speech, the actual term "nanotechnology" would not be

Nanoparticles for Biomedical Applications. https://doi.org/10.1016/B978-0-12-816662-8.00001-1

used until 1974 by Norio Tanaguchi, where he defined nanotechnology as being able to manipulate a single nanoscale object.[9]

In the early to mid 1980s, the development of the scanning tunneling microscope[10] by Binning and Rohrer (both at IBM) and the atomic force microscope[11] by Binning allowed the imaging of surfaces with atomic resolution. The imaging of atoms with the scanning tunneling microscope later led to the placement of atoms in particular positions, famously spelling out IBM using xenon atoms in 1990[12] and marking the beginning of the realization of nanotechnology. Also in the early 1980s, K. Eric Drexler at the Massachusetts Institute of Technology was developing an alternative vision for nanotechnology based on bottom-up nanotechnology or molecular engineering that focused heavily on biological mechanisms such as protein design.[13] This vision inspired by Feynman's 1959 speech led to the first book on nanotechnology[14] titled "*Engines of Creation: The Coming Era of Nanotechnology*" published in 1986 and the creation of the first organization dedicated to the development of nanotechnology, the Foresight Institute that same year. In 1985, Kroto, Heath, and Smalley from Rice University discovered the 60 carbon atom structure known as Buckminsterfullerene,[15] or colloquially the "Buckyball."

In the 1990s, the field would continue to grow, leading to the creation of the first journal dedicated to the subject titled "Nanotechnology," published by IOP Publishing in the United Kingdom and the introduction of the term "Nanomedicine" in a book coauthored by Drexler. The scientific advancements in the field continued to flourish, including different types of nanoparticles described in this book, such as the discovery of the carbon nanotube in 1991[16] (described in Chapter 14) or the discovery of the polyelectrolyte complex micelle (polyion complex micelle) by Kataoka in 1995[17] (described in Chapter 20).

Eventually, the enthusiasm and promise of nanotechnology would begin permeating the political sphere, leading to the creation of the Interagency Working Group on Nanotechnology in 1998, which catalyzed the National Nanotechnology Initiative in the United States in 2000.[18] Similar initiatives would begin around the globe, such as the Canadian National Institute for Nanotechnology formed in 2001. These surges in funding would bring many new developments to the field, particularly in the context of medicine. The United States National Institute of Health National Cancer Institute launched an alliance for nanotechnology in cancer in 2004, establishing multiinstitutional collaboration, research, training, and characterization centers. These Centers of Cancer Nanotechnology Excellence are scheduled to lose funding in 2020, claiming not lack of interest in the field but the transition of nanotechnology from an emerging field to a more established field.[19]

Nobel laureate Paul Ehrlich introduced the concept of targeted therapy or "magic bullets" that can go specifically to their intended cellular target without harming healthy tissue in the early 1900s.[20] This concept was later merged with nanotechnology into the concept of the targeted nanoparticle. The term "nanoparticle" itself began appearing in scientific publications in 1978 and, interestingly, the sole publications in 1978 and 1979 containing the word nanoparticle also contained the word "Medicine" or "Medical" (Fig. 1.1). The publication in 1978 analyzed the in vivo distribution of 400 nm gelatin nanoparticles. However, nanoparticle research was being conducted in the late 1960s and early 1970s using different terms such as "nanopellet" or "nanocapsule".[21] In addition, lipid-based nanoparticles called "liposomes" (described in Chapter 10) were discovered in the 1960s by Alec Bangham when attempting to image lipids using negative staining electron microscopy.[22] Nanoparticle research has grown tremendously throughout the years, and the proportion of nanoparticle research dedicated to the medical field is significant, as illustrated in Fig. 1.1. The remainder of this book will outline recent developments in the field of nanoparticles for biomedical applications.

Chapters 2–9 and 22 describe fundamental concepts that can be applied to a variety of nanoparticle types. Chapter 2 describes nanoparticle integrity, protein corona, and colloidal stability in biological environments. Chapter 3 describes different targeting mechanisms and targeting ligands used for nanoparticles, while Chapter 5 analyzes how size, shape, particle rigidity, and blood hemodynamics affect targeting. Chapter 4 describes passive targeting techniques specifically in the context of leaky vasculature in cancer applications. Chapter 6 describes different methods to administer nanoparticles, such as parenteral, pulmonary, nasal, oral, transdermal, and ocular. Chapter 7 describes the different surface, en-route, and cellular barriers that nanoparticles face once entering the body, and the design challenges introduced by these barriers. Chapter 8 describes how to perform and interpret pharmacokinetic studies of nanoparticles to facilitate their approval in the clinic. Chapter 9 describes common methods of characterizing nanoparticles such as electron microscopy and light-scattering techniques. Chapter 22 discusses how the emerging field of artificial intelligence can play a role in optimizing combinatorial nanoparticle therapies for oncology and infectious diseases.

Chapters 10–21 describe different types of nanoparticles and their applications in a biomedical context. Chapter 10 describes the design and fabrication of different liposomes. Chapter 11 describes proteinaceous cages, called virus-like particles. Chapter 12 discusses gold nanoparticles and their application in photothermal therapy, surgery, and imaging. Chapter 13 discusses magnetic nanoparticles and their clinical and emerging applications. Chapter 14 describes carbon-based nanoparticles such as fullerenes, nanotubes, and nanodiamonds. Chapter 15

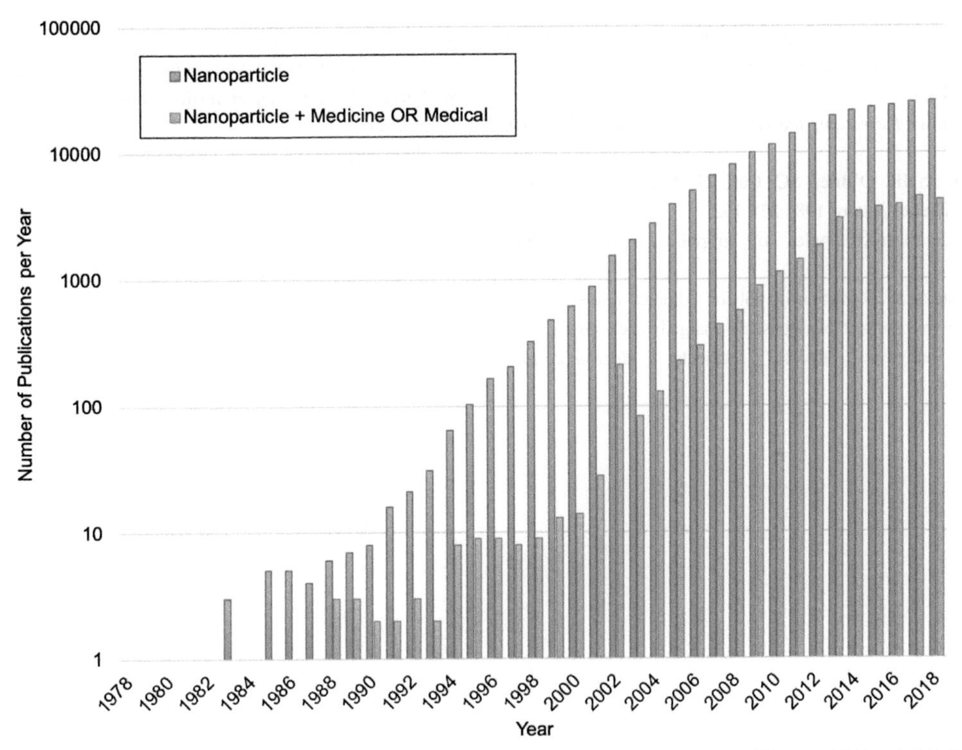

FIGURE 1.1 Publications containing the word "Nanoparticle" (Blue) and publications containing the word "Nanoparticle" and "Medicine" or "Medical" (Orange) between the years of 1978 and 2018. Analysis done using Web of Science. Please note the logarithmic y-axis.

describes quantum dots and their applications in sensing, imaging, and therapeutic delivery. Chapter 16 describes silica nanoparticles with specific pores called mesoporous silica nanoparticles. Chapter 17 describes cerium oxide nanoparticles and their role as redox modulators. Chapter 18 describes a variety of polymeric nanoparticles such as nanoshells, nanospheres, polyplexes, polymersomes, and dendrimers. Chapters 19 and 20 describe self-assembled nanoparticles. Chapter 19 focuses on self-assembly using hydrophobic interactions, such as peptide amphiphile micelles. Chapter 20 focuses on electrostatic-driven self-assembly such as bulk and nanoscale polyelectrolyte complexes and layer by layer assemblies. Chapter 21 focuses on nanoemulsions and their design for biomedical applications. The nanoparticle varieties discussed in this book represent some of the most promising for translation to the clinic.

Overall, this book is a collection of different topics that are fundamental to the design and application of nanoparticles in biomedicine and that are written by experts in the nanomedicine field. This book is intended to provide a broad understanding of the field of nanoparticles and nanomedicine for newcomers and established biomedical researchers. It is our intention that this book will also be suitable as a textbook for advanced coursework in the field of nanoparticles for biomedical applications.

References

1. Roco MC. The long view of nanotechnology development: the National Nanotechnology Initiative at 10 years. *J Nanoparticle Res* 2011;**13**:427–45.
2. Gubala V, Johnston LJ, Liu Z, Krug H, Moore CJ, Ober CK, Schwenk M, Vert M. Engineered nanomaterials and human health: part 1. Preparation, functionalization and characterization (IUPAC Technical Report). *Pure Appl Chem* 2018;**90**:1283–324.
3. Faivre D, Schüler D. Magnetotactic bacteria and magnetosomes. *Chem Rev* 2008;**108**:4875–98.
4. Srinivasarao M. Nano-optics in the biological world: beetles, butterflies, birds, and moths. *Chem Rev* 1999;**99**:1935–61.
5. Freestone I, Meeks N, Sax M, Higgitt C. The lycurgus cup — a Roman nanotechnology. *Gold Bull* 2007;**40**:270–7.
6. Faraday M. On the relations of gold and other metals to light. In: *Proceedings of the Royal Society of London*; 1857.
7. Mie G. Beiträge zur Optik trüber Medien, speziell kolloidaler Metallösungen. *Ann Phys* 1908;**330**:377–445.
8. Feynman RP. *There's plenty of Room at the bottom*. Engineering and Science; 1960. p. 22–36.
9. Mulvaney P. Nanoscience vs nanotechnology—defining the field. *ACS Nano* 2015;**9**:2215–7.
10. Binnig G, Rohrer H. Scanning tunneling microscopy—from birth to adolescence. *Rev Mod Phys* 1987;**59**:615.
11. Binnig G, Quate CF, Gerber C. Atomic force microscope. *Phys Rev Lett* 1986;**56**:930–3.
12. Eigler DM, Schweizer E. Positioning single atoms with a scanning tunnelling microscope. *Nature* 1990;**344**:524–6.

13. Drexler KE. Molecular engineering: an approach to the development of general capabilities for molecular manipulation. *Proc Natl Acad Sci USA* 1981;**78**:5275–8.
14. Eric KD. *Engines of creation: the coming era of nanotechnology*. 1986.
15. Kroto HW, Heath JR, O'Brien SC, Curl RF, Smalley RE. C 60 : buckminsterfullerene. *Nature* 1985;**318**:162.
16. Iijima S. Helical microtubules of graphitic carbon. *Nature* 1991;**354**:56.
17. Harada A, Kataoka K. Formation of polyion complex micelles in an aqueous milieu from a pair of oppositely-charged block copolymers with poly (ethylene glycol) segments. *Macromolecules* 1995;**28**:5294–9.
18. National Research Council. *Small wonders, endless frontiers: a review of the National Nanotechnology Initiative*. 2002.
19. Service R. U.S. cancer institute cancels nanotech research centers. *Science* 2019.
20. Strebhardt K, Ullrich A. Paul Ehrlich's magic bullet concept: 100 years of progress. *Nat Rev Cancer* 2008;**8**:473–80.
21. KREUTER J. Nanoparticles—a historical perspective. *Int J Pharm* 2007;**331**:1–10.
22. Bangham AD, Horne RW. Negative staining of phospholipids and their structural modification by surface-active agents as observed in the electron microscope. *J Mol Biol* 1964;**8**:660–8.

Chapter 2

Nanoparticle behavior and stability in biological environments

Raquel Martínez[1], María F. Navarro Poupard[1], Aitor Álvarez[1], Enrica Soprano[1], Martina Migliavacca[1], Carolina Carrillo-Carrión[1], Ester Polo[1], Beatriz Pelaz[1,2] and Pablo del Pino[1]

[1]*Centro Singular de Investigación en Química Biolóxica e Materiais Moleculares (CiQUS), Departamento de Física de Partículas, Universidade de Santiago de Compostela, Santiago de Compostela, Spain;* [2]*Centro Singular de Investigación en Química Biolóxica e Materiais Moleculares (CiQUS), Departamento de Química Inorgánica, Universidade de Santiago de Compostela Santiago de Compostela, Spain*

2.1 Introduction

Since the initial progress in the field of interfacing inorganic nanoparticles (NPs) with biological settings (biomolecules, biofluids, cells, and animal models), our knowledge about how the individual physicochemical properties of NPs become affected by such bionanointerfacing has greatly evolved.[1,2] Numerous reports have addressed, with varying degrees of comprehensiveness, the influence of NP parameters such as size,[3] shape,[4] charge,[5] colloidal stability,[6] corrosion,[7] stiffness,[8] and so forth, on interactions with molecules, living cells, and animal models.[9,10] The motivation is twofold: first, engineered nanomaterials have raised great expectations for health, including applications as contrast agents, drug nanocarriers, and mediators for hyperthermia and photodynamic therapy[2]; second, nanomaterials may be also released unintentionally, for instance, through mechanical wear or chemical powder waste, and therefore, they are subject of health concerns.[9]

The typical sizes of NPs lay between molecules and bulk materials, that is, within the size range of organelles and proteins, with which they share one important feature: aggregation and loss of colloidal stability negatively affect their function. In the case of proteins, aggregation typically leads to critical conformational changes such as amyloidosis,[11,12] whereas in the case of NPs, it may result in precipitation, reshaping, corrosion, and most importantly, loss of the intended physicochemical properties, such as optoelectronic, magnetic, or catalytic capabilities.[13] Ultimately, preserving the original size, shape, structure, composition, and state of aggregation of NPs when they are immersed in biological environments, at least for a specific time required to achieve the NP-dependent intended use, is essential to maintain the NP's function and avoid potential unwanted effects.[14]

On the other hand, NP degradation (as in breaking down NPs to smaller building blocks such as atoms, clusters, and molecules) may become useful for drug release applications and/or to avoid long-term accumulation inside living subjects such as cells or animals, thereby positively impacting on the NP biocompatibility.[15] We should also acknowledge, in any case, that some NP-based applications benefit of biomolecule-driven aggregation and/or self-assembly processes,[16] mostly in the biosensing area, including colorimetric sensors, surface-enhanced Raman scattering, and magnetic relaxation switching.

In this chapter, NP behavior and stability in the context of biology and medicine will be addressed (see Fig. 2.1). Toward this end, first, we will provide the most important concepts and considerations to the fabrication and characterization of NPs for intended use in biological milieu; secondly, we will briefly expose and discuss several case examples of relevance in the field of bionanotechnology. Herein, for the sake of brevity, we will exclusively approach engineered NPs obtained by bottom-up fabrication methods. We believe that such NPs are the most adequate models to deal with the topic in question, owing to their homogeneity in terms of physicochemical properties, thereby allowing for correlating model NPs with their behavior in biological settings.

2.2 General considerations on the fabrication of nanoparticles

In the following section, we briefly introduce some general concepts and approaches, which may be useful to design different NPs with robust biostability. For the reader interested in further details, we recommend a highly comprehensive

Nanoparticles for Biomedical Applications. https://doi.org/10.1016/B978-0-12-816662-8.00002-3

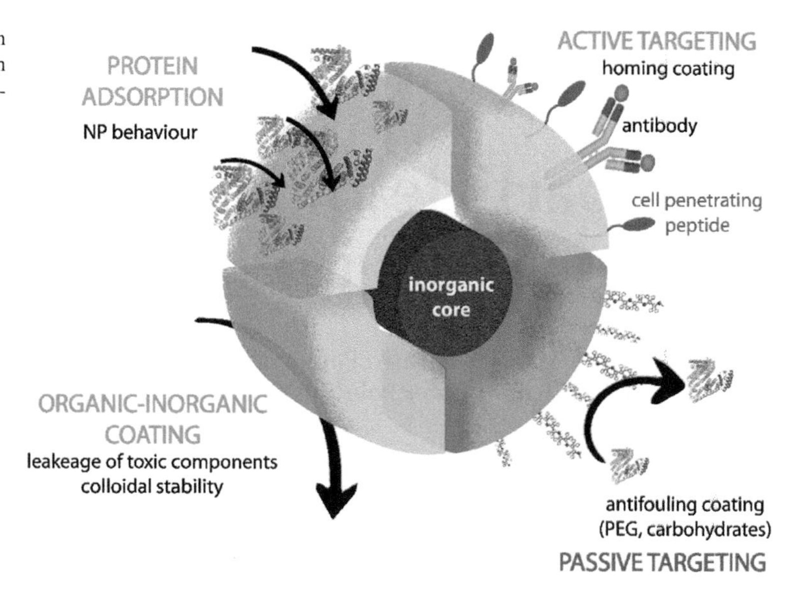

FIGURE 2.1 Nanoparticle (NP) behavior and stability in biological settings are governed by different properties, such as protein corona, functionalization, and NP surface interactions with the surrounding media.

protocol article[17] and a handful of reviews,[9,10,14,18,19] recently published by some of us (among others).

2.2.1 Synthesis of inorganic nanoparticles

The synthesis of NPs has greatly developed in the past two decades. Currently, fine control over the size, shape, structure, and composition of the final products can be readily achieved by different well-established wet-chemistry synthetic methods (both in aqueous and in organic solvents); importantly, such methods are highly reproducible in any advanced chemistry laboratory.[20]

It is well known that the size, shape, composition, structure (that is, core–shell, element doping, and so forth), and monodispersity dictate the physicochemical properties of NPs. These factors are particularly critical when referring to plasmonic, magnetic, photoemissive, and catalytic NPs.[13] In the case of plasmonic NPs (e.g., gold, silver, copper, and/or aluminum), such factors determine the position of the localized surface plasmon resonance (LSPR) bands, photothermal capabilities, and near- and far-field scattering processes, among others[16]; in the case of magnetic NPs (e.g., magnetite, maghemite, doped ferrites, and iron), the characteristics of their hysteresis loop (that is, coercive and saturation fields, and magnetization) will be dictated by such factors[21]; for photoemissive NPs (e.g., quantum dots [QDs], up- or downconversion NPs, or nanoperovskites), the photoemission intensity and wavelength, and their quantum yield (QY) are influenced by such morpho/structural characteristics[22]; lastly, the performance of heterogeneous nanocatalysts (e.g., palladium, copper, gold, ruthenium, or platinum) is influenced by crystal structure, valence state, and coating of their surfaces.[23]

For the vast majority of wet-chemical synthetic routes to produce NPs, some common aspects may be outlined: (1) metal or metal oxide precursors are dispersed in a solvent (polar, nonpolar, or mixtures); (2) temperature of the solvent and/or the addition of a reducing agent dictates when nuclei (precursors of the NPs) start to grow; (3) the addition of surfactants, linkers or capping molecules, influences shape and size; (4) the absolute and relative concentration of reactants, as well as heating ramps during the NP growth, influence the final size and shape. Ultimately, after their synthesis and purification, usually by centrifugal precipitation, one obtains a colloidal dispersion of NPs coated by a shell (e.g., purely organic, silica, MOF), which provides the NPs with steric or ionic hindrance and thereby with colloidal stability; otherwise, NPs would aggregate or collapse into the corresponding bulk materials.

2.2.2 Surface modification (functionalization)

Independently of whether the NPs are produced in aqueous media or in organic solvents, the stabilizing shell after the synthesis is in most of the cases insufficient to stabilize the NP in biological media, in which high ionic strengths, polarity, pH values, and the coexistence of polyelectrolytes, biomolecules, and biomacromolecules in high concentration may trigger NP precipitation, NP reshaping, and in some cases, NP degradation. Thus, further chemical surface engineering (in the following referred to as functionalization) is typically required to warrant colloidal stability in such media.[19] After the synthetic and purification processes, the produced NPs do not present pristine surfaces (that is, they are not "naked"); they may be considered core–shell inorganic–organic nanostructures. Briefly, the stabilizing shell may provide two types of stabilization mechanisms: (1) electrostatic repulsion by charged species (for instance, citric acid, compounds containing carboxylic or amine groups, polyelectrolytes, or polymers) and/or (2) steric hindrance (e.g., polyether derivatives, proteins, gelatin, MOF-based shells, silica shells). Thus, the original surfactant (as coating after the synthesis and purification steps) is typically exchanged or modified to enhance their colloidal stability in biological settings. One should keep in mind that biological relevant pH values range from the extracellular neutral environment (pH $\sim$7) to the acidic lysosomes (pH $\sim$4.5); thus, if the NPs are stabilized by charged groups, these should remain charged during operation at biological pH values. In Table 2.1, a selection of common NP stabilizers is provided together with a selection of the corresponding references for each case.

2.3 Characterization of colloidal stability

In general, engineered NPs for bioapplications are expected to behave like macromolecules dispersed in solution; that is, they should not sediment or aggregate or disintegrate or reshape when they are exposed to biological settings.[57] Therefore, a proper characterization of engineered NPs in different biological media should be mandatory, if one aims to understand the interaction and functioning of such NPs in the presence of biomolecules, or inside living cells or animals. To this aim, several characterization techniques may be used in parallel. In the following, we briefly discuss the most common ones, typically available (if not all, most of them) in any laboratory devoted to nanobiotechnology.

2.3.1 Dynamic light scattering and laser Doppler anemometry

Particle analyzers such as the Malvern's Zetasizer family and the Horiba's nanoPartica family, among others, allow for determining the hydrodynamic diameter d_h and zeta potential (typically denoted ζ-potential) of NPs dispersed in solution. As an alternative to dynamic light scattering (DLS) analyzers in which the extracted d_h is based on time-dependent scattering intensity fluctuations (correlogram), nanoparticle tracking analyzers (NTAs, such as the ZetaView or the Nanosight families) directly provide information about d_h from individual NPs; that is, although both techniques measure Brownian motion (diffusion constant) in solution, NTA raw data provide number-weighted d_h distributions, whereas DLS experimentally provides intensity-weighted distributions, which after deconvolution can be expressed in number-weighted size distributions. For the interested reader, other less common techniques for particle size analysis can be used, including analytical ultracentrifugation, differential centrifugal sedimentation, or asymmetric-flow field-flow fractionation (AF4).[58–60]

The number-weighted hydrodynamic size typically exceeds the size obtained by electron microscopy due to the NP surface hydration. Let us consider polymer-coated NPs; in general, polymer coatings collapse onto the NPs surface after sample drying onto substrates used for transmission electron microscopy (TEM) or scanning electron microscopy. Thus, extracting useful information about the colloidal state of NPs from electron microscopy data is challenging, when not impossible, due to NP aggregation during the sample preparation. One can rarely find examples in which TEM (using negative staining to resolve the morphology of the organic shell) and DLS data can be directly compared; among these rare examples, we have recently reported on a 2D library of PEGylated Au NPs,[8] which was used to correlate some of their basic physicochemical properties (such as size, ζ-potential, hydrophilicity, elasticity, and catalytic activity) with their interaction with cells (see Fig. 2.2). In this example, diameters extracted from negative staining TEM micrographs of the core–shell Au-NP/PEG shells were similar to the hydrodynamic diameters as obtained from the number distribution with DLS.

Laser Doppler anemometry (LDA), typically performed in aqueous solutions with a known pH, provides information about how a particle moves under the influence of an applied electric field; therefore, the ζ-potential is also referred to as electrokinetic potential. Although the interpretation of LDA data is more complex,[61] stated in simple terms, ζ-potential values are normally related to the net charge of an NP in solution under those specific conditions. Commonly, values above $\pm$30 mV have been considered as requirement for colloidal stability. Nevertheless, this last assumption is not a universal truth. The isoelectric point of the NPs can be also determined by LDA, performing titration experiments in which the case examples are recorded against pH.

The combination of DLS and LDA allows for extracting valuable information regarding the colloidal stability of NPs in complex media. For instance, as a routine characterization, the evolution of the hydrodynamic diameter (d_h) and ζ-potential of NPs over time in relevant biological media such as phosphate buffer saline (PBS), cell media with or without fetal bovine serum (FBS), and antibiotics is becoming more and more usual (see Section 7).

2.3.2 UV-Vis spectroscopy

The absorbance spectra of solutions of NPs provide meaningful insights about their colloidal state. This fast, ultrasensitive, affordable, and reliable technique is typically used to characterize plasmonic NPs, as changes in their LSPR bands are directly related to changes in the dispersion media (i.e., polarity) and more importantly, to the NPs aggregation state induced, for instance, by ionic screening (e.g., salts present in the medium) or by the presence of proteins, charged polymers, or other

TABLE 2.1 Common materials used to form robust coatings around nanoparticles (NPs), aiming enhanced colloidal stability.

NP stabilizer[§]	Original surfactant[◆]	Inorganic core	Diameter/length (nm)	References
PEG	Citrate	Au (spherical)	13–28	8,24,25
	CTAB	Au (rods)	33–100	26,27
	Sulfate	Au (triangular plates)	100–160	28
	SDS	Ag (spherical)	4	29,30
PMA	Dodecanethiol	Au (spherical)	2–6	31,32
	PEG/dodecylamine	Au (spherical/rod)	20–100	33,34
	PEG/dodecylamine	Ag (triangular nanoplates)	70	33
	SDS	Ag (spherical)	4	30
	Oleylamine/dodecylamine	Iron oxides (spherical)	4–90	21,35–37
	TOPO	QDs (CdSe, CdS, etc.)	2–7	36,38,39
	Oleic acid	Upconverting NPs (spherical)	15–30	40,41
	Oleic acid	ZnO (spherical)	7	6
PVP	Citrate	Au (spherical)	13–28	34
	CTAB	Au (rods)	33–100	
	Oleate	Upconverting NPs (spherical)	20	42
LbL (polyelectrolytes)	Citrate	Au (spherical)	20–100	43
	CTAB	Au (rods)	500	43
pDA	Citrate	Au (spherical)	50	44
	PEG	Au (rods)	44	45
	Citrate	Iron oxide (spherical)	19–240	46
Proteins (BSA, HRP, etc.)	Citrate	Au (spherical)	15–19	47,48
		Fe_3O_4 (spherical)	n.d.	49
	CTAB	Au (rods)	100	50
Silica	APS	Au (sphere)	15	51
	CTAB	Au (rods)	50	52
	Oleic acid	Iron oxide (spherical)	5	53
	PVP	Upconverting NPs (spherical)	20	42
MOFs (ZIF-8 based)	CTAB	Au (nanostars)	120	7,54,55
	PVP	Au (spherical)	13–30	56
	PVP	Ag (cubic)	160	56
MUA	TOAB	Au (spherical)	3–7	31
	SDS	Ag (spherical)	4	29,30

[§] *PEG*, polyethylene glycol; *PMA*, poly[isobutylene–alt–maleic anhydride]–graft–dodecyl; *PVP*, polyvinylpyrrolidone; *LbL*, layer-by-layer; *pDA*, poly-dopamine; *BSA*, bovine serum albumin; *HRP*, horseradish peroxidase; *MOFs*, metal organic frameworks; *ZIF-8*, zeolitic imidazolate framework; *MUA*, mercaptoundecanoic acid.

[◆] *CTAB*, cetyltrimethylammonium bromide; *SDS*, sodium S-dodecylthiosulfate; *PEG*, polyethylene glycol; *TOPO*, tri-n-octylphosphine oxide; *APS*, (3-aminopropyl)trimethoxysilane; *PVP*, polyvinylpyrrolidone; *TOAB*, tetraoctylammonium bromide.

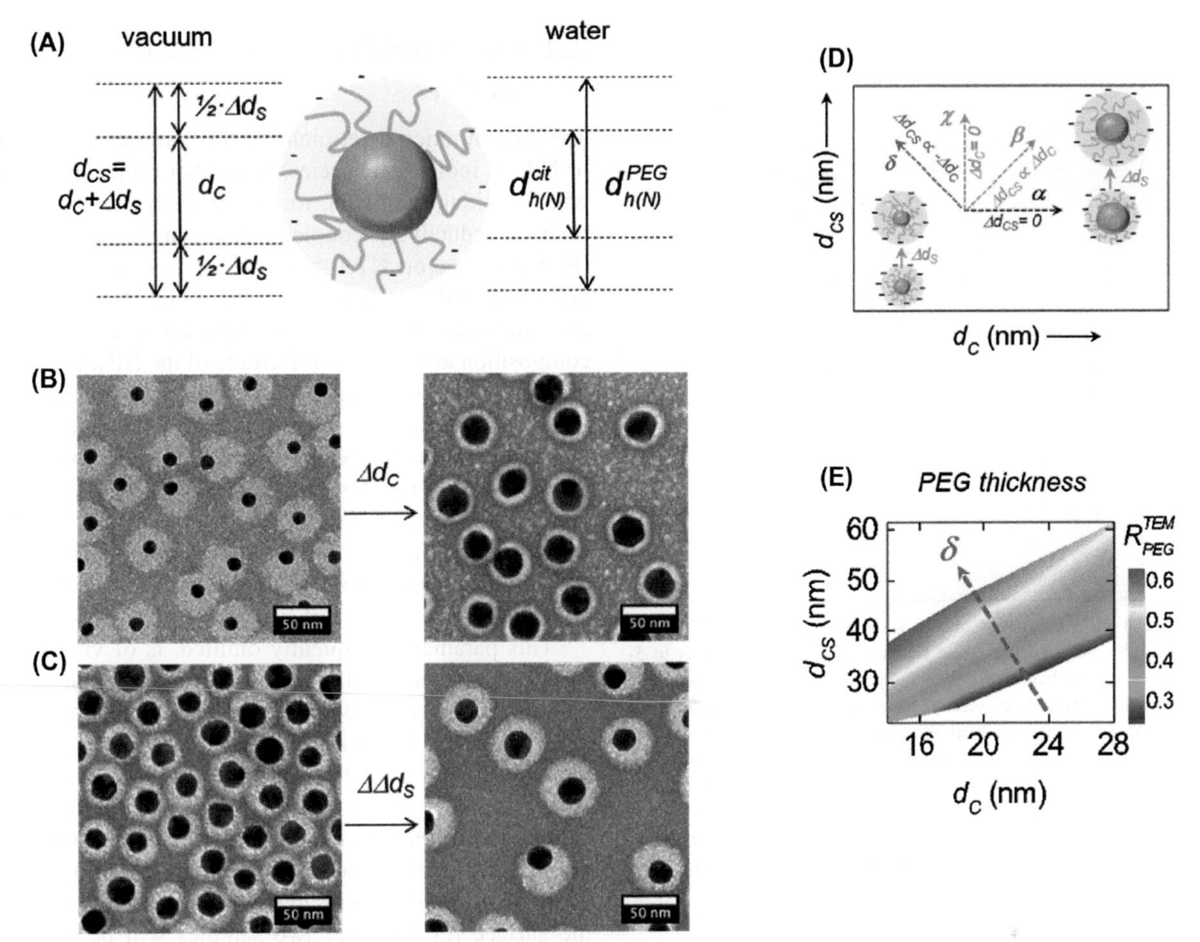

FIGURE 2.2 (A) PEGylated Au nanoparticles (NPs), showing different properties in vacuum and in solution. d_C and d_{CS} refer to the diameters of the Au cores and of the cores with the PEG shell (the core—shell system), respectively, as determined by transmission electron microscopy (TEM). $d_{h(N)}^{cit}$ and $d_{h(N)}^{PEG}$ refer to the hydrodynamic diameters as obtained from the number distribution with DLS of the originally citric acid stabilized Au NPs before PEGylation (that is, PEG coating) and of the PEGylated NPs, respectively. (B) Negative staining TEM images of two types of PEGylated NPs are shown, in which d_C increases, whereas d_{CS} is kept constant at ca. 38 nm. (C) Negative staining TEM images of two types of PEGylated NPs are shown, in which d_{CS} increases, whereas d_C is kept constant at ca. 23 nm. Scale bar: 50 nm. (D) Different variables related to the size of the PEGylated Au NPs. (E) Heatmap of the proportion of PEG in the NP size (R_{PEG}^{TEM}). *Adapted with permission from del Pino, P. et al. Basic physicochemical properties of polyethylene glycol coated gold nanoparticles that determine their interaction with cells.* Angew Chem Int Ed *2016;***55***:5483—5487.*

biomolecules.[62] Also, as in solutions of nucleic acids, dyes, or in general, any UV-Vis active molecule, absorbance at NP-type specific wavelengths can be used to determine NP concentration in solution (using the corresponding calibration curves).[8] Moreover, this technique can be used with nonplasmonic NPs since aggregation induces an absorbance broad peak in the NIR due to scattering produced by the NP aggregates.[63]

2.3.3 Gel electrophoresis

This technique based on the use of a polymeric matrix, typically agarose, allows to get valuable information about the colloidal stability of the NPs and even of the surface modifications introduced after functionalization.[17,64] In general, highly concentrated solutions of NPs are placed in the gel's lane entry; the porosity of the gel is controlled by the percentage of the agarose (typically in the range of 1%—2% in buffer). Upon a voltage application, the NPs will move to the cathode or the anode depending on their charge; negative and positive ones will migrate to the anode and cathode, respectively. That said, only colloidally stable NPs will be able to move inside the gel. This is due to the required use of rich electrolyte buffers (e.g., tris/borate/EDTA—TBE 0.5x), in which the presence of salts induces aggregation of nonstable NPs in the lane entry; such aggregates will, in general, not migrate inside the shell or produce smearing. Notice that in case of monodisperse, colloidally stable NPs, one expects narrow migration bands (the

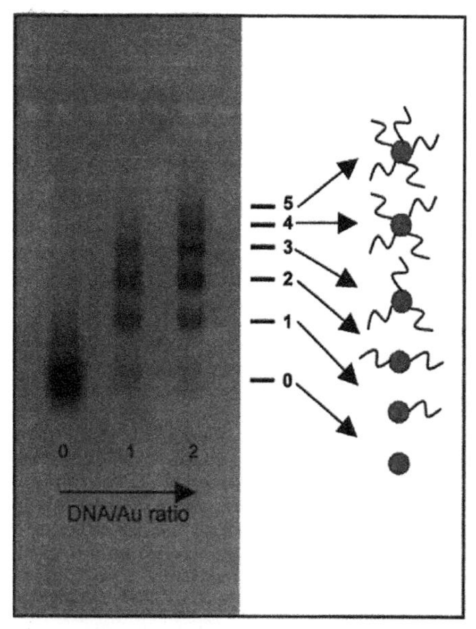

FIGURE 2.3 Electrophoretic mobility of 5 nm Au/100b HS-ssDNA conjugates (3% gel). The first lane (left to the right) corresponds to 5-nm particles (single band). When ~1 equivalent of DNA is added to the Au particles (second lane), discrete bands appear (namely **0**, **1**, **2**, **3**,...). When the DNA amount is doubled (third lane), the intensity of the discrete bands changes and additional retarded bands appear (**4**, **5**). Because of the discrete character, each band can be directly assigned to a unique number of DNA strands per particle. *Reproduced with permission from Zanchet, D, Micheel, C, Parak, WJ, Gerion, D, Alivisatos, AP. Electrophoretic isolation of discrete Au nanocrystal/DNA conjugates.* Nano Lett *2001;1:32–35.*

narrower the band, the higher the degree of NP monodispersity). Polydisperse or nonhomogeneously functionalized NPs will produce smearing or distinct bands. For instance, gel electrophoresis has been used to determine the number of ligands per NP (see Fig. 2.3).

2.3.4 Size exclusion chromatography

Size chromatograms of NPs provide valuable information about both the NP size of the sample and their colloidal stability. Moreover, the comparison of their elution time with that of proteins or polymers with a known size can be used to determine their hydrodynamic radius.[17,66] Alternatively, size exclusion columns (e.g., PD-10 desalting columns packed with Sephadex G-25 resin) allows for rapid buffer exchange, desalting, and removal of small contaminants (salts, dyes, surfactants, radioactive labels) from NP solutions using gravity flow; that is, NPs will not be retained in the Sephadex resin, whereas nonattached molecules will be delayed, thereby allowing for purification of NP products.

For more information about this and other complementary techniques for characterization of NP colloidal stability, see the protocol article by Hühn et al.[17]

2.4 Concentration determination: dose matters

The concentration determination (i.e., atomic species and/or NPs as individual species) is another critical parameter when working with NPs, for which analytical techniques such as inductively coupled plasma mass spectrometry (ICP-MS) and/or NTA are typically used. As already described, NPs are hybrid systems built of an inorganic core stabilized by an organic shell. Ideally, the specific composition and molecular formula of the NPs, that is, the precise number of ligands and number of inorganic atoms forming the inorganic core should be known. However, this information has been solely accurately reported for small particles or clusters, such as Au-NPs with core diameter ~3 nm, stabilized by chains of the synthetic amino acid tiopronin.[67] Yet the complexity in determining the specific composition of NPs increases with both the NP size and the number of ligands.

This parameter, frequently omitted, is of vital importance to interpret colloidal stability results since NP corrosion (that is, leaking of atoms and/or surfactants) directly induces biological effects, including cytotoxicity, oxidative stress, genotoxicity, and immunotoxicity.[68,69] As an example, considering NPs with the same inorganic core composition, the active surface is directly related to the square radius. So, when comparing NPs with radius r, 2r, or 4r, the surface and, therefore, the atoms located on the surface for the latter two samples will be 4 and 16 times the ones located onto the surface for the smaller NP (r). The number of surface atoms is critical when the NPs exhibit catalytic properties or if they can suffer from degradation processes triggered on their surface. Similar examples can be provided considering the NPs volume and, thus, the number of NPs that are contained within the same mass of material.

One of the most extended ways of expressing NP dosage is milligrams of material per milliliter of solution (mg/mL). However, the conversion of the mg/mL concentrations to molarities (mol of NPs per L) provides a more easily comparable metric, allowing for a more rational comparison of the results. Using this nomenclature, NPs may be considered as molecules. The approximate determination of the inorganic NP molecular weights is relatively straightforward by considering their dimensions (volume of a single NP) and the density of the bulk material from what they are made of. Then, providing different metrics of the dosage used would help to extract more comprehensive data from the analysis and to compare results obtained by different authors in different laboratories and using different methodologies. For more detailed information about this, the reader is referred to previous work.[30,70]

2.5 Determination of the protein corona

The formation of a layer of adsorbed proteins onto the surface of NPs exposed to protein containing media is among the most crucial factors influencing the interaction of NPs with living matter, and therefore, it may determine the biological fate of NPs as well as their colloidal properties (see Fig. 2.4). This protein layer named protein corona has been subject of intense research during the last decade,[71] originally initiated by the group of K. Dawson.[72–74] When the complexity of the biological fluid is higher than just proteins, that is, any biological fluid or supplemented cell media, other molecules beside proteins such as sugars, or lipids, can also be adsorbed onto the NPs. In those cases, the term biomolecular corona can be used instead of protein corona.[75]

A deeper knowledge about the identity of the adsorbed proteins, their abundance, and their orientation should shed some light in understanding the mechanisms by which the NPs are recognized by cells, both in vivo and in vitro.[76] The capability of the proteins to interact with a particular NP model is determined by their affinity constant. However, the complexity of the media, in which a huge amount of nonbounded proteins among other compounds are available and ready to interact with the NPs, leads to a dynamic behavior of the corona, where the composition is a result of a competition equilibria between the affinities of the media components. Of course, this dynamic nature hinders its straightforward characterization.

Another challenging issue is that the actual isolation of the NPs with the corresponding corona (for instance, by centrifugation, SEC, electrophoresis) alters this equilibrium, and therefore the corona identity.[71] Only few techniques are able to study the in situ corona without a previous purification step, such as fluorescence correlation spectroscopy (FCS),[71,77] flow cytometry,[78] diffusion-ordered nuclear magnetic resonance (NMR) spectroscopy,[79] nanoparticle tracking analysis (NTA),[80] and isothermal titration calorimetry.[27,72] However, such studies are still rare. Importantly, to extract quantifiable data (e.g., dissociation constants, d_h) from these techniques, studies are usually restricted to model proteins (e.g., albumin, transferrin, fibrinogen, immunoglobulins, low-density lipoproteins). To our knowledge, examples of non–optics-based methods for exploring the corona formation in situ are virtually nonexisting; one exception was recently reported by Carril et al., in which NPs are labeled with ^{19}F and their diffusion coefficient measured using ^{19}F diffusion-ordered NMR spectroscopy. ^{19}F diffusion NMR measurements of hydrodynamic radii allowed for in situ characterization of NPs in complex environments by quantification of protein adsorption to the surface of NPs, as determined by increase in hydrodynamic radius (see Fig. 2.5).[79]

As shown above in Fig. 2.5, by evaluating the size of the NPs upon the dispersion in protein containing media, information regarding the protein corona formation can also be obtained. Of course, the size of the NPs should be small enough to be able to distinguish the protein-coated NPs from the noncoated ones and from the measurement error. The size increment for particles bigger than 50 nm caused by the formation of a protein layer will be roughly in the same order of magnitude of measurement errors from DLS, NTA, FCS, or NMR. Therefore, such studies are limited to relatively small NPs. Notice, however, that in the ultrasmall

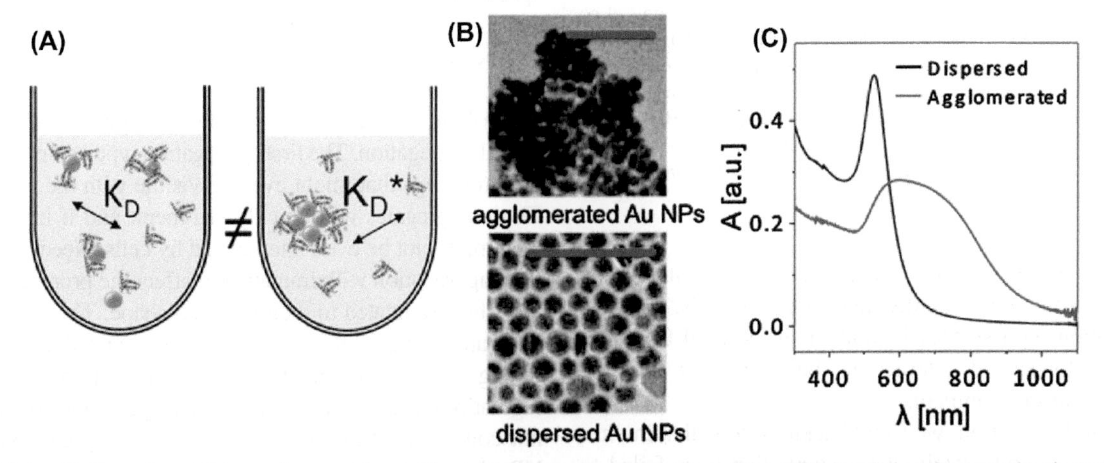

FIGURE 2.4 (A) Formation of the protein corona is sensitive to the dispersion of the nanoparticles (NPs) in solution, for example, via steric effects; dissociation equilibrium coefficient K_D is given by the ratio of the off- to on-rates for protein binding to the NPs. (B) If dried NPs (in this case, gold NPs of ca. $d_c = 15$ nm in core diameter) are observed to form agglomerates in transmission electron microscopy imaging (scale bars are 100 nm in both micrographs), they are usually also agglomerated in solution. (C) Agglomeration in solution can be observed with UV/Vis absorption spectroscopy, in which the absorption A is plotted versus the wavelength λ. *Reproduced with permission from Del Pino, P. et al. Protein corona formation around nanoparticles - from the past to the future.* Mater Horizons *2014; 1:301–313 (2014) with permission from The Royal Society of Chemistry.*

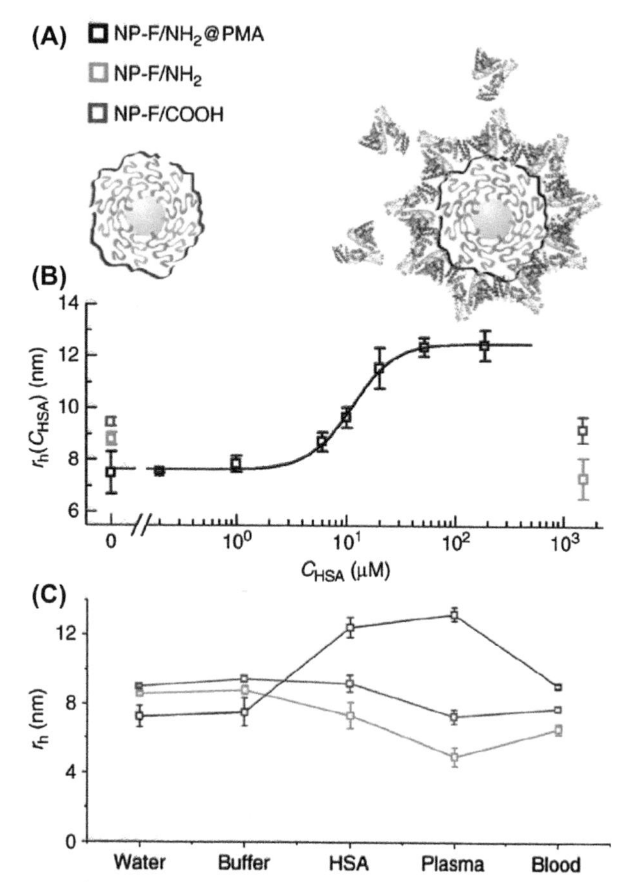

FIGURE 2.5 A) Size increase in the presence of human serum albumin (HSA) for three types of ^{19}F-labeled nanoparticles (NPs). (B) Hydrodynamic radii $r_h \pm$ standard deviation (from at least three measurements) as measured in situ (i.e., under equilibrium with excess proteins present in solution) for the three types of NPs in the presence of increasing concentrations c_{HSA} of HSA in PBS, and the corresponding fit based on the Hill's model for the case of NP-F/NH_2@PMA, which was the only NP type that underwent an increase of size due to protein adsorption. In the case of NP-F/NH_2 and NP-F/COOH, no protein adsorption in terms of no significant change in hydrodynamic radius was observed. (C) Size measurements in different media. Hydrodynamic radii $r_h \pm$ standard deviation (from at least two measurements) as measured for the three types of NPs: in water, aqueous buffer (HEPES or PBS), in the presence of HSA (under saturation conditions), in isolated plasma, and in blood. *Reproduced with permission from Carril, M. et al. In situ detection of the protein corona in complex environments.* Nat Commun *2017;8:1542.*

NP size range (1−3 nm in diameter), the identity of the protein corona may rapidly fluctuate[81]; that is, size (in combination with surface identity) may be used to nearly eliminate long-lived interactions between NPs and the biomolecular environment.

Last in this section, we should acknowledge that in vitro studies concerning protein corona formation have failed to minimally reproduce commonly observed in vivo phenomena.[82–85] Therefore, recent articles have shifted the focus toward in vivo protein corona formation, for which, in general, after circulation for varying time periods in living animals, NPs are extracted for protein corona analysis.

2.6 Stability in biologically relevant media

The stability of engineered NPs measured in biologically relevant media, such as high ionic strength buffers, protein-supplemented media, cell media, or plasma, provides a more accurate scenario than measurement in plain water; such measurements illustrate the actual features of the NP dispersion that will dictate their interaction with cells or living organisms. In the literature, thousands of different protocols to decorate the NP surface are available. However, not all of them are suitable for all the NPs. For example, using ligands that contain reactive groups that will preferentially react with a specific material, for example, gold and thiolated molecules, ensures a strong ligand−NP interaction that will enhance the NP stability. Yet, this strong interaction might not be enough if the ligand length is too short compared with the NP size or if the ligand hydrophilicity is low. So, a rational selection of the elements that compose our nanomaterial is required. Furthermore, perfectly stable NPs in water or in low salt content aqueous solutions can suffer from an impaired stability once they are in a harsher, more complex environment, as the biological media are. The charge losses induced by screening processes[86,87] and the unspecific protein adsorption, as discussed above, are two of the major inducers of NP aggregation. We should also acknowledge that protein adsorption (i.e., protein corona) may also stabilize NPs in biological media. That said, NP aggregation is not the only process that affect the NP stability in these media; for instance, leaking of metal ions due to redox reactions, the production of reactive oxidative species, and processes of ligand replacement can also occur, among others. These processes that directly affect NP integrity will be discussed in Section 7. Regarding the NP aggregation state, obviously, having completely aggregated NPs that are not colloidally stable and rapidly precipitate, differs from partial aggregation. The first aggregation type will produce big NP groupings that might even be visible with the naked eye. Those aggregates will quickly sediment, and if big enough, they might not be even internalized by cells. Needless to say, such aggregation will dramatically affect the properties of the NPs that are related to their size and shape. The fact that the NPs are dramatically, irreversibly aggregated can lead to wrong conclusions and therefore to misinterpret their cell regulation capabilities; specially, if the aggregation of the NP is not considered. More important than the aggregation of the NPs that can be detected just at plain sight is the partial aggregation, which produces aggregates that can only be observed using techniques such as DLS. For plasmonic NPs, the formation of such aggregates as discussed above can be detected easily by a change in the color solution; however, many other NPs do not exhibit this property. Partial aggregation in solutions of TiO_2, ZnO, silica, or iron oxide NPs will not be visible without a proper analysis, for instance, by DLS.[6,88]

The routine characterization of the aggregation state in media such as PBS, HEPES, or other biological relevant buffers at the biological pH range, protein containing media such PBS with BSA or FBS, and cell media with and without supplements (i.e., FBS, antibiotics, and essential amino acids), among others, should be considered as a fundamental physicochemical characterization of nanomaterials.

2.7 Correlating basic physicochemical properties with nanoparticle behavior in biological settings

For a long time, an ideal nanocarrier has been considered as one that among other properties should be able to avoid unspecific protein adsorption. Evading the formation of the corona provides the nanocarrier with longer circulation times, thereby enhancing the success rate to achieve efficient targeting.[85] Toward this end, PEGylation of NPs is the most common strategy. This approach was described in the 1950s and 1960s for PEGylated surfaces.[89,90] This ability of PEG chains to prevent protein adsorption has been widely explored in vitro and in vivo; it is well known that PEG shells prevent the opsonization of NPs.[91] However, the PEGylation of NPs modifies more than just one physicochemical property; the hydrodynamic size is also increased, the surface charge is reduced, and normally, the colloidal stability is enhanced.[77] On this note, we reported that PEGylated NPs with longer PEG chains presented higher hydrophobicities than NPs PEGylated with shorter chains.[8] Not only does the PEG length play a role, but also the grafting density controls the stealth capabilities of PEG shells.[92,93] We also demonstrated that, in most of the cases, the PEGylation of NPs is not fully capable of preventing the unspecific adsorption of proteins.[77] Indeed, Schöttler et al. reported that protein adsorption is required to create the stealth effect of PEGylated nanocarriers.[94]

Usually, the differences in protein adsorption have been associated to changes in the surface charge, NP curvature, size, or shape.[93] For instance, it has been reported that ultrasmall NPs (diameter < 3 nm) may not acquire a resilient protein corona.[81] However, the difficulties to relate the results obtained in different studies, when varying the NP model, have led to the researchers to carry out more systematic studies. On this note, we have prepared a series of NPs libraries in which an individual physicochemical property is modified, whereas others are kept constant.[8,77,95] These studies have clarified that any parameter in an exclusive basis is not solely responsible for the final behavior of NPs in biological settings. That is, the stability of the NPs in complex media is the result of the contribution of several factors as already mentioned. Despite great efforts achieved during the last decade to correlate protein corona formation with NP physicochemical properties, many unresolved fundamental questions remain.[96] The unspecific adsorption of proteins is driven by several entangled NP features such as the NP net charge,[97] the hydrophobicity/hydrophilicity of the NPs,[8] the local surface charge (for instance, the distribution of the charged groups in zwitterionic polymers),[98] the functional groups or ligands attached to the NP surface,[93] and the colloidal stability.[59] Other parameters are defined by the proteins themselves such as the protein concentration, the protein affinity, or the protein conformation[99]; finally, the media also contribute with parameters such as the pH, the salt concentration, or the temperature.[100,101]

We want to acknowledge that building a designed fusion protein corona onto NPs (what the authors called protein corona shield nanoparticle) has been recently reported to minimize interactions with serum proteins, thereby preventing the clearance of NPs by macrophages, while ensuring systematic targeting functions in vitro and in vivo.[102]

Lastly in this section, we want to emphasize that the general term NP refers to an enormously heterogeneous group of materials, as the term protein refers to an enormously heterogeneous group of macromolecules composed of amino acids. Therefore, as in proteins, we cannot expect to extract universal rules from examples focused on correlating some NP physicochemical properties with NP behavior in biological settings. As in current proteomics studies, we may advance toward more comprehensive studies (large-scale study of NPs), with the general aim of building a "nanomics" analogous to proteomics.

2.8 Degradation in biological settings

Unspecific protein adsorption is among the most relevant processes that NPs suffer in biological settings; however, it is not the only one. The components of biological media include dissolved oxygen and other potential oxidative agents that can affect the integrity of the NP core, leading to ion leaking and thus NP corrosion. Manifold articles have reported on the induced toxicity of NPs due to these processes. In the case of silver NPs, the ion leaking process has been extensively used as antibacterial[103] and to induce controlled toxicity in cancer cells.[104] In the case of Cd-containing QDs, release of Cd ions upon QD corrosion in biological settings, and its toxic effects, has been well studied in the past two decades.[105] In general, the uncontrolled NP degradation upon biological corrosion is unwanted. NPs can also trigger region of species production in biological settings,[106] which has been used as an

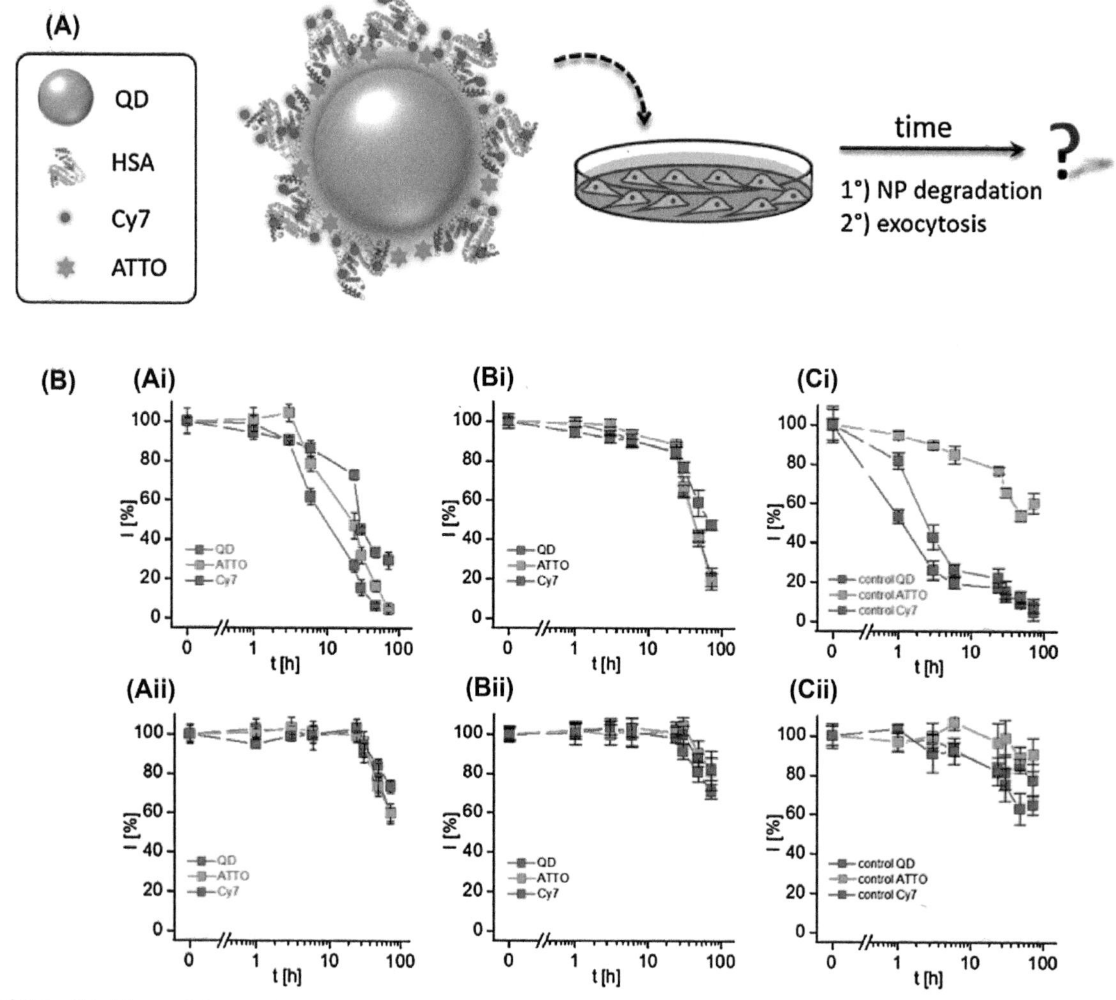

FIGURE 2.6 (A) Scheme of the experimental setup. Cells are loaded with nanoparticles (NPs), which are composed out of three fluorescence-labeled components: QDs, PMA-ATTO, and HSA-Cy7. The NP degradation over time and the subsequent exocytosis of the different components are the processes under study. (B) Time-dependent decrease in intracellular fluorescence due to NPs, which had been internalized by HeLa cells, as obtained by flow cytometry analysis. Two types of NPs were studied: (A) HSA-Cy7 adsorbed to QDs, i.e., PMA-ATTO-QD@$(\text{HSA-Cy7})_{\text{ads}}$, (B) HSA-Cy7 cross-linked to QDs, i.e., PMA-ATTO-QD@$(\text{HSA-Cy7})_{\text{cov}}$, and (C) control samples (PMA-QD, PMA-ATTO, HSA-Cy7). Data were derived by cells grown under (1) normal conditions or (2) inhibiting conditions. The graphs represent the normalized intensity values per cell, calculated as $I\,[\%] = I(t)\,[\text{a.u.}]/I(t=0)\,[\text{a.u.}]$, of each label as a function of follow-up times t. Error bars correspond to the standard deviation (SD) from three independent experiments. *Reproduced with permission from Carrillo-Carrion, C. et al. Triple-labeling of polymer-coated quantum dots and adsorbed proteins for tracing their fate in cell cultures.* ACS Nano *2019;13:4631–4639.*

advantage, for instance, in photodynamic therapy. However, this is totally unwanted in most situations at extra- and intracellular levels.

Recently, the need to better understand the biological fate of NPs in vivo has helped to understand that upon cell internalization, NPs may be affected by different degradation processes. It is worth underlining that understanding such degradation process is even more critical in the case of working with intrinsically toxic elements, as for example, Cd-containing QDs. In general, after internalization in cells by endocytic processes, NPs will end up in the endo/lysosomal system of cells, and therefore, they will be submitted to an acidic environment and enzyme digestion processes. We cannot forget that enzymes are also present in cell media and the nature and abundance of these enzymes will vary with the cellular type and the tissue location. For instance, the enzymatic composition in lungs is different than that of the spleen, liver, and so forth. These differences are very important in tumors, which may be used as a perk for enzyme-controlled drug release.[107]

Kreyling et al. reported the in vitro and in vivo enzymatic degradation of polymer-coated gold NPs.[32] In this example, the degradation in vivo induced different accumulation and excretion pathways of the inorganic NPs

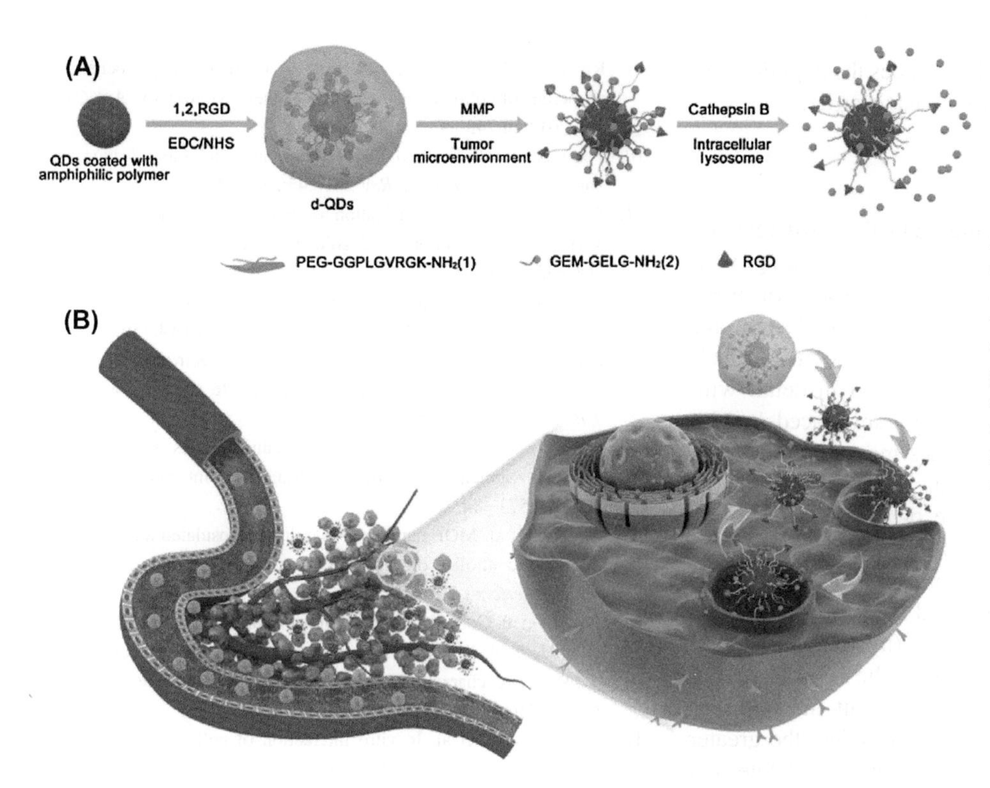

FIGURE 2.7 Dual enzymatic reaction-assisted gemcitabine (GEM) nanovectors were used to achieve multistage tumor cell targeting and efficient drug release during the GEM-transporting process. (A) Schematic illustration of the preparation of nanovectors and their enzyme-sensitive behavior. (B) Schematic illustration of the nanovectors delivering GEM to pancreatic cancer cells. *Reproduced with permission from Han, H. et al. Dual enzymatic reaction-assisted gemcitabine delivery systems for programmed pancreatic cancer therapy.* ACS Nano *2017;11:1281–1291.*

cores and the corresponding polymer coatings (i.e., organic shells). This was induced by the degradation of amide bonds, which was an essential part of this particular polymeric shell. Some potential enzymes were identified in vitro, and a similar enzymatic degradation was hypothesized in vivo. The results reported by Kreyling et al. specifically highlight the loss of integrity of the biomolecules attached to the NP surface, such as antibodies, carbohydrates, and peptides, which typically are aimed to carry out targeting functions. On the same note, Zhu et al. explored a library of enzymes for degradation of the chemical bonds formed by click chemistry, which were used to attach fluorophores (reporters) to a polymeric shell acting as NP coating.[108]

Similarly, Parak et al. studied the in vitro NP integrity upon internalization by cells of polymer-coated CdSe/ZnS QDs modified with a model protein corona (i.e., an outer shell of HSA protein molecules, either adsorbed or chemically linked to the surface of the polymer-coated QD).[109] In this work, a combination of flow cytometry and confocal microscopy was proposed as methodological approach for analyzing individually the exocytosis of the different parts of the NP, and such data were correlated with the degradation of the different components inside living cells (see Fig. 2.6). For that, the NP was triple fluorescence labeled: the QD core having intrinsic fluorescence, the polymer shell labeled with a fluorescent organic dye, and the HSA labeled with another dye. Results indicated that HSA was partly transported with the underlying polymer-coated QDs into cells, which is imperative if the attached protein is working as a targeting unit as well as in the case of therapeutic proteins aimed to be delivered inside cells. Moreover, upon desorption of proteins, those initially adsorbed to the QDs remained longer inside cells compared with free proteins. Part of the polymer shell was released from the QDs by enzymatic degradation, probably by degradation of amide bonds as found previously by Kreyling et al.,[32] but importantly, such polymer shell degradation was on a slower time scale than protein desorption. The significance of this work is to remark that when designing an engineered NP for a specific intended use, one should keep in mind two facts: (1) NPs do not remain a constant entity once they interact with living matter and (2) different NP components can have different pharmacokinetics and biodistribution.

Understanding how enzymatic NP degradation processes work has allowed for the development of more efficient nanocarriers. Han et al. reported a nanovector for pancreas cancer targeting (see Fig. 2.7).[107] This vector was modified with a shell that degrades sequentially to finally induce the gemcitabine (GEM) release inside the tumoral pancreatic cells. A stealth PEG layer was added to the nanocarrier to increase their blood circulation time. However, this PEG shell was attached through a metalloproteinase 9 (MM-9) cleavable bond to an RGD peptide. Thus, NPs that were in the tumoral region lost the PEG shell, allowing the peptide to drive the NPs inside the tumoral cells, where cathepsin B degrades the peptide bond by which GEM was attached to the nanocarrier.

2.9 Conclusions

In this chapter, we aimed to highlight the most relevant factors that should be considered when working with engineered NPs in biological settings. Some of these considerations are solely related to the NP design, for example, how to select the stability forces to ensure their colloidal stability. However, as discussed in detail with several case examples, once the NPs are placed in biological media, the scenario becomes more complex. The unspecific protein adsorption can seriously impair the stability of the NPs; the presence of salts and oxidative species can also trigger unwanted processes; the enzymes present in the biological environment can drive some degradation/corrosion processes and other factors such as pH changes; or oxygen concentration (hypoxia, in tumors) can also affect to the biological fate of the NPs. That said, the more knowledge we can gather about the physico-chemical features of NPs in biological milieu, the greater the capability for us to predict their biological fate and even to convert some of the expected degradation biological processes into advantages. This knowledge can be the key to the development of fully functional, predictable NPs, solving some of the major current limitations of nanomedicines, such as targeting and a spatiotemporal controlled drug release.

References

1. Pelaz B, et al. The state of nanoparticle-based nanoscience and biotechnology: progress, promises, and challenges. *ACS Nano* 2012;**6**:8468–83.
2. Pelaz B, et al. Diverse applications of nanomedicine. *ACS Nano* 2017;**11**:2313–81.
3. Li K, Schneider M. Quantitative evaluation and visualization of size effect on cellular uptake of gold nanoparticles by multiphoton imaging-UV/Vis spectroscopic analysis. *J Biomed Opt* 2014;**19**(1–11):11.
4. Chithrani BD, Chan WCW. Elucidating the mechanism of cellular uptake and removal of protein-coated gold nanoparticles of different sizes and shapes. *Nano Lett* 2007;**7**:1542–50.
5. Zhang L, et al. Softer zwitterionic nanogels for longer circulation and lower splenic accumulation. *ACS Nano* 2012;**6**:6681–6.
6. Abdelmonem AM, et al. Charge and agglomeration dependent in vitro uptake and cytotoxicity of zinc oxide nanoparticles. *J Inorg Biochem* 2015;**153**:334–8.
7. Carrillo-Carrion C, et al. Aqueous stable gold nanostar/ZIF-8 nanocomposites for light-triggered release of active cargo inside living cells. *Angew Chem Int Ed Engl* 2019;**58**:7078–82.
8. del Pino P, et al. Basic physicochemical properties of polyethylene glycol coated gold nanoparticles that determine their interaction with cells. *Angew Chem Int Ed* 2016;**55**:5483–7.
9. Rivera-Gil P, et al. The challenge to relate the physicochemical properties of colloidal nanoparticles to their cytotoxicity. *Acc Chem Res* 2013;**46**:743–9.
10. Feliu N, et al. In vivo degeneration and the fate of inorganic nanoparticles. *Chem Soc Rev* 2016;**45**:2440–57.
11. Fernández C, et al. Nucleation of amyloid oligomers by RepA-WH1-prionoid-functionalized gold nanorods. *Angew Chem Int Ed* 2016;**55**:11237–41.
12. Eisele YS, et al. Targeting protein aggregation for the treatment of degenerative diseases. *Nat Rev Drug Discov* 2015;**14**:759.
13. del Pino P. Tailoring the interplay between electromagnetic fields and nanomaterials toward applications in life sciences: a review. *J Biomed Opt* 2014;**19**.
14. Pelaz B, et al. Interfacing engineered nanoparticles with biological systems: anticipating adverse NanoBio interactions. *Small* 2013;**9**:1573–84.
15. Chen X, et al. MOF nanoparticles with encapsulated autophagy inhibitor in controlled drug delivery system for antitumor. *ACS Appl Mater Interfaces* 2018;**10**:2328–37.
16. Polo E, et al. Colloidal bioplasmonics. *Nano Today* 2018;**20**:58–73.
17. Hühn J, et al. Selected standard protocols for the synthesis, phase transfer, and characterization of inorganic colloidal nanoparticles. *Chem Mater* 2017;**29**:399–461.
18. Nazarenus M, et al. In vitro interaction of colloidal nanoparticles with mammalian cells: what have we learned thus far? *Beilstein J Nanotechnol* 2014;**5**:1477–90.
19. Fratila RM, Mitchell SG, del Pino P, Grazu V, de la Fuente JM. Strategies for the biofunctionalization of gold and iron oxide nanoparticles. *Langmuir* 2014;**30**:15057–71.
20. Parak WJ. Complex colloidal assembly. *Science* 2011;**334**:1359–60.
21. Zhang Q, et al. Model driven optimization of magnetic anisotropy of exchange-coupled core-shell ferrite nanoparticles for maximal hysteretic loss. *Chem Mater* 2015;**27**:7380–7.
22. Ashraf S, et al. Fluorescence-based ion-sensing with colloidal particles. *Curr Opin Pharmacol* 2014;**18**:98–103.
23. Gavia DJ, Shon Y-S. Catalytic properties of unsupported palladium nanoparticle surfaces capped with small organic ligands. *ChemCatChem* 2015;**7**:892–900.
24. Yang F, et al. Real-time, label-free monitoring of cell viability based on cell adhesion measurements with an atomic force microscope. *J Nanobiotechnol* 2017;**15**:23.
25. Conde J, et al. Design of multifunctional gold nanoparticles for in vitro and in vivo gene silencing. *ACS Nano* 2012;**6**:8316–24.
26. Alkilany AM, Yaseen AIB, Park J, Eller JR, Murphy CJ. Facile phase transfer of gold nanoparticles from aqueous solution to organic solvents with thiolated poly(ethylene glycol). *RSC Adv* 2014;**4**:52676–9.
27. Polo E, et al. Photothermal effects on protein adsorption dynamics of PEGylated gold nanorods. *Appl Mater Today* 2019;**15**:599–604.
28. Pelaz B, et al. Tailoring the synthesis and heating ability of gold nanoprisms for bioapplications. *Langmuir* 2012;**28**:8965–70.
29. Caballero-Díaz E, et al. The toxicity of silver nanoparticles depends on their uptake by cells and thus on their surface chemistry. *Part Part Syst Charact* 2013;**30**:1079–85.
30. Manshian BB, et al. High-content imaging and gene expression approaches to unravel the effect of surface functionality on cellular interactions of silver nanoparticles. *ACS Nano* 2015;**9**:10431–44.

31. Ma X, et al. Colloidal gold nanoparticles induce changes in cellular and subcellular morphology. *ACS Nano* 2017;**11**:7807–20.
32. Kreyling WG, et al. In vivo integrity of polymer-coated gold nanoparticles. *Nat Nanotechnol* 2015;**10**:619.
33. Soliman MG, Pelaz B, Parak WJ, del Pino P. Phase transfer and polymer coating methods toward improving the stability of metallic nanoparticles for biological applications. *Chem Mater* 2015;**27**:990–7.
34. Xu M, et al. How entanglement of different physicochemical properties complicates the prediction of in vitro and in vivo interactions of gold nanoparticles. *ACS Nano* 2018;**12**:10104–13.
35. Munshi R, et al. Magnetothermal genetic deep brain stimulation of motor behaviors in awake, freely moving mice. *Elife* 2017;**6**:e27069.
36. Ali Z, et al. Multifunctional nanoparticles for dual imaging. *Anal Chem* 2011;**83**:2877–82.
37. Joris F, et al. The impact of species and cell type on the nanosafety profile of iron oxide nanoparticles in neural cells. *J Nanobiotechnol* 2016;**14**:69.
38. Manshian BB, et al. Evaluation of quantum dot cytotoxicity: interpretation of nanoparticle concentrations versus intracellular nanoparticle numbers. *Nanotoxicology* 2016;**10**:1318–28.
39. Zhang F, et al. Polymer-coated nanoparticles: a universal tool for biolabelling experiments. *Small* 2011;**7**:3113–27.
40. Dukhno O, et al. Quantitative assessment of energy transfer in upconverting nanoparticles grafted with organic dyes. *Nanoscale* 2017;**9**:11994–2004.
41. Wilhelm S, et al. Water dispersible upconverting nanoparticles: effects of surface modification on their luminescence and colloidal stability. *Nanoscale* 2015;**7**:1403–10.
42. Johnson NJJ, Sangeetha NM, Boyer J-C, van Veggel FCJM. Facile ligand-exchange with polyvinylpyrrolidone and subsequent silica coating of hydrophobic upconverting β-NaYF4:Yb3+/Er3+ nanoparticles. *Nanoscale* 2010;**2**:771–7.
43. Yu X, et al. Distance control in-between plasmonic nanoparticles via biological and polymeric spacers. *Nano Today* 2013;**8**:480–93.
44. Liu X, et al. Mussel-inspired polydopamine: a biocompatible and ultrastable coating for nanoparticles in vivo. *ACS Nano* 2013;**7**:9384–95.
45. Khlebtsov BN, Burov AM, Pylaev TE, Khlebtsov NG. Polydopamine-coated Au nanorods for targeted fluorescent cell imaging and photothermal therapy. *Beilstein J Nanotechnol* 2019;**10**:794–803.
46. Adnan NNM, et al. Exploiting the versatility of polydopamine-coated nanoparticles to deliver nitric oxide and combat bacterial biofilm. *Macromol Rapid Commun* 2018;**39**:1800159.
47. Chanana M, Rivera_Gil P, Correa-Duarte MA, Liz-Marzán LM, Parak WJ. Physicochemical properties of protein-coated gold nanoparticles in biological fluids and cells before and after proteolytic digestion. *Angew Chem Int Ed* 2013;**52**:4179–83.
48. Strozyk MS, Chanana M, Pastoriza-Santos I, Pérez-Juste J, Liz-Marzán LM. Protein/polymer-based dual-responsive gold nanoparticles with pH-dependent thermal sensitivity. *Adv Funct Mater* 2012;**22**:1436–44.
49. Männel MJ, et al. Catalytically active protein coatings: toward enzymatic cascade reactions at the intercolloidal level. *ACS Catal* 2017;**7**:1664–72.
50. Tebbe M, Kuttner C, Männel M, Fery A, Chanana M. Colloidally stable and surfactant-free protein-coated gold nanorods in biological media. *ACS Appl Mater Interfaces* 2015;**7**:5984–91.
51. Liz-Marzán LM, Giersig M, Mulvaney P. Synthesis of nanosized Gold–Silica Core–Shell particles. *Langmuir* 1996;**12**:4329–35.
52. Pastoriza-Santos I, Pérez-Juste J, Liz-Marzán LM. Silica-coating and hydrophobation of CTAB-stabilized gold nanorods. *Chem Mater* 2006;**18**:2465–7.
53. Vogt C, et al. High quality and tuneable silica shell–magnetic core nanoparticles. *J Nanoparticle Res* 2010;**12**:1137–47.
54. Zheng G, et al. Shape control in ZIF-8 nanocrystals and metal nanoparticles@ZIF-8 heterostructures. *Nanoscale* 2017;**9**:16645–51.
55. Zheng G, et al. Encapsulation of single plasmonic nanoparticles within ZIF-8 and SERS analysis of the MOF flexibility. *Small* 2016;**12**:3935–43.
56. Lu G, et al. Imparting functionality to a metal–organic framework material by controlled nanoparticle encapsulation. *Nat Chem* 2012;**4**:310–6.
57. Moore TL, et al. Nanoparticle colloidal stability in cell culture media and impact on cellular interactions. *Chem Soc Rev* 2015;**44**:6287–305.
58. Caputo F, Clogston J, Calzolai L, Rösslein M, Prina-Mello A. Measuring particle size distribution of nanoparticle enabled medicinal products, the joint view of EUNCL and NCI-NCL. A step by step approach combining orthogonal measurements with increasing complexity. *J Control Release* 2019;**299**:31–43.
59. Johnston BD, et al. Colloidal stability and surface chemistry are key factors for the composition of the protein corona of inorganic gold nanoparticles. *Adv Funct Mater* 2017;**27**:1701956.
60. Fissan H, Ristig S, Kaminski H, Asbach C, Epple M. Comparison of different characterization methods for nanoparticle dispersions before and after aerosolization. *Anal Methods* 2014;**6**:7324–34.
61. Bhattacharjee S. In relation to the following article "DLS and zeta potential — what they are and what they are not? *J Control Release* 2016;**235**:337–51. J. Control Release 2016;238:311–312.
62. Borghei Y-S, et al. Visual detection of cancer cells by colorimetric aptasensor based on aggregation of gold nanoparticles induced by DNA hybridization. *Anal Chim Acta* 2016;**904**:92–7.
63. Liu T-M, Conde J, Lipiński T, Bednarkiewicz A, Huang C-C. Revisiting the classification of NIR-absorbing/emitting nanomaterials for in vivo bioapplications. *NPG Asia Mater* 2016;**8**:e295.
64. Sperling RA, Pellegrino T, Li JK, Chang WH, Parak WJ. Electrophoretic separation of nanoparticles with a discrete number of functional groups. *Adv Funct Mater* 2006;**16**:943–8.
65. Zanchet D, Micheel CM, Parak WJ, Gerion D, Alivisatos AP. Electrophoretic isolation of discrete Au nanocrystal/DNA conjugates. *Nano Lett* 2001;**1**:32–5.
66. Sperling RA, et al. Size determination of (Bio)conjugated water-soluble colloidal Nanoparticles: a comparison of different techniques. *J Phys Chem C* 2007;**111**:11552–9.
67. Templeton AC, Chen S, Gross SM, Murray RW. Water-soluble, isolable gold clusters protected by tiopronin and coenzyme a monolayers. *Langmuir* 1999;**15**:66–76.
68. L'Azou B, et al. Comparative cytotoxicity of cadmium forms (CdCl2, CdO, CdS micro- and nanoparticles) in renal cells. *Toxicol Res* 2014;**3**:32–41.
69. Völker C, Kämpken I, Boedicker C, Oehlmann J, Oetken M. Toxicity of silver nanoparticles and ionic silver: comparison of adverse effects and potential toxicity mechanisms in the freshwater clam Sphaerium corneum. *Nanotoxicology* 2015;**9**:677–85.

70. Feliu N, et al. Nanoparticle dosagea nontrivial task of utmost importance for quantitative nanosafety research. *Wiley Interdiscip Rev Nanomed Nanobiotechnoly* 2016;**8**:479–92.
71. Del Pino P, et al. Protein corona formation around nanoparticles - from the past to the future. *Mater Horizons* 2014;**1**:301–13.
72. Cedervall T, et al. Understanding the nanoparticle–protein corona using methods to quantify exchange rates and affinities of proteins for nanoparticles. *Proc Natl Acad Sci* 2007;**104**:2050–5.
73. Lundqvist M, et al. Nanoparticle size and surface properties determine the protein corona with possible implications for biological impacts. *Proc Natl Acad Sci USA* 2008;**105**:14265–70.
74. Monopoli MP, Bombelli FB, Dawson KA. Nanobiotechnology: nanoparticle coronas take shape. *Nat Nanotechnol* 2011;**6**:11–2.
75. Gianneli M, et al. Label-free in-flow detection of receptor recognition motifs on the biomolecular corona of nanoparticles. *Nanoscale* 2018;**10**:5474–81.
76. Polo E, Collado M, Pelaz B, del Pino P. Advances toward more efficient targeted delivery of nanoparticles in vivo: understanding interactions between nanoparticles and cells. *ACS Nano* 2017;**11**:2397–402.
77. Pelaz B, et al. Surface functionalization of nanoparticles with polyethylene glycol: effects on protein adsorption and cellular uptake. *ACS Nano* 2015;**9**:6996–7008.
78. Lo Giudice MC, Herda LM, Polo E, Dawson KA. In situ characterization of nanoparticle biomolecular interactions in complex biological media by flow cytometry 2016;**7**:13475.
79. Carril M, et al. In situ detection of the protein corona in complex environments. *Nat Commun* 2017;**8**:1542.
80. Wohlleben W. Validity range of centrifuges for the regulation of nanomaterials: from classification to as-tested coronas. *J Nanoparticle Res* 2012;**14**:1300.
81. Boselli L, Polo E, Castagnola V, Dawson KA. Regimes of biomolecular ultrasmall nanoparticle interactions. *Angew Chem Int Ed* 2017;**56**:4215–8.
82. Hadjidemetriou M, et al. The human in vivo biomolecule corona onto PEGylated liposomes: a proof-of-concept clinical study. *Adv Mater* 2019;**31**:1803335.
83. Chen F, et al. Complement proteins bind to nanoparticle protein corona and undergo dynamic exchange in vivo. *Nat Nanotechnol* 2016;**12**:387.
84. Corbo C, et al. Unveiling the in vivo protein corona of circulating leukocyte-like carriers. *ACS Nano* 2017;**11**:3262–73.
85. Bertrand N, et al. Mechanistic understanding of in vivo protein corona formation on polymeric nanoparticles and impact on pharmacokinetics. *Nat Commun* 2017;**8**:777.
86. Puertas AM, de las Nieves FJ. Colloidal stability of polymer colloids with variable surface charge. *J Colloid Interface Sci* 1999;**216**:221–9.
87. Loeb J. The influence of electrolytes on the cataphoretic charge of colloidal particles and the stability of their suspensions. *J Gen Physiol* 1923;**5**:395.
88. Manshian BB, et al. The role of intracellular trafficking of CdSe/ZnS QDs on their consequent toxicity profile. *J Nanobiotechnol* 2017;**15**:45.
89. Vroman L. Effect of adsorbed proteins on the wettability of hydrophilic and hydrophobic solids. *Nature* 1962;**196**:476–7.
90. Bangham AD, Pethica BA, Seaman GVF. The charged groups at the interface of some blood cells. *Biochem J* 1958;**69**:12–9.
91. Pozzi D, et al. Effect of polyethyleneglycol (PEG) chain length on the bio–nano-interactions between PEGylated lipid nanoparticles and biological fluids: from nanostructure to uptake in cancer cells. *Nanoscale* 2014;**6**:2782–92.
92. Dai Q, Walkey C, Chan WCW. Polyethylene glycol backfilling mitigates the negative impact of the protein corona on nanoparticle cell targeting. *Angew Chem Int Ed* 2014;**53**:5093–6.
93. Walkey CD, Chan WCW. Understanding and controlling the interaction of nanomaterials with proteins in a physiological environment. *Chem Soc Rev* 2012;**41**:2780–99.
94. Schöttler S, et al. Protein adsorption is required for stealth effect of poly(ethylene glycol)- and poly(phosphoester)-coated nanocarriers. *Nat Nanotechnol* 2016;**11**:372–7.
95. Colombo M, et al. Tumour homing and therapeutic effect of colloidal nanoparticles depend on the number of attached antibodies. *Nat Commun* 2016;**7**:13818.
96. Hadjidemetriou M, Kostarelos K. Evolution of the nanoparticle corona. *Nat Nanotechnol* 2017;**12**:288.
97. Hühn D, et al. Polymer-coated nanoparticles interacting with proteins and cells: focusing on the sign of the net charge. *ACS Nano* 2013;**7**:3253–63.
98. Safavi-Sohi R, et al. Bypassing protein corona issue on active targeting: zwitterionic coatings dictate specific interactions of targeting moieties and cell receptors. *ACS Appl Mater Interfaces* 2016;**8**:22808–18.
99. Lesniak A, et al. Serum heat inactivation affects protein corona composition and nanoparticle uptake. *Biomaterials* 2010;**31**:9511–8.
100. Casals E, Pfaller T, Duschl A, Oostingh GJ, Puntes V. Time evolution of the nanoparticle protein corona. *ACS Nano* 2010;**4**:3623–32.
101. Mahmoudi M, et al. Temperature: the “ignored” factor at the NanoBio interface. *ACS Nano* 2013;**7**:6555–62.
102. Oh JY, et al. Cloaking nanoparticles with protein corona shield for targeted drug delivery. *Nat Commun* 2018;**9**:4548.
103. Hajipour MJ, et al. Antibacterial properties of nanoparticles. *Trends Biotechnol* 2012;**30**:499–511.
104. AshaRani PV, Low Kah Mun G, Hande MP, Valiyaveettil S. Cytotoxicity and genotoxicity of silver nanoparticles in human cells. *ACS Nano* 2009;**3**:279–90.
105. Kirchner C, et al. Cytotoxicity of colloidal CdSe and CdSe/ZnS nanoparticles. *Nano Lett* 2005;**5**:331–8.
106. Xia T, et al. Comparison of the mechanism of toxicity of zinc oxide and cerium oxide nanoparticles based on dissolution and oxidative stress properties. *ACS Nano* 2008;**2**:2121–34.
107. Han H, et al. Dual enzymatic reaction-assisted gemcitabine delivery systems for programmed pancreatic cancer therapy. *ACS Nano* 2017;**11**:1281–91.
108. Zhu L, Pelaz B, Chakraborty I, Parak WJ. Investigating possible enzymatic degradation on polymer shells around inorganic nanoparticles. *Int J Mol Sci* 2019;**20**:935.
109. Carrillo-Carrion C, et al. Triple-labeling of polymer-coated quantum dots and adsorbed proteins for tracing their fate in cell cultures. *ACS Nano* 2019;**13**:4631–9.

Chapter 3

Active targeting and transport

Aria W. Tarudji and Forrest M. Kievit
University of Nebraska, Department of Biological Systems Engineering, Lincoln, NE, United States

3.1 Introduction

In the biomedical field, nanoparticles (NPs) are mainly used in drug delivery, imaging, and theranostics—the ability of NPs to act as both a therapeutic and diagnostic tool. One of the most well-known examples of nanomaterials in medical use is Doxil, a liposomal NP that carries doxorubicin, a standard chemotherapeutic agent used for breast and other types of cancers. Doxil was developed to take advantage of the leakiness of blood vessels in tumors that allow it to permeate into the cancer tissue before releasing the drug as well as being retained in the tumor because of the lack of lymphatic drainage. This so-called enhanced permeability and retention (EPR) effect that is utilized by many developed NP systems is considered as passive targeting approach (see Chapter 4). On the other hand, active targeting relies on the specific binding of targeting ligands on the surface of the NPs to target cell receptors. Some of the typical active targeting ligands used are antibodies, proteins, peptides, aptamers, small molecules, and natural polymers. Each ligand contains advantages and disadvantages in altering the physicochemical properties of the NPs because of ligand size and charge, binding affinity and avidity, specificity, conjugation mechanism, and cost of production.

Active targeting is often used to increase the delivery rate, accumulation, and retention of the NPs inside the targeted tissue, which allows better drug release and more effective drug delivery. However, active targeting should not be thought of as actively seeking out target tissue as with a heat-seeking missile. Rather, actively targeted NPs still fully distribute throughout the body but only accumulate and are retained more efficiently in target tissues as with walking along a beach scattered with landmines where the landmine only goes off when contacted. More importantly, active targeting increases the selectivity of internalization and endocytosis by specific cells, improves target tissue distribution, and increases the permeability of biological membranes by targeting an active transporter of the barrier (e.g., blood−brain barrier [BBB] and blood−testes barrier).[1−7] This has been shown in various elegant studies with tumor targeting where total tumor accumulation was not affected by the presence of a targeting agent on the surface of the NP, but the targeting agent did enhance distribution throughout the tumor as well as intracellular delivery.[8−11] Moreover, since actively targeted NPs do not solely depend on EPR, actively targeted NPs allow targeting of hematological malignancies,[12,13] small metastatic tumors,[14] neurodegenerative disorders,[15−17] and other diseases that do not show the EPR effect.

The nanosize of NPs (typically 5−200 nm) results in an extraordinarily high surface-area-to-volume ratio, which can lead to upward of a square meter of surface area per milligram of NP. The high surface-area-to-volume ratio allows for relatively large quantities of active targeting ligands to be conjugated or adsorbed onto the NP surface. Targeting ligands in close proximity to one another on the NPs surface can lead to a higher binding affinity to target cells through the multivalent effect, where the binding strength between NPs and targeted tissue is stronger than individual ligands to the tissue.[18,19] The concentration of ligands mounted on the NPs affects the total affinity binding of ligands. For example, Poon et al. showed that there is a decrease in the dissociation constant, K_D, indicating an increase in binding affinity, when there are more folates on the surface of the NPs.[19] Additionally, Hong et al. found a similar multivalent effect using generation-5 dendrimers conjugated with folic acid, where an increase of up to 15,200-fold was observed when compared with the K_D of free folic acid binding.[20] However, there appears to be a limit to this multivalent effect. As ligand concentration on the surface of the NP is too concentrated, steric binding interference begins to prevent binding of targeting ligand to antigen, resulting in reduced binding affinities.[19]

Despite extensive research with actively targeted NPs, there has not been any active targeting NP system used clinically. Some have shown safety and efficacy in phase 1

Nanoparticles for Biomedical Applications. https://doi.org/10.1016/B978-0-12-816662-8.00003-5

and phase 2 clinical trials, but none have passed large, multicenter phase 3 clinical trials.[21] In this chapter, we describe the physical phenomena behind active targeting mechanisms and place them within the context of actively targeted NPs. We provide examples of how these different strategies are used for active targeting of NPs to various diseases.

3.2 The strength of molecular interactions

Binding affinity is the strength of a molecule to bind with a targeted counterpart molecule. Every molecule has a binding affinity with other molecules as can be observed with many docking simulation studies in a two-molecule system. However, in the real world, these two molecules are surrounded by other large and small molecules and a high concentration of water (~55 M). Therefore, the binding affinity of an active targeting agent to a targeted molecule must be stronger than the binding affinity with nonspecific molecules. The interaction between active targeting and targeted molecules can be through various chemical forces, including the hydrophobic effect, ionic bond, hydrogen bond, and van der Waals interactions (Table 3.1). Van der Waals forces are the weakest among the chemical interactions, having a binding energy of 4 kJ/mol, just above the 2.6 kJ/mol of average kinetic energy of a molecule in solution at 37°C.[22] Even though the cumulative strength of van der Waals forces increases when there are more atoms to interact, the van der Waals forces are easily overcome by the other forces and bonds. Moreover, the small interacting surface area between a targeting and targeted molecule reduces the van der Waals forces significantly. For example, the binding site of an antibody is usually only over several amino acids, or 0.4–8 nm^2.Van der Waals forces also work across a short range of approximately 0.5 nm because of the exponential decay as the distance increases. Furthermore, van der Waals forces become repulsive closer than 0.4 nm apart. The second weakest bond energy is the hydrogen bond. Hydrogen bonds occur in an interaction between an oxygen or nitrogen atom with a hydrogen atom, which is formed by the polarity difference between oxygen or nitrogen and hydrogen. The hydrogen bond usually occurs at a distance of 0.15–0.5 nm.[23] However, in aqueous solutions, the hydrogen bond between targeting and targeted molecules issignificantly weakened as both form hydrogen bonds with the surrounding solvent. The ionic bond, on the other hand, is stronger in the ability to interact and attract an oppositely charged atom. An ionic bond works across a much larger distance and can reach up to 10 nm apart. The hydrophobic effect significantly helps the targeting ability as water molecules in aqueous solutions interact with hydrophobic molecules less than with water or other hydrophilic molecules. The interaction range of hydrophobic molecules is less than 10 nm and decays exponentially with distance. The high surface-area-to-volume ratio of NPs also generates a high surface energy, around 7.6–454 J/m^2 depending on the size, shape, and material of the NP, which can lead to nonspecific binding to nontarget molecules. Therefore, any targeting agent must have a binding energy that is greater than the surface energy of the NP to provide successful active targeting. Depending on the NP, the surface energy can be substantial, so the NP must be adequately coated with a biocompatible polymer such as polyethylene glycol (PEG) to reduce this surface energy and allow for active targeting.

The binding between the targeting and the targeted molecules is initialized when the molecules are around 10 nm apart. The ionic interaction brings the molecules closer until the secondary bonds, which act in the shorter range, such as hydrophobic interactions, hydrogen bonds, and van der Waals forces, pull them together. Even though the primary ionic bond is strong at long-range interactions, both primary and secondary bonds are essential in keeping both molecules together because the total binding energy of primary and secondary bonds is usually much higher than the binding energy of the primary bond alone.[23] On the other hand, the same attraction mechanisms are also formed with other molecules, which often cause nonspecific binding and NP surface energy–generated protein corona around the NPs that can potentially overwhelm specific

TABLE 3.1 Various types of binding energy between two molecules in a solution.

Bond	Energy (kJ/mol)	Length of interaction (nm)
Ion-dipole	20	10
Hydrogen	20	0.15–0.5
Hydrophobic	<40	10
Van der Waals	4	0.4–0.6
Average molecular kinetic energy in solution	2.6	
Nanoparticle surface energy	7.6–454	

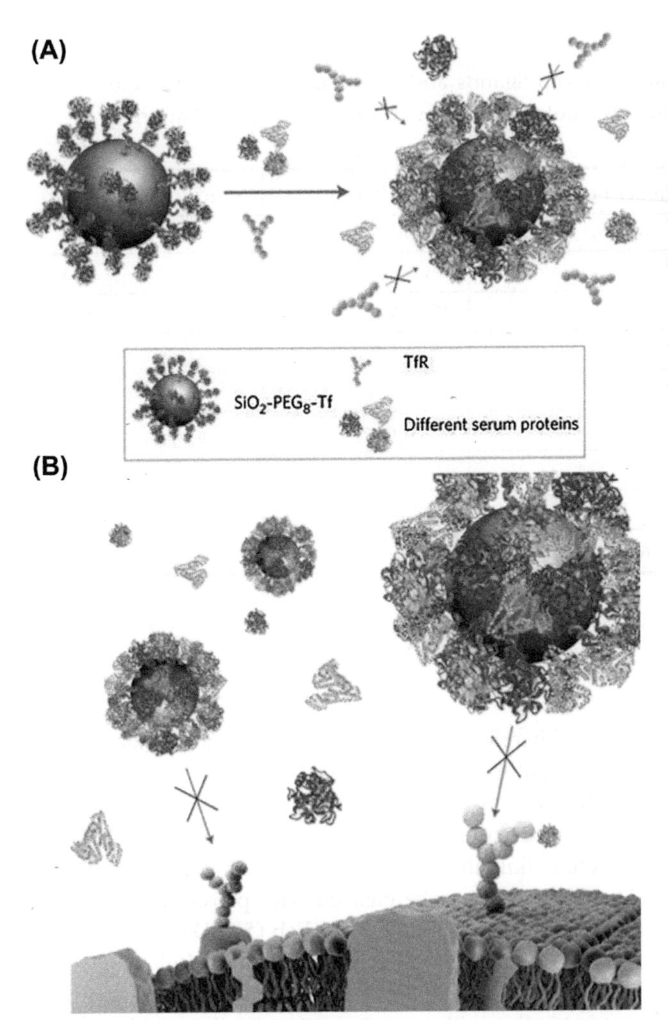

FIGURE 3.1 Opsonization of SiO_2-PEG-transferrin nanoparticlesurface blocking the binding with (A) free transferrin receptor and (B) transferrin receptor on cell surface.[24] *Credit: Reproduced with permission from Anna S et al.: Transferrin-functionalized nanoparticles lose their targeting capabilities when a biomolecule corona adsorbs on the surface.* Nat Nanotechnol *8:137–143, 2013.*

TABLE 3.2 Effect of nanoparticle physicochemical properties on surface binding energy.

Property	Effect on corona coverage and thickness
Size	Inversely proportional
Aspect ratio	Directly proportional
Zeta potential	Directly (both + and −) proportional
Hydrophobicity	Directly proportional
Surface roughness	Directly proportional

ligand–antigen interactions (Fig. 3.1).[24] Therefore, the combined specificity of targeting agents and the ability of NPs to prevent corona formation are both crucial.

Blood plasma contains a large amount of proteins, biomolecules, cells, and salt, which interact with one another and readily adsorb on the surface of NPs to form opsonins, which are recognized by the immune system for removal. The opsonins on the surface of NPs form the corona, where the thickness is directly proportional to the surface energy of the NP. The surface energy of a bare, uncoated NP is affected by physicochemical parameters such as size, shape, surface charge, and hydrophobicity, as summarized in Table 3.2. The surface-area-to-volume ratio of an NP is one of the main factors affecting corona formation on the surface of NPs because surface energy is directly proportional with surface area. Smaller NPs have higher surface area per mass of NP and thus show greater corona formation as compared with larger NPs.[25] Nonspherical NPs have a higher surface-area-to-volume ratio than spherical NPs so they show more corona formation compared with that of spherical NPs.[26] Furthermore, NPs with a rough surface have a greater surface-area-to-volume ratio as compared with NPs with a smooth surface and thus show more corona formation and thickness as compared withsmooth NPs. A higher degree of hydrophobicity on the surface of an NP also affects the corona formation because of the relatively strong binding energy associated with hydrophobic binding in aqueous solution.[25] The surface charge of an NP also affects corona formation through ionic interactions that attract and binds opsonins to the surface of NPs.[27] Corona formation also negatively affects the physicochemical properties of the NPs and leads to a reduction in blood circulation half-life. Furthermore, the corona will often cover the targeting agents on the surface of the NP so they can no longer bind with their target molecules, reducing the effectiveness of the NPs *in vivo*.[24] PEG is also used to reduce opsonin binding on the NPs by both reducing the surface energy of the NP and through steric hindrance. As a result, PEG was found to increase the half-life of circulating NPs inside the blood.[28]

3.3 Targeting agents

Targeting agents are one of the main components in actively targeted NPs. Most ligands utilize 3D structure, charge, and hydrophobicity, which complement its targeted molecules to increase the binding specificity. Various ligands are utilized in actively targeted NPs with a wide range of molecular weights, targeting specificities, and manufacturing costs (Table 3.3). Each ligand has its own advantages and disadvantages for its use in actively targeted NPs.

TABLE 3.3 Comparison of molecular weight, binding affinity between ligands and targeted molecules, half-life in blood circulation, targeting specificity, and manufacturing cost between different targeting agents that are commonly used in actively targeted nanoparticles.

Targeting agents	Molecular weight (kDa)	Binding affinity range (K_D)	Blood half-life	Specificity	Cost
Antibody (IgG)	150	10^{-7}–10^{-13} M	15–30 days	+++	$$$
F(ab')$_2$	110	10^{-5}–10^{-11} M	Several days	+++	$$$$
F(ab)	50	10^{-5}–10^{-11} M	30 min	+++	$$
scFV	28	10^{-5}-10^{-11} M	10–30 min	+++	$$
Aptamers	5–50	10^{-7}–10^{-11} M	5–10 min	+++	$$
Peptides	1.5–50	10^{-9}–10^{-12} M	4–15 min	+++	$$
Protein	80	10^{-7}–10^{-15} M	10–20 days	++	$$
Carbohydrate	0.2–100	10^{-3}–10^{-5} M	Minutes to hours	++	$$
Vitamin	0.3–1.4	10^{-9}–10^{-11} M	Hours to days	++	$

+: the targeting specificity of ligands relative to one another (+ = not specific, ++ = moderately specific, +++ = very specific).
$: the estimated production costs of targeting ligands determined from various commercial sources ($ = <USD0.25/μmol, $$ = USD0.25–5/μmol, $$$ = USD5–10/μmol, $$$$= > USD10/μmol).

3.3.1 Antibody/antibody fragment

Antibodies (Abs) are one of the earliest and most commonly used ligands for actively targeted NPs. Abs are a specific type of protein produced in B cells that bind to target antigens as part of the body's adaptive immune system. Here, we consider Abs separate from proteins since Abs are widely used in NP targeting studies because of their high specificity, strong affinity, and a wide variety of available targets.

There are five major classes of antibodies or immunoglobulins (Ig) that are produced in mammals: IgA, IgD, IgE, IgG, and IgM, all made up of combinations of heavy chains (50 kDa or 440 amino acids each) and light chains (25 kDa or 220 amino acids each).[29–33] The most common Ig used in active targeting is IgG.[31,32] IgG is the dominant class of human Ig and consists of two identical light chains and two identical heavy chains that are held together by several disulfide bonds between cysteines to form a 150 kDa molecule (Table 3.3). The heavy and light chains each contain three complementary-determining regions, located at the N-termini of Abs. These complementary-determining regions have the most variable amino acid combinations to complement the specific target antigen and also provide a very strong avidity in the range of 10^{-7}–10^{-13} M (Table 3.3).[34] The C-termini of Abs contain a fragment crystallizable region (Fc), which has a high affinity toward leukocytes. The structure of Abs allows the Abs to recognize and bind to the antigen of pathogen or cell, whereas the Fc region remains accessible for leukocyte binding and subsequent phagocytosis of the target pathogen or cell. Therefore, the orientation of Ab attachment to NPs is important to ensure functionality.

NPs with Fc regions facing outward can be recognized and phagocytosed by leukocytes. One possibility to overcome this limitation is by removing the Fc region from the Ab. Whole Ab can be cleaved with pepsin and papain to produce F(ab')$_2$ (110 kDa) and Fab (50 kDa), respectively. F(ab')$_2$ can also be cleaved by dithiothreitol to generate Fab' (55 kDa). Since the variable region is the most crucial part in binding with an antigen, the cleaving of Ab does not eliminate the binding ability of Ab fragments. Moreover, work has been done with a single chain of the variable fragment (scFv, 25 kDa) to only keep the variable region while having much smaller molecules than the whole Ab or Ab fragments (Fig. 3.2).[33,35,36]

F(ab')$_2$ and full Abs ($K_D = 6.9 \times 10^{-9}$ M) have binding affinities up to 100 times stronger than the binding affinities of Fab and scFv ($K_D = 6 \times 10^{-7}$ M and 5.9×10^{-7} M, respectively).[37] F(ab')$_2$ and Abs have two binding regions, whereas Fab and scFv only have one binding region; thus, the lack of a multivalent effect may account for some of this loss in binding affinity or increase in K_D. This was shown empirically by utilizing high-speed atomic force microscopy. Preiner et al.[38] found that whole Abs showed bipedal stochastic walking on a surface of regularly spaced epitopes until the Abs found two antigens, within a 6–12 nm range, which perfectly aligned with both binding regions of the Ab. Conversely, monovalent Fab fragments might rotate on the same antigen until it found the same orientation and stand still. The multivalent effect might need to be considered when designing the density of

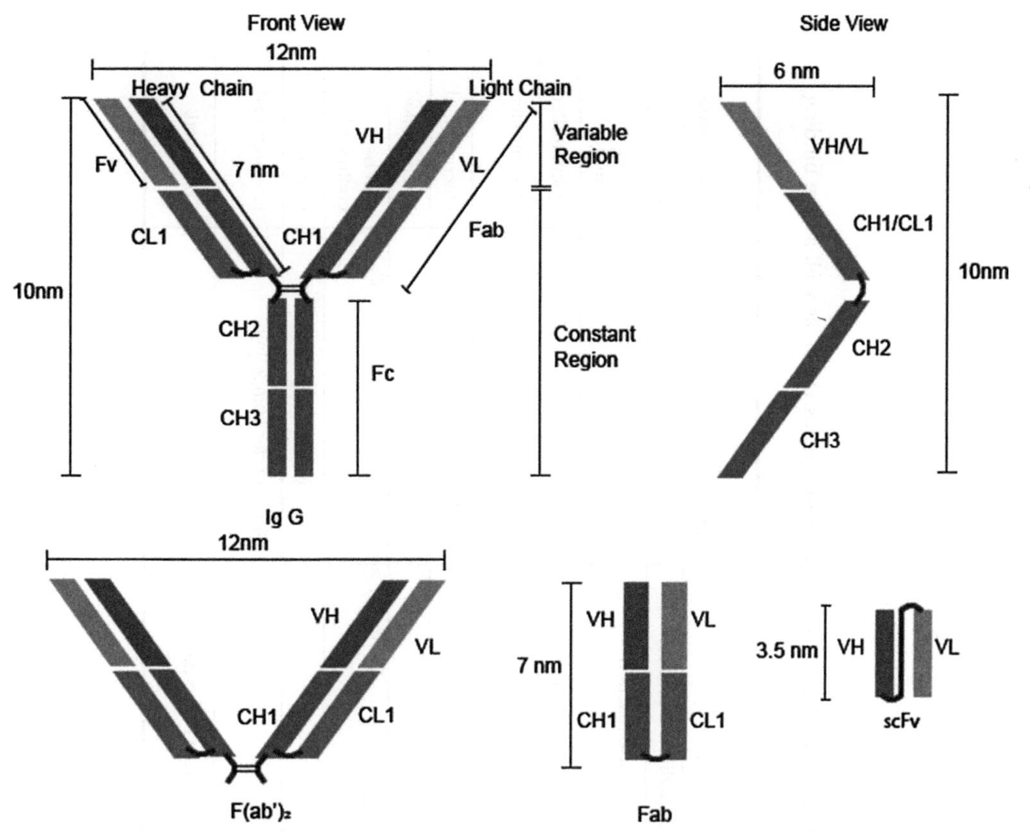

FIGURE 3.2 An illustration showing the shape and dimension of Ab and Ab fragments from both front and side views.

Abs and Ab fragments on the NP surface because suboptimal distance and geometric constraint destabilize multiple binding.[38–41]

The specificity and high affinity of Abs to bind with antigens combined with the ability of NPs as a delivery vehicle and imaging agent have brought many opportunities and breakthroughs in biomedicine. Therefore, the conjugation of Abs onto the surface of NPs has been widely studied, such as Ab-NP conjugation strategy, the density of Ab on NPs surface,[39–41] and controlled orientation of Ab on the surface.[42]

Abs possess a large number of functional groups that can be conjugated to NPs. These include carboxylic acid groups (glutamic and aspartic acids), amine groups (lysine, asparagine, and glutamine), and thiol groups (cysteine). However, the spread of these amino acids along the Abs results in an uncontrollable orientation of conjugated Ab on NP. NPs containing a random orientation of Abs resulted in a 10-fold reduction in antigen-binding affinity compared with NPs where the Ab-binding regions all faced outward.[43] Therefore, various conjugation strategies for Ab attachment on NPs result in different abilities to control orientation as outlined below.

3.3.2 Several common covalent-binding reactions

- Carboxylic acid and primary amine reaction:

An amide bond is a stable linkage formed by the condensation reaction of a carboxylic acid and a primary amine, usually through a carbodiimide reaction (Table 3.4). Carbodiimide reactions often utilize 1-ethyl-3-(3-dimethylaminopropyl)carbodiimide (EDC) to form an intermediate ester bond before being substituted by a primary amine group. An amide bond can also be formed by activating primary alcohol groups on Abs (serine, threonine) or NPs with p-toluenesulfonyl chloride to become amine reactive. An advantage of the amide bond is that no modification on the Ab is required, reducing the risk of loss in reactivity and denaturation. One of the limitations is the inability to control the orientation of the Ab on NP because of the distribution of carboxylic acid and amine groups throughout the Ab. The Ab might link to more than one NP, to more than one site of the same NP, or even linkage to NP on the variable region, which can block Ab binding to targeted molecules. Therefore, the ratio of reactants must be carefully controlled.

- Schiff base reaction:

A reaction between an aldehyde and primary amine forms an imine bond, a Schiff base. Typically, NPs are activated with aldehyde groups such as by reaction with excess glutaraldehyde. Another way of binding Ab to NP

TABLE 3.4 Commonly used linkage, functional group, and chemical reactions to bind antibodies (Abs) with nanoparticles (NPs), as well as the binding stability and Abs orientation on the surface of the NPs.

Type of bond	Linkage	Conjugated functional group	Commonly used reaction	Linkage stability	Abs orientation
Covalent	Amide bond	Primary amine–carboxylic acid	Carbodiimide reaction	Stable	Uncontrolled
	Imine bond	Hydrazide/hydrazine–aldehyde/ketone	Schiff base reaction	Labile under acid condition	Can be controlled
	Thioether bond	Thiol–maleimide	Michael reaction	Stable	Uncontrolled
	Disulfide bond	Thiol–thiol		Labile under reducing conditions	Uncontrolled
	Dative bond	Thiol–metal		Stable	Uncontrolled
	Triazole ring	Azide–alkyne	Click chemistry	Stable	Uncontrolled
Noncovalent	Biotin–avidin	Biotin–avidin Biotin–streptavidin		Stable	Can be controlled
	Protein A and G	Protein A/G–Ab Fc region		Labile under competing Abs	Controlled
	Ionic bond (physioadsorption)			Labile under competing opsonins	Uncontrolled
	Nucleotide-binding site–indole	Nucleotide-binding site–indole	Ultraviolet free radical		Controlled

with Schiff base is to utilize hydrazide or hydrazine functional group (R−NH−NH_2) with aldehyde or ketone to form a hydrazone bond (Table 3.4).

While these conjugation reactions do not ensure a well-oriented Ab, the mild oxidation of vicinal hydroxyl groups with sodium periodate on carbohydrate residues to become aldehyde groups can result in oriented Ab conjugation.[44] This takes advantage of the fact that carbohydrate residues on Abs are specifically located on the Fc region. As an example, an oxidized Ab was conjugated to a hydrazide group of a bifunctional PEG that also contains a dithiolaromatic group. The dithiolaromatic group was then used to bind to the surface of a gold NP through a covalent bond between sulfur and gold atom.[44]

- Thiol reaction:

Although thiols are present on Abs, they are involved in intramolecular disulfide bridges within the native Ab. Hence, these disulfide bridges must first be reduced to make thiols available for reaction. Conversely, free thiols can be introduced onto Abs by reaction with amine groups, such as with using Traut's reagent. Free thiols on Abs can be used to conjugate to NPs through disulfide or thioether bonds (Table 3.4). Typically, disulfide bonds are not used because they are difficult to control and often lead to cross-linking between NPs. On the other hand, thioethers can be formed with maleimide-activated NPs as well as through Michael addition reactions with aldehydes on the NP, with efficiency up to 95%−99%.[45] Abs with activated thiol groups can also create a covalent bond to metal NPs (*e.g.*, gold NPs), which is often called a dative bond where the bond was formed through electron from the metal atom shared to the thiol group (Table 3.4). For example, Abs were reduced with tris(2-carboxyethyl) phosphine, a weak reducing agent that allows more specific disulfide bond reduction on Ab, which are then available for dative binding to the gold NPs.[46] However, the reduction method might be too harsh to the Ab that it might damage the Ab tertiary structure and reduce the binding activity of Ab significantly when compared withthe carbodiimide reaction and ionic interaction.[46] Similar to the formation of an amide bond or a Schiff base, the orientation of Abs on the NPs is also difficult to control using these thiol reactions.

- Click chemistries:

Click chemistries are a set of reactions that are highly specific, stereospecific, efficient, easily performed, reactive in easily removed solvents and eliminate the need for chromatography to remove byproducts. These reactions might require a catalyst, a substance involved in a chemical reaction that increases the reaction rate but is not consumed in the overall reaction. Copper is a typical catalyst used in click chemistry between an azide functional group (N_3) and an alkyne functional group (Table 3.4). Click reactions to conjugate Abs to NPs have been shown to be fivefold to eightfold more efficient than amide reactions.[47,48] Nevertheless, Ab orientation on the NPs is still difficult to control.

3.3.3 Several common non-covalent bindings

- Avidin−biotin:

The specific binding between avidin and biotin is one of the strongest known non-covalent bonds ($K_D \sim 10^{-15}$ M) (Table 3.4). Avidin is a glycoprotein with four subunits, which can bind to up to four biotins. An advantage of this reaction is that avidin can be introduced directly into the Ab backbone in the Fc region through genetic engineering of hybridomas, in vitro cell cultures that produce Abs. The resulting fusion protein can then be attached to biotinylated NPs with well-controlled orientation and stoichiometry.

- Proteins A and G:

Protein A and protein G are proteins utilized by *Staphylococcus aureus* and *Streptococcus C40*, respectively. Both protein A and protein G are able to bind and neutralize Ab from immune recognition, as they specifically bind to the Fc region of IgG. This has provided the opportunity to utilize these proteins to control Ab orientation on NPs (Table 3.4). Up to 95% of protein A on the surface of cyanoacrylic NPs was found to bind with Ab during the conjugation reaction.[49] However, *in vivo* studies were disappointing where Ab conjugated NPs accumulated mostly in the liver and spleen. The adsorption of excess protein in blood serum might compete with protein A, which can break the binding between Ab and protein A.[50]

- Physioadsorption:

Adsorption of Abs on the NP surface was one of the earliest studied attachment techniques. Ab-bound phospholipid-based NPs were prepared by merely adding the ligand to the NPs solution. If the phospholipid charge was neutral, 4%−40% of the IgG bound to the liposomal NP. When anionic phospholipids were used, the binding of Ab to NP was about 50% higher than that of neutral phospholipids.[51] These results suggest that Ab adsorption on liposomal NPs depends on the hydrophobicity, as well as the ionic charge of the liposome NP (Table 3.4). Ab-bound liposomal NPs increased the antigen binding by 30%−50% compared with free Ab.[51] However, adsorbed Abs might be exchanged by stronger binding opsonins in the blood, potentially decreasing the effectiveness of the Ab-NP.

- Others:

A small indole molecule can be entrapped into the nucleotide-binding site of Ab ($K_D = 1-8\ \mu M$) with the help of ultraviolet light (Table 3.4). The nucleotide-binding site allows specific site and orientation of Ab on the NP surface.[52] Utilizing the nucleotide-binding site of Ab increased NP binding and sensitivity toward antigen significantly as compared with a carbodiimide reaction, ionic interaction, and thiol bond.[46]

Despite the advantages of Abs as a targeting ligand, its large size can significantly increase the hydrodynamic size of small NPs. For example, 12.5 nm NPs increase in size to 25 nm after being conjugated with Abs.[46] The production cost of Ab is also very expensive because of the need for live animal hosts to produce titers. Mammalian cell culture can be used as a potentially cheaper method but requires significant numbers of cells to generate useable quantities of Ab. $F(ab')_2$ is derived from whole Ab with further purification, which makes the production cost of $F(ab')_2$ even more expensive than the production cost of the whole Ab. Even though Fab can be derived from whole Ab, similar to $F(ab)'_2$ production, Fab and scFv can also be produced from bacteria, which grow much faster and in higher densities than mammalian cell culture and can reduce the production cost of Fab and scFv.

3.3.4 Aptamers

Beyond their use for storing and expressing the genetic code, nucleic acids (DNA and RNA) form two- and three-dimensional structures, which are more stable than linear oligonucleotides. Oligonucleotides are well-known for their double-stranded helical structures and their single-stranded hairpin structures. However, these are not the only three-dimensional structures of oligonucleotides. For example, a thrombin-binding aptamer is a G-quadruplex structure formed by the stacks of planar guanine tetrads (Fig. 3.3), where molecular structure of the thrombin-binding aptamer was determined by NMR spectroscopy and X-ray crystallography.[55] The natural use of oligonucleotides to bind with other molecules is very limited; however, random arrangements and panning of oligonucleotides have led to the evolution of oligonucleotide-based targeting ligands. The randomly arranged oligonucleotide sequences are called aptamers, which means: to fit.[56]

An early and widely used method to produce aptamers is through SELEX (Systematic Evolution of Ligands by Exponential enrichment), which was developed in 1990.[57] In the same year, an independent study found a specific three-dimensional structure of RNA that was able to bind with a small molecule.[56] SELEX produces aptamers of 20–100 oligonucleotides, with molecular weights of 5–50 kDa (Table 3.3). The process of SELEX usually goes through 8–20 panning steps from a large pool of aptamers (10^{13}–10^{15} aptamer sequences) until only several high-affinity aptamers toward targeted molecule are obtained at the end of the cycles.

Similar to Abs, aptamers can bind to various antigens, such as inorganic molecules, small organic molecules, proteins, peptides, carbohydrates, antibiotics, whole cells, and even organisms, with high specificity and selectivity. The interactions between aptamers and antigens are usually based on electrostatic interactions, hydrophilic interactions, and complementary shapes. The multivalent effect can also be exploited with aptamer-modified NPs to increase binding affinity. This was shown using a dimer aptamer composed of two aptamers (15-mer and 29-mer thrombin aptamers linked by a flexible linker), which bind two different sites on thrombin. The dimer aptamer decreased the K_D 10-fold when compared with the K_D of the 15-mer thrombin aptamer itself.[58] A similar effect was found with multiple different aptamer sequences on a single NP. Multitargeted NPs were able to accumulate on the targeted molecule at a higher level than NPs modified with a single aptamer sequence.[59]

Another advantage of aptamers is that they can be engineered to have multiple regions with different functions such as to promote entrapment inside an NP. For example, phosphorothioate-modified DNA bases were used to give a hydrophobic characteristic to the aptamers while a tumor targeting sequence was kept hydrophilic.[60] This allowed the active targeting domain to be exposed on the surface of the NP while entrapping the hydrophobic domain inside the NP during NP synthesis. The entrapped aptamer was able to improve accumulation of the targeted NPs on lung cancer cells grown subcutaneously in nude mice.

One of the limitations of aptamers is the high serum nuclease activity in blood that can quickly degrade nucleotides or aptamers—unmodified nucleotides have stability half-lives of as short as 2 min in blood serum (Table 3.3).[61] These very short half-lives can be overcome by chemical modifications of the aptamer backbone such as capping the 3′-terminus to prevent 3′-exonuclease activity, which is much higher than 5′-exonuclease activity in serum. Another strategy is to create enantiomer nucleotide backbones (L-ribose and L-deoxyribose), which also reduces nuclease degradation.[62] Despite the adaptability of aptamers, their binding is typically limited toward hydrophobic and negativelycharged antigens. Aptamers are very hydrophilic, and the phosphate backbone is negatively charged; therefore, the difference between hydrophobicity–hydrophilicity characteristics of antigen and aptamers weakens the binding because of the

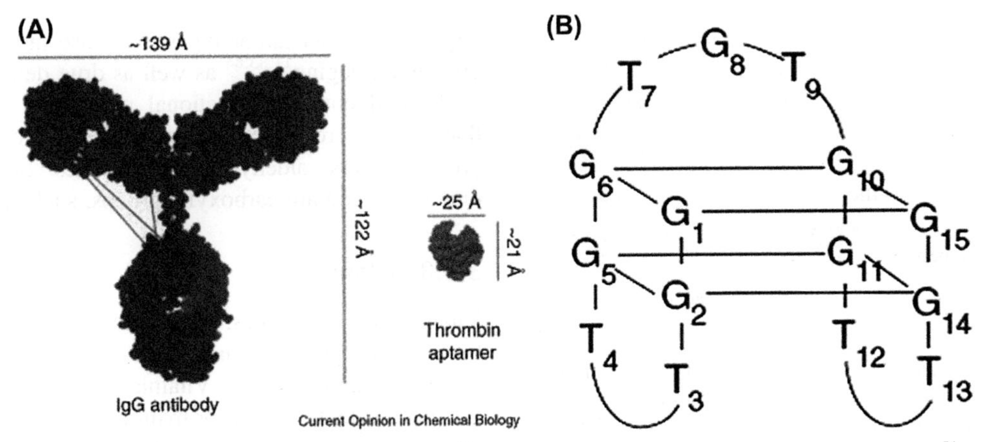

FIGURE 3.3 (A) Size comparison between Ab and thrombin aptamer[53] and (B) chemical structure of thrombin-binding aptamer.[54] *Credit: Reproduced with permission from Jennifer FL et al.: Aptamer therapeutics advance,* Curr Opin Chem Biol *10:282–289, 2006; and Baobin C et al.: Stability and bioactivity of thrombin binding aptamers modified with D-/l-isothymidine in the loop regions,* Org Biomol Chem *12:8866–8876, 2014.*

hydrophobic force preventing hydrogen bonding to occur. Likewise, if the antigen is negatively charged, there will be a repulsive ionic interaction between the antigen and aptamer.

3.3.5 Proteins

Similar to Abs, proteins also contain functional groups on their N- and C-termini, as well as the amino acid building blocks. Transferrin has been extensively used as a targeting protein on the surface of NPs because of its ability to target the transferrin receptor, which is upregulated in many types of cancer cells. One of the advantages using proteins is the higher molecular weight compared withthe other ligands (*e.g.*, MW of transferrin is 80 kDa), which significantly increase the circulation time of the protein in the blood (Table 3.3). One of the most common conjugations of transferrin to NPs is through carbodiimides reaction to form an amide bond. For example, transferrin conjugated to PEG–liposomal NPs wasused to target disseminated gastric cancer cells through an intraperitoneal injection.[63] The transferrin-targeted NPs had higher uptake and penetration into solid tumor tissue, which resulted in a higher survival rate in a human xenograft mouse model as compared with control NPs without transferrin.[63] In another study, transferrin-targeted NPs were found to penetrate hepatic and cervical tumor spheroids much more than the free drug and non-targeted NPs.[64]

However, the competition between proteins on NPs and the excess protein in the blood plasma might reduce the targeting ability of protein targeting NPs toward the protein receptors.[64,65]

3.3.6 Peptides

Peptides can be thought of as very small proteins, as they consist of a short chain of amino acids and can be conjugated to NP in a similar conjugation technique as Ab conjugation to NP. The conjugation site and the availability of the active site for binding with antigen are also important when considering peptide conjugation strategies. On the other hand, peptides are similar to nucleic acid aptamers as most peptides are easily synthesized in the lab and bind with a specific target. Peptide sequences can be discovered through multiround panning processes using phage display technology.[67] Peptides can also be engineered to have similar active binding sites with antibodies and proteins. The binding affinities of peptides are comparable withthe binding affinities of antibody fragments, which are in the nanomolar range. Peptides can be designed with multiple binding sites to take advantage of the multivalent effect, which increases the binding affinity of the peptides to the antigens (Fig. 3.4).[66]

Arginine–glycine–aspartate (RGD) tripeptide and its derivatives are well-known for their ability to bind to integrins, the binding proteins of cells with the extracellular matrix. Integrins are often upregulated in solid tumors; hence many tumor-targeted NPs have relied on RGD-based peptides as a targeting agent.[68–72] To increase binding affinity and specificity to $\alpha_5\beta_1$ integrin, which is overexpressed on breast, prostate, rectal, and colon cancers, a multivalent peptide containing GRGDSP and PHSRN subunits was developed.[73,74] From the crystal structure, GRGDSP and PHSRN peptides are able to bind on the same face of fibronectin 3.5 nm apart.[75] RGD domain of the GRGDSP is a well-known component to interact with fibronectin, whereas PHSRN peptides arethe synergy region that increases the avidity between targeting peptides and fibronectin. This multivalent peptide was attached to the surface of a liposomal/micellar NP carrying doxorubicin to improve delivery into colon cancer cells. As a result, the multivalent peptide sequence was able to improve the delivery rate as compared with the NPs targeted with GRGDSP alone.[74]

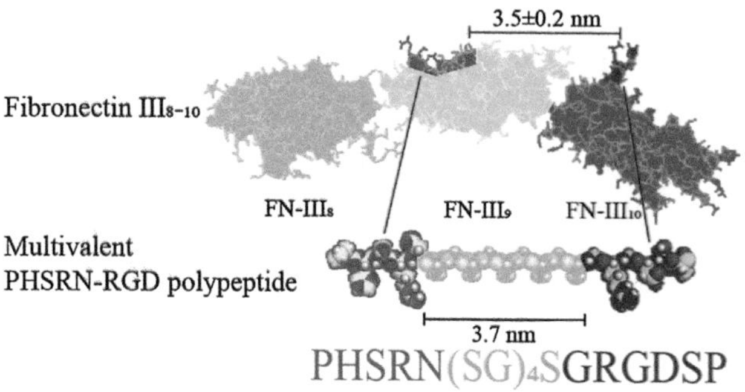

3.5±0.2 nm
Fibronectin III8-10
FN-III8 FN-III9 FN-III10
Multivalent PHSRN-RGD polypeptide
3.7 nm
PHSRN(SG)4SGRGDSP

FIGURE 3.4 Two binding sites of a polypeptides chain of GRGDSP and PSHRN increase the binding specificity and avidity toward fibronectin III on the repeats 9 and 10, compared with the individual binding sites. *Inspired by Kokkoli E.*[66]

However, peptides have several disadvantages such as cleaving and degradation of peptides exposed on the surface of NPs by serum protease in the blood plasma, which reduce the effectiveness of peptide targeting. Fortunately, the stability of peptides in blood plasma can be improved by adding cysteines to form disulfide bonds generating a more stable cyclic peptide, blocking the C- and N-terminus, utilizing D-amino acids backbones, or using synthetic amino acids that are incompatible with proteases.[76–78] The small size of peptides also makes them prone to kidney clearance (MW = 1.5−50 kDa) (Table 3.3), which can be overcome by conjugating peptides to NPs.

3.3.7 Carbohydrates

Carbohydrates consist of carbon, hydrogen, and oxygen, and sometimes phosphorus, sulfur, and nitrogen atoms. There are three types of carbohydrates: monosaccharides, disaccharides, and polysaccharides. Monosaccharides are the simplest form of carbohydrates, such as glucose, fructose, and galactose, and are usually the building blocks of the more complex carbohydrates. Disaccharides comprise two monosaccharides, such as sucrose (glucose and fructose), lactose (glucose and galactose), and maltose (glucose and glucose). Polysaccharides and oligosaccharides are a chain of sugars with three or more monosaccharides and can be linear (such as with amylose) or branched (such as with glycogen). Therefore, the molecular weight and blood circulation half-life of carbohydrates widely varied, with molecular weights of 0.2−100 kDa and blood circulation half-lives of minutes to hours (Table 3.3).

Many cancer cells overexpress the CD44 cellsurface marker, which binds to hyaluronic acid (HA), a glycosaminoglycan component of the extracellular matrix. HA has garnered significant attention as it can be conjugated to the NP surface as a targeting agent similar with other ligands,[79–81] and it can also be utilized as the HA-based NP building block reducing the need for secondary conjugations.[11,82–86] HA-based NPs have been used for targeting various tumor types in mouse models for intraoperative imaging[11,83,84] as well as drug delivery.[82,85,86]

Several common functional groups on carbohydrates that can be readily conjugated are hydroxyl (alcohol) groups, ethers, aldehydes, and ketones. Some carbohydrates also contain carboxylic groups, such as in HA.

3.3.8 Vitamins

Vitamins are molecules, which are essential for the body but are not part of minerals, essential fatty acids, and essential amino acids. Vitamins can be hydrophobic (vitamin A, D, E, and K) or hydrophilic (vitamin B and C). Almost every tissue has vitamin receptors, but some tumors and specific tissues often overexpressed vitamin receptors, which allows for vitamins to be used in actively targeted NPs.

Two of the most utilized vitamins in actively targeted NPs are folate (vitamin B9) and vitamin B12. Folate is required for biosynthesis of purines and pyrimidines. Even though the folate receptor availability on the normal cells is limited, folate receptors are commonly overexpressed on the surface of activated myeloid cells and tumor cells, such as ovarian, lung, breast, and brain cancers.[87,88] On the other hand, vitamin B12 is often used in active targeting for intestine absorption, as vitamin B12 promotes receptor-mediated endocytosis to go through the intestine endothelial cells into the blood vessel.[89–92]

Vitamin B12 is much larger (1355 Da) than other vitamins (*e.g.*, folate is 441 Da) (Table 3.3). Therefore, vitamin B12 needs a specific pathway to be absorbed in the intestine. In the small intestine, vitamin B12 interacts with intrinsic factor protein, which helps to bind to intrinsic factor receptor and is absorbed through the intestinal wall.

Folate, on the other hand, has a carboxylic acid group that is readily conjugated with an amine group and other functional groups. The conjugation of folate on the carboxylic acid also does not affect the K_D of folate to the folate receptor, as the terminal carboxylic group is more reactive for conjugation. There are two folate receptors, FR-α ($K_D \sim 10^{-11}$) and FR-β ($K_D \sim 10^{-9}$) (Table 3.3).[93] FR-α is overexpressed on 40% of human cancers and has limited expression in normal cells. On the other hand, FR-β is upregulated in activated myeloid cells, such as 70% of acute myeloid leukemia cells.[94,95] Folate is also stable, is inexpensive, promotes rapid internalization into tumor cells, is readily conjugated, and is nonimmunogenic.

Vitamins as targeting agents offer high specificity to their respective receptors ($K_D = 10^{-9}-10^{-11}$ M),[93] non-immunogenicity, as well as ease of production leading to very low costs (Table 3.3). However, vitamin-modified NPs have similar disadvantages as protein-targeting NPs, in which excess vitamins in the body might compete with vitamin-modified NPs to bind with the specific receptor,[96–99] reducing the targeting ability. Moreover, the expression of vitamin receptors (e.g., folate receptor) on the surface of multiple cell types, such as activated myeloid cells and tumor cells, might cause off-targeting using vitamin-targeting NPs.

3.4 Active targeting strategies for various diseases

NPs have been widely studied over the past few decades in the biomedical field. However, most studies have focused on cancer, which has led to the formation of a substantial body of literature on understanding the effects of physicochemical, molecular, and active targeting properties of NPs in tumor tissues and the body. Fortunately, much of this literature, such as ligand conjugation techniques, physicochemical properties of NPs that increase blood circulation half-life, and strategies that improve tissue penetration, can be translated to use in other diseases. Even though cancer is still one of the most focused research areas of NPs, the utility of NPs in non-neoplastic diseases has begun to gain attention. This includes the use of the active targeting ability of NPs to increase transmembrane penetration, accumulation in non-EPR diseases, and more selective and specific therapeutics delivery and imaging. Here, focus is given to studies that have pre-clinical mechanistic data.

3.4.1 Cancer

Cancer is an unregulated cell growth usually caused by mutations in cell growth signaling and receptor regulatory proteins. Cancer is well-known for its EPR effect compared with healthy tissues because of uncontrolled angiogenesis and lack of lymphatic drainage. Therefore, passive targeting NPs (see Chapter 4) are able to show a significant result in cancer therapy. However, active targeting can still improve NP delivery in EPR cancers. A series of studies found that active targeting did not increase the accumulation of NPs in EPR tumors, which was dominated by the EPR effect, but distribution throughout the tumor and delivery into cells was increased with active targeting.[8–10,100,101] These results showed the importance of active targeting in improving NP delivery even in tumors where the EPR effect allows for passive NP targeting. Active targeting is even more critical in cancers that do not have an EPR effect such as some hematological malignancies,[102–106] small metastatic tumors,[107–110] and circulating tumor cells.[111] In these cases, active targeting is required for specific binding to these cells. For example, Ab-modified iron oxide NPs targeted to the HER2/neu receptor were able to bind to breast cancer metastases to the liver, lungs, brain, and bone marrow in a transgenic mouse model, whereas IgG control-modified NPs showed no uptake into these cells.[14] Active Ab-mediated targeting of NPs to tumors can be further enhanced when NPs are loaded with chemotherapeutic agents. Chemotherapy loading into the active targeted NPs reduced the immune response against these PEG-coated NPs, allowing for increased tumor delivery compared with the active targeted NPs without chemotherapy loading.[112] The reduction in the immune response was a result of the cytotoxicity of the chemotherapy agent to both adaptive and innate immune cells, which blocked any subsequent immune response.[112]

Leukemia is a hematological malignancy that does not form a solid tumor despite some evidence of EPR observed in bone marrow[103]; hence, there is no EPR effect that NPs can exploit. Therefore, actively targeted NPs might be ideal in targeting leukemia cells to reduce the toxicity of systemic therapies. On acute myeloid leukemia, epidermal growth factor receptor (EGFR) is often overexpressed, which can readily be targeted by an anti-EGFR Ab, aptamer, or peptide. In one study, anti-EGFR Ab was biotinylated to allow for attachment to NeutrAvidin-modified mesoporous silica NPs (MSNs).[13] Active targeted NPs were able to specifically bind to and be internalized by EGFR-expressing leukemia cell both in vitro and in an *ex ovo* model. Following this, chemotherapy-loaded, anti-EGFR Ab-targeted MSNs showed active targeting-mediated cell kill in leukemia cells both *in vitro* and in a mouse model, which improved survival.[113]

The GE11 peptide, an EGF mimetic, has been conjugated to various NPs for active targeting of EGFR-overexpressing tumors.[114–117] However, the internalization mechanism for NPs modified with the artificial GE11 peptide is different from that of those modified with natural EGF.[118] Single particle tracking revealed EGF-modified NPs were rapidly internalized into EGFR-expressing cells *in vitro*, showing 80% internalization within 10 min. On the other hand, GE11-modified NPs took 4 h to reach the same level of internalization as EGF-modified NPs, while non-targeted NPs reached only 31% internalization. The difference in internalization between NPs targeted with EGF and GE11 was found to be a result of EGFR activation with native EGF, which promoted rapid internalization, whereas EGFR was not activated by GE11.[118] This is one example of how the choice of active targeting agent on the surface of an NP can alter target cell uptake.

3.4.2 Atherosclerosis

Atherosclerosis is the leading cause of cardiovascular disease, in which chronic, inflammatory lipid-rich plaques and cholesterol particles accumulate within the artery wall. The inflamed endothelial cells are also prone to leakiness, which can result in an EPR-like effect. Therefore, NPs are suitable to be used in passive drug delivery and diagnosis of atherosclerosis.[119–122] While passive targeting of atherosclerotic plaques can be achieved with NPs depending on the permeability of the vessel wall,[123] active targeting is expected to achieve higher penetration into the plaque and internalization into target cells. Several ligands have been used in active targeting of atherosclerosis, such as vascular cell adhesion molecule-1 (VCAM-1),[124,125] monocyte chemoattractant protein-1 (MCP-1),[126] interleukin-10 (IL-10),[127] and E-selectin,[128] in hopes of improving therapeutic delivery and retention to reduce plaque size and inflammation. These active targeted NPs showed higher accumulation rates within the plaques and significantly longer retention times to potentially improve therapeutic delivery. HA NPs have also been used for active targeting of inflammatory cells in plaques since the inflammatory process requires HA-immune cell interactions.[129] HA can also act as a therapeutic since nanoformulated HA has been shown to act as an anti-inflammatory.[130] Thus, the HA provided the building blocks to achieve the NP size needed for passive accumulation, active targeting to promote target cell-specific interactions, and therapy by providing atheroprotective effects.[129]

3.4.3 Kidney disease

Chronic kidney disease is a state of reduced kidney function that can lead to various other health complications such as stroke, hypertension, and liver dysfunction. Small molecule therapeutics have been hindered by poor circulation times, which requires high doses to be delivered leading to off-target side effects and even lethality. Thus, active targeted NPs have been developed using a kidney-targeting peptide $(KKEEE)_3K$ to specifically bind to megalin, a cell surface receptor on renal tubule cells, through multivalent display.[131] NPs slightly larger than the 10 nm cutoff of glomerular filtration were used and showed selective accumulation on renal proximal tubule cells *in vitro*. In healthy mice, active targeted NPs showed significantly higher kidney accumulation than non-targeted NPs, suggesting the use of active targeting for kidney disease.[131]

3.4.4 Neurological disorders

Neurological disorders encompass various diseases, including brain cancer, traumatic brain injury (TBI), stroke, neuroinflammation, and progressive neurodegenerative diseases such as Alzheimer's and Parkinson's disease. The treatment of neurological disorders is especially challenging because of the sensitivity and importance of the brain to survival as well as the BBB, which prevents the passive accumulation of delivered therapies into the brain (also see Chapter 7). Whereaspassive targeting of NPs is possible for disorders where the BBB is significantly disrupted such as in brain cancer[132] and TBI,[133–138] active targeting is required in disorders where BBB integrity is intact. Targets typically include transmembrane ligands to act as a Trojan horse to gain access into the brain through receptor-mediated transcytosis across the BBB. These include receptors for transferrin,[3,139–141] lactoferrin,[2,142,143] and possibly RAGE (receptor for advanced glycation end products), which is overexpressed on diseased brain microvascular cells,[144] or tight junction proteins.

The rabies virus glycoprotein peptide (RVG29, TYIWMPENPRPGTPCDIFTNSRGKRASNG) was developed to cross the BBB by taking advantage of the pathway exploited by the neurotropic rabies virus, either through nicotinic acetylcholine receptor (nAchR) or GABA receptor binding. RVG29 conjugated to generation-5 PAMAM dendrimers through bifunctional PEG accumulated in all regions of the mouse brain significantly higher than the nontargeting NPs.[145] Similar results have been found in other RVG29 active-targeting NPs where receptor-mediated transcytosis across the BBB increased brain delivery of various therapeutics to improve treatment in mouse models of Alzheimer's disease and Parkinson's disease.[17,146–148]

RVG29-conjugated NPs have been utilized for active targeting toward TBI.[15] TBI is an injury that results from a primary impact to the brain followed by the secondary release of biochemicals such as reactive oxygen species (ROS), glutamate, calcium, and lipid peroxidation products that can cause long-term neuroinflammation and neurodegeneration for years following the injury. A transportan–RVG29 peptide complex was developed to form a micelle, where anti-caspase-3 siRNA was entrapped inside the cationic micelle. As a result, RVG29 significantly increased the micelle accumulation in a mouse model of TBI compared withcontrol peptide and resulted in decreased caspase-3 production in target neurons.[15]

Neuroinflammation increases expression of vascular cell adhesion molecule-1 (VCAM-1) on brain endothelial cells, which is an ideal target of active NP targeting. NPs targeted to VCAM-1 with Abs or peptides have been used for imaging specific regions of neuroinflammation.[149,150] Similar strategies have been used with the platelet–endothelial cell adhesion molecule (PECAM-1), which is also overexpressed on brain endothelial cells as a result of neuroinflammation. NPs actively targeted to PECAM-1 show improved brain delivery as compared with control NPs.[151] This could improve diagnostic information and provide a platform for therapeutic delivery.

3.4.5 Rheumatic inflammation

Rheumatoid arthritis (RA) is a chronic inflammatory disease where macrophages are chronically activated and degrade bone and cartilage around joints. While methotrexate (MTX) is one of the most common and effective therapeutics for RA treatment, its prolonged use is accompanied by drug resistance and adverse side effects. Therefore, active targeted NPs could help improve the site-specific delivery of MTX. Activated macrophages express the folate receptor,[152] FR-β, which opens the opportunity for folate surface modification of NPs. As an example, an MTX-encapsulated folate–PEG–lipid NP was developed where folate was covalently conjugated to the PEG on the surface of the NP to achieve higher uptake into lipopolysaccharide-activated RAW264.7 cells as compared with non-targeted NPs showing the specificity toward activated cells. Similarly, folate and MTX surface-decorated dendrimers have been used for improved active *in vivo* delivery to inflamed joints.[153,154]

As another target, synovial fibroblasts in RA highly activate nuclear factor-kappa B (NF-κB), leading to inflammation. The HAP-1 peptide is able to specifically bind to synovial fibroblasts offering the ability for active NP targeting. Encapsulated NEMO-binding domain peptide, which inactivates NF-kB, within a HAP-1-coated NP, showed accumulation enhancement on SF compared with non-targeted NP, as well as a reduction in both histological score and pro-inflammatory signaling compared with control NPs.[155]

3.4.6 Diabetes

Diabetes is a condition where the body cannot regulate blood glucose level, which can be a result of either the pancreas producing little to no insulin (type I diabetes) or the body not responding to insulin (type II diabetes). Insulin monitoring and injection remain the most effective treatment for diabetes patients to regulate the level of blood glucose. Therefore, more patient-friendly approaches for insulin delivery are desirable for a better control glucose levels and improve patient compliance. NPs offer a means for active transport out of the gastrointestinal tract to allow for oral delivery of therapeutics.[156–158]

Vitamin B12 is absorbed in the ileum of the small intestine for active transcytosis across the epithelial barrier into the blood. Therefore, attaching vitamin B12 to the surface of NPs can provide an active targeting mechanism to gain access to systemic circulation across the epithelial barrier.[159] In one study, insulin-entrapped calcium phosphate NPs were coated with chitosan conjugated to vitamin B12 to allow for active transcytosis across the epithelium.[89] In diabetic rats, active targeted NPs increased the oral bioavailability of insulin 4.3-fold as compared with non-targeted NPs, which extended the therapeutic response to insulin as compared with standard subcutaneous injection of insulin.[89] Transferrin can also be used for active targeting in the intestines to promote NP uptake, transcytosis across the epithelial barrier, and insulin absorption to achieve a therapeutic response.[160] To target goblet cells, which are responsible for mucus production in the intestines and transcytosis into the blood, NPs have been modified with the CSK (CSKSSDYQC) targeting peptide and were found to enhance absorption of delivered insulin.[161–163]

3.5 Conclusions and future outlook

Various actively targeted NPs have been developed using various NP materials, NP sizes, ligands, conjugation techniques, antigens, and targeted tissues. Actively targeted NPs have also shown promising results in *in vitro* and *in vivo* studies for improving the selectivity and specificity of accumulation and drug efficacy in targeted tissues compared with those of passive targeting NPs. Some actively targeted NPs have also been found to increase permeation across biological barriers (described in more detail in Chapter 7) such as the BBB and intestinal barrier. Active targeting is crucial for NP delivery to diseases that do not show an EPR effect. However, despite the growing interest and the prospect of actively targeted NPs in the biomedical field, as well as numerous clinical trials, there is currently no approved actively targeted NP used clinically. The diversity in the surface marker expressed by targeted tissue between individuals, complicated synthesis of actively targeted NPs, and difficulty in upscaling production hinder the translation of actively targeted NPs into widespread clinical use. On the other hand, the exponential improvement in technologies, such as better diagnostic tools for preselection of patients who would respond to the therapies, might be helpful in pushing actively targeted NPs into the market in the future.

References

1. Han L, Cai Q, Tian D, et al. Targeted drug delivery to ischemic stroke via chlorotoxin-anchored, lexiscan-loaded nanoparticles. *Nanomed-Nanotechnol* 2016;**12**(7):1833–42.
2. Hu K, Shi Y, Jiang W, Han J, Huang S, Jiang X. Lactoferrin conjugated PEG-PLGA nanoparticles for brain delivery: preparation, characterization and efficacy in Parkinson's disease. *Int J Pharm* 2011;**415**(1–2):273–83.
3. Karatas H, Aktas Y, Gursoy-Ozdemir Y, et al. A nanomedicine transports a peptide caspase-3 inhibitor across the blood-brain barrier and provides neuroprotection. *J Neurosci* 2009;**29**(44):13761–9.
4. Tang X, Liang Y, Zhu Y, et al. Anti-transferrin receptor-modified amphotericin B-loaded PLA-PEG nanoparticles cure Candidal meningitis and reduce drug toxicity. *Int J Nanomedicine* 2015;**10**:6227–41.
5. Li J, Wang F, Sun D, Wang R. A review of the ligands and related targeting strategies for active targeting of paclitaxel to tumours. *J Drug Target* 2016;**24**(7):590–602.
6. Xu K, Wang H, Liu L, et al. Efficacy of CG(3)R(6)TAT nanoparticles self-assembled from a novel antimicrobial peptide for the

treatment of Candida albicans meningitis in rabbits. *Chemotherapy* 2011;**57**(5):417–25.
7. Zhao H, Bao XJ, Wang RZ, et al. Postacute ischemia vascular endothelial growth factor transfer by transferrin-targeted liposomes attenuates ischemic brain injury after experimental stroke in rats. *Hum Gene Ther* 2011;**22**(2):207–15.
8. Choi CH, Alabi CA, Webster P, Davis ME. Mechanism of active targeting in solid tumors with transferrin-containing gold nanoparticles. *Proc Natl Acad Sci U S A* 2010;**107**(3):1235–40.
9. Kievit FM, Veiseh O, Fang C, et al. Chlorotoxin labeled magnetic nanovectors for targeted gene delivery to glioma. *ACS Nano* 2010;**4**(8):4587–94.
10. Kirpotin DB, Drummond DC, Shao Y, et al. Antibody targeting of long-circulating lipidic nanoparticles does not increase tumor localization but does increase internalization in animal models. *Cancer Res* 2006;**66**(13):6732–40.
11. Souchek JJ, Wojtynek NE, Payne WM, et al. Hyaluronic acid formulation of near infrared fluorophores optimizes surgical imaging in a prostate tumor xenograft. *Acta Biomater* 2018;**75**:323–33.
12. Lu Y, Wu J, Wu J, et al. Role of formulation composition in folate receptor-targeted liposomal doxorubicin delivery to acute myelogenous leukemia cells. *Mol Pharm* 2007;**4**(5):707–12.
13. Durfee PN, Lin YS, Dunphy DR, et al. Mesoporous silica nanoparticle-supported lipid bilayers (protocells) for active targeting and delivery to individual leukemia cells. *ACS Nano* 2016;**10**(9):8325–45.
14. Kievit FM, Stephen ZR, Veiseh O, et al. Targeting of primary breast cancers and metastases in a transgenic mouse model using rationally designed multifunctional SPIONs. *ACS Nano* 2012;**6**(3):2591–601.
15. Kwon EJ, Skalak M, Lo Bu R, Bhatia SN. Neuron-targeted nanoparticle for siRNA delivery to traumatic brain Injuries. *ACS Nano* 2016;**10**(8):7926–33.
16. Kwon HJ, Cha MY, Kim D, et al. Mitochondria-targeting ceria nanoparticles as antioxidants for alzheimer's disease. *ACS Nano* 2016;**10**(2):2860–70.
17. You L, Wang J, Liu T, et al. Targeted brain delivery of rabies virus glycoprotein 29-modified deferoxamine-loaded nanoparticles reverses functional deficits in Parkinsonian mice. *ACS Nano* 2018;**12**(5):4123–39.
18. Kitov PI, Bundle DR. On the nature of the multivalency Effect: a thermodynamic model. *J Am Chem Soc* 2003;**125**(52):16271–84.
19. Poon Z, Chen S, Engler AC, et al. Ligand-clustered "patchy" nanoparticles for modulated cellular uptake and in vivo tumor targeting. *Angew Chem Int Ed Engl* 2010;**49**(40):7266–70.
20. Hong S, Leroueil PR, Majoros IJ, Orr BG, Baker Jr JR, Banaszak Holl MM. The binding avidity of a nanoparticle-based multivalent targeted drug delivery platform. *Chem Biol* 2007;**14**(1):107–15.
21. Rosenblum D, Joshi N, Tao W, Karp JM, Peer D. Progress and challenges towards targeted delivery of cancer therapeutics. *Nat Commun* 2018;**9**(1):1410.
22. Chapter 4 - biophysical principles. In: Pollard TD, Earnshaw WC, Lippincott-Schwartz J, Johnson GT, editors. *Cell Biology*. 3rd ed. Elsevier; 2017. p. 53–62.
23. van Oss CJ, Good RJ, Chaudhury MK. Nature of the antigen-antibody interaction. Primary and secondary bonds: optimal conditions for association and dissociation. *J Chromatography* 1986;**376**:111–9.
24. Salvati A, Pitek AS, Monopoli MP, et al. Transferrin-functionalized nanoparticles lose their targeting capabilities when a biomolecule corona adsorbs on the surface. *Nat Nanotechnol* 2013;**8**(2):137–43.
25. Lindman S, Lynch I, Thulin E, Nilsson H, Dawson KA, Linse S. Systematic investigation of the thermodynamics of HSA adsorption to N-iso-propylacrylamide/N-tert-butylacrylamide copolymer nanoparticles. Effects of particle size and hydrophobicity. *Nano Lett* 2007;**7**(4):914–20.
26. Gagner JE, Lopez MD, Dordick JS, Siegel RW. Effect of gold nanoparticle morphology on adsorbed protein structure and function. *Biomaterials* 2011;**32**(29):7241–52.
27. Roser M, Fischer D, Kissel T. Surface-modified biodegradable albumin nano- and microspheres. II: effect of surface charges on in vitro phagocytosis and biodistribution in rats. *Eur J Pharm Biopharm* 1998;**46**(3):255–63.
28. Maruyama K, Takizawa T, Yuda T, Kennel SJ, Huang L, Iwatsuru M. Targetability of novel immunoliposomes modified with amphipathic poly(ethylene glycol)s conjugated at their distal terminals to monoclonal antibodies. *Biochim Biophys Acta* 1995;**1234**(1):74–80.
29. Stanfield RL, Wilson IA. Antibody molecular structure. In: *Therapeutic monoclonal antibodies*; 2009.
30. Bazak R, Houri M, El Achy S, Kamel S, Refaat T. Cancer active targeting by nanoparticles: a comprehensive review of literature. *J Cancer Res Clin Oncol* 2015;**141**(5):769–84.
31. Crivianu-Gaita V, Thompson M. Aptamers, antibody scFv, and antibody Fab' fragments: an overview and comparison of three of the most versatile biosensor biorecognition elements. *Biosens Bioelectron* 2016;**85**:32–45.
32. Ulbrich K, Holá K, Šubr V, Bakandritsos A, Tuček J, Zbořil R. Targeted drug delivery with polymers and magnetic nanoparticles: covalent and noncovalentapproaches, release control, and clinical studies. *Chem Rev* 2016;**116**(9):5338–431.
33. Richards DA, Maruani A, Chudasama V. Antibody fragments as nanoparticle targeting ligands: a step in the right direction. *Chem Sci* 2017;**8**(1):63–77.
34. Ernst RE, High KN, Glass TR, Zhao Q. Determination of equilibrium dissociation constants. In: *Therapeutic monoclonal antibodies*; 2009.
35. Rodrigo G, Gruvegard M, Van Alstine JM. Antibody fragments and their purification by protein L affinity chromatography. *Antibodies* 2015;**4**(3):259–77.
36. Pietersz GA, Wang XW, Yap ML, Lim B, Peter K. Therapeutic targeting in nanomedicine: the future lies in recombinant antibodies. *Nanomed-Nanotechnol.* 2017;**12**(15):1873–89.
37. Muller-Loennies S, MacKenzie CR, Patenaude SI, et al. Characterization of high affinity monoclonal antibodies specific for chlamydial lipopolysaccharide. *Glycobiology* 2000;**10**(2):121–30.
38. Preiner J, Kodera N, Tang JL, et al. IgGs are made for walking on bacterial and viral surfaces. *Nat Commun* 2014;**5**.
39. Byzova NA, Safenkova IV, Slutskaya ES, Zherdev AV, Dzantiev BB. Less is more: acomparison of antibody-gold nanoparticle conjugates of different ratios. *Bioconjugate Chem* 2017;**28**(11):2737–46.
40. Malaspina DC, Longo G, Szleifer I. Behavior of ligand binding assays with crowded surfaces: molecular model of antigen capture by antibody-conjugated nanoparticles. *PLoS One* 2017;**12**(9).

41. Saha B, Evers TH, Prins MWJ. How antibody surface coverage on nanoparticles determines the activity and kinetics of antigen capturing for biosensing. *Anal Chem* 2014;**86**(16):8158–66.
42. Mazzucchelli S, Colombo M, De Palma C, et al. Single-domain protein A-engineered magnetic nanoparticles: toward a universal strategy to site-specific labeling of antibodies for targeted detection of tumor cells. *ACS Nano* 2010;**4**(10):5693–702.
43. Lo YS, Nam DH, So HM, et al. Oriented immobilization of antibody fragments on Ni-decorated single-walled carbon nanotube devices. *ACS Nano* 2009;**3**(11):3649–55.
44. Kumar S, Aaron J, Sokolov K. Directional conjugation of antibodies to nanoparticles for synthesis of multiplexed optical contrast agents with both delivery and targeting moieties. *Nat Protoc* 2008;**3**(2):314–20.
45. Zhai J, Scoble JA, Li N, et al. Epidermal growth factor receptor-targeted lipid nanoparticles retain self-assembled nanostructures and provide high specificity. *Nanoscale* 2015;**7**(7):2905–13.
46. Mustafaoglu N, Kiziltepe T, Bilgicer B. Site-specific conjugation of an antibody on a gold nanoparticle surface for one-step diagnosis of prostate specific antigen with dynamic light scattering. *Nanoscale* 2017;**9**(25):8684–94.
47. Jeong S, Park JY, Cha MG, et al. Highly robust and optimized conjugation of antibodies to nanoparticles using quantitatively validated protocols. *Nanoscale* 2017;**9**(7):2548–55.
48. Thorek DLJ, Elias DR, Tsourkas A. Comparative analysis of nanoparticle-antibody conjugations: carbodiimide versus click chemistry. *Mol Imaging* 2009;**8**(4):221–9.
49. Kubiak C, Manil L, Couvreur P. Sorptive properties of antibodies onto cyanoacrylic nanoparticles. *Int J Pharm* 1988;**41**(3):181–7.
50. Illum L, Jones PDE, Baldwin RW, Davis SS. Tissue distribution of poly(Hexyl 2-Cyanoacrylate) nanoparticles coated with monoclonal-antibodies in mice bearing human-tumor xenografts. *J Pharmacol Exp Ther* 1984;**230**(3):733–6.
51. Huang L, Kennel SJ. Binding of immunoglobulin-G to phospholipid-vesicles by sonication. *Biochemistry* 1979;**18**(9):1702–7.
52. Handlogten MW, Kiziltepe T, Moustakas DT, Bilgicer B. Design of a heterobivalent ligand to inhibit IgE clustering on mast cells. *Chem Biol* 2011;**18**(9):1179–88.
53. Lee JF, Stovall GM, Ellington AD. Aptamer therapeutics advance. *Curr Opin Chem Biol* 2006;**10**(3):282–9.
54. Cai B, Yang X, Sun L, et al. Stability and bioactivity of thrombin binding aptamers modified with D-/L-isothymidine in the loop regions. *Org Biomol Chem* 2014;**12**(44):8866–76.
55. Collie GW, Parkinson GN. The application of DNA and RNA G-quadruplexes to therapeutic medicines. *Chem Soc Rev* 2011;**40**(12):5867–92.
56. Ellington AD, Szostak JW. In vitro selection of RNA molecules that bind specific ligands. *Nature* 1990;**346**:818.
57. Tuerk C, Gold L. Systematic evolution of ligands by exponential enrichment: RNA ligands to bacteriophage T4 DNA polymerase. *Science* 1990;**249**(4968):505–10.
58. Hasegawa H, Taira KI, Sode K, Ikebukuro K. Improvement of aptamer affinity by dimerization. *Sensors* 2008;**8**(2):1090–8.
59. Medley CD, Bamrungsap S, Tan W, Smith JE. Aptamer-conjugated nanoparticles for cancer cell detection. *Anal Chem* 2011;**83**(3):727–34.
60. Zhang C, Ji X, Zhang Y, et al. One-pot synthesized aptamer-functionalized CdTe:Zn^{2+} quantum dots for tumor-targeted fluorescence imaging in vitro and in vivo. *Anal Chem* 2013;**85**(12):5843–9.
61. Griffin LC, Tidmarsh GF, Bock LC, Toole JJ, Leung LL. In vivo anticoagulant properties of a novel nucleotide-based thrombin inhibitor and demonstration of regional anticoagulation in extracorporeal circuits. *Blood* 1993;**81**(12):3271–6.
62. Klussmann S, Nolte A, Bald R, Erdmann VA, Furste JP. Mirror-image RNA that binds D-adenosine. *Nat Biotechnol* 1996;**14**(9):1112–5.
63. Iinuma H, Maruyama K, Okinaga K, et al. Intracellular targeting therapy of cisplatin-encapsulated transferrin-polyethylene glycol liposome on peritoneal dissemination of gastric cancer. *Int J Cancer* 2002;**99**(1):130–7.
64. Kumari P, Rompicharla SVK, Muddineti OS, Ghosh B, Biswas S. Transferrin-anchored poly(lactide) based micelles to improve anticancer activity of curcumin in hepatic and cervical cancer cell monolayers and 3D spheroids. *Int J Biol Macromol* 2018;**116**:1196–213.
65. Jhaveri A, Deshpande P, Pattni B, Torchilin V. Transferrin-targeted, resveratrol-loaded liposomes for the treatment of glioblastoma. *J Control Release* 2018;**277**:89–101.
66. Kokkoli E. *Engineering biomimetic peptides for targeted drug delivery*. Washington, DC: The National Academies Press; 2011.
67. Rahim A, Coutelle C, Harbottle R. High-throughput Pyrosequencing of a phage display library for the identification of enriched target-specific peptides. *Biotechniques* 2003;**35**(2):317–20. 322, 324.
68. Mei L, Fu L, Shi KR, et al. Increased tumor targeted delivery using a multistage liposome system functionalized with RGD, TAT and cleavable PEG. *Int J Pharm* 2014;**468**(1–2):26–38.
69. Ge ZS, Chen QX, Osada K, et al. Targeted gene delivery by polyplex micelles with crowded PEG palisade and cRGD moiety for systemic treatment of pancreatic tumors. *Biomaterials* 2014;**35**(10):3416–26.
70. Schleich N, Po C, Jacobs D, et al. Comparison of active, passive and magnetic targeting to tumors of multifunctional paclitaxel/SPIO-loaded nanoparticles for tumor imaging and therapy. *J Control Release* 2014;**194**:82–91.
71. Babu A, Amreddy N, Muralidharan R, et al. Chemodrug delivery using integrin-targeted PLGA-Chitosan nanoparticle for lung cancer therapy. *Sci Rep* 2017;**7**.
72. Huang KZ, Duan NJ, Zhang CM, Mo R, Hua ZC. Improved antitumor activity of TRAIL fusion protein via formation of self-assembling nanoparticle. *Sci Rep* 2017;**7**.
73. Mardilovich A, Craig JA, McCammon MQ, Garg A, Kokkoli E. Design of a novel fibronectin-mimetic peptide-amphiphile for functionalized biomaterials. *Langmuir* 2006;**22**(7):3259–64.
74. Pangburn TO, Bates FS, Kokkoli E. Polymersomes functionalized via "click" chemistry with the fibronectin mimetic peptides PR_b and GRGDSP for targeted delivery to cells with different levels of alpha(5)beta(1) expression. *Soft Matter* 2012;**8**(16):4449–61.
75. Leahy DJ, Aukhil I, Erickson HP. 2.0 A crystal structure of a four-domain segment of human fibronectin encompassing the RGD loop and synergy region. *Cell* 1996;**84**(1):155–64.
76. Werle M, Bernkop-Schnurch A. Strategies to improve plasma half life time of peptide and protein drugs. *Amino Acids* 2006;**30**(4):351–67.

77. Fosgerau K, Hoffmann T. Peptide therapeutics: current status and future directions. *Drug Discov Today* 2015;**20**(1):122–8.
78. Mathur D, Prakash S, Anand P, et al. PEPlife: a repository of the half-life of peptides. *Sci Rep* 2016;**6**.
79. Ricci V, Zonari D, Cannito S, et al. Hyaluronated mesoporous silica nanoparticles for active targeting: influence of conjugation method and hyaluronic acid molecular weight on the nanovector properties. *J Colloid Interface Sci* 2018;**516**:484–97.
80. Tian ZF, Liu JW, Li N, Garamus VM, Zou AH. Hyaluronic acid-coated liposome for active targeting on CD44 expressing tumors. *J Nanopart Res* 2018;**20**(9).
81. Liu YY, Qiao LN, Zhang SP, et al. Dual pH-responsive multifunctional nanoparticles for targeted treatment of breast cancer by combining immunotherapy and chemotherapy. *Acta Biomater* 2018;**66**:310–24.
82. Hill TK, Davis AL, Wheeler FB, et al. Development of a self-assembled nanoparticle formulation of Orlistat, Nano-ORL, with increased cytotoxicity against human tumor cell lines. *Mol Pharm* 2016;**13**(3):720–8.
83. Hill TK, Kelkar SS, Wojtynek NE, et al. Near infrared fluorescent nanoparticles derived from hyaluronic acid improve tumor contrast for image-guided surgery. *Theranostics* 2016;**6**(13):2314–28.
84. Kelkar SS, Hill TK, Marini FC, Mohs AM. Near infrared fluorescent nanoparticles based on hyaluronic acid: self-assembly, optical properties, and cell interaction. *Acta Biomater* 2016;**36**:112–21.
85. Souchek JJ, Davis AL, Hill TK, et al. Combination treatment with Orlistat-containing nanoparticles and taxanes is synergistic and enhances microtubule stability in taxane-resistant prostate cancer cells. *Mol Cancer Ther* 2017;**16**(9):1819–30.
86. Zhong L, Xu L, Liu Y, et al. Transformative hyaluronic acid-based active targeting supramolecular nanoplatform improve long circulation and enhance cellular uptake in cancer therapy. *Acta Pharm Sin B* 2019;**9**(2):397–409.
87. Parker N, Turk MJ, Westrick E, Lewis JD, Low PS, Leamon CP. Folate receptor expression in carcinomas and normal tissues determined by a quantitative radioligand binding assay. *Anal Biochem* 2005;**338**(2):284–93.
88. Cheung A, Bax HJ, Josephs DH, et al. Targeting folate receptor alpha for cancer treatment. *Oncotarget* 2016;**7**(32):52553–74.
89. Verma A, Sharma S, Gupta PK, et al. Vitamin B12 functionalized layer by layer calcium phosphate nanoparticles: a mucoadhesive and pH responsive carrier for improved oral delivery of insulin. *Acta Biomater* 2016;**31**:288–300.
90. Allen RH, Seetharam B, Podell E, Alpers DH. Effect of proteolytic enzymes on the binding of cobalamin to R protein and intrinsic factor.In vitro evidence that a failure to partially degrade R protein is responsible for cobalamin malabsorption in pancreatic insufficiency. *J Clin Invest* 1978;**61**(1):47–54.
91. Fowler R, Vllasaliu D, Trillo FF, et al. Nanoparticle transport in epithelial cells: pathway switching through bioconjugation. *Small* 2013;**9**(19):3282–94.
92. Wang J, Tan J, Luo J, et al. Enhancement of scutellarin oral delivery efficacy by vitamin B12-modified amphiphilic chitosan derivatives to treat type II diabetes induced-retinopathy. *J Nanobiotechnology* 2017;**15**(1):18.
93. Wibowo AS, Singh M, Reeder KM, et al. Structures of human folate receptors reveal biological trafficking states and diversity in folate and antifolate recognition. *Proc Natl Acad Sci USA* 2013;**110**(38):15180–8.
94. Antony AC. The biological chemistry of folate receptors. *Blood* 1992;**79**(11):2807–20.
95. Low PS, Kularatne SA. Folate-targeted therapeutic and imaging agents for cancer. *Curr Opin Chem Biol* 2009;**13**(3):256–62.
96. Jin H, Pi J, Yang F, et al. Folate-chitosan nanoparticles loaded with ursolic acid confer anti-breast cancer activities in vitro and in vivo. *Sci Rep-Uk* 2016;**6**.
97. Nakamura T, Kawano K, Shiraishi K, Yokoyama M, Maitani Y. Folate-targeted gadolinium-lipid-based nanoparticles as a bimodal contrast agent for tumor fluorescent and magnetic resonance imaging. *Biol Pharm Bull* 2014;**37**(4):521–7.
98. Patil YB, Toti US, Khdair A, Ma L, Panyam J. Single-step surface functionalization of polymeric nanoparticles for targeted drug delivery. *Biomaterials* 2009;**30**(5):859–66.
99. Li H, Liu Y, Chen LH, et al. Folate receptor-targeted lipid-albumin nanoparticles (F-LAN) for therapeutic delivery of an Akt1 antisense oligonucleotide. *J Drug Target* 2018;**26**(5–6):466–73.
100. Bartlett DW, Su H, Hildebrandt IJ, Weber WA, Davis ME. Impact of tumor-specific targeting on the biodistribution and efficacy of siRNA nanoparticles measured by multimodality in vivo imaging. *Proc Natl Acad Sci U S A* 2007;**104**(39):15549–54.
101. Wang X, Li J, Wang Y, et al. HFT-T, a targeting nanoparticle, enhances specific delivery of paclitaxel to folate receptor-positive tumors. *ACS Nano* 2009;**3**(10):3165–74.
102. Guo J, Russell EG, Darcy R, et al. Antibody-targeted cyclodextrin-based nanoparticles for siRNA delivery in the treatment of acute myeloid leukemia: physicochemical characteristics, in vitro mechanistic studies, and ex vivo patient derived therapeutic efficacy. *Mol Pharm* 2017;**14**(3):940–52.
103. Deshantri AK, Moreira AV, Ecker V, et al. Nanomedicines for the treatment of hematological malignancies. *J Control Release* 2018;**287**:194–215.
104. Samir A, Elgamal BM, Gabr H, Sabaawy HE. Nanotechnology applications in hematological malignancies. *Oncol Rep* 2015;**34**(3):1097–105.
105. Vinhas R, Mendes R, Fernandes AR, Baptista PV. Nanoparticles-emerging potential for managing leukemia and lymphoma. *Front Bioeng Biotechnol* 2017;**5**:79.
106. de la Puente P, Azab AK. Nanoparticle delivery systems, general approaches, and their implementation in multiple myeloma. *Eur J Haematol* 2017;**98**(6):529–41.
107. Sun H, Su J, Meng Q, et al. Cancer-cell-biomimetic nanoparticles for targeted therapy of homotypic tumors. *Adv Mater* 2016;**28**(43):9581–8.
108. Xiong J, Feng JL, Qiu LH, et al. SDF-1-loaded PLGA nanoparticles for the targeted photoacoustic imaging and photothermal therapy of metastatic lymph nodes in tongue squamous cell carcinoma. *Int J Pharm* 2019;**554**:93–104.
109. Wada H, Zheng JZ, Gregor A, et al. Intraoperative near-infrared fluorescence-guided peripheral lung tumor localization in rabbit models. *Ann Thorac Surg* 2019;**107**(1):248–56.
110. Li Y, Xiao Y, Lin H-P, et al. In vivo β-catenin attenuation by the integrin α5-targeting nano-delivery strategy suppresses triple negative breast cancer stemness and metastasis. *Biomaterials* 2019;**188**:160–72.

111. Li JH, Sharkey CC, Huang DT, King MR. Nanobiotechnology for the therapeutic targeting of cancer cells in blood. *Cell Mol Bioeng* 2015;**8**(1):137−50.
112. Yang E, Qian W, Cao Z, et al. Theranostic nanoparticles carrying doxorubicin attenuate targeting ligand specific antibody responses following systemic delivery. *Theranostics* 2015;**5**(1):43−61.
113. Mandal T, Beck M, Kirsten N, Linden M, Buske C. Targeting murine leukemic stem cells by antibody functionalized mesoporous silica nanoparticles. *Sci Rep* 2018;**8**(1):989.
114. Colzani B, Speranza G, Dorati R, et al. Design of smart GE11-PLGA/PEG-PLGA blend nanoparticulate platforms for parenteral administration of hydrophilic macromolecular drugs: synthesis, preparation and in vitro/ex vivo characterization. *Int J Pharm* 2016;**511**(2):1112−23.
115. Milane L, Duan Z, Amiji M. Therapeutic efficacy and safety of paclitaxel/lonidamine loaded EGFR-targeted nanoparticles for the treatment of multi-drug resistant cancer. *PLoS One* 2011;**6**(9):e24075.
116. Milane L, Duan ZF, Amiji M. Pharmacokinetics and biodistribution of lonidamine/paclitaxel loaded, EGFR-targeted nanoparticles in an orthotopic animal model of multi-drug resistant breast cancer. *Nanomed-Nanotechnol* 2011;**7**(4):435−44.
117. Chariou PL, Lee KL, Wen AM, Gulati NM, Stewart PL, Steinmetz NF. Detection and imaging of aggressive cancer cells using an epidermal growth factor receptor (EGFR)-Targeted filamentous plant virus-based nanoparticle. *Bioconjugate Chem* 2015;**26**(2):262−9.
118. Mickler FM, Mockl L, Ruthardt N, Ogris M, Wagner E, Brauchle C. Tuning nanoparticle uptake: live-cell imaging reveals two distinct endocytosis mechanisms mediated by natural and artificial EGFR targeting ligand. *Nano Lett* 2012;**12**(7):3417−23.
119. Wang Y, Li L, Zhao W, et al. Targeted therapy of atherosclerosis by a broad-spectrum reactive oxygen species scavenging nanoparticle with intrinsic anti-inflammatory activity. *ACS Nano* 2018;**12**(9):8943−60.
120. Tang J, Lobatto ME, Hassing L, et al. Inhibiting macrophage proliferation suppresses atherosclerotic plaque inflammation. *Sci Adv* 2015;**1**(3).
121. Liang M, Tan H, Zhou J, et al. Bioengineered H-ferritin nanocages for quantitative imaging of vulnerable plaques in atherosclerosis. *ACS Nano* 2018;**12**(9):9300−8.
122. Duivenvoorden R, Tang J, Cormode DP, et al. A statin-loaded reconstituted high-density lipoprotein nanoparticle inhibits atherosclerotic plaque inflammation. *Nat Commun* 2014;**5**:3065.
123. Lobatto ME, Calcagno C, Millon A, et al. Atherosclerotic plaque targeting mechanism of long-circulating nanoparticles established by multimodal imaging. *ACS Nano* 2015;**9**(2):1837−47.
124. Iiyama K, Hajra L, Iiyama M, et al. Patterns of vascular cell adhesion molecule-1 and intercellular adhesion molecule-1 expression in rabbit and mouse atherosclerotic lesions and at sites predisposed to lesion formation. *Circ Res* 1999;**85**(2):199−207.
125. Bruckman MA, Jiang K, Simpson EJ, et al. Dual-modal magnetic resonance and fluorescence imaging of atherosclerotic plaques in vivo using VCAM-1 targeted tobacco mosaic virus. *Nano Lett* 2014;**14**(3):1551−8.
126. Kao CW, Wu PT, Liao MY, et al. Magnetic nanoparticles conjugated with peptides derived from monocyte chemoattractant protein-1 as a tool for targeting atherosclerosis. *Pharmaceutics* 2018;**10**(2).
127. Kamaly N, Fredman G, Fojas JJ, et al. Targeted interleukin-10 nanotherapeutics developed with a microfluidic chip enhance resolution of inflammation in advanced atherosclerosis. *ACS Nano* 2016;**10**(5):5280−92.
128. Ma S, Tian XY, Zhang Y, et al. E-selectin-targeting delivery of microRNAs by microparticles ameliorates endothelial inflammation and atherosclerosis. *Sci Rep* 2016;**6**:22910.
129. Beldman TJ, Senders ML, Alaarg A, et al. Hyaluronan nanoparticles selectively target plaque-associated macrophages and improve plaque stability in atherosclerosis. *ACS Nano* 2017;**11**(6):5785−99.
130. Stern R, Asari AA, Sugahara KN. Hyaluronan fragments: an information-rich system. *Eur J Cell Biol* 2006;**85**(8):699−715.
131. Wang J, Poon C, Chin D, et al. Design and in vivo characterization of kidney-targeting multimodal micelles for renal drug delivery. *Nano Res* 2018;**11**(10):5584−95.
132. Karim R, Palazzo C, Evrard B, Piel G. Nanocarriers for the treatment of glioblastoma multiforme: current state-of-the-art. *J Control Release* 2016;**227**:23−37.
133. Xu JL, Ypma M, Chiarelli PA, et al. Theranostic oxygen reactive polymers for treatment of traumatic brain injury. *Adv Funct Mater* 2016;**26**(23):4124−33.
134. Yoo D, Magsam AW, Kelly AM, Stayton PS, Kievit FM, Convertine AJ. Core-cross-linked nanoparticles reduce neuroinflammation and improve outcome in a mouse model of traumatic brain injury. *ACS Nano* 2017;**11**(9):8600−11.
135. Bharadwaj VN, Lifshitz J, Adelson PD, Kodibagkar VD, Stabenfeldt SE. Temporal assessment of nanoparticle accumulation after experimental brain injury: effect of particle size. *Sci Rep* 2016;**6**:29988.
136. Bharadwaj VN, Nguyen DT, Kodibagkar VD, Stabenfeldt SE. Nanoparticle-based therapeutics for brain injury. *Adv Healthc Mater* 2018;**7**(1).
137. Bharadwaj VN, Rowe RK, Harrison J, et al. Blood-brainbarrier disruption dictates nanoparticle accumulation following experimental brain injury. *Nanomed-Nanotechnol* 2018;**14**(7):2155−66.
138. Boyd BJ, Galle A, Daglas M, Rosenfeld JV, Medcalf R. Traumatic brain injury opens blood-brain barrier to stealth liposomes via an enhanced permeability and retention (EPR)-like effect. *J Drug Target* 2015;**23**(9):847−53.
139. Liu ZY, Gao XL, Kang T, et al. B6 peptide-modified PEG-PLA nanoparticles for enhanced brain delivery of neuroprotective peptide. *Bioconjugate Chem* 2013;**24**(6):997−1007.
140. Loureiro JA, Gomes B, Fricker G, Coelho MAN, Rocha S, Pereira MC. Cellular uptake of PLGA nanoparticles targeted with anti-amyloid and anti-transferrin receptor antibodies for Alzheimer's disease treatment. *Colloids Surf B Biointerfaces* 2016;**145**:8−13.
141. Loureiro JA, Andrade S, Duarte A, et al. Resveratrol and grape extract-loaded solid lipid nanoparticles for the treatment of alzheimer's disease. *Molecules* 2017;**22**(2).
142. Huang RQ, Han L, Li JH, et al. Neuroprotection in a 6-hydroxydopamine-lesioned Parkinson model using lactoferrin-modified nanoparticles. *J Gene Med* 2009;**11**(9):754−63.
143. Huang RQ, Ke WL, Liu Y, et al. Gene therapy using lactoferrin-modified nanoparticles in a rotenone-induced chronic Parkinson model. *J Neurol Sci* 2010;**290**(1−2):123−30.
144. Deane R, Du Yan S, Submamaryan RK, et al. RAGE mediates amyloid-beta peptide transport across the blood-brain barrier and accumulation in brain. *Nat Med* 2003;**9**(7):907−13.

145. Liu Y, Huang R, Han L, et al. Brain-targeting gene delivery and cellular internalization mechanisms for modified rabies virus glycoprotein RVG29 nanoparticles. *Biomaterials* 2009;**30**(25):4195–202.
146. Gong C, Li XN, Xu LL, Zhang YH. Target delivery of a gene into the brain using the RVG29-oligoarginine peptide. *Biomaterials* 2012;**33**(12):3456–63.
147. Kim JY, Choi WI, Kim YH, Tae G. Brain-targeted delivery of protein using chitosan- and RVG peptide-conjugated, pluronic-based nano-carrier. *Biomaterials* 2013;**34**(4):1170–8.
148. Liu Y, Guo YB, An S, et al. Targeting caspase-3 as dual therapeutic benefits by RNAi facilitating brain-targeted nanoparticles in a rat model of Parkinson's disease. *PLoS One* 2013;**8**(5).
149. Montagne A, Gauberti M, Macrez R, et al. Ultra-sensitive molecular MRI of cerebrovascular cell activation enables early detection of chronic central nervous system disorders. *Neuroimage* 2012;**63**(2):760–70.
150. Garello F, Pagoto A, Arena F, et al. MRI visualization of neuro-inflammation using VCAM-1 targeted paramagnetic micelles. *Nanomed Nanotechnol Biol Med* 2018;**14**(7):2341–50.
151. Dan M, Cochran DB, Yokel RA, Dziubla TD. Binding, transcytosis and biodistribution of anti-PECAM-1 iron oxide nanoparticles for brain-targeted delivery. *PLoS One* 2013;**8**(11).
152. Zhao J, Zhao M, Yu C, et al. Multifunctional folate receptor-targeting and pH-responsive nanocarriers loaded with methotrexate for treatment of rheumatoid arthritis. *Int J Nanomedicine* 2017;**12**:6735–46.
153. Chandrasekar D, Sistla R, Ahmad FJ, Khar RK, Diwan PV. Folate coupled poly(ethyleneglycol) conjugates of anionic poly(amidoamine) dendrimer for inflammatory tissue specific drug delivery. *J Biomed Mater Res A* 2007;**82**(1):92–103.
154. Thomas TP, Goonewardena SN, Majoros IJ, et al. Folate-targeted nanoparticles show efficacy in the treatment of inflammatory arthritis. *Arthritis Rheum* 2011;**63**(9):2671–80.
155. You C, Zu J, Liu X, et al. Synovial fibroblast-targeting liposomes encapsulating an NF-kappaB-blocking peptide ameliorates zymosan-induced synovial inflammation. *J Cell Mol Med* 2018;**22**(4):2449–57.
156. Maisel K, Ensign L, Reddy M, Cone R, Hanes J. Effect of surface chemistry on nanoparticle interaction with gastrointestinal mucus and distribution in the gastrointestinal tract following oral and rectal administration in the mouse. *J Control Release* 2015;**197**:48–57.
157. Ensign LM, Cone R, Hanes J. Oral drug delivery with polymeric nanoparticles: the gastrointestinal mucus barriers. *Adv Drug Deliver Rev* 2012;**64**(6):557–70.
158. Ball RL, Bajaj P, Whitehead KA. Oral delivery of siRNA lipid nanoparticles: fate in the GI tract. *Sci Rep* 2018;**8**.
159. Francis MF, Cristea M, Winnik FM. Exploiting the vitamin B12 pathway to enhance oral drug delivery via polymeric micelles. *Biomacromolecules* 2005;**6**(5):2462–7.
160. Zhu X, Wu J, Shan W, et al. Polymeric nanoparticles amenable to simultaneous installation of exterior targeting and interior therapeutic proteins. *Angew Chem Int Ed Engl* 2016;**55**(10):3309–12.
161. Jin Y, Song Y, Zhu X, et al. Goblet cell-targeting nanoparticles for oral insulin delivery and the influence of mucus on insulin transport. *Biomaterials* 2012;**33**(5):1573–82.
162. Zhang J, Zhu X, Jin Y, Shan W, Huang Y. Mechanism study of cellular uptake and tight junction opening mediated by goblet cell-specific trimethyl chitosan nanoparticles. *Mol Pharm* 2014;**11**(5):1520–32.
163. Zhang P, Xu Y, Zhu X, Huang Y. Goblet cell targeting nanoparticle containing drug-loaded micelle cores for oral delivery of insulin. *Int J Pharm* 2015;**496**(2):993–1005.

Chapter 4

Passive targeting in nanomedicine: fundamental concepts, body interactions, and clinical potential

Steven M. Narum[1,b], Tram Le[1,b], Dao P. Le[1], Joanne C. Lee[1], Nathan D. Donahue[1], Wen Yang[1] and Stefan Wilhelm[1,2,a]

[1]*Stephenson School of Biomedical Engineering, University of Oklahoma, Norman, OK, United States;* [2]*Stephenson Cancer Center, Oklahoma City, OK, United States*

4.1 Introduction

Over the past few decades, researchers have been designing and applying nanoparticles for diagnosis and treatment of diseases inside the body. These *in vivo* biomedical applications of nanoparticles represent a major research area within the continuously growing field of nanomedicine.[1] While it is a fascinating concept to use systemically administered nanoparticles inside the body for medical applications, development and clinical translation of nanomedicines are challenging. One of these challenges is delivery.[2] Direct and efficient delivery of administered nanoparticles to diseased tissues and cells is required for most nanomedicines to ensure accurate diagnosis and effective treatment. However, biological barriers within the body, such as the mononuclear phagocyte system (MPS), limit nanoparticle delivery to diseased sites.[3]

To address this nanoparticle delivery challenge, researchers have been working on so-called "targeting" strategies.[4] The goal of these strategies is to deliver nanoparticles preferentially to diseased tissues while minimizing their accumulation in healthy organs and cells. Such targeted delivery approaches may have several clinical benefits, including (1) reduced treatment-related side effects; (2) improved imaging and diagnosis; and (3) enhanced therapeutic outcomes.

In this chapter, we focus on passive nanoparticle targeting strategies in the context of solid tumor management. This chapter begins with a brief introduction of nanomedicine (see Section 4.2), after which the journey of administered nanoparticles en route to malignant tissues and cells in the body is briefly explored (see Section 4.3). Section 4.4 provides a concise description of active and passive nanoparticle targeting strategies. In Section 4.5, we discuss fundamental concepts of passive nanoparticle targeting, including pathophysiological characteristics of solid tumors and nanoparticle design rules. Section 4.6 briefly explores limitations of passive nanoparticle targeting, and Section 4.7 explains nanoparticle—body interactions and biological barriers. We focus on clinical potential and relevance of passively targeted cancer nanomedicines in Section 4.8 and conclude our chapter with an outlook on how to further exploit the potential of this technology for biomedical applications (see Section 4.9).

4.2 What is "nanomedicine"?

Nanomedicine can be broadly defined as the biomedical and clinical applications of rationally engineered nanoscale materials with typical dimensions between 1 and 100 nm.[5] Materials in this nanoscale size regime are referred to as nanoparticles. Nanoparticles exhibit unique optical,[6] magnetic,[7] and biological properties[8] that are usually not observed in their corresponding bulk materials. Researchers are able to synthesize nanoparticles from inorganic (e.g., semiconductor quantum dots,[9] upconversion nanoparticles,[10] and iron oxide nanoparticles[11]) and organic materials (e.g., liposomes,[12] dendrimers,[13] and polymeric nanoparticles[14]) with defined physicochemical properties, including nanoparticle size, shape, and surface chemistry. Such high tunability of material properties allows

a ORCID: orcid.org/0000-0003-2167-6221.
b Authors contributed equally to this work.

Nanoparticles for Biomedical Applications. https://doi.org/10.1016/B978-0-12-816662-8.00004-7

researchers to engineer nanoparticles with unique capabilities for biomedical and clinical use. For example, nanoparticles can be synthesized to function as drug delivery vehicles for therapeutic applications or as imaging contrast agents for medical imaging and diagnosis. Application of these rationally engineered nanoparticles for cancer management is referred to as cancer nanomedicine.[15]

Medical applications of nanoparticles as carriers for therapeutic agents require encapsulation and/or surface modification strategies. Researchers can load nanoparticles with a variety of therapeutic agents, including small molecule drugs, chemotherapeutics, peptides, antibodies, and nucleic acid–based drugs. This can improve solubility and bioavailability of drugs *in vivo* and potentially lead to better therapeutic efficacy against diseased cells compared with administration of free drugs.[16,17] Combination of therapeutic and diagnostic capabilities into one nanoparticle is also possible, and such nanoparticles are referred to as "theranostic" nanoparticles in the literature.[18,19] To exert their intended biomedical function, diagnostic, therapeutic, and theranostic nanoparticles are typically administered via systemic administration.

4.3 Systemic nanomedicine and the journey of administered nanoparticles in the body

Systemic administration, i.e., administering nanoparticles directly into the body's circulatory system, is a frequently used approach in nanomedicine. The rationale for systemic nanomedicine is that intravenously (i.v.) administered nanoparticles transport directly with the bloodstream throughout the body and may eventually reach diseased tissues, such as a primary solid tumor or metastatic lesions. Upon accumulation, nanoparticles will exert their deliberate biomedical function in these diseased tissues (Fig. 4.1A).

Before i.v. administered nanoparticles reach malignant sites in the body, several key steps occur. First, exposure of nanoparticles to blood leads to formation of a so-called

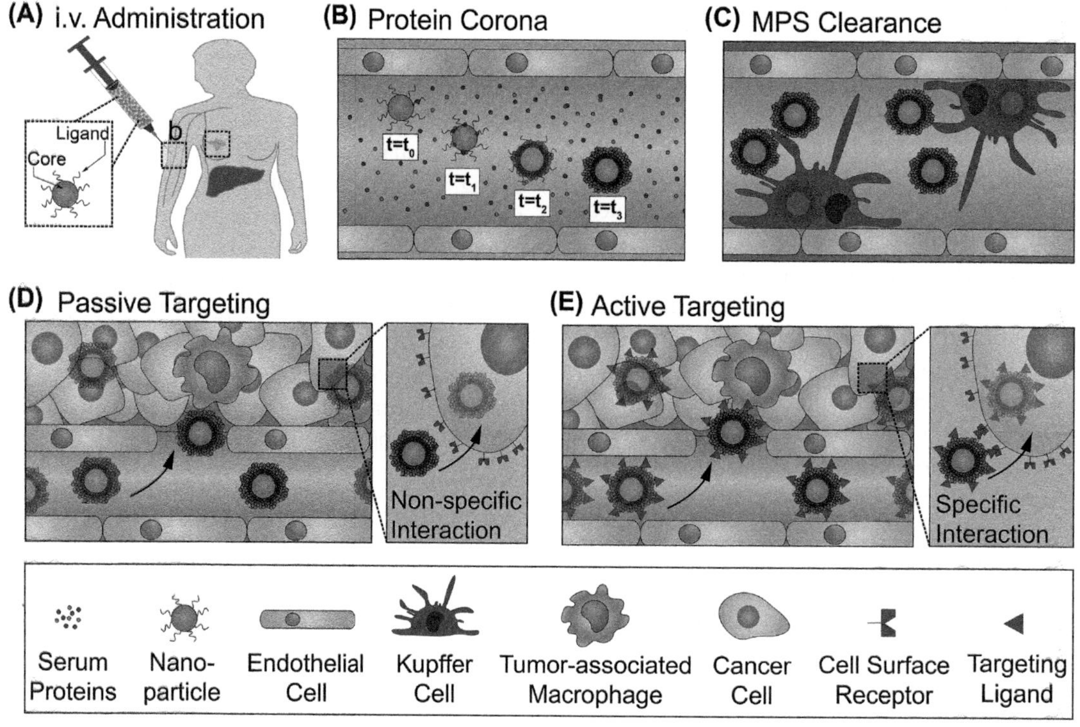

FIGURE 4.1 Schematic overview representing biological barriers and transport mechanisms of systemically administered nanoparticles in biomedical applications. (A) Systemic (intravenous, i.v.) administration of engineered nanoparticles into the circulatory system is a commonly used administration route in biomedicine. Engineered nanoparticles typically comprise organic and/or inorganic nanoscale core materials. The nanoparticle core is often surface modified with organic polymers and ligand molecules. (B) Protein corona formation is a dynamic process, which starts immediately upon i.v. administration into the circulatory system. The nanoparticle protein corona changes dynamically over time. (C) Cells of the mononuclear phagocyte system (MPS), such as liver macrophages (Kupffer cells), may line the luminal surface of liver sinusoid blood vessels. Kupffer cells have been reported to remove opsonized nanoparticles quantitatively from the bloodstream. (D) The passive targeting mechanism suggests nanoparticle transport through interendothelial gaps (paracellular transport) of compromised blood vessels. In cancer nanomedicine, nonspecific interaction with tumor cells may occur upon paracellular nanoparticle transport. (E) Ligand-coated nanoparticles follow the same transport pathway as passively targeted nanoparticles. In contrast to passive targeting nanoparticles, ligand-coated nanoparticles may then interact specifically with tumor cells, potentially leading to increased nanoparticle retention and improved cell uptake.

protein corona that covers the nanoparticle surface (Fig. 4.1B). Certain proteins within the corona, called opsonins, may then direct nanoparticles to phagocytic cells in organs of the MPS. Major MPS organs include the liver and spleen. Liver macrophages, called Kupffer cells, are one type of phagocytic MPS cells. They can remove nanoparticles efficiently and in large quantity from the bloodstream (Fig. 4.1C).[20,21] Consequently, nanoparticles will not be able to accumulate within solid tumors once they have been engulfed by MPS cells and removed from the blood. Therefore, organs and cells of the MPS represent major biological barriers that significantly limit nanoparticle blood circulation times and delivery. Nanoparticles need to overcome these biological barriers for efficient delivery to diseased sites.

Crossing the tumor endothelium is another key step in the journey of nanoparticles from the administration site to diseased tissues *in vivo*. It has been reported in the literature that the vascular wall of tumor blood vessels is compromised.[21a] In contrast to healthy blood vessels, tumor blood vessels may exhibit specific pathological characteristics that nanoparticles exploit during accumulation within cancerous tissues.[22] Briefly, systemically administered nanoparticles may transport from the tumor blood vessel lumen through interendothelial gaps into the tumor interstitial space.[23] This is a fundamental mechanism for both passive and active nanoparticle targeting (Fig. 4.1D and E).[24,25]

4.4 Active versus passive nanoparticle targeting strategies

The literature divides targeted nanoparticle delivery strategies into two major categories: (1) passive and (2) active targeting.[24] The goal of these targeting strategies is to deliver nanoparticles and their therapeutic/diagnostic payloads preferentially to diseased tissues while minimizing nanoparticle accumulation in healthy organs and cells. Although we focus on passive targeting in this chapter, the fundamental mechanisms of nanoparticle accumulation within malignant tissues are similar for both strategies. In cancer nanomedicine, both targeting strategies exploit a tumor's pathophysiological characteristics for nanoparticle accumulation. In addition, researchers use empirically derived nanoparticle design rules with the intention to improve tumor delivery (Fig. 4.1D and E).

In contrast to passive targeting nanoparticles, active targeting nanoparticles are engineered with specific nanoparticle surface ligands (Fig. 4.1E).[26] These surface ligands are referred to as targeting ligands. Typical examples of targeting ligands are biomolecules, including nucleic acids, antibodies, and peptides. Such biomolecules can recognize and bind to specific cell surface receptors on cancerous cells with high affinity.[24] Hence, active targeting approaches in nanomedicine are rationally designed strategies to exploit specific biomolecular interactions that may occur between nanoparticle surface ligands and cell surface receptors. In comparison with passive targeting, the underlying rationale for the use of active targeting is twofold: (1) improved retention of passively accumulated nanoparticles at diseased sites as a result of specific interaction between surface ligands and cell surface receptors, and (2) increased specific interaction of nanoparticles with targeted diseased cells while minimizing nontargeted nanoparticle−cell interactions (Fig. 4.1E).[27]

4.5 Fundamental concepts of passive targeting strategies

The term "passive targeting" has been widely used in nanomedicine to describe findings related to accumulation of nanoparticles in solid tumors. Upon i.v. administration of nanoscale materials, Matsumura and Maeda reported in 1986 two key observations that represent the foundation of passive nanoparticle targeting.[28] The first observation was spontaneous accumulation of administered macromolecular drug carriers in areas of solid tumors with leaky vasculature. The second observation was retention of intratumoral nanoparticles due to compromised lymphatic drainage. Together, these observations form the basis of a concept termed "enhanced permeability and retention (EPR) effect."[29]

Passive targeting and EPR effect are closely related. To better understand this relationship, we will briefly discuss the pathophysiology of tumor vasculature that enables enhanced vascular permeability.

One of the hallmarks of metabolically active cancers is sustained angiogenesis, i.e., formation of new blood vessels and neovasculature.[30,31] This provides a nutrient and oxygen supply to tumors and helps with removing metabolic waste products. Chronically activated angiogenesis, however, may lead to formation of highly abnormal tumor vessels.[22] Such blood vessels often exhibit a chaotic and disorganized course, branch irregularly, and are structurally different from healthy vessels (Fig. 4.2A).[32−35]

Dvorak and coworkers identified six distinctly different types of tumor blood vessels with characteristic architectures (Fig. 4.2A).[35] These different vessels are referred to as (1) feeding artery; (2) mother vessel; (3) glomeruloid microvascular proliferation (GMP); (4) vascular malformation; (5) capillary; and (6) draining vein. The first angiogenic tumor blood vessel type is called "mother vessel," which forms from existing normal venules and capillaries. Mother vessels are characterized by (1) thin layer of flattened endothelial cells; (2) disrupted basement membrane; and (3) little or no pericyte cell coverage. These

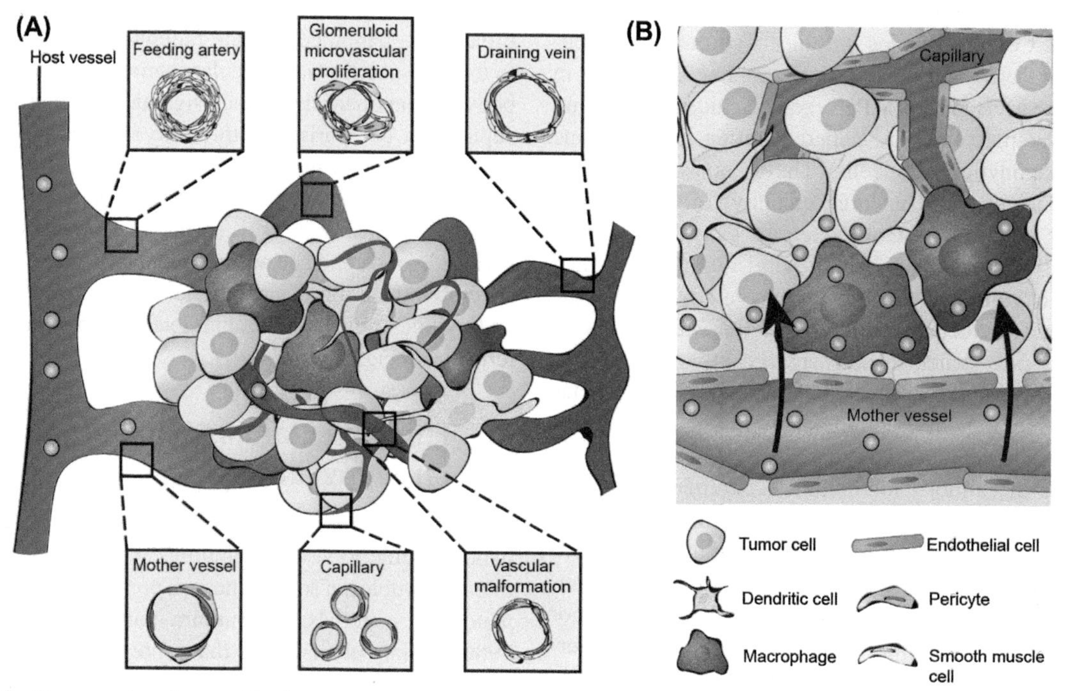

FIGURE 4.2 Heterogeneity of tumor blood vessels, nanoparticle extravasation mechanism, and pathological features of tumor endothelium. (A) Schematic representation of six different types of tumor blood vessels identified by Dvorak and coworkers: (i) feeding arteries; (ii) mother vessels; (iii) glomeruloid microvascular proliferations (GMPs); (iv) vascular malformations; (v) capillaries; and (vi) draining veins. (B) According to the EPR effect, nanoparticles extravasate from tumor blood vessels via passive diffusion through interendothelial gaps. This transport route is referred to as paracellular transport pathway. *Modified with permission from Wilhelm S. et al. Analysis of nanoparticle delivery to tumours.* Nature Reviews Materials *2016;1, 2016:14.*

features contribute to the abnormal hyperpermeability of mother vessels to plasma proteins and likely to nanoparticles (Fig. 4.2B). In addition, mother vessels and GMPs are typical examples of tumor blood vessels that may exhibit interendothelial gaps.[32,36,37] Such gaps between endothelial cells increase the leakiness of tumor vasculature. The size of these gaps can range from a few nanometers to several hundred nanometers, as reported from the analysis of mouse tumor models.[23] In addition to discontinuous endothelium with gaps and pores, mother vessels may also exhibit fenestrated endothelium, which may allow nanoparticle extravasation.[38]

Extravasation is a term used to describe the transport of i.v. administered nanoparticles from the lumen of tumor blood vessels into the tumor interstitium. If extravasation of nanoparticles occurs through interendothelial gaps, the underlying transport pathway is referred to as paracellular route, i.e., transport through gaps between adjacent endothelial cells (Fig. 4.2B).[39] The paracellular route is a passive transport mechanism and requires a nanoparticle concentration gradient between blood and tumor interstitium. This concentration difference then drives nanoparticles passively (mostly by diffusion) across the endothelium and facilitates nanoparticle tumor accumulation (Fig. 4.2B).[40] Since a large enough concentration gradient is required to enable nanoparticle diffusion across the endothelium, high nanoparticle bolus doses and long blood circulation times of administered nanoparticles may increase the efficiency of this passive tumor targeting mechanism.[41]

The EPR effect suggests that administered nanoparticles can accumulate in solid tumors with discontinuous endothelium if the following nanoparticle design criteria are met: (1) smaller nanoparticle size than the cutoff size of tumor interendothelial gaps, and (2) long blood circulation times of nanoparticles. The rationale for long nanoparticle blood circulation times is to increase the chance for paracellular nanoparticle extravasation. The longer the i.v. administered nanoparticles are able to remain in the bloodstream at high concentrations, the higher the chance for paracellular nanoparticle transport into the tumor. Both active and passive nanoparticle targeting strategies are designed to exploit the EPR effect for tumor delivery, i.e., both targeting strategies use concentration-dependent passive paracellular transport across discontinuous endothelium for nanoparticle tumor accumulation (Figs. 4.1D,E, and 4.2B).

Another key principle of nanoparticle targeting is nanoparticle retention within the tumor space. Nanoparticle retention occurs due to poor lymphatic drainage of solid tumors.[42] In normal tissues, the lymphatic system drains excess fluid from the tissue to maintain an interstitial fluid balance.[43] In solid tumors, however, lymphatic vessels are compressed by the high density of continuously proliferating cancer cells, which may cause the collapse of these vessels and can lead to the poor infiltration of lymphocytes.[44,44a] Collapsed lymphatic vessels are no longer able to efficiently drain fluid from the tumor tissue, which may result in elevated interstitial fluid pressures inside tumor tissues.[43] Nanoparticle tumor retention due to impaired lymphatic drainage is a key concept of the EPR effect and may be observed to a similar extent for both passive and active targeting nanoparticles.

Besides solid tumors, the EPR effect is also found in atherosclerosis, which is associated with chronic inflammation of arterial blood vessels. This opens the possibility to target inflamed tissue sites of atherosclerosis with nanoparticles.[45,46] Researchers have used nanoparticles to image and treat atherosclerotic plaques.[42–44] Similar to nanoparticle extravasation mechanisms in solid tumors, atherosclerotic plaques may exhibit mirconeovasculature that is permeable to systemically administered nanoparticles.[46] Atherosclerotic plaques form by deposition of lipids, cholesterol, calcium, cellular waste products, and other compounds on the inner walls of arterial blood vessels.[46] Nanoparticles may be transported through leaky vasculature of atherosclerotic plaques into the tissue interstitium, where they accumulate over time as a result of underdeveloped lymphatics.[46] To probe and model translocation of poly(D,L-lactide-*co*-glycolide) PLGA-based nanoparticles in atherosclerotic endothelium, Langer *et al.* reported in 2014 an *in vitro* model based on an endothelialized microfluidic chip.[47] In the future, such *in vitro* models may provide key insights in nanoparticle transport mechanisms with clinical relevance to help overcome endothelial barriers. Results from these studies may lead to new nanoparticle design principles for *in vivo* applications in diagnosis and treatment of atherosclerotic plaques and solid tumors.

4.6 Limitations of passive nanoparticle targeting

According to the EPR effect, solid tumors exhibit pathophysiological features, including leaky vasculature and impaired lymphatic drainage that may facilitate nanoparticle targeting. These features may theoretically result in enhanced vascular permeability and retention of nanoparticles within tumors. However, it is important to mention that the extent of the EPR effect can vary substantially between and within tumors.[48,49] Solid tumors are highly heterogeneous with large variability of vascular permeability, lymphatic drainage, blood perfusion rates, interstitial tissue pressures, extracellular matrix (ECM) density, and ECM composition.[50–52] All of these factors may individually and/or collectively affect EPR. While the EPR effect has been derived based on observations in mouse tumor models, the extent to which EPR occurs in humans is controversial and subject to debate.[53–55] Current data suggest that the EPR effect is highly variable across and within individual tumors.[56]

Even for the same tumor, the extent of vascular permeability, lymphatic drainage, and even blood perfusion rates of existing tumor vessels may vary significantly for different tumor areas. This intratumoral heterogeneity suggests that EPR may be highly variable within the same tumor, which impedes uniform distribution of nanoparticles throughout the tumor tissue.[57] The resulting heterogeneous intratumoral nanoparticle and drug distribution may lessen therapeutic effects and may lead to resistance of cancer cells to chemotherapeutics.

The idea of passive nanoparticle targeting suggests that rationally designed nanomedicines may exploit EPR features for tumor accumulation. Since the proposal of the EPR effect in the mid-1980s, passive targeting has evolved into a key rationale for developing nanoscale therapeutic and diagnostic agents for cancer management. However, it should be emphasized that passive targeting does not necessarily result in quantitative and efficient tumor delivery of administered nanoparticles. A recent meta-analysis of preclinical studies published between 2005 and 2015 reported that only about 1% of the injected nanoparticle dose (median value) accumulates within solid tumors of mouse models.[38] The majority of administered nanoparticles interact with nonmalignant cells and accumulate in healthy organs such as the liver and spleen rather than in "targeted" cancerous tissues.[21] The potential reasons for nanoparticle accumulation in healthy organs will be discussed in the next section, where we focus on nanoparticle body interactions and biological barriers that impede efficient nanoparticle delivery.

4.7 Nanoparticle–body interactions and biological barriers

Nanomedicines may provide improved clinical benefits if nanoparticles are able to reach diseased sites in the body efficiently and effectively.[24] However, achieving efficient and targeted nanoparticle *in vivo* delivery requires a better fundamental understanding of how administered nanoparticles and biological systems interact. These interactions are referred to as "nano–bio" interactions in the literature and are highly complex and multiparametric.[58] Nano–bio interactions occur on multiple different scales that range from biomolecular and cellular to tissue and system levels (Fig. 4.1B and C).[59] The fate of administered nanoparticles in the body is eventually determined by these multilevel nano–bio interactions.[60] In this section, we discuss nanoparticle–body interactions and corresponding biological barriers categorized into three major types: (1) nanoparticle–blood interactions; (2) nanoparticle–MPS interactions; and (3) nanoparticle–kidney interactions. We conclude the section with a brief discussion of nanoparticle design strategies to control nano–bio interactions and to overcome biological barriers.

4.7.1 Nanoparticle–blood interactions

Upon i.v. administration, nanoparticles interact with cellular and acellular components of the blood.[61] As nanoparticles get transported with the bloodstream, they may be engulfed by circulating blood cells, such as circulating monocytes and other phagocytes.[62,63] In addition, serum proteins and other biomolecules within the bloodstream adsorb onto the nanoparticle surface (Figs. 4.1B and 4.3A).[61] This protein/biomolecule adsorption leads to the formation of a so-called protein corona (or biomolecular corona), which is an energetically favorable biochemical process.[64–70] The literature differentiates the nanoparticle protein corona into two compartments: (1) hard protein corona and (2) soft protein corona (Fig. 4.3A).[71,72] Whereas the hard corona typically comprises tightly bound surface proteins, the soft corona is more dynamic and allows exchange of surface proteins with lower binding affinity over time (Fig. 4.3A).[73,74] Recent studies have investigated the dynamic changes of the protein corona *in vivo* and how they affect the biological fate of nanoparticles.[75,76]

Nanoparticle protein corona formation is one of the most important and most complex nano–bio interactions. Its importance stems from the fact that formation and presence of a protein corona change the synthetic identity of nanoparticles into a biological identity[66,77,78] (Fig. 4.3B). The synthetic identity refers to intentionally engineered physicochemical properties of nanoparticles that include nanoparticle size, shape, surface chemistry, and surface functional groups.[79] The new biological identity determines the physiological response and biological fate of nanoparticles *in vivo*. For example, certain proteins called opsonins within the protein corona may be recognized by phagocytic cells in the liver,[80] which may then lead to liver accumulation of opsonized nanoparticles as a result of phagocytic cell uptake.[20,21] The nanoparticle protein corona can also change nanoparticle aggregation state and surface charge, which may further affect the biological fate of nanoparticles in the body.[64,78]

As shown schematically in Fig. 4.3C–F, nanoparticle protein corona formation may affect their intratumoral targeting capabilities. Once intentionally engineered active targeting nanoparticles accumulate in the tumor space, they may lose their binding specificity toward targeted cells as a result of nanoparticle protein corona formation (Fig. 4.3E and F). The reason for this is that the nanoparticle protein corona may sterically hinder specific ligand–receptor interactions. Targeting surface ligands may get buried within the protein corona.[81] For passive and active targeting nanoparticles, protein corona formation may direct nanoparticles to off-target cells, such as tumor-associated macrophages (TAMs) and other immune cells within the tumor microenvironment (Fig. 4.3C–F).[82,83,83a]

4.7.2 Nanoparticle–MPS interactions

Off-target nanoparticle accumulation due to protein corona formation does not just occur inside a tumor. The body itself has a network of MPS organs and immune cells in place that effectively remove foreign nanomaterials from the bloodstream (Fig. 4.4).[84] These organs include the liver, spleen, lymph nodes, skin, bone marrow, and other organs with resident phagocytic macrophages.[85] These resident macrophages are typically derived from circulating monocytes and may exhibit a range of phenotypical diversity.[86]

Biodistribution analyses have shown that accumulation of nanoparticles in MPS organs and cells is a universal phenomenon, which has been observed for different types of materials, such as micelles and polymeric nanoparticles, liposomes, carbon nanotubes, quantum dots, and gold nanoparticles.[87–90] This off-target nanoparticle accumulation in MPS organs is a significant challenge for the development and clinical translation of nanomedicines, as it impedes efficient delivery of nanoparticles to diseased sites. In addition, MPS accumulation of nanoparticles may cause severe toxicity-related side effects, particularly in organs such as the liver and spleen.[91]

Fig. 4.4 summarizes nanoparticle interactions with the liver. Tsoi et al. reported that when blood enters liver sinusoids, its fluid velocity decreases by approximately 1000-fold compared withblood velocities in arteries and veins in systemic circulation.[85] Reduced blood velocity within the liver sinusoid is in part responsible for increased nanoparticle uptake by phagocytic cells near the vascular inlet. Besides the relative location of cells within the liver sinusoidal microarchitecture, a cell's phenotype, nanoparticle internalization, and dissociation kinetics are also important factors that determine nanoparticle–cell interactions in the liver. In addition, immune cells, such as hepatic B cells, have been shown to interact with hard nanoparticles as efficiently as Kupffer cells and liver sinusoidal endothelial cells.[85] It has been suggested that Kupffer cells recognize opsonins within the nanoparticle protein corona via scavenger receptors.[92] This molecular recognition may then trigger nanoparticle uptake into macrophages. While organic nanoparticles can be more readily degraded and eliminated upon accumulation in MPS cells, inorganic nanoparticles can reside in these cells

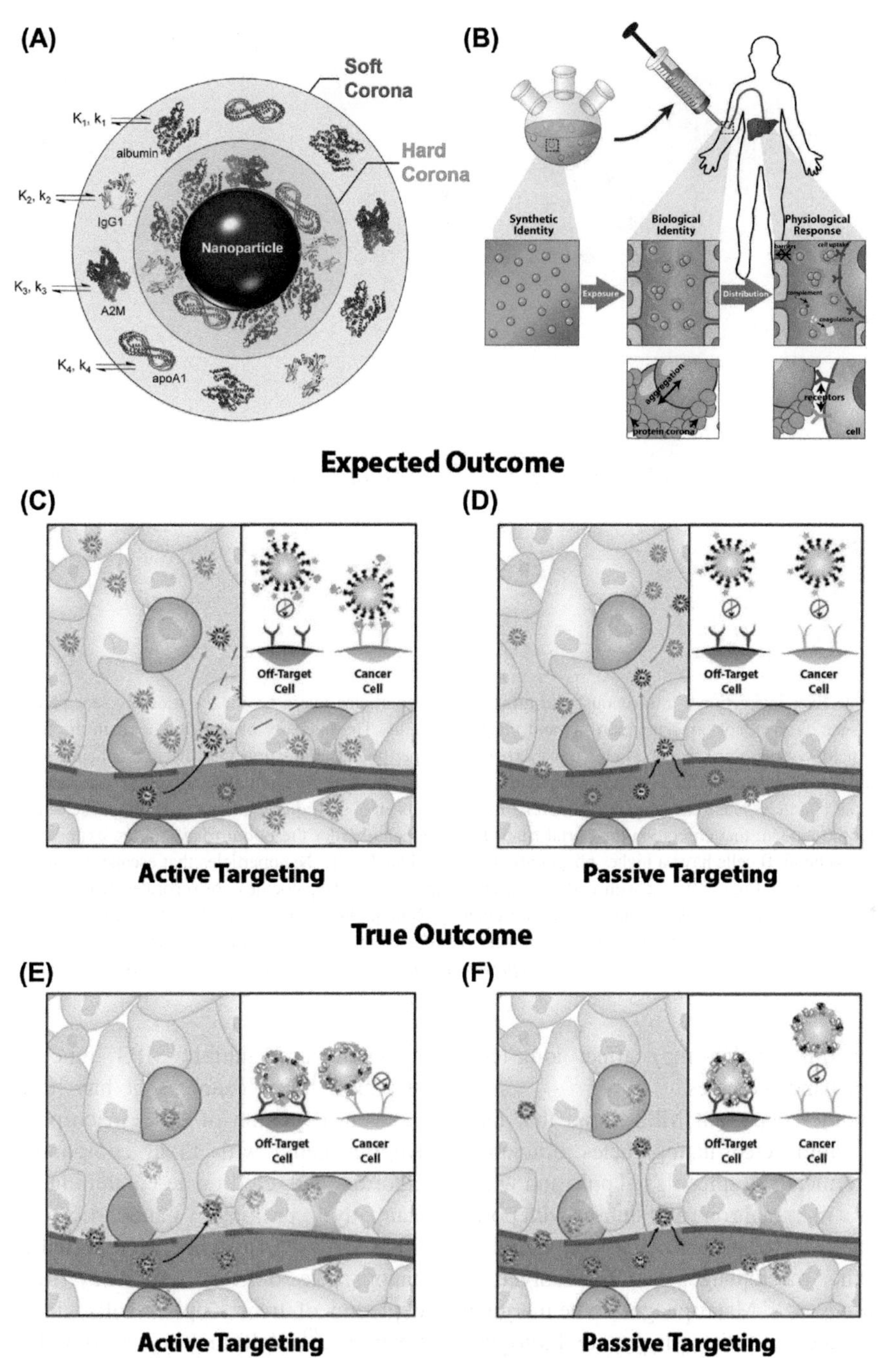

FIGURE 4.3 Nanoparticle–blood interactions and protein corona formation. (A) Protein corona formation is a dynamic process. The adsorption of proteins on the nanoparticle surface is a kinetic (k) and thermodynamic (K) function of individual protein properties and nanoparticle physicochemical characteristics. The protein corona can be classified into (i) hard corona (high-affinity proteins with strong binding) and (ii) soft corona (low-affinity proteins with weak binding). (B) Upon intravenous administration, blood serum proteins adsorb on the nanoparticle surface. This changes the rationally engineered synthetic identity of nanoparticles into a biological identity. This new biological identity is presented to the body and determines nanoparticle interactions with cells, tissues, and organs. (C–F) Protein corona formation may affect cancer cell targeting capabilities of nanoparticles. Active and passive targeting nanoparticles may enter the tumor interstitium through interendothelial gaps according to the EPR effect. (C,D) In a hypothetical situation without nanoparticle protein corona formation, ligand-functionalized active targeting nanoparticles may interact with specific cell surface receptors on targeted cancer cells to facilitate receptor-mediated endocytosis for selective nanoparticle cell uptake. Passive targeting nanoparticles do not exhibit specific cell interactions. (E,F) Upon formation of a protein corona, active targeting nanoparticles may lose their specific targeting capabilities, as protein corona formation masks surface-bound ligands. Both active and passive targeting nanoparticles may show nonspecific cellular uptake that is enabled by the protein corona. *(A) Modified with permission from Fleischer, CC, Payne CK. Nanoparticle–cell interactions: molecular structure of the protein corona and cellular outcomes. Accounts Chem Res 2014;47:2651–2659. (E &F) Panels b–f modified with permission from Lazarovits J, Chen Y, Sykes EA, Chan WC. Nanoparticle-blood interactions: the implications on solid tumour targeting.* Chem Commun Camb Engl *2015;**51**:2756–2767.*

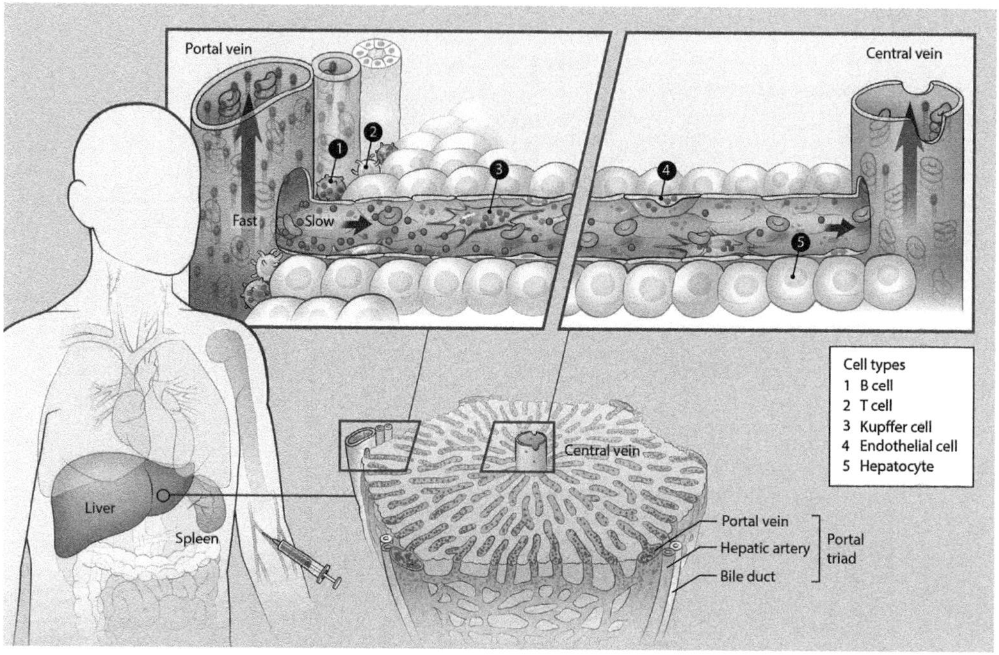

FIGURE 4.4 Nanoparticle liver interactions. Intravenously administered nanoparticles interact with the mononuclear phagocyte system (MPS). The MPS consists of organs, such as liver, spleen, bone marrow, and phagocytic cells. The intensity of the blue color in the figure indicates the extent of nanoparticle uptake within MPS organs. As nanoparticles transport from the peripheral circulation into the liver, their velocity reduces 1000-fold. In consequence, nanoparticles could interact with a variety of hepatic cell types, resulting in gradual nanoparticle clearance from the bloodstream. A concentration gradient of nanoparticles along the length of the liver sinusoid has been observed. The number of nanoparticles leaving the liver through the central vein is lower than the amount that enters via the portal triad. B and T cells border the portal triad and are exposed to a high concentration of incoming nanoparticles. In general, B cells have a higher phagocytic potential than T cells. Nanoparticles that escape the first set of cellular interactions transport along the liver sinusoid and may interact with endothelial and Kupffer cells. Hepatocytes are separated from the blood vessel by a layer of fenestrated endothelium and do not seem to take up nanoparticles efficiently. Nanoparticles that escape blood clearance during a pass through the liver return to the systemic circulation via the central vein and may ultimately return back into the liver (or another MPS organ). This process may repeat itself until nanoparticle clearance from the bloodstream is complete. *Reproduced with permission from Chan WC. Nanomedicine 2.0.* Accounts Chem Res *2017;50:627–632.*

for long periods of time, which may affect long-term toxicity and safety of nanomedicines.[93]

The spleen is another important MPS organ that may clear systemically administered nanoparticles efficiently from the blood. Anatomically, a spleen's red pulp and white pulp are separated by a marginal zone and sinuses with pores of ~3 μm (Fig. 4.5).[94] The red pulp accounts for ~75% of the spleen. It contains macrophages and is involved in degradation of erythrocytes.[86] Macrophages in the marginal zone, splenic B cells, and dendritic cells provide biological barriers against pathogens.[95] Macrophages within the white pulp are involved in innate immunity and clearing of apoptotic cells and may remove circulating nanoparticles.[96] Overall, splenic macrophages have been shown to exhibit lower phagocytic potency toward circulating nanoparticles compared with liver macrophages, such as Kupffer cells.[84] Nanoparticles with sizes larger than 200 nm in diameter are typically more likely to be cleared by splenic macrophages, whereas liver macrophages interact more strongly with smaller nanoparticles (100 nm or less).[97]

To reduce MPS sequestration of systemically administered nanoparticles, researchers have explored strategies to modulate and inhibit MPS functions and phagocytic response.[21] For example, it has been demonstrated that transient depletion of MPS macrophages, such as hepatic Kupffer cells, with toxic compounds (e.g., gadolinium chloride and clodronate-containing liposomes) can substantially prolong nanoparticle blood circulation times.[20,98–100] Tavares et al. reported 18–150 times greater nanoparticle delivery efficiency to solid tumors upon depletion of liver Kupffer cells via clodronate–liposome treatment.[20] Wolfram *et al.* used a chloroquine-based liver preconditioning strategy to reduce nanoparticle accumulation in the liver by temporarily inhibiting phagocytosis of Kupffer cells.[101] Overwhelming MPS cells by administering large bolus doses of organic and inorganic nanoparticles is another approach to saturate the phagocytic response of Kupffer cells.[102–104] This approach does not require depletion and elimination of macrophages to reduce nanoparticle uptake by the MPS. While most of these examples focus on modulation and inhibition of the liver, it will be important to systematically assess how other MPS organs (e.g., spleen, lymph nodes, skin, bone marrow, and other organs and tissues) individually and collectively

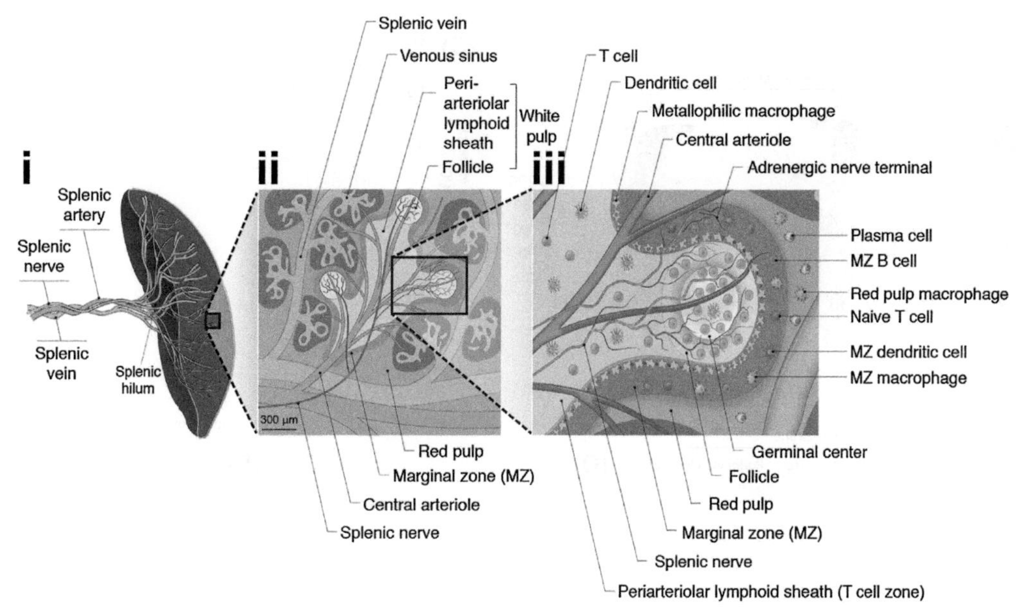

FIGURE 4.5 Spleen anatomy and microarchitecture. (i) Gross schematic illustration of the spleen. The splenic vein directs filtered blood from the spleen back into recirculation. (ii) Schematic of major zones within the spleen, including nonlymphoid red pulp, which filters blood, and the lymphoid white pulp, comprised of the periarteriolar lymphoid sheath and follicles. (iii) Microarchitecture of spleen with specific cell types. *Modified with permission from Noble B, Brennan FH, Popovich PG. The spleen as a neuroimmune interface after spinal cord injury.* J Neuroimmunol *2018.*

contribute to nanoparticle sequestration and elimination.[20,20a] A better fundamental understanding of nanoparticle–MPS interactions from a whole-organ perspective to cellular and molecular levels may allow researchers to design nanoparticles that are potentially able to overcome MPS biological barriers for more efficient nanoparticle delivery to diseased sites.

4.7.3 Nanoparticle–kidney interactions

Kidneys are major organs for clearance and elimination of nanoparticles through blood filtration.[105] Blood enters the kidney through paired renal arteries and exits through paired renal veins. Kidneys comprise three main anatomical regions: (1) renal cortex; (2) medulla; and (3) pelvis. In cortex and medulla, nephrons are basic structural units that contain the renal corpuscle, through which blood is transported into glomeruli. Increased blood pressure within the glomerular cavity causes filtration of fluid, solutes, and waste into the Bowman's space. Unfiltered fluid is transported back into the main bloodstream via efferent arterioles. Filtered fluid that may contain waste products, solutes, and nanoparticles flows from the Bowman's space into proximal tubules. The luminal surface of these tubules is covered with densely packed microvilli that balance secretion into urine and reabsorption.[105]

Nanoparticle filtration within the kidney occurs along the glomerular filtration membrane (GFM, Fig. 4.6). This membrane consists of four major structural units: (1) endothelial glycocalyx; (2) endothelial cells; (3) glomerular basement membrane (GBM); and (4) podocytes. The endothelial glycocalyx has been reported to help in the retention of proteins.[106] The GFM endothelium exhibits fenestrations 70–90 nm in size, where as the GBM exhibits pores with sizes of 2–8 nm. Podocytes that cover the GBM face toward the Bowman's space. The podocyte layer has a pore size of 4–11 nm. This four-layer anatomical architecture controls renal filtration and clearance of materials not only by size but also by charge (Fig. 4.6).[107–109]

The kidney filtration threshold for inorganic nanoparticles has been reported to be 5.5 nm.[110] For proteins and soft macromolecules, studies have shown that those materials with hydrodynamic diameter (HD) slightly larger than 6 nm can still be renally cleared and eliminated.[105] This has been attributed to the mechanical deformation capabilities of these soft organic nanomaterials in comparison with more rigid inorganic nanoparticles.[109] Nanoparticles with sizes larger than the renal filtration cutoff are more likely to interact with MPS organs and cells than kidneys.[21] However, non–renal-clearable nanoparticles with sizes smaller than 100 nm can still interact with the glomerulus but will not be able to cross the GBM for elimination into urine (Fig. 4.6A and B).[105]

A recent study by Zheng *et al.* reported that the GFM acts as a nanoparticle-size "bandpass" filter (Fig. 4.6C–E).[111] For the GFM, the following trends for size-dependent renal clearance of nanoparticles have been reported: (1) HD > 100 nm: minimal nanoparticle transport across endothelium; (2) HD = 6–100 nm: able to transport through endothelium but blocked by GBM; (3)

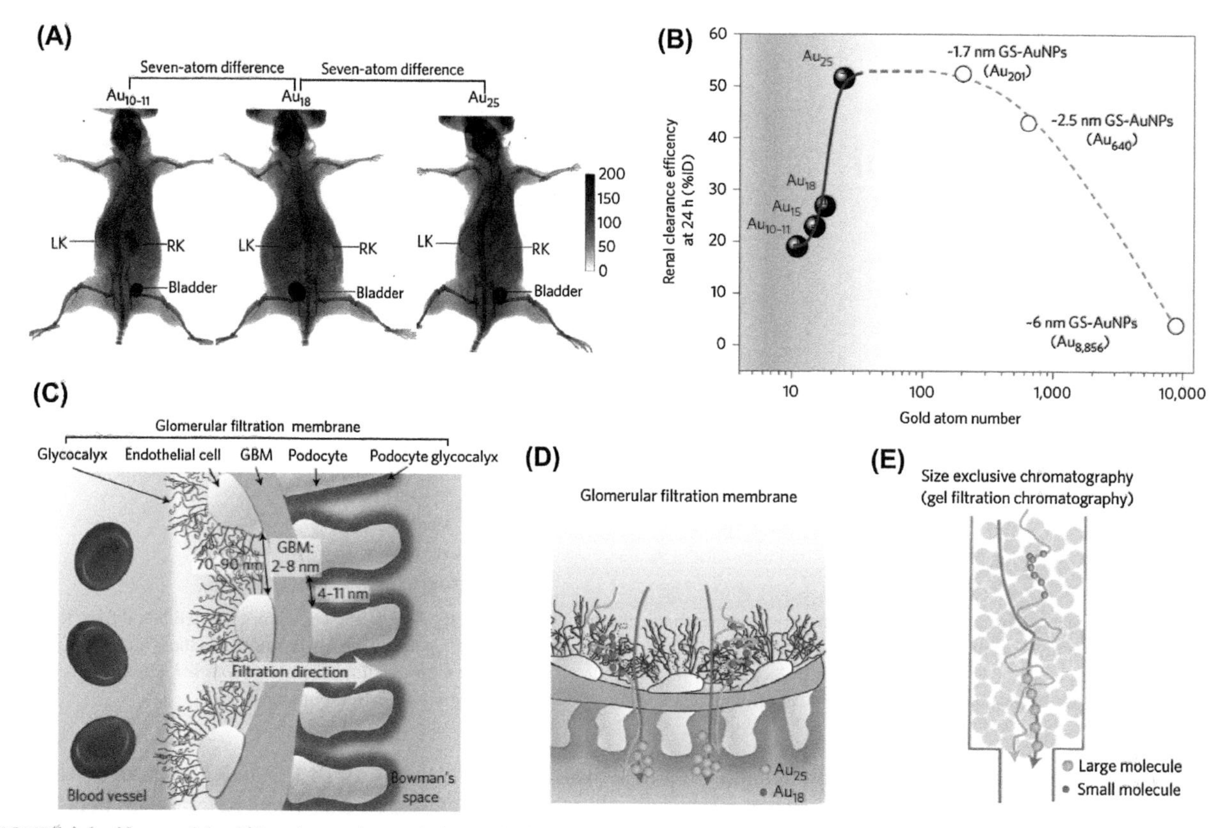

FIGURE 4.6 Nanoparticle–kidney interactions and glomerular filtration of nanoparticles. (A) Whole-body X-ray-based biodistribution images of mice 40 min post intravenous administration of gold nanoclusters (AuNCs) Au_{10-11}, Au_{18}, or Au_{25}. Kidney retention time increased in the following order: $Au_{10-11} > Au_{18} > Au_{25}$. LK, left kidney; RK, right kidney. (B) Renal clearance efficiencies in percentage of the injected dose (%ID) unit of Au_{10-11}, Au_{15}, Au_{18}, and Au_{25}, 1.7 nm (Au_{201}), 2.5 nm (Au_{640}), and 6 nm (Au_{8856}) glutathione-coated AuNCs/AuNPs at 24 h p.i. versus number of gold atoms. Importantly, for AuNCs < Au_{25}, the renal clearance efficiency decreased exponentially with decreasing number of gold atoms per AuNCs. (C) The glomerular filtration membrane (GFM) consists of an endothelial glycocalyx, endothelial cells, the glomerular basement membrane (GBM), and podocytes. (C)–(E). The GFM exhibits capabilities similar to a size "bandpass" filter for nanoparticles. Nanoparticles with a hydrodynamic diameter (HD) > 100 nm cannot transport through the endothelium. Nanoparticles with HD = 6–100 nm cannot cross the GBM. Nanoparticles with HD between 2 and 6 nm can traverse the GFM. In general, smaller nanoparticles will cross the GFM faster than larger ones. Nanoparticles with HD between 1 and 2 nm cross the membrane with similar velocity and efficiency. Nanoparticles with HD < 1 nm physically interact with the endothelial glycocalyx, resulting in inverse size-dependent glomerular filtration. In general, smaller nanoparticles clear more slowly than larger ones. *Modified with permission from Du B, et al. Glomerular barrier behaves as an atomically precise bandpass filter in a sub-nanometre regime.* Nat Nanotechnol. *2017;12.*

HD = 2–6 nm: size-dependent nanoparticle interactions with GBM and podocytes—smaller nanoparticles are cleared faster than larger nanoparticles; (4) HD = 1–2 nm: these materials exhibit comparable renal clearance characteristics with those nanoparticles with HD 2–6 nm; and (5) HD < 1 nm: these materials interact substantially with glycocalyx, which decreases renal clearance efficiency of nanoparticles with decreasing size (Fig. 4.6B).[105] In addition to size-dependent renal clearance, there is also nanoparticle surface charge dependence.[107,108] The GFM glycocalyx is overall negatively charged. In consequence, renal nanoparticle clearance rates decrease in the following order: positively charged nanoparticles > neutral nanoparticles > negatively charged nanoparticles.[105]

In summary, the renal system represents a nanoparticle size and charge-dependent biological barrier for administered nanomedicines. This barrier may be able to significantly reduce blood circulation times of small nanoparticles. Ultimately, this may impede efficient delivery of nanoparticles to diseased tissues.

4.7.4 Controlling nano–bio interactions through nanoparticle design

Efficient and targeted delivery of nanoparticles to diseased sites is a major quest in nanomedicine research. Researchers have been able to develop nanomaterial design strategies that allow, to a certain extent, the control of *in vivo* fate of nanomedicines by modulating nano–bio interactions.[3] One of these strategies is nanoparticle surface modification with antifouling polymers, such as poly(ethylene glycol), i.e., PEG.[112,113] Nanoparticle surface modification with PEG is referred to as PEGylation. PEGylation reduces nonspecific serum protein adsorption onto the nanoparticle surface and therefore reduces the formation of a protein corona.[64,65] This in turn may increase nanoparticle blood circulation times and theoretically increase passive and active targeting capabilities of PEGylated nanoparticles and ligand-conjugated nanoparticles.[114]

To mitigate the negative effect of protein corona formation on active targeting, Dai *et al.* developed a PEG surface modification strategy for antibody-decorated gold nanoparticles.[81] Antibodies, such as the FDA-approved HER2 targeting monoclonal antibody Trastuzumab (Herceptin), are conjugated with 5-kDa PEG. This PEG linker is then covalently attached to the gold nanoparticle surface via sulfur–gold interactions at a density of <0.1 antibodies per square nanometer of nanoparticle surface area. The remaining nanoparticle surface is then backfilled with shorter 2-kDa methoxy-terminated PEG. This PEG backfilling strategy significantly reduces nonspecific serum protein adsorption and maximizes specific antibody—cell surface receptor interactions.[81]

Other strategies to reduce nanoparticle protein corona formation include the use of zwitterionic polymers as surface ligands.[115,116] A different and highly innovative approach to reduce MPS uptake of nanoparticles is by covering the nanoparticles with cell membranes derived from erythrocytes, leukocytes, or thrombocytes.[117,118] This camouflaging strategy can help in the reduction of nanoparticle MPS clearance from the bloodstream and increase nanoparticle blood circulation times.[119] Discher *et al.* reported a biologically inspired nanoparticle surface engineering strategy to minimize MPS recognition and clearance of nanoparticles. They demonstrated that nanoparticles showed reduced uptake by phagocytic cells for improved drug delivery when the nanoparticle surface was decorated with minimal "self"-peptides, such as CD47 peptides.[120]

In summary, nanoparticle surface engineering strategies allow reduction in protein corona formation and MPS clearance by reducing nonspecific protein adsorption onto the nanoparticle surface. However, these strategies cannot completely passivate the nanoparticle surface and may not fully prevent protein adsorption. This opens up many opportunities for researchers to focus on better chemical and biological nanoparticle surface engineering strategies. The goals of these strategies may be manifold, including (1) minimizing nanoparticle protein corona formation; (2) reducing nanoparticle MPS interactions; (3) controlling nano–bio interactions; and (4) improving nanoparticle delivery to targeted tissues and cells in the body.

4.8 Clinical potential of passive nanoparticle targeting

Passive and active nanoparticle targeting strategies are extensively used in preclinical research. In contrast to clinical research, which involves human subjects, preclinical research involves studies in tissue culture and animal models. While the concept of "active nanoparticle targeting" has generated significant interest with >1500 preclinical publications on this topic between 2007 and 2017, there are currently no FDA-approved active targeting cancer nanotherapeutics.[82,121] In 2016, seven active targeting nanoparticle cancer formulations were in early clinical trials (phase I and phase II) according to a survey by Chan *et al.*[121] These data highlight that, while active targeting is an attractive idea, significant challenges exist with delivering nanoparticles to tumors and cancer cells. One of these challenges is to deliver nanoparticles *in vivo* in adequate quantities to their intended diseased tissue destinations.[122] Research by Chan *et al.* has demonstrated that overall median nanoparticle delivery efficiencies to solid tumors in preclinical studies reach only approximately 1% of the injected nanoparticle dose.[38] Importantly, the nanoparticle delivery efficiency to malignant cells in a solid tumor has been reported to be about 500 times lower ($<0.002\%$ID) with similar efficiencies for passive and active targeting nanoparticles.[82] This indicates that the majority of nanoparticles that reach a tumor do not interact with tumor cells. In addition, intratumoral nanoparticles are more likely to interact with TAMs and other off-target cells in the tumor rather than malignant cells.[82,83]

Active targeting strategies have not yet translated into FDA-approved cancer nanotherapeutics. The current list of FDA-approved cancer nanotherapeutics comprises five liposome-based and one protein-based formulations (Table 4.1).[15,123] These formulations have been designed with the goal to exploit passive nanoparticle targeting strategies and do not exhibit active targeting surface ligands. The first cancer nanotherapeutic received FDA approval in 1995 and was introduced into the market as Doxil.[124,125] Doxil is a liposomal formulation of the small-molecule cancer drug doxorubicin. Doxil liposomes have been formulated with PEG surface ligands to increase blood circulation times by reducing MPS interactions. Therefore, Doxil is a typical example of a cancer nanotherapeutic formulation that exploits the fundamental concepts of passive nanoparticle targeting for improved nanoparticle tumor delivery.[17]

In summary, passive targeting has high clinical relevance in nanomedicine. All FDA-approved nanoformulations are based on passive targeting design principles. While active targeting nanoparticles are intensively explored and applied in preclinical research, only few of them have entered clinical trial phases. It is important to note that none of the current FDA-approved cancer nanotherapeutics uses active targeting strategies for enhanced tumor accumulation or cell targeting specificity.

TABLE 4.1 FDA-approved cancer nanotherapeutics.

Generic name and/or proprietary name	Nanoparticle type	Active pharmaceutical ingredient (API)	Type of cancer	Year of FDA approval	Refs
Liposomal doxorubicin (Doxil)	Liposome	Doxorubicin	HIV-related Kaposi sarcoma, ovarian cancer, and multiple myeloma	1995	17
Liposomal daunorubicin (DaunoXome)	Liposome	Daunorubicin	HIV-related Kaposi sarcoma	1996	126
Nab-paclitaxel (Abraxane)	Albumin nanoparticles	Paclitaxel	Breast, lung, and pancreatic cancer	2005	127
Liposomal vincristine (Marqibo)	Liposome	Vincristine sulfate	Acute lymphoblastic leukemia	2012	128
Liposomal irinotecan (Onivyde or MM-398)	Liposome	Irinotecan	Postgemcitabine metastatic pancreatic cancer	2015	129
Liposomal cytarabine-daunorubicin (Vyxeos or CPX-351)	Liposome	Cytarabine and daunorubicin (5:1)	High-risk acute myeloid leukemia	2017	123

4.9 Perspective and conclusion

Effective and efficient delivery of drugs and imaging contrast agents to tumors in the body is one of the major challenges in cancer treatment and diagnosis. Strategies that allow specific delivery of chemotherapeutic drugs to diseased tissues while avoiding healthy organs and cells are needed. Current nanomedicines are designed to address these clinical needs. Researchers have been engineering nanoparticles with active and passive targeting capabilities. However, the current list of FDA-approved cancer nanotherapeutics comprises only passive targeting nanoparticles (Table 4.1). Most of these formulations have received FDA approval because they showed favorable toxicity profiles in comparison with administration of free drug rather than improved overall survival.[130]

One of the potential reasons for why it is so challenging to translate cancer nanomedicines into the clinic is the current gap between preclinical animal models and human subjects.[130a] While preclinical animal tumor models may exhibit EPR, its prevalence in tumors of human subjects may be substantially different. The extent of EPR for human tumors is a controversial topic due to significant intratumoral and interpatient variability.[29,49,131] This variability makes it challenging to select cancer patients who may benefit from treatment with cancer nanomedicines. To address this challenge, a recent clinical trial quantified tumor accumulation of administered ferumoxytol (iron oxide nanoparticle) as a marker to predict tumor treatment response to a liposomal irinotecan formulation (MM-398). Preliminary results indicate positive correlation between tumor size reduction (i.e., tumor shrinkage) as a result of MM-398 treatment and ferumoxytol levels in tumors for a small group of patients.[132] These results are encouraging as they may suggest that researchers could preselect patients who are more likely to benefit from nanomedicine to improve overall therapeutic outcomes.[133]

Another challenge in preclinical research is that commonly used fast-growing animal tumor models do not recapitulate the majority of solid tumors in humans in terms of pathophysiology and EPR.[24] Therefore, animal tumor models that better resemble human tumor pathology are needed.[134,135] The variability of tumors is a major concern when developing nanoparticles for cancer applications. A recent study by Sykes *et al.* demonstrated that physicochemical properties of nanoparticles can be optimized according to a tumor's pathophysiology to improve nanoparticle tumor accumulation and therapeutic effects.[136] While this study used preclinical animal models, it suggests that there may be a need to tailor nanoparticle design to a patient's individual cancer characteristics, including cancer type and stage. This may open opportunities for personalized cancer nanomedicine, which may be combined in the future with companion diagnostics and imaging to preselect patient groups with improved likelihood for nanomedicine-based treatment response.

The development of personalized nanomedicine requires deep understanding of nano–bio interactions.[136a] Biological processes and mechanisms involved in the biodistribution and intratumoral distribution of nanoparticles need to be further investigated to guide the design of nanomedicines.[4] To this end, Chan *et al.* have applied 3D optical microscopy as a new tool with the ultimate goal to image the intratumoral distribution of nanoparticles on a whole-tissue level with subcellular resolution.[137–139] High-resolution volumetric optical imaging results can be further supported by single cell analytical approaches, including flow cytometry, fluorescence-activated cell sorting, and single-cell elemental analysis (for example, single-cell inductively coupled plasma mass spectrometry, SC-ICP-MS[140]). Quantitative imaging studies and single-cellbioanalysis may be used to inform the engineering of nanoparticles with optimal intratumoral distribution and cellular interaction.[140a]

While EPR has become a blanket term that incorporates a large number of complex biological processes,[4] engineering of nanomedicines with EPR as the only nanoparticle design rationale may be outdated. As discussed in this chapter, passive and active targeting nanoparticles rely on passive paracellular transport across the endothelium for tumor accumulation. This is a fundamental paradigm of the EPR effect. However, studies have emphasized the high intratumoral and intertumoral variability that may raise concerns about its significance.[27] While paracellular extravasation of nanoparticles has been the key concept for designing nanomedicines over the past few decades, recent research suggests the possibility for transcellular extravasation pathways.[141,142] Specifically, caveolae-mediated pathways across tumor endothelium as reported by Schnitzer *et al.* may be intriguing new concepts of nanoparticle delivery to tumors.[39,143] In addition, the use of iRGD peptides as shown by Ruoslahti and coworkers may open transcytosis pathways for nanomedicines to cross the tumor endothelial barrier.[144–146] Research by Dvorak *et al.* suggests a different transcellular pathway for nanoparticles. A network of grouped and interlinked cytoplasmic vesicles and vacuoles, termed vesiculovacuolar organelle may be exploited for efficient nanoparticle delivery into tumors.[38,147,148] These transcellular pathways may open up new strategies for nanoparticle tumor delivery and may shift the EPR paradigm toward a transcellular nanoparticle tumor delivery mechanism. However, more research is needed to better evaluate the significance and impact of these transcellular pathways for cancer nanomedicine.[38]

In summary, the concept of passive nanoparticle targeting has allowed the design and clinical translation of nanomedicines for systemic use in patients. The current collection of FDA-approved cancer nanotherapeutics exploits the fundamental concepts of passive targeting, which highlights the clinical potential of this technology. However, the true promise of nanomedicine has yet to be fulfilled. Current nanoparticle targeting strategies do not allow full control over biodistribution and cellular interactions of nanomedicines.[148a] More research is needed to better understand nano–bio interactions, systemic nanoparticle transport, and delivery of nanoparticles to targeted sites in the body. Further fundamental research studies with the aim to elucidate biological mechanisms and processes of nanoparticles *in vivo* may guide the design and development of future nanomedicines. This improved fundamental understanding may enable researches to achieve the true goal of nanomedicine, that is, substantial improvements in patient survivals and significant clinical benefits.

Acknowledgments

The authors thank Dr. Dai for assistance with illustrations and Ms. Xuan for manuscript proofreading. The work has been supported by the Vice President for Research of the University of Oklahoma (Junior Faculty Fellowship, JFF).

References

1. Pelaz B, et al. Diverse applications of nanomedicine. *ACS Nano* 2017;**11**:2313–81.
2. Torrice M. Does nanomedicine have a delivery problem? *ACS Central Sci* 2016;**2**:434–7.
3. Blanco E, Shen H, Ferrari M. Principles of nanoparticle design for overcoming biological barriers to drug delivery. *Nat Biotechnol* 2015;**33**:941–51.
4. Bertrand N, Wu J, Xu X, Kamaly N, Farokhzad OC. Cancer nanotechnology: the impact of passive and active targeting in the era of modern cancer biology. *Adv Drug Deliver Rev* 2014;**66**:2–25.
5. Kim B, Rutka JT, Chan W. Nanomedicine. *New Engl J Medicine* 2010;**363**:2434–43.
6. Boisselier E, Astruc D. Gold nanoparticles in nanomedicine: preparations, imaging, diagnostics, therapies and toxicity. *Chem Soc Rev* 2009;**38**:1759–82.
7. Gobbo OL, Sjaastad K, Radomski MW, Volkov Y, Prina-Mello A. Magnetic nanoparticles in cancer theranostics. *Theranostics* 2015;**5**: 1249–63.
8. Cutler JI, Auyeung E, Mirkin CA. Spherical nucleic acids. *J Am Chem Soc* 2012;**134**:1376–91.
9. Chan WC, Nie S. Quantum dot bioconjugates for ultrasensitive nonisotopic detection. *Science* 1998;**281**:2016–8.
10. Wilhelm S. Perspectives for upconverting nanoparticles. *ACS Nano* 2017. https://doi.org/10.1021/acsnano.7b0712.
11. Spinowitz BS, et al. Ferumoxytol for treating iron deficiency anemia in CKD. *J Am Soc Nephrol* 2008;**19**:1599–605.
12. Allen TM, Cullis PR. Liposomal drug delivery systems: from concept to clinical applications. *Adv Drug Deliver Rev* 2013;**65**:36–48.
13. Menjoge AR, Kannan RM, Tomalia DA. Dendrimer-based drug and imaging conjugates: design considerations for nanomedical applications. *Drug Discov Today* 2010;**15**:171–85.
14. Elsabahy M, Wooley KL. Design of polymeric nanoparticles for biomedical delivery applications. *Chem Soc Rev* 2012;**41**:2545–61.
15. Shi J, Kantoff PW, Wooster R, Farokhzad OC. Cancer nanomedicine: progress, challenges and opportunities. *Nat Rev Cancer* 2016;**17**. nrc.2016.108.
16. Wais U, Jackson AW, He T, Zhang H. Nanoformulation and encapsulation approaches for poorly water-soluble drug nanoparticles. *Nanoscale* 2015;**8**:1746–69.
17. Barenholz Y. Doxil® — the first FDA-approved nano-drug: lessons learned. *J Control Release* 2012;**160**:117–34.

18. Xie J, Lee S, Chen X. Nanoparticle-based theranostic agents. *Adv Drug Deliver Rev* 2010;**62**:1064–79.
19. Chen H, Zhang W, Zhu G, Xie J, Chen X. Rethinking cancer nanotheranostics. *Nat Rev Mater* 2017;**2**. natrevmats201724.
20. Tavares AJ, et al. Effect of removing Kupffer cells on nanoparticle tumor delivery. *Proc National Acad Sci* 2017;**114**:E10871–80.
20a Poon W, Zhang Y-N, Ouyang B, Kingston BR, Wu JLY, Wilhelm S, Chan WCW. *ACS Nano* 2019;**13**(5):5785–98. https://doi.org/10.1021/acsnano.9b01383.
21. Zhang Y-N, Poon W, Tavares AJ, McGilvray ID, Chan W. Nanoparticle–liver interactions: cellular uptake and hepatobiliary elimination. *J Control Release* 2016;**240**:332–48.
21a Hobbs SK, Monsky WL, Yuan F, Roberts WG, Griffith L, Torchilin VP, Jain RK. Regulation of transport pathways in tumor vessels: role of tumor type and microenvironment. *Proceedings of the National Academy of Sciences* 1998;**95**(8):4607–12.
22. Carmeliet P, Jain RK. Angiogenesis in cancer and other diseases. *Nature* 2000;**407**. 35025220.
23. Hobbs SK, et al. Regulation of transport pathways in tumor vessels: role of tumor type and microenvironment. *Proc National Acad Sci* 1998;**95**:4607–12.
24. Rosenblum D, Joshi N, Tao W, Karp JM, Peer D. Progress and challenges towards targeted delivery of cancer therapeutics. *Nat Commun* 2018;**9**:1410.
25. Li R, Zheng K, Yuan C, Chen Z, Huang M. Be active or not: the relative contribution of active and passive tumor targeting of nanomaterials. *Nanotheranostics* 2017;**1**:346–57.
26. Sykes EA, Chen J, Zheng G, Chan W. Investigating the impact of nanoparticle size on active and passive tumor targeting efficiency. *ACS Nano* 2014;**8**:5696–706.
27. Bae Y, Park K. Targeted drug delivery to tumors: myths, reality and possibility. *J Control Release* 2011;**153**:198–205.
28. Matsumura Y, Maeda H. A new concept for macromolecular therapeutics in cancer chemotherapy: mechanism of tumoritropic accumulation of proteins and the antitumor agent smancs. *Cancer Research* 1986;**46**:6387–92.
29. Fang J, Nakamura H, Maeda H. The EPR effect: unique features of tumor blood vessels for drug delivery, factors involved, and limitations and augmentation of the effect. *Adv Drug Deliver Rev* 2011;**63**:136–51.
30. Hanahan D, Weinberg RA. Hallmarks of cancer: the next generation. *Cell* 2011;**144**.
31. Hanahan D, Weinberg RA. The hallmarks of cancer. *Cell* 2000;**100**.
32. Nagy J, Chang S-H, Shih S-C, Dvorak A, Dvorak H. Heterogeneity of the tumor vasculature. *Semin Thromb Hemost* 2010;**36**:321–31.
33. Nagy J, Chang S-H, orak A, Dvorak H. Why are tumour blood vessels abnormal and why is it important to know? *Brit J Cancer* 2009;**100**:6604929.
34. Dvorak HF. How tumors make bad blood vessels and stroma. *Am J Pathology* 2003;**162**:1747–57.
35. Dvorak H, Nagy J, Dvorak J, orak A. Identification and characterization of the blood vessels of solid tumors that are leaky to circulating macromolecules. *Am J Pathology* 1988;**133**:95–109.
36. Nagy JA, Benjamin L, Zeng H, Dvorak AM, Dvorak HF. Vascular permeability, vascular hyperpermeability and angiogenesis. *Angiogenesis* 2008;**11**:109–19.
37. Nagy JA, Dvorak AM, Dvorak HF. Vascular hyperpermeability, angiogenesis, and stroma generation. *Cold Spring Harb Perspect Med* 2012;**2**:a006544.
38. Wilhelm S, et al. Analysis of nanoparticle delivery to tumours. *Nature Rev Mater* 2016;**1**. natrevmats201614.
39. Kim SM, Faix PH, Schnitzer JE. Overcoming key biological barriers to cancer drug delivery and efficacy. *J Control Release* 2017;**267**:15–30.
40. Chrastina A, Massey KA, Schnitzer JE. Overcoming in vivo barriers to targeted nanodelivery. *Wiley Interdiscip Rev Nanomed Nanobiotechnol* 2011;**3**:421–37.
41. Moghimi S, Hunter A, Murray J. Long-circulating and target-specific nanoparticles: theory to practice. *Pharmacol Rev* 2001;**53**:283–318.
42. Wickline SA, Neubauer AM, Winter PM, Caruthers SD, Lanza GM. Molecular imaging and therapy of atherosclerosis with targeted nanoparticles. *J Magn Reson Imaging* 2007;**25**:667–80.
43. Fredman G, et al. Targeted nanoparticles containing the proresolving peptide Ac2-26 protect against advanced atherosclerosis in hypercholesterolemic mice. *Sci Transl Med* 2015;**7**.
44. Lobatto ME, et al. Atherosclerotic plaque targeting mechanism of long-circulating nanoparticles established by multimodal imaging. *ACS Nano* 2015;**9**:1837–47.
44a Bordry N, Broggi MAS, de Jonge K, Schaeuble K, Gannon PO, Foukas PG, Danenberg E, Romano E, Baumgaertner P, Fankhauser M, Wald N, Cagnon L, Abed-Maillard S, El Hajjami HM, Murray T, Ioannidou K, Letovanec I, Yan P, Michielin O, Matter M, Swartz MA, Speiser DE. Lymphatic vessel density is associated with CD8+ T cell infiltration and immunosuppressive factors in human melanoma. *Oncoimmunology* 2018;**7**. https://doi.org/10.1080/2162402X.2018.1462878.
45. Moulton KS, et al. Loss of collagen XVIII enhances neovascularization and vascular permeability in atherosclerosis. *Circulation* 2004;**110**:1330–6.
46. Barua S, Mitragotri S. Challenges associated with penetration of nanoparticles across cell and tissue barriers: a review of current status and future prospects. *Nano Today* 2014;**9**:223–43.
47. Kim Y, et al. Probing nanoparticle translocation across the permeable endothelium in experimental atherosclerosis. *Proc National Acad Sci* 2014;**111**:1078–83.
48. Prabhakar U, et al. Challenges and key considerations of the enhanced permeability and retention effect for nanomedicine drug delivery in oncology. *Cancer Res* 2013;**73**:2412–7.
49. Kobayashi H, Watanabe R, Choyke PL. Improving conventional enhanced permeability and retention (EPR) effects; what is the appropriate target? *Theranostics* 2013;**4**:81–9.
50. Gerlinger M, et al. Intratumor heterogeneity and branched evolution revealed by multiregion sequencing. *New Engl J Medicine* 2012;**366**:883–92.
51. Fisher R, Pusztai L, Swanton C. Cancer heterogeneity: implications for targeted therapeutics. *British journal of cancer* 2013;**108**.
52. Crockford A, Jamal-Hanjani M, Hicks J, Swanton C. Implications of intratumour heterogeneity for treatment stratification. *J Pathology* 2014;**232**:264–73.
53. Björnmalm M, Thurecht KJ, Michael M, ott A, Caruso F. Bridging bio–nano science and cancer nanomedicine. *ACS Nano* 2017. https://doi.org/10.1021/acsnano.7b0485.
54. Nel A, Ruoslahti E, Meng H. New insights into "permeability" as in the enhanced permeability and retention effect of cancer nanotherapeutics. *ACS Nano* 2017;**11**:9567–9.
55. van der Meel R, Lammers T, Hennink WE. Cancer nanomedicines: oversold or underappreciated? *Expert Opin Drug Del* 2016. https://doi.org/10.1080/17425247.2017.126234.
56. Ramanathan RK, et al. Correlation between ferumoxytol uptake in tumor lesions by MRI and response to nanoliposomal irinotecan in patients with advanced solid tumors: a pilot study. *Clin Cancer Res* 2017;**23**:3638–48.

57. Ekdawi SN, et al. Spatial and temporal mapping of heterogeneity in liposome uptake and microvascular distribution in an orthotopic tumor xenograft model. *J Control Release* 2015;**207**:101–11.
58. Nel AE, et al. Understanding biophysicochemical interactions at the nano–bio interface. *Nat Mater* 2009;**8**:543–57.
59. Lai ZW, Yan Y, Caruso F, Nice EC. Emerging techniques in proteomics for probing nano–bio interactions. *ACS Nano* 2012;**6**:10438–48.
60. von Roemeling C, Jiang W, Chan CK, Weissman IL, Kim B. Breaking down the barriers to precision cancer nanomedicine. *Trends Biotechnol* 2017;**35**:159–71.
61. Lazarovits J, Chen Y, Sykes EA, Chan WC. Nanoparticle-blood interactions: the implications on solid tumour targeting. *Chem Commun* 2015;**51**:2756–67.
62. Baumann D, et al. Complex encounters: nanoparticles in whole blood and their uptake into different types of white blood cells. *Nanomed* 2013;**8**:699–713.
63. Rothen-Rutishauser BM, Schürch S, Haenni B, Kapp N, Gehr P. Interaction of fine particles and nanoparticles with red blood cells visualized with advanced microscopic techniques. *Environ Sci Technol* 2006;**40**:4353–9.
64. Walkey CD, et al. Protein corona fingerprinting predicts the cellular interaction of gold and silver nanoparticles. *ACS Nano* 2014;**8**: 2439–55.
65. Walkey CD, Olsen JB, Guo H, Emili A, Chan WC. Nanoparticle size and surface chemistry determine serum protein adsorption and macrophage uptake. *J Am Chem Soc* 2012;**134**:2139–47.
66. Walkey CD, Chan WC. Understanding and controlling the interaction of nanomaterials with proteins in a physiological environment. *Chem Soc Rev* 2011;**41**:2780–99.
67. Ritz S, et al. Protein corona of nanoparticles: distinct proteins regulate the cellular uptake. *Biomacromolecules* 2015;**16**:1311–21.
68. Tenzer S, et al. Nanoparticle size is a critical physicochemical determinant of the human blood plasma corona: a comprehensive quantitative proteomic analysis. *ACS Nano* 2011;**5**:7155–67.
69. Cedervall T, et al. Understanding the nanoparticle–protein corona using methods to quantify exchange rates and affinities of proteins for nanoparticles. *Proc National Acad Sci* 2007;**104**:2050–5.
70. Lundqvist M, et al. Nanoparticle size and surface properties determine the protein corona with possible implications for biological impacts. *Proc Natl Acad Sci* 2008;**105**:14265–70.
71. Winzen S, et al. Complementary analysis of the hard and soft protein corona: sample preparation critically effects corona composition. *Nanoscale* 2015;**7**:2992–3001.
72. Liu W, et al. Protein corona formation for nanomaterials and proteins of a similar size: hard or soft corona? *Nanoscale* 2012;**5**: 1658–68.
73. Lundqvist M, et al. The evolution of the protein corona around nanoparticles: a test study. *ACS Nano* 2011;**5**:7503–9.
74. Casals E, Pfaller T, Duschl A, Oostingh G, Puntes V. Time evolution of the nanoparticle protein corona. *ACS Nano* 2010;**4**:3623–32.
75. Bertrand N, et al. Mechanistic understanding of in vivo protein corona formation on polymeric nanoparticles and impact on pharmacokinetics. *Nat Commun* 2017;**8**:777.
76. Chen F, et al. Complement proteins bind to nanoparticle protein corona and undergo dynamic exchange in vivo. *Nat Nanotechnol* 2017;**12**:387.
77. Monopoli MP, Åberg C, Salvati A, Dawson KA. Biomolecular coronas provide the biological identity of nanosized materials. *Nat Nanotechnol* 2012;**7**:779.
78. Albanese A, et al. Secreted biomolecules alter the biological identity and cellular interactions of nanoparticles. *ACS Nano* 2014;**8**: 5515–26.
79. Albanese A, Tang PS, Chan W. The effect of nanoparticle size, shape, and surface chemistry on biological systems. *Annu Rev Biomed Eng* 2012;**14**:1–16.
80. Murphy K, Weaver C. *Janeway's immunobiology*. 2016.
81. Dai Q, Walkey C, Chan WC. Polyethylene glycol backfilling mitigates the negative impact of the protein corona on nanoparticle cell targeting. *Angewandte Chemie Int Ed* 2014;**53**:5093–6.
82. Dai Q, et al. Quantifying the ligand-coated nanoparticle delivery to cancer cells in solid tumours. *ACS Nano* 2018;**12**:8423–35.
83. Miller MA, et al. Tumour-associated macrophages act as a slow-release reservoir of nano-therapeutic Pt (IV) pro-drug. *Nat Commun* 2015;**6**.
83a. Huai Y, Hossen MN, Wilhelm S, Bhattacharya R, Mukherjee P. Nanoparticle Interactions with the Tumor Microenvironment. *Bioconjugate chemistry* 2019;**30**(9):2247–63.
84. Gustafson H, Holt-Casper D, Grainger DW, Ghandehari H. Nanoparticle uptake: the phagocyte problem. *Nano Today* 2015;**10**: 487–510.
85. Tsoi KM, et al. Mechanism of hard-nanomaterial clearance by the liver. *Nat Mater* 2016;**15**:1212–21.
86. Gordon S, Taylor PR. Monocyte and macrophage heterogeneity. *Nat Rev Immunol* 2005;**5**:953.
87. Zhang C, et al. Pharmacokinetics, biodistribution, efficacy and safety of N-octyl-O-sulfate chitosan micelles loaded with paclitaxel. *Biomaterials* 2008;**29**:1233–41.
88. Fonge H, Huang H, Scollard D, Reilly RM, Allen C. Influence of formulation variables on the biodistribution of multifunctional block copolymer micelles. *J Control Release* 2012;**157**:366–74.
89. Ye L, et al. A pilot study in non-human primates shows no adverse response to intravenous injection of quantum dots. *Nat Nanotechnol* 2012;**7**:453.
90. Jong WH, et al. Particle size-dependent organ distribution of gold nanoparticles after intravenous administration. *Biomaterials* 2008;**29**:1912–9.
91. Sanvicens N, Marco PM. Multifunctional nanoparticles – properties and prospects for their use in human medicine. *Trends Biotechnol* 2008;**26**:425–33.
92. Wang H, Wu L, Reinhard BM. Scavenger receptor mediated endocytosis of silver nanoparticles into J774A.1 macrophages is heterogeneous. *ACS Nano* 2012;**6**:7122–32.
93. Fischer HC, Hauck TS, Gómez-Aristizábal A, Chan WC. Exploring primary liver macrophages for studying quantum dot interactions with biological systems. *Adv Mater* 2010;**22**:2520–4.
94. Huang S, et al. In vivo splenic clearance correlates with in vitro deformability of red blood cells from plasmodium yoelii-infected mice. *Infect Immun* 2014;**82**:2532–41.
95. Noble B, Brennan FH, Popovich PG. The spleen as a neuro-immune interface after spinal cord injury. *J Neuroimmunol* **321**, 2018, 1–11.
96. Davies LC, Jenkins SJ, Allen JE, Taylor PR. Tissue-resident macrophages. *Nat Immunol* 2013;**14**:986–95.

97. Cataldi M, Vigliotti C, Mosca T, Cammarota M, Capone D. Emerging role of the spleen in the pharmacokinetics of monoclonal antibodies, nanoparticles and exosomes. *Int J Mol Sci* 2017;**18**:1249.
98. Rooijen N, Sanders A. Liposome mediated depletion of macrophages: mechanism of action, preparation of liposomes and applications. *J Immunol Methods* 1994;**174**:83–93.
99. Rooijen VN. The liposome-mediated macrophage 'suicide' technique. *J Immunol Methods* 1989;**124**:1–6.
100. Rüttinger D, Vollmar B, Wanner GA, Messmer K. In vivo assessment of hepatic alterations following gadolinium chloride-induced Kupffer cell blockade. *J Hepatol* 1996;**25**:960–7.
101. Wolfram J, et al. A chloroquine-induced macrophage-preconditioning strategy for improved nanodelivery. *Sci Rep* 2017;**7**:13738.
102. Kao YJ, Juliano RL. Interactions of liposomes with the reticuloendothelial system effects of reticuloendothelial blockade on the clearance of large unilamellar vesicles. *Biochim Biophys Acta* 1981;**677**:453–61.
103. itt R, et al. Liposomal blockade of the reticuloendothelial system: improved tumor imaging with small unilamellar vesicles. *Science* 1983;**220**:502–5.
104. Liu T, Choi H, Zhou R, Chen I-W. RES blockade: a strategy for boosting efficiency of nanoparticle drug. *Nano Today* 2015;**10**.
105. Du B, Yu M, Zheng J. Transport and interactions of nanoparticles in the kidneys. *Nat Rev Mater* 2018;**3**:1–17.
106. Singh A, et al. Glomerular endothelial glycocalyx constitutes a barrier to protein permeability. *J Am Soc Nephrol* 2007;**18**:2885–93.
107. Tay M, Comper W, Singh A. Charge selectivity in kidney ultrafiltration is associated with glomerular uptake of transport probes. *Am J Physiol-renal* 1991;**260**:F549–54.
108. Comper WD, Glasgow EF. Charge selectivity in kidney ultrafiltration. *Kidney Int* 1995;**47**:1242–51.
109. Tencer J, Frick I-M, Öquist BW, Alm P, Rippe B. Size-selectivity of the glomerular barrier to high molecular weight proteins: upper size limitations of shunt pathways. *Kidney Int* 1998;**53**:709–15.
110. Choi H, et al. Renal clearance of quantum dots. *Nat Biotechnol* 2007;**25**.
111. Du B, et al. Glomerular barrier behaves as an atomically precise bandpass filter in a sub-nanometre regime. *Nat Nanotechnol* 2017;**12**. nnano.2017.170.
112. Klibanov AL, Maruyama K, Torchilin VP, Huang L. Amphipathic polyethyleneglycols effectively prolong the circulation time of liposomes. *Febs Lett* 1990;**268**:235–7.
113. Gref R, et al. Biodegradable long-circulating polymeric nanospheres. *Science* 1994;**263**:1600–3.
114. Kirpotin DB, et al. Antibody targeting of long-circulating lipidic nanoparticles does not increase tumor localization but does increase internalization in animal models. *Cancer Res* 2006;**66**:6732–40.
115. Moyano DF, et al. Fabrication of corona-free nanoparticles with tunable hydrophobicity. *ACS Nano* 2014;**8**:6748–55.
116. García K, et al. Zwitterionic-coated "stealth" nanoparticles for biomedical applications: recent advances in countering biomolecular corona formation and uptake by the mononuclear phagocyte system. *Small* 2014;**10**:2516–29.
117. Hu C-MJ, et al. Erythrocyte membrane-camouflaged polymeric nanoparticles as a biomimetic delivery platform. *Proc National Acad Sci* 2011;**108**:10980–5.
118. Hu C-MJ, et al. Nanoparticle biointerfacing by platelet membrane cloaking. *Nature* 2015;**526**.
119. Luk BT, Zhang L. Cell membrane-camouflaged nanoparticles for drug delivery. *J Control Release* 2015;**220**:600–7.
120. Rodriguez PL, et al. Minimal 'self' peptides that inhibit phagocytic clearance and enhance delivery of nanoparticles. *Science* 2013;**339**:971–5.
121. Wilhelm S, Tavares AJ, Chan WC. Reply to "Evaluation of nanomedicines: stick to the basics". *Nature Reviews Materials* 2016;**1**.
122. Jain RK. Vascular and interstitial barriers to delivery of therapeutic agents in tumors. *Cancer Metast Rev* 1990;**9**:253–66.
123. Lancet JE, et al. Final results of a phase III randomized trial of CPX-351 versus 7+3 in older patients with newly diagnosed high risk (secondary) AML. *J Clin Oncol* 2016;**34**. 7000–7000.
124. Gabizon A, et al. Prolonged circulation time and enhanced accumulation in malignant exudates of doxorubicin encapsulated in polyethylene-glycol coated liposomes. *Cancer Res* 1994;**54**: 987–92.
125. Gabizon A, Shmeeda H, Barenholz Y. Pharmacokinetics of pegylated liposomal doxorubicin. *Clin Pharmacokinet* 2003;**42**: 419–36.
126. Gill P, et al. Randomized phase III trial of liposomal daunorubicin versus doxorubicin, bleomycin, and vincristine in AIDS-related Kaposi's sarcoma. *J Clin Oncol* 1996;**14**:2353–64.
127. Gradishar WJ, et al. Phase III trial of nanoparticle albumin-bound paclitaxel compared with polyethylated castor oil–based paclitaxel in women with breast cancer. *J Clin Oncol* 2005;**23**:7794–803.
128. Silverman JA, Deitcher SR. Marqibo® (vincristine sulfate liposome injection) improves the pharmacokinetics and pharmacodynamics of vincristine. *Cancer Chemoth Pharm* 2013;**71**:555–64.
129. Jr, F. C., Grapsa D, Syrigos KN, Saif M. The safety and efficacy of Onivyde (irinotecan liposome injection) for the treatment of metastatic pancreatic cancer following gemcitabine-based therapy. *Expert Rev Anticanc* 2016;**16**:697–703.
130. Petersen GH, Alzghari SK, Chee W, Sankari SS, La-Beck NM. Meta-analysis of clinical and preclinical studies comparing the anticancer efficacy of liposomal versus conventional non-liposomal doxorubicin. *J Control Release* 2016;**232**:255–64.
130a Leong HS, Butler KS, Brinker CJ, Azzawi M, Conlan S, Dufès C, Owen A, Rannard S, Scott C, Chen C, Dobrovolskaia MA. On the issue of transparency and reproducibility in nanomedicine. *Nature nanotechnology* 2019;**14**(7):629.
131. Maeda H, Nakamura H, Fang J. The EPR effect for macromolecular drug delivery to solid tumors: improvement of tumor uptake, lowering of systemic toxicity, and distinct tumor imaging in vivo. *Adv Drug Deliver Rev* 2013;**65**:71–9.
132. Ramanathan RK, et al. *Abstract CT224: Pilot Study in Patients With Advanced Solid Tumors to Evaluate Feasibility of Ferumoxytol (FMX) as Tumor Imaging Agent Prior to MM-398, a Nanoliposomal Irinotecan (nal-IRI)*. 2014.
133. Miller MA, Arlauckas S, Weissleder R. Prediction of anti-cancer nanotherapy efficacy by imaging. *Nanotheranostics* 2017;**1**: 296–312.
134. Day C-P, Merlino G, Van Dyke T. Preclinical mouse cancer models: a maze of opportunities and challenges. *Cell* 2015;**163**:39–53.
135. Olson B, Li Y, Lin Y, Liu ET, Patnaik A. Mouse models for cancer immunotherapy research. *Cancer Discov* 2018;**8**:1358–65.
136. Sykes EA, et al. Tailoring nanoparticle designs to target cancer based on tumor pathophysiology. *Proc Natl Acad Sci* 2016;**113.9**:E1142–51.

136a Lazarovits J, Chen YY, Song F, Ngo W, Tavares AJ, Zhang YN, Audet J, Tang B, Lin Q, Tleugabulova MC, Wilhelm S. Synthesis of Patient-Specific Nanomaterials. *Nano letters* 2018;**19**(1):116–23.
137. Syed A, et al. Three-dimensional imaging of transparent tissues via metal nanoparticle labeling. *J Am Chem Soc* 2017;**139**:9961–71.
138. Sindhwani S, Syed A, Wilhelm S, Chan WC. Exploring passive clearing for 3D optical imaging of nanoparticles in intact tissues. *Bioconjugate Chem* 2016;**28**:253–9.
139. Sindhwani S, et al. Three-dimensional optical mapping of nanoparticle distribution in intact tissues. *ACS Nano* 2016;**10**:5468–78.
140. Wilhelm S, Bensen RC, Kothapali NR, Burgett AWG, Merrifield R, Stephan C. Quantification of gold nanoparticle uptake into cancer cells using single cell ICPMS. *PerkinElmer Appl. Note.* 2018:1–4.
140a Donahue ND, Acar H, Wilhelm S. Concepts of nanoparticle cellular uptake, intracellular trafficking, and kinetics in nanomedicine. *Advanced drug delivery reviews* 2019. https://doi.org/10.1016/j.addr.2019.04.008.
141. Wang Z, Tiruppathi C, Cho J, Minshall RD, Malik AB. Delivery of nanoparticle-complexed drugs across the vascular endothelial barrier via caveolae. *IUBMB Life* 2011;**63**:659–67.
142. Wang Z, Tiruppathi C, Minshall RD, Malik AB. Size and dynamics of caveolae studied using nanoparticles in living endothelial cells. *ACS Nano* 2009;**3**:4110–6.
143. Oh P, et al. In vivo proteomic imaging analysis of caveolae reveals pumping system to penetrate solid tumors. *Nat Med* 2014;**20**:1062–8.
144. Ruoslahti E. Tumor penetrating peptides for improved drug delivery. *Adv Drug Deliver Rev* 2017;**110**:3–12.
145. Sugahara KN, et al. Tumor-Penetrating iRGD peptide inhibits metastasis. *Mol Cancer Ther* 2015;**14**:120–8.
146. Sugahara KN, et al. Coadministration of a tumor-penetrating peptide enhances the efficacy of cancer drugs. *Science* 2010;**328**.
147. Dvorak AM, Feng D. The vesiculo–vacuolar organelle (VVO): a new endothelial cell permeability organelle. *J Histochem Cytochem* 2000;**49**:419–31.
148. Dvorak A, et al. The vesiculo-vacuolar organelle (VVO): a distinct endothelial cell structure that provides a transcellular pathway for macromolecular extravasation. *J Leukocyte Biol* 1996;**59**:100–15.
148a Leong HS, Butler KS, Brinker CJ, Azzawi M, Conlan S, Dufès C, Owen A, Rannard S, Scott C, Chen C, Dobrovolskaia MA. On the issue of transparency and reproducibility in nanomedicine. *Nature nanotechnology* 2019;**14**(7):629.
149. Fleischer CC, Payne CK. Nanoparticle–cell interactions: molecular structure of the protein corona and cellular outcomes. *Accounts Chem Res* 2014;**47**:2651–9.
150. Chan WC. Nanomedicine 2.0. *Accounts Chem Res* 2017;**50**:627–32.

Chapter 5

Effects of shape, rigidity, size, and flow on targeting

Hanieh Safari[1], Jonathan Kin-Hun Lee[1] and Omolola Eniola-Adefeso[1,2,3]
[1]Department of Chemical Engineering, University of Michigan, Ann Arbor, MI, United States; [2]Department of Biomedical Engineering, University of Michigan, Ann Arbor, MI, United States; [3]Macromolecular Science and Engineering Program, University of Michigan, Ann Arbor, MI, United States

5.1 Introduction

Targeted drug delivery encompasses a range of approaches that allow for specific, local delivery of an active pharmaceutical ingredient (API) to a diseased tissue with the primary goal of increasing drug efficacy while minimizing systemic side effects.[1] Targeted delivery systems typically utilize particulate carriers with the API loaded within the carrier matrix or core and delivered into the body via injection into the bloodstream. Once in the blood, different factors will interfere with the efficacy of the targeted carriers. These interfering factors include the mononuclear phagocyte system (MPS),[2] plasma proteins,[3] blood shear flow,[4,5] an undesired burst or a delayed release of the API, and the inefficient localization of the particles to the target site.[6,7] Thus, different aspects of the particle design need to be optimized to maximize the functionality of these delivery vehicles. This chapter discusses how the size, shape, and rigidity of the particles can be manipulated to improve their targeting efficacy and how blood flow parameters, e.g., hemodynamics, can be utilized to make each of the discussed systems more efficient.

5.2 Effect of the size and shape on targeting

Two of the most significant design parameters known to dictate the effectiveness of particle carriers in the bloodstream are their size and shape. The size and shape of the particles affect their circulation time,[8,9] the clearance rate of the particles from the body,[2,10] protein corona formation on their surface,[11] margination and binding to the vascular wall,[7,12] drug release profile,[13] and thus, their efficiency in treating the targeted disease.[14] In this section, we discuss the effect of these two parameters on the different aspects of targeting mentioned above.

5.2.1 Effect of the particle size and shape on their immune clearance and circulation time

Upon being introduced into circulation, drug carriers are subjected to clearance from the bloodstream by white blood cells or different organs. The rate of this clearance is dependent on the particle size and shape and also defines the *in vivo* circulation time of the particles in the bloodstream. Depending on the application, an increase or decrease in carrier accumulation in a specific organ and uptake by white blood cells may be desirable and tailoring the particle size and shape can help achieve these goals. Thus, it is crucial to understand how these carrier physical characteristics will affect each of the performance parameters mentioned above. In this section, we summarize the results of numerous studies on the clearance of particles of different sizes by the reticuloendothelial system.

Phagocytosis, cellular eating, of particulate carriers is one of the parameters affected by the size and the shape of the drug carriers. Phagocytosis of particles by granulocytes is a two-step process where the phagocytes first attach to particles and then internalize them.[10] A pioneering study by Champion et al. showed that the size is a significant factor for the attachment of the microspheres to rat alveolar macrophages. Spheres of 2–3 μm diameter were shown to have maximum phagocytosis rate,[10] which is attributed to the enhanced attachment of the particles of this size range to the rat macrophages while the rate of the internalization was not affected by the particle size.[10] In general, different

Nanoparticles for Biomedical Applications. https://doi.org/10.1016/B978-0-12-816662-8.00005-9

studies using macrophages from various species have shown that a specific particle size exists where the phagocytosis of the particles is maximized. This maximum particle size is reported to occur at 1–2 μm for the mouse peritoneal macrophages[15] and at around 1 μm for human monocyte-derived macrophages.[16] The presence of this maximum is attributed to the ruffled surface of the macrophages, where the height of the hemispherical membrane protrusions and the distance between them dictate the optimum size for maximized phagocytosis (Fig. 5.1).[10]

The particle shape is another factor that strongly affects the phagocytosis of the particles. Generally, several studies have demonstrated that elongated particles will have reduced uptake by macrophages. Champion et al. reported for the first time that the uptake of the particles by alveolar macrophages is dependent on their shape and surface curvature. Macrophages were shown not to internalize particles if contacting particles via their flat, low curvature side.[2] The same group reported that worm-like particles with aspect ratios >20 would escape phagocytosis by rat alveolar macrophages (Fig. 5.2).[17] Another study also confirmed that prolate ellipsoids have lower internalization by macrophages despite having a higher attachment rate to these cells.[18] Computer simulations have also confirmed the trend of the reduced phagocytosis of elongated particles, predicting that elongated particles coming into contact with the lipid bilayer of the cells through their lower curvature side will require longer times for translocation.[19] Unfortunately, the bulk of studies studying the effect of particle shape on phagocytosis have focused on experimental assays on macrophages in culture media. Thus, the impact of the size and shape of the particles on their uptake by other phagocyte cells, including neutrophils, remains unclear. A recent report by Kelley et al. demonstrating the effect of particle surface PEGylation on the phagocytosis of targeted particles by primary human neutrophils shows an opposite trend than what was previously observed for macrophages.[20] Thus, it is possible that the reported trend for the particle shape on macrophages may not translate to other phagocytes.

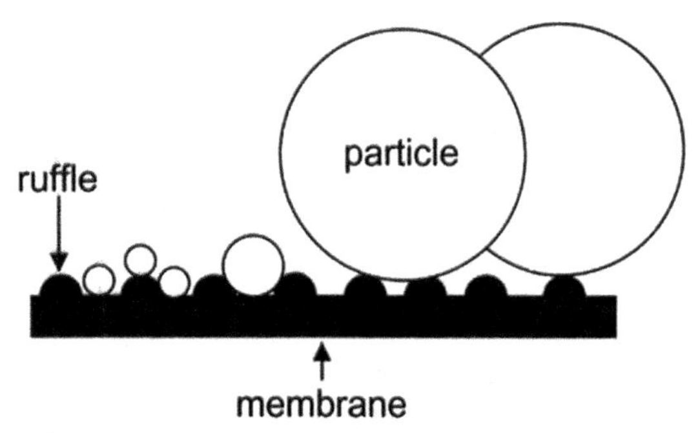

FIGURE 5.1 Schematic of the ruffled structure of macrophages. Midsized particles can make three contact points with the cell membrane compared with the two points for the smaller and larger particles, which enhances their uptake by macrophages.[10]

Biodistribution is yet another *in vivo* parameter of particulate carriers that can be profoundly affected by their size. Liver, spleen, lungs, kidneys, and heart are the primary organs, in which particles are reported to accumulate.[9] The main clearance mechanism in the liver is their uptake by the Kupffer cells, which are the resident macrophages in the liver.[21] As discussed in the previous paragraph, the uptake of nanoparticles by macrophages increases with the increase in their size. Thus, we can conclude that increasing the size of nanoparticles will increase their accumulation in the liver.[22] Indeed, a study of the *in vivo* biodistribution of the mesoporous nanoparticles between the sizes of 80 and 360 nm shows that increasing the particle size increases their accumulation in the liver.[9] In the spleen, filtration is a primary contributor to particle clearance in addition to phagocytosis by macrophages.[21] Particles larger than 200 nm are presumed to be efficiently trapped by spleen filtration.[23] A log–log relationship has been reported for the uptake of particles by the spleen, where increasing their size increases their splenic clearance.[21] For the kidneys, the size of particulate carriers needs to be less than 6 nm to enable renal clearance.[24,25] Interestingly, the observed trend of an increase in entrapment of the particles with increasing particle size is reversed for larger particles in the micrometer size ranges. For example, the percentage of the injected dosage of silica beads in the size range of 700 nm and 3 μm found in different organs decreased with an increase in the particle size in a tumor-bearing mouse model, i.e., a lower number of particles are cleared by the reticuloendothelial system, RES, organs for the larger sizes.[26]

The particle shape also influences the biodistribution of particle carriers in different organs. For example, the use of high aspect ratio particles can help particulate carriers to avoid clearance by the spleen.[23] In this approach, elongated particles with major axis sizes as high as 18 μm can avoid the spleen filtration if their minor axis dimension is kept below the spleen pore size.[27] As discussed above, if the dimensions of the particles are below the kidney filtration limit of 6 nm, they will go through renal clearance. Thus, utilizing nonspherical particles, which have one dimension of larger than the 6 nm cutoff limit, can help to avoid renal clearance of the smaller carriers.[27] As a result of the lower uptake of the high aspect ratio particles by macrophages, increasing their aspect ratio helps decrease their accumulation in the liver as well.[27] In general, we can conclude from different studies that increasing the aspect ratio of the carriers can be a helpful strategy for lowering their uptake by the different RES organs.

Due to the influence of the particle size and shape on the phagocytosis rate and their accumulation in different organs, the circulation time of particulate carriers in blood is

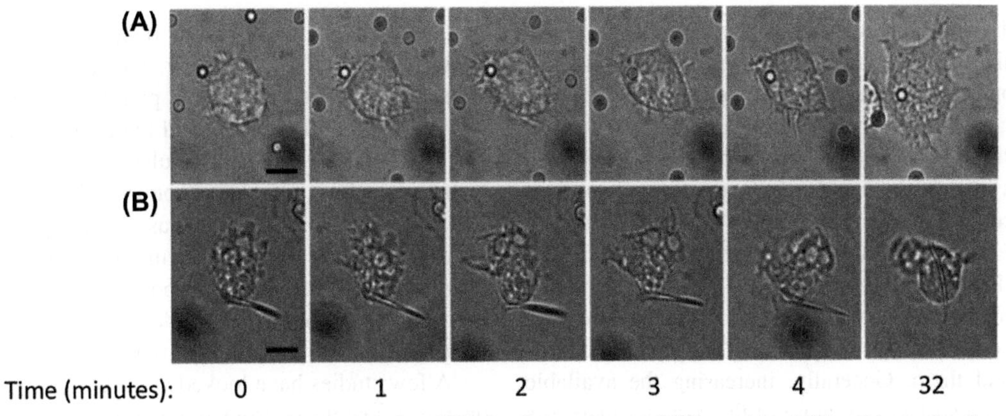

FIGURE 5.2 Time-lapse video microscopy clips at 0, 1, 2, 3, 4, and 32 min after attachment of different shaped PS particles to alveolar macrophages for (A) 3 μm spheres and (B) worms. As it can be seen, macrophages can attach to the side of the worm but would not be able to internalize it.[17]

also a function of their size and shape. Particles should be large enough to avoid renal filtration and small enough to prevent their clearance by RES organs to have extended blood circulation.[28] The spherical size of 10–200 nm has been reported to be the optimum range in this respect.[28] Different studies have also reported longer circulation time of the high aspect ratio particles, including nanorods and filomicelles, which can be concluded that it is due to their lower entrapment in and uptake by RES organs and macrophages, respectively.[8,23,27]

In summary, size and shape affect the circulation time and the tissue/organ accumulation of particulate carriers. Thus, the drug carriers can be custom-designed to either increase or decrease their circulation time or target them to a specific organ of interest.

5.2.2 Effect of the particle size and shape on protein corona formation

Particles rapidly adsorb plasma proteins onto their surface upon coming into contact with blood. This protein adsorption results in the formation of a protein corona around the nano/microparticles, which will modify their physicochemical property and bioavailability and, ultimately, determine the host immune response.[29,30] As a result, different factors that alter the identity of the protein corona on particulate carriers should be carefully studied for improving their efficacy. The quantity and quality of the proteins adsorbed onto a particle surface is a function of their surface curvature and thus is dependent on their size and shape.[31,32] In this section, we focus on explaining the influence of the size and shape of particulate carriers on their protein profile.

Studies with gold nanoparticles have confirmed the reduction in the amount and number of bound proteins on the surface of the nanoparticles with an increase in their size, which is a consequence of the higher surface curvature for the smaller particles.[11] The composition of the protein corona of the gold nanoparticles has also been shown to be size dependent. For example, gold nanoparticles decorated with polyethylene glycol (PEG) were demonstrated to have a lower extent of serum protein adsorption onto their surface with an increase in the particle size.[32] This protein adsorption trend with gold nanoparticle size is an outcome of the higher surface curvature of the smaller nanoparticles, which creates available free space between the PEG chains and lowers the thermodynamic barrier for protein adsorption.[32] When silica nanoparticles were used, the binding affinities of different plasma proteins were found to be dependent on the nanoparticle size. Lipoprotein clustering had increased binding to smaller particles, while prothrombin or the actin regulatory protein gelsolin preferentially bound to larger particles.[30] For polystyrene particles of different sizes and surface charges, it was demonstrated that the presence of a difference in the corona for nanoparticles of different sizes is dependent on their surface charge. Different sized particles did not show any difference in the composition of their corona when they were neutrally charged.[31] However, significant differences were observed in the composition of the protein coronas of negatively and positively charged polystyrene particles of different sizes.[31]

Particle shape has also been reported to alter the plasma protein corona formation on nanoparticles. For titanium dioxide (TiO_2) nanoparticles, the composition of the corona is dependent on their shape. Immunoglobulin M (IgM) and immunoglobulin G (IgG) were among the major bound proteins on nanorods, whereas fibrinogen was the primary protein existing in the corona of the nanotubes.[33] Mesoporous silica nanorods and nanospheres have also been investigated to observe the effect of morphology on the adsorption of albumin, γ-globulin, and fibrinogen proteins on these nanoparticles.[34] This study reported that decreasing the surface curvature of the particles will reduce the initial adsorption rate of the proteins onto their surface. However, this trend is reversed for the proteins that have a rod shape conformation, such as fibrinogen.[34] When *in vivo* protein corona of gold nanorods and nanostars was studied after circulation in rodents, the total amount of the adsorbed proteins was more significant for nanostars because of their larger surface area.[35] The total number of the proteins is a result of the interplay between both the size and the shape of the particles.[35]

In summary, the size and shape of the particles are significant, contributing factors to the protein corona formed around them. Generally, increasing the available surface area and surface curvature of the particles increases the total amount of the proteins adsorbed on the particle surface. However, the composition of the adsorbed proteins as well as the extent and rate of the protein adsorption is a result of the interplay between the size, shape, material composition, the surface charge, and the conformation of the protein of interest and should be studied for different carriers independently.

5.2.3 Effect of the shape and size on the drug release profile

The release profile of the loaded drug from particles is an essential factor that can affect the drug carrier targeting efficacy. Numerous studies have suggested that the release kinetics of particulate carriers is a consequence of their size. However, the effects of the size on the drug release kinetics of carriers are highly dependent on the mechanism, which controls the release kinetics. When we have diffusion-controlled release, which is the dominant mechanism in the initial burst release phase, decreasing the particle size has been shown to increase the drug release rate in different studies.[13] This can be attributed to the increased surface area to volume ratio and, thus, swelling rate for smaller particles leading to a higher diffusion rate of the drug (Fig. 5.3A).[13,36,38,39] However, the release kinetics in the slower degradation-controlled phase is dependent on the particle fabrication process and their internal structure. For particles made by the emulsion–solvent–evaporation technique, which is the most common fabrication technique for polymeric particles, it has been demonstrated that smaller particles will have a more intact inner structure, whereas larger particles look porous inside.[38] Thus, larger particles will exhibit a faster degradation rate and quicker release of the cargo in the degradation-controlled phase.[38]

A few studies have looked at the effect of particle shape on the drug release from polymeric particles. For a fixed total drug loading and size, the particles with a larger surface area to volume ratio will have the fastest release.[40] This result has been confirmed for poly(lactic-co-glycolic acid) (PLGA) particles. For the Nile Red–loaded PLGA particles, rod-shaped carriers had a faster release profile compared with the spheres of the same volume (Fig. 5.3B).[37] Thus, shifting toward the nonspherical shapes and increasing the aspect ratio of particles is a viable approach to increase their drug release rate.

The results of the discussed studies have demonstrated that decreasing the surface area to volume ratio of the micro/nanoparticles will extend their release profile when the diffusion-controlled release mechanism is dominant. However, further investigations are required to fully understand how modifying the size and shape of the particles will change their release profile when other mechanisms control the release of the cargo.

5.2.4 Effect of the size and shape on margination and vascular binding

For vascular targeting applications, particulate carriers need to be able to marginate out of the red blood cell, RBC, core

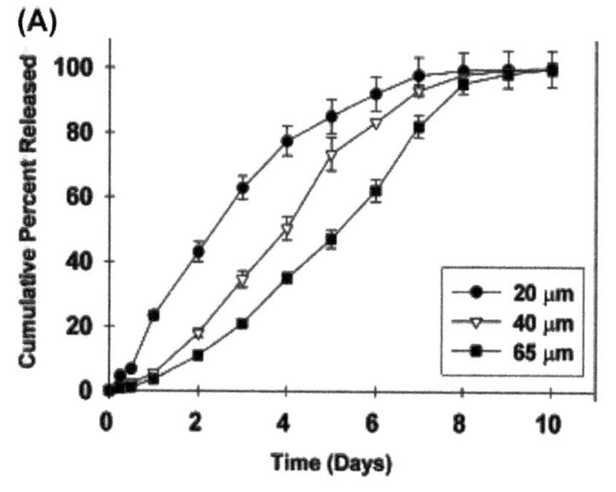

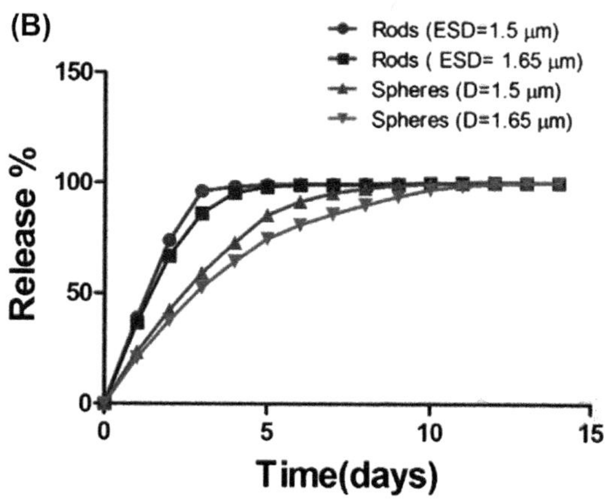

FIGURE 5.3 (A) Effect of particle size on the release profile of poly(lactide-glycolide) (PLG) microspheres.[36] (B) Effect of shape on release profile of poly(lactic-co-glycolic acid) (PLGA) rods and spheres of the same equivalent spherical diameter (ESD).[37] Smaller particles and elongated rod-shaped particles have a faster release due to their increased surface area to volume ratio.

to the cell-free layer near the vascular wall to bind effectively. Different theoretical and experimental studies have shown this margination, and binding is dependent on the size and shape of the particles. This dependence is discussed in this section further.

Several models of blood flow have demonstrated that increasing the size of the particles will improve their margination, and generally, microparticles will have better margination compared with nanoparticles.[41,42] *In vitro* assays using a parallel plate flow chamber have demonstrated that nanospheres have minimum adhesion to inflamed endothelium in human blood. These assays suggest that 2–5 μm particles are the optimum size for targeting the vascular wall (Fig. 5.4).[12] The results have also been confirmed via *in vivo* experiments in $ApoE^{-/-}$-deficient mice, an atherosclerotic murine model, where 2-μm particles show 2.3- to 3.5-fold higher adhesion in different regions of aorta compared with 500-nm particles.[43]

Particle shape is also another major contributor to the margination and adhesion trend of particulate carriers. Simulation studies modeling blood flow have shown that despite having similar or lower margination, ellipsoidal particles will have improved adhesion to the vascular wall due to their slower rotational dynamics near the wall,[41,42] which has also been confirmed in different experimental studies. *In vitro* experiments using a parallel plate flow chamber have demonstrated that increasing the aspect ratio of the microparticles increases their adhesion to the human umbilical vein endothelial cells (HUVECs) in shear flow. This increase in adhesion with a higher particle aspect ratio is more pronounced for larger particles. However, for nanoparticles, no significant difference is observed between particles of different aspect ratios.[7] Follow-up confocal studies show that despite having increased binding, rod localization to the cell-free layer remains the same as that of spheres.[7] Thus, the observed increased adhesion of the rods can be attributed to their increased contact area with the wall, having a higher total number of targeting ligands when the ligand density is fixed, and reduced drag forces acting to detach them from the wall.[7] These results were confirmed by *in vivo* experiments validating the increased adhesion of microrods compared with the spheres of the same volume in inflamed mouse aortae, whereas nanorods and nanospheres did not show any significant difference in their adhesion (Fig. 5.5).[44]

To summarize, different *in vitro* and *in vivo* studies have verified the margination, and binding of microparticles is higher than nanoparticles and it is maximized at diameters of around 2–5 μm. Thus, changing the particle shape can be a useful strategy to improve the binding of the particles, especially larger particles and higher aspect ratios.

5.2.5 Effect of the size and shape on the uptake of the particles by tumor cells

Cancer has been one of the leading causes of death worldwide, and the delivery of therapeutics to tumor tissue remains a fundamental challenge in the field. Thus, one of the main areas of focus for the usage of drug carrier particles is in the treatment of cancer. For a carrier to have a therapeutic effect on the tumor lesions, it must penetrate deep into the tumor tissue. In this section, we will discuss how the modification of the size and shape of the particles will influence their efficiency for the treatment of tumors.

Many research groups have explored two principal mechanisms for explaining the concept of particle uptake in tumors. The first approach is passive targeting, involving the usage of the enhanced permeation and retention (EPR) effect. The gap between the endothelial cells of tumor blood vessels leads to increased permeability of tumor

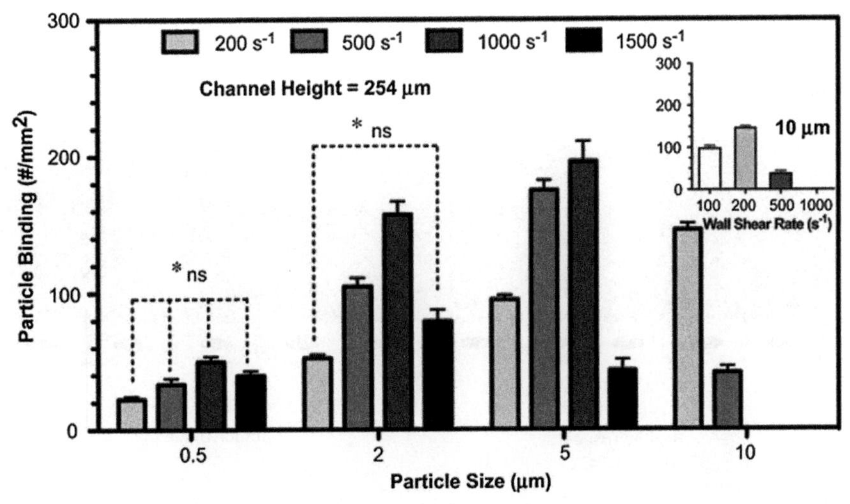

FIGURE 5.4 *In vitro* binding of particles of different sizes in parallel plate flow chamber at different shear rates. As represented, 2–5 μm particles have maximum binding in different shear rates.[12]

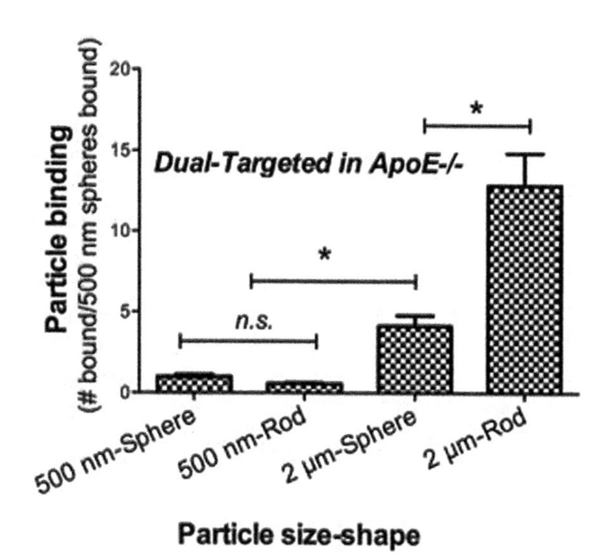

FIGURE 5.5 Binding of targeted rods and spheres of different sizes to the ApoE$^{-/-}$ mouse aorta.[44] As it can be seen, the binding is significantly higher for microrods compared with spheres of the same size.

vasculature in comparison with normal tissues. This change in the microenvironment makes the supply of oxygen and nutrition to tumor tissue possible. This leaky tumor vasculature has been utilized as a strategy to deliver drugs and therapeutics to tumors (Fig. 5.6).[45] The other approach, active targeting, involves conjugating targeting ligands on the surface of the nanoparticles, which allows binding to the specific receptors expressed on the surface of the tumor cells. The targeted carriers then deliver their drug cargo after binding to the tumor tissue. There are two dominant mechanisms in this regard for tumor targeting. Particles can bind to the receptors expressed on the surface of the cells with receptor-mediated endocytosis, and they can then penetrate deeper into the tissue via transcytosis pathways.[46]

Particulate carriers need to be in the nanosized range to take advantage of the EPR effect. It is believed that particles in the 10–200 nm spherical size range can be used to penetrate and accumulate in the tumor tissue via the leaky vasculature.[14] Thus, size is an important parameter that needs to be considered when designing nanoparticles for tumor targeting. He et al. used polymeric nanoparticles grafted with carboxymethyl chitosan to study the tumor uptake of the nanoparticles in H-22 tumor-bearing mice. Their results showed that decreasing the size of the nanoparticles increases their distribution in tumor tissue.[22] Another study used hyaluronic acid (HA) nanoparticles for targeting receptors in tumor-bearing mice. *In vivo* fluorescent imaging of the animal and *ex vivo* NIR imaging after organ removal both confirmed that the decrease in the size of the nanoparticles would increase their accumulation in tumor tissue.[47] Multistage delivery systems can be used to design particles, which are not only able to avoid the renal clearance but also capable of penetrating deep into the tumor tissue. With this consideration in mind, Wong and coworkers have developed a multistage nanodelivery system that changes size in different stages of tumor targeting. Initially, 100 nm particles pass through the leaky tumor regions by utilizing the EPR effect. Then, the particles shrink to 10 nm, allowing for penetration into dense tumor vasculature, which is not achievable by larger particles. *In vitro* experiments utilizing activation of MMP-2, a protease highly expressed in the tumor microenvironment, for degrading particles have shown that this system can penetrate deep into tumor tissues.[48]

Particle shape is again another design parameter that can affect the uptake of the particles by cancerous cells and their accumulation in the tumor tissue. It has been reported that mesoporous silica nanorods will be taken up at a greater extent by HeLa cells compared with spheres. The maximum uptake

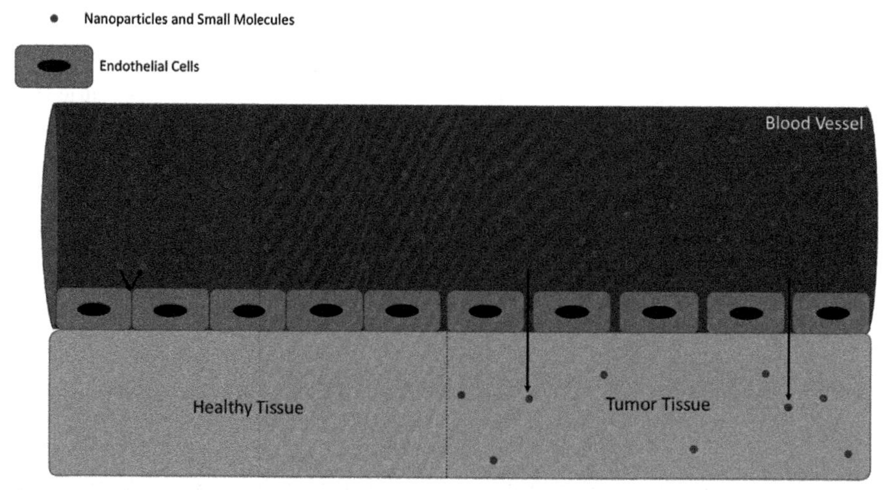

FIGURE 5.6 Schematic representation of the enhanced permeation and retention (EPR) effect. Nanoparticles and small molecules can accumulate in the tumor site through the leaky vasculature.

was observed for the aspect ratio of ~2.1–2.5 and had the highest cytotoxic efficiency for delivering chemotherapy agents.[49] Studying uptake of the differently shaped particles using human melanoma cells has also demonstrated that increasing the aspect ratio of the particles will increase their internalization rate and extent, leading to a higher impact on cellular function.[50] A similar impact of the aspect ratio of particles has been reported for HeLa Cells.[51] It is noteworthy that the reported effects of particle aspect ratio on particle internalization by cancer cells are the opposite of the trend observed for particle uptake by phagocytic cells, where increasing their aspect ratio lowers their uptake by macrophages.[2] The prolonged circulation of the elongated particles combined with their drift to the vessel wall has also been reported in several studies to increase their accumulation in the tumor site presumably via the EPR effect.[8,51] It is also said that utilizing nonspherical particles will enhance the specific accumulation and lower the nonspecific binding to the target site of the diseased tumor endothelium as well as more significant inhibition of the cancerous cell growth.[52,53]

To summarize, when considering targeting tumor tissues for the treatment of different cancers, particle size and shape are parameters that need to be carefully studied to design the most efficient delivery system. We need to find the optimum size and shape of the particles, which can efficiently localize and penetrate deep into the tissue while being able to avoid immune clearance.

5.3 Effect of the carrier rigidity on targeting

While size and shape are well-established design parameters for targeted drug carriers, particle modulus has only recently been investigated as a potential physical parameter for facilitating targeted drug delivery processes.[54] With advancements in particle fabrication methods, different types of materials have been used to vary particle modulus, such as hydrogels made of materials such as PEG, polyacrylamide, and lipid shell PLGA.[55–58]

One of the factors that affects the targeting efficacy of particles is their collisions with RBCs. RBCs, with a modulus of approximately 26 kPa, tend to localize in the center of blood vessels.[59] Conversely, white blood cells (WBCs) and platelets, with moduli of two to five times that of RBCs, tend to localize near the endothelium in the RBC-free layer.[60,61] Thus, targeted particles with varying modulus are presumed to exhibit similar margination behavior. Indeed, simulations of rigid and deformable carriers indicate that at low shear rates, both types of particles have nearly the same propensity for margination, with deformable particles slightly outperforming their rigid counterparts.[62] However, they also show that this trend reverses at higher shear, where the rigid particles marginate better than the soft ones. This phenomenon is attributed to the increased deformation of the soft particles, which leads to an increase in lift force that drives a particle away from the wall, consistent with RBC behavior.

Experiments performed with 2 μm PEG hydrogel particles corroborate findings by the study as mentioned above. Here, targeted PEG particles with moduli varying from 23 to 500 kPa in whole blood were perfused over activated HUVEC in a flow chamber.[58] Their ability to bind to an activated endothelium was evaluated *in vitro* and *in vivo*. It was found that particles with lower moduli bound more effectively to the endothelium than stiffer particles at low shear rates. As the shear rate increased, the more rigid particles outperformed the soft particles by about two to threefold. These findings indicate that for targeted particles, the modulus must be considered in the ability of particle carriers to marginate to the endothelium to effectively deliver therapeutics to the tissue of interest.

Particle modulus has also been associated with cellular uptake. In a different study, core–shell nanoparticles were fabricated with a PLGA core and a lipid shell.[55] Two types of particles were manufactured, a stiffer particle with a core and shell (P-L NPs), and a softer particle with a layer of water in between (P-W-L NPs). When incubated with HeLa cells, the stiffer P-L NPs were found to be more readily internalized than their soft counterparts. Molecular dynamics (MD) simulations of these particles revealed that as a cellular membrane wraps around a particle, softer particles can deform into an ellipsoidal shape, whereas stiffer particles retain their spherical shape. The energy required for a membrane to wrap around an ellipsoidal particle was found to be about 30% higher than for a spherical particle. A similar study using monolayer and bilayer lipid–polymer hybrid particles found that in a cervical carcinoma xenograft model, the stiffer monolayer particles reduced tumor size to a greater extent than the bilayer particles due to enhanced uptake by cancer cells.[56] Thus, the increase in uptake can be partly attributed to the energetically favorable shape of a rigid particle for cellular internalization.

However, this increased propensity for cellular internalization can also lead to increased removal by macrophages. Indeed, uptake studies have shown that stiffer particles are taken up at a higher rate than deformable ones.[63,64] This increased uptake leads to a decrease in circulation time of targeted particles, which reduces the targeting efficiency. Particles that are quickly cleared from the body have fewer opportunities to bind to the targeted tissue than those that can circulate the body for longer times. While rigid particles were found to bind to an inflamed endothelium at higher efficiencies than deformable particles, this trend was reversed when particles were injected in vivo in a murine model.[58] It was found that more deformable particles adhered to an inflamed mouse mesentery than rigid particles, attributed to the longer circulation time of the deformable particles, and conversely, the faster clearance time of the rigid particles (Fig. 5.7).

However, there have been some studies that contradict this trend of increased uptake with increasing particle rigidity. In a study using particles fabricated from diethyl acrylate (DEA) and 2-hydroxyethyl methacrylate (HEMA), it was found that macrophage uptake of these DEA-HEMA particles was not, in fact, highest for the most rigid particles.[57] Instead, particles with intermediate moduli were taken up at a higher rate than at either extreme. These differences in uptake are associated with the different mechanisms by which they enter the cell. Softer particles are primarily taken up via clathrate-mediated endocytosis; conversely, rigid particles are taken up via micropinocytosis and phagocytosis. Particles of intermediate modulus are more likely to be internalized due to their ability to participate in both mechanisms.

Particle modulus is an important physical parameter to consider in the context of targeted drug carriers, but its effects on targeting efficiency have yet to be thoroughly characterized. However, based on work done thus far, there are competing factors to mediate. Increased rigidity (18–211 kPa) tends to enhance margination and uptake by relevant tissue cells, including endothelial and cancer cells. However, this increased uptake extends to macrophages, decreasing circulation time and reducing opportunities for particles to localize and bind to their target. It has typically been seen that softer particles have a longer circulation time than rigid particles. Some studies, however, have found that intermediate moduli, between very soft and stiff particles, are more likely to be taken up by macrophages. Such nuances in the effects of modulus on particle targeting need to be further explored to understand and optimize drug carrier design for efficient targeting fully.

5.4 Effect of flow on targeting

Once injected, particles will need to navigate through the bloodstream and bind to the vascular wall or extravasate into different tissues. The blood flow regime and the shear rate are dependent on the blood vessel of interest, including capillaries, small venules, and arteries.[65,66] Thus, different studies have investigated how this difference in flow pattern will contribute to the targeting characteristics of the drug carriers.

For vascular-targeted particles, it has been demonstrated that the adhesion of microparticles to endothelial cells in a flow chamber will increase with increasing wall shear rate (WSR) up to a critical wall shear rate WSR_{crit}. Beyond this critical level, the adhesion level reduces with increasing WSR. The magnitude of the WSR_{crit} decreases with increasing particle size.[12] This drop in the adhesion level beyond the critical shear rate has been attributed to the detaching hemodynamic forces.[12] The improvement in the particle adhesion with increasing the shear rate below WSR_{crit} is the consequence of the increase in particle flux when the shear rate is raised.[12] It has also been reported that the rolling velocity of the targeted microspheres will increase at higher wall shear rates,[67] which can translate to lower adhesion probability in high shears when the total particle flux is fixed. This shear-enhanced binding behavior of the nanoparticles has been validated by simulation studies as well. Simulations have shown that shear force will decrease the free energy of the system until reaching a threshold shear value beyond which the free energy will increase with raising the shear. This result translates to a biphasic binding behavior where increasing the shear will increase the endothelial binding of the particles up to the point of the threshold shear after which the binding will decrease with increasing shear force.[68] The results of this

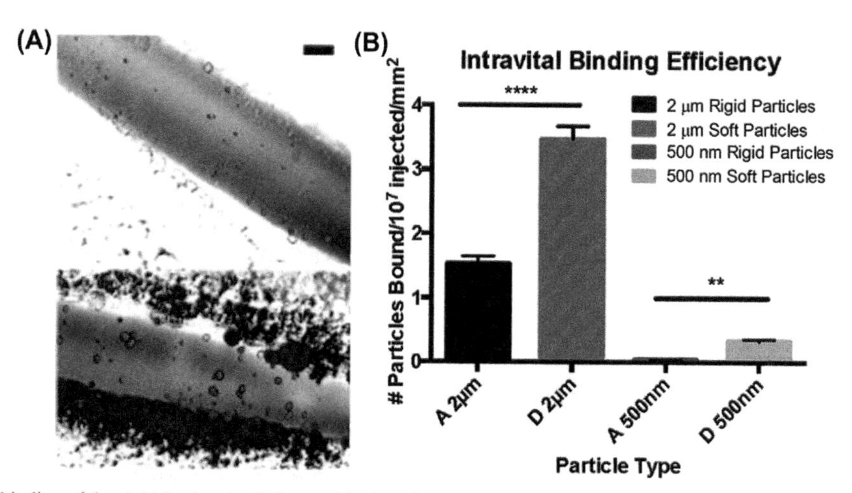

FIGURE 5.7 (A) The binding of the rigid (top) and soft (bottom) hydrogels to the inflamed mouse mesentery. (B) Quantified binding of the rigid (A) and soft (D) particles to the mouse mesentery.[58]

study show the agreement between the computational and experimental studies. When particle adhesion in disturbed flow was tested, microspheres bound at a higher level in pulsatile flow compared with laminar flow at the same shear rate. However, the observed trend of the adhesion level as a function of particle size in pulsatile flow has been the same as the trend observed in laminar flow.[12]

Another parameter that can be affected by the exposure of the cells to flow is the expression level of the inflammatory markers by the activated endothelial cells. Interleukin 1 beta (IL-1β)—induced E-selectin expression by endothelial cells has been shown to be enhanced by laminar shear compared with static conditions.[69] The peak expression time point is also extended by exposure of the cells to shear. The leukocyte binding levels were also improved when the endothelial cells are activated in presence of shear.[69] However, when the cells were activated with tumor necrosis factor alpha (TNFα), shear-enhanced E-selectin expression was observed only for intermediate timepoints.[70] While shear preconditioning has been reported to enhance the expression levels of E-selectin with shear-IL-1 β activation,[69] it has been reported to downregulate the expression level when activation was induced by TNFα.[70] In addition, the expression of some genes on the surface of the endothelial cells has been shown to be affected by their exposure to shear flow. Studies have demonstrated that the expression of the genes involved in endothelial cell survival, angiogenesis, and vascular remodeling is upregulated in endothelial cells by their exposure to laminar flow while the expression of the proinflammatory and prothrombotic genes is downregulated as a consequence.[71] The results of different studies suggest that exposure to the shear stress will change the expression level of different inflammatory markers and genes on the endothelial cells. However, the upregulation or downregulation of these markers is dependent on the signaling pathway involved and has to be studied independently for each of these markers.

Another consequence of the exposure to shear flow is its impact on the uptake of the nanocarriers by endothelial cells. The bulk of studies of the impact of particle size and shape on phagocytosis and endocytosis have been under static conditions, which does not account for the shear environment of blood flow. The endocytosis of the nanocarriers (NCs) coated by antibodies (Abs) to cell adhesion molecules is impacted by the flow. Generally, the internalization of the Abs/NCs with a restricted range of avidity to endothelial cells is stimulated by exposure to laminar flow compared with static conditions.[72] Similarly, it has also been demonstrated that the uptake of the quantum dots (QDs) and functionalized gold nanoparticles by endothelial cells will be significantly elevated by exposure to shear.[4,73] Interestingly enough, the shear stress has been shown to reduce the nonspecific uptake of the gold nanoparticles under flow conditions when the endothelial cells are exposed to unfunctionalized nanoparticles.[4] These results demonstrate that the increased uptake of the targeted nanoparticles in the presence of flow is probably a consequence of their altered interaction with the inflammatory receptors on the surface of the activated cells. It has been hypothesized that the increased internalization of the nanoparticles under shear stress can be attributed to either engagement of the higher number of the endocytic receptors on the surface of the cells by rolling of the carrier or enhanced mechanical stimulus on the cells.[74]

The elevated shear stress at diseased sites with abnormalities such as stenotic sites can be used for specific delivery of the drugs to the target site. Particles can be custom-designed and used for shear-activated targeting to release their drug cargo only under the elevated shear of the target site.[75] Liposomes, extracellular vesicles including exosomes, nanoemulsions, microcapsules, and hydrogels are the typical types of particles that can be used as shear-sensitive drug carriers.[75]

To summarize, the findings of different studies have demonstrated that flow and blood hemodynamics can be a major contributor to the performance of targeted carriers. As discussed in the paragraphs above, the expression level of the inflammatory markers on the surface of the endothelial cells, internalization, and adhesion level of the carriers to the vascular wall cells will all be impacted by the presence of shear force. Thus, the flow component on the performance of drug carriers should be carefully studied when designing a drug carrier. In addition, shear force can also be used as a trigger for the local release of drug cargo in the diseased site by designing shear-sensitive drug carriers.

5.5 Summary

In this chapter, we expanded our knowledge of how particle design parameters such as size, shape, and rigidity will affect their performance as drug carriers and how this performance is affected by the presence of blood flow. We learned how particle size and shape would impact the phagocytosis rate and clearance of the particles by each of the RES organs and their circulation time. We understood how modifying the size and the shape of the particles will change their protein corona and drug release profile, their margination, and adhesion to the vascular wall, and their efficiency in treating tumor lesions. Next, we looked upon the rigidity to see how changing the moduli of the particles will change each of the mentioned parameters. The last section was about understanding the blood flow and hemodynamics and its impact on targeting. We discussed how the presence of the wall shear rate will change the adhesion profile of particles, expression levels of different markers on their surface, their internalization by cells, and their release characteristics. To design a drug carrier for clinical applications, all of the aforementioned parameters need to be carefully considered to maximize the efficiency of the carrier system in the treatment of the disease model of interest.

The field of targeted drug delivery is expanding quickly, and new particulate delivery systems are being designed every day. However, there remain challenges restricting their efficacy and transition into clinics. For instance, the effects of a physical parameter on different stages of carrier targeting can be counterproductive to each other. For these purposes, the development of novel particle types such as two-stage delivery systems can be a solution. Furthermore, computational models can be helpful to predict the optimum range of size, shape, and rigidity. Importantly, the effects of the different design parameters on the functionality of particulate carriers should be explicitly studied for each disease model, as the target site significantly determines the desired size, shape, and modulus of the carriers. Besides, when designing the particles, it should be considered that for many cases, in vivo data obtained in animal models may not entirely reflect and predict the results in clinical settings. This can be a consequence of the differences in the composition blood, and anatomy of humans and mice, the most common laboratory animal, or the fact that many of the patients might be suffering from more than one disorder simultaneously, which complicates the performance of therapeutic carriers. Despite all these challenges, particulate targeted delivery systems are a promising approach and have the potential to improve the treatment status of different disorders, including cancer and cardiovascular disease.

References

1. Singh R, Lillard Jr JW. Nanoparticle-based targeted drug delivery. *Exp Mol Pathol* 2009;**86**:215–23. https://doi.org/10.1016/j.yexmp.2008.12.004.
2. Champion JA, Mitragotri S. Role of target geometry in phagocytosis. *Proc Natl Acad Sci* 2006;**103**(13):4930–4. https://doi.org/10.1073/pnas.0600997103.
3. Namdee K, Sobczynski DJ, Onyskiw PJ, Eniola-adefeso O. Differential impact of plasma proteins on the adhesion efficiency of vascular-targeted carriers (VTCs) in blood of common laboratory animals. *Bioconjugate Chem* 2015;**26**:2419–28. https://doi.org/10.1021/acs.bioconjchem.5b00474.
4. Klingberg H, Loft S, Oddershede LB, Møller P. The influence of flow, shear stress and adhesion molecule targeting on gold nanoparticle uptake in human endothelial cells. *Nanoscale* 2015;**7**(26):11409–19. https://doi.org/10.1039/c5nr01467k.
5. Doshi N, Prabhakarpandian B, Rea-ramsey A, Pant K, Sundaram S, Mitragotri S. Flow and adhesion of drug carriers in blood vessels depend on their shape : a study using model synthetic microvascular networks. *J Control Release* 2010;**146**:196–200. https://doi.org/10.1016/j.jconrel.2010.04.007.
6. Maeda H, Nakamura H, Fang J. The EPR effect for macromolecular drug delivery to solid tumors: improvement of tumor uptake, lowering of systemic toxicity, and distinct tumor imaging in vivo. *Adv Drug Deliv Rev* 2013;**65**:71–9. https://doi.org/10.1016/j.addr.2012.10.002.
7. Thompson AJ, Mastria EM, Eniola-Adefeso O. The margination propensity of ellipsoidal micro/nanoparticles to the endothelium in human blood flow. *Biomaterials* 2013;**34**:5863–71. https://doi.org/10.1016/j.biomaterials.2013.04.011.
8. Janát-amsbury MM, Ray A, Peterson CM, Ghandehari H. Geometry and surface characteristics of gold nanoparticles influence their biodistribution and uptake by macrophages. *Eur J Pharm Biopharm* 2011;**77**(3):417–23. https://doi.org/10.1016/j.ejpb.2010.11.010.
9. He Q, Zhang Z, Gao F, Li Y, Shi J. In vivo biodistribution and urinary excretion of mesoporous silica nanoparticles : effects of particle size and PEGylation. *Small* 2011;**7**(2):271–80. https://doi.org/10.1002/smll.201001459.
10. Champion JA, Walker A, Mitragotri S. Role of particle size in phagocytosis of polymeric microspheres. *Pharm Res* 2008;**25**(8):1815–21. https://doi.org/10.1007/s11095-008-9562-y.
11. Schäffler M, Semmler-Behnke M, Sarioglu H, Takenaka S, Wenk A, Schleh C, et al. Serum protein identification and quantification of the corona of 5, 15 and 80 nm gold nanoparticles. *Nanotechnology* 2013;**24**. https://doi.org/10.1088/0957-4484/24/26/265103.
12. Charoenphol P, Huang RB, Eniola-Adefeso O. Potential role of size and hemodynamics in the efficacy of vascular-targeted spherical drug carriers. *Biomaterials* 2010;**31**(6):1392–402. https://doi.org/10.1016/j.biomaterials.2009.11.007.
13. Golomb G, Fisher P, Rahamim E. The relationship between drug release rate, particle size and swelling of silicone matrices. *J Control Release* 1990;**12**:121–32.
14. Kobayashi H, Watanabe R, Choyke PL. Improving conventional enhanced permeability and retention (EPR) Effects ; what is the appropriate target ? *Theranostics* 2014;**4**(1). https://doi.org/10.7150/thno.7193.
15. Tabata Y, Ikada Y. Effect of the size and surface charge of polymer microspheres on their phagocytosis by macrophage. *Biomaterials* 1988;**9**:356–62.
16. Chikaura H, Nakashima Y, Fujiwara Y, Komohara Y, Takeya M, Nakanishi Y. Effect of particle size on biological response by human monocyte-derived macrophages. *Biosur Biotribol* 2016;**2**(1):18–25. https://doi.org/10.1016/j.bsbt.2016.02.003.
17. Champion JA, Mitragotri S. Shape induced inhibition of phagocytosis of polymer particles. *Pharm Res* 2009;**26**(1):244–9. https://doi.org/10.1007/s11095-008-9626-z.
18. Sharma G, Valenta DT, Altman Y, et al. Polymer particle shape independently influences binding and internalization by macrophages. *J Control Release* 2010;**147**(3):408–12. https://doi.org/10.1016/j.jconrel.2010.07.116.
19. Yang K, Ma YQ. Computer simulation of the translocation of nanoparticles with different shapes across a lipid bilayer. *Nat Nanotechnol* 2010;**5**:579. https://doi.org/10.1038/nnano.2010.141.
20. Kelley WJ, Fromen CA, Lopez-cazares G, Eniola-adefeso O. PEGylation of model drug carriers enhances phagocytosis by primary human neutrophils. *Acta Biomater* 2018;**79**:283–93. https://doi.org/10.1016/j.actbio.2018.09.001.
21. Moghimi SM, Porter CJH, Muir IS, Illum L, Davis SS. Non-phagocytic uptake of intravenously injected microspheres in rat spleen : influence of particle size and hydrophilic coating. *Biochem Biophys Res Commun* 1991;**177**(2):861–6.

22. He C, Hu Y, Yin L, Tang C, Yin C. Effects of particle size and surface charge on cellular uptake and biodistribution of polymeric nanoparticles. *Biomaterials* 2010;**31**(13):3657–66. https://doi.org/10.1016/j.biomaterials.2010.01.065.
23. Fish MB, Thompson AJ, Fromen CA, Eniola-adefeso O. Emergence and utility of nonspherical particles in biomedicine. *Ind Eng Chem Res* 2015;**54**:4043–59. https://doi.org/10.1021/ie504452j.
24. Longmire M, Choyke PL, Kobayashi H. Clearance properties of nano-sized particles and molecules as imaging agents : considerations and caveats. *Nanomedicine* 2008;**3**(5):703–17.
25. Hirn S, Semmler-behnke M, Schleh C, et al. Particle size-dependent and surface charge-dependent biodistribution of gold nanoparticles after intravenous administration. *Eur J Pharm Biopharm* 2011;**77**(3):407–16. https://doi.org/10.1016/j.ejpb.2010.12.029.
26. Decuzzi P, Godin B, Tanaka T, et al. Size and shape effects in the biodistribution of intravascularly injected particles. *J Control Release* 2010;**141**(3):320–7. https://doi.org/10.1016/j.jconrel.2009.10.014.
27. Geng YAN, Dalhaimer P, Cai S, et al. Shape effects of filaments versus spherical particles in flow and drug delivery. *Nat Nanotechnol* 2007;**2**(4):249–55. https://doi.org/10.1038/nnano.2007.70.
28. Yoo JW, Chambers E, Mitragotri S. Factors that control the circulation time of nanoparticles in blood : challenges, solutions and future prospects. *Curr Pharm Des* 2010;**16**:2298–307.
29. Maiolo D, Del Pino P, Metrangolo P, Parak WJ, Baldelli Bombelli F. Nanomedicine delivery: does protein corona route to the target or off road? *Nanomedicine* 2015;**10**(21):3231–47.
30. Tenzer S, Docter D, Rosfa S, et al. Nanoparticle size is a critical physicochemical determinant of the human blood plasma corona: a comprehensive quantitative proteomic analysis. *ACS Nano* 2011;**5**(9):7155–67. https://doi.org/10.1021/nn201950e.
31. Lundqvist M, Stigler J, Elia G, Lynch I, Cedervall T, Dawson KA. Nanoparticle size and surface properties determine the protein corona with possible implications for biological impacts. *Proc Natl Acad Sci* 2008;**105**(38):14265–70. https://doi.org/10.1073/pnas.0805135105.
32. Walkey CD, Olsen JB, Guo H, Emili A, Chan WC. Nanoparticle size and surface chemistry determine serum protein adsorption and macrophage uptake. *J Am Chem Soc* 2012;**134**:2139–47. https://doi.org/10.1021/ja2084338.
33. Deng ZJ, Mortimer G, Schiller T, Musumeci A, Martin D, Minchin RF. Differential plasma protein binding to metal oxide nanoparticles. *Nanotechnology* 2009;**20**:455101. https://doi.org/10.1088/0957-4484/20/45/455101.
34. Ma Z, Bai J, Wang Y, Jiang X. Impact of shape and pore size of mesoporous silica nanoparticles on serum protein adsorption and RBCs hemolysis. *ACS Appl Mater Interfaces* 2014;**6**:2431–8.
35. García-álvarez R, Hadjidemetriou M, Sánchez-iglesias A, Liz-marzán LM, Kostarelos K. In vivo formation of protein corona on gold nanoparticles. The effect of their size and shape. *Nanoscale* 2018;**10**:1256–64. https://doi.org/10.1039/c7nr08322j.
36. Berkland C, King M, Cox A, Kim KK, Pack DW. Precise control of PLG microsphere size provides enhanced control of drug release rate. *J Control Release* 2002;**82**:137–47.
37. Safari H, Adili R, Holinstat M, Eniola-Adefeso O. Modified two-step emulsion solvent evaporation technique for fabricating biodegradable rod-shaped particles in the submicron size range. *J Colloid Interface Sci* 2018;**518**:174–83. https://doi.org/10.1016/j.jcis.2018.02.030.
38. Lin X, Yang H, Su L, Yang Z, Tang X. Effect of size on the in vitro/in vivo drug release and degradation of exenatide-loaded PLGA microspheres. *J Drug Deliv Sci Technol* 2018;**45**:346–56. https://doi.org/10.1016/j.jddst.2018.03.024.
39. Chen W, Palazzo A, Hennink WE, Kok RJ. Effect of particle size on drug loading and release kinetics of gefitinib-loaded PLGA microspheres. *Mol Pharm* 2017;**14**:459–67. https://doi.org/10.1021/acs.molpharmaceut.6b00896.
40. Fattahi P, Borhan A, Abidian MR. Microencapsulation of chemotherapeutics into monodisperse and tunable biodegradable polymers via electrified liquid jets: control of size, shape, and drug release. *Adv Mater* 2013;**25**:4555–60. https://doi.org/10.1002/adma.201301033.
41. Müller K, Fedosov DA, Gompper G. Margination of micro- and nano-particles in blood flow and its effect on drug delivery. *Sci Rep* 2014;**4**:4871. https://doi.org/10.1038/srep04871.
42. Cooley M, Sarode A, Hoore M, Fedosov DA, Mitragotri S, Gupta AS. Influence of particle size and shape on their margination and wall-adhesion: implications in drug delivery vehicle design across nano-to-micro scale. *Nanoscale* 2018;**10**(32):15350–64. https://doi.org/10.1039/C8NR04042G.
43. Charoenphol P, Mocherla S, Bouis D, Namdee K, Pinsky DJ, Eniola-Adefeso O. Targeting therapeutics to the vascular wall in atherosclerosis-carrier size matters. *Atherosclerosis* 2011;**217**(2):364–70.
44. Namdee K, Thompson AJ, Golinski A, Mocherla S, Bouis D, Eniola-Adefeso O. In vivo evaluation of vascular-targeted spheroidal microparticles for imaging and drug delivery application in atherosclerosis. *Atherosclerosis* 2014;**237**(1):279–86. https://doi.org/10.1016/j.atherosclerosis.2014.09.025.
45. Fang J, Nakamura H, Maeda H. The EPR effect: unique features of tumor blood vessels for drug delivery, factors involved, and limitations and augmentation of the effect. *Adv Drug Deliv Rev* 2011;**63**(3):136–51. https://doi.org/10.1016/j.addr.2010.04.009.
46. Danhier F, Feron O, Préat V. To exploit the tumor microenvironment: passive and active tumor targeting of nanocarriers for anti-cancer drug delivery. *J Control Release* 2010;**148**:135–46. https://doi.org/10.1016/j.jconrel.2010.08.027.
47. Choi KY, Chung H, Min KH, et al. Self-assembled hyaluronic acid nanoparticles for active tumor targeting. *Biomaterials* 2010;**31**(1):106–14. https://doi.org/10.1016/j.biomaterials.2009.09.030.
48. Wong C, Stylianopoulos T, Cui J, et al. Multistage nanoparticle delivery system for deep penetration into tumor tissue. *Proc Natl Acad Sci* 2011;**108**(6):2426–31. https://doi.org/10.1073/pnas.1103909108.
49. Meng H, Yang S, Li Z, et al. Aspect ratio determines the quantity of mesoporous silica nanoparticle uptake by a small GTPase-dependent macropinocytosis mechanism. *ACS Nano* 2011;**5**(6):4434–47. https://doi.org/10.1021/nn103344k.
50. Huang X, Teng X, Chen D, Tang F, He J. The effect of the shape of mesoporous silica nanoparticles on cellular uptake and cell function. *Biomaterials* 2010;**31**(3):438–48. https://doi.org/10.1016/j.biomaterials.2009.09.060.
51. Venkataraman S, Hedrick JL, Ong YZ, et al. The effects of polymeric nanostructure shape on drug delivery. *Adv Drug Deliv Rev* 2011;**63**(14–15):1228–46. https://doi.org/10.1016/j.addr.2011.06.016.
52. Kolhar P, Anselmo AC, Gupta V, et al. Using shape effects to target antibody-coated nanoparticles to lung and brain endothelium. *Proc Natl Acad Sci* 2013;**110**(26):10753–8. http://www.pnas.org/content/110/26/10753.short.
53. Barua S, Yoo JW, Kolhar P, Wakankar A, Gokarn YR, Mitragotri S. Particle shape enhances specificity of antibody-displaying

nanoparticles. *Proc Natl Acad Sci* 2013;**110**(9):3270–5. https://doi.org/10.1073/pnas.1216893110/-/DCSupplemental. www.pnas.org/cgi/doi/10.1073/pnas.1216893110.
54. Anselmo AC, Mitragotri S. Impact of particle elasticity on particle-based drug delivery systems. *Adv Drug Deliv Rev* 2017;**108**:51–67. https://doi.org/10.1016/j.addr.2016.01.007.
55. Sun J, Zhang L, Wang J, et al. Tunable rigidity of (polymeric core) –(lipid shell) nanoparticles for regulated cellular uptake. *Adv Mater* 2015;**27**:1402–7. https://doi.org/10.1002/adma.201404788.
56. Zhang L, Feng Q, Wang J, et al. Microfluidic synthesis of hybrid nanoparticles with controlled lipid layers : understanding flexibility-regulated cell-nanoparticle interactions. *ACS Nano* 2015;**9**(10):9912–21. https://doi.org/10.1021/acsnano.5b05792.
57. Banquy X, Suarez F, Argaw A, et al. Effect of mechanical properties of hydrogel nanoparticles on macrophage cell uptake. *Soft Matter* 2009;**5**(20):3984–91. https://doi.org/10.1039/b821583a.
58. Fish MB, Fromen CA, Lopez-cazares G, et al. Exploring deformable particles in vascular-targeted drug delivery: softer is only sometimes better. *Biomaterials* 2017;**124**:169–79. https://doi.org/10.1016/j.biomaterials.2017.02.002.
59. Dulinska I, Targosz M, Strojny W, et al. Stiffness of normal and pathological erythrocytes studied by means of atomic force microscopy. *J Biochem Biophys Methods* 2006;**66**:1–11. https://doi.org/10.1016/j.jbbm.2005.11.003.
60. Zhou ZL, Hui TH, Tang B, Ngan AHW. Accurate measurement of stiffness of leukemia cells and leukocytes using an optical trap by a rate-jump method. *RCS Adv* 2014;**4**:8453. https://doi.org/10.1039/c3ra45835k.
61. Radmacher M, Fritz M, Kacher CM, Cleveland JP, Hansma PK. Measuring the viscoelastic properties of human platelets with the atomic force microscope. *Biophys J* 1996;**70**(1):556–67. https://doi.org/10.1016/S0006-3495(96)79602-9.
62. Müller K, Fedosov DA, Gompper G. Understanding particle margination in blood flow – a step toward optimized drug delivery systems. *Med Eng Phys* 2016;**38**:2–10. https://doi.org/10.1016/j.medengphy.2015.08.009.
63. Anselmo AC, Zhang M, Kumar S, et al. Elasticity of nanoparticles influences their blood circulation, phagocytosis, endocytosis, and targeting. *ACS Nano* 2015;**9**(3):3169–77. https://doi.org/10.1021/acsnano.5b00147.
64. Beningo KA, Wang YL. Fc-receptor-mediated phagocytosis is regulated by mechanical properties of the target. *J Cell Sci* 2002;**115**(4):849–56.
65. Nagaoka T, Yoshida A. Noninvasive evaluation of wall shear stress on retinal microcirculation in humans. *Investig Ophthalmol Vis Sci* 2006;**47**(3):1113–9. https://doi.org/10.1167/iovs.05-0218.
66. Koutsiaris AG, Tachmitzi SV, Batis N, et al. Volume flow and wall shear stress quantification in the human conjunctival capillaries and post-capillary venules in vivo. *Biorheology* 2007;**44**(5–6):375–86.
67. Greenberg AW, Brunk DK, Hammer DA. Cell-free rolling mediated by L-selectin and sialyl Lewis(x) reveals the shear threshold effect. *Biophys J* 2000;**79**(5):2391–402. https://doi.org/10.1016/S0006-3495(00)76484-8.
68. Liu J, Agrawal NJ, Calderon A, Ayyaswamy PS, Eckmann DM, Radhakrishnan R. Multivalent binding of nanocarrier to endothelial cells under shear flow. *Biophys J* 2011;**101**(2):319–26. https://doi.org/10.1016/j.bpj.2011.05.063.
69. Huang RB, Eniola-Adefeso O. Shear stress modulation of IL-1β-induced E-selectin expression in human endothelial cells. *PLoS One* 2012;**7**(2):e31874. https://doi.org/10.1371/journal.pone.0031874.
70. Huang RB, Gonzalez AL, Eniola-Adefeso O. Laminar shear stress elicit distinct endothelial cell e-selectin expression pattern via TNFα and IL-1β activation. *Biotechnol Bioeng* 2013;**110**(3):999–1003. https://doi.org/10.1002/bit.24746.
71. Chen BP, Li YS, Zhao Y, et al. DNA microarray analysis of gene expression in endothelial cells in response to 24-h shear stress. *Physiol Genomics* 2001;**7**(1):55–63. http://www.ncbi.nlm.nih.gov/pubmed/11595792.
72. Han J, Shuvaev VV, Davies PF, Eckmann DM, Muro S, Muzykantov VR. Flow shear stress differentially regulates endothelial uptake of nanocarriers targeted to distinct epitopes of PECAM-1. *J Control Release* 2015;**210**:39–47. https://doi.org/10.1016/j.jconrel.2015.05.006.
73. Samuel SP, Jain N, O'Dowd F, et al. Multifactorial determinants that govern nanoparticle uptake by human endothelial cells under flow. *Int J Nanomed* 2012;**7**:2943–56.
74. Han J, Zern BJ, Shuvaev VV, Davies PF, Muro S, Muzykantov V. Acute and chronic shear stress differently regulate endothelial internalization of nanocarriers targeted to platelet-endothelial cell adhesion molecule-1. *ACS Nano* 2012;**6**(10):8824–36. https://doi.org/10.1021/nn302687n.
75. Xia Y, Shi CY, Xiong W, Hou XL, Fang JG, Wang WQ. Shear stress-sensitive carriers for localized drug delivery. *Curr Pharm Des* 2016;**22**(38):5855–67. https://doi.org/10.2174/1381612822666160628081419.

Chapter 6

Routes of administration for nanocarriers

Nishan K. Shah[1], Elisa A. Torrico Guzmán[2], Zimeng Wang[3] and Samantha A. Meenach[1,2]

[1]*Department of Biomedical and Pharmaceutical Sciences, College of Pharmacy, University of Rhode Island, Kingston, RI, United States;* [2]*Department of Chemical Engineering, College of Engineering, University of Rhode Island, Kingston, RI, United States;* [3]*Phosphorex Inc., Hopkinton, MA, United States*

6.1 Introduction

The development of nanoparticle (NP)-based drug delivery systems has been continuously expanding in scope and interest over the past several decades owing to their many advantages in multiple applications, including targeted delivery of therapeutics to specific organs and tissues, controlled release of therapeutics, avoidance of immune response and/or cellular uptake, improved pharmacokinetic profiles, enhanced therapeutic efficacy, and safety, among others. Nanocarriers have been explored in many administration routes, including, but not limited to, parenteral, pulmonary, nasal, oral, transdermal, and ocular routes (as seen in Fig. 6.1), which are the most commonly investigated. The delivery of therapeutics using nanocarriers is often associated with intravenous (parenteral) delivery, but naturally this has expanded into many other delivery systems. Interestingly, each delivery route involves its own physiological barriers (whether cellular or noncellular) and delivery challenges. In addition, each administration route offers advantages and opportunities. Overall, this chapter contains a brief overview into each administration route with respect to nanocarrier drug delivery and applications (see Table 6.1) and serves as a starting point and stepping stone for further in-depth exploration into the varied and interested challenges and opportunities associated with each.

6.2 Parenteral delivery

Parenteral delivery is the administration of a therapeutic that goes through biological tissues directly to blood vessels, organs, or tissues.[1,2] This type of delivery offers advantages, including high bioavailability, and in some cases, exceptional therapeutic absorption.[1,3] This method can be utilized for patients who cannot take oral formulations due to limitations (e.g., sickness, obstruction, loss of consciousness, etc.). These routes of administration are often favorable for patients experiencing disease states that require immediate therapy and for drug monitoring by medical personnel.[1,4–7] The types of parenteral delivery routes that will be discussed in this chapter, including intravenous, intramuscular, intraperitoneal, and subcutaneous routes (Fig. 6.2A).

6.2.1 Intravenous delivery

Aside from oral administration, intravenous (IV) delivery is the most commonly used route of administration in the clinic and involves the delivery of nanocarriers into veins.[8] Dosing is performed using either bolus or infusion delivery. The fate of IV-delivered nanocarriers is based on the physical makeup of the product (active ingredient and excipients). Alternations to the product and its characteristics will determine overall outcomes. Products administered by IV administration are subject to numerous biological challenges that stem from their physical characteristics, including size, charge, shape, and surface modifications.[9,10] Within the body, nanocarriers are subject to protein adsorption, rapid elimination by the reticuloendothelial system (RES), unwanted tissue deposition, and restricted access by biological barriers.[1,11,12] Size plays a key role in the biological elimination of nanocarriers, where carriers <10 nm are small enough to be filtered and cleared by renal clearance, whereas carriers >200 nm are susceptible to the RES, leading to a decrease in therapy.[12] Charge also plays a key role in the interactions of nanocarriers with circulating proteins and phagocytotic cells.[13,14] Highly negative carriers are susceptible to macrophage uptake, whereas positively charged products are likely to aggregate with circulation proteins and cellular membranes and are often toxic. Therefore, neutrally charged formulations are usually overall favorable, unless a specific biological action utilizing charge is desired (i.e., macrophage uptake).[9,13,14] Surface modifications will also have a significant impact on

Nanoparticles for Biomedical Applications. https://doi.org/10.1016/B978-0-12-816662-8.00006-0

TABLE 6.1 Sample nanocarrier formulations based on route of delivery, nanocarrier type, disease and/or application, and development state.

Route of delivery	Type of nanocarrier	Drug(s) and disease/application	State	Reference
IV	Liposomes	Doxil; cancer	In vitro, in vivo, FDA-approved	8,11
IV	Various NPs	Taxane therapeutics; cancer	In vitro, in vivo, FDA-approved	7
IV	PLGA	Carboplatin; cancer	In vitro, in vivo	171
IV	Nanocrystal	Paclitaxel; cancer	In vitro, in vivo	172
IV	PLGA NP	Docetaxel; cancer	In vitro, in vivo	12
IP	PLGA	shRNA; cancer	In vitro, in vivo	2,170
IP	Inorganic material	Gold nanoshells; cancer	In vitro, in vivo	34
IP	Nanocrystal	Paclitaxel; cancer	In vitro, in vivo	31
IP	Inorganic material	Iron oxide nanoworms; peptide targeting agent	In vitro, in vivo	25
IP	Inorganic material	Gold nanorods; cancer	In vitro, in vivo	38
IM	Nanocrystals	Paliperidone palmitate; antipsychotic	In vitro, in vivo FDA-approved	46
IM	PLGA	Tat protein; vaccine	In vitro, in vivo	47
IM	Solid lipid NPs	Irinotecan; cancer	In vitro, in vivo	40
IM	PLGA	Progesterone; hormone therapy	In vitro, in vivo	45
IM	Protamine	Recombinant surface antigen; hepatitis B	In vitro, in vivo	43
SC	PLGA NP	Rifampicin, isoniazide; tuberculosis	In vitro, in vivo	61
SC	PLGA NP	Doxycycline; lymphatic filariasis	In vitro, in vivo	51
SC	PLGA NP	Gemcitabine; cancer	In vitro, in vivo	54
SC	PLGA NP	Ramizol; gastrointestinal *Clostridium difficile*–associated disease	In vitro, in vivo	41
SC	Chitosan–plasmid DNA NP	PDGF-BB and FGF-2 genes; inflammatory diseases	In vitro, in vivo	58
Pulmonary	Chitosan NP	Insulin (systemic); diabetes	In vivo	89
Pulmonary	Ab-decorated liposomes	Triptolide; cancer	In vitro, in vivo	21
Pulmonary	Magnetic Fe_3O_4 in PLGA NP	Quercetin; lung cancer and imaging	In vitro	173
Pulmonary	Peptide–micelle hybrid NP	Fasudil; pulmonary arterial hypertension	In vitro, in vivo	174
Pulmonary	SLNP	Quorum sensing inhibitor; infections	In vitro	175
Nasal	Chitosan–PLGA NP	Desvenlafaxine; antidepressant	In vivo	176
Nasal	Chitosan NP	Antigen ovalbumin; vaccines	In vitro, in vivo	177
Nasal	Nanoemulsion	Saquinavir mesylate; neuro-AIDS	Ex vivo, in vivo	178
Nasal	Micelles	Quantum dots; nose-to-brain delivery	In vivo	179
Nasal	Liposomes	Tacrine brain delivery; Alzheimer's	In vitro	180
Oral	Nanocrystals	Rapamune; Tricor; hypercholesterolemia Emend; antiemetic	In vitro, in vivo, FDA-approved	8,74,181

Continued

TABLE 6.1 Sample nanocarrier formulations based on route of delivery, nanocarrier type, disease and/or application, and development state.—cont'd

Route of delivery	Type of nanocarrier	Drug(s) and disease/application	State	Reference
Oral	PLGA NP	Insulin; biologics *Helicobacter pylori* vaccine; vaccine	In vitro, in vivo	70,71,77,182
Oral	PLGA	Epirubicin; antineoplastic	In vitro, in vivo	183
Oral	Solid lipid NPs	Domperidone; nausea and vomiting	In vitro, in vivo	76
Oral	PLGA	Ibuprofen; antiinflammatory	In vitro, in vivo	77
TD	Transferosomal gels with iodophor	Insulin (systemic); diabetes	In vitro, in vivo	184
TD	Lipid NP	Lutein; skin protectant	In vitro, ex vivo	185
TD	QD with various surface charges	Imaging	Ex vivo	186
TD	PLGA NP	Indomethacin; antiinflammatory	Ex vivo	187
TD	Chitosan NP	Minoxidil sulfate; androgenic alopecia	In vitro	188
Ocular	Liposomes	Brinzolamide; glaucoma	In vitro, in vivo	189
Ocular	Lipid NP	N-palmitoylethanolamide; inflammation	In vitro, in vivo	157,158
Ocular	PLGA NP	Memantine; glaucoma	In vitro, in vivo	190
Ocular	Alginate	Daptomycin; MRSA	In vitro, in vivo	168
Ocular	Lipid–polymer hybrid NP	Moxifloxacin; antibiotic	In vitro, in vivo	191

IM, intramuscular; *IP*, intraperitoneal; *IV*, intravenous; *NP*, nanoparticle; *NSCLC*, non–small-cell lung cancer; *PLGA*, poly(lactic-co-glycolic) acid; *SC*, subcutaneous; *TD*, transdermal.

the biological end-point of nanocarriers.[9,15,16] Numerous studies have shown unfavorable pharmacokinetic (PK) profiles and unwanted deposition based on the lack of targeting or other forms of modification.[11,12,17] Although there is evidence to support nanocarrier shape plays a role in biological interactions, research is still ongoing.[18]

The major advantage of IV administration is based on the direct delivery of products into circulation,[6] which allows for increased bioavailability. In comparison with IV delivery, orally administered carriers are exposed to enzymes that cause degradation of drugs, acidic pH, and mucus. IV administration of products avoids complications related to degradation, allowing for more effective delivery of sensitive carriers.[3,6] In addition, IV delivery is advantageous for carriers that require careful drug monitoring.[1,11,19]

6.2.1.1 Applications

Finding ways to predict biological outcomes of nanocarriers in vitro has been a subject of interest for many years. For example, one study investigated the interactions of nanocarriers and blood components and showed a simple yet detailed method to measure the influence of protein adsorption, coagulation, complement activation, and hemolysis on nanocarrier characteristics.[10] Another study utilized centrifugation as a method to examine cellular membrane binding and disruption in the characteristics of nanocarriers.[20] The development of in vitro experiments such as these can provide time and cost-efficient ways to predict outcomes of nanocarriers in vivo. In addition, research on the impact of surface modification of nanocarriers has been a subject of interest to increase the targetability of nanocarriers, to increase pharmacokinetic profiles and decrease side effects. The most successful modification to date is antibody (Ab) conjugation, and clinical trials exploring Ab-functionalized nanocarriers are underway.[11]

Both polymeric and liposomal nanocarriers used for chemotherapy have had some success in the clinic and are primarily administered via IV, and the majority of FDA-approved liposomal formulations are administered via IV.[21] Improvement of PK profiles compared with drug suspensions and a decrease in toxicity have been major advantages of chemotherapeutic nanocarriers.[1] Furthermore, the enhanced permeability and retention (EPR) effect is another benefit of IV administration. The proposed mechanism is based on "leaky" blood vessels present in and around tumors, which

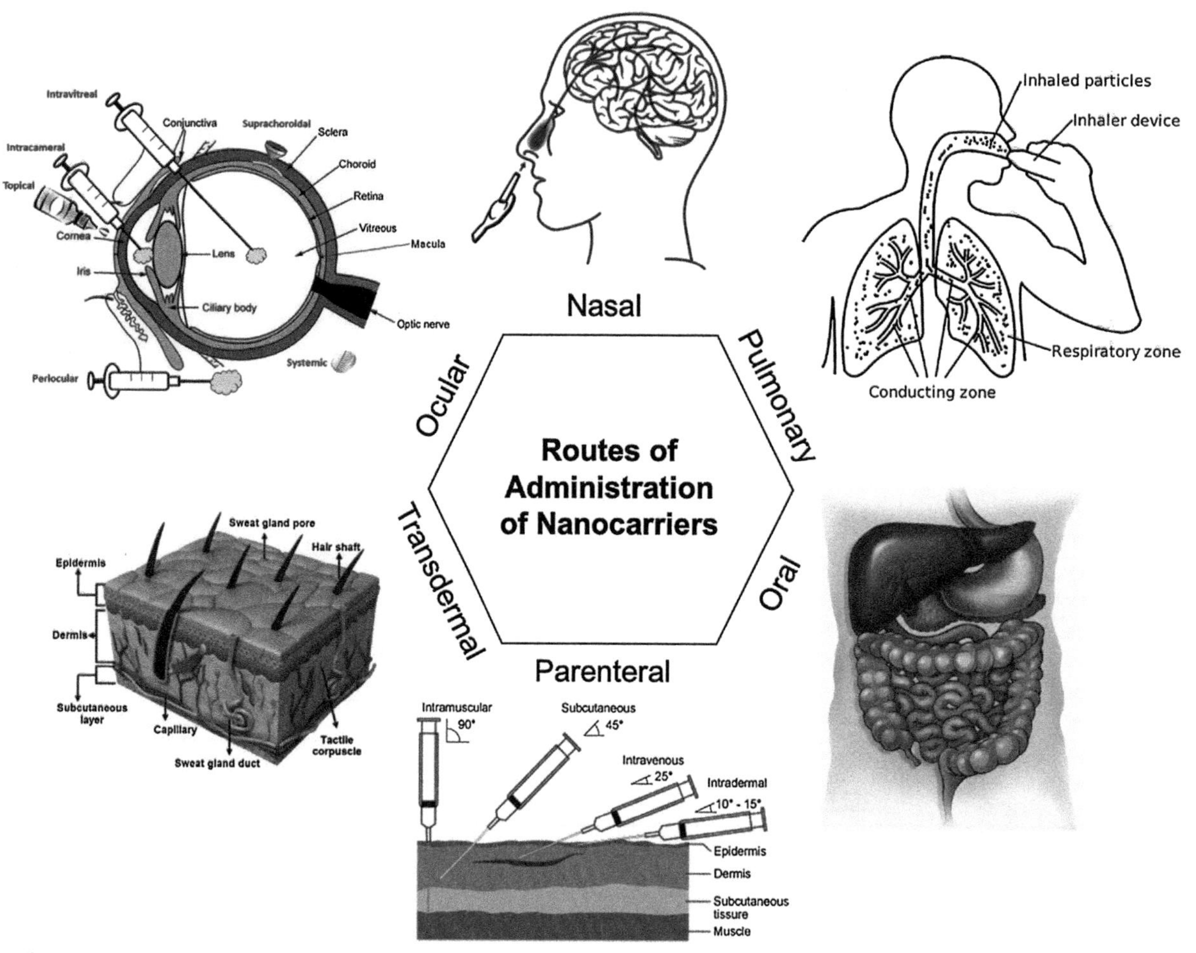

FIGURE 6.1 Overview schematic of routes of administration for nanocarriers to be discussed, including ocular, nasal, pulmonary, oral, transdermal, and parenteral delivery routes. *Adopted from Ahmed TA, Aljaeid BM. Preparation, characterization, and potential application of chitosan, chitosan derivatives, and chitosan metal nanoparticles in pharmaceutical drug delivery.* Drug Des Devel Ther *2016;**10**:483–507; Daniher DI, Zhu J. Dry powder platform for pulmonary drug delivery.* Particuology *2008;**6**:225–238; Future MR.* Nasal drug delivery market 2018 scope by spray and nebulizers delivery technologies with leading companies profiles – ME&A forecast till 2022*; 2018; Lee H, Song C, Baik S, Kim D, Hyeon T, Kim DH. Device-assisted transdermal drug delivery.* Adv Drug Deliv Rev *2018;**127**:35–45;* Overview of gastrointestinal tract*; 2018.*

allow for nanosized material to more readily reach the tumor tissue and exert their therapeutic action.[7,11,19,22] To facilitate EPR, nanocarriers are often coated with a hydrophilic, neutral polymer that can allow the nanocarrier avoiding protein aggregation on the surface of the carrier, reducing clearance in the RES.[8,19,23] Poly(ethylene glycol) (PEG) is the most widely used hydrophilic polymer for NP coatings,[12,17] and PEG coatings are used in several FDA-approved nanomedicine formulations (e.g., Doxil).[21,23] Another FDA-approved cancer nanocarrier formulation is Abraxane, a third-generation paclitaxel (PTX) delivery formulation that consists of PTX bound to human serum albumin, the most common circulation protein.[7,21] Abraxane has shown significant improvements in administration time (decrease from 3 h to 30 min), as well as improvements in critical PK characteristics in comparison with Taxol, the commonly used PTX formulation.[7]

6.2.1.2 Obstacles and opportunities

IV administration is one of the most widely used administration routes and the main administration route for anticancer therapeutics.[7,11,22] Despite widespread studies investigating colloidal science and biological interactions,[10,20,24] more studies are needed to further identify and counter potential hazards of IV-delivered nanocarriers. Other obstacles to consider are more technical. Scale-up synthesis and high-throughput screening methods need to be designed to combat the issue of supply and time–cost investment. An example of this includes product shortage, such as the current Doxil shortage, which needs to be avoided.[11] Based on the major obstacles, there are plenty of opportunities for the design of high-throughput screening methods, scale-up manufacturing, and predictive tools.

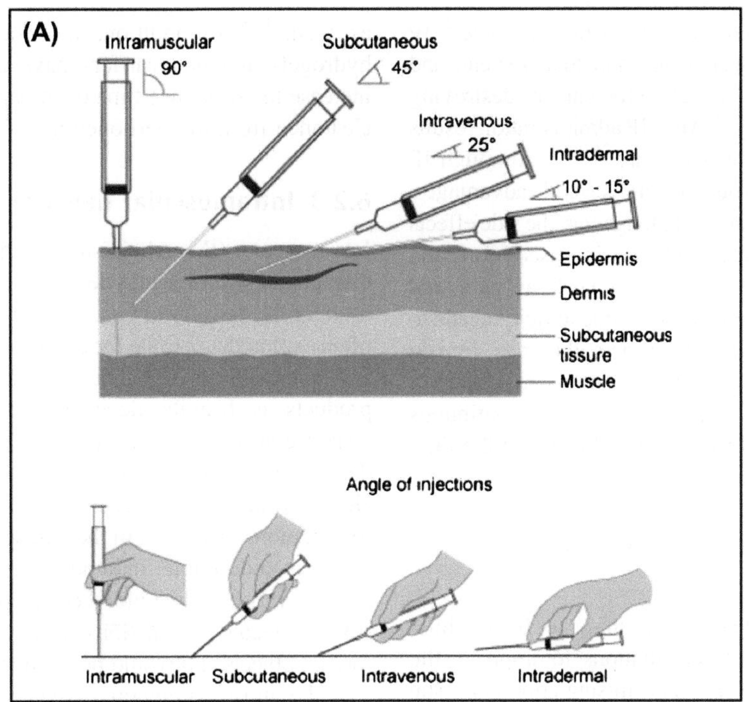

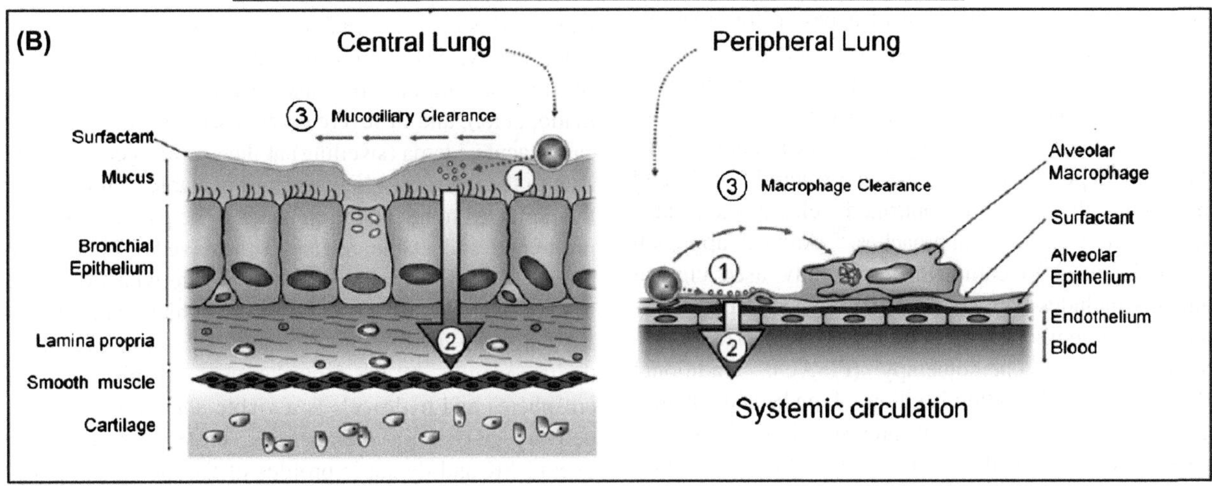

FIGURE 6.2 (A) Routes and delivery locations for parenteral delivery of therapeutics or nanocarriers, including intramuscular, subcutaneous, intravenous, and intradermal delivery methods. (B) Cellular and noncellular pulmonary barriers for nanocarriers, including those present in the central lung/upper airways (bronchial) and peripheral/lower airways (alveoli). *Adapted from Ahmed TA, Aljaeid BM. Preparation, characterization, and potential application of chitosan, chitosan derivatives, and chitosan metal nanoparticles in pharmaceutical drug delivery.* Drug Des Devel Ther *2016;**10**:483–507 and de Carvalho CS, Daum N, Lehr C-M. Carrier interactions with the biological barriers of the lung: advanced in vitro models and challenges for pulmonary drug delivery.* Adv Drug Deliv Rev *2014;**75**:129–140.*

6.2.2 Intraperitoneal delivery

Intraperitoneal (IP) delivery involves the delivery of therapeutics to the peritoneum cavity to increase local concentrations.[25] The major use of IP delivery has been for the treatment of peritoneal cancers. The fate of nanocarriers administered via the IP route is highly dependent on the localization of the malignant tissue and the deposition of the administered product in relation to vital organs.[26] IP administration generally during or postsurgery[27] and deposition of nanocarriers are initially localized at the administration site, while deviation from the site is affected by the physical characteristics and surface modifications of the formulation and the dynamics of the site itself, including fluid dynamics, gravity, presence of mucus, etc.[28]

In addition to avoiding the stomach, intestines, and first-pass metabolism, the major advantage of IP delivery is the superior level of treatment over IV administration, likely due to the close proximity of therapeutics to malignant tissue.[27] IP delivery has been used in the clinic for more than 50 years and has demonstrated that it is very efficient in destroying cancerous tissue postsurgery.[29] Also, IP administration results in reduced levels of systemic exposure.[26,29,30] Although IP administration of nanocarriers offers several advantages, challenges are inevitable. Major challenges are the side effects associated with IP delivery, including pain, discomfort, and systemic toxicity.[31] While side effects such as pain and discomfort are likely unavoidable, systemic toxicity needs to be addressed by designing nanocarriers that can remain localized. Also, traditional chemotherapeutics are subject to short residence times and require frequent or continuous administration, which can increase side effects and the likelihood of toxicity.[29,31,32]

6.2.2.1 Applications, obstacles, and opportunities

To address some of challenges pertaining to IP administration, the development of formulations to improve the localization of IP therapeutics is a promising approach. One such method is the development of adhesive formulations that can adhere to the peritoneum, such as chitosan-coated nanocarriers.[32] Another method would be the inclusion of nanocarriers in biological mimics, such as hydrogels.[29,31] Nanocarriers with targeting ligands, which include antibodies and peptides, are also being explored,[25,33,34] and formulations that exhibit controlled release have also shown promise as novel approaches.[29] Another approach that can be used to complement currently used clinical treatments includes nanocarrier-driven hyperthermic intraperitoneal chemotherapy (HIPEC) and pressurized intraperitoneal aerosol chemotherapy (PIPAC). Traditional HIPEC involves the administration of preheated chemotherapeutic solution to a site of interest.[27] In doing so, the increased temperature allows for increased drug penetration and therapeutic efficacy.[25,28,34] Clinically, HIPEC has shown to increase the survival rate when used in conjunction with surgery.[35] PIPAC, a newer treatment option, utilizes the nebulization of therapeutic solutions (both raw drug and formulations) using CO_2.[28,34,36] To assist in both HIPEC and PIPAC, nanocarriers not only can be used to control solution and tissue heating but can also increase drug deposition via passive and active targeting.[28,34,36,37] As of 2017, NP formulations developed for the treatment of IP-related cancers are in clinical trials.[28] A phase I study of IP-administered formulated paclitaxel (Nanotox) showed higher and prolonged drug levels within the peritoneum, resulting in minimal toxicity and systemic drug exposure following six doses of Nanotax administered for six cycles.[30] A form of HIPEC that utilizes nanocarriers through the use of external heating of inorganic materials to enhance delivery and penetration is currently being studied as well.[34,38] In addition, bioadhesive systems such as hydrogels and nanocarriers have also shown promise to increase the residence time of therapeutics and decrease NP clearance from the peritoneum.[29,31,32]

6.2.3 Intramuscular delivery

Intramuscular (IM) administration involves the delivery of a therapeutic within a muscle and is the most common route used for the delivery of vaccines.[39] In addition, IM delivery is often explored as a route for depot products such as hydrogels and microspheres.[40,41] The deposition of IM-administered products is heavily dependent on the overall immune response at the delivery site. With respect to the use of IM delivery for vaccines, immune responses are preferred.[42,43] However, an immune response following administration of formulations that result in the extended release of small molecules is undesirable. Inflammation can result in the recruitment of various white blood cells, which can pose a threat to small molecule formulations, as they would be recognized as foreign objects and would be engulfed.[44]

Like most parenteral delivery systems, invasiveness, pain, and stress are major drawbacks for IM delivery. Additionally, IM administration can be associated with severe pain, immune responses (rashes, erythema, inflammation, etc.), and in severe cases, tissue necrosis.[45] In most cases, acute edema (swelling) at the site of injection occurs. Due to the interest in long-acting injectables with IM being the preferred route, attention needs to be paid to ensure that prolonged and stable release is achieved for the desired time.[41,45] Generally, the major challenge with IM delivery lies in water-soluble therapeutics, which can result in challenges in dissolution, degradation, and uptake of both the therapeutic and the formulation.[44] IM injection of microspheres and hydrogels is a viable alternative to the oral delivery of certain therapeutics, thereby increasing the overall PK and dynamic profiles of the therapeutics, while decreasing the likelihood of systemic side effects.[2,46] Additionally, IM-administered depot injections can allow for the modulation of dosing regimens by decreasing the dosing frequency.

6.2.3.1 Applications, obstacles, and opportunities

Although there are drawbacks concerning patient compliance and biological responses with IM delivery, vaccine and biological therapeutic research is heavily dependent on this type of delivery.[42,44] As a result, a significant portion of IM delivery-related research is devoted to improving the sustained release and biological responses of newly developed vaccines and other biological therapeutics.[43,47] This interest is mainly due to the advantageous changes in PK and dynamic profiles of nanocarrier formulations, as well as the significant decrease in dosing frequency.[2,41,46] Another novel use of nanocarriers in IM delivery is the development of adjuvants, which are entities that work to increase antigen uptake and promote dendritic cells to initiate an immune response.[48] Aside from vaccine products, there are very few products using IM for the delivery of small molecules. Microspheres are the main form of technology used for sustained drug release for these applications.[41,46] Currently, there are no FDA-approved nanoscale IM formulations, and the future of IM delivery is dependent on extending the time between doses of both small and large molecule therapeutics.

6.2.4 Subcutaneous delivery

Subcutaneous (SC) administration involves the delivery of therapeutics into the interstitial area underlying the epidermis via injection. The interstitial area under the skin primarily comprises negatively charged glycosaminoglycan and collagen fibers, which provides a relatively slow and steady absorption rate of molecules, owing to reduced blood flow.[49] Conventional SC formulations include aqueous solutions, oily solutions, suspensions, and simple emulsions of therapeutics. To modify the release profile of compounds, they can be encapsulated into particle or implant-based formulations. Particle-based delivery systems can also be applied for lymph-targeting delivery.[50]

The fate of nanocarriers delivered through the SC route depends on the particle properties and the injection location.[51] Particle size is the key factor in determining the final absorption route. Particles <10 nm tend to be absorbed via the capillaries draining from the injection site, where they then go into systemic circulation. Particles 10–100 nm in diameter move through the interstitium and are taken up directly into the lymphatic system. Particles >100 nm show low capability of diffusion through the water channel within the interstitium (also around 100 nm). As a result, the larger particles mostly retain at the injection site and form a depot. During particle diffusion through interstitium, charge and hydrophilicity play important roles, as they influence the interaction between particles and interstitial compounds. Furthermore, the driving force of particle transport into lymph is fluid flow from the interstitium to the lymphatics, which varies in different locations. Correspondingly, the variation of injection site also affects the lymphatic transport by changing the fluid flow and pressure surrounding the formulation.[51–54]

6.2.4.1 Applications and advantages

SC administration of therapeutics is widely applied to obtain higher bioavailability, modify the release profile to allow for longer systemic exposure, or serve as an alternative dosing route when oral delivery is not applicable.[50] Various nanocarrier-based SC formulations have been developed to deliver therapeutics such as anticancer drugs,[54] antibiotics,[41] HIV drugs,[55] peptide hormones,[56] anticoagulants,[57] protein drugs,[58] mRNA,[59] and immunosuppressive antirheumatic drugs.[60] Such nanocarrier-based formulations have been developed for the treatment of pancreatic, non–small-cell lung, breast, ovarian cancers,[54] gastrointestinal (GI) *Clostridium difficile*–associated diseases,[41] tuberculosis,[61] lymphatic filariasis,[51] venous thrombosis,[57] inflammatory diseases,[58] rheumatoid arthritis,[60] and the prevention of HIV-1 vaginal transmission.[8] The function of these particular nanocarriers can be divided into three aspects, including (1) the formation of depots at the injection site to provide sustained release of therapeutics,[41,54–57,60,61] (2) the application of particles 70–11 nm in diameter for lymphatic system targeting,[51,60] or (3) systemic delivery of nanocarriers via the SC route.[59]

Compared with other parenteral routes such as IV and IM administration, SC administration is typically convenient to patients. First, it is often less painful and less time-consuming, which improves patient compliance. Furthermore, it is easy to do and suitable for self-administration, which reduces the total cost of treatment.[53,62] In addition, nanocarrier formulations delivered via the SC route provide protection for the therapeutic and result in prolonged release, thereby reducing dosing frequency, improved safety and efficiency, and targeted delivery of therapeutics.[51]

6.3 Oral delivery

Oral administration of therapeutics is by far the most common route of administration, owing to its simplicity and high patient compliance.[63] It involves the ingestion of a therapeutic followed by transition throughout the GI tract before undergoing first-pass metabolism and systemic delivery.[3,6,8,63] Orally administered products are exposed to barriers in the GI tract that include gastric acid, mucus, enzymes, and the epithelial lining.[64–66] Upon initial consumption, products that transition to the stomach will be subject to its acidic environment, enzymes, and stomach mucosa. Following the stomach, the product will be subjected to further pH changes, enzymes, and significantly more mucosa.[67] Upon exposure to the enzymes in the environment, initial breakdown of the formulation and encapsulated therapeutic can ensue, leading to destruction of the formulation and potentially the encapsulated therapy. pH changes may induce changes in the ionization state of the therapy, which can inhibit absorption. Both stomach and intestinal mucosa function to prevent the absorption of foreign material into the bloodstream.[68] As a result, both unencapsulated therapies and nanocarriers will have to either adhere to the mucus, fully transport through to allow for systemic absorption, or will be destroyed.[69]

6.3.1 Current challenges and advantages

The major challenge in oral delivery are the barriers that are present in the GI tract, particularly for biological therapeutics (Fig. 6.3B).[6,65] Most biological therapeutics (vaccines, peptides, proteins, etc.) are subject to enzymatic degradation and denaturation in acidic conditions, making it virtually impossible to deliver them without protection.[65,67,70,71] Like biological molecules, small molecules may be subject to enzymatic degradation as well as degradation via continual pH changes. Another consideration for small molecules is drug transporters, including those related to cellular uptake and efflux.[6,63] In either case, the interaction of small molecules with drug transporters will likely alter the bioavailability of the therapeutic. In addition, mucus is an obstacle that must be considered.[63] Due to its complex matrices, mucus has the ability to slow down or completely inhibit particle transport and drug absorption, making treatment difficult, and using particle engineering to overcome this limitation is challenging.[63,72,73] Physicochemically, it is important that the properties of the carriers are heavily considered before particle engineering begins for optimal formulation design.[6] Since 70% of all newly discovered small molecules are poorly water soluble, and macromolecule therapeutics are likely to be destroyed in the GI tract, oral delivery of nanocarriers offer advantages, including protection of the cargo and pH-dependent release.[74,75] In addition, the PK characteristics of therapeutics become more favorable.[75,76] Proper formulation design may allow for increased drug loading, allowing for a decrease in dosing regimen with respect to time and dosage.[65,77,78]

6.3.2 Applications

A number of formulations have shown promise for increasing adhesion to mucosa, increased drug penetration, sustained release, and successful delivery of biological therapeutics.[63,64,69,71,79–81] Much of the research has involved the use of lipids, PLGA, and various grades of Eudragit, all of which are known to withstand some of the obstacles of the GI tract.[6,67,68,70,78,82] To this same extent, nanocrystal formulations, which are FDA-approved for oral delivery, are considered a viable approach for oral delivery of small molecule therapeutics.[6,63,74] Many of the FDA-approved nanoscale products are nanocrystals or liposomes. Nanocrystals not only improve PK profiles of therapeutics but also increase the drug loading and improve the release and dissolution kinetics through increased surface area to volume ratio.[8,11,21,61] Their popularity is based on the use of nearly 100% drug in the product itself, as well as the well-established methods of production and history of success.

6.3.3 Obstacles and opportunities

Due to the high use of oral delivery as an administration route, there is still a high level of promise in designing nanotechnologies for oral drug delivery. However, formulations need to be designed to overcome biological barriers present in the GI tract. The use of acid-resistant polymers that are also biocompatible stands as an exceptional route to consider when designing oral delivery systems. Nanocrystals, although widely used, remain as a promising approach for small molecule therapeutics. Given the history

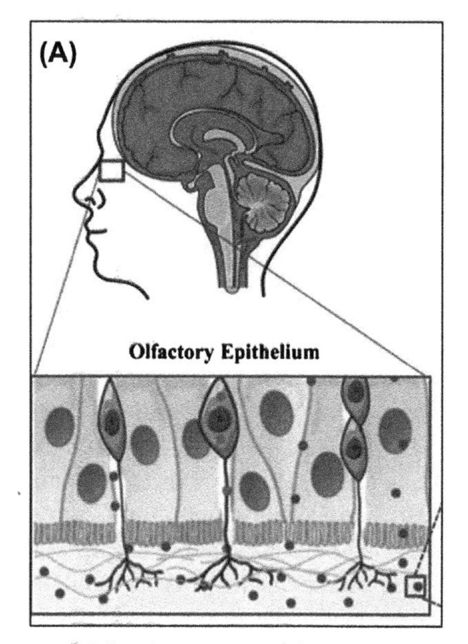

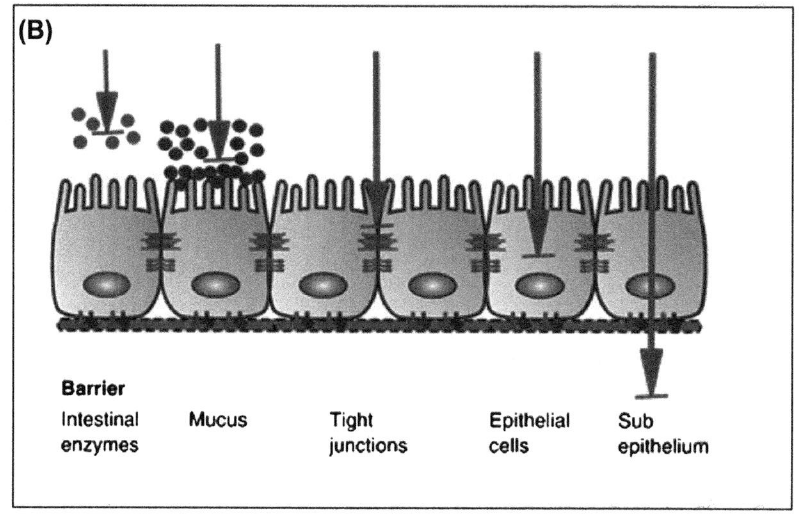

FIGURE 6.3 (A) Overview of the olfactory epithelium involved in nasal drug delivery and the proximity to the brain and central nervous system. (B) Gastrointestinal barriers associated with oral drug delivery. *Adapted from Samaridou E, Alonso MJ. Nose-to-brain peptide delivery – the potential of nanotechnology.* Bioorganic Me Chem *2018;**26**:2888–2905 and Lundquist P, Artursson P. Oral absorption of peptides and nanoparticles across the human intestine: opportunities, limitations and studies in human tissues.* Adv Drug Deliv Rev *2016.*

of success as well as the continual development of new therapeutics, it is likely that nanocrystals will be a suggested formulation design for oral delivery.

6.4 Pulmonary delivery

In recent years, pulmonary delivery has attracted growing interest in the research community for its advantages over other delivery systems to treat local diseases in the lungs and respiratory tract such as asthma and chronic obstructive pulmonary diseases[83] as well as systemic delivery of therapeutics via the pulmonary route.[84] The local treatment of pulmonary diseases provides high concentration of a drug at the site by directly delivering it to the lung. As a result, a lower overall dose is required, thereby reducing systemic side effects. Due to the high surface area in the lungs, systemic delivery can be attained via the alveoli, where the drug is absorbed into the bloodstream; therefore, a rapid onset of action can be achieved, and the first-pass metabolism is avoided.

Internally, the lungs are divided into bronchi, bronchioles, and smaller air passages that include the alveoli, blood vessels, and lymph tissue. The main function of the lungs is to exchange oxygen and carbon dioxide, which occurs in the alveoli. There are more than 300 million alveoli in the lungs, with a combined surface area of about 100 m^2, thin alveolar epithelium (0.1−0.2 μm), and high membrane permeability, which enables an efficient mass transfer, providing a route for systemic delivery of therapeutics.[85,86] The alveolar surface is coated by a film of pulmonary surfactant, a mixture of lipids, and proteins. The resulting surfactant is secreted and recycled by type II pneumocytes and cleared by alveolar macrophages,[87] reduces the surface tension in the lungs, and represents the first barrier against pathogens.[88] In the upper airways, the epithelium is covered by mucus that is produced by goblet cells. In addition, the bronchial surface contains ciliated columnar cells, which are responsible for mucociliary clearance, Clara cells that produce electron-dense granules, and a surfactant lipoprotein that intervenes in ion transport.[87]

6.4.1 Delivery devices

The three major types of inhalers used for pulmonary delivery are metered dose inhalers (MDIs), nebulizers, and dry powder inhalers (DPIs). The mechanisms of delivery and the formulation requirements are different for each type. MDIs are pressurized vessels that rely on the driving force of the propellant to atomize droplets containing drug and excipients, where the drugs are either solutions or particulate suspensions. Nebulizers deliver liquid medication in a steady stream of droplets of 1−5 μm and can deliver larger doses compared with other inhalers but may also require longer times.[89] Nebulizers produce ultrafine droplets with high polydispersity, which make them unsuitable for the delivery of larger particles (bigger than the droplet size) to the lungs.[85] DPIs are breath-activated devices that deliver medication in the form of a dry powder directly to the airways. During administration, a capsule containing a set dose of drug in the form of microparticles is punctured, and these particles are aerosolized.[90] Particles delivered using DPIs tend to agglomerate due to hygroscopic phenomena and electrostatic interactions, which reduce aerosolization performance.[85] Overall, DPIs are preferred over other devices owing to the promise of physical stability of the formulation in solid form and because they are portable and easy to use and can be applied to a wide variety of active ingredients and dose weights.[91,92] Overall, all three of these device types could be used to deliver nanocarrier formulations.

6.4.2 Particle fate

Particle deposition in the lungs is governed by the aerodynamic diameter of the particles and occurs by one of the following mechanisms: inertial impaction, sedimentation, or diffusion. NPs deposit by diffusion due to Brownian motion, and this deposition can be enhanced by breath-holding (reduction of airflow). Aggregates of NPs into microparticles (i.e., nanocomposite microparticles) allow for deposition via impaction and sedimentation mechanisms. Once the microsized particles deposit in the airways, they dissociate back into NPs.[32,33] Inhalable particles can be categorized into different sizes, including coarse (≥5 μm), fine (0.5−5 μm), or ultrafine (≤0.5 μm). Coarse carriers collide with the upper airways (trachea and large bronchi) and deposit by impaction, fine particles can reach the lower lung airways by sedimentation, and ultrafine particles can deposit throughout the respiratory tract, reaching the alveoli by diffusion.[86,93]

Another parameter that can influence the particle deposition in the lungs is the electrostatic charge that occurs in most of the inhalers during the aerosolization process. Fine particles can acquire charge via electron exchange due to the different surface potential when they are in contact to each other or to the walls of the device.[94] This effect may be not be desired for systemic delivery of the drugs, which requires particles to reach the alveolar epithelium.[95] Nanocarriers can be cleared from the lungs via endocytotic mechanisms, which involves pinocytosis and phagocytosis, which reduce the efficacy of these formulations.[96] The clearance of particles depends on their deposition location. In the upper airways, particles are removed by the mucociliary escalator. Once mucus entraps foreign particles, cilia beat in a coordinated direction and transport them to the larynx where the particles can be coughed up or swallowed. Most insoluble particles larger than 6 μm are eliminated by mucociliary clearance.[97] Smaller particles that reached the alveoli are uptaken by alveolar macrophages. In general, nanocarrier clearance and uptake will be also affected by parameters such as the encapsulated drug properties, type of NP, size and surface coating, and interaction of the nanocarrier with cells. The cellular and noncellular barriers that nanocarriers may face can be seen in Fig. 6.2B.

6.4.3 Applications

Inhalation therapy of nanomedicines enables the delivery of drugs within the lungs for the treatment of pulmonary diseases such as lung cancer,[98] cystic fibrosis–related infections,[99] and pulmonary hypertension,[100] among others. The pulmonary delivery of peptide and proteins represents a great potential for the treatment for both local and systemic diseases such as diabetes and thrombosis. Gene delivery[101] and vaccines are other applications of pulmonary inhalation. Examples of drug-loaded carriers such as lipids, solid lipid NPs, and polymeric NPs for diverse applications are reviewed elsewhere.[102] Several studies are ongoing that apply pulmonary delivery for different drugs using different carriers. Table 6.1 shows additional examples of pulmonary delivery applications. In a recent study, liposomes functionalized with phosphatidic acid and an ApoE-derived peptide (mApoE-PA-LIP) were delivered to the brain of Alzheimer's disease mice via the pulmonary administration, showing a significant decrease in the total brain beta-amyloid compared with untreated mice and suggesting a potential application of inhalation therapy for brain delivery of NP.[103]

6.4.4 Challenges and advantages

The pulmonary route offers advantages in the delivery of poorly water-soluble compounds that cannot be achieved via parenteral or oral delivery.[86] Since the lungs have limited intra- and extracellular drug–enzyme activities, the bioavailability of the drug can be enhanced compared with other delivery routes. In addition, the dosage amount can be reduced, leading to a decreased systemic toxicity.[104] A high adsorption rate and the rapid onset of action are possible due to the thin epithelial monolayer (0.1–0.4 μm) and large surface area of the alveoli.[93] Parameters to consider to ensure effective delivery in the lungs include (1) deposition and localization of drugs to a targeted area or cells, (2) ability to escape mucociliary clearance, (3) penetration through mucus, (4) transport across epithelial cells to reach the bloodstream, (5) low entrapment and interaction of formulations in biofilms, (6) modified or reduced phagocytic activity of alveolar macrophages, and (7) minimal protein–carrier interactions.[85,97] To address the design challenges relevant to pulmonary delivery, it is important to focus on both the physicochemical properties of carriers, such as surface chemistry, charge, hydrophilicity, and the pulmonary barriers such as cilia, mucus, and macrophages that limit the localization, penetration, and adsorption of carriers.[105]

Interactions between nanocarriers and cells are of particular interest because the properties of the carriers as well as the physiological environment influence nanocarrier uptake and biological response to the delivered drug.[96] Cationic hydrogel rod-shaped NP resulted in increased uptake in lung dendritic cells and promoted a superior immune response, avoiding extensive alveolar microphages (AMs) clearance, whereas the anionic NPs were preferentially uptaken by AM and found to be immunologically inert.[106] In another study, cationic PS NPs showed faster and higher uptake in alveolar epithelial model cells, whereas anionic PS NPs had a significant uptake and translocation through the monolayer for systemic delivery application. In another example, PEGylated polyaspartamide–polylactide-based NPs demonstrated the ability to enhance the diffusion through cystic fibrosis artificial mucus avoiding interactions with mucus components compared with unPEGylated NPs.[107,108] The limited number of FDA-approved excipients for inhalation, which include sugars, lipids, and small PEGs, among others, represents a limitation in the development of new formulations for pulmonary delivery, and use of new excipients will require further safety and toxicity studies.[107,109] Additives for pulmonary administration also influence the effectiveness and potential toxicity of inhalation formulations, which has been reviewed in Pilcer and Amighi's work.[110]

6.4.5 Future opportunities

The challenges involved in effective pulmonary delivery have resulted in strong interest in developing formulations that can overcome physiological and biological barriers. Studies involving nanocarriers that allow for mucus penetration include the surface modification with PEG-based coatings, as reviewed by Huckaby et al.[111] The potential use of other mucus-inert biomaterials such as polysarcosine, polyglycydol, etc., and mucolytic agents such as papain and human DNase (rhDNase), among others, has been reviewed elsewhere.[112,113] Other surface modifications for the enhancement of peptide or protein absorption are of great interest, as evaluated in the conjugation of liposomes to germ agglutinin that increased the association of liposomes to alveolar epithelial cells in vitro and in vivo.[114] The carrier interactions with biological barriers and in vitro pulmonary models for more accurate evaluations represent fields under exploration, as seen in the review by de Souza Carvalho et al.[115] Overall, the potential for pulmonary nanocarrier formulations is endless and ongoing.

6.5 Nasal delivery

While oral delivery and parenteral delivery are common routes of administration, nasal delivery has been widely investigated in recent years for the administration of formulations that have poor stability in GI fluids. The nasal route offers potential advantages in bioavailability, patient compliance, and improved immune response with respect to vaccines compared with the other routes. Therapies administered intranasally can be absorbed by the highly vascularized mucosa of the nose, which reduces degradation of the agents and increases the onset of action avoiding passage through the GI tract and liver. Nasal delivery also has the advantage in allowing contact with the blood–brain barrier (BBB), allowing the delivery of active compounds to the central nervous system.[116,117] Nanocarriers such as liposomes, polymeric NPs, carbon nanotubes, nanoemulsions, nanogels, quantum dots combined with enzymatic inhibitors, nasal absorption enhancers, or/and mucoadhesives such as chitosan have been evaluated to improve stability and permeation of nasal formulations and to circumvent biological barriers to improve absorption in the nasal cavity.[118]

Formulations for nasal delivery are typically administered by droppers and metered spray pumps. The majority of liquid formulations uses sprays, which offer more anterior drug deposition than nasal drops, thereby decreasing the clearance of the drug.[119] However, the nasal region is often considered a poor site for topical and systemic delivery.[118] The dosing necessary to avoid irritation and cytotoxicity is limited to 25–150 μL, so the development of efficient devices for new and expensive drugs is required to increase the bioavailability and patient compliance to ensure the efficacy of the treatment. Further characteristics and performance of current nasal drug delivery devices in a clinical perspective are reviewed elsewhere.[120]

6.5.1 Particle fate

The nasal cavity comprises three regions, including the nasal vestibule, respiratory, and olfactory regions, with a total surface area of 150 cm^2 in adults. It also contains nasal-associated lymphoid tissue situated mainly in the nasopharynx[121] and keratinized stratified squamous epithelium in the anterior region. The inferior region is covered by hairs known as vibrissae, which can arrest and trap inspired particles. Posteriorly, the respiratory epithelium contains a nonkeratinizing stratified squamous and ciliated epithelium rich in goblet cells that secrete mucus.[122] These secretions make the surface sticky to trap foreign particles. The site of drug deposition in the nose is highly dependent on the dosage form, as mentioned earlier. Therapies deposited near the nasopharynx area may cause irritation and an unpleasant taste, which reduces the patient compliance. When the therapies are deposited in the anterior portion of the nose, adsorption is drastically reduced, representing a problem for the delivery of drugs and vaccines.

The olfactory epithelium (see Fig. 6.3A) represents only 5% of the total nasal cavity but provides a direct route to the brain.[123] Particles >10 μm tend to accumulate in the upper respiratory region, and carriers <500 nm are transported to the lungs. Only particles in the range of 5–7 μm accumulate in the nasal cavity.[119] It is expected that nanocarriers are uptaken by cells by endocytosis, where particles 100–500 nm in diameter are transported by transcellular routes and 10-nm particles are transported paracellularly.[121] The diameter of tight junctions in the nasal cavity is 3.9–8.4 Å,[124] so particles require an adsorption enhancers to increase penetration through the cells. Different approaches have been studied to enhance the transport, penetration, and absorption of nanocarriers. Chitosan-based NPs have shown improvement of drug transport from the nose to brain due to their mucoadhesive properties and ability to open tight junctions in the olfactory epithelia.[125] PEGylation has been applied in formulations to increase the stability and transport through the mucus. PEG–PLA NPs loaded with the antigen tetanus toxoid for vaccine delivery showed enhanced particle stability in mucosal fluids that facilitated the transport of the antigen and showed a long-lasting immune response.[126]

6.5.2 Applications

Nasal delivery has been widely used for topical and systemic delivery of therapeutics, and the delivery of agents in controlled, engineered nanocarriers is gaining increasing interest. The nasal mucosa represents the first contact of inhaled antigens. For this reason, it has been extensively studied for vaccine delivery, especially for respiratory infections. For example, the influenza vaccine can be delivered by the nasal route and shows enhanced immune response due to promoted absorption with chitosan.[127] For example, a nasal vaccination of HBsAg absorbed in poly-ε-caprolactone (PCL)/chitosan NP was evaluated for the hepatitis B virus, showing a significant immune response in mice nasal secretions, which is believed to be enhanced by the cationic mucoadhesive nature of chitosan.[128] In another study, an antigen of mycobacterium tuberculosis and MPLA (monophosphoryl lipid A) as adjuvant were coentrapped in PLGA:DDA (dimethyl dioctadecylammonium bromide) hybrid NP and evaluated in animal models showing efficient mucosal and systemic responses for tuberculosis vaccination.[129] A comprehensive review of nasal nanovaccines based on the type of nanomaterial can be found elsewhere.[130]

Brain delivery via nasal administration is of interest, as nanocarriers can bypass the BBB when absorbed by the olfactory epithelium. Nasal administration of lactoferrin-modified PEG-PLGA NPs has been evaluated for efficient intranasal delivery of rotigotine to the brain to treat Parkinson's disease.[131] Polysorbate 80 polystyrene NPs showed greater penetration into the epithelial cell layer with no tissue damage in porcine olfactory epithelium for CNS targeting for neurological diseases.[132] Table 6.1 shows additional applications for nasal delivery. Nanocarriers used for nose-to-brain targeting for the treatment of neurodegenerative disorders are reviewed elsewhere.[133]

6.5.3 Challenges, advantages, and limitations

The physiological and histological characteristics of the nasal cavity provide an option for rapid systemic drug absorption and quick onset of action. Intranasal absorption evades the GI and hepatic enzymatic degradation, which allow for the delivery of macromolecules, and it enhances therapeutics bioavailability compared with compounds delivered to GI tract. The noninvasive, painless nature of this route makes it practical for patient compliance.[116,118] Mucociliary clearance has a negative impact on nanocarrier bioavailability, representing the main limitation for effective drug delivery and transport via nasal route. The absorption responses of free drugs are often mirrored in nanocarriers with similar physicochemical characteristics. The challenges in producing effective formulations include increasing bioavailability for systemic applications, mucus and cell layer penetration enhancement, successful bypass of the BBB for brain delivery, and to have a high uptake for vaccines or topical delivery.

6.5.4 Future opportunities

Although nasal delivery has been applied for topical delivery of free drugs for the treatment of chronic allergies, mucosa inflammation, and persistent rhinosinusitis, the use of nanocarriers may enhance the properties of such formulations. Systemic delivery is another potential application, as the rapid absorption and onset of action make this route of delivery crucial for intense, acute pain and for the management of severe conditions such as seizures, cardiovascular attacks, and nauseas. Research on the application of nanocarriers for nasal delivery is ongoing to take advantage of this particular route and its advantageous physiological characteristics by the surface modification of nanocarriers for different applications. The imaging and diagnosis application of NP-mediated for brain delivery have been reviewed using different routes of administration,[134] and definitely, nasal delivery could serve as a potential route for such applications. More studies that evaluate particle–particle interactions as well as particle–cell interactions to better understand the mechanisms of absorption and uptake using different surface modifications are required.

6.6 Transdermal delivery

Transdermal delivery has been extensively used for the treatment of skin disorders mainly because of advantages such as the high surface area of skin, minimal or no pain, and high patient compliance. Current technologies involving the use of nanocarriers and patches have extended the range of applications of the dermal route for topical and systemic drug delivery systems. Formulations for transdermal delivery are frequently found in the form of creams, ointments, lotions, and patches, where skin permeation is enhanced by the low molecular weight of compounds and the use of lipophilic drugs at low doses.[135] Nanosized colloidal particles such as liposomes, micelles, polymeric NPs, and inorganic particles have been studied to overcome the primary barrier for this delivery route—the stratum corneum in the skin. The encapsulation of compounds in nanocarriers not only improves the penetration and absorption through the skin but also protects the agents from degradation and offers controlled release from the carrier.[136] To benefit from all the advantages of dermal delivery, it will require the investigation of newer ways to enhance the skin penetration of larger hydrophilic drugs and macromolecules for treatment of diseases and vaccination applications.[135]

6.6.1 Particle fate

The skin is a biologically active and multifunctional and is often called the largest organ in the body. Its stratified structure contains two layers—the epidermis and dermis. The main objectives in the administration of agents to the skin include treatment of disorders of the skin and to deliver the drugs to other tissues. The stratum corneum limits drug diffusion to the inner layer into the body and is considered the sole penetration pathway for topically applied substances. Particles can be absorbed by single or combined routes, including between the cells of the stratum corneum (intercellular), across the corneal cellular layer (transcellular), and into the concavity of a hair follicle (follicular), including interactions with sweat glands or skin furrows as seen in Fig. 6.4A.[137] Through the follicular route, particles can either penetrate to the dermis or accumulate for increased drug release. The pathway chosen is likely dependent on particle size, charge, material, and morphology.[135] The tight junctions in the stratum corneum create a water tight barrier that is impermeable for most drugs that are both above 500 kDa and hydrophilic,[138]

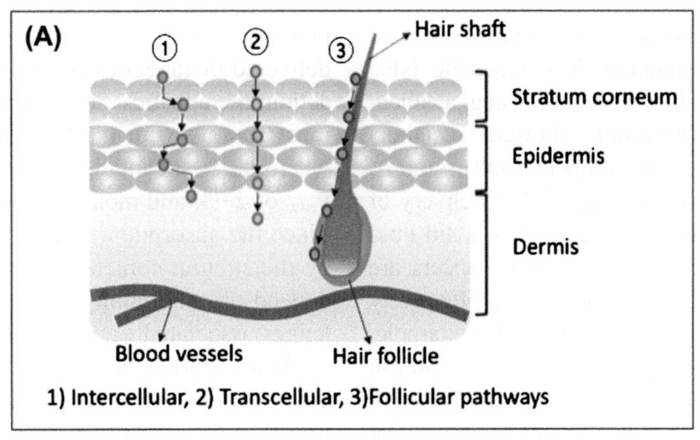

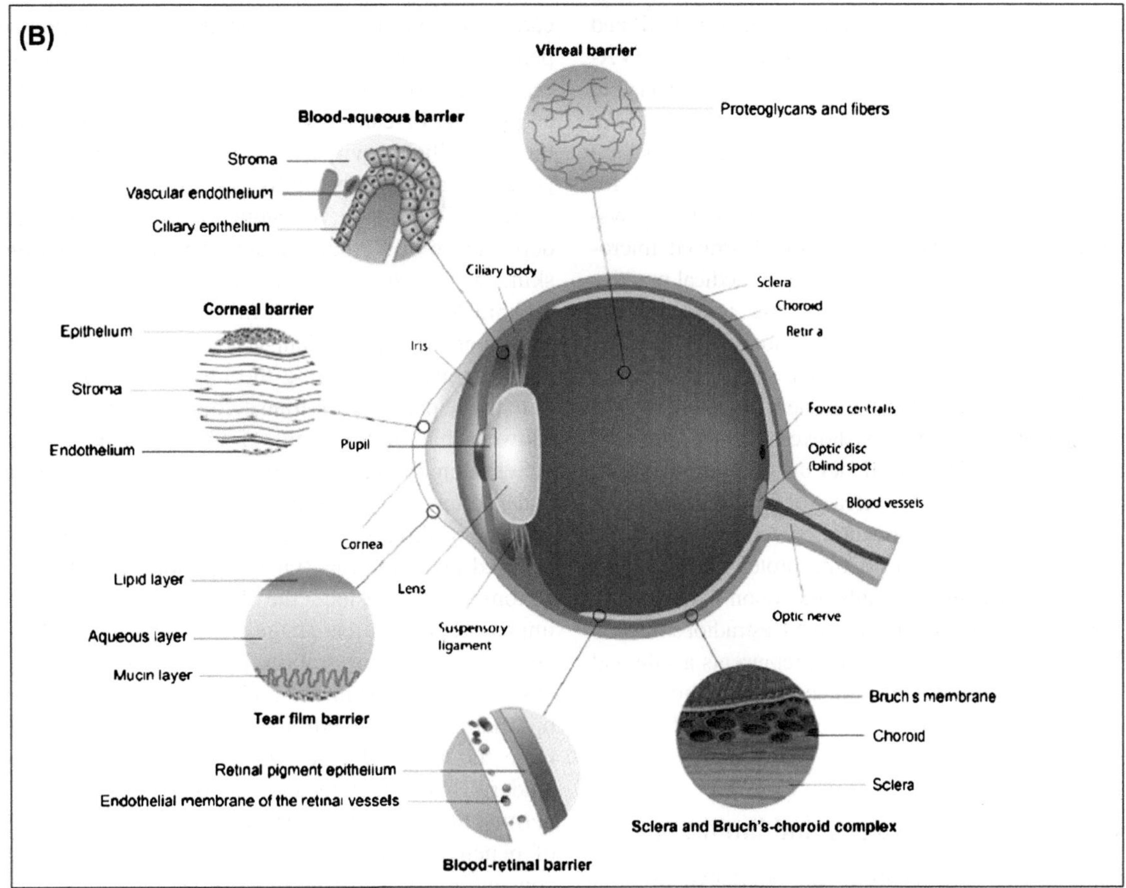

FIGURE 6.4 (A) Pathways of particle transport associated with transdermal drug delivery and (B) physiological barriers present during ocular drug delivery. *Adapted from Yu M, Wu J, Shi J, Farokhzad OC. Nanotechnology for protein delivery: overview and perspectives.* J Control Release *2016;**240**:24–37 and Huang D, Chen YS, Rupenthal ID. Overcoming ocular drug delivery barriers through the use of physical forces.* Adv Drug Deliv Rev *2018;**126**:96–112.*

which makes difficult for particles and drugs to penetrate. Permeation to the dermis allows the drugs to interact with keratinocytes and immunologically active cells that can translocate them to lymphatic and blood vessels in the dermis, providing a route for systemic circulation.[137]

6.6.2 Applications

Dermal and transdermal routes of nanocarriers have been applied for local delivery, antiseptic creams, gene delivery, vaccines, treatment of hair disorders, nanodiagnostics, and systemic delivery. Nanocarriers used include liposomes, solid lipid NPs, polymeric NPs, quantum dots, magnetic NPs, etc.[139] Topical delivery of all-trans-retinol using a silica-coated lecithin/oleylamine emulsion showed sustained release and improved stability of the compound and promoted skin retention evaluated in porcine skin.[140] The delivery of local anesthetics to the skin based on liposomes, solid lipid NPs, hydrogels, and patches, as permeation enhancers are reviewed by de Araujo.[141] These NPs have been effectively delivered using matches as well as microneedles. For example, an antimicrobial wound dressing patch, using ethyl cellulose as matrix membrane, was fabricated with a colloidal suspension of silver NPs and diethyl phthalate as the plasticizer. The patch showed no interaction between the matrix and NP and presented a controlled release of silver over 12 h.[142] PVA-based polymer films were studied for dermal delivery of macromolecules and NPs upon physical stimulus of laser microporation into pig skin, demonstrating that a microporation–patch combination could be an option for cutaneous immunization.[143] Transdermal drug delivery systems that utilize transcutaneous patches of arrayed microneedles have attracted increasing interest in medical practice as an alternative method to hypodermic injection. For example, anti-PD-1 was encapsulated along with glucose oxidase in hyaluronic acid combined with pH-sensitive dextran NP microneedle (MN) transdermal patch for the treatment of melanoma. The study showed enhanced immune response in mouse melanoma model using induced release from MN as opposed to passive release or free aPD1 injection dose.[144] Current designs, fabrication, materials, and use of polymeric microneedles for transdermal protein delivery have been reviewed elsewhere.[145] Finally, the lotion-like formulation for transdermal delivery of micellar NP estradiol emulsion (MNPEE), an FDA-approved product, represents a safe and effective commercial validation of nanocarrier technology for transdermal hormone therapy.[146] More examples can be found in Table 6.1.

6.6.3 Challenges, advantages, and limitations

In dermal delivery, therapeutics can be delivered at a controlled rate, which minimizes frequent dosing administration and results in lower infections rates, which lead to increased patient acceptance and compliance.[119,136,147] Even though there are advantages of dermal delivery, it also has limitations, some of them associated with penetration and enzymatic barriers. In addition, not all the drugs are suitable for transdermal delivery. Molecules with high molecular weights have a hard time penetrating the layers of the skin. Also, some formulations and patches can cause irritation and sensitization, leading to discomfort of patients. Because of slow release and adsorption, dermally delivered therapeutics are not suitable for the rapid onset of action therapeutics. Therapeutics with high permeability must comply with the low dose/high permeability factor, where the best candidates have a dose less than 10 mg, log $P_{o/w}$ of 2–3, and molecular weight less than 400 Da.[148,149] Since the absorption of drugs in the skin is highly limited by the stratum corneum, advances in transdermal delivery depend on their ability to overcome the barriers and challenges associated to permeation and skin irritation.

Many studies have shown that physicochemical properties such as lipophilicity, particle size, charge, morphology, and material composition are impact nanocarrier penetration in the skin.[135] Alternation of the penetration pathways has drawn increased interest in the case of hydrophilic compounds and macromolecules such as proteins or carrier systems. Evidence also shows that the hair follicle cavity can act as targeted site for enhanced penetration and absorption of topically applied substances.[139] A study by Shim et al.[150] showed the size dependence of NP penetration when applied to guinea pig skin, where 40-nm NPs diffused 1.5-fold more than 130 nm NPs. Interestingly, in this same study, they evaluated penetration into hair-less guinea pig skin and found no difference, suggesting the importance of the hair follicle in the pathway for transdermal delivery. Some studies showed that pretreatment of the skin can enhance the penetration of nanocarriers.[151] In this study, ultrasound and sodium lauryl sulfate were used as pretreatments on guinea pig skin, which greatly enhanced the penetration of charged quantum dots (QDs). In addition, among the two cationic QDs tested, the least cationic one showed improved penetration, suggesting that an optimal charge is needed for skin penetration. Due to the uncertain quantity absorbed in the skin for each particular formulation, the optimal dose to be administered is highly dependent on understanding of the penetration rate through the epidermis and translocation to the blood vessels in the dermis. Studies that can provide information about the rate of penetration and diffusion are ongoing to correlate to concentrations available in the systemic circulation.[147]

6.6.4 Future opportunities

Novel techniques and engineered drug formulations are necessary to overcome the skin barriers for dermal delivery. The enhancement in permeation and reduction of skin irritation would enlarge the market for hydrophilic compounds, macromolecules, and conventional drugs for new therapeutic applications in dermal delivery.[152] The challenges faced in this route of delivery open the opportunity for more targeted delivery of nanocarriers to hair follicle openings, as they show a promising pathway for local and systemic delivery.[153]

6.7 Ocular delivery

Ocular drug delivery involves the administration of therapeutics to the eye. Ocular drug delivery systems remain to be one of the more challenging products to develop, given the complexity of the eye.[154,155] Ocularly administered formulations face a variety of fates and barriers (see Fig. 6.4B) that are heavily dependent on the adsorption of the systems to the cornea in addition to transport through the cornea.[156,157] Once adsorbed to the cornea, products will engage in passive or transporter-mediated diffusion.[155,156] Diffusion and penetration of drugs into the multiple layers of the eye is also reliant on the polarity of the system. Prior to diffusion through the cornea, products must initially diffuse through the tear film barrier, which consists of lipid, aqueous, and mucosal layers.[158] The cornea (or corneal barrier) itself is made up of epithelial, stroma, and endothelial cells.[159] The combined barriers create an alternating polarity obstacle, making diffusion a significant challenge.[158,160] Nanotechnologies that are lipid based and oil/water emulsion based have shown the greatest level of promise in ocular delivery due to their ability to diffuse through the multipolar layering while possessing the abilities to adhere to both the mucus layer of the tear film barrier and the cornea.[155,158,160]

6.7.1 Current challenges and advantages

Due to the complex anatomy of the eye, many challenges arise when developing ocular systems. Traditionally, administration of therapeutics to the eye is either topical, systemic, or periocular. Topically administered products (i.e., eye drops) involve approximately 90% of all ocular products.[160–162] Drainage, blinking, and lacrimation all stand as major challenges for topically administered products. However, once topical products are administered to the eye, they interact with the cornea immediately. Reflex blinking and tear formation become obstacles, as the product needs to withstand both sheering force and lubricated movement.[163,164] Additionally, a mucosal layer also exists and functions similarly to mucus in both the GI and pulmonary tracts.[158,160,163] Aside from the cornea, both the blood–aqueous–barrier and blood–retinal–barrier exist, making the transport of drugs heavily dependent on their polarity.[160,163,165] In total, it is estimated that less than 5% of an administered drug will successfully be absorbed through the cornea and that 0.001% of an administered drug will reach the posterior region, making treatment of posterior diseases even more difficult.[166,167] Although intravitreal and subconjunctival administration are useable routes of drug administration that provide a high concentration of drug localization, due to the frequent dosing required to maintain a relevant concentration of the therapeutic, they are not considered to be viable options.[166,168] The major advantage of ocular drug delivery systems is the localized administration of the therapeutic to the eye.[156,169] Although the anatomy and dynamic environment of the eye pose numerous obstacles, localized delivery has shown decreased systemic side effects and increased therapeutic outcomes in comparison with systemic administration of therapeutics for ocular diseases.[155]

6.7.2 Applications

Research in ocular drug delivery has involved the use of hydrogel systems and nanotechnology. Hydrogel systems have been a major interest, primarily due to their longevity once administered (i.e., contact lenses). Hydrogel systems that are mucoadhesive (chitosan), biocompatible (Eudragit, PLGA), and/or biodegradable (alginate) are able to withstand some of the initial mechanical obstacles when first administered.[163] Nanotechnologies, having a size advantage, are able to diffuse through the multiple layers of the eye to reach their intended site, if designed correctly.[168] Studies suggest that lipid-based carriers show the greatest level of promise for ocular delivery systems, likely due to their ability to initially penetrate the cornea.[158,166] Additionally, lipid–polymer hybrid NPs have shown equal amounts of promise. In some studies, hydrogels and nanotechnologies have been combined to form a depot system that utilizes the structural integrity of the hydrogel with the penetration capabilities of nanotechnologies.[161,168,170] Currently, only a few nanoscale products exist for the treatment of ocular diseases. A major focus has been on the use of lipid-based formulations to aid in the transport across the cornea. Additionally, cationic products have been used to increase the adsorption to the cornea via electrostatic interactions. However, most lipid-based ocular products currently on market are used to treat dry eye syndrome. Ocular products, in general, are solutions or suspensions and range from antiinflammatory to antibiotic products.[8,11]

6.8 Conclusions

Nanocarriers offer many exciting opportunities and advantages for drug delivery applications across a variety of administration routes. As mentioned previously, each administration route comes with its own positive attributes, challenges, and barriers and the successful implementation of nanocarriers in the given applications will only be possible with careful design and particle engineering. One must consider not only the nanocarrier properties, materials, and loaded therapeutics but also the cellular and noncellular barriers present in the administration route, safety and ease of delivery, efficacy in vitro and in vivo, and stability of the particles. Overall, the utilization of nanocarriers offers exciting and virtually unlimited opportunities for the treatment of a multitude of diseases and the exploration of new diagnostics modalities.

References

1. Gulati N, Gupta H. *Parenteral drug Delivery: a review*. 2011. p. 133–45.
2. Shi Y, Li L. Current advances in sustained-release systems for parenteral drug delivery. *Expert Opin Drug Deliv* 2005;**2**:1039–58.
3. Teekamp N, Duque LF, Frijlink HW, Hinrichs WL, Olinga P. Production methods and stabilization strategies for polymer-based nanoparticles and microparticles for parenteral delivery of peptides and proteins. *Expert Opin Drug Deliv* 2015;**12**:1311–31.
4. Almeida AJ, Souto E. Solid lipid nanoparticles as a drug delivery system for peptides and proteins. *Adv Drug Deliv Rev* 2007;**59**:478–90.
5. Gamazo C, Prior S, Concepción Lecároz M, Vitas AI, Campanero MA, Pérez G, Gonzalez D, Blanco-Prieto MJ. Biodegradable gentamicin delivery systems for parenteral use for the treatment of intracellular bacterial infections. *Expert Opin Drug Deliv* 2007;**4**:677–88.
6. Luo C, Sun J, Du Y, He Z. Emerging integrated nanohybrid drug delivery systems to facilitate the intravenous-to-oral switch in cancer chemotherapy. *J Control Release* 2014;**176**:94–103.
7. Reddy LH, Bazile D. Drug delivery design for intravenous route with integrated physicochemistry, pharmacokinetics and pharmacodynamics: illustration with the case of taxane therapeutics. *Adv Drug Deliv Rev* 2014;**71**:34–57.
8. Bobo D, Robinson KJ, Islam J, Thurecht KJ, Corrie SR. Nanoparticle-based medicines: a review of FDA-approved materials and clinical trials to date. *Pharm Res* 2016;**33**:2373–87.
9. Albanese A, Tang PS, Chan WCW. The effect of nanoparticle size, shape, and surface chemistry on biological systems. *Annu Rev Biomed Eng* 2012;**14**:1–16.
10. Fornaguera C, Calderó G, Mitjans M, Vinardell MP, Solans C, Vauthier C. Interactions of PLGA nanoparticles with blood components: protein adsorption, coagulation, activation of the complement system and hemolysis studies. *Nanoscale* 2015;**7**(14):6045–58.
11. Anselmo AC, Mitragotri S. Nanoparticles in the clinic. *Bioeng Transl Med* 2016;**1**:10–29.
12. Rafiei P, Haddadi A. Docetaxel-loaded PLGA and PLGA-PEG nanoparticles for intravenous application: pharmacokinetics and biodistribution profile. *Int J Nanomed* 2017;**12**:935–47.
13. Honary S, Zahir F. Effect of zeta potential on the properties of nano-drug delivery systems - a review (Part 1). *Trop J Pharm Res* 2013;**12**:255–64.
14. Honary S, Zahir F. Effect of zeta potential on the properties of nano - drug delivery systems - a review (part 2). *Trop J Pharm Al Res* 2013;**12**:265–73.
15. Bagalkot V, Deiuliis JA, Rajagopalan S, Maiseyeu A. "Eat me" imaging and therapy. *Adv Drug Deliv Rev* 2016;**99**:2–11.
16. Qie Y, Yuan H, von Roemeling CA, Chen Y, Liu X, Shih KD, Knight JA, Tun HW, Wharen RE, Jiang W, Kim BY. Surface modification of nanoparticles enables selective evasion of phagocytic clearance by distinct macrophage phenotypes. *Sci Rep* 2016;**6**:26269.
17. Suk JS, Xu Q, Kim N, Hanes J, Ensign LM. PEGylation as a strategy for improving nanoparticle-based drug and gene delivery. *Adv Drug Deliv Rev* 2016;**99**:28–51.
18. Gratton SEA, Ropp PA, Pohlhaus PD, Luft JC, Madden VJ, Napier ME, Desimone JM. The effect of particle design on cellular internalization pathways. *Proc Natl Acad Sci U S A* 2008;**105**.
19. Ajorlou E, Khosroushahi AY. Trends on polymer- and lipid-based nanostructures for parenteral drug delivery to tumors. *Cancer Chemother Pharmacol* 2017;**79**:251–65.
20. Xi A, Bothun GD. Centrifugation-based assay for examining nanoparticle-lipid membrane binding and disruption. *Analyst* 2014;**139**(5):973–81.
21. Ventola CL. Progress in nanomedicine: approved and investigational nanodrugs. *PT* 2017;**42**:742–55.
22. Gupta N, Hatoum H, Dy GK. First line treatment of advanced non-small-cell lung cancer - specific focus on albumin bound paclitaxel. *Int J Nanomed* 2014;**9**:209–21.
23. Tyagi P, Subramony JA. Nanotherapeutics in oral and parenteral drug delivery: key learnings and future outlooks as we think small. *J Control Release* 2018;**272**:159–68.
24. Oliveira CL, Veiga F, Varela C, Roleira F, Tavares E, Silveira I, Ribeiro AJ. Characterization of polymeric nanoparticles for intravenous delivery: focus on stability. *Colloids Surf B Biointerfaces* 2017;**150**:326–33.
25. Hunt H, Simón-Gracia L, Tobi A, Teesalu T, Kotamraju VR, Sharma S, Sugahara KN, Ruoslahti E, Teesalu T, Nigul M, Sugahara KN. Targeting of p32 in peritoneal carcinomatosis with intraperitoneal linTT1 peptide-guided pro-apoptotic nanoparticles. *J Control Release* 2017;**260**:142–53.
26. Colby AH, Oberlies NH, Pearce CJ, Herrera VLM, Colson YL, Grinstaff MW. Nanoparticle drug-delivery systems for peritoneal cancers: a case study of the design, characterization and development of the expansile nanoparticle. *Wiley Interdiscip Rev Nanomed Nanobiotechnol* 2017;**9**:1–20.
27. Dakwar GR, Zagato E, Delanghe J, Hobel S, Aigner A, Denys H, Braeckmans K, Ceelen W, De Smedt SC, Remaut K. Colloidal stability of nano-sized particles in the peritoneal fluid: towards optimizing drug delivery systems for intraperitoneal therapy. *Acta Biomater* 2014;**10**(7):2965–75.
28. Nowacki M, Peterson M, Kloskowski T, McCabe E, Guiral DC, Polom K, Pietkun K, Zegarska B, Pokrywczynska M, Drewa T, Roviello F, Medina EA, Habib SL, Zegarski W. *Nanoparticle as a novel tool in hyperthermic intraperitoneal and pressurized intra-peritoneal aerosol chemotheprapy to treat patients with peritoneal carcinomatosis*. Oncotarget; 2017.
29. Xu S, Fan H, Yin L, Zhang J, Dong A, Deng L, Tang H. Thermosensitive hydrogel system assembled by PTX-loaded copolymer nanoparticles for sustained intraperitoneal chemotherapy of peritoneal carcinomatosis. *Eur J Pharm Biopharm* 2016;**104**:251–9.
30. Williamson SK, Johnson GA, Maulhardt HA, Moore KM, McMeekin DS, Schulz TK, Reed GA, Roby KF, MacKay CB, Smith HJ, Weir SJ, Wick JA, Markman M, Dizerega GS, Baltezor MJ, Espinosa J, Decedue CJ. A phase i study of intraperitoneal nanoparticulate paclitaxel (Nanotax®) in patients with peritoneal malignancies. *Cancer Chemother Pharmacol* 2015;**75**:1075–87.

31. Sun B, Taha MS, Ramsey B, Torregrosa-Allen S, Elzey BD, Yeo Y. Intraperitoneal chemotherapy of ovarian cancer by hydrogel depot of paclitaxel nanocrystals. *J Control Release* 2016;**235**:91–8.
32. Deng Y, Yang F, Cocco E, Song E, Zhang J, Cui J, Mohideen M, Bellone S, Santin AD, Saltzman WM. Improved i.p. drug delivery with bioadhesive nanoparticles. *Proc Natl Acad Sci* 2016;**113**:11453–8.
33. Dasa SSK, Diakova G, Suzuki R, Mills AM, Gutknecht MF, Klibanov AL, Slack-Davis JK, Kelly KA. Plectin-targeted liposomes enhance the therapeutic efficacy of a PARP inhibitor in the treatment of ovarian cancer. *Theranostics* 2018;**8**(10):2782–98.
34. Wu C-C, Yang Y-C, Hsu Y-T, Wu T-C, Hung C-F, Huang J-T, Chang C-L. Nanoparticle-induced intraperitoneal hyperthermia and targeted photoablation in treating ovarian cancer. *Oncotarget* 2015;**6**:26861–75.
35. Ye H, Karim AA, Loh XJ. Current treatment options and drug delivery systems as potential therapeutic agents for ovarian cancer: a review. *Mater Sci Eng C* 2015;**45**:609–19.
36. Mikolajczyk A, Khosrawipour V, Schubert J, Chaudhry H, Pigazzi A, Khosrawipour T. Particle stability during pressurized intra-peritoneal aerosol chemotherapy (PIPAC). *Anticancer Res* 2018;**38**:4645–9.
37. Solaß W, Giger-Pabst U, Zieren J, Reymond MA. Pressurized intraperitoneal aerosol chemotherapy (PIPAC): occupational health and safety aspects. *Ann Surg Oncol* 2013;**20**:3504–11.
38. Bagley AF, Hill S, Rogers GS, Bhatia SN. Plasmonic photothermal heating of intraperitoneal tumors through the use of an implanted near-infrared source. *ACS Nano* 2013;**7**:8089–97.
39. Vaccine Recommendations and Guidelines of the ACIP; (n.d.). https://www.Cdc.Gov/Vaccines/Hcp/Acip-Recs/General-Recs/Administration.Html.
40. ud Din F, Kim DW, Choi JY, Thapa RK, Mustapha O, Kim DS, Oh YK, Ku SK, Youn YS, Oh KT, Yong CS, Kim JO, Choi HG. Irinotecan-loaded double-reversible thermogel with improved antitumor efficacy without initial burst effect and toxicity for intramuscular administration. *Acta Biomater* 2017;**54**:239–48.
41. Wright L, Rao S, Thomas N, Boulos RA, Prestidge CA. Ramizol®encapsulation into extended release PLGA micro- and nanoparticle systems for subcutaneous and intramuscular administration: in vitro and in vivo evaluation. *Drug Dev Ind Pharm* 2018;**44**:1451–7.
42. Dewangan HK, Pandey T, Maurya L, Singh S. Rational design and evaluation of HBsAg polymeric nanoparticles as antigen delivery carriers. *Int J Biol Macromol* 2018;**111**:804–12.
43. Gonzalez-Aramundiz JV, Peleteiro Olmedo M, Gonzalez-Fernandez A, Alonso Fernandez MJ, Csaba NS. Protamine-based nanoparticles as new antigen delivery systems. *Eur J Pharm Biopharm* 2015;**97**:51–9.
44. Darville N, Van Heerden M, Erkens T, De Jonghe S, Vynckier A, De Meulder M, Vermeulen A, Sterkens P, Annaert P, Van Den Mooter G. Modeling the time course of the tissue responses to intramuscular long-acting paliperidone palmitate nano-/microcrystals and polystyrene microspheres in the rat. *Toxicol Pathol* 2016;**44**:189–210.
45. Xie B, Liu Y, Guo Y, Zhang E, Pu C, He H, Yin T, Tang X. Progesterone PLGA/mPEG-PLGA hybrid nanoparticle sustained-release system by intramuscular injection. *Pharm Res* 2018;**35**(3):62.
46. Darville N, Van Heerden M, Vynckier A, De Meulder M, Sterkens P, Annaert P, Van Den Mooter G. Intramuscular administration of paliperidone palmitate extended-release injectable microsuspension induces a subclinical inflammatory reaction modulating the pharmacokinetics in rats. *J Pharm Sci* 2014;**103**:2072–87.
47. Caputo A, Castaldello A, Brocca-Cofano E, Voltan R, Bortolazzi F, Altavilla G, Sparnacci K, Laus M, Tondelli L, Gavioli R, Ensoli B. Induction of humoral and enhanced cellular immune responses by novel core-shell nanosphere- and microsphere-based vaccine formulations following systemic and mucosal administration. *Vaccine* 2009;**27**:3605–15.
48. Lu F, Mencia A, Bi L, Taylor A, Yao Y, HogenEsch H. Dendrimer-like alpha-d-glucan nanoparticles activate dendritic cells and are effective vaccine adjuvants. *J Control Release* 2015;**204**:51–9.
49. Ogston-Tuck S. Subcutaneous injection technique: an evidence-based approach. *Nurs Stand* 2014;**29**:53–8.
50. McLennan DN, Porter CJH, Charman SA. Subcutaneous drug delivery and the role of the lymphatics. *Drug Discov Today Technol* 2005;**2**:89–96.
51. Singh Y, Srinivas A, Gangwar M, Meher JG, Misra-Bhattacharya S, Chourasia MK. Subcutaneously administered ultrafine PLGA nanoparticles containing doxycycline hydrochloride target lymphatic filarial parasites. *Mol Pharm* 2016;**13**:2084–94.
52. Trevaskis NL, Kaminskas LM, Porter CJH. From sewer to saviour-targeting the lymphatic system to promote drug exposure and activity. *Nat Rev Drug Discov* 2015;**14**:781–803.
53. Viola M, Sequeira J, Seiça R, Veiga F, Serra J, Santos AC, Ribeiro AJ. Subcutaneous delivery of monoclonal antibodies: how do we get there? *J Control Release* 2018;**286**:301–14.
54. Zhu S, Li X, Lansakara-P DSP, Kumar A, Cui Z. A nanoparticle depot formulation of 4-(N)-stearoyl gemcitabine shows a strong antitumour activity. *J Pharm Pharmacol* 2013;**65**:236–42.
55. Mandal S, Prathipati PK, Kang G, Zhou Y, Yuan Z, Fan W, Li Q, Destache CJ. Tenofovir alafenamide and elvitegravir loaded nanoparticles for long-acting prevention of HIV-1 vaginal transmission. *Aids* 2017;**31**:469–76.
56. Gautier JC, Grangier JL, Barbier A, Dupont P, Dussossoy D, Pastor G, Couvreur P. Biodegradable nanoparticles for subcutaneous administration of growth hormone releasing factor (hGRF). *J Control Release* 1992;**20**:67–77.
57. Jogala S, Chinnala KM, Aukunuru J. Novel subcutaneous sustained release nanoparticles encapsulating low molecular weight heparin (LMWH): preparation, characterization and evaluation. *Int J Pharm Pharm Sci* 2016;**8**:264–8.
58. Jean M, Smaoui F, Lavertu M, Méthot S, Bouhdoud L, Buschmann MD, Merzouki A. Chitosan-plasmid nanoparticle formulations for IM and SC delivery of recombinant FGF-2 and PDGF-BB or generation of antibodies. *Gene Ther* 2009;**16**:1097–110.
59. Schumann C, Nguyen DX, Norgard M, Bortnyak Y, Korzun T, Chan S, St Lorenz A, Moses AS, Albarqi HA, Wong L, Michaelis K, Zhu X, Alani AWG, Taratula OR, Krasnow S, Marks DL, Taratula O. Increasing lean muscle mass in mice via nanoparticle-mediated hepatic delivery of follistatin mRNA. *Theranostics* 2018;**8**:5276–88.
60. Parvathy S,.Sreeja CN,.Vidhya V, Nimitha V. Leflunomide loaded solid lipid nanoparticle in rheumatoid 2017;**9**:29681–29706.
61. Pandey R, Khuller GK. Subcutaneous nanoparticle-based antitubercular chemotherapy in an experimental model. *J Antimicrob Chemother* 2004;**54**:266–8.

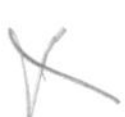

62. Turner MR, V Balu-Iyer S. Challenges and opportunities for the subcutaneous delivery of therapeutic proteins. *J Pharm Sci* 2018;**107**:1247–60.
63. Date AA, Hanes J, Ensign LM. Nanoparticles for oral delivery: design, evaluation and state-of-the-art. *J Control Release* 2016;**240**:504–26.
64. Khutoryanskiy VV. Beyond PEGylation: alternative surface-modification of nanoparticles with mucus-inert biomaterials. *Adv Drug Deliv Rev* 2017;**124**:140–9.
65. Lundquist P, Artursson P. Oral absorption of peptides and nanoparticles across the human intestine: opportunities, limitations and studies in human tissues. *Adv Drug Deliv Rev* 2016;**106**(Pt B):256–76.
66. Yu F, Li Y, Liu CS, Chen Q, Wang GH, Guo W, Wu XE, Li DH, Wu WD, Chen XD. Enteric-coated capsules filled with mono-disperse micro-particles containing PLGA-lipid-PEG nanoparticles for oral delivery of insulin. *Int J Pharm* 2015;**484**(1-2):181–91.
67. Alai MS, Lin WJ, Pingale SS. Application of polymeric nanoparticles and micelles in insulin oral delivery. *J Food Drug Anal* 2015;**23**(3):351–8.
68. García-Díaz M, Foged C, Nielsen HM. Improved insulin loading in poly(lactic-co-glycolic) acid (PLGA) nanoparticles upon self-assembly with lipids. *Int J Pharm* 2015;**482**(102):84–91.
69. Liu Y, Yang T, Wei S, Zhou C, Lan Y, Cao A, Yang J, Wang W. Mucus adhesion- and penetration-enhanced liposomes for paclitaxel oral delivery. *Int J Pharm* 2018;**537**(1-2):245–56.
70. Malathi S, Nandhakumar P, Pandiyan V, Webster TJ, Balasubramanian S. Novel PLGA-based nanoparticles for the oral delivery of insulin. *Int J Nanomedicine* 2015;**10**:2207–18.
71. Tan Z, Liu W, Liu H, Li C, Zhang Y, Meng X, Tang T, Xi T, Xing Y. Oral *Helicobacter pylori* vaccine-encapsulated acid-resistant HP55/PLGA nanoparticles promote immune protection. *Eur J Pharm Biopharm* 2017;**111**:33–43.
72. Crater JS, Carrier RL. Barrier properties of gastrointestinal mucus to nanoparticle transport. *Macromol Biosci* 2010;**10**:1473–83.
73. Lock JY, Carlson TL, Carrier RL. Mucus models to evaluate the diffusion of drugs and particles. *Adv Drug Deliv Rev* 2017;**124**:34–49.
74. Junghanns JUAH, Müller RH. Nanocrystal technology, drug delivery and clinical applications. *Int J Nanomedicine* 2008;**3**:295–309.
75. Lucio D, Martínez-Ohárriz MC, Gu Z, He Y, Aranaz P, Vizmanos JL, Irache JM. Cyclodextrin-grafted poly(anhydride) nanoparticles for oral glibenclamide administration. In vivo evaluation using *C. elegans*. *Int J Pharm* 2018;**547**(1-2):97–105.
76. Shazly GA, Alshehri S, Ibrahim MA, Tawfeek HM, Razik JA, Hassan YA, Shakeel F. Development of domperidone solid lipid nanoparticles: in vitro and in vivo characterization. *AAPS PharmSciTech* 2018.
77. Lozoya-Agullo I, Araújo F, González-Álvarez I, Merino-Sanjuán M, González-Álvarez M, Bermejo M, Sarmento B. PLGA nanoparticles are effective to control the colonic release and absorption on ibuprofen. *Eur J Pharm Sci* 2018;**115**:119–25.
78. Wang J, Li L, Wu L, Sun B, Du Y, Sun J, Wang Y, Fu Q, Zhang P, He Z. Development of novel self-assembled ES-PLGA hybrid nanoparticles for improving oral absorption of doxorubicin hydrochloride by P-gp inhibition: in vitro and in vivo evaluation. *Eur J Pharm Sci* 2017;**99**:185–92.
79. El-Say KM, El-Sawy HS. Polymeric nanoparticles: promising platform for drug delivery. *Int J Pharm* 2017;**528**:675–91.
80. Fabiano A, Piras AM, Uccello-Barretta G, Balzano F, Cesari A, Testai L, Citi V, Zambito Y. Impact of mucoadhesive polymeric nanoparticulate systems on oral bioavailability of a macromolecular model drug. *Eur J Pharm Biopharm* 2018;**130**:281–9.
81. Tian H, He Z, Sun C, Yang C, Zhao P, Liu L, Leong KW, Mao HQ, Liu Z, Chen Y. Uniform core-shell nanoparticles with thiolated hyaluronic acid coating to enhance oral delivery of insulin. *Adv Healthc Mater* 2018;**7**(17):e1800285.
82. Zhao M, Lee SH, Song JG, Kim HY, Han HK. Enhanced oral absorption of sorafenib via the layer-by-layer deposition of a pH-sensitive polymer and glycol chitosan on the liposome. *Int J Pharm* 2018;**544**(1):14–20.
83. Yhee JY, Im J, Nho RS. Advanced therapeutic strategies for chronic lung disease using nanoparticle-based drug delivery. *J Clin Med* 2016;**5**:82.
84. Al-Qadi S, Grenha A, Carrion-Recio D, Seijo B, Remuñan-Lopez C. Microencapsulated chitosan nanoparticles for pulmonary protein delivery: in vivo evaluation of insulin-loaded formulations. *J Control Release* 2012;**157**:383–90.
85. Bailey MM, Berkland CJ. Nanoparticle formulations in pulmonary drug delivery. *Med Res Rev* 2009;**29**:196–212.
86. Ngan CL, Asmawi AA. Lipid-based pulmonary delivery system: a review and future considerations of formulation strategies and limitations. *Drug Deliv Transl Res* 2018;**8**:1527–44.
87. Standring S, Gray H. *Gray's anatomy: the anatomical basis of clinical practice*. Edinburgh: Churchill Livingstone/Elsevier; 2008 [Chapter 57].
88. Echaide M, Autilio C, Arroyo R, Perez-Gil J. Restoring pulmonary surfactant membranes and films at the respiratory surface. *Biochim Biophys Acta Biomembr* 2017;**1859**:1725–39.
89. Ibrahim M, Verma R, Garcia-Contreras L. Inhalation drug delivery devices: technology update. *Med Devices* 2015;**8**:131–9.
90. Callard preedy E, Prokopovich P. 2 - history of inhaler devices. In: Prokopovich P, editor. *Inhaler devices*. Woodhead Publishing; 2013. p. 13–28.
91. Ali M. Chapter 9 – pulmonary drug delivery. In: Kulkarni VS, editor. *Handb. non-invasive drug deliv. syst.* Boston: William Andrew Publishing; 2010. p. 209–46.
92. Javadzadeh Y, Yaqoubi S. Chapter 20 – therapeutic nanostructures for pulmonary drug delivery. In: Andronescu E, Grumezescu AM, editors. *Nanostructures drug deliv.* Elsevier; 2017. p. 619–38.
93. Yang W, Peters JI, Williams RO. Inhaled nanoparticles—a current review. *Int J Pharm* 2008;**356**:239–47.
94. Karner S, Anne N. The impact of electrostatic charge in pharmaceutical powders with specific focus on inhalation-powders. *J Aerosol Sci* 2011;**42**:428–45.
95. Patil JS, Sarasija S. Pulmonary drug delivery strategies: a concise, systematic review. *Lung India* 2012;**29**:44–9.
96. Kuhn DA, Vanhecke D, Michen B, Blank F, Gehr P, Petri-Fink A, Rothen-Rutishauser B. Different endocytotic uptake mechanisms for nanoparticles in epithelial cells and macrophages. *Beilstein J Nanotechnol* 2014;**5**:1625–36.
97. Lee W-H, Loo C-Y, Traini D, Young PM. Inhalation of nanoparticle-based drug for lung cancer treatment: advantages and challenges. *Asian J Pharm Sci* 2015;**10**:481–9.

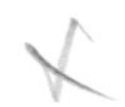

98. Youngren-Ortiz SR, Hill DB, Hoffmann PR, Morris KR, Barrett EG, Forest MG, Chougule MB. Development of optimized, inhalable, gemcitabine-loaded Gelatin nanocarriers for lung cancer. *J Aerosol Med Pulm Drug Deliv* 2017;**30**:299–321.
99. Gunday Tureli N, Torge A, Juntke J, Schwarz BC, Schneider-Daum N, Tureli AE, Lehr CM, Schneider M. Ciprofloxacin-loaded PLGA nanoparticles against cystic fibrosis *P. aeruginosa* lung infections. *Eur J Pharm Biopharm* 2017;**117**:363–71.
100. Makled S, Nafee N, Boraie N. Nebulized solid lipid nanoparticles for the potential treatment of pulmonary hypertension via targeted delivery of phosphodiesterase-5-inhibitor. *Int J Pharm* 2017;**517**:312–21.
101. Fernández Fernández E, Santos-Carballal B, de Santi C, Ramsey JM, MacLoughlin R, Cryan S-A, Greene CM. Biopolymer-based nanoparticles for cystic fibrosis lung gene therapy studies. *Mater (Basel, Switzerland)* 2018;**11**:122.
102. Mansour HM, Rhee YS, Wu X. Nanomedicine in pulmonary delivery. *Int J Nanomedicine* 2009;**4**:299–319.
103. Sancini G, Dal Magro R, Ornaghi F, Balducci C, Forloni G, Gobbi M, Salmona M, Re F. Pulmonary administration of functionalized nanoparticles significantly reduces beta-amyloid in the brain of an Alzheimer's disease murine model. *Nano Res* 2016;**9**:2190–201.
104. Loira-pastoriza C, Todoroff J, Vanbever R. Delivery strategies for sustained drug release in the lungs. *Adv Drug Deliv Rev* 2014;**75**:81–91.
105. Ruge CA, Kirch J, Lehr C-M. Pulmonary drug delivery: from generating aerosols to overcoming biological barriers—therapeutic possibilities and technological challenges. *Lancet Respir Med* 2013;**1**:402–13.
106. Fromen CA, Rahhal TB, Robbins GR, Kai MP, Shen TW, Luft JC, DeSimone JM. Nanoparticle surface charge impacts distribution, uptake and lymph node trafficking by pulmonary antigen-presenting cells. *Nanomedicine* 2016;**12**:677–87.
107. Craparo EF, Porsio B, Sardo C, Giammona G, Cavallaro G. Pegylated polyaspartamide-polylactide-based nanoparticles penetrating cystic fibrosis artificial mucus. *Biomacromolecules* 2016;**17**:767–77.
108. Thorley AJ, Ruenraroengsak P, Potter TE, Tetley TD. Critical determinants of uptake and translocation of nanoparticles by the human pulmonary alveolar epithelium. *ACS Nano* 2014;**8**:11778–117789.
109. Healy AM, Amaro MI, Paluch KJ, Tajber L. Dry powders for oral inhalation free of lactose carrier particles. *Adv Drug Deliv Rev* 2014;**75**:32–52.
110. Depreter F, Pilcer G, Amighi K. Inhaled proteins: challenges and perspectives. *Int J Pharm* 2013;**447**:251–80.
111. Huckaby JT, Lai SK. PEGylation for enhancing nanoparticle diffusion in mucus. *Adv Drug Deliv Rev* 2018;**124**:125–39.
112. V Khutoryanskiy V. Beyond PEGylation: alternative surface-modification of nanoparticles with mucus-inert biomaterials. *Adv Drug Deliv Rev* 2018;**124**:140–9.
113. Liu M, Zhang J, Shan W, Huang Y. Developments of mucus penetrating nanoparticles. *Asian J Pharm Sci* 2015;**10**:275–82.
114. Murata M, Yonamine T, Tanaka S, Tahara K, Tozuka Y, Takeuchi H. Surface modification of liposomes using polymer-wheat germ agglutinin conjugates to improve the absorption of peptide drugs by pulmonary administration. *J Pharm Sci* 2013;**102**:1281–9.
115. de Carvalho CS, Daum N, Lehr C-M. Carrier interactions with the biological barriers of the lung: advanced in vitro models and challenges for pulmonary drug delivery. *Adv Drug Deliv Rev* 2014;**75**:129–40.
116. Pires A, Fortuna A, Alves G, Falcao A. Intranasal drug delivery: how, why and what for? *J Pharm Pharm Sci* 2009;**12**:288–311.
117. Turker S, Onur E, Ozer Y. Nasal route and drug delivery systems. *Pharm World Sci* 2004;**26**:137–42.
118. Kumar A, Pandey AN, Jain SK. Nasal-nanotechnology: revolution for efficient therapeutics delivery. *Drug Deliv* 2016;**23**:671–83.
119. Patel A, Patel M, Yang X, Mitra AK. Recent advances in protein and Peptide drug delivery: a special emphasis on polymeric nanoparticles. *Protein Pept Lett* 2014;**21**:1102–20.
120. Djupesland PG. Nasal drug delivery devices: characteristics and performance in a clinical perspective-a review. *Drug Deliv Transl Res* 2013;**3**:42–62.
121. Illum L. Nanoparticulate systems for nasal delivery of drugs: a real improvement over simple systems? *J Pharm Sci* 2007;**96**:473–83.
122. Strandring S, Gray H. *Gray's anatomy: the anatomical basis of clinical practice*. Edinburgh. 2008 [Chapter 32].
123. Illum L. Is nose-to-brain transport of drugs in man a reality? *J Pharm Pharmacol* 2004;**56**:3–17.
124. Hayashi M, Hirasawa T, Muraoka T, Shiga M, Awazu S. Comparison of water influx and sieving coefficient in rat jejunal, rectal and nasal absorptions of antipyrine. *Chem Pharm Bull (Tokyo)* 1985;**33**:2149–52.
125. Casettari L, Illum L. Chitosan in nasal delivery systems for therapeutic drugs. *J Control Release* 2014;**190**:189–200.
126. Vila A, Sanchez A, Evora C, Soriano I, Vila Jato JL, Alonso MJ. PEG-PLA nanoparticles as carriers for nasal vaccine delivery. *J Aerosol Med* 2004;**17**:174–85.
127. Illum L, Jabbal-Gill I, Hinchcliffe M, Fisher AN, Davis SS. Chitosan as a novel nasal delivery system for vaccines. *Adv Drug Deliv Rev* 2001;**51**:81–96.
128. Jesus S, Soares E, Costa J, Borchard G, Borges O. Immune response elicited by an intranasally delivered HBsAg low-dose adsorbed to poly-ε-caprolactone based nanoparticles. *Int J Pharm* 2016;**504**:59–69.
129. Khademi F, Derakhshan M, Yousefi-Avarvand A, Najafi A, Tafaghodi M. A novel antigen of *Mycobacterium tuberculosis* and MPLA adjuvant co-entrapped into PLGA:DDA hybrid nanoparticles stimulates mucosal and systemic immunity. *Microb Pathog* 2018;**125**:507–13.
130. Bernocchi B, Carpentier R, Betbeder D. Nasal nanovaccines. *Int J Pharm* 2017;**530**:128–38.
131. Bi C, Wang A, Chu Y, Liu S, Mu H, Liu W, Wu Z, Sun K, Li Y. Intranasal delivery of rotigotine to the brain with lactoferrin-modified PEG-PLGA nanoparticles for Parkinson's disease treatment. *Int J Nanomedicine* 2016;**11**:6547–59.
132. Mistry A, Stolnik S, Illum L. Nose-to-Brain delivery: investigation of the transport of nanoparticles with different surface characteristics and sizes in excised porcine olfactory epithelium. *Mol Pharm* 2015;**12**:2755–66.
133. Md S, Bhattmisra SK, Zeeshan F, Shahzad N, Mujtaba MA, Srikanth Meka V, Radhakrishnan A, Kesharwani P, Baboota S, Ali J. Nano-carrier enabled drug delivery systems for nose to brain

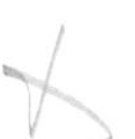

targeting for the treatment of neurodegenerative disorders. *J Drug Deliv Sci Technol* 2018;**43**:295−310.
134. Yang H. Nanoparticle-mediated brain-specific drug delivery, imaging, and diagnosis. *Pharm Res* 2010;**27**:1759−71.
135. Palmer BC, DeLouise LA. Nanoparticle-enabled transdermal drug delivery systems for enhanced dose control and tissue targeting. *Molecules* 2016;**21**.
136. Tomoda K, Makino K. Chapter 7 - nanoparticles for transdermal drug delivery system (TDDS). In: Ohshima H, Makino K, editors. *Colloid interface sci. Pharm. Res. Dev.* Amsterdam: Elsevier; 2014. p. 131−47.
137. Sewell MJ, Burkhart CN, Morrell DS. Dermatological pharmacology. In: Brunton LL, Hilal-Dandan R, Knollmann BC, editors. *Goodman & Gilman's pharmacol. basis ther.* New York, NY: McGraw-Hill Education; 2017. 13e.
138. Bos JD, Meinardi MM. The 500 Dalton rule for the skin penetration of chemical compounds and drugs. *Exp Dermatol* 2000;**9**:165−9.
139. Papakostas D, Rancan F, Sterry W, Blume-Peytavi U, Vogt A. Nanoparticles in dermatology. *Arch Dermatol Res* 2011;**303**:533−50.
140. Eskandar NG, Simovic S, Prestidge CA. Nanoparticle coated emulsions as novel dermal delivery vehicles. *Curr Drug Deliv* 2009;**6**:367−73.
141. de Araújo DR, da Silva DC, Barbosa RM, Franz-Montan M, Cereda CMS, Padula C, Santi P, de Paula E. Strategies for delivering local anesthetics to the skin: focus on liposomes, solid lipid nanoparticles, hydrogels and patches. *Expert Opin Drug Deliv* 2013;**10**:1551−63.
142. Suksaeree J, Thuengernthong A, Pongpichayasiri K, Maneewattanapinyo P, Settharaksa S, Pichayakorn W. Formulation and evaluation of matrix type transdermal patch containing silver nanoparticles. *J Polym Environ* 2018;**26**:4369−75.
143. Engelke L, Winter G, Engert J. Application of water-soluble polyvinyl alcohol-based film patches on laser microporated skin facilitates intradermal macromolecule and nanoparticle delivery. *Eur J Pharm Biopharm* 2018;**128**:119−30.
144. Wang C, Ye Y, Hochu GM, Sadeghifar H, Gu Z. Enhanced cancer immunotherapy by microneedle patch-assisted delivery of anti-PD1 antibody. *Nano Lett* 2016;**16**:2334−40.
145. Ye Y, Yu J, Wen D, Kahkoska AR, Gu Z. Polymeric microneedles for transdermal protein delivery. *Adv Drug Deliv Rev* 2018;**127**:106−18.
146. Valenzuela P, Simon JA. Nanoparticle delivery for transdermal HRT. *Maturitas* 2012;**73**:74−80.
147. Weiser JR, Saltzman WM. Controlled release for local delivery of drugs: barriers and models. *J Control Release* 2014;**190**:664−73.
148. Ranade V, Cannon J. *Drug delivery systems.* CRC Press; 2011.
149. Nanoparticles for dermal and transdermal drug delivery. In: Uchechi O, Ogbonna J, Attama A, Sezer A, editors. *Application of nanotechnology in drug delivery*; 2014.
150. Shim J, Seok Kang H, Park W-S, Han S-H, Kim J, Chang I-S. Transdermal delivery of mixnoxidil with block copolymer nanoparticles. *J Control Release* 2004;**97**:477−84.
151. Lopez RF, Seto JE, Blankschtein D, Langer R. Enhancing the transdermal delivery of rigid nanoparticles using the simultaneous application of ultrasound and sodium lauryl sulfate. *Biomaterials* 2011;**32**:933−41.
152. Paudel KS, Milewski M, Swadley CL, Brogden NK, Ghosh P, Stinchcomb AL. Challenges and opportunities in dermal/transdermal delivery. *Ther Deliv* 2010;**1**:109−31.
153. Prow TW, Grice JE, Lin LL, Faye R, Butler M, Becker W, Wurm EMT, Yoong C, Robertson TA, Soyer HP, Roberts MS. Nanoparticles and microparticles for skin drug delivery. *Adv Drug Deliv Rev* 2011;**63**:470−91.
154. Peynshaert K, Devoldere J, De Smedt SC, Remaut K. In vitro and ex vivo models to study drug delivery barriers in the posterior segment of the eye. *Adv Drug Deliv Rev* 2018;**126**:44−57.
155. Reimondez-Troitiño S, Csaba N, Alonso MJ, De La Fuente M. Nanotherapies for the treatment of ocular diseases. *Eur J Pharm Biopharm* 2015;**95**:279−93.
156. Gaudana R, Ananthula HK, Parenky A, Mitra AK. Ocular drug delivery. *AAPS J* 2010;**12**(3):348−60.
157. Puglia C, Blasi P, Ostacolo C, Sommella E, Bucolo C, Platania CBM, Romano GL, Geraci F, Drago F, Santonocito D, Albertini B, Campiglia P, Puglisi G, Pignatello R. Innovative nanoparticles enhance N-palmitoylethanolamide intraocular delivery. *Front Pharmacol* 2018;**9**:285.
158. Alvarez-Trabado J, Diebold Y, Sanchez A. Designing lipid nanoparticles for topical ocular drug delivery. *Int J Pharm* 2017;**532**(1):204−17.
159. Wang J, Zhao F, Liu R, Chen J, Zhang Q, Lao R, Wang Z, Jin X, Liu C. Novel cationic lipid nanoparticles as an ophthalmic delivery system for multicomponent drugs: development, characterization, in vitro permeation, in vivo pharmacokinetic, and molecular dynamics studies. *Int J Nanomed* 2017;**12**:8115−27.
160. Gan L, Wang J, Jiang M, Bartlett H, Ouyang D, Eperjesi F, Liu J, Gan Y. Recent advances in topical ophthalmic drug delivery with lipid-based nanocarriers. *Drug Discov Today* 2013;**18**(5-6):290−307.
161. Åhlén M, Tummala GK, Mihranyan A. Nanoparticle-loaded hydrogels as a pathway for enzyme-triggered drug release in ophthalmic applications. *Int J Pharm* 2018;**536**(1):73−81.
162. Lee CH, Li YJ, Huang CC, Lai JY. Poly(ε-caprolactone) nanocapsule carriers with sustained drug release: single dose for long-term glaucoma treatment. *Nanoscale* 2017;**9**(32):11754−64.
163. Imperiale JC, Acosta GB, Sosnik A. Polymer-based carriers for ophthalmic drug delivery. *J Control Release* 2018;**285**:106−41.
164. Salama AH, Mahmoud AA, Kamel R. A novel method for preparing surface-modified fluocinolone acetonide loaded PLGA nanoparticles for ocular use: in vitro and in vivo evaluations. *AAPS PharmSciTech* 2016;**17**(5):1159−72.
165. Janagam DR, Wu L, Lowe TL. Nanoparticles for drug delivery to the anterior segment of the eye. *Adv Drug Deliv Rev* 2016;**122**:31−64.
166. Nguyen H, Eng S, Ngo T, Dass CR. Delivery of therapeutics for deep-seated ocular conditions − status quo. *J Pharm Pharmacol* 2018;**70**(8):994−1001.
167. Rodríguez Villanueva J, Rodríguez Villanueva L, Guzmán Navarro M. Pharmaceutical technology can turn a traditional drug, dexamethasone into a first-line ocular medicine. A global perspective and future trends. *Int J Pharm* 2017;**516**:342−51.
168. Costa JR, Silva NC, Sarmento B, Pintado M. Potential chitosan-coated alginate nanoparticles for ocular delivery of daptomycin. *Eur J Clin Microbiol Infect Dis* 2015;**34**(6):1255−62.

169. Kamaleddin MA. Nano-ophthalmology: applications and considerations. *Nanomed Nanotechnol Biol Med* 2017;**13**(4):1459–72.
170. Shi Z, Li SK, Charoenputtakun P, Liu CY, Jasinski D, Guo P. RNA nanoparticle distribution and clearance in the eye after subconjunctival injection with and without thermosensitive hydrogels. *J Control Release* 2018;**270**:14–22.
171. Jose S, Juna BC, Cinu TA, Jyoti H, Aleykutty NA. Carboplatin loaded Surface modified PLGA nanoparticles: optimization, characterization, and in vivo brain targeting studies. *Colloids Surf B Biointerfaces* 2016.
172. Hollis CP, Weiss HL, Leggas M, Evers BM, Gemeinhart RA, Li T. Biodistribution and bioimaging studies of hybrid paclitaxel nanocrystals: lessons learned of the EPR effect and image-guided drug delivery. *J Control Release* 2013;**172**:12–21.
173. Verma NK, Crosbie-Staunton K, Satti A, Gallagher S, Ryan KB, Doody T, McAtamney C, MacLoughlin R, Galvin P, Burke CS, Volkov Y, Gun'ko YK. Magnetic core-shell nanoparticles for drug delivery by nebulization. *J Nanobiotechnol* 2013;**11**:1–12.
174. Gupta N, Ibrahim HM, Ahsan F. Peptide–micelle hybrids containing fasudil for targeted delivery to the pulmonary arteries and arterioles to treat pulmonary arterial hypertension. *J Pharm Sci* 2014;**103**:3743–53.
175. Nafee N, Husari A, Maurer CK, Lu C, de Rossi C, Steinbach A, Hartmann RW, Lehr C-M, Schneider M. Antibiotic-free nanotherapeutics: ultra-small, mucus-penetrating solid lipid nanoparticles enhance the pulmonary delivery and anti-virulence efficacy of novel quorum sensing inhibitors. *J Control Release* 2014;**192**:131–40.
176. Tong G-F, Qin N, Sun L-W. Development and evaluation of Desvenlafaxine loaded PLGA-chitosan nanoparticles for brain delivery. *Saudi Pharm J* 2017;**25**:844–51.
177. Amidi M, Romeijn SG, Borchard G, Junginger HE, Hennink WE, Jiskoot W. Preparation and characterization of protein-loaded N-trimethyl chitosan nanoparticles as nasal delivery system. *J Control Release* 2006;**111**:107–16.
178. Mahajan HS, Mahajan MS, Nerkar PP, Agrawal A. Nanoemulsion-based intranasal drug delivery system of saquinavir mesylate for brain targeting. *Drug Deliv* 2014;**21**:148–54.
179. Hopkins LE, Patchin ES, Chiu P-L, Brandenberger C, Smiley-Jewell S, Pinkerton KE. Nose-to-brain transport of aerosolised quantum dots following acute exposure. *Nanotoxicology* 2014;**8**:885–93.
180. Corace G, Angeloni C, Malaguti M, Hrelia S, Stein PC, Brandl M, Gotti R, Luppi B. Multifunctional liposomes for nasal delivery of the anti-Alzheimer drug tacrine hydrochloride. *J Liposome Res* 2014;**24**:323–35.
181. Augustine R, Ashkenazi DL, Arzi RS, Zlobin V, Shofti R, Sosnik A. Nanoparticle-in-microparticle oral drug delivery system of a clinically relevant darunavir/ritonavir antiretroviral combination. *Acta Biomater* 2018;**74**:344–59.
182. Chaves LL, Costa Lima SA, Vieira ACC, Barreiros L, Segundo MA, Ferreira D, Sarmento B, Reis S. Development of PLGA nanoparticles loaded with clofazimine for oral delivery: assessment of formulation variables and intestinal permeability. *Eur J Pharm Sci* 2018;**112**:28–37.
183. Tariq M, Alam MA, Singh AT, Iqbal Z, Panda AK, Talegaonkar S. Biodegradable polymeric nanoparticles for oral delivery of epirubicin: In vitro, ex vivo, and in vivo investigations. *Colloids Surf B Biointerfaces* 2015.
184. Marwah H, Garg T, Rath G, Goyal AK. Development of transferosomal gel for trans-dermal delivery of insulin using iodine complex. *Drug Deliv* 2016;**23**:1636–44.
185. Mitri K, Shegokar R, Gohla S, Anselmi C, Muller RH. Lipid nanocarriers for dermal delivery of lutein: preparation, characterization, stability and performance. *Int J Pharm* 2011;**414**:267–75.
186. Ryman-Rasmussen JP, Riviere JE, Monteiro-Riviere NA. Penetration of intact skin by quantum dots with diverse physicochemical properties. *Toxicol Sci* 2006;**91**:159–65.
187. Takeuchi I, Suzuki T, Makino K. Skin permeability and transdermal delivery route of 50-nm indomethacin-loaded PLGA nanoparticles. *Colloids Surfaces B Biointerfaces* 2017;**159**:312–7.
188. Matos BN, Reis TA, Gratieri T, Gelfuso GM. Chitosan nanoparticles for targeting and sustaining minoxidil sulphate delivery to hair follicles. *Int J Biol Macromol* 2015;**75**:225–9.
189. Li H, Liu Y, Zhang Y, Fang D, Xu B, Zhang L, Chen T, Ren K, Nie Y, Yao S, Song X. Liposomes as a novel ocular delivery system for Brinzolamide: in vitro and in vivo studies. *AAPS PharmSciTech* 2016;**17**(3):710–7.
190. Sánchez-López E, Egea MA, Davis BM, Guo L, Espina M, Silva AM, Calpena AC, Souto EMB, Ravindran N, Ettcheto M, Camins A, García ML, Cordeiro MF. Memantine-loaded PEGylated biodegradable nanoparticles for the treatment of glaucoma. *Small* 2018;**14**(2).
191. Liu D, Lian Y, Fang Q, Liu L, Zhang J, Li J. Hyaluronic-acid-modified lipid-polymer hybrid nanoparticles as an efficient ocular delivery platform for moxifloxacin hydrochloride. *Int J Biol Macromol* 2018;**116**:1023–36.
192. Ahmed TA, Aljaeid BM. Preparation, characterization, and potential application of chitosan, chitosan derivatives, and chitosan metal nanoparticles in pharmaceutical drug delivery. *Drug Des Devel Ther* 2016;**10**:483–507.
193. Daniher DI, Zhu J. Dry powder platform for pulmonary drug delivery. *Particuology* 2008;**6**:225–38.
194. Future MR. *Nasal drug delivery market 2018 scope by spray and nebulizers delivery technologies with leading companies profiles – ME&A forecast till 2022*. 2018.
195. Lee H, Song C, Baik S, Kim D, Hyeon T, Kim DH. Device-assisted transdermal drug delivery. *Adv Drug Deliv Rev* 2018;**127**:35–45.
196. *Overview of gastrointestinal tract*. 2018.
197. Samaridou E, Alonso MJ. Nose-to-brain peptide delivery – the potential of nanotechnology. *Bioorganic Med Chem* 2018;**26**:2888–905.
198. Yu M, Wu J, Shi J, Farokhzad OC. Nanotechnology for protein delivery: overview and perspectives. *J Control Release* 2016;**240**:24–37.
199. Huang D, Chen YS, Rupenthal ID. Overcoming ocular drug delivery barriers through the use of physical forces. *Adv Drug Deliv Rev* 2018;**126**:96–112.

Chapter 7

Challenges and barriers

Elizabeth Nance[1,2,3,4] and Michael McKenna[1]

[1]*Department of Chemical Engineering, University of Washington, Seattle, WA, United States;* [2]*Department of Radiology, University of Washington, Seattle WA, United States;* [3]*Center on Human Development and Disability, University of Washington, Seattle, WA, United States;* [4]*Molecular Engineering and Sciences Institute, University of Washington, Seattle, WA, United States*

7.1 Overview

Depending on the route of administration, the intended target site, and the desired action of a therapeutic, a nanoparticle delivery vehicle must overcome a multitude of barriers to have the intended on-target, on-site effect. This chapter focuses on these barriers, which are broadly grouped into surface, en-route, and cellular barriers. En-route barriers are further subdivided into (1) the barriers that exist in the process of nanoparticle absorption across an epithelium to transport to an endothelial barrier and (2) the barriers that exist for a nanoparticle to passage across an endothelial barrier to a target cell within an organ. This chapter also discusses the challenges presented by the physical and physiological barriers at each step of a nanoparticle's route to a target site. Lastly, we highlight key findings in the field for how nanoparticles can be designed to overcome these barriers.

7.2 Surface barriers

Nanoparticles administered into the human body via transdermal, oral, inhalation, intranasal, ocular, vaginal, or rectal delivery first encounter an epithelial layer. The ability of a nanoparticle to deliver an active drug molecule to a site for absorption often requires traversing this epithelial layer. This passage can be hampered by hostile environments, for example, as resembled in the intestinal tract lumen where there is high enzymatic and hydrolytic activity.

7.2.1 Skin

For transdermal nanodrug delivery systems, the first barrier encountered is the skin. The human skin is the largest organ in our body, with a surface area of 1.8–2.0 m^2 in the average adult. It is composed of three main layers: the epidermis, dermis, and hypodermis (subcutaneous layer).[1] The skin protects the body against environmental factors and regulates heat and water loss from the body. For drug delivery, the skin is an important route when topical, regional, and systemic effects are desired, and it is also useful for avoiding hepatic first-pass metabolism.[2] Drug permeation through the skin is usually limited by the stratum corneum, which is about 15–20 cell layers thick. Nanoparticles applied topically to the skin can access several routes of delivery, which include passage (1) across the intact stratum corneum, (2) through the hair follicles with the associated sebaceous glands, or (3) via the sweat glands.[3]

The most used and investigated nanocarriers for dermal/transdermal drug delivery include liposomes, transfersomes, ethosomes, niosomes, dendrimers, lipid and polymer nanoparticles, and nanoemulsions. However, transdermal delivery systems have been limited to certain carriers of a range of size, molecular weight, lipophilicity, and charge preference. To overcome the skin barrier, hydrophilic molecules diffuse predominantly "laterally" along surfaces of the less abundant water-filled interlamellar spaces or use the free space between a lamella and a corneocyte outer membrane. Transcellular diffusion is generally considered minimal for transdermal drug transport.[4] In regions of narrow aqueous transepidermal pathways, the presence of poor cellular and intercellular lipid packing coincides with wrinkles on the skin surface, and they are the sites of lowest skin resistance to the transport of hydrophilic entities. Transport through the follicles has recently become of greater interest, although follicular orifices occupy only 0.1% of the total skin surface area.[5] Investigations in ex vivo porcine skin and in vivo human skin have revealed that polystyrene nanoparticles

Nanoparticles for Biomedical Applications. https://doi.org/10.1016/B978-0-12-816662-8.00007-2

accumulate preferentially in the follicular openings in both species.[6–8] This distribution was increased in a time-dependent manner, and follicular localization was favored by smaller particle sizes. The current consensus in the field is that nanoparticles smaller than 20 nm can penetrate or permeate intact skin, while nanoparticles between 20 and 45 nm can penetrate damaged skin.[9] Larger particles can be translocated or may be stored in skin appendages.[2,9]

The skin carries a negative surface charge due to the presence of phosphatidylcholine and negatively charged groups on carbohydrates found in mammalian cells. Therefore, cationic compounds have a positive effect on skin permeation and nanoparticles with predominant positive charge would promote transdermal permeation.[10] Shape has also been identified as a factor that influences skin penetration. Rod-shaped particles have shown higher permeation in the skin than spherical particles.[11] Additional favorable physicochemical characteristics for transdermal delivery include a molecular weight less than approximately 500 Da and an affinity for both lipophilic and hydrophilic phases.[12]

7.2.2 Luminal space in the gastrointestinal and respiratory tracts

Nanoparticles administered to the respiratory or gastrointestinal tracts interact first with the luminal fluid. The luminal fluid is in contact with the surface of the mucus and varies in volume, dynamics, and composition. The luminal fluid in the small intestine is a dynamic mixture of enzymes, lipids, bile, bacteria, and cellular debris, with significant changes to the composition following food intake.[13] All of these components can interact with or influence the stability of a nanoparticle, altering the physicochemical properties of the nanoparticle. Further, the volume of the luminal fluid may affect the dissolution and distribution of the nanotherapeutic to the underlying mucosal layer. Importantly, the presence of enzymes in the luminal fluid can degrade a nanoparticle and the drug carried within the nanoparticle, prior to reaching the drug's site of action. The use of enteric coatings on nanoparticle formulations can provide protection from enzymatic degradation while transiting the gastrointestinal or respiratory tracts.[14]

7.2.3 Passage across the mucosal layer to underlying epithelium

For delivery to the nose, lung, eye, vaginal tract, rectum, or gastrointestinal tract, or administration methods that access these organs (e.g., intranasal, inhalation, oral delivery), a nanoparticle will encounter a mucosal layer prior to reaching the underlying epithelium.[15–18] The mucus constitutes a complex barrier to diffusion of nanoparticles toward the epithelial surface. Mucus is a viscoelastic hydrogel composed of large glycoproteins, predominantly of the mucin family.[19,20] Mucus production amounts to an average of 1 kg/day in an adult human. Mucus serves as an adhesive barrier to most foreign entities and also introduces steric hindrance and enzymatic activity that can impede or degrade a delivery vehicle.[19] The barrier properties, as discussed in this section, are variable throughout the body (Table 7.1) and also vary with patient age and health condition. The current understanding of the barrier properties of mucus are discussed in a recent review[21] and include an expert analysis on the effect on transport and therapeutic outcome.

The ability of nanoparticles to overcome the mucosal barrier and penetrate the mucosal layer has been extensively studied in recent years.[18,21,39,40] In general, the use of multiple particle tracking has shown that mucus has a pore cutoff size of 500 nm.[41] Spherical nanoparticles larger than 500 nm become sterically trapped, independent of surface chemistry. For smaller particles, surface chemistry can significantly impact nanoparticle mobility, retention, and transport to the underlying epithelium.[41–43] Mucus can bind nanoparticles and proteins via hydrophobic interactions.[44] Charged groups of the mucin proteins can also interact with charged particles and immobilize them in mucus.[45] The charge density in the mucus mesh depends on local ionic strength and pH. Under hypertonic conditions, charge interactions between mucus and particles will be partially shielded by ions in the fluid, reducing interactions below the levels seen in hypotonic fluids.[45] Negatively charged carboxylate- and sulfate-modified particles showed a higher transport rate than near neutral or positively charged amine-modified particles. The amine nanoparticle transport is limited by particle aggregation and electrostatic adhesive interaction with mucin fibers. The interactions of particle and mucus made by electrostatic–ionic interactions, van der Waals interactions, hydrophobic forces, and hydrogen bonding also influence nanoparticle retention at the mucosal surface.

7.2.3.1 Eye

In the eye, the cornea and conjunctiva epithelia are covered by surface mucins. Ocular mucins are both secreted and cell surface-associated, and are distributed throughout the corneal and conjunctival epithelia, goblet cells, and the lacrimal apparatus.[15] They have heterogeneous functions at the ocular surface including (1) clearance of allergens, pathogens, and debris; (2) lubrication; (3) antimicrobial activity; (4) surface protection against abrasive stress (boundary lubrication); and (5) formation of an apical cell surface barrier.[15,46] A topically applied drug delivery system can be rapidly removed from the ocular surface through blinking, which shears anything off the tear film

TABLE 7.1 Overview of properties of mucus that influence nanoparticle penetration and retention, where reported in literature.

Type of mucus	Average thickness (μm)	Reported thicknesses (μm)	Clearance time	Clearance rate (mm/min)	pH
Respiratory			10–20 min[22]	2–10[22–24]	
Nasal			8–9 min[25]	5–11[24]	6. 5[26]
Airway	15 [27]	7–30[28,29]		1–4[23]	7.0–9.0 (Trachea)[30]
Bronchial	55 [31]	50–60[31]		2–3[24]	7.0–9.0[30]
Gastrointestinal			2–6 h (Mouth to colon)[32]		
Gastric	189 [17]	160–200[17]			1.0–2.0[32,33]
Duodenum	170 [17]	140–200[17]			2.5–6[32,33]
Jejunum	123 [17]	115–125[17]			4.5–6.5[32,33]
Ileum	480 [17]	400–500[17]			7.0–8.0[32]
Colonic	830 [17]	700–900[17]	~Hours to days (for oral administration route)[32]		7.0–8.0[32]
Ocular			5–10 min[34]		7.0–7.4[32,35]
Mucus layer	0.035 [36]	0.02–0.05[36]			
Tear film	5 [37]	3–7[37]		1 μL/min34	~Slightly basic[36]
Female cervical vaginal tract			~1–3 h[18]		3.5–4.5 (Healthy women)[38] 5.4–8.2 (Infertile women)[18]

The values for the average and reported thickness of mucus are total thickness, which includes the thickness of both the loosely adherent and firmly adherent layers.

layer of the eye and results in a short drug retention time.[34] The flow of lacrimal fluid moves the drug to the nasolacrimal duct from the ocular surface in a few minutes, with a lacrimal turnover rate of approximately 1 μL/min.[47] Typically, less than 5% of the drug administered is retained on the ocular surface as a result of the corneal epithelium barrier and nasolacrimal duct drainage.[48,49] The cornea itself is approximately 500 μm thick.[50] The healthy corneal epithelium is lipophilic in nature with tight junctions, which leads to limitation of the permeation of hydrophilic molecules.[51] Chitosan has been the most widely explored nanoparticle coating to increase residence time in the precorneal region.[52] For intravitreal delivery, poly(ethylene glycol) (PEG) coatings on nanoparticles can increase distribution and retention in the eye.[53] For posterior segment delivery, nanoparticle residence time and localization depend on the size and surface properties. Particles in the range of 20–2000 nm have been retained at the site of administration for at least 2 months.[54,55] Positively charged nanoparticles can penetrate the vitreal barrier and reach the inner limiting membrane of the eye.[56] Negatively charged particles can penetrate the whole retina and reach the outer retinal layers such as the photoreceptor layer and the retinal pigment epithelium (RPE). In the presence of disease, negatively charged particles can reach even further to the choroid region due to disruption of the RPE.[57]

7.2.3.2 Nose

Nasal delivery has conventionally been restricted to topically or locally acting therapeutic agents for the treatment of a nasal issue. More recently, nasal delivery has received increased attention as a substitute for oral and parenteral routes for several systemic therapeutic agents. The volume and surface area of the human nasal cavity is 15–20 mL and 150–200 cm^2, respectively.[58] The nasal mucosa lines the entire nasal cavity from the nostrils to the pharynx. A dynamic layer of mucus overlies the nasal epithelium (the outermost layer of cells of the nasal mucosa). The nasal submucosa underlies the basement membrane. This layer is made up of glands, mucus, nerves, an extensive network of blood vessels, and cellular elements like blood plasma. The entire mucosa is highly concentrated with blood vessels and contains large venouslike spaces.[59] Nanoparticles have been used for intranasal vaccine delivery,[60] to induce systemic and mucosal immunity, and for treatment of neurological disorders.[61] Although studies identifying particle size are not conclusive, the most commonly used size ranges are 40–200 nm.[62] Cationic particles increase residence time in the nasal cavity compared to anionic platforms. Cationic chitosan nanoparticles and polymer nanoparticles have demonstrated the ability to cross epithelium via tight junction disruption, and uptake in the brain.[63,64] However, cationic phospholipid nanoparticles used for vaccine delivery have not taken up in the brain, or crossed airway epithelium,[65] suggesting that nanoparticle composition might play a role in transport across the nasal mucosal barrier.

7.2.3.3 Lung

An inhaled nanotherapeutic in the lungs encounters airway surfaces lined by ciliated epithelial cells and covered with an airway surface layer. The airway surface layer has a mucus layer that entraps inhaled particles and foreign pathogens, and a low viscosity periciliary layer (PCL) that lubricates airway surfaces and facilitates ciliary beating for efficient mucus clearance.[16,24] Normal respiratory mucus is composed of ~1% mucins, ~1% salt, ~1% other proteins, and ~97% water.[66,67] The hydration status of respiratory mucus is principally regulated by the export of Cl^- through the cystic fibrosis (CF) transmembrane conductance regulator (CFTR) and Ca^{+2}-activated chloride channels, and by the influx of Na^+ through the epithelial Na^+ channel.[68] By regulating these two processes, the epithelium controls the amount of water on the airway surface, which influences the thickness of the mucosal barrier. In normal, healthy lungs, after secretion and hydration of mucins, a thin layer of mucus (e.g., 2–5 μm thick in the trachea) is formed above the cilia from the bronchioles to the upper airway to protect the epithelium. The thickness of this mucosal layer is altered in the presence of disease, which can significantly impair nanoparticle transport to the airway epithelium.[27,28] Inhalation of drug-loaded nanoparticles has been a promising approach for the treatment of diseases such as asthma, chronic obstructive pulmonary disease, CF, and lung cancer. Nanoparticles with a primary or agglomerate particle size between 10 and 100 nm will deposit more efficiently in the alveolar region compared to particles with an agglomerate particle size between 100 and 1000 nm.[69–72] A large body of literature has focused on making nanoparticles mucoadhesive through the incorporation of cationic or thiolated surfaces that interact with negatively charged glycosylated or cysteine-rich hydrophobic domains of airway mucin fibers. Additionally, nanoparticle formulations with hydrophobic core polymers could interact with mucins through hydrophobic interactions. Nanoparticles that are mucoadhesive were thought to be retained for longer duration in the lungs due to the ability of these charged nanoparticles to change mucus rheology through multivalent mucus–particle interactions, which decreases mucociliary clearance (MCC) rates.[73] However, mucoadhesive nanoparticles are unable to reach the underlying epithelium due to entrapment in the mucus gel layer, which is rapidly cleared. Therefore, more recent findings have focused on the penetration and retention of nanoparticles that are mucus-penetrating.[40] Mucus-penetrating particles possess a dense brush layer of PEG on the particle surface.[74–76] When particles are mucus-penetrating, they can reach the underlying PCL that is cleared less rapidly and diffuse to the epithelial surface.

7.2.3.4 Gastrointestinal tract

Following oral delivery, a nanotherapeutic will encounter a heterogenous mucosal environment as it transits through the gastrointestinal (GI) tract. The thickness of mucus layer in the human intestine ranges from 100 to 900 μm (gastric compartment to colon) and consists of an outer, loosely adherent layer, and an inner, thinner, and more strongly adherent layer. The inner, strongly adherent layer has been estimated to be 116 μm thick in the colon.[17,41,77] The outer loosely attached layer is thinner in the small intestine (~100–170 μm) but thicker in the colon (600–800 μm).[17,41,78] In the intestinal tract, the ionic strength, ionic composition, and pH have all been shown to vary significantly depending on the location in the intestine, feeding status, and meal contents. Osmolality and ionic strength can fluctuate from hypotonic to isotonic to hypertonic within short distances in the gut after a meal.[79] Therefore, for orally delivered nanotherapeutics, particle interactions with the mucosal layers will depend partially on, among other factors, feeding state. Gut transit time will also play a role in nanoparticle transport across the mucosal layer because the GI tract is continuously motile and in various stages of activity.[80] As discussed in Section 7.2.3.7, gut transit time varies across species, therefore translation of results for nanoparticle retention from one study to the next should take into account the species and model used for the specified study.

Although there are many different sites within the GI that might be targeted with nanotherapeutics, there are general considerations that apply to the ability of nanoparticles to overcome or interact with the mucosal layer throughout the GI tract. There is a size limit to cross the intestinal mucosal barrier because the range of mesh pore spacing of the mucus is 50–1800 nm.[81] Hydrophobicity and surface charge play a key role in interaction with GI mucus. Particles with hydrophobic surfaces are generally considered mucoadhesive. Similarly, particles with positive surfaces, such as those coated or made with chitosan, show increased interaction and adherence to the luminal mucus gel.[82] Additionally, as with delivery to the lung, mucus-penetrating particles have shown greater ability to reach the underlying adherent layer, diffuse to the epithelial surface, and transverse the epithelium to reach systemic circulation.[83] Given the wide range of conditions in the GI tract, design of nanoparticles to leverage transport to a specific region of the GI tract should be considered. The reader is referred to several excellent reviews that discuss the various barriers, including gut transit time and feed state, to developing drugs for effective oral delivery.[39,84–87] For recent developments in targeting nanoparticles to specific sites in the GI tract, the reader is referred to a review by Ensign et al.[88]

7.2.3.5 Vaginal tract

In the vaginal tract, cervicovaginal mucus (CVM) can have a significant impact on the penetration, distribution, and residence time of nanoparticle-based systems for vaginal drug delivery applications. Mucus produced at the cervix bathes and coats the vaginal walls, mixing with vaginal epithelial cells and vaginal transudate, and serves as a physical barrier to protect the vagina against infection. Outside the period of ovulation, the composition of CVM is composed mostly of water (~90%–95%) with gel-forming glycoproteins, lipids, soluble proteins, enzymes, and various immune factors.[19] During ovulation, cervical mucus becomes watery and mucin proteins align to allow sperm to pass more readily through the cervix into the uterus. However, ovulatory mucus is produced in more copious amounts, thus facilitating clearance and impeding drug absorption. Mucins in CVM from nonovulatory women and women on hormonal contraceptives form a tight meshwork, acting as a barrier to protect the epithelium.[89] Nonovulatory human CVM was recently found to have pores in the range of 50–1800 nm, with an average of 340 ± 70 nm.[81]

7.2.3.6 Colorectal delivery

For certain applications, such as treatment of colorectal cancer and colitis, or rectal protection against sexually transmitted diseases, colorectal delivery may be utilized. Additionally, colorectal delivery can allow drugs to reach systemic circulation without degradation due to stomach acid or digestive enzymes and avoids the hepatic first-pass metabolism, discussed in Section 7.3.1. The colon absorbs 1.4–1.8 L of water per day, a process which is driven by active transport.[86] A wide range of nanoparticles sizes, from 100 to 500 nm are capable of penetrating the colorectal mucosal barrier,[83] as long as the particles are mucus-penetrating. Interestingly, what might be a more important factor than the nanoparticle design is the tonicity in which the nanoparticles are delivered. Further studies by Maisel et al. show that the ion composition of the fluid significantly affects nanoparticle penetration across the colorectal mucosal layer.[90] Nanoparticle retention and distribution was improved when nanoparticles were administered in moderately hypotonic enemas, whereas hypertonic and isotonic enemas reduced retention and limited distribution, even of mucus-penetrating particles, in colorectal tissue.[90]

7.2.3.7 Mucosal variance across species

Many nanotherapeutics are tested preclinically in animal models. Therefore, it is important to acknowledge the mucus barrier shows large species variation. In the nose, the total mucosal area is correlated to the nasal surface area. The nasal surface area: body weight ratio of humans is 2.5 cm^2/kg, whereas in animals it ranges from 7.7 to 46 cm^2/kg for rats, rabbits, pigs, dogs, and monkeys.[91] In the GI, the rat intestinal mucus layer is 10-fold thicker or more in all segments of the intestine compared to the thickness in humans.[17,81,92] The variation in mucosal barrier properties and GI transit time differs species to species. The rat and mouse have a long GI transit time of 20–30 h, whereas the canine is approximately 6–8 h.[32] In the vaginal tract, the immunological and hormonal differences between murine models and humans alter the barrier properties of the mucosal layer,[39] as well. Each of these species-based differences can introduce a translational barrier for nanotherapeutics that must overcome the mucosal layer to be effective.

7.2.4 Mucociliary clearance

The understanding of mucus layer thickness, function, and clearance times at various mucosal surfaces is important to the development of nanoparticles, since they must penetrate mucus at rates markedly faster than mucus renewal and clearance in order to overcome the barrier. Mucus is continuously secreted, then shed and discarded or digested and recycled. The fastest turnover is typically observed at surfaces with the thinnest mucus layer. In the eye, the tear turnover rate under normal physiological conditions is in the range of 13%–20% per minute, leading to nearly complete clearance of most molecules and particulates from the eye within minutes.[93] In the nose, cilia lining epithelium coated with nasal mucosa create motions which drain mucus from the nasal passage to the throat, where the mucus is swallowed and digested by stomach enzymes. The activity level of cilia in the nasal cavity is dependent on temperature, where in cold temperatures cilia become less active. The mucus flow rate is about 7–12 mm per minute, and the mucus layer is renewed approximately every 20 min.[22,94,95] In the respiratory tract, the coordinated interaction of the mucus layer and PCL on the surface of the respiratory tract results in mucociliary clearance (MCC). MCC rates of 100–300 μm/s have been measured in the human trachea,[23] and the luminal gel layer of respiratory tract mucus is replaced every 10–20 min, leading to efficient clearance of inhaled particulates.[22] The sol phase of respiratory mucus is thought to be cleared much less rapidly than the more solidlike luminal gel layer. In the GI, peristaltic forces lead to quick turnover times of the mucus, on the order of 4–6 h.[96–98] In the vagina, mucus is cleared by intra-abdominal pressure as well as abdominal motions, which squeeze the walls of the vagina together.[99] The typical clearance time in the human cervical vaginal tract remains unclear, but is likely on the order of a few hours. Therefore, due to these differences in MCC along with differences in mucosal properties, the design of a nanoparticle to overcome mucosal barrier properties and mucosal clearance is dependent on target location and necessary site of action.

7.2.5 Absorption across an epithelial layer

If the target site requires access to systemic circulation, nanoparticles must absorb across the epithelium. Nanoparticle design factors that influence absorption across an epithelium include (1) physical and chemical stability of the particles and drug at the mucosal site, (2) residence times in regions of particle uptake, (3) interaction with mucosal contents and (4) transport through mucus, as discussed previously in this chapter, and (5) adhesion to epithelial surfaces. Nanoparticles can permeate across an epithelium by translocation via the tightly regulated narrow paracellular space, or by transport first through the apical plasma membrane (for intracellular delivery).[100,101] There is some evidence to support transport through the basolateral part of the plasma membrane (for transcellular delivery) to reach systemic circulation.[102] General mechanisms of nanoparticle uptake in cells are discussed in Section 7.4.

7.3 En-route barriers

Once a nanotherapeutic has absorbed across an epithelial layer it passes into systemic circulation. However, if administered orally, a nanoparticle must first overcome the first-pass effect. In this section, we will cover barriers introduced by the first-pass effect, circulation, passage across an endothelial layer, and transit through a tissue extracellular space (ECS) (Fig. 7.1).

7.3.1 First-pass effect following oral delivery

Extensive hepatic first-pass metabolism is one of the principal reasons for poor oral bioavailability of drugs. Hepatic first-pass (referred to as first-pass effect or first-pass metabolism) occurs when a drug absorbed from the GI tract is metabolized by enzymes within the liver to their water-soluble form, which facilitates excretion through the kidneys.[103] Enzymes that can act on a drug are GI lumen enzymes, gut wall enzymes, bacterial enzymes, and hepatic enzymes. Metabolism of a drug to its water-soluble form prevents the required amount of drug to reach systemic circulation, which can result in the need for higher doses of drug to achieve a minimum effective plasma concentration.

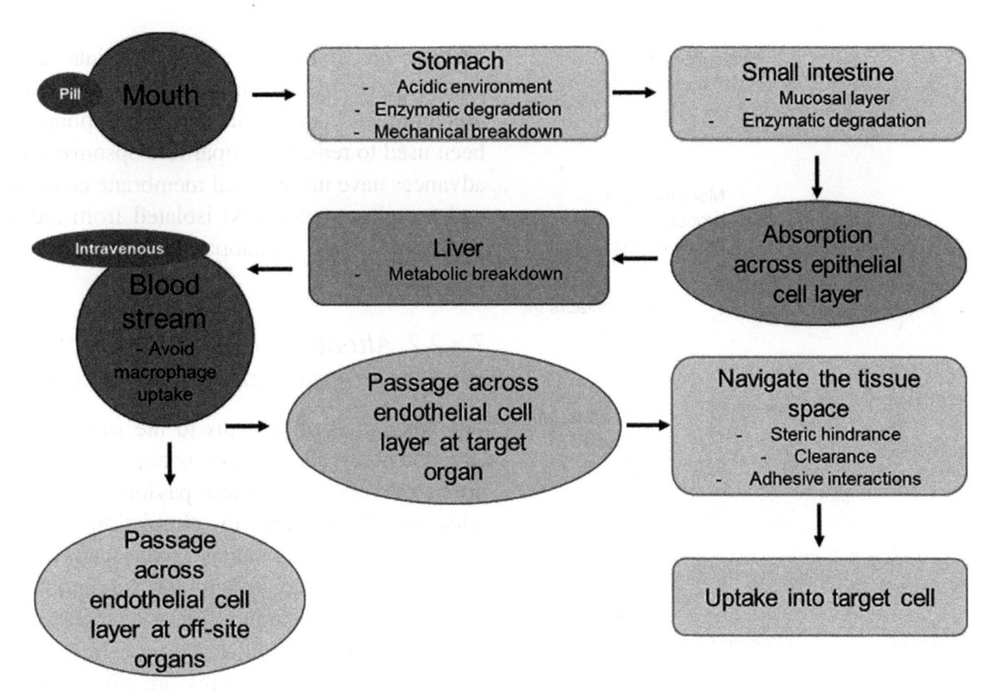

FIGURE 7.1 Overview of biological barriers encountered by a nanoparticle when administered orally or through a route that reaches systemic administration.

When this happens, dose-related side effects can occur—the resulting metabolites may possess equal pharmacological activity or may have modified activity leading to increased or decreased effect, and the metabolites produced can be toxic compared to the parent drug. Nanoparticles have been commonly used to overcome the first-pass metabolism of most drugs through protection of the drug from enzymatic degradation by incorporation into the nanoparticle core, or through the use of surface coatings.[88] Surface coatings can decrease hepatic first-pass clearance by increasing transport in Peyer's patches, small patches of lymphatic tissue in the intestine, or uptake in M-cells, specialized epithelial cells associated with the immune system in the gut.[85,104] Using nanoparticles to target the intestinal lymphatic system can be useful for improving oral bioavailability of drugs that are susceptible to a high-degree of first-pass metabolism, such as steroids.[105–108]

7.3.2 Circulation

A large amount of focus in the nanotechnology field has centered around the barriers faced when nanoparticles are administered to or reach systemic circulation. These barriers include opsonization and subsequent sequestration by the mononuclear phagocyte system (MPS) (also referred to as the reticuloendothelial system (RES)), nonspecific distribution, hemorheological or blood vessel flow limitations, pressure gradients, enzymatic degradation, and cellular internalization.[109,110] Additionally, while in circulation, nanoparticles can become destabilized, have leakage or displacement of cargo, undergo degradation or disassembly, or have premature detachment of target ligands.[111] Nanoparticle size and surface chemistry or surface coating are the most common properties to tune to increase circulation time and reduce opsonization and MPS clearance. For example, highly cationic nanoparticles are rapidly cleared from circulation to a greater extent than anionic nanoparticles.[112] Neutral nanoparticles, as well as those with a slight negative charge, show significantly prolonged circulating half-lives.[113] Nanoparticle circulation studies have defined optimal size ranges to avoid excretion from filtration through the liver, spleen, and kidney. Generally, smaller than 10 nm unmodified nanoparticles are filtered by the kidney,[114] nanoparticles between 10 and 200 nm are captured by Kupffer cells in the liver and splenic macrophages,[115] and particles larger than 200 nm are retained in the red pulp of the spleen.[115–117] In addition, some studies have suggested that nanoparticles should be greater than 120 nm to avoid nanoparticle entrapment in the disse and hepatic parenchymal space.[118]

7.3.2.1 Nanoparticle opsonization and the mononuclear phagocyte system

The MPS consists of a system of phagocytic cells, predominantly resident macrophages, in the spleen, lymph nodes, and liver (Fig. 7.2). The MPS can sequester nanoparticles immediately after systemic injection.[119] Sequestration can occur when nanoparticles become opsonized. Opsonization involves the adsorption of plasma proteins,

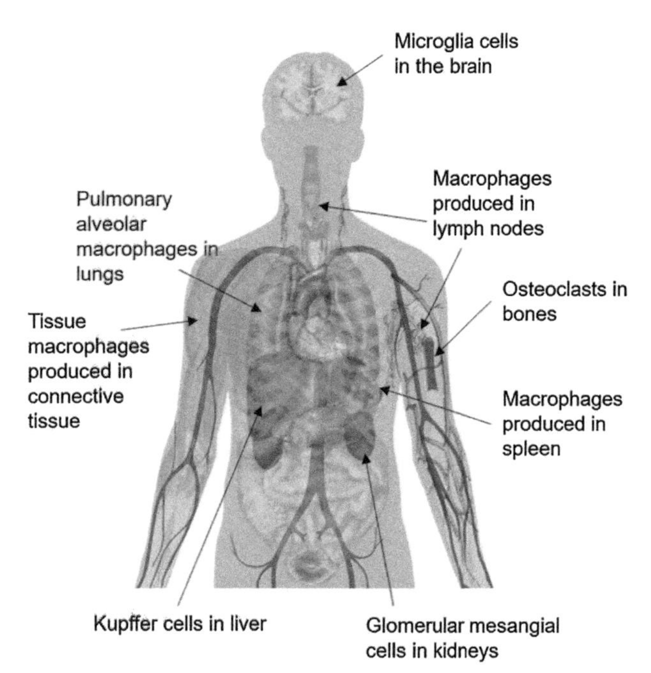

FIGURE 7.2 Phagocytic cells that can internalize nanoparticles in circulation or in tissue.

including immunoglobulins, complement proteins, albumin, apolipoprotein, and fibrinogen, onto the surface of circulating nanoparticles.[120] There are many factors that can influence the process of opsonization, including nanoparticle size, surface charge, hydrophobicity, and surface chemistry.[121] Once proteins are adsorbed to the surface of a nanoparticle, the nanoparticle can undergo attachment to specific receptors on the surface of phagocytes, which leads to nanoparticle internalization. Nanoparticles are then transported to phagosomes and fused with lysosomes.[122] Opsonization can mask active-targeting ligands on the surface of nanoparticles, resulting in a reduction in specificity. The opsonization of nanoparticles and subsequent clearance by MPS could also initiate severe immunological reactions.

Opsonization can be reduced or avoided through controlling the surface coating of nanoparticles. For example, PEG has been widely utilized to shield particle surfaces from protein interaction,[123] effectively making them stealthlike in the body. PEG is a biocompatible, hydrophilic, biologically inert polymer that has been approved by the US Food and Drug Administration (FDA) for internal use, for a number of applications. PEGylation involves the grafting of PEG to the surface of nanoparticles. Ethylene glycol units form tight associations with water molecules, leading to formation of a hydrating layer[124] that hinders protein adsorption and subsequent clearance by the MPS. The density of PEG engraftment on the surface of nanoparticles can affect the effectiveness of the PEG layer.[75,125] While PEG is the most commonly utilized polymer for coating nanoparticles, other materials including polaxamers, polyvinyl alcohol, poly(amino acid)s, and polysaccharides[126] and zwitterionic compounds[127] have also been used to reduce nanoparticle opsonization. More recent advances have utilized cell membrane coatings (both lipidic and protein components) isolated from red blood cells or leukocytes on nanoparticles to reduce protein adsorption.[128,129]

7.3.2.2 Alterations of nanoparticle physicochemical properties in circulation

The adsorption of proteins to the surface of nanoparticles can potentially destabilize nanoparticles and lead to the premature release of their payloads.[130] When a drug is released prematurely in circulation, it eliminates the favorable pharmacokinetics of the nanocarrier and is then available to induce toxicity or susceptible to enzymatic degradation and clearance. Plasma proteins can also bind to or displace the encapsulated drug. The abilities of proteins to destabilize nanostructures are often measured and can vary protein to protein.[131] For example, polymeric micelles (e.g., PEG-b-poly(propyl methacrylate-co-methacrylic acid)/poly(amidoamine) and PEG-b-poly(D,L-lactide)) were tested with a series of proteins (e.g., albumin, α- and β-globulins, γ-globulins). Although most proteins were found to contribute to micelle destabilization, a more significant effect was observed for α- and β-globulins.[130] However, destabilization of nanoparticles may also result from interactions with other components in blood (e.g., blood cells) and the degradation of the polymeric constituents of the nanoparticle through hydrolysis or enzymatic activity.[132]

7.3.2.3 Blood vessel flow limitations and pressure gradients

Blood vasculature varies throughout the body based on blood flow needs and nutrient demand of tissues. The properties of blood vessels influence nanoparticle flow and partitioning to the endothelial surface. The capillary is the smallest of the blood vessels, ranging from 5 to 40 μm in diameter.[133] The capillary has a high surface area to volume ratio, maximizing the potential for blood–tissue exchange. Furthermore, the vessel walls of most capillaries in the body consist of an endothelial cell layer, just one-cell thick, thereby minimizing transport times across the vessel wall.[134] There is a hydrostatic pressure that exists between capillary and tissue, and an osmotic pressure that is the difference in protein concentration in blood and the interstitial space. The net difference in these two pressures causes fluid flow from capillaries into tissue, driving convective transport of macromolecules into the interstitial space.[135] Blood flow is dependent on the volume of blood, viscosity of blood (as determined by composition), blood vessel length and diameter, and blood vessel curvature and branching, all of which can be influenced by age and health status.[136] Blood flowing within blood vessels is composed of blood cells, which make up 45% of total blood volume and are primarily red blood cells. Red blood cells accumulate preferentially within the center of the blood vessel, creating a cell-free layer closer to the endothelium, leading to small particle accumulation in this space.[137]

7.3.2.4 Nanoparticle margination in blood flow

In addition to blood vessel and blood flow characteristics, nanoparticle fluid dynamics in blood vessels is an important nanoparticle design consideration. In particular, margination dynamics influences nanoparticle association with vessel walls, which favors particle–cell binding and receptor–ligand interactions in active targeting strategies and enables extravasation through the fenestrated vasculature in most target organs. Margination is the lateral drift of nanoparticles to endothelial walls and has been shown to be influenced by nanoparticle size and shape.[138] Larger nanoparticles are subjected to a greater magnitude of drag force from fluid flow, which leads to lower interaction with blood vessel endothelium. Spherical geometries exhibit minimal lateral drift and are less likely to marginate to vessel walls and establish contact/binding points with endothelial cells. Nonspherical nanoparticles are more prone to tumbling and oscillatory effects in vasculature, which increases the likelihood of nanoparticle–cell wall contact and potential extravasation through fenestrations in vasculature.[139] Recent research has begun to explore the role of particle stiffness on nanoparticle margination in blood flow. Discher et al. have shown that increased flexibility of nanoparticles can increase circulation, through avoiding interaction and uptake by macrophages.[140] Top-down particle fabrication approaches, such as Particle Replication in Nonwetting Templates (PRINT), nanoimprint lithography, and thermostretched template–induced methods are providing ways to control nanoparticle stiffness.[141,142] From these techniques, the field has generally found that "soft" nanoparticles have longer circulation times in vivo compared to "hard" nanoparticles.[143,144]

7.3.3 Splenic clearance

Nanoparticles in blood circulation are susceptible to splenic filtration. The structure of the spleen enables the removal of older erythrocytes from the blood circulation as well as blood-borne microorganisms, cellular debris, and nanoparticles.[145] Many of these entities are captured by splenic macrophages in the marginal zone of the spleen. The maximal slit size in the spleen is estimated between 200 and 500 nm in width, but the spleen can also filter nanoparticles smaller than 100 nm.[132] Some studies have shown this can lead to a higher uptake of nanoparticles per unit mass than nanoparticle uptake in the liver.[117,146,147] Nanoparticles larger than 100–200 nm are incapable of crossing the endothelial slit of splenic sinuses, and instead are filtered off and retained in the red pulp. In the red pulp, these nanoparticles are internalized by red pulp macrophages and slowly destroyed.[115,116] Particle removal by splenic filtration tends to increase with size and is maximal for particles larger than 400 nm.[117,148] As nanoparticle size increases, Kupffer cell capture decreases, and splenic capture is enhanced.

7.3.4 Renal clearance

The kidney is capable of rapidly removing molecules from the vascular compartment with minimal catabolism or breakdown. Nanoparticles smaller than 10 nm can be excreted by renal clearance in the kidney, with smaller nanoparticles exhibiting faster excretion rates.[114] The renal molecular weight cutoff size is ~48 kDa (for some polymers such as PEG and dextran). Circulating nanoparticles will enter the glomerular capillary bed via the afferent arteriole. This bed is composed of three layers, including the fenestrated endothelium, the glomerular basement membrane (GBM) which is negatively charged, and podocyte extensions of glomerular epithelial cells.[149] Glomerular filtrate flows through the fenestrate, across the GBM, and through filtration slits formed by the spaces between podocyte extensions. This filtration slit introduces the primary size barrier for nanoparticles and has a pore size of 4.5–5 nm.[114] Nanoparticles that are less than 6 nm can be freely filtered, independent of molecular charge. Filtration of particles in the range of 6–8 nm is dependent on charge interactions between the particle and the negative charges of the GBM.[150] Based on this, positive particles are more readily filtered than negatively charged particles of equal size. Particles larger than 8 nm do not undergo glomerular filtration. Following glomerular filtration, nanoparticles enter the proximal tubule of the kidney where they can be resorbed into the luminal space for excretion. However, the brush border of the proximal tubule epithelial cells is negatively charged, so positively charged nanoparticles are more readily resorbed compared to negatively charged nanoparticles.[151,152]

7.3.5 Hepatic clearance

For nanoparticles that do not undergo renal or splenic clearance, the hepatobiliary system represents the primary route of excretion. The liver serves as a site of phagocytosis, catabolism, and biliary excretion of circulating nanoparticles.[153] Nanoparticles in the size range of 10–200 nm can be rapidly captured by the liver. Phagocytosis mainly occurs through uptake by Kupffer cells, which have ciliated borders and stellate branches that act as mechanical traps for the removal of nanoparticles in blood.[114] Kupffer cells possess receptors for selective endocytosis of opsonized particles, including receptors for complement proteins. In addition to Kupffer cells, hepatocytes can clear nanoparticles via endocytosis and enzymatic breakdown. Hepatocytes are within the pathway for biliary excretion, and therefore particles processed by these cells are potentially excreted into the bile.[151] Kupffer cells are part of the MPS and rely exclusively on intracellular degradation for particle removal. Nanoparticles that are excreted via the biliary system are catabolized through hepatocytes. However, the phagocytic capacity of hepatocytes is much less than that of Kupffer cells. Interestingly, although uptake of particles from the blood to the liver may occur relatively quickly, hepatic processing and biliary excretion of these particles is relatively slow, often resulting in prolonged retention of NPs within the liver parenchyma itself.[114]

7.3.6 Endothelial barriers

Blood vessels throughout the body vary slightly in structure, but share the same general features. Importantly, in all blood vessels, an intact layer of healthy endothelial cells is essential for normal blood vessel function. Endothelial cell barrier function is attributed to the close alignment of endothelial cells in the vessel wall such that movement of water, proteins, and blood cells between the intravascular and interstitial compartments is controlled.[154] The endothelial barrier is formed by a layer of endothelial cells joined laterally by cell–cell junctions. The basolateral aspect of this layer is attached to a basement membrane composed of collagen, fibronectin, laminin, and glycosaminoglycans (GAGs). The permeability of blood endothelium is multifold, and the restrictiveness of transport depends on the organ, whether the endothelium is continuous or noncontinuous, and whether it is fenestrated or not.

7.3.6.1 General endothelium structure

Blood endothelium can be fenestrated, meaning the endothelial layer contains small holes, approximately 60–80 nm in diameter,[155] that allow diffusion of molecules and proteins.[156] Blood endothelium can also be discontinuous, with larger gaps than in fenestrated endothelium.[157] Discontinuous endothelia are found primarily in the liver and spleen where large macromolecules must easily cross the endothelium.[158] Similar to other epithelia, endothelial cells rest on a basement membrane. The basement membrane of endothelium provides structural support and also inhibits diffusion due to the presence of negatively charged domains on proteoglycans. The thickness of the basement membrane does vary throughout the body.[159]

Nanoparticles can penetrate the endothelium through several pathways. Depending on size, particles can passively diffuse through fenestrations or gaps in fenestrated or discontinuous endothelial layers.[160] Additionally, nanoparticles can passage across endothelial layers through transcellular, paracellular, or receptor-mediated pathways.[161] Paracellular transport occurs between endothelium cells, and transcellular transport occurs through endothelial cells. Nanoparticles can be actively targeted by grafting the surface or the shell of the nanocarriers with specific ligands or antibodies to molecules expressed on the endothelium. More recently, researchers have found that nanoparticles in the size range of 50–100 nm, a common size used for drug delivery, can take advantage of the transcellular caveolar pathway to traffic across endothelium.[162,163] In the presence of disease, the endothelium can become injured or dysfunctional, which can lead to discontinuities or breaks in the endothelial lining. The disruption of normal endothelial function and structure can lead to increased passive transport of nanoparticles across the endothelium.[154,164]

7.3.6.2 Blood–retinal barrier

The blood–retinal barrier (BRB) is a specialized transport barrier between the blood and the retina that has tight junctions between the monolayer of retinal pigmented epithelial cells and retinal capillary endothelial cells of the retinal circulation.[165] As a result of the anatomic position of the BRB, it effectively limits the transportation of molecules from the choroidal blood circulation to the posterior segment of the eye.[48] Moreover, the BRB also plays an important role in controlling the environment of the neural retina compared to the high blood flow and leaky walls of choroidal vasculature. In the choroidal vasculature, molecules easily enter into the choroidal extracellular gap, but have difficulty passing through the retinal pigmented epithelial layer.[166] Therefore, nanoparticle design would need to be tailored toward the specific barriers based on the intended site of action in the eye.

7.3.6.3 Blood–brain barrier

One of the most restrictive and exclusive barriers in the body is the blood–brain barrier (BBB). The BBB is a description of the structural interface that exists between the brain tissue and circulating blood. The BBB is continuous and not fenestrated.[167] There are about 400 miles of blood vessels in the adult brain, and almost all of these vessels consist of a layer of endothelial cells that line the capillary wall, with pericytes embedded in the basement membrane of the capillary, and astrocyte end-feet ensheathing the capillary.[168] The astrocytes provide biochemical support to the endothelial cells, which in part regulates vasodilation and constriction of the blood vessels. Paracellular transport is utilized for ions and solutes that depend on a gradient of concentration. Transcellular transport of lipophilic molecules occurs primarily via passive diffusion. The balance between paracellular–transcellular transport is often the metric used to define the degree of permeability in a healthy BBB.[169] Hydrophilic molecules, like proteins and peptides, rely on specific transport through interaction with specific receptors on the surface of endothelial layers. Importantly, the brain endothelium expresses a family of efflux pumps, known as ATP-binding cassette transporters that can actively efflux foreign entities, including nanoparticles, into the blood.[170]

Nanoparticle physicochemical properties can be tailored toward a mechanism of passage across the BBB. It is generally thought that nanoparticles must be low molecular weight and lipophilic or amphiphilic to passively cross the BBB. Nanoparticles can pass through brain endothelial cells via transcytosis, accessed by activating receptors for transferrin and low-density lipoproteins.[171–173] Active targeting of these receptors has been achieved with peptides, proteins, or antibodies conjugated to the surface of nanoparticles. One well-studied mechanism for transport across the BBB is nanoparticles coated with polysorbate 80 (P80, also known as Tween 80). Nanoparticles coated with P80 absorb apolipoprotein E to the surface, which induces a receptor-mediated transcytosis process across the brain endothelium.[174,175] Other surfactants and surface coatings are being studied to determine if similar mechanisms occur. Additionally, targeting ligands such as transferrin have been commonly used to increase uptake across the BBB.[176] Nanoparticles can be transported through endothelial cells by endocytosis, as well, where content can be released in the cytoplasm and then exocytosed to the endothelium abluminal (brain parenchyma) side.[177] There are also recent findings that show nanoparticles can open tight junctions between endothelial cells, which leads to localized permeabilization of the BBB.[178] In the presence of injury or disease, the BBB is often impaired, which can result in increased nanoparticle uptake,[179–182] although the mechanism of this uptake is still being explored.

7.3.7 Extracellular matrix navigation

Once the barriers associated with endothelium have been overcome or bypassed, or if the route of administration is direct injection into the tissue of interest, nanoparticles must then be able to navigate the spaces that exist between cells to achieve sufficient distribution and induce a therapeutic outcome in distant diseased cells. There are multiple obstacles that can limit the effectiveness of this extracellular transport, including the tortuous geometry of ECSs, interactions with cellular surfaces, and interactions with the extracellular matrix (ECM). The ECM is a highly heterogeneous network of proteins and macromolecules that come together to form meshlike structures between cells.[183,184] This network presents both steric and adhesive barriers to any drug delivery vehicle attempting to travel the ECS. Sterically, the ECM hinders free movement by presenting additional physical structures that must be navigated. Adhesive interactions are brought about by the transient binding of nanoparticles to ECM-associated components or nonspecific interactions with fixed charges on the ECM. To better understand how these physical and adhesive interactions come about, it is important to have a grasp of both ECM composition and structure.

7.3.7.1 ECM Composition

The composition of the ECM is highly variable, both spatially—from tissue to tissue and even within tissues—and temporally—differing throughout development, disease progression, and wound healing.[184–188] This fluidity relates directly to the tissue-specific functions of the ECM and the roles it plays in pathological processes and wound healing. The dynamic nature of the ECM makes it impossible to define a constant chemical makeup. However, there does exist some underlying compositional principles that transcend all ECM structures. In general, the ECM is composed of some combination of two main classes of macromolecules: fibrous proteins and proteoglycans.[187–189]

Fibrous proteins (including collagens, elastin, fibronectin, and laminins) constitute the main structural elements of the ECM, providing tensile strength, regulating cell adhesion, and directing tissue development.[184,190,191] Collagen, the most abundant of these proteins, possesses the ability to assemble into supramolecular complexes, such as fibrils and networks, depending on the resident tissue and the current needs of the local cellular environment.[192] Collagen fibers possess a near-neutral surface charge at physiological pH and thus predominantly act as physical barriers to extracellular nanoparticle transport.

Proteoglycans are composed of GAG chains covalently linked to a specific protein core (with the exception of hyaluronic acid) and form the basis of higher order ECM structures. The primary functions of proteoglycans (providing compressive resistance and trafficking cellular signals) can be attributed to the hydrodynamic and biochemical characteristics of their GAG components. GAGs are long, negatively charged, linear chains of disaccharide repeats. The fixed negative charges present on GAGs allow them to attract positively charged ions and form osmotically driven hydration layers. These hydrodynamic properties are utilized for specific roles in multiple tissues and are known to be abundant in cartilage and

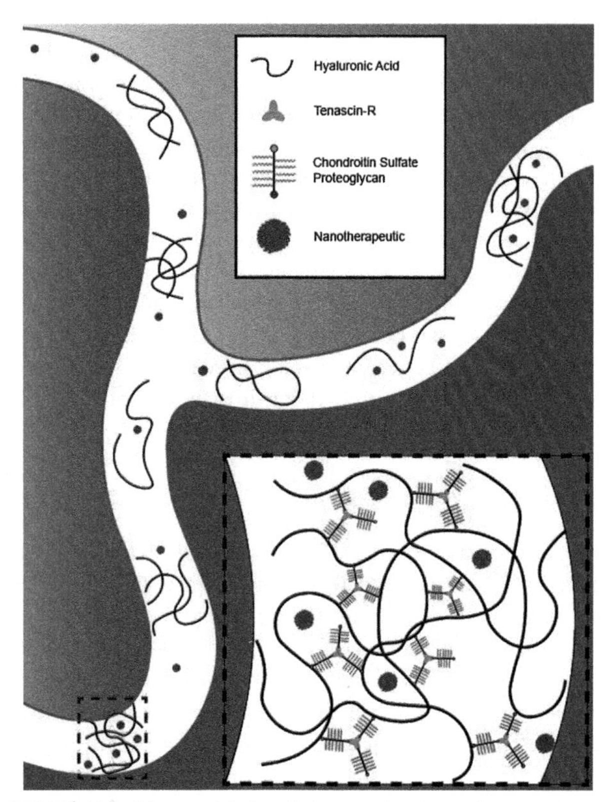

FIGURE 7.3 Nanoparticle-based therapeutics (orange) attempting to navigate the extracellular matrix (ECM) of the brain. The ECM of the brain is composed of hyaluronic acid, chondroitin sulfate proteoglycans, and glycoproteins such as tenascin-R.

neural ECM.[193,194] As noted, the ECM of the brain is a good example of a matrix rich in proteoglycans. Brain ECM is composed primarily of a hyaluronic acid backbone cross-linked by chondroitin sulfate proteoglycans (a distinct class of proteoglycans) and glycoproteins, such as tenascin R (Fig. 7.3). Any nanoparticle-based drug delivery vehicles attempting to navigate the brain ECM, such as those depicted in Fig. 7.3 (displayed as orange spheres), are consequently subject to potential repulsive or attractive forces brought about by electrostatic interactions with negative charges present on the chondroitin sulfate GAG chains, as well as hydrophobic interactions with proteoglycan core proteins. Similar to the previously mentioned fibrous proteins, proteoglycans also present steric obstructions to free nanoparticle movement within the ECS, while also altering local viscosity gradients. The extent at which these physical and adhesive interactions interplay is dependent on the ECM structure.

7.3.7.2 ECM Structure

Due to the variation in ECM composition and function throughout the body, the ECM can take on a wide range of structures. In load-bearing tendons, for example, the ECM can assemble with highly ordered and specialized axial and longitudinal organization.[195,196] On the other end of the spectrum, the ECM can be entirely amorphous. Typically, GAG-rich structures, such as the ECM of loose connective tissue, take on a fluidlike state.[194,197] ECM components can either be bound to cells or free floating within the ECS, depending on both the local composition and cellular environment.[183] As an additional layer of complexity, ECM structures can change frequently and are known to rearrange in the presence of disease, throughout development, and during aging.[187,188]

The ECM presents a unique challenge to any nanoparticle attempting to move within the ECSs of tissue environments. The composition of the ECM can alter local viscosity regimes, and its presence can lead to an enhanced drag on any particles subject to steric interactions with its structure. It also presents additional obstructions that must either be navigated through or steered around, increasing the mean free path a particle must take to travel a given distance. Nanoparticles are also prone to adhesive interactions with the ECM. These interactions are brought about by electrostatic and hydrophobic interactions with various components of the ECM. Collectively, these steric and adhesive barriers can significantly hinder the tissue penetrative ability of particles and should always be accounted for when developing nanoparticle-based therapeutics.

7.4 Cellular barriers

In many cases, nanoparticles must internalize into cells to have the intended therapeutic effect. When this is the case, nanoparticles must cross the cell membrane, traffic within the cell to the target intracellular compartment, and release the payload in a timely fashion, while avoiding premature degradation or exocytosis. In this section, we will discuss common cellular uptake mechanisms, and trafficking in and toward intracellular compartments to target subcellular organelles.

7.4.1 Uptake mechanisms

Nanoparticles must traverse the cell membrane lipid bilayer, which is typically 4 nm thick. Low molecular weight (<1 kDa), hydrophobic molecules are capable of simple diffusion through the lipid bilayer membrane of cells; however, microscale and nanoscale supramolecular constructs require active uptake mechanisms. Nanoparticle surface charge is a major determinant of cellular internalization, with charge-based uptake highly dependent on cell type. With different surface modifications, nanoparticles can be taken up via specific (receptor-mediated) endocytosis or nonspecific endocytosis.[198] Additionally, size,[199] shape,[200] and particle rigidity[201] are key parameters, especially for internalization of nanoparticles via phagocytosis.

It is important to note that the use of PEG to overcome previously discussed barriers can often hinder or limit nanoparticle interactions with cell membranes, reducing total nanoparticle uptake. Recent research has focused on the incorporation of labile bonds in the PEG chain, so that nanoparticles become unPEGylated upon reaching the target cells.[202] This can be controlled to lead to increased rates of membrane destabilization, transport of the loaded cargo inside the cells, and release of the nanoparticle from the endosome.[203]

Nanoparticles can uptake into cells via several mechanisms. Phagocytosis is mainly conducted by specialized mammalian cells (like monocytes, macrophages, and neutrophils) as discussed previously in the chapter, and referenced in Fig. 7.2. Phagocytosis occurs for particles that have undergone opsonization or for solid particles with diameters >750 nm.[204] In this case, the cell membrane forms an internal phagosome containing the nanoparticle. Phagocytic cells, particularly macrophages, tend to show a strong preference for rigid particles. Shape also influences nanoparticle internalization in phagocytic cells, based on the aspect ratio of the particle when it first comes into contact with a cell.[205,206] Several studies have demonstrated the ability of a macrophage to internalize an ellipsoid particle within a few minutes when the cell contacts the pointed first, whereas the same ellipsoid particle takes over 12 h to internalize if the cell contacts the flat side first.[205] The mechanism of this effect originates in the complexity of the actin structure required to initiate uptake and was, to an extent, independent of particle size.

Endocytosis is a form of active transport in which a cell takes in objects by enclosing them in vesicles or vacuoles pinched off from its cytoplasmic membrane. The known endocytic processes that enclose nanoparticles in membrane vesicles in an energy-dependent manner are mainly via phagocytosis, pinocytosis, and caveolae-dependent or clathrin-mediated endocytosis.[207,208] Smaller particles ranging from a few to several hundred nanometers are internalized by pinocytosis or macropinocytosis, which occurs in almost all cell types.[209] Macropinocytosis involves fluid-phase uptake via membrane protrusions on the cell surface, and often occurs for particles larger than several hundred nanometers. Energy-dependent clathrin-mediated endocytosis is probably the primary characterized mechanism for the cellular uptake of nanoparticles, in which cargo is deposited in small endocytic vesicles (usual diameter < 100 nm) that fuse with early endosomes. Nanoparticles can also uptake via caveolin-mediated endocytosis, which involves specific receptor binding.[102,163,207] Caveolae/lipid rafts, consisting of plasma membrane invaginations of 50–80 nm in size, contain cholesterol, sphingolipids, and caveolins. For endothelial cells, the caveolae-mediated endocytosis is the important cellular uptake pathway for nanoparticles. More recently, a plethora of additional mechanisms have emerged that use clathrin- and caveolin-independent pathways, many of them relying on the cholesterol-dependent clustering of lipid-anchored proteins into diverse microdomains. It is important to remember that the heterogeneity of nanoparticle surfaces and potential polydispersity in nanoparticle size will require multiple uptake pathways to be involved in internalization in the cell.

7.4.2 Intracellular trafficking

Phagosomes formed from internalization of nanoparticles via phagocytosis are ferried through the cytoplasm. Actin becomes depolymerized from the phagosome, allowing the vacuole membrane to become accessible to early endosomes.[210] The vacuolar membrane will mature through a series of fusion and fission events, eventually fusing with late endosomes and ultimately lysosomes to form a phagolysosome. This process can take anywhere from a half hour to several hours depending on the surface properties of the ingested particle.[211]

Once a nanoparticle is internalized via macropinocytosis, clathrin-mediated endocytosis and caveolae-mediated endocytosis, the nanoparticle will then be trafficked within the cell. Macropinocytosis leads to the formation of a macropinosome, which is thought to eventually fuse with lysosomes or recycle its content to the surface. Clathrin-mediated endocytosis of a nanocarrier leads to the formation of an early endosome, which is acidified and fuses with prelysosomal vesicles containing enzymes.[208] This gives rise to a late endosome and then a lysosome, an acidic and enzyme-rich environment prone to nanocarrier and drug degradation. Unless a lysosomal delivery is desired, strategies for cytosolic drug delivery by this route focus on the drug escape from the endosome as early as possible. Caveolae-mediated endocytosis of a nanocarrier gives rise to a caveolar vesicle that can be delivered to a caveosome, avoiding a degradative acidic and enzyme-rich environment.

Internalization mechanisms and intracellular trafficking introduce additional barriers to effective therapeutic delivery with nanoparticles, given the harsh and highly degradative endosomal and lysosomal environments. Therefore, research has focused on strategies aimed at promoting endosomal escape or lysosomal avoidance altogether.[132] Several innovative "charge-conversion" strategies aimed at site-specifically switching the charge of nanoparticles in response to environmental stimuli, such as pH, have been utilized for protein-based nanocarriers,[212] polymers, and liposomes. Membrane-destabilizing peptides have been used to induce endosomal escape. Cationic polymers, such as poly(ethylene imine) (PEI) and poly (L-lysine) (PLL), have also been incorporated in nanoparticle design to release therapeutics from endosomal compartments. The cationic charge of the nanoparticle interacts with the outer negatively charged surface of the endosomal membrane, resulting in membrane flipping and consequent destabilization.[213] The proton-sponge effect has been induced by polymers containing protonatable secondary and/or tertiary amine groups. With these polymers, protons are absorbed, which results in an influx of water into the endosomal compartment that leads the compartment to swell. With continual swelling, the endosomal compartment eventually ruptures, releasing its contents.[214]

7.4.3 Translocation to intracellular organelle

Incorporating multiple intracellular stimulus and tailored physiochemical materials properties of nanoparticles can release the drug to the intracellular organelles, such as cytosol, nucleus, mitochondria, Golgi, and endoplasmic reticulum (ER).[198] However, nanoparticles utilized for gene therapy face additional challenges. These include instability of the genetic material RNA and DNA-based therapies, and in the specific case of plasmid DNA, the need to translocate into the nucleus. Endosomal compartmentalization can degrade genetic material, but DNA that does survive endosomal escape can still be degraded by cytoplasmic nucleases. Nanoparticle encapsulation of DNA can help avoid early degradation, but will still need to enter the nucleus to be therapeutically effective. The nuclear envelope encases the cell genome and consists of a structure that is fluid with the ER. Nuclear pore complexes are locations where the inner and outer membranes of this envelope fuse together and are the sites of macromolecule trafficking for molecules smaller than 40 kDa in molecular weight. Therefore, most nucleic acid delivery systems are impermeable through nuclear pore complexes due to their large size.[215] To facilitate nuclear targeting through active transport, nuclear localization signal peptides have been developed to allow DNA nuclear entry. These peptides are short clusters of amino acids that can bind to DNA either through noncovalent electrostatic interaction or by covalent attachment, thereby increasing their entry into the nucleus and subsequent therapeutic benefit within the cell.

7.4.4 Exocytosis

While cellular uptake of nanoparticles is well researched, less is known about the elimination of nanoparticles from cells. Current techniques are often limited in differentiating between excretion of nanoparticles and degradation of nanoparticles. Studies that have explored cellular excretion mechanisms vary depending on the cell type and the nanoparticle type. Macrophages can exocytose up to 44% of iron oxide nanoparticles that are 15 nm or 30 nm in size within 7 days of internalization.[216] However, HeLa cells can rapidly exocytose 50% of 8 nm quantum dots within 100 min.[217] In general, exocytosis has been higher for smaller spherical particles.[218] Exocytosis of single-walled carbon nanotubes and gold nanoparticles suggests that an optimum size for exocytosis is 25 nm. Spherical particles are exocytosed less readily than rodlike particles, indicating a role for shape to play in this process, as well.[218] An extensive review of nanoparticle exocytosis discusses the effect of physicochemical properties and nanoparticle surface modifications of mechanisms of nanoparticle excretion from cells.[219]

7.5 Conclusions

There are many competing design considerations that influence a nanoparticle's path in vivo and eventual fate. To take into account the multiple interacting aspects of physiology and nanomaterial properties, the direction of nanoparticle applications should move toward the use of design mapping.[179,220] Synthesis of pathophysiological barriers and nanoparticle physicochemical properties into a broader system view creates an integrated approach to future work using nanotechnology to treat various diseases.

References

1. Proksch E, Brandner JM, Jensen JM. The skin: an indispensable barrier. *Exp Dermatol* 2008;**17**(12):1063–72.
2. Palmer BC, DeLouise LA. Nanoparticle-enabled transdermal drug delivery systems for enhanced dose control and tissue targeting. *Molecules* 2016;**21**(12).
3. Baroli B, et al. Penetration of metallic nanoparticles in human full-thickness skin. *J Investig Dermatol* 2007;**127**(7):1701–12.
4. Cevc G, Vierl U. Nanotechnology and the transdermal route: a state of the art review and critical appraisal. *J Control Release* 2010;**141**(3):277–99.
5. Hung CF, et al. Cutaneous penetration of soft nanoparticles via photodamaged skin: lipid-based and polymer-based nanocarriers for drug delivery. *Eur J Pharm Biopharm* 2015;**94**:94–105.
6. Alvarez-Roman R, et al. Visualization of skin penetration using confocal laser scanning microscopy. *Eur J Pharm Biopharm* 2004;**58**(2):301–16.
7. Alvarez-Roman R, et al. Skin penetration and distribution of polymeric nanoparticles. *J Control Release* 2004;**99**(1):53–62.
8. Toll R, et al. Penetration profile of microspheres in follicular targeting of terminal hair follicles. *J Investig Dermatol* 2004;**123**(1):168–76.
9. Lademann J, et al. Hair follicles–an efficient storage and penetration pathway for topically applied substances. Summary of recent results obtained at the Center of Experimental and Applied Cutaneous Physiology, Charite -Universitatsmedizin Berlin, Germany. *Skin Pharmacol Physiol* 2008;**21**(3):150–5.
10. Okora Uchechi JDNO, Attama AA. Nanoparticles for dermal and transdermal drug delivery. In: Sezer AD, editor. *Application of nanotechnology in drug delivery*. IntechOpen; 2014.

11. Fernandes R, et al. Interactions of skin with gold nanoparticles of different surface charge, shape, and functionality. *Small* 2015;**11**(6):713–21.
12. Mota AH, et al. Broad overview of engineering of functional nanosystems for skin delivery. *Int J Pharm* 2017;**532**(2):710–28.
13. Lemme MAMaA. Examination of the composition of the luminal fluid in the small intestine of broilers and absorption of amino acids under various ambient temperatures measured in vivo. *Int J Poult Sci* 2008;**7**(3):223–33.
14. Lundquist P, Artursson P. Oral absorption of peptides and nanoparticles across the human intestine: opportunities, limitations and studies in human tissues. *Adv Drug Deliv Rev* 2016;**106**(Pt B):256–76.
15. Mantelli F, Argueso P. Functions of ocular surface mucins in health and disease. *Curr Opin Allergy Clin Immunol* 2008;**8**(5):477–83.
16. Knowles MR, Boucher RC. Mucus clearance as a primary innate defense mechanism for mammalian airways. *J Clin Investig* 2002;**109**(5):571–7.
17. Atuma C, et al. The adherent gastrointestinal mucus gel layer: thickness and physical state in vivo. *Am J Physiol Gastrointest Liver Physiol* 2001;**280**(5):G922–9.
18. Ensign LM, Cone R, Hanes J. Nanoparticle-based drug delivery to the vagina: a review. *J Control Release* 2014;**190**:500–14.
19. Cone RA. Barrier properties of mucus. *Adv Drug Deliv Rev* 2009;**61**(2):75–85.
20. Boegh M, Nielsen HM. Mucus as a barrier to drug delivery - understanding and mimicking the barrier properties. *Basic Clin Pharmacol Toxicol* 2015;**116**(3):179–86.
21. Murgia X, et al. The role of mucus on drug transport and its potential to affect therapeutic outcomes. *Adv Drug Deliv Rev* 2018;**124**:82–97.
22. Ali MS, Pearson JP. Upper airway mucin gene expression: a review. *The Laryngoscope* 2007;**117**(5):932–8.
23. Wanner A. Alteration of tracheal mucociliary transport in airway disease. Effect of pharmacologic agents. *Chest* 1981;**80**(6 Suppl. l):867–70.
24. Wanner A, Salathe M, O'Riordan TG. Mucociliary clearance in the airways. *Am J Respir Crit Care Med* 1996;**154**(6 Pt 1):1868–902.
25. Schuhl JF. Nasal mucociliary clearance in perennial rhinitis. *J Investig Allergol Clin Immunol* 1995;**5**(6):333–6.
26. Washington N, et al. Determination of baseline human nasal pH and the effect of intranasally administered buffers. *Int J Pharm* 2000;**198**(2):139–46.
27. Clunes MT, Boucher RC. Cystic fibrosis: the mechanisms of pathogenesis of an inherited lung disorder. *Drug Discov Today Dis Mech* 2007;**4**(2):63–72.
28. Matsui H, et al. Evidence for periciliary liquid layer depletion, not abnormal ion composition, in the pathogenesis of cystic fibrosis airways disease. *Cell* 1998;**95**(7):1005–15.
29. Tarran R, et al. The relative roles of passive surface forces and active ion transport in the modulation of airway surface liquid volume and composition. *J Gen Physiol* 2001;**118**(2):223–36.
30. Clary-Meinesz C, et al. Influence of external pH on ciliary beat frequency in human bronchi and bronchioles. *Eur Respir J* 1998;**11**(2):330–3.
31. Verkman AS, Song Y, Thiagarajah JR. Role of airway surface liquid and submucosal glands in cystic fibrosis lung disease. *Am J Physiol Cell Physiol* 2003;**284**(1):C2–15.
32. Gruber P, Longer MA, Robinson JR. Some biological issues in oral, controlled drug delivery. *Adv Drug Deliv Rev* 1987;**1**(1):1–18.
33. Ovesen L, et al. Intraluminal pH in the stomach, duodenum, and proximal jejunum in normal subjects and patients with exocrine pancreatic insufficiency. *Gastroenterology* 1986;**90**(4):958–62.
34. Schoenwald RD. Ocular drug delivery. Pharmacokinetic considerations. *Clin Pharmacokinet* 1990;**18**(4):255–69.
35. Bonanno JA, Polse KA. Measurement of in vivo human corneal stromal pH: open and closed eyes. *Investig Ophthalmol Vis Sci* 1987;**28**(3):522–30.
36. King-Smith PE, et al. The thickness of the tear film. *Curr Eye Res* 2004;**29**(4–5):357–68.
37. Holly FJ. Formation and rupture of the tear film. *Exp Eye Res* 1973;**15**(5):515–25.
38. Clarke MA, et al. A large, population-based study of age-related associations between vaginal pH and human papillomavirus infection. *BMC Infect Dis* 2012;**12**:33.
39. Ensign LM, Cone R, Hanes J. Oral drug delivery with polymeric nanoparticles: the gastrointestinal mucus barriers. *Adv Drug Deliv Rev* 2012;**64**(6):557–70.
40. Schneider CS, et al. Nanoparticles that do not adhere to mucus provide uniform and long-lasting drug delivery to airways following inhalation. *Sci Adv* 2017;**3**(4).
41. Lai SK, Wang YY, Hanes J. Mucus-penetrating nanoparticles for drug and gene delivery to mucosal tissues. *Adv Drug Deliv Rev* 2009;**61**(2):158–71.
42. Dawson M, et al. Transport of polymeric nanoparticle gene carriers in gastric mucus. *Biotechnol Prog* 2004;**20**(3):851–7.
43. Crater JS, Carrier RL. Barrier properties of gastrointestinal mucus to nanoparticle transport. *Macromol Biosci* 2010;**10**(12):1473–83.
44. Griffiths PC, et al. Probing the interaction of nanoparticles with mucin for drug delivery applications using dynamic light scattering. *Eur J Pharm Biopharm* 2015;**97**(Pt A):218–22.
45. Lieleg O, Vladescu I, Ribbeck K. Characterization of particle translocation through mucin hydrogels. *Biophys J* 2010;**98**(9):1782–9.
46. Mantelli F, Mauris J, Argueso P. The ocular surface epithelial barrier and other mechanisms of mucosal protection: from allergy to infectious diseases. *Curr Opin Allergy Clin Immunol* 2013;**13**(5):563–8.
47. Tomlinson A, Doane MG, McFadyen A. Inputs and outputs of the lacrimal system: review of production and evaporative loss. *Ocul Surf* 2009;**7**(4):186–98.
48. Gaudana R, et al. Ocular drug delivery. *AAPS J* 2010;**12**(3):348–60.
49. Gaudana R, et al. Recent perspectives in ocular drug delivery. *Pharm Res* 2009;**26**(5):1197–216.
50. Doughty MJ, Zaman ML. Human corneal thickness and its impact on intraocular pressure measures: a review and meta-analysis approach. *Surv Ophthalmol* 2000;**44**(5):367–408.
51. Patel A, et al. Ocular drug delivery systems: an overview. *World J Pharmacol* 2013;**2**(2):47–64.
52. Bhatta RS, et al. Mucoadhesive nanoparticles for prolonged ocular delivery of natamycin: in vitro and pharmacokinetics studies. *Int J Pharm* 2012;**432**(1–2):105–12.
53. Xu Q, et al. Nanoparticle diffusion in, and microrheology of, the bovine vitreous ex vivo. *J Control Release* 2013;**167**(1):76–84.

54. Amrite AC, et al. Effect of circulation on the disposition and ocular tissue distribution of 20 nm nanoparticles after periocular administration. *Mol Vis* 2008;**14**:150–60.
55. Amrite AC, Kompella UB. Size-dependent disposition of nanoparticles and microparticles following subconjunctival administration. *J Pharm Pharmacol* 2005;**57**(12):1555–63.
56. Koo H, et al. The movement of self-assembled amphiphilic polymeric nanoparticles in the vitreous and retina after intravitreal injection. *Biomaterials* 2012;**33**(12):3485–93.
57. Kim H, Robinson SB, Csaky KG. Investigating the movement of intravitreal human serum albumin nanoparticles in the vitreous and retina. *Pharm Res* 2009;**26**(2):329–37.
58. Kapoor M, Cloyd JC, Siegel RA. A review of intranasal formulations for the treatment of seizure emergencies. *J Control Release* 2016;**237**:147–59.
59. Beule AG. Physiology and pathophysiology of respiratory mucosa of the nose and the paranasal sinuses. *GMS Curr Top Otorhinolaryngol, Head Neck Surg* 2010;**9**:Doc07.
60. Marasini N, Skwarczynski M, Toth I. Intranasal delivery of nanoparticle-based vaccines. *Ther Deliv* 2017;**8**(3):151–67.
61. Costa C, et al. Nose-to-brain delivery of lipid-based nanosystems for epileptic seizures and anxiety crisis. *J Control Release* 2019;**295**:187–200.
62. Feng Y, et al. An update on the role of nanovehicles in nose-to-brain drug delivery. *Drug Discov Today* 2018;**23**(5):1079–88.
63. Dombu CY, et al. Characterization of endocytosis and exocytosis of cationic nanoparticles in airway epithelium cells. *Nanotechnology* 2010;**21**(35):355102.
64. Sonaje K, et al. Opening of epithelial tight junctions and enhancement of paracellular permeation by chitosan: microscopic, ultrastructural, and computed-tomographic observations. *Mol Pharm* 2012;**9**(5):1271–9.
65. Bernocchi B, et al. Mechanisms allowing protein delivery in nasal mucosa using NPL nanoparticles. *J Control Release* 2016;**232**:42–50.
66. Matthews LW, et al. Studies on pulmonary secretions. I. The overall chemical composition of pulmonary secretions from patients with cystic fibrosis, bronchiectasis, and laryngectomy. *Am Rev Respir Dis* 1963;**88**:199–204.
67. Hamed R, Fiegel J. Synthetic tracheal mucus with native rheological and surface tension properties. *J Biomed Mater Res A* 2014;**102**(6):1788–98.
68. Tarran R, et al. Normal and cystic fibrosis airway surface liquid homeostasis. The effects of phasic shear stress and viral infections. *J Biol Chem* 2005;**280**(42):35751–9.
69. Carvalho TC, Peters JI, Williams 3rd RO. Influence of particle size on regional lung deposition–what evidence is there? *Int J Pharm* 2011;**406**(1–2):1–10.
70. Braakhuis HM, et al. Physicochemical characteristics of nanomaterials that affect pulmonary inflammation. *Part Fibre Toxicol* 2014;**11**:18.
71. Cassee FR, et al. Particle size-dependent total mass deposition in lungs determines inhalation toxicity of cadmium chloride aerosols in rats. Application of a multiple path dosimetry model. *Arch Toxicol* 2002;**76**(5–6):277–86.
72. Geiser M, Kreyling WG. Deposition and biokinetics of inhaled nanoparticles. *Part Fibre Toxicol* 2010;**7**:2.
73. Alpar HO, et al. Biodegradable mucoadhesive particulates for nasal and pulmonary antigen and DNA delivery. *Adv Drug Deliv Rev* 2005;**57**(3):411–30.
74. Xu Q, et al. Scalable method to produce biodegradable nanoparticles that rapidly penetrate human mucus. *J Control Release* 2013;**170**(2):279–86.
75. Xu Q, et al. Impact of surface polyethylene glycol (PEG) density on biodegradable nanoparticle transport in mucus ex vivo and distribution in vivo. *ACS Nano* 2015;**9**(9):9217–27.
76. Huckaby JT, Lai SK. PEGylation for enhancing nanoparticle diffusion in mucus. *Adv Drug Deliv Rev* 2018;**124**:125–39.
77. van der Waaij LA, et al. Bacterial population analysis of human colon and terminal ileum biopsies with 16S rRNA-based fluorescent probes: commensal bacteria live in suspension and have no direct contact with epithelial cells. *Inflamm Bowel Dis* 2005;**11**(10):865–71.
78. Pelaseyed T, et al. The mucus and mucins of the goblet cells and enterocytes provide the first defense line of the gastrointestinal tract and interact with the immune system. *Immunol Rev* 2014;**260**(1):8–20.
79. Fordtran JS, Locklear TW. Ionic constituents and osmolality of gastric and small-intestinal fluids after eating. *Am J Dig Dis* 1966;**11**(7):503–21.
80. Soybel DI. Anatomy and physiology of the stomach. *Surg Clin N Am* 2005;**85**(5):875–94 [v].
81. Lai SK, et al. Nanoparticles reveal that human cervicovaginal mucus is riddled with pores larger than viruses. *Proc Natl Acad Sci USA* 2010;**107**(2):598–603.
82. Chen D, et al. Comparative study of Pluronic((R)) F127-modified liposomes and chitosan-modified liposomes for mucus penetration and oral absorption of Cyclosporine A in rats. *Int J Pharm* 2013;**449**(1–2):1–9.
83. Maisel K, et al. Effect of surface chemistry on nanoparticle interaction with gastrointestinal mucus and distribution in the gastrointestinal tract following oral and rectal administration in the mouse. *J Control Release* 2015;**197**:48–57.
84. Pawar VK, et al. Targeting of gastrointestinal tract for amended delivery of protein/peptide therapeutics: strategies and industrial perspectives. *J Control Release* 2014;**196**:168–83.
85. Pridgen EM, Alexis F, Farokhzad OC. Polymeric nanoparticle drug delivery technologies for oral delivery applications. *Expert Opin Drug Deliv* 2015;**12**(9):1459–73.
86. Hunter AC, et al. Polymeric particulate technologies for oral drug delivery and targeting: a pathophysiological perspective. *Nanomedicine* 2012;**8**(Suppl. 1):S5–20.
87. Smart AL, Gaisford S, Basit AW. Oral peptide and protein delivery: intestinal obstacles and commercial prospects. *Expert Opin Drug Deliv* 2014;**11**(8):1323–35.
88. Date AA, Hanes J, Ensign LM. Nanoparticles for oral delivery: design, evaluation and state-of-the-art. *J Control Release* 2016;**240**:504–26.
89. Odeblad E. The functional structure of human cervical mucus. *Acta Obstet Gynecol Scand* 1968;**47**:57–79.
90. Maisel K, et al. Enema ion compositions for enhancing colorectal drug delivery. *J Control Release* 2015;**209**:280–7.
91. Suman JD. Current understanding of nasal morphology and physiology as a drug delivery target. *Drug Deliv Transl Res* 2013;**3**(1):4–15.

92. Hansson GC, Johansson ME. The inner of the two Muc2 mucin-dependent mucus layers in colon is devoid of bacteria. *Gut Microb* 2010;**1**(1):51–4.
93. Liu S, et al. Prolonged ocular retention of mucoadhesive nanoparticle eye drop formulation enables treatment of eye diseases using significantly reduced dosage. *Mol Pharm* 2016;**13**(9):2897–905.
94. Saketkhoo K, Januszkiewicz A, Sackner MA. Effects of drinking hot water, cold water, and chicken soup on nasal mucus velocity and nasal airflow resistance. *Chest* 1978;**74**(4):408–10.
95. Mainardes RM, et al. Liposomes and micro/nanoparticles as colloidal carriers for nasal drug delivery. *Curr Drug Deliv* 2006;**3**(3):275–85.
96. Allemann E, Leroux J, Gurny R. Polymeric nano- and microparticles for the oral delivery of peptides and peptidomimetics. *Adv Drug Deliv Rev* 1998;**34**(2–3):171–89.
97. Galindo-Rodriguez SA, et al. Polymeric nanoparticles for oral delivery of drugs and vaccines: a critical evaluation of in vivo studies. *Crit Rev Ther Drug Carrier Syst* 2005;**22**(5):419–64.
98. Lehr Claus-Michael, Poelma Fred GJ, Junginger Hans E, Tukker Josef J. An estimate of turnover time of intestinal mucus gel layer in the rat in situ loop. *Int J Pharm* 1991;**70**(3):235–40.
99. Kieweg SL, Katz DF. Squeezing flows of vaginal gel formulations relevant to microbicide drug delivery. *J Biomech Eng* 2006;**128**(4):540–53.
100. Wang Z, et al. CuO nanoparticle interaction with human epithelial cells: cellular uptake, location, export, and genotoxicity. *Chem Res Toxicol* 2012;**25**(7):1512–21.
101. He B, et al. The transport pathways of polymer nanoparticles in MDCK epithelial cells. *Biomaterials* 2013;**34**(17):4309–26.
102. Bannunah AM, et al. Mechanisms of nanoparticle internalization and transport across an intestinal epithelial cell model: effect of size and surface charge. *Mol Pharm* 2014;**11**(12):4363–73.
103. Pond SM, Tozer TN. First-pass elimination. Basic concepts and clinical consequences. *Clin Pharmacokinet* 1984;**9**(1):1–25.
104. des Rieux A, et al. Nanoparticles as potential oral delivery systems of proteins and vaccines: a mechanistic approach. *J Control Release* 2006;**116**(1):1–27.
105. Cai S, et al. Lymphatic drug delivery using engineered liposomes and solid lipid nanoparticles. *Adv Drug Deliv Rev* 2011;**63**(10–11):901–8.
106. Trevaskis NL, Kaminskas LM, Porter CJ. From sewer to saviour - targeting the lymphatic system to promote drug exposure and activity. *Nat Rev Drug Discov* 2015;**14**(11):781–803.
107. Chaudhary S, et al. Recent approaches of lipid-based delivery system for lymphatic targeting via oral route. *J Drug Target* 2014;**22**(10):871–82.
108. Singh I, et al. Lymphatic system: a prospective area for advanced targeting of particulate drug carriers. *Expert Opin Drug Deliv* 2014;**11**(2):211–29.
109. Storm G, Belliot SO, Daemen T, Lasic DD. Surface modification of nanoparticles to oppose uptake by the mononuclear phagocyte system. *Adv Drug Deliv Rev* 1995;**17**:31–48.
110. Owens 3rd DE, Peppas NA. Opsonization, biodistribution, and pharmacokinetics of polymeric nanoparticles. *Int J Pharm* 2006;**307**(1):93–102.
111. Elsabahy M, Wooley KL. Design of polymeric nanoparticles for biomedical applications. *Chem Soc Rev* 2013;**41**(7):2545–61.
112. Arvizo RR, et al. Modulating pharmacokinetics, tumor uptake and biodistribution by engineered nanoparticles. *PLoS One* 2011;**6**(9):e24374.
113. Alexis F, et al. Factors affecting the clearance and biodistribution of polymeric nanoparticles. *Mol Pharm* 2008;**5**(4):505–15.
114. Choi HS, et al. Renal clearance of quantum dots. *Nat Biotechnol* 2007;**25**(10):1165–70.
115. Moghimi SM, Hunter AC, Andresen TL. Factors controlling nanoparticle pharmacokinetics: an integrated analysis and perspective. *Annu Rev Pharmacol Toxicol* 2012;**52**:481–503.
116. Moghimi SM, et al. An investigation of the filtration capacity and the fate of large filtered sterically-stabilized microspheres in rat spleen. *Biochim Biophys Acta* 1993;**1157**(3):233–40.
117. Moghimi SM, et al. Non-phagocytic uptake of intravenously injected microspheres in rat spleen: influence of particle size and hydrophilic coating. *Biochem Biophys Res Commun* 1991;**177**(2):861–6.
118. Moghimi SM, Hunter AC, Murray JC. Long-circulating and target-specific nanoparticles: theory to practice. *Pharmacol Rev* 2001;**53**(2):283–318.
119. Patel HM, Moghimi SM. Serum-mediated recognition of liposomes by phagocytic cells of the reticuloendothelial system - the concept of tissue specificity. *Adv Drug Deliv Rev* 1998;**32**(1–2):45–60.
120. Tenzer S, et al. Rapid formation of plasma protein corona critically affects nanoparticle pathophysiology. *Nat Nanotechnol* 2013;**8**(10):772–81.
121. Nel AE, et al. Understanding biophysicochemical interactions at the nano-bio interface. *Nat Mater* 2009;**8**(7):543–57.
122. Sahay G, Alakhova DY, Kabanov AV. Endocytosis of nanomedicines. *J Control Release* 2010;**145**(3):182–95.
123. Gref R, et al. Biodegradable long-circulating polymeric nanospheres. *Science* 1994;**263**(5153):1600–3.
124. Harris JM, Chess RB. Effect of pegylation on pharmaceuticals. *Nat Rev Drug Discov* 2003;**2**(3):214–21.
125. Perry JL, et al. PEGylated PRINT nanoparticles: the impact of PEG density on protein binding, macrophage association, biodistribution, and pharmacokinetics. *Nano Lett* 2012;**12**(10):5304–10.
126. Guo S, Huang L. Nanoparticles escaping RES and endosome: challenges for siRNA delivery for cancer therapy. *J Nanomater* 2011;**2011**:12.
127. Zhang L, et al. Softer zwitterionic nanogels for longer circulation and lower splenic accumulation. *ACS Nano* 2012;**6**(8):6681–6.
128. Parodi A, et al. Synthetic nanoparticles functionalized with biomimetic leukocyte membranes possess cell-like functions. *Nat Nanotechnol* 2013;**8**(1):61–8.
129. Hu CM, et al. Erythrocyte membrane-camouflaged polymeric nanoparticles as a biomimetic delivery platform. *Proc Natl Acad Sci USA* 2011;**108**(27):10980–5.
130. Elsabahy M, Wooley KL. Design of polymeric nanoparticles for biomedical delivery applications. *Chem Soc Rev* 2012;**41**(7):2545–61.
131. Chen H, et al. Fast release of lipophilic agents from circulating PEG-PDLLA micelles revealed by in vivo forster resonance energy transfer imaging. *Langmuir* 2008;**24**(10):5213–7.
132. Blanco E, Shen H, Ferrari M. Principles of nanoparticle design for overcoming biological barriers to drug delivery. *Nat Biotechnol* 2015;**33**(9):941–51.

133. Popel AS, Johnson PC. Microcirculation and hemorheology. *Annu Rev Fluid Mech* 2005;**37**:43–69.
134. Fullstone G, et al. Modelling the transport of nanoparticles under blood flow using an agent-based approach. *Sci Rep* 2015;**5**:10649.
135. Wiig H, Swartz MA. Interstitial fluid and lymph formation and transport: physiological regulation and roles in inflammation and cancer. *Physiol Rev* 2012;**92**(3):1005–60.
136. Gomez-Garcia MJ, et al. Nanoparticle localization in blood vessels: dependence on fluid shear stress, flow disturbances, and flow-induced changes in endothelial physiology. *Nanoscale* 2018;**10**(32):15249–61.
137. Ye H, Zhen Z, Yu L, Wei M, Li Y. Manipulating nanoparticle transport within blood flow through external forces: an exemplar of mechanics in nanomedicine. *Proc Math Phys Eng Sci* 2018:474.
138. Muller K, Fedosov DA, Gompper G. Margination of micro- and nano-particles in blood flow and its effect on drug delivery. *Sci Rep* 2014;**4**:4871.
139. Muller K, Fedosov DA, Gompper G. Understanding particle margination in blood flow – a step toward optimized drug delivery systems. *Med Eng Phys* 2016;**38**(1):2–10.
140. Geng Y, et al. Shape effects of filaments versus spherical particles in flow and drug delivery. *Nat Nanotechnol* 2007;**2**(4):249–55.
141. Wang Y, et al. Generation of a library of particles having controlled sizes and shapes via the mechanical elongation of master templates. *Langmuir* 2011;**27**(2):524–8.
142. Tao L, et al. Lithographically defined uniform worm-shaped polymeric nanoparticles. *Nanotechnology* 2010;**21**(9):095301.
143. Merkel TJ, et al. Using mechanobiological mimicry of red blood cells to extend circulation times of hydrogel microparticles. *Proc Natl Acad Sci USA* 2011;**108**(2):586–91.
144. Doshi N, et al. Red blood cell-mimicking synthetic biomaterial particles. *Proc Natl Acad Sci USA* 2009;**106**(51):21495–9.
145. Cataldi M, et al. Emerging role of the spleen in the pharmacokinetics of monoclonal antibodies, nanoparticles and exosomes. *Int J Mol Sci* 2017;**18**(6).
146. Perrault SD, et al. Mediating tumor targeting efficiency of nanoparticles through design. *Nano Lett* 2009;**9**(5):1909–15.
147. Zhang G, et al. Influence of anchoring ligands and particle size on the colloidal stability and in vivo biodistribution of polyethylene glycol-coated gold nanoparticles in tumor-xenografted mice. *Biomaterials* 2009;**30**(10):1928–36.
148. Demoy M, et al. In vitro evaluation of nanoparticles spleen capture. *Life Sci* 1999;**64**(15):1329–37.
149. Deen WM, Lazzara MJ, Myers BD. Structural determinants of glomerular permeability. *Am J Physiol Renal Physiol* 2001;**281**(4):F579–96.
150. Zhang XD, et al. In vivo renal clearance, biodistribution, toxicity of gold nanoclusters. *Biomaterials* 2012;**33**(18):4628–38.
151. Longmire M, Choyke PL, Kobayashi H. Clearance properties of nano-sized particles and molecules as imaging agents: considerations and caveats. *Nanomedicine* 2008;**3**(5):703–17.
152. Ohlson M, Sorensson J, Haraldsson B. A gel-membrane model of glomerular charge and size selectivity in series. *Am J Physiol Renal Physiol* 2001;**280**(3):F396–405.
153. Kuntz E, K.H D. *Hepatology: principles and practice: history, morphology, biochemistry, diagnostics, clinic, therapy*. 2nd ed., vol. 3. Springer; 2006.
154. Rodrigues SF, Granger DN. Blood cells and endothelial barrier function. *Tissue Barriers* 2015;**3**(1–2):e978720.
155. Favero G, et al. Endothelium and its alterations in cardiovascular diseases: life style intervention. *BioMed Res Int* 2014;**2014**:801896.
156. Levick JR, Smaje LH. An analysis of the permeability of a fenestra. *Microvasc Res* 1987;**33**(2):233–56.
157. Aird WC. Phenotypic heterogeneity of the endothelium: i. Structure, function, and mechanisms. *Circ Res* 2007;**100**(2):158–73.
158. Wisse E. An electron microscopic study of the fenestrated endothelial lining of rat liver sinusoids. *J Ultrastruct Res* 1970;**31**(1):125–50.
159. Morrissey MA, Sherwood DR. An active role for basement membrane assembly and modification in tissue sculpting. *J Cell Sci* 2015;**128**(9):1661–8.
160. Kim Y, et al. Probing nanoparticle translocation across the permeable endothelium in experimental atherosclerosis. *Proc Natl Acad Sci USA* 2014;**111**(3):1078–83.
161. Xu S, et al. Targeting receptor-mediated endocytotic pathways with nanoparticles: rationale and advances. *Adv Drug Deliv Rev* 2013;**65**(1):121–38.
162. Wang Z, Malik AB. Nanoparticles squeezing across the blood-endothelial barrier via caveolae. *Ther Deliv* 2013;**4**(2):131–3.
163. Voigt J, Christensen J, Shastri VP. Differential uptake of nanoparticles by endothelial cells through polyelectrolytes with affinity for caveolae. *Proc Natl Acad Sci USA* 2014;**111**(8):2942–7.
164. Ye H, et al. Manipulating nanoparticle transport within blood flow through external forces: an exemplar of mechanics in nanomedicine. *Proc Math Phys Eng Sci* 2018;**474**(2211):20170845.
165. Achouri D, et al. Recent advances in ocular drug delivery. *Drug Dev Ind Pharm* 2013;**39**(11):1599–617.
166. Tomi M, Hosoya K. The role of blood-ocular barrier transporters in retinal drug disposition: an overview. *Expert Opin Drug Metabol Toxicol* 2010;**6**(9):1111–24.
167. Gregoire N. The blood-brain barrier. *J Neuroradiol* 1989;**16**(3):238–50.
168. Abbott NJ, et al. Structure and function of the blood-brain barrier. *Neurobiol Dis* 2010;**37**(1):13–25.
169. Wolburg H, Lippoldt A. Tight junctions of the blood-brain barrier: development, composition and regulation. *Vasc Pharmacol* 2002;**38**(6):323–37.
170. Kooij G, et al. The role of ATP-binding cassette transporters in neuro-inflammation: relevance for bioactive lipids. *Front Pharmacol* 2012;**3**:74.
171. Yemisci M, et al. Systemically administered brain-targeted nanoparticles transport peptides across the blood-brain barrier and provide neuroprotection. *J Cereb Blood Flow Metab* 2015;**35**(3):469–75.
172. Song Q, et al. Lipoprotein-based nanoparticles rescue the memory loss of mice with Alzheimer's disease by accelerating the clearance of amyloid-beta. *ACS Nano* 2014;**8**(3):2345–59.
173. Gao X, et al. Overcoming the blood-brain barrier for delivering drugs into the brain by using adenosine receptor nanoagonist. *ACS Nano* 2014;**8**(4):3678–89.
174. Kreuter J. Influence of the surface properties on nanoparticle-mediated transport of drugs to the brain. *J Nanosci Nanotechnol* 2004;**4**(5):484–8.
175. Kreuter J. Mechanism of polymeric nanoparticle-based drug transport across the blood-brain barrier (BBB). *J Microencapsul* 2013;**30**(1):49–54.

176. Wiley DT, et al. Transcytosis and brain uptake of transferrin-containing nanoparticles by tuning avidity to transferrin receptor. *Proc Natl Acad Sci USA* 2013;**110**(21):8662–7.
177. Kong SD, et al. Magnetic targeting of nanoparticles across the intact blood-brain barrier. *J Control Release* 2012;**164**(1):49–57.
178. Koffie RM, et al. Nanoparticles enhance brain delivery of blood-brain barrier-impermeable probes for in vivo optical and magnetic resonance imaging. *Proc Natl Acad Sci USA* 2011;**108**(46):18837–42.
179. Curtis C, et al. Systems-level thinking for nanoparticle-mediated therapeutic delivery to neurological diseases. *Wiley Interdiscip Rev Nanomed Nanobiotechnol* 2017;**9**(2).
180. Nance E, et al. Systemic dendrimer-drug treatment of ischemia-induced neonatal white matter injury. *J Control Release* 2015;**214**:112–20.
181. Nance E, et al. Nanoscale effects in dendrimer-mediated targeting of neuroinflammation. *Biomaterials* 2016;**101**:96–107.
182. Joseph A, Wood T, Chen C-C, Corry K, Snyder JM, Juul SE, Parikh P, Nance E. Curcumin-loaded polymeric nanoparticles for neuroprotection in neonatal rats with hypoxic-ischemic encephalopathy. *Nano Research* 2018;**11**(10):5670–88.
183. Dityatev A, Seidenbecher CI, Schachner M. Compartmentalization from the outside: the extracellular matrix and functional microdomains in the brain. *Trends Neurosci* 2010;**33**(11):503–12.
184. Mouw JK, Ou G, Weaver VM. Extracellular matrix assembly: a multiscale deconstruction. *Nat Rev Mol Cell Biol* 2014;**15**(12):771–85.
185. Hay ED. Extracellular matrix alters epithelial differentiation. *Curr Opin Cell Biol* 1993;**5**(6):1029–35.
186. Lu P, et al. Extracellular matrix degradation and remodeling in development and disease. *Cold Spring Harb Perspect Biol* 2011;**3**(12).
187. Mecham RP. Overview of extracellular matrix. *Curr Protoc Cell Biol* 2001 [Chapter 10]: p. Unit 10 1.
188. Sonbol HS. Extracellular matrix remodeling in human disease. *J Microsc Ultrastruct* 2018;**6**(3):123–8.
189. Frantz C, Stewart KM, Weaver VM. The extracellular matrix at a glance. *J Cell Sci* 2010;**123**(Pt 24):4195–200.
190. Birk DE, et al. Collagen fibrillogenesis in situ: fibril segments become long fibrils as the developing tendon matures. *Dev Dynam* 1997;**208**(3):291–8.
191. Zhang G, et al. Development of tendon structure and function: regulation of collagen fibrillogenesis. *J Musculoskelet Neuronal Interact* 2005;**5**(1):5–21.
192. Sasaki N, Odajima S. Elongation mechanism of collagen fibrils and force-strain relations of tendon at each level of structural hierarchy. *J Biomech* 1996;**29**(9):1131–6.
193. Bandtlow CE, Zimmermann DR. Proteoglycans in the developing brain: new conceptual insights for old proteins. *Physiol Rev* 2000;**80**(4):1267–90.
194. Knudson CB, Knudson W. Cartilage proteoglycans. *Semin Cell Dev Biol* 2001;**12**(2):69–78.
195. Kannus P. Structure of the tendon connective tissue. *Scand J Med Sci Sport* 2000;**10**(6):312–20.
196. Wang JH. Mechanobiology of tendon. *J Biomech* 2006;**39**(9):1563–82.
197. Chen Q, et al. Cartilage matrix protein: expression patterns in chicken, mouse, and human. *Ann N Y Acad Sci* 1996;**785**:238–40.
198. Yameen B, et al. Insight into nanoparticle cellular uptake and intracellular targeting. *J Control Release* 2014;**190**:485–99.
199. Chithrani BD, Ghazani AA, Chan WC. Determining the size and shape dependence of gold nanoparticle uptake into mammalian cells. *Nano Lett* 2006;**6**(4):662–8.
200. Xie X, et al. The effect of shape on cellular uptake of gold nanoparticles in the forms of stars, rods, and triangles. *Sci Rep* 2017;**7**(1):3827.
201. Sun J, et al. Tunable rigidity of (polymeric core)-(lipid shell) nanoparticles for regulated cellular uptake. *Adv Mater* 2015;**27**(8):1402–7.
202. Fang Y, et al. Cleavable PEGylation: a strategy for overcoming the "PEG dilemma" in efficient drug delivery. *Drug Deliv* 2017;**24**(Suppl. 1):22–32.
203. Xu M, et al. PEG-detachable polymeric micelles self-assembled from amphiphilic copolymers for tumor-acidity-triggered drug delivery and controlled release. *ACS Appl Mater Interfaces* 2019.
204. Champion JA, Walker A, Mitragotri S. Role of particle size in phagocytosis of polymeric microspheres. *Pharm Res* 2008;**25**(8):1815–21.
205. Champion JA, Mitragotri S. Role of target geometry in phagocytosis. *Proc Natl Acad Sci USA* 2006;**103**(13):4930–4.
206. Paul D, et al. Phagocytosis dynamics depends on target shape. *Biophys J* 2013;**105**(5):1143–50.
207. Hillaireau H, Couvreur P. Nanocarriers' entry into the cell: relevance to drug delivery. *Cell Mol Life Sci* 2009;**66**(17):2873–96.
208. Zhang S, Gao H, Bao G. Physical principles of nanoparticle cellular endocytosis. *ACS Nano* 2015;**9**(9):8655–71.
209. Kuhn DA, et al. Different endocytotic uptake mechanisms for nanoparticles in epithelial cells and macrophages. *Beilstein J Nanotechnol* 2014;**5**:1625–36.
210. Swanson JA, Baer SC. Phagocytosis by zippers and triggers. *Trends Cell Biol* 1995;**5**(3):89–93.
211. Aderem A, Underhill DM. Mechanisms of phagocytosis in macrophages. *Annu Rev Immunol* 1999;**17**:593–623.
212. Lee Y, et al. A protein nanocarrier from charge-conversion polymer in response to endosomal pH. *J Am Chem Soc* 2007;**129**(17):5362–3.
213. Wasungu L, Hoekstra D. Cationic lipids, lipoplexes and intracellular delivery of genes. *J Control Release* 2006;**116**(2):255–64.
214. Chou LY, Ming K, Chan WC. Strategies for the intracellular delivery of nanoparticles. *Chem Soc Rev* 2011;**40**(1):233–45.
215. Terry LJ, Shows EB, Wente SR. Crossing the nuclear envelope: hierarchical regulation of nucleocytoplasmic transport. *Science* 2007;**318**(5855):1412–6.
216. Serda RE, et al. Logic-embedded vectors for intracellular partitioning, endosomal escape, and exocytosis of nanoparticles. *Small* 2010;**6**(23):2691–700.
217. Jiang X, et al. Endo- and exocytosis of zwitterionic quantum dot nanoparticles by live HeLa cells. *ACS Nano* 2010;**4**(11):6787–97.
218. Chithrani BD, Chan WC. Elucidating the mechanism of cellular uptake and removal of protein-coated gold nanoparticles of different sizes and shapes. *Nano Lett* 2007;**7**(6):1542–50.
219. Sakhtianchi R, et al. Exocytosis of nanoparticles from cells: role in cellular retention and toxicity. *Adv Colloid Interface Sci* 2013;**201–202**:18–29.
220. Sun W, Hu Q, Ji W, Wright G, Gu Z. Leveraging physiology for precision drug delivery. *Physiol Rev* 2017;**97**(1):189–225.

Chapter 8

A pharmacokinetics primer for preclinical nanomedicine research

Hao Guo[1] and John Andrew MacKay[1,2,3]

[1]*Department of Pharmacology and Pharmaceutical Sciences, School of Pharmacy, University of Southern California, Los Angeles, CA, United States;* [2]*Department of Biomedical Engineering, Viterbi School of Engineering, University of Southern California, Los Angeles, CA, United States;* [3]*Department of Ophthalmology, Roski Eye Institute, Keck School of Medicine, University of Southern California, Los Angeles, CA, United States*

Variables studied in this chapter:

C_{max} Maximum blood concentration
t_{max} Time to achieve maximum blood concentration
CL clearance
V volume of distribution
V_{ss} Volume of distribution at steady state
AUC Area under the curve
AUMC area under the moment curve
MRT mean residence time
MAT mean absorption time
F bioavailability.
$t_{1/2}$ Half-life
$t_{1/2,\ terminal}$ Terminal half-life
$t_{1/2,\ abs}$ Absorption half-life
$t_{1/2,\ elim}$ Elimination half-life
$t_{1/2,\ dist}$ Distribution half-life

8.1 Introduction

As suggested by its linguistic roots in Greek, pharmacokinetics (PK) involves the characterization of the use of drugs "pharmakeia" and their motion "kinetikos" in the body. PK was developed because pharmacists realized that timing of the appearance and disappearance of drugs in the body would determine their dose, frequency, and route of administration. Thus, scholars and practitioners of pharmacy began collecting blood-based samples as a function of time after dose and standardizing methods for their interpretation. A primary endpoint for most first-in-humans phase I clinical trials is to produce a PK profile after a single, safe dose.[1,2] With estimates of human PK parameters, it becomes possible to evaluate therapeutically relevant, multidose regimens during subsequent clinical trials. A reasonable PK profile can mean several things. For example, the half-life must be sufficient that the patient can take it at reasonable intervals without trough concentrations too low to maintain therapy. During peak concentrations following dosing, the drug concentration must remain below pharmacodynamically acceptable limits for acute and chronic toxicity. Alternatively, the extent of absorption for an extravascular dose (including oral and subcutaneous administration) should be high enough to limit dose-to-dose variability in blood levels and toxicity. Unless efficacy is of remarkable benefit to the patient, drug candidates that fail to have a clinically relevant half-life and oral bioavailability usually do not succeed. While there remains deep PK expertise within major pharmaceutical companies, better dissemination of PK expertise is required to academic groups developing early-stage nanoparticles, like those shown in Fig. 8.1.

Throughout the 1970–2000s, a number of attempts were made to develop drug carriers, which by their nature would change the PK profile of a drug to that of the carrier. A common rationale was that the drug carrier could increase the therapeutic index,[3] making drugs more potent and/or safer. The most successful examples are liposomes, into which more than 10 different small molecules have been entrapped and approved by the US Food and Drug Administration.[4] Optimized liposomes do a good job of retaining and then releasing active drugs; furthermore, they force encapsulated/engrafted drugs to adopt the PK of the liposomes. Since liposomes cannot typically be administered orally, it was important that their dose frequency remain on the order of once a week. This requires that liposomes have an $\sim$2 day half-life in humans,[5] which they achieved. It took 20 years of research and development to achieve this in liposomes, which was facilitated by grafting an optimal polymer (polyethylene glycol), at the optimal molecular weight ($\sim$2000 Da), at the optimal surface grafting density ($\sim$5% by mol lipid).[4] During the 2000s,

Nanoparticles for Biomedical Applications. https://doi.org/10.1016/B978-0-12-816662-8.00008-4

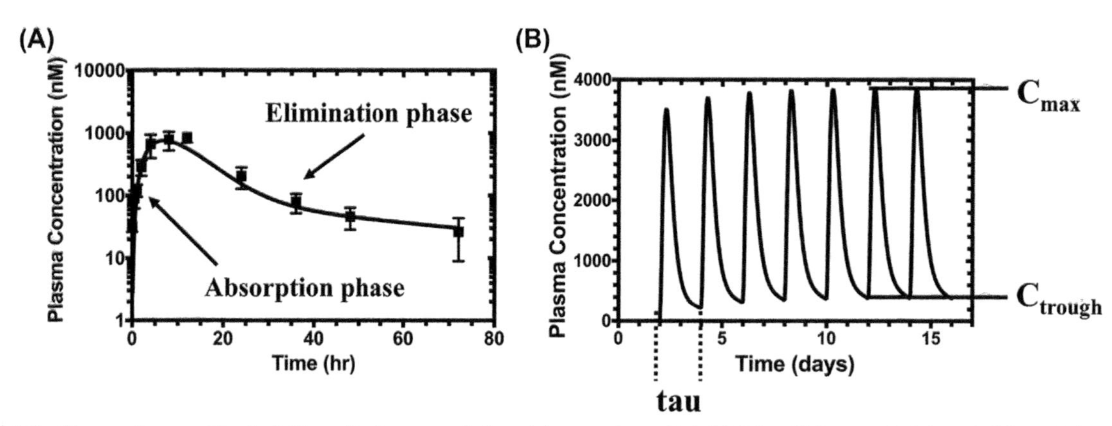

FIGURE 8.1 Plasma pharmacokinetic (PK) profile for a protein-based drug carrier, called CA192, which was administered SC to mice. (A) After a single dose, the formulation exhibited both an absorption and distribution phase before settling into an elimination phase with a terminal half-life of ~24 hr. (B) A modeling approach was used to estimate how plasma concentrations would appear over time during multiple dosing at 48 hr intervals (tau). C_{max} and C_{trough} are indicated. *Data extracted from Guo, H., et al., A novel elastin-like polypeptide drug carrier for cyclosporine A improves tear flow in a mouse model of Sjögren's syndrome. J Control Release, 2018. 292: p. 183–195.*

the conviction spread that many other materials and architectures would make capable drug carriers and "nanomedicine" entered the lexicon. During this period, drug delivery technologies expanded well beyond schools of pharmacy and major pharmaceutical companies, where traditional expertise in PK resided. Biologists, bioengineers, chemists, chemical engineers, and electrical engineers have developed numerous technologies, as detailed in this book and elsewhere. These range from implantable digitally operated pumps, bioerodable wafers,[6] PEGylated proteins,[7] sterically shielded liposomes,[4] antibody–drug conjugates,[8] and other nanoparticles.[9]

The purpose of this chapter is to quickly orient scholars investigating preclinical nanoparticles to the design and analysis of PK studies. Based on personal observations, reputable academic journals commonly peer review or even publish PK studies that fail to collect adequate time points, to calculate basic PK parameters, or to use simple models of drug disposition. It is common to see PK studies reduced to the observation that the concentrations for one formulation remain higher than another, which essentially removes kinetics from the analysis. Why does this matter? Unlike the nonlinear, indirect connections between drug regimen and its pharmacodynamic effect, the tools to relate drug regimen to blood concentrations of nanoparticles over time are very effective. When those profiles are used to estimate established PK parameters, structure–function studies will reveal significant strengths and weaknesses of emerging nanoparticles. Such studies should be used to interpret and optimize the nanoparticle physicochemistry (size, shape, surface chemistry, rate of drug release, ligand grafting density, etc.) to reach dosing regimens sufficient for therapeutic end points. In this way, scholars of early-stage nanoparticles can maximize the likelihood of developing approved nanomedicines.

8.1.1 Inputs to a pharmacokinetic study

The inputs to a PK study are concentration–time profiles, which represent nanoparticle concentration in the plasma, serum, or whole blood. Whole blood contains ~42% hematocrit, which typically excludes nanoparticles. When blood samples are allowed to clot, blood cells and clotting factors can be removed by centrifugation, and the supernatant is defined as serum. Nanoparticles that bind blood cells or clotting factors may thus have lower concentrations than in whole blood. When blood is prevented from clotting, usually through the chelation of divalent cations and heparin, the blood cells can be removed by centrifugation and the supernatant is defined as plasma. Thus, plasma contains albumin, immunoglobulins, lipoproteins, clotting factors, and complement. All of the above factors may interact to different extents with nanoparticles. As these interactions raise or lower the observed sample concentrations, they will also affect estimates of PK parameters. For this reason, it is important to consider and identify the method for collecting blood samples.

To establish reliable PK parameter estimates, samples must be collected at sufficiently placed time points. In the absence of prior information about a nanoparticle, time points may be spread at factors of 2 (e.g., 0, 0.5, 1, 2, 4, 8, 16, 32, 64 hr) to capture both absorption/distribution phases with a short half-life and terminal phases with a longer half-life. In subsequent studies, time points can be removed or added such that each log-linear phase is covered by three to four time points ranging over about three half-lives. While the planning and collection of this data is critical, these concentration–time profiles only constitute an input to a PK study. Having determined these concentration–time profiles, the prudent investigator must next estimate output parameters, statistically compare these between formulations, and place these in the context of approved drugs and scientific literature.

8.1.2 Half-life

One potential output of a PK study is half-life, which is a familiar concept to many scholars. Half-life is a useful way to characterize first-order processes throughout the chemical, physical, electrical, biological, and even economic worlds. First-order processes can be easily identified by semilog plots as a function of time, whereby log-linear regions can be fit by an exponential growth or decay to estimate the half-life. PK processes often reveal half-lives, which can predict how a dose regimen will affect nanoparticle levels in the body. Dose too high and side effects dominate. Dose too infrequently and periods pass with subtherapeutic drug concentrations. Yet, calculation of blood half-life alone is inadequate to compare formulations. Observed PK profiles in the blood reflect multiple half-lives related to absorption, distribution, metabolism, and excretion (ADME) (Fig. 8.2A). Absorption includes transfer of nanoparticles at a site of introduction to its detection in blood samples. Distribution includes the reversible transfer of nanoparticles from blood into other tissues, which fill and release over time like a reservoir. Metabolism includes processes that irreversibly modify the nanoparticle from one species to another, keeping in mind that nanoparticle metabolites exhibit their own PK profiles in the body. Excretion includes irreversible transfer of nanoparticles from the body into urine or feces. Each of these processes takes time. If the dose were directly introduced into any one of these compartments, its concentration at that site often exhibits a constant, unique half-life (Fig. 8.2B). In contrast, the PK profile in the blood reflects contributions from all ADME processes. Even the terminal blood half-life following IV administration depends on processes of distribution and elimination (metabolism and/or excretion). A reasonable goal of a PK study might be to study a parameter specific to one ADME process and its structure–activity relationship with the nanoparticle. Since half-life is neither specific for, nor solely dependent on any particular ADME process, other PK parameters are recommended to evaluate structure–function studies of a nanoparticle.

8.1.3 Clearance

Arguably, the most important PK parameter for any nanoparticle (or cargo) is clearance, *Cl*. Like half-life, clearance is a constant that is independent of the time points selected for analysis. While observed half-lives are interrelated functions of all four ADME processes, clearance only quantifies processes that irreversibly eliminate the nanoparticle from blood. Since clearance isolates the effects of distribution (and absorption) from those of elimination (metabolism and excretion), PK studies are well-served by estimating this parameter. This chapter describes multiple ways to estimate clearance; however, its specific mathematical definition is as follows:

$$\text{Rate of drug elimination from the body} = Cl\,C(t) \quad (8.1)$$

This essentially states that the loss of the nanoparticle (or its cargo) in the body with respect to time is proportional to the measured concentration in a blood sample, $C(t)$. An important assumption is that the capacity to clear the nanoparticle is a first-order, nonsaturable process. For a first-order process, no matter how high the concentration, the rate of drug elimination can always increase. Though there are exceptions, this is a reasonable assumption for many small molecule drugs and nanoparticles near their intended doses. A nanoparticle that results in the same clearance at different doses is said to follow linear PK.

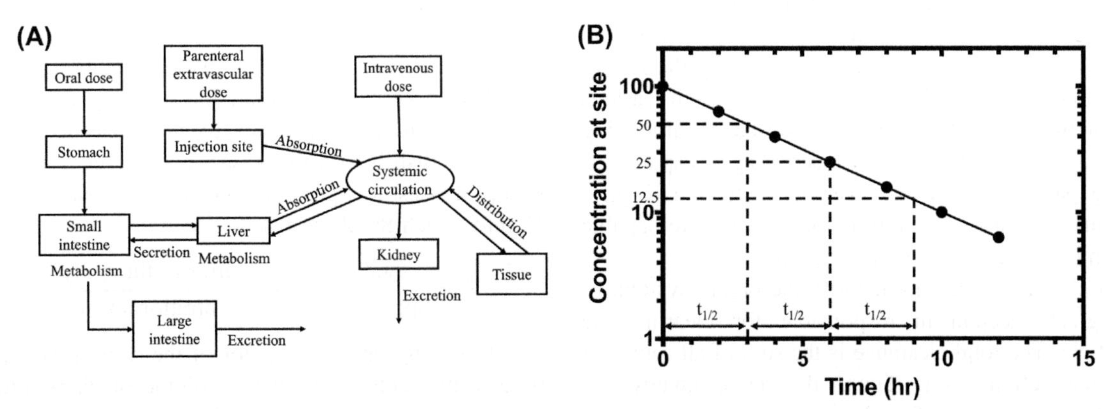

FIGURE 8.2 (A) Summary of important sites of mass transfer involved in absorption, distribution, metabolism, and excretion (ADME) processes after different routes of administration. The pharmacokinetic (PK) profile observed in systemic circulation (blood) results from mass balances around all ADME processes relevant to the site of administration. (B) For first-order ADME processes, the nanoparticle concentration driving each isolated flux falls by a constant half-life over time. Following a log-linear decay, this representative profile has a half-life of 3 hr. Different ADME processes will have different half-lives.

Inspection of Eq. 8.1 reveals that Cl has units of volume per time. Clearance scales with the size of the clearance organs, and therefore with the size of the organism. As such, it is common to normalize clearance to body weight or surface area. This can be useful in comparing subjects of different size, age, or species. Clearance estimates are immediately useful because they allow the calculation of a maintenance dose, MD, which will maintain an average target concentration, C_{target}, over multiple doses at steady state:

$$MD = \frac{tau\ Cl\ C_{target}}{F} \tag{8.2}$$

Where the bioavailability, F, represents the total absorbed dose ($F = 1$ for an IV bolus), and *tau* represents the time interval between doses. When designing a dosing regimen for a novel nanoparticle, calculation of a maintenance dose can help achieve target blood concentrations, which may be guided by *in vitro* cell-based or biochemical assays.

When nanoparticle clearance is determined only from blood and without inspecting measures of flux into particular organs, this is more accurately described as total clearance. The major two clearance organs are the kidney and the liver, and one or both play a major role in the clearance of nanoparticles. Many small molecule drugs have sufficient permeability or specificity to transport into hepatocytes, where they may be metabolized and/or excreted into the bile. Due to larger size, nanoparticles generally have low membrane permeability and instead become substrates for active internalization into liver cells through receptor-mediated endocytosis, macropinocytosis, or phagocytosis. Nanoparticles in the ~10–100 nm size range can diffuse through fenestrations of the basement membrane supporting the liver sinusoidal endothelial cells.[10] This slows transport to hepatocytes due to the size dependence of a Fickian diffusion constant and to a reduction in "permeable" surface area through fenestrations. Another significant complication, nanoparticles undergo opsonization by factors in blood that form a protein corona.[11] This corona tags them for capture by the reticuloendothelial system (RES). Distributed through various organs of the body, the RES is composed of circulating monocytes and resident tissue macrophages capable of engulfing particulates. In the liver, these are the Kupffer cells. Thus, within liver, multiple mechanisms are capable of clearing nanoparticles and their cargo.

Total clearance does not identify the organ, system, or physiological mechanism responsible for clearing the nanoparticle. The total clearance is the sum of all routes of nanoparticle elimination. Thus, if one estimates the contribution of a specific clearance mechanism, it is possible to estimate how significant each clearance mechanism is to the overall PK as follows:

$$Cl = Cl_{renal} + Cl_{hepatic} + Cl_{RES,nonhepatic} + Cl_{other} \tag{8.3}$$

For particles larger than the glomerular filtration cutoff (~5–10 nm), the renal clearance, Cl_{renal}, is typically low, such that hepatic clearance dominates. In contrast, small proteins, polymers, micelles, and inorganic nanoparticles may have very significant renal clearance. As suggested, $Cl_{hepatic}$, can represent accumulation in hepatocytes, direct capture by Kupffer cells, or binding to other cell types. Other tissues within the RES may also accumulate/retain/degrade nanoparticles through $Cl_{RES,\ nonhepatic}$. Having identified the total nanoparticle clearance, it may be possible to determine the significance of individual clearance mechanisms. By identifying which mechanism of elimination dominates clearance for a particular nanoparticle, effort can be focused on blocking that specific mechanism. This could more systematically reduce the nanoparticle clearance, increase the observed half-life, increase intervals between doses, and enhance therapeutic effects.

8.1.4 Volume of distribution

As a nanoparticle moves around the body, there are a number of places it may go before it is irreversibly cleared. It may bind tissues or blood cells, making its apparent concentration in the plasma lower. It may associate with plasma proteins or lipoproteins, while remaining concentrated in the plasma. Many drugs partition rapidly away from the plasma, such that observed plasma concentrations are much lower than would be expected by dilution into the available plasma volume, which is approximately 0.05 mL/g body weight for a rodent.[12] In addition, many drugs partition slowly enough to observe a distribution phase in their PK profile before they follow a log-linear terminal phase. In either case, distribution processes decrease plasma concentrations, which decreases the driving force to engage a pharmacological target. This also decreases concentrations passing through clearance organs, which lowers rate of drug clearance (Eq. 8.1) and can result in a longer terminal half-life. So, a nanoparticle with a significant distribution component could have a very long half-life, albeit concentrations too low to support efficacy. To account for distribution processes, as distinct from elimination processes, it is possible to calculate apparent volumes, V, into which the drug distributes:

$$V = \frac{\text{total amount of drug in the body}}{\text{apparent drug concentration in blood}} \tag{8.4}$$

Depending on the behavior of the drug, there are multiple further definitions of the volume of distribution. For example, immediately after a bolus dose to the vascular compartment, the drug concentration is measurable and in rapid equilibrium. By either taking a concentration immediately after dosing or by extrapolating back to time zero, it is possible to estimate V. Many drugs and nanoparticles have delayed distribution processes, which causes concentrations at later times to fall to lower levels then captured by the initial volume of distribution. For these drugs, it may be useful to calculate an apparent volume at steady state, V_{ss}. Volume of distribution estimates are immediately useful because they allow the calculation of a loading dose, LD, which can immediately bring a drug to a target concentration, C_{target}:

$$LD = \frac{V\ C_{target}}{F} \tag{8.5}$$

Where the bioavailability, F, represents the total absorbed dose. Estimation of a LD may be necessary to optimize therapies using nanoparticles with long half-lives, because the PK concentration profiles will not rise to steady-state levels for approximately four half-lives. Thus, nanoparticles with a long half-life, like an antibody–drug conjugate, may benefit from an initial loading dose.

8.2 Quantifying sample concentrations

Across assayed PK time points, the concentration of the nanoparticle and/or any critical cargo should be assessed. The analytical technique must be sensitive and accurate enough to estimate reliable concentrations in biological solutions. Concentrations below the limit of detection of an assay should be excluded from log-linear fitting because baseline signal will not decrease over time. Fitting data beyond the limit of detection will artifactually increase the nanoparticle half-life in the terminal phase. In addition, for any label attached to a nanoparticle, it is important that the free label be completely removed prior to administration and it is also important that biological factors do not lead to premature separation from the label. The following techniques are commonly useful to evaluate nanoparticle PK.

8.2.1 Fluorescence

Fluorescence is a sensitive and adaptable method for studying the PK profiles of nanoparticles as illustrated in Fig. 8.3. Fluorescence is the emission of light when excited electrons transition back to the ground state and can be detected by microplate assays in concentrations down to ~10 nM. Fluorophores span a range of sizes from small molecules, to recombinant proteins, to quantum dot (Qdots) nanoparticles. Among these, wavelengths of excitation and emission can vary from the ultraviolet (UV) to the infrared (IR) range of the electromagnetic spectrum.[13] While whole blood contains significant hemoglobin, diluted plasma has low absorption of excitation wavelengths or background from autofluorescent species that contribute to emission of fluorescent samples. Chemically conjugated fluorophores can be used as reporters enabling the detection and quantification of polymers, proteins, micelles, liposomes, and other nanoparticles of interest. Organic fluorophores, such as rhodamine and fluorescein, have generally useful properties in nanoparticle PK. More so than for small molecule drugs, nanoparticles are large enough that low levels of fluorophore modification are less likely to significantly alter the PK profile. Protein-fluorophores (green fluorescent protein) are perhaps less useful due to their lack of stability and higher molecular weight. Nanoparticle labels such as Qdots have excellent fluorescent properties; however, their sizes rival the size of many potential nanomedicines, which increase the likelihood that their properties may affect the observed PK profile.[14] For all fluorophores, the coupling of the labels to the target proteins could compromise their plasma stability as well as the biochemical functions of peptides and proteins.

8.2.2 Radiotracers

Radiolabeling enables accurate quantitative determination of very low amount of target macromolecules, making it a reliable method to trace biotherapeutics throughout the body during a PK study. Some commonly used radionuclides for peptide and protein studies include ^{3}H, ^{125}I, ^{14}C, ^{35}S, and ^{32}P.[15] Radioactive labels can be introduced into the macromolecules during biosynthesis, i.e., recombinant protein expression, or after biosynthesis through chemical modification of amino acids side chains. In addition to high sensitivity, a major advantage of radiolabeling is that it need

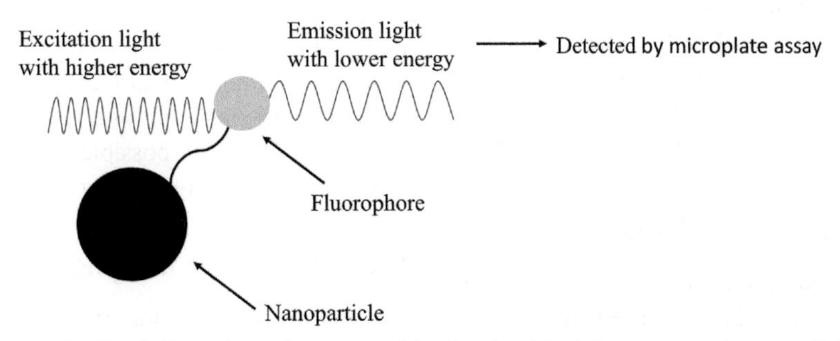

FIGURE 8.3 Fluorescent tags can be chemically conjugated to nanoparticles that absorb/emit lower energy photons, which can be quantified accurately over a range of low concentrations. Using validated microplate assays, plasma samples may be assayed to estimate nanoparticle concentration at different time points.

not modify the molecular structure, which can make the nanoparticle chemically identical to their unlabeled analogues.[16] From a research perspective, exposure to radiation is more highly regulated, which necessities specialized facilities and personnel trained in PK studies using radioisotopes. Despite the fact that radiotracers are the gold-standard for following nanoparticles over the widest dynamic range, their need for added protective measures remains a limitation to their broader use in nanoparticle PK.

8.2.3 Enzyme-linked immunosorbent assay (ELISA)

ELISA is another widely used technique for quantification of blood concentrations. Target molecules are first immobilized on a solid surface by passive binding or capture through antibody recognition. Detection is accomplished by measuring the activity of enzyme which is preconjugated to a highly specific detection antibody through chromogenic reaction. Two commonly used enzyme labels are horseradish peroxidase (HRP) and alkaline phosphatase (AP). ELISA is known for high specificity and sensitivity. However, performing an ELISA involves at least one antibody with specificity for a particular antigen, which restricts ELISA to nanoparticles that have validated antibodies. A recognition sequence may be genetically or chemically conjugated to the biotherapeutic under investigation to enable the use of commercially available antibodies; however, like other labeling approaches, this may alter their original activity and PK parameters.

8.2.4 Mass spectrometry

Liquid chromatography-mass spectrometry (LC-MS) is another quantitative analytical technique broadly applied in PK studies, combining the resolving power of liquid chromatography (LC) with the detection specificity of mass spectrometry (MS). LC-MS has the ability to quantify multiple analytes simultaneously with high selectivity and sensitivity. Just like other quantification methods, LC-MS has its own disadvantages. In addition to high operational cost, LC-MS has significant interlaboratory variability[17] due to the absence of standardized LC-MS method validation guidelines and documents.[18] LC-MS is especially powerful at detecting the PK for drugs which may be cargo on nanoparticles as well as protein and polymeric nanoparticles.

8.2.5 Obtaining samples from blood

There are multiple methods for collecting blood samples, which largely depend on the volume and sensitivity of the assay for the nanoparticle and cargo. Generally it is better to develop a full PK profile within each subject. For studies in mice with relatively small blood volumes, this may not be possible. For this reason, rats are often the species of choice for evaluating PK studies.

Cardiac puncture is a terminal procedure which can be applied to both mice and rats under deep anesthesia, allowing the collection of a single, good quality, and large volume of blood (up to 1 mL from mouse and 15 mL from rat) from the experimental animals.[19] This method can be performed through a ventral, left lateral, or open approach. For studies in mice, this approach may be necessary for the evaluation of larger volumes using LC-MS.

Tail venipuncture can be performed multiple times to collect small volume of blood (20 μL–0.2 mL from mice and 0.1–2 mL from rats) from incision with sterile scalpel blades of the tail vein.[20] With approval by an Institutional Animal Care and Use Committee (IACUC), it may be possible to obtain up to eight samples over a 24 hr period. In particular, when using this approach with mice, it is helpful to immediately dilute the whole blood into a volume of heparinized saline. Upon centrifugation, this yields plasma, which can be corrected for its dilution factor. This approach works well for fluorescence and radiotracers.

Retro-orbital sampling can be performed in both rats and mice by penetrating a capillary into the retro-orbital sinus to collect medium to large volume of blood (up to 0.5 mL). Retro-orbital bleeding should only be used under general anesthesia or as a terminal procedure because it causes "more than minimal or transient pain and distress" according to Animal Research Advisory Committee (ARAC).[21] The use of a topical ophthalmic anesthetic before bleeding is also recommended. Repeated blood sampling via this route is not recommended.

Indwelling catheter. The use of temporary or surgical cannulation methods should be considered when continuous and multiple sampling in the experimental animal is required.[22] Temporary cannulation is usually made in the tail vein through a nonsurgical procedure, which can only be used for a few hours. Surgical cannulation, on the other hand, is usually done in the femoral artery, femoral vein, carotid artery, jugular vein, vena cava, and dorsal aorta, requiring proper anesthesia and analgesia to minimize the pain. After cannulation, animals should be single housed in a large and spacious cage. Blood sample may be collected over 24 hr at the volume of 0.1–0.2 mL/sample from surgical cannula. The surgical cannula needs to be flushed with an anticoagulant after every blood withdraw. For preclinical PK, it is possible to purchase rats that already have been surgically catheterized.

8.2.6 Molecular imaging

The miniaturized version of positron emission tomography (PET), named as microPET, has been widely used in preclinical pharmacokinetic study with small animals to noninvasively acquire quantitative and repetitive images of radiolabeled biopharmaceutics and depict their spatial distribution, which is then aligned with 3D anatomic images obtained by a computed tomography (CT) scanner. The use of microPET-CT is restricted by the difficult handling of radioactive materials; however, for calibrated studies, the accuracy of quantification rivals that of gamma counting plasma samples. Thus, by fitting the signal from a tissue that mostly represents the blood volume, such as the heart, it is possible to obtain useful PK data related to both blood half-lives and also the clearance to the liver and kidneys.[23] Alternatively, optical imaging modalities are available to track the distribution of biomaterials prelabeled with bioluminescent and fluorescent reporters; however, their quantification is more challenging due to scattering and attenuation of signal through tissues. 3D tomography also is available in more recent optical imaging modalities. Similar to microPET, when used in combination with other tomographic technologies such as magnetic resonance imaging (MRI) or CT, the optimal images can also be correlated with anatomical context.

8.3 Noncompartmental parameter estimation

Compartmental and noncompartmental analyses are two common approaches to understand the PK properties of nanoparticles. Compartmental modeling assumes the body is composed of a certain number of kinetically homogeneous interconnected compartments. The established model can be used to predict drug concentrations at any time points and, therefore, optimize the dosing regimen.[24] On the other hand, noncompartmental analysis is model-independent. In comparison with compartment modeling, noncompartmental analysis is more robust, especially when estimating the PK parameters using fewer time points. In addition to providing key parameters to compare between formulations, the clearance and volume of distribution estimates can be used to develop maintenance doses and loading doses, respectively. The remainder of Section 8.3 introduces equations used to determine noncompartmental parameters.

8.3.1 Terminal half-life

Terminal half-life is defined as the time required to reduce the blood sample concentration by half after absorption and distribution phases have ended. If sufficient time points are collected, the PK profile will often adopt a log-linear decay, and this fraction of the dataset $C_z(t)$ can be fit using nonlinear regression to the following:

$$C_z(t) = C_z(0)\, e^{-\lambda_z t} = C_z(0)\, e^{-\frac{\ln(2)t}{t_{1/2}}} \tag{8.6}$$

In the above equations, λ_z is the apparent terminal rate constant and $t_{1/2}$ is the respective terminal half-life. $C_z(0)$ represents the y-intercept of this curve, which may be significantly lower than the observed initial concentration following the IV dose of a nanoparticle.

8.3.2 Area under the curve

Area under the curve (AUC) is the definite integral in the nanoparticle blood concentration versus time profile, representing the total drug exposure across time. AUC can be used to determine a number of parameters, most importantly clearance, bioavailability, and mean residence time. First, the AUC extending from the last time point obtained, n, until infinity can be estimated assuming the profile will continue to follow a monoexponential decline at the terminal half-life estimated above as follows:

$$AUC_{n-\infty} = \frac{C_n}{\lambda_z} \tag{8.7}$$

Where C_n is the last concentration determined at the last time point. Second, to determine the AUC from the time of the dose until the end of the collected time points, the "trapezoid method" can be used. The idea is to divide the plasma drug concentration over time profile into trapezoids between each time point. Summing up these areas allows an estimate of the AUC. Based on trapezoidal method and Eq. 8.7, the total AUC can thus be calculated as below:

$$AUC_{0-\infty} = \sum_{i=0}^{i=n}\left[\frac{(C_i + C_{i+1})(t_{i+1} - t_i)}{2}\right] + \frac{C_n}{\lambda_z} \tag{8.8}$$

Summation of all of the individual trapezoids and terminal contribution, thus allows estimation of the AUC (Fig. 8.4).

8.3.3 Bioavailability

Due to incomplete absorption from an extravascular dose as well as first-pass metabolism from oral administration, only a certain fraction of a dose may reach circulation. For small molecule drugs, oral and/or subcutaneous bioavailability can be high (F ~ 1). Many nanoparticles have low bioavailability, which is due to their low permeability and slow diffusion constant. Bioavailability can be estimated as the ratio of the AUC following an extravascular dose, D_{EV}, to an intravenous dose, D_{IV}:

$$F = \frac{AUC_{EV}}{D_{EV}} \frac{D_{IV}}{AUC_{IV}} \tag{8.9}$$

This bioavailability represents the total absorbed dose with respect to an IV dose. For low bioavailability nanoparticles, it may be necessary to use higher extravascular doses to reach similar concentration levels in blood samples. This definition can be used to estimate any extravascular bioavailability, including intramuscular injection

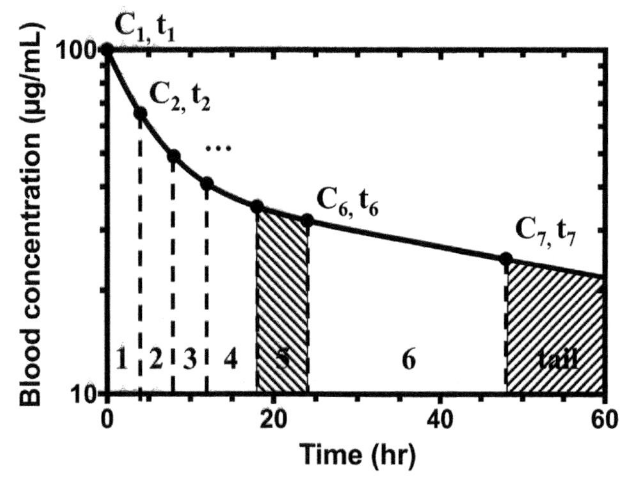

FIGURE 8.4 The complete area under the curve (AUC) for any pharmacokinetic (PK) profile can be estimated using the trapezoid rule between each data point added to the AUC following the last time point (Eq. 8.8). For example, the "tail" contribution, $AUC_{7-\infty}$, can be estimated as C_7/λ_z (Eq. 8.7), where λ_z is estimated by fitting the terminal log-linear data points to Eq. 8.6. The remaining areas between each data point can be estimated using the trapezoid rule. For example, trapezoid #5 has an area of $(C_5+C_6)(t_6\text{-}t_5)\div 2$.

(IM), oral administration (PO), and subcutaneous administration (SC).

8.3.4 Clearance

As the most fundamentally important PK parameter measuring the body's capacity to clear drug from the blood, clearance accounts for elimination by metabolism or excretion. Under all routes of administration, clearance can be calculated as follows:

$$\frac{Cl}{F} = \frac{D}{AUC} \tag{8.10}$$

For IV administration, the bioavailability, F, is 1 or 100%. As the dose, D, is known by the investigator, estimation of total clearance for an IV bolus of a nanoparticle requires only an accurate estimate of the AUC as described above (Eq. 8.8).

8.3.5 Area under the moment curve

If the concentration versus time data are again multiplied by time, the area under the "first statistical moment" (AUMC) is obtained. The first moment at each time point can be calculated by multiplying the time by the blood sample concentration. Making use of the trapezoidal method again and adding the contribution to AUMC following the last observed time point, the AUMC can be estimated as follows:

$$AUMC_{0-\infty} = \sum_{i=0}^{i=n}\left[\frac{(t_iC_i + t_{i+1}C_{i+1})(t_{i+1} - t_i)}{2}\right] + \frac{t_nC_n}{\lambda_z} + \frac{C_n}{\lambda_z^2} \tag{8.11}$$

This parameter is useful to estimate several additional PK parameters, including the mean residence time and the volume of distribution at steady state.

8.3.6 Mean residence time

Upon administration, drug molecules distribute throughout the body and reside in the body for various periods. Mean residence time (MRT) is the average amount of time a nanoparticle will reside in the body:

$$MRT = \frac{AUMC}{AUC} \tag{8.12}$$

The MRT can be directly estimated from any nanoparticle PK profile simply by dividing the AUMC by the AUC.

8.3.7 Mean absorption time

All extravascular doses (IM, PO, SC, *etc.*) have an absorption phase before the nanoparticle enters the circulatory system. Mean absorption time (MAT) is the average amount of time drug molecules take to appear in blood samples. It can be calculated by subtracting the MRT of IV dose from the MRT of an extravascular dose as follows:

$$MAT = MRT_{EV} - MRT_{IV} \tag{8.13}$$

The MAT is thus a useful measure of how long it takes for a nanoparticle formulation to be absorbed. In contrast, bioavailability (Eq. 8.9) measures the total extent to which a nanoparticle is absorbed.

8.3.8 Volume of distribution

The extent of drug distribution is quantified by the apparent volume of distribution V, which as described above is the amount of drug in the body divided by the concentration of drug observed in a blood sample. One way to estimate V is based on the initial concentration observed after administering a known dose, D_{IV}, of drug by IV administration:

$$V = \frac{D_{IV}}{C_0} \tag{8.14}$$

C_0 is the drug concentration immediately after dosing. Notably, V is an apparent volume, which for many small molecules greatly exceeds the physical volume of blood or even the body itself. In contrast, due to their high hydrodynamic radius and steric stabilization, many nanoparticles dilute only into the pool of available plasma. Thus, nanoparticles often have very low volumes of distribution compared to many small molecule drugs. The lower bound on V is the total volume of blood or plasma in the subject.

8.3.9 Volume at steady state

The volume of distribution at steady state (V_{ss}) is defined as the volume of distribution when pseudoequilibrium between blood circulation and tissue accumulation is reached, which can be estimated as follows:

$$\frac{V_{ss}}{F} = Cl\,MRT = \frac{D\,AUMC}{AUC^2} \quad (8.15)$$

V_{ss} is always equal to or greater than V; therefore, if a dose, D, is needed to reach a target concentration (Eq. 8.5), the volume at steady state will always yield a higher loading dose than the initial volume of distribution. This elevates blood concentrations to a greater extent immediately after the first dose, which may be problematic if a nanoparticle exhibits a dose-limiting acute toxicity in the central pool of blood. Thus, using the initial volume of distribution to estimate a loading dose yields more conservative peak nanoparticle levels but may require a longer delay to achieve steady-state effects in pharmacological target tissues.

8.4 Compartmental modeling of parameters

While noncompartmental analysis described above is an excellent strategy for quantifying and comparing relevant PK parameters for nanoparticles, it cannot predict the expected blood levels under different doses, dose intervals, routes of administration, or make other helpful predictions. An alternative is to apply a model based on mass balances around one or more "compartments." One of these compartments will represent the location of the sample, and the other compartments may represent sites of drug absorption, target tissues, clearance organs, or unspecified tissues. To make solutions tractable, the assumption is usually made that fluxes between compartments are either first or zero order processes. The solution of these models requires either analytically solving or numerically integrating a system of linear differential equations, which is beyond the scope of this chapter. Compartmental PK modeling can estimate many of the same parameters as noncompartmental analysis. In addition, compartmental models can estimate concentrations at time points not assayed. Through the principle of "superposition," the solution for single dose can be added sequentially together in time to estimate the profile for a multidose regimen. There are a number of analytical solutions for common PK cases; however, compartmental modeling can also make use of computational packages that do not require an analytical solution to fit or predict PK profiles. In the remainder of this section, three very common compartmental models for a bolus dose will be examined: (i) elimination of an IV dose for a drug with one-compartment PK; (ii) distribution and elimination of an IV dose for a drug exhibiting two-compartment PK; and (iii) the absorption and elimination of an extravascular dose for a drug exhibiting one-compartment PK.

8.4.1 One-compartment IV bolus

For the simplest case after an IV dose, D_{IV}, some drugs and nanoparticles behave as if they were introduced into a single, well-mixed compartment. For example, due to its rapid decline below detectable conditions, the non-PEGylated hydrogel nanoparticle discussed in Section 8.6.4 fits well into a one-compartment model.[25] The model assumes the bolus mixes instantaneously into a single compartment, that observed concentrations reflect an apparent volume of distribution, V, and that a single flux accounts for total drug clearance, via a first-order rate constant, k_{elim} (Fig. 8.5A). Due to the additivity of

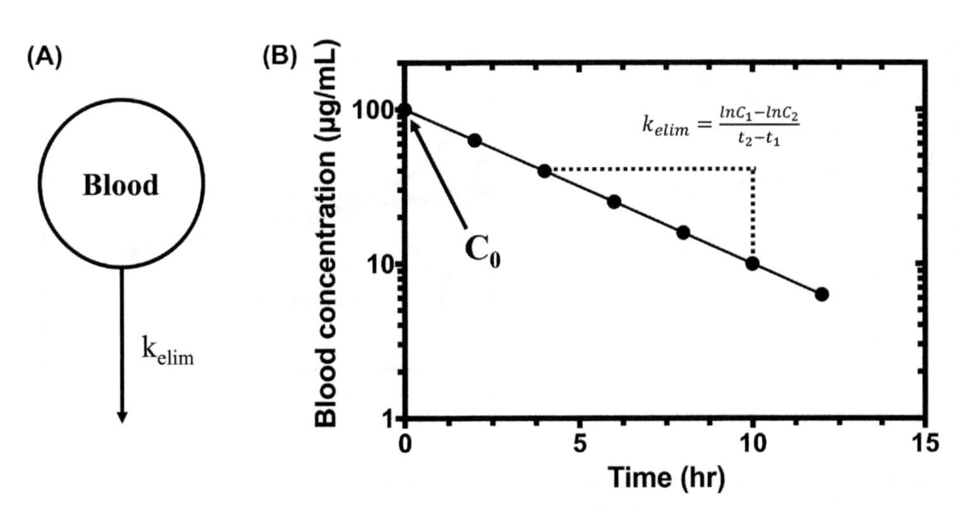

FIGURE 8.5 (A) Model depiction for an IV bolus with one-compartment behavior; (B) A representative pharmacokinetic (PK) profile of a one-compartment model. On a semilog scale, the blood concentration decreases by a straight line, which indicates it is well-fit to a single exponential decay with a slope of $-k_{elim}$.

clearance (Eq. 8.3), this flux is the sum of multiple mechanisms of clearance. Based on these assumptions, a mass balance integrates into the following solution:

$$C(t) = C_0\, e^{-k_{elim}t} = \frac{D_{IV}}{V} e^{-k_{elim}t} \qquad (8.16)$$

When PK data are plotted on a semilog scale and fit to the above equation, the y-intercept gives an estimate of C_0, from which V can be estimated (Eq. 8.14). As a first-order process, the flux arrow leaving the blood compartment has the definition:

$$\text{rate of loss from compartment} = k_{elim}\, X(t) = k_{elim}\, V\, C(t) \qquad (8.17)$$

Recognizing the rate of loss from the compartment must equal the defined rate of clearance from the body (Eq. 8.1) leads to the useful relationship:

$$Cl = k_{elim} V \qquad (8.18)$$

The above holds for all compartmental models with a single, first-order flux representing clearance from a blood compartment with an apparent volume of distribution, V. It should be noted that direct integration of Eq. 8.16 from time zero until infinity results in an AUC as follows:

$$AUC = \int_{t=0}^{t=\infty} C_0\, e^{-k_{elim}t} dt = \frac{C_0}{k_{elim}} \qquad (8.19)$$

Which using Eq. 8.10 estimates the same Cl as Eq. 8.18. Finally, it is useful to relate the half-life to the k_{elim}, Cl, and V, which can be obtained by substituting the relationship of a half-life into Eq. 8.18:

$$t_{1/2,\ elim} = \frac{\ln(2)}{k_{elim}} = \frac{\ln(2)\, V}{Cl} \qquad (8.20)$$

This relationship shows that even under constant clearance, an increase in the volume of distribution has the direct effect of increasing the half-life. Thus, when comparing related nanoparticles, it is only possible to state that an increase in observed half-life means that clearance has decreased if the volume of distribution remains unchanged. This is why it is important to calculate clearance and volume of distribution, in addition to the half-life.

8.4.2 Two-compartment IV bolus

While some drugs and optimized nanoparticles fit the one-compartment model quite well, this is not generally the case. Specific examples of structure–function studies for nanoparticles that fail to fit one-compartment models are found below in Sections 8.6.1, 8.6.3 and 8.6.4, such as liposomes, antibodies, and PEGylated hydrogel nanoparticles.[25–27] To visualize deviations from the one-compartment behavior, PK profiles should always be plotted with the Y-axis concentration on a log scale. Semilog plotting makes it easy to determine if the nanoparticle follows a single log-linear decay (Eq. 8.16) or if another model is required. If the semilog plot clearly shows a rapid early decline in concentration, followed by a slower, log-linear elimination phase then the PK profile may be better described by two-compartment model (Fig. 8.6A). In addition to the assumptions of the one-compartment model, the two-compartment model assumes that there is a second "tissue" compartment that serves as a reservoir for material being transferred from the blood compartment. This tissue compartment is filled and drained by first-order fluxes with constants, k_{12}, and k_{21}, respectively. Based on these assumptions, a mass balance integrates into a solution of the following form:

$$C(t) = Ae^{-\alpha t} + Be^{-\beta t} \qquad (8.21)$$

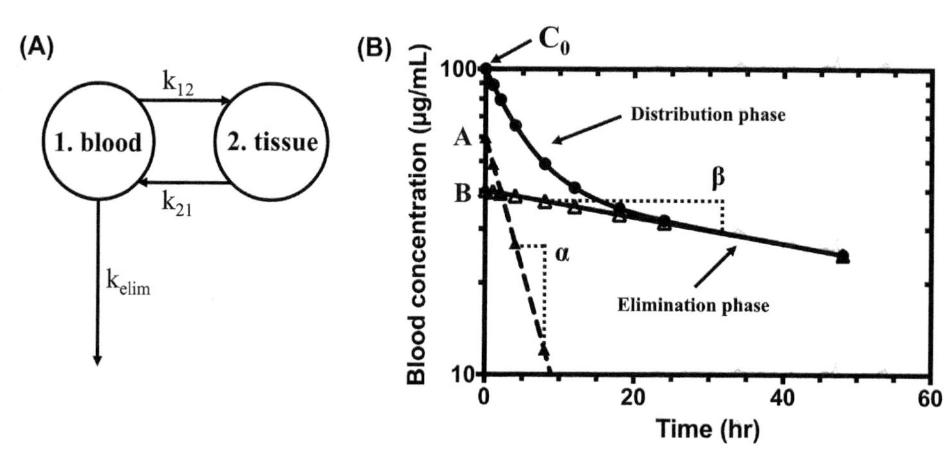

FIGURE 8.6 (A) Model depiction for an IV bolus with two-compartment behavior; (B) A representative pharmacokinetic (PK) profile of a two-compartment model. The blood concentration follows two-phase exponential decay with both distribution and elimination phases. Following an IV bolus, material in the blood compartment begins to distribute to the tissue compartment. After the flux from blood to tissue and tissue to blood equalizes, the profile enters an elimination phase, which can be recognized as a straight line on semilog plot. A best-fit line with intercept B and slope β can be fit to the elimination phase. Subtraction of the elimination phase contribution during the distribution phase generates residuals, which can then be plotted as a "residual" line representing with Y-intercept of A and slope α.

Where "macroconstants" A, B, α, and β can be fit with nonlinear graphing software (Fig. 8.6B). If defined such that α is greater than β, then the distribution half-life can be determined as:

$$t_{1/2,\,dist} = \frac{\ln(2)}{\alpha} \tag{8.22}$$

and the observable elimination half-life as:

$$t_{1/2,\,elim} = \frac{\ln(2)}{\beta} \tag{8.23}$$

Direct integration of Eq. 8.21 from time zero until infinity results in an AUC as follows:

$$AUC = \int_{t=0}^{t=\infty} \left(Ae^{-\alpha t} + Be^{-\beta t}\right)dt = \frac{A}{\alpha} + \frac{B}{\beta} \tag{8.24}$$

Which using Eq. 8.10 can be used to estimate *Cl*.

At time zero, Eq. 8.21 simplifies to:

$$C_0 = A + B \tag{8.25}$$

Using this relationship and Eq. 8.14 allows the estimation of the apparent volume of distribution specific to the blood sample compartment, V_1:

$$V_1 = \frac{D_{IV}}{A + B} \tag{8.26}$$

Eq. 8.18, which also applies to the two-compartment model, can be rearranged as follows:

$$k_{elim} = \frac{Cl}{V_1} \tag{8.27}$$

Estimates for *Cl* and V_1, can be used to estimate k_{elim}, which is equivalent to the single elimination flux constant described in the one-compartment model above. Based on their mathematical relationship, α, β, and k_{elim} cannot equal to one another. Thus, the observed half-life of elimination does not have the same value as the estimated half-life of the flux associated with clearance. While its derivation is beyond the scope of this chapter, the relationship between macroconstants (α, β) and the "microconstants" (k_{elim}, k_{12}, k_{21}) is defined so that they simultaneously satisfy both of the following relationships:

$$\alpha + \beta = k_{elim} + k_{12} + k_{21} \text{ and } \alpha\beta = k_{elim}k_{21} \tag{8.28}$$

Rearranging the above equations, it is possible to first estimate:

$$k_{21} = \frac{\alpha\beta}{k_{elim}} \tag{8.29}$$

and then:

$$k_{12} = \alpha + \beta - k_{elim} - k_{21} \tag{8.30}$$

Thus, it is possible to estimate all of the microconstants for the two-compartment model by first fitting the PK profile to the biexponential (Eq. 8.21). The remaining macroconstants, A and B, are compound parameters, which depend on a number of other parameters as follows:

$$A = \frac{D_{IV}(\alpha - k_{21})}{V_1(\alpha - \beta)} \tag{8.31}$$

and

$$B = \frac{D_{IV}(k_{21} - \beta)}{V_1(\alpha - \beta)} \tag{8.32}$$

For a one-compartment nanoparticle, the entire PK profile may be accurately fit by just four or five accurate time points spaced over two to three half-lives. In contrast, for a two-compartment nanoparticle with both distribution and elimination phases, it is important to collect at least three to four time points centered around the distribution half-life as well as three to four time points more broadly centered around the elimination half-life. Additional time points are essential, because the biexponential equation has four independent parameters (Eq. 8.21), which for four or fewer time points leaves no degrees of freedom to fit the model. Having accurately estimated all four macroconstants, it is then possible to estimate the microconstants, the clearance, and the volume of distribution stepwise in the order presented above. With these parameters, investigators can ask how changing the nanoparticle's physicochemical properties might specifically affect the PK profile. A striking feature of many nanoparticle PK profiles is how they often have volumes of distribution nearly as low as the blood or plasma volume.[25–31] However, even those formulations with significant two-compartment behavior are associated with a decrease in AUC, increase in clearance, and overall lower blood concentrations. Thus, adopting specific modifications to the nanoparticle that resists either clearance or extensive two-compartment distribution may be needed to achieve therapeutic end points in preclinical models.

8.4.3 One-compartment extravascular bolus

Many preclinical PK studies of nanoparticles explore only IV administration. There are excellent reasons for this, as a clear understanding of the IV disposition of the nanoparticle should precede any other route of administration. There are also excellent reasons to study extravascular delivery. For example, oral administration could allow patients to easily take nanomedicines by pill. Even if oral administration is not feasible, the avoidance of IV administration would advance nanomedicines. Subcutaneous administration offers easier patient self-administration, nanomedicine access to the lymphatics, and extension of the MRT in the blood compartment through extended

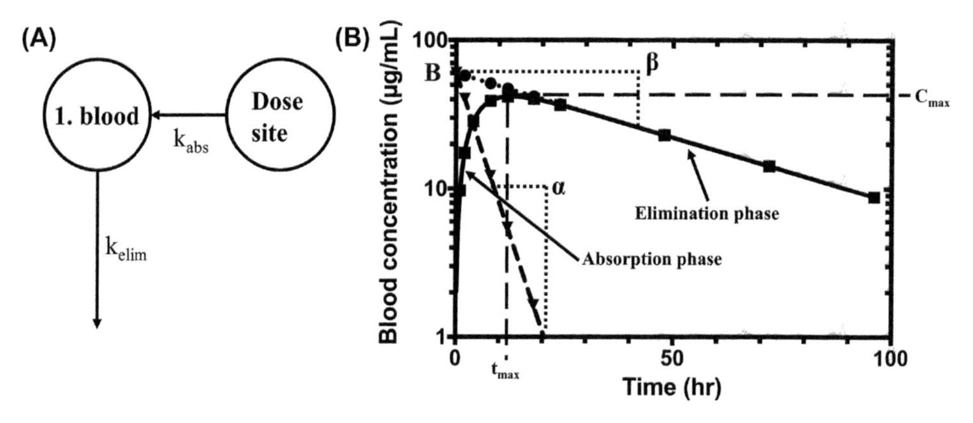

FIGURE 8.7 (A) Model depiction for an extravascular bolus for a drug with one-compartment behavior; (B) A representative pharmacokinetic (PK) profile of the one-compartment extravascular bolus model. Following an extravascular dose, material in the absorption site starts entering the blood compartment. After the absorption phase ends, the profile enters an elimination phase, which can be recognized as a straight line on the semilog plot. A best-fit line with intercept B and slope β can be fit to the terminal "elimination" phase. Subtraction of the early absorption phase data from the contribution of the elimination phase generates residuals that plot as a log-linear line with Y-intercept of B and slope α. If elimination is faster than absorption, then $k_{elim} = \alpha$ and $k_{abs} = \beta$; however, if absorption is faster than elimination then $k_{elim} = \beta$ and $k_{abs} = \alpha$. This has consequences for interpreting the PK for oral and SC doses of nanoparticles.

release. As in prior sections, simple compartmental models can be derived for an extravascular bolus of a drug that exhibits one-compartment PK (Fig. 8.7A). A compartment representing the dose site has been included, which could represent a subcutaneous pocket, the GI tract, or the peritoneal cavity. The key assumptions of this model are that the extravascular bolus, D_{EV}, appears instantaneously in the dose site, that drug is absorbed by a first-order process with constant k_{abs}, that only a fraction of the dose, F, reaches detection in the blood sample compartment, that the concentrations observed in the blood sample compartment reflect an apparent volume of distribution, V, and that total clearance is accounted for by a first-order process with rate constant, k_{elim}. Another important assumption of this model is that k_{elim} is not equal to k_{abs}. Based on these assumptions, mass balances can be solved as follows:

$$C(t) = \frac{F\,D_{EV}k_{abs}}{V(k_{abs} - k_{elim})}\left(e^{-k_{elim}t} - e^{-k_{abs}t}\right) \tag{8.33}$$

To fit this equation to an absorption PK profile, the following form can be used:

$$C(t) = B\left(e^{-\beta t} - e^{-\alpha t}\right) \tag{8.34}$$

Integration of the above equation from zero to infinity allows estimation of the AUC as follows:

$$AUC = \int_{t=0}^{t=\infty} \left(Be^{-\beta t} - Be^{-\alpha t}\right)dt = \frac{B}{\beta} - \frac{B}{\alpha} \tag{8.35}$$

There are two ways to interpret data fit to equation 8.33. Since k_{elim} and k_{abs} cannot be equal for this solution, one of the two processes must have a longer half-life. Thus, the process with the longer half-life remains a significant contribution at the terminal phase of the PK profile. Conversely, the process with the shorter half-life will decay nearly to zero by the terminal phase. From an extravascular PK profile alone, it is impossible to determine whether the terminal half-life reflects either k_{elim} or k_{abs}. If an IV one-compartment PK profile for the same nanomedicine has already been quantified, then the k_{elim} and V will be known. Based on this knowledge, it may be possible to interpret Eq. 8.34 by one of two approximations.

First, if absorption kinetics are faster than elimination ($k_{abs} >> k_{elim}$) then:

$$k_{abs} = \alpha \text{ and } k_{elim} = \beta \tag{8.36}$$

Using the fit parameter B from Eq. 8.34, the volume of distribution divided by bioavailability can be estimated:

$$\frac{V}{F} = \frac{D_{EV}k_{abs}}{B(k_{abs} - k_{elim})} \tag{8.37}$$

Alternatively, if absorption is slower than elimination ($k_{abs} << k_{elim}$) then:

$$k_{abs} = \beta \text{ and } k_{elim} = \alpha \tag{8.38}$$

Using the fit parameter B, the volume of distribution divided by bioavailability can be estimated:

$$\frac{V}{F} = \frac{D_{EV}k_{abs}}{B(k_{elim} - k_{abs})} \tag{8.39}$$

For either approximation, substituting the dose D_{EV} into Eq. 8.10 then allows estimation of the clearance divided by bioavailability:

$$\frac{Cl}{F} = \frac{D_{EV}}{AUC} \tag{8.40}$$

The absorption half-life can be determined as:

$$t_{1/2,\,abs} = \frac{\ln(2)}{k_{abs}} \tag{8.41}$$

The elimination half-life can be estimated as:

$$t_{1/2,\,elim} = \frac{\ln(2)}{k_{elim}} \tag{8.42}$$

By solving the time where the first derivative of equation 8.33 becomes equal to zero, it is possible to calculate the time until the peak concentration is reached:

$$t_{max} = \frac{\ln\left(\frac{k_{abs}}{k_{elim}}\right)}{(k_{abs} - k_{elim})} \tag{8.43}$$

Note that the time until the maximum concentration is independent of the dose, volume of distribution, or bioavailability. It only depends on the absorption and elimination rate constants. To estimate the peak concentration, C_{max}, one only needs to substitute the t_{max} into Eq. 8.33. Lastly, it is important to note that analysis of an extravascular PK profile by itself allows only the determination of *V/F* and *Cl/F*. It is impossible to determine the absolute *V* or *Cl* unless the bioavailability is known. Bioavailability would need to be determined by comparison with an IV dataset for the same nanoparticle.

8.5 Interpreting the PK of drug carriers

Drug carriers are sometimes designed to prolong the blood circulation and improve PK properties of small molecule drugs, which might enhance potency while diminishing systemic toxicity. The modulatory effect of a drug carrier needs to be validated by comparing the drug and carrier PK profiles. Through monitoring carrier and drug PK simultaneously post administration, actionable information regarding drug release kinetics and mechanism can be obtained.

8.5.1 Renal filtration cutoff

The glomerular capillary wall is composed of three layers: endothelium, glomerular basement membrane (GBM), and podocyte extensions of glomerular epithelial cells.[32] The endothelium is fenestrated, allowing free filtration. The spaces between podocyte extensions constitute the primary size barrier with a physiologic pore size of 4.5–5 nm. Consistent with this size range, the molecular weight cutoff for macromolecules is thought to be 30–50 kDa. Nanoparticles <6 nm are usually small enough to undergo free glomerular filtration; however, nanoparticles >8 nm do not filter through the GBM due to the size limit. Drug carriers exceeding that limit have significantly lower renal elimination and thus longer circulation half-life. Also, the highly negatively charged GBM makes it easier for positively charged molecules to filter relative to those negatively charged ones, which are repelled by the GBM due to charge–charge repulsion. Charge–charge interaction is especially important for those macromolecules with sizes around the renal filtration size cutoff. These observations inspired various nanoparticle architectures that decrease both renal and total clearance.

8.5.2 Absorption from extravascular administration

SC administration may outperform IV administration in several aspects, including ease of administration, high patient compliance, low risk of systemic infection, and, in some cases, prolonged drug exposure.[33] However, the bioavailability of SC administered therapeutics may be limited by incomplete absorption. In addition, biotherapeutics with different MW reach the systemic circulation via different routes. Compounds with MW less than or equal to 16 kDa usually enter the systemic circulation through blood capillaries, while biotherapeutics with higher MW have to be transported through the interstitial fluid. They are taken up into lymphatic capillaries draining the injection site and eventually are channeled back into the circulatory system.[34] In addition, extracellular matrix (ECM) maintains a negatively charged environment for interstitial fluid, which may delay the absorption of positively charged macromolecules in comparison with negatively charged macromolecules with similar MW.

Oral dosage, due to its convenience, cost-effectiveness, and high patient compliance, is often the preferred route of administration. Orally administered drugs need to be absorbed by the small intestinal tract before entering the systemic circulation. The incomplete absorption and first-pass elimination greatly constrain the bioavailability of orally administered nanoparticles, often ranging from 1% to 5%. Strategies to increase the magnitude and reproducibility for the oral bioavailability of nanoparticles would overcome major barriers to their use. Incidentally, were orally bioavailable nanoparticles developed that could be taken daily, they might not require a 2-day half-life in humans, which as indicated above enabled parenteral/IV administration of clinically approved liposomes.[5]

8.5.3 Opsonization and capture by the reticuloendothelial system

Opsonization is the process through which nanocarriers or foreign organisms are tagged with opsonin proteins, thereby making them easily recognizable to phagocytes. Nanoparticles have been shown to be readily opsonized upon entering the blood circulation and rapidly taken up by the reticuloendothelial system (RES) consisting of phagocytic cells such as monocytes and macrophages. But neutrally charged particles, including zwitterionic species, have much lower opsonization rate than charged nanoparticles.[35] To reduce opsonization, different shielding groups blocking electrostatic and hydrophobic interactions, such as polysaccharides (dextrans) and polyethylene glycols (PEGs), have been broadly investigated.[36] Strategies to reduce opsonization will remain essential to maintain the PK properties of nanoparticles.

8.6 Structure–function studies to optimize pharmacokinetic parameters

8.6.1 The effect of particle size distribution

Liposomes composed of bovine brain sphingomyelin-phosphatidylcholine (SM-PC), 4:1 M ratio, were used to deliver [^{14}C] sucrose, as a hydrophilic tracer.[26] Three different methods were used to formulate liposomes, which generate different distributions of particle sizes. The small unilamellar vesicles (SUVs) are the smallest and least polydisperse. The reverse phase evaporation vesicles (REVs) are intermediate in size. In contrast, the multilamellar vesicles (MLVs) are large and polydisperse. Their PK profiles were compared in rats and replotted here in terms of concentration *vs.* time (Fig. 8.8). All three liposomes significantly reduce the clearance compared to free sucrose. Despite having identical surface properties, the small size of the SUV promotes the highest blood concentrations, highest AUC, lowest clearance, and lowest volume at steady state (Table 8.1). All liposome diameters are well above the renal filtration cutoff, which prevents rapid filtration. However, the larger MLV, being more subject to opsonization and RES clearance, exhibit substantially higher clearance. For the MLV, nearly 88% of their biexponential fit follows a fast-distribution half-life of 0.3 hr. Accumulation in organs of the RES is partially supported by higher liver and spleen accumulation. In contrast, all three liposome formulations maintain similar elimination half-lives. These data demonstrate the critical importance of reaching the window of 10–100 nm to develop clinically relevant nanoparticles.

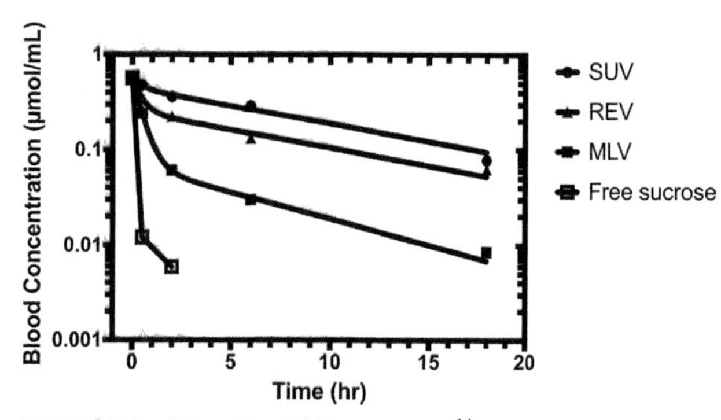

FIGURE 8.8 Whole blood PK profile for [^{14}C] sucrose entrapped into sphingomyelin–phosphocholine liposomes with different sizes, which were administered IV to rats. Small unilamellar vesicles (SUVs) lack a distribution phase, have the highest area under the curve (AUC), and the longest terminal half-life. Reverse phase evaporation vesicles (REVs) have a more significant distribution phase, which reduces their AUC even though they have a similar terminal half-life. Multilamellar vesicles (MLVs) have a very significant distribution phase, which greatly reduces their AUC; however, they too have a similar terminal half-life. Free sucrose has a 3 hr half-life; therefore, the majority of signal remaining in the liposome samples is a reasonable estimate of liposome-entrapped label. *Data extracted from Allen, T. and J. Everest, Effect of liposome size and drug release properties on pharmacokinetics of encapsulated drug in rats. J Pharmacol Exp Ther, 1983. 226(2): p. 539–544.*

8.6.2 Surface charge

Surface charge is another important consideration in the optimization of nanoparticle PK. In this case,[30] through chemical modification, authors generated four types of gold nanoparticles (AuNPs) with different surface charges, albeit consistent hydrodynamic radii of 9–10 nm: neutral (TEGOH), positive (TTMA), negative (TCOOH), and zwitterionic (TZwit). The PK profiles of these four nanoparticles were determined after IV administration (Fig. 8.9). PK parameters are summarized in Table 8.2. Some parameters were calculated in the original publication; however, the remainder have been estimated based on extracted data. Zwitterionic and neutral AuNPs clearly have the optimal PK profiles relative to charged particles, with higher drug exposure, longer MRTs, and slower elimination. Charged particles, on the other hand, get eliminated rapidly. Being more subject to opsonization, charged particles, especially positively charged particles, are more likely to be eliminated rapidly by RES clearance.[35] Also, the positively charged (TTMA) particles exhibit a greater distribution phase and volume of distribution at steady state, which may reflect their adsorption to the negatively charged glycocalyx. Clearly, the PK of these nanoparticles benefits greatly from maintaining charge neutrality.

8.6.3 Hydrophobicity

Antibody–drug conjugates (ADCs), which combine the specificity of an IgG antibody and the potency of small molecule therapeutics attached via a chemical linker, can greatly improve the PK profile of small molecule drugs due to their ability recycle back out of hepatocytes via the neonatal Fc receptor (FcRn). Even so, excessive hydrophobicity contributed by the linker appears to induce a PK penalty. In this study, different ADCs with the same antibody backbone (h1F6) were compared with different linkers (linker 1, 2, and 3).[27] Using hydrophobic interaction chromatography, the hydrophobicity of different ADCs was sequenced as h1F6-1> h1F6-2> h1F6-3> h1F6. Then a PK study was performed as shown in Fig. 8.10. Based on these data, the PK parameters have been summarized in Table 8.3. In comparison to other nanoparticles, antibodies are exceptional drug carriers with clearance (0.01–0.05 mL/hr) a

TABLE 8.1 Size-dependent pharmacokinetic (PK) parameters of [^{14}C] sucrose liposomes following IV administration to rats.

Parameters (Unit)	Small unilamellar vesicles (SUVs)	Reverse-phase evaporation Vesicles (REVs)	Multilamellar vesicles (MLVs)	Free sucrose
Hydrodynamic diameter (nm)	20–100	100–400	200–3000	N/A
AUC (μmol/mL hr)	5.1	3.6	0.9	0.2
$AUMC$ (μmol/mL hr^2)	43.9	49.6	5.1	0.07
MRT (hr)	8.5	13.9	5.5	0.4
$t_{1/2,\ terminal}$ (hr)	6.3	11.2	6.6	1.5
V_{ss} (mL)	13.2	31.2	47.6	17.8
Cl (mL/hr)	1.6	2.2	8.7	46.6
Liver/spleen at 0.5 h (% of injected dose)	8.6 ± 3.2	29.6 ± 3.2	50.5 ± 11.2	N/A
Model used	Two-compartment IV bolus			N/A
A (μmol/mL)	0.13	0.32	0.50	
B (μmol/mL)	0.45	0.25	0.07	
α (hr^{-1})	1.93	2.17	2.10	
β (hr^{-1})	0.07	0.09	0.13	
$t_{1/2,\ dist}$ (hr)	0.4	0.3	0.3	
$t_{1/2,\ elim}$ (hr)	9.9	7.7	5.3	
AUC (μmol/mL hr)	6.5	2.9	0.8	
V_1 (mL)	13.8	14.0	14.0	
Cl (mL/hr)	1.2	2.7	10.3	
k_{elim} (hr^{-1})	0.09	0.19	0.73	
k_{12} (hr^{-1})	0.40	1.06	1.12	
k_{21} (hr^{-1})	1.51	1.00	0.37	

AUC, area under the curve; AUMC, area under the moment curve; MRT, mean residence time.
Dose: 8 μmol of phosphocholine administered to 200 g rats. Blood volume, V_1, estimated 7% of body weight.
Mean ± SD.
Data interpreted from Allen, T. and J. Everest, Effect of liposome size and drug release properties on pharmacokinetics of encapsulated drug in rats. J Pharmacol Exp Ther, 1983. 226(2): p. 539–544.

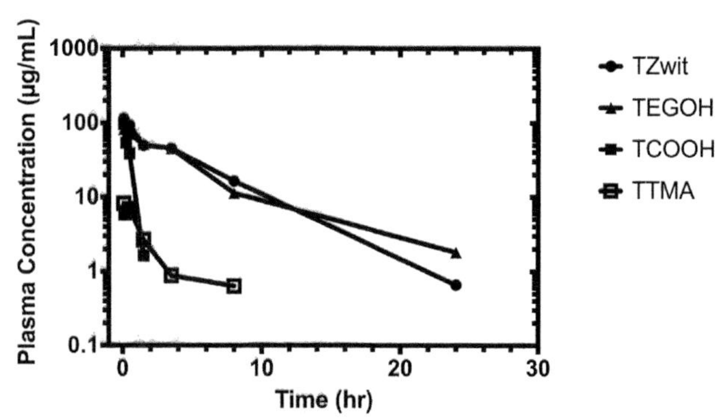

FIGURE 8.9 Plasma concentration over time profiles of gold nanoparticles (AuNPs) with different surface charges were depicted after injected IV in mice. Highly charged nanoparticles coated with thioalkyl tetra(ethylene glycol)ated trimethylammonium (TTMA) and thioalkyl tetra(ethylene glycol)ated carboxylate ligands (TCOOH) exhibit the most severe distribution phase upon administration and short terminal half-life, which leads to the lowest AUC. Negatively charged TCOOH slightly outperforms positively charged TTMA due to slower redistribution. Nanoparticles coated with neutral thioalkyl tetra(ethylene glycol)ated (11-Mercaptoundecyl)tetra(ethylene glycol) (TEGOH) and zwitterionic thioalkyl tetra(ethylene glycol)ated zwitterionic ligands (TZwit) demonstrate more optimal pharmacokinetic (PK) profiles with milder distribution phases, longer terminal half-lives, and thus significantly higher area under the curve (AUC). *Data extracted from Arvizo, R.R., et al., Modulating pharmacokinetics, tumor uptake and biodistribution by engineered nanoparticles. PLoS One, 2011. 6(9): p. e24374.*

8.6.4 Density and thickness of shielding layer

Blocking the electrostatic and hydrophobic interactions has the potential to help nanoparticles evade the uptake by RES and thus prolong circulation time. The mostly investigated shielding group is poly(ethylene glycol) (PEG). Better stealth has been reported by increasing the surface density of PEG. In this case, PRINT hydrogel nanoparticles were coated with PEG into two different conformations: brush and mushroom, by high-density PEG and low-density PEG, respectively.[25] As shown in Fig. 8.11, the PK properties of these two confirmations were compared, with non-PEGylated nanoparticles as a negative control. Authors utilized two-compartmental modeling to calculate PK parameters, as summarized in Table 8.4. PEGylation significantly decreased the clearance, prolonged the circulation period, and increased the total exposure compared with non-PEGylated nanoparticles. Notably, the high-density brush confirmation has superior shielding effect than low-density mushroom confirmation, yielding better PK performance.

8.6.5 Serum albumin binding

In addition to IgG, serum albumin can also undergo FcRn-mediated recycling, avoiding lysosome degradation and

TABLE 8.2 Surface charge–dependent pharmacokinetic (PK) parameters of gold nanoparticles following IV administration to mice.

	Surface charge			
Parameters (Unit)	TEGOH	TZwit	TTMA	TCOOH
Zeta potential (mV)	−1.1	−2.0	+24.4	−37.9
AUC (μg/mL hr)	436,080	486,819	10,318	45,682
AUMC (μg/mL hr^2)	2,449,506	2,240,577	8551	19,111
MRT (hr)	5.6	4.6	0.8	0.4
$t_{1/2,\ terminal}$ (hr)	6.0	3.4	0.7	0.2
V (mL)	1.9	1.5	21.1	2.3
V_{ss} (mL)	1.8	1.5	14.0	2.1
Cl (mL/hr)	0.4	0.3	16.9	4.9

AUC, Area under the curve; *AUMC*, Area under the moment curve; *MRT*, Mean residence time.
Dose: TEGOH 160 mg, TTMA 174 mg, TCOOH 224 mg, TZwit 167 mg to mice.
Data interpreted from Arvizo, R.R., et al., Modulating pharmacokinetics, tumor uptake and biodistribution by engineered nanoparticles. PLoS One, 2011. 6(9): p. e24374.

magnitude lower than observed for other optimized nanoparticles (0.1–0.5 mL/hr) in mice. Their avoidance of renal filtration and RES clearance is critical. Even so, the evidence suggests that the linker chemistry can play a large role in harnessing the innate ability of IgG antibodies to recycle back out of hepatocytes and avoid clearance.

achieving longer circulation half-life. Another case reported that introducing an albumin-binding domain (ABD) to a vaccine carrier, termed as iTEP, significantly improved its PK profile.[31] The serum concentration over time profiles of iTEP and ABD-iTEP administered subcutaneously were compared and depicted in Fig. 8.12. As summarized in

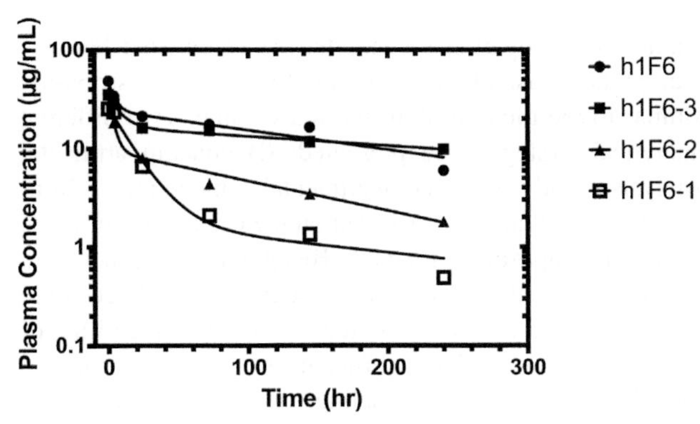

FIGURE 8.10 The plasma concentration versus time profiles of antibodies with different hydrophobicity after IV administration into mice. Unconjugated h1F6 and least hydrophobic conjugate h1F6-3 have the highest area under the curve (AUC), due to milder distribution phases and longer terminal half-lives. Along with the increment in hydrophobicity (h1F6-3→h1F6-2→h1F6-1), the distribution phase gets intensified and the terminal half-life gets shortened, causing an AUC reduction. *Data extracted from Lyon, R.P., et al., Reducing hydrophobicity of homogeneous antibody-drug conjugates improves pharmacokinetics and therapeutic index. Nat Biotechnol, 2015. 33(7): p. 733.*

Table 8.5, fusing to ABD significantly reduced the clearance of iTEP by 50%, yielding a four-fold higher AUC. Thus, strategies to hijack natural biological mechanisms used by proteins abundant in the blood appear to be excellent candidates for enhancing the PK of nanoparticles.

8.7 Conclusion

A clinically relevant PK profile is essential to develop therapeutic nanoparticles. This should be achieved through structure–function optimization of PK parameters discussed above. The most important PK parameters include clearance, volume of distribution, half-life, and bioavailability in cases of extravascular administration. These parameters can be estimated based on blood-based concentrations *vs.* time as inputs, which must be collected at the correct time and assayed using accurate and precise methods. Nanoparticle and/or cargo concentration in biological solutions can then be quantified by fluorescence, radioactivity, ELISA, and mass spectrometry. Optimal PK

TABLE 8.3 Linker-dependent pharmacokinetic (PK) parameters of antibody–drug conjugates following IV administration to mice.

	ADCs with different linker hydrophobicity			
Parameters (Unit)	h1F6	h1F6-3	h1F6-2	h1F-1
AUC (µg/mL hr)	4546	8723	1482	873
AUMC (µg/mL hr^2)	556,854	4,529,965	193,531	53,294
MRT (hr)	122	519	131	61
$t_{1/2,\ terminal}$ (hr)	66	375	103	66
V (mL)	0.9	1.3	1.2	1.8
V_{ss} (mL)	1.2	2.7	4.0	3.1
Cl (mL/hr)	0.01	0.005	0.03	0.05
Model used	Two-compartment IV bolus			
A (µg/mL)	24.3	18.8	28.0	24.8
B (µg/mL)	24.3	16.6	9.5	1.8
α (hr^{-1})	0.214	0.114	0.277	0.059
β (hr^{-1})	0.005	0.002	0.007	0.004
$t_{1/2,\ dist}$ (hr)	3.2	6.1	2.5	11.7
$t_{1/2,\ elim}$ (hr)	139	347	99	173
AUC (µg/mL hr)	4974	8465	1458	870
V_1 (mL)	0.9	1.3	1.2	1.7
Cl (mL/hr)	0.009	0.005	0.031	0.052
k_{elim} (hr^{-1})	0.010	0.004	0.026	0.031
k_{12} (hr^{-1})	0.100	0.057	0.183	0.025
k_{21} (hr^{-1})	0.110	0.055	0.075	0.008

ADC, Antibody–drug conjugate; *AUC*, Area under the curve; *AUMC*, Area under the moment curve; *MRT*, Mean residence time.
Dose: 45 µg of antibody. The calculation is based on the assumption that 4–6wk old female BALB/c mice have an average body weight of 15g.
Data interpreted from Lyon, R.P., et al., Reducing hydrophobicity of homogeneous antibody-drug conjugates improves pharmacokinetics and therapeutic index. Nat Biotechnol, 2015. 33(7): p. 733.

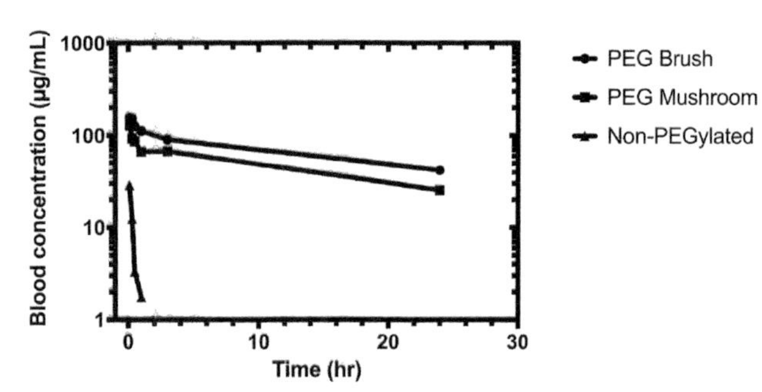

FIGURE 8.11 Blood concentration of nanoparticles with different polyethylene glycol (PEG) shielding density over time after IV administration in mice. PEGylated nanoparticles, in comparison with the non-PEGylated one, have notably milder distribution phases, longer terminal half-lives, and thus significantly higher area under the curve (AUC). But high-density PEG appears to have better shielding effect, which results in lower distribution to "tissue" compartment. Therefore, PEG brush has higher AUC than PEG mushroom. *Data extracted from Perry, J.L., et al., PEGylated PRINT nanoparticles: the impact of PEG density on protein binding, macrophage association, biodistribution, and pharmacokinetics. Nano Letters, 2012. 12(10): p. 5304-5310.*

studies of nanoparticles can often be recognized because nanoparticles usually have an initial volume of distribution similar to the total blood or plasma volume. Two different analytical strategies are presented: (i) noncompartmental analysis and (ii) compartmental modeling. Noncompartmental analysis is based on the calculation of AUC using the trapezoidal method. Being model-independent, noncompartmental analysis is sometimes considered more robust when the timing, number, and reproducibility of concentration may be insufficient to fit an appropriate model. Compartmental modeling, on the other hand, can predict nanoparticle concentrations, which may be useful to design multidose regimens. For nanoparticles, unsatisfactory PK properties can arise from low hydrodynamic radius, which leads to increased renal clearance and larger distribution effects. Optimal nanoparticles are typically charge neutral, because either positive or negative surfaces increase clearance. Optimal nanoparticles also benefit from steric shielding, which reduces opsonization and clearance

TABLE 8.4 PEG-density dependent pharmacokinetic (PK) parameters among PRINT nanoparticles following IV administration in mice.

	Shielding density		
Parameters (Unit)	PEG brush	PEG mushroom	Non-PEGylated
PEG_{5k} density (number/nm)	0.083 ± 0.006	0.028 ± 0.002	0
AUC (µg/mL hr)	2863	1726	8.3
AUMC (µg/mL hr^2)	73,189	33,544	4.5
MRT (hr)	25.6	19.4	0.5
$t_{1/2,\ terminal}$ (hr)	19.0	14.9	0.5
V (mL)	1.5	1.4	4.8
V_{ss} (mL)	2.2	2.4	14.3
Cl (mL/hr)	0.087	0.126	26.2
Model used	Two-compartment		One-compartment
A (µg/mL)	65.8	103.3	N/A
B (µg/mL)	100.0	74.2	N/A
α (hr^{-1})	1.50	5.01	N/A
β (hr^{-1})	0.04	0.04	N/A
$t_{1/2,\ dist}$ (hr)	0.46	0.14	N/A
$t_{1/2,\ elim}$ (hr)	19.3	15.8	0.2
AUC (µg/mL hr)	2823	1706	10
V_1 (mL)	1.5	1.2	4.8
Cl (mL/hr)	0.088	0.127	21.72
k_{elim} (hr^{-1})	0.059	0.104	4.524
k_{12} (hr^{-1})	0.559	2.830	N/A
k_{21} (hr^{-1})	0.921	2.119	N/A

AUC, area under the curve; AUMC, area under the moment curve; MRT, mean residence time; PEG, polyethylene glycol.
Dose: non-PEGylated 218.5 µg, PEG mushroom 217 µg, PEG brush 248.6 µg.
Data interpreted from Perry, J.L., et al., PEGylated PRINT nanoparticles: the impact of PEG density on protein binding, macrophage association, biodistribution, and pharmacokinetics. Nano Letters, 2012. 12(10): p. 5304–5310.

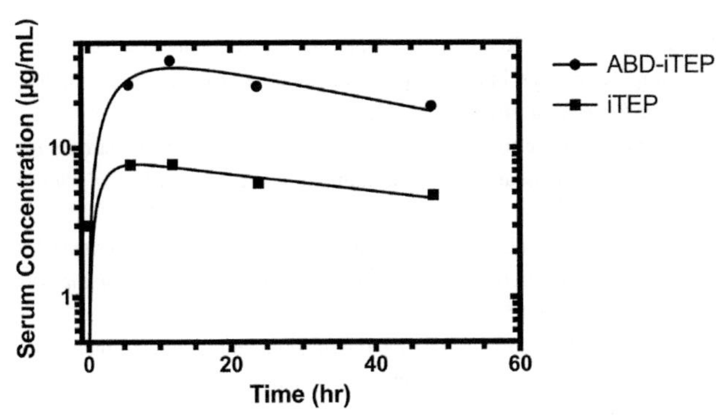

FIGURE 8.12 Serum concentration of vaccine carriers with or without albumin binding capability over time after SC administration to mice. Terminal half-life was only slightly altered with the addition of albumin-binding domain (ABD), which likely results from delayed absorption from the site of injection. Due to this, ABD-iTEP (immune-tolerant elastin-like polypeptide) has clearly higher area under the curve (AUC) than iTEP. This can be explained by lower tissue distribution (lower V_{ss}) and reduced clearance achieved by the albumin-binding capability. In the absence of IV data, it is not clear if the ABD had an effect on bioavailability, which may also be responsible for the elevated levels observed. Concentration at time 0 was assumed to be 3 ug/mL to be presented within this log10-scale Y-axis. *Data extracted from Wang, P., et al., An albumin-binding polypeptide both targets cytotoxic T lymphocyte vaccines to lymph nodes and boosts vaccine presentation by dendritic cells. Theranostics, 2018. 8(1): p. 223.*

TABLE 8.5 Albumin-binding dependent pharmacokinetic (PK) parameters for immune-tolerant elastin-like polypeptides (iTEPs) administered SC to mice.

Parameters (unit)	ABD-iTEP	iTEP
AUC (µg/mL hr)	2685	897
AUMC (µg/mL hr^2)	214,659	113,659
MRT (hr)	80	127
$t_{1/2,\ terminal}$ (hr)	54	88
V_{ss}/F (mL)	2.6	10.4
Cl/F (mL/hr)	0.03	0.08
Model used	One-compartment extravascular bolus	
B (µg/mL)	49.7	8.7
k_{abs} (hr^{-1})	0.209	0.559
k_{elim} (hr^{-1})	0.022	0.013
$t_{1/2,\ abs}$ (hr)	3	1
$t_{1/2,\ elim}$ (hr)	32	51
AUC (µg/mL hr)	2021	654
V/F(mL)	2.0	8.7
Cl/F (mL/hr)	0.044	0.113
t_{max} (hr)	12.0	6.9
C_{max} (µg/mL)	34.1	7.8

ABD, albumin-binding domain; AUC, area under the curve; AUMC, area under the moment curve; MRT, mean residence time. Dose: 89.1 µg of ABD-iTEP and 73.8 µg of iTEP per mouse. The compartmental model fit was interpreted assuming that $k_{abs} >> k_{elim}$.
Data interpreted from Wang, P., et al., An albumin-binding polypeptide both targets cytotoxic T lymphocyte vaccines to lymph nodes and boosts vaccine presentation by dendritic cells. Theranostics, 2018. 8(1): p. 223.

by the RES. Examples of nanoparticle structure–function studies evaluating several of these variables are presented and reanalyzed using the approaches described.

Acknowledgment

Authors would like to thank the University of Southern California (USC), the National Institute of Health R01 EY026635 to JAM, RO1 GM114839 to JAM, and the Gavin S. Herbert Endowed Chair of Pharmaceutical Sciences.

References

1. Olmos D, et al. Safety, pharmacokinetics, and preliminary activity of the anti-IGF-1R antibody figitumumab (CP-751,871) in patients with sarcoma and Ewing's sarcoma: a phase 1 expansion cohort study. *Lancet Oncol* 2010;**11**(2):129–35.
2. Wilson WH, et al. Navitoclax, a targeted high-affinity inhibitor of BCL-2, in lymphoid malignancies: a phase 1 dose-escalation study of safety, pharmacokinetics, pharmacodynamics, and antitumour activity. *Lancet Oncol* 2010;**11**(12):1149–59.
3. Papahadjopoulos D, et al. Sterically stabilized liposomes: improvements in pharmacokinetics and antitumor therapeutic efficacy. *Proc Natl Acad Sci USA* 1991;**88**(24):11460–4.
4. Allen TM, Cullis PR. Liposomal drug delivery systems: from concept to clinical applications. *Adv Drug Deliv Rev* 2013;**65**(1):36–48.
5. Gabizon A, Shmeeda H, Barenholz Y. Pharmacokinetics of pegylated liposomal doxorubicin. *Clin Pharmacokinet* 2003;**42**(5):419–36.
6. Voskerician G, et al. Biocompatibility and biofouling of MEMS drug delivery devices. *Biomaterials* 2003;**24**(11):1959–67.
7. Veronese FM. Peptide and protein PEGylation: a review of problems and solutions. *Biomaterials* 2001;**22**(5):405–17.
8. Wu AM, Senter PD. Arming antibodies: prospects and challenges for immunoconjugates. *Nat Biotechnol* 2005;**23**(9):1137.
9. Giljohann DA, et al. Gold nanoparticles for biology and medicine. *Angew Chem Int Ed* 2010;**49**(19):3280–94.
10. Braet F, Wisse E. Structural and functional aspects of liver sinusoidal endothelial cell fenestrae: a review. *Comp Hepatol* 2002;**1**(1):1.
11. Owens III DE, Peppas NA. Opsonization, biodistribution, and pharmacokinetics of polymeric nanoparticles. *Int J Pharm* 2006;**307**(1):93–102.
12. Lee H, Blaufox M. Blood volume in the rat. *J Nucl Med* 1985;**26**(1):72–6.
13. Gonçalves MST. Fluorescent labeling of biomolecules with organic probes. *Chem Rev* 2008;**109**(1):190–212.
14. Toseland CP. Fluorescent labeling and modification of proteins. *Journal of chemical biology* 2013;**6**(3):85–95.

15. Patel AC, Matthewson SR. *Radiolabeling of peptides and proteins. Molecular biomethods handbook*. Springer; 1998. 411-411.
16. Holtzhauer M. *Basic methods for the biochemical lab*. 2006.
17. Christians U, et al. Impact of laboratory practices on interlaboratory variability in therapeutic drug monitoring of immunosuppressive drugs. *Ther Drug Monit* 2015;**37**(6):718–24.
18. Clarke W, Rhea JM, Molinaro R. Challenges in implementing clinical liquid chromatography–tandem mass spectrometry methods–seeing the light at the end of the tunnel. *J Mass Spectrom* 2013;**48**(7):755–67.
19. Adeghe A-H, Cohen J. A better method for terminal bleeding of mice. *Lab Anim* 1986;**20**(1):70–2.
20. Omaye S, et al. Simple method for bleeding the unanaesthetized rat by tail venipuncture. *Lab Anim* 1987;**21**(3):261–4.
21. Health NIo. *Guidelines for survival bleeding of mice and rats*. 2012.
22. Parasuraman S, Raveendran R, Kesavan R. Blood sample collection in small laboratory animals. *J Pharmacol Pharmacother* 2010;**1**(2):87.
23. Janib SM, et al. Kinetic quantification of protein polymer nanoparticles using non-invasive imaging. *Integrative Biology* 2012;**5**(1):183–94.
24. Guo H, et al. A novel elastin-like polypeptide drug carrier for cyclosporine A improves tear flow in a mouse model of Sjögren's syndrome. *J Control Release* 2018;**292**:183–95.
25. Perry JL, et al. PEGylated PRINT nanoparticles: the impact of PEG density on protein binding, macrophage association, biodistribution, and pharmacokinetics. *Nano Letters* 2012;**12**(10):5304–10.
26. Allen T, Everest J. Effect of liposome size and drug release properties on pharmacokinetics of encapsulated drug in rats. *J Pharmacol Exp Ther* 1983;**226**(2):539–44.
27. Lyon RP, et al. Reducing hydrophobicity of homogeneous antibody-drug conjugates improves pharmacokinetics and therapeutic index. *Nat Biotechnol* 2015;**33**(7):733.
28. Lee C, et al. Berunda polypeptides: Bi-headed rapamycin carriers for subcutaneous treatment of autoimmune dry eye disease. *Mol Pharm* 2019.
29. Banskota S, et al. Long circulating genetically encoded intrinsically disordered zwitterionic polypeptides for drug delivery. *Biomaterials* 2019;**192**:475–85.
30. Arvizo RR, et al. Modulating pharmacokinetics, tumor uptake and biodistribution by engineered nanoparticles. *PLoS One* 2011;**6**(9):e24374.
31. Wang P, et al. An albumin-binding polypeptide both targets cytotoxic T lymphocyte vaccines to lymph nodes and boosts vaccine presentation by dendritic cells. *Theranostics* 2018;**8**(1):223.
32. Longmire M, Choyke PL, Kobayashi H. *Clearance properties of nano-sized particles and molecules as imaging agents: considerations and caveats*. 2008.
33. McDonald TA, et al. Subcutaneous administration of biotherapeutics: current experience in animal models. *Curr Opin Mol Ther* 2010;**12**(4):461–70.
34. Richter WF, Bhansali SG, Morris ME. Mechanistic determinants of biotherapeutics absorption following SC administration. *AAPS J* 2012;**14**(3):559–70.
35. Roser M, Fischer D, Kissel T. Surface-modified biodegradable albumin nano-and microspheres. II: effect of surface charges on in vitro phagocytosis and biodistribution in rats. *Eur J Pharm Biopharm* 1998;**46**(3):255–63.
36. Nie S. Understanding and overcoming major barriers in cancer nanomedicine. *Nanomedicine* 2010;**5**(4):523–8.

Chapter 9

Nanoparticle characterization techniques

Jos Campbell[1,2], Sean Burkitt[1,2], Natalie Dong[1,2] and Cristina Zavaleta[1,2]
[1]*Department of Biomedical Engineering, University of Southern California, Los Angeles, CA, United States;* [2]*Michelson Center for Convergent Biosciences, Los Angeles, CA, United States*

9.1 Introduction

Understanding the interaction of nanomaterials with biological systems remains a complex problem that can be difficult to probe directly. Researchers must treat animal models as partially understood black boxes where many of the factors that affect the pharmacokinetics and biodistribution of nanoparticles are inferred via assay after the fact. For these findings to be useful, it is imperative to accurately characterize the physiochemical properties of the nanoparticles so that the effects of minor changes to the materials can be correlated with relevant assay outcomes. To that end, this chapter will attempt to cover the primary considerations, techniques, and caveats of the methods used to understand nanoparticles and how their properties influence their applications.

One thing that must be considered is that a sample of a nanoparticle material is not homogenous and will be polydisperse to some degree. There is no single size, shape, or surface charge value that can be given, only an average of the population, and in the case of surface charge, it is relative to its environment. To this end, it must be understood that the error in the measurement is proportional to the heterogeneity of the particles, which is why a great deal of focus has been spent in developing methods to produce monodisperse particles. Not only is it important from a characterization standpoint, but if some variable changes drastically through your population (size for example), the researcher does not know which part of their population is responsible for the observed result.

Nanomaterials vary widely in their composition depending on which functions they must fulfill. Various metals can provide imaging contrast, whereas organic compounds can impart specificity in biological interactions or enable the particles to deliver drug molecules to the target tissues. The specific elemental makeup and purity can significantly affect the performance of a nanoparticle; for example, the cadmium:selenium ratio in a quantum dot sample must be carefully controlled to ensure high-quality fluorescence signal. Elemental compositions are often measured using various X-ray techniques or more traditional chemical analysis processes, such as atomic absorption spectroscopy or inductively coupled plasma mass spectrometry (ICP-MS). Crystallographic structure is important especially when intending to fabricate a multilayered nanoparticle; the crystallographic morphology can help or hinder the attachment of hard layers of other metals or soft layers of proteins or polymers. Certain crystallographic sites present as especially charged regions on the surface of a particle that may act as catalytic hotspots or can be used to selectively bind protective molecules. This effect can be used in the fabrication of gold nanorods where a structure directing agent such as cetyltrimethylammonium bromide (CTAB) can be manipulated by reaction conditions to bias deposition of new gold into specific lattice planes giving the particle a selective growth axis.[1] Crystallographic information is usually collected via X-ray or electron diffraction techniques.

The size, shape, surface charge, and concentration of a nanoparticle formulation has profound implications on particle uptake, biodistribution, or payload carrying efficiency.[2] The immense surface area-to-volume ratio of particles on the nanoscale is responsible for many of their characteristic advantages; hence, slight changes in these features can lead to significant variance in biodistribution, cellular toxicity, uptake, and retention times. Correctly tuning the surface charge allows researchers to selectively avoid or target specific cell types, cell wall features, or tissues.[3] These characteristics are usually measured with a selection of techniques, including electron microscopy, dynamic light scattering, zeta potential measurements, nanoparticle tracking analysis (NTA), or variations of Coulter counting.

Polydispersity is a natural feature of nearly all nanomaterials, as no two particles are exactly the same no matter how well they have been fabricated. Given that as a percentage, a few hundred atoms is a much larger proportion

Nanoparticles for Biomedical Applications. https://doi.org/10.1016/B978-0-12-816662-8.00009-6

of total volume on the nanoparticle scale; this can lead to small subpopulations of a sample overcontributing to an experimental result, or a small subset may hide an otherwise valuable observation. A great deal of effort has been focused on developing methods of particle fabrication such that the polydispersity is kept as low as possible to ensure conclusions drawn from experiments truly reflect the behavior of the average particle of that sample. Polydispersity occurs in nearly every material property of a nanoparticle: size, shape, charge, surface chemistry, crystal structure, and surface area. There is no single technique to measure each property relative to every other, and each must be measured independently.

We emphasize again that there is no single technique that can tell you everything you want to know about a nanoparticle, and every method used provides one piece of the puzzle, and therefore in every case, you must use multiple techniques. A thorough understanding of a particle sample comes from a series of carefully chosen characterization experiments that build on previous data sets to create the most accurate picture of the particle being investigated. The following sections are intended to describe these techniques in general, how and when they are used, and what caveats must be considered when interpreting the data.

9.2 Electron microscopy

Some of the most useful techniques for nanoparticle characterization come from variations of electron microscopy (EM). The value of many EM techniques is greater for "hard" particles such as those based on metals as it provides fairly absolute characterization of particle size, crystallographic structure, or elemental composition. Sample preparation for "soft" particles, such as liposomes, micelles, polymeric, or dendrimer particles, are more difficult to prepare devoid of artifacts, as their significantly lower density can make them more difficult, but not impossible to characterize. A comprehensive guide to the techniques and applications of the many varieties of instruments would fill the average bookshelf. So instead, we will discuss some of the more important points to consider and how this family of techniques and instruments can shine a light on the nanoscale world.

There is a hard limit to the maximum resolution of any microscopic observation using visible light microscopy. The ability to distinguish between two separate objects next to each other is tied directly to the wavelength of the light being used to make the observation. If the distance between the structures is less than half the wavelength of the light being used, the two objects cannot be resolved and will appear as a single structure.[4] This concept was proposed by Ernst Karl Abbe in 1873 who outlined the relationship with the below equation, where d is feature size, λ the wavelength, n the refractive index within the imaging medium, and θ the half angle subtended by the objective lens.[4]

$$d = \frac{\lambda}{2n \sin \theta} \tag{9.1}$$

Therefore, given that visible light, at its shortest, has a wavelength of $\sim$400 nm, if you wish to resolve structures at less than 200 nm, you need to use light with a shorter wavelength. This is where high-energy electron beams with wavelengths in the range of angstroms (0.1 nm) become useful.[5]

Electron microscopes operate in two primary ways, either by transmitting the beam directly through the sample via transmission electron microscopy (TEM) or rastering the beam across the surface of the sample and collecting the scattered electrons via scanning electron microscopy (SEM). Each method has its drawbacks and specific applications, but in both cases, an electron beam is emitted from a filament, usually tungsten, and manipulated toward the sample via a system of magnetic lenses. Given that both cases result in a sample being bombarded with high-energy electrons that interact with the sample, not only can we use these techniques to observe structures at this minute scale, but specific interactions of the beam with the sample can reveal detailed elemental information. This allows researchers not only to see nanometer scale structures but also to ask, what are they made of?

Electron microscopes can use several techniques to probe the elemental configuration of a sample. Primarily, this is accomplished using electron diffraction (ED), electron energy loss spectroscopy (EELS), and energy-dispersive X-ray (EDX) sometimes called (EDS, EDXS, XEDS, or EDXMA). Both TEM and SEM can utilize similar techniques; however, SEM is the only instrument able to examine "large" 3D structures. TEM is restricted to obtaining information on smaller, thinner structures (sub-100 nm) due to the need for the beam to penetrate through the sample, making it feasible for analyzing the crystallographic structure of single particles and the elemental distribution within them. SEM is far more capable at examining groups of particles or surface mapping materials from 100 nm and up. A variant of TEM, scanning transmission electron microscopy (STEM), can make use of the exceptional resolution of TEM but is more specialized for elemental analysis. In STEM, the beam of a TEM is rastered across the thin sample section to create a map of spectroscopic information in the form of either EELS or EDX information. STEM units, like many other variations, are usually accessories to standard TEM systems.[5]

TEM is unable to interrogate bulk samples, but it is used to view samples that can be prepared in either very thin slices via ultramicrotomy or particles that can be drop cast onto the sample grids. The sample is visualized as a projected shadow on a phosphorescent screen or is projected directly onto a digital camera. Structural information about particle size or crystallographic/elemental information can be obtained. High-resolution transmission electron microscope (HRTEM) instruments are even able to produce images of the lattices of atoms that form the materials.

SEM would be used when the researcher is examining the surface of a sample with 10–20 nm features and a total sample area of 1 cm^2 (samples can be much larger depending on the chamber setup). While TEM would be used to examine down to subnanometer features like lattice fringes of a single particle with an upper image size of around 300^2 μm. Almost all the beautiful submicron microscope pictures of insect skin or microchips you may have seen have been collected using SEM and post-processed in software to attribute color to elemental or structural image components.[6] This is because SEM is capable of capturing much wider field images, and because it is only interrogating the surface, it is able to produce images that retain three-dimensional depth.

An electron microscope of any kind is not the sort of instrument you expect to find in a normal lab. Due to their expensive nature, technical complexity, and support requirements, these instruments are usually part of a core facility where researchers can book time usually for a fee, and in some cases, the actual driving of the instrument is restricted to a technician. This is more often the case with TEM, as SEM is a far more robust technique with nearly fully automated instruments driven by computers being increasingly common. Typically, a user can achieve basic operations on an SEM after about an hour of instruction, and core facilities usually have a microscopist on duty so any questions or problems that arise can be promptly tended to.

Given that the resolution of a TEM is significantly greater than that of SEM, there are some additional considerations in its operation. Often a similar hour-long training session is needed for a new user, but unlike SEM, there are several things a user can do on a TEM that can cause significant damage or extended instrument downtime by making a small mistake during normal operation. Improper sample loading can introduce gas to the beamline column or, more concerning, can introduce contaminants to the column that cannot be easily removed. More commonly, it is easy to "lose" the beam when adjusting for higher resolution images. This is typically more of an annoyance but may take a technician a while to fix. For this reason, TEM users are not usually considered "trained" until many hours of operation have been logged. In the case of HRTEM instruments, a normal user will almost never operate the instrument without a significant amount of training and logged hours on more basic TEM instruments.

When analyzing nanoparticles, electron microscopy has difficulty with "soft" materials, such as proteins, lipids, polymers, or any component that forms a monolayer on the surface of a nanoparticle surface. This is due to the electron interaction volume (Fig. 9.1) of the high-energy electron beam and the methods the various instruments use to collect data. Methods of limiting these shortcomings include reducing the acceleration voltage and raising the pressure within the sample chamber to avoid sample outgassing, as is used in environmental scanning electron microscopes (ESEMs); however, higher pressure and lower voltage add significant limitations to the resolution of the images. Other methods to image these low-density materials include uranyl acetate staining processes for lipids enabling the visualization of liposomes or exosome structures.[7] Methods for both positive and negative staining of samples are available, uranyl acetate being an example of both a positive and negative stain. In positive staining, deposition of uranium to the surface of structures within the sample add significant density granting image contrast. Negative staining is used to visualize samples by adding a layer of amorphous electron-dense stain compound. The sample can then be visualized as a less dense region than the surrounding area.[8]

One of the most significant developments in electron microscopy for nanoparticle characterization has come from the advent of cryogenic electron microscopy (CryoEM). Recent developments in CryoEM have reduced the level of artifacts caused by the usually arduous dehydration and resin imbedding process used to prepare samples, such as cells, capsules, or micelles. This enables researchers to examine these fragile samples with minimal structural artifacts without the need for resin embedding and ultramicrotome sectioning.

Understanding the electron interaction volume of the incident beam is critical in understanding the experimental data being collected from a sample.[9] Illustrated in Fig. 9.1, the electron interaction volume is the volume of sample material that the beam is interacting with while it is generating sample data. The total volume and depth scales with incident angle of the beam, sample density, and acceleration voltage, with the latter two variables having the greatest effect. The differing regions of the interaction volume give rise to specific signal dependent on the mechanism of interaction to generate those signals. Few backscatter electrons are collected from deeper than 500 nm, whereas the majority of the secondary electrons are generated from the upper 5–50 nm. This means that selecting for different beam interaction products, auger or backscatter electrons, or characteristic X-rays provides not just differing information about the same point but also information from differing depths of the sample.

9.2.1 Transmission electron microscopy)

If you were to replace the light waves in an optical microscope with electrons and change the glass optical lenses

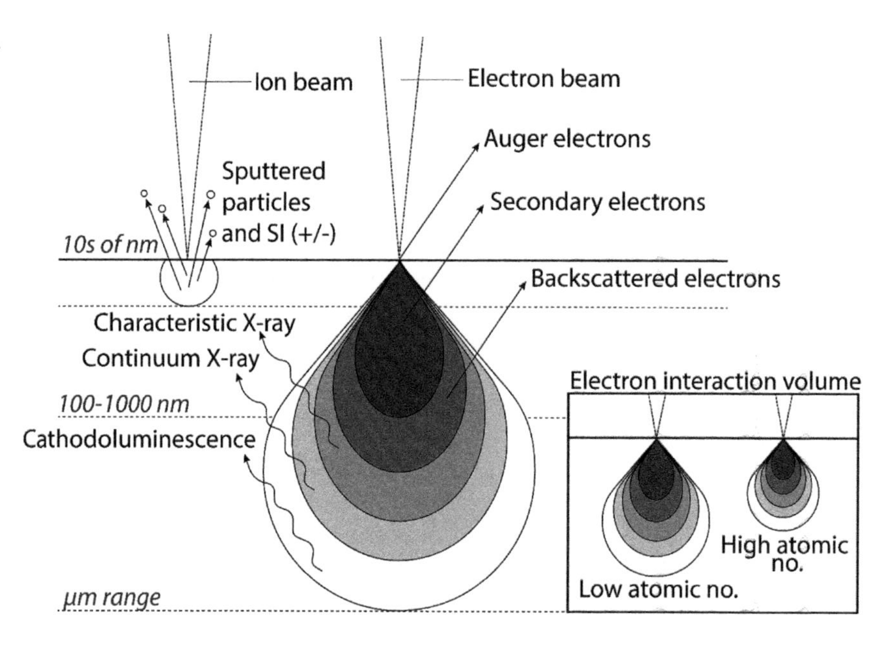

FIGURE 9.1 Electron interaction volume. Illustration by Cheryl Chan.

for magnetic fields, you would find yourself with an instrument that is fairly close to the structure of a TEM. TEM instruments are typically a tall column with the electron gun at the top and a phosphorescent imaging plate and/or CCD camera at the base (see Fig. 9.2. The sample is inserted into the beam about two-thirds of the way along the beamline. The sample is mounted on a (usually copper) metal grid disk, and a thin film of carbon is usually deposited on the mesh. Many variations of different metal types or film style combinations can be used to fulfill various applications or support different sample types. Should the user need to examine a sample with the least possible interference, either for maximal resolution or to avoid the carbon film contributing to the elemental signal, a style of film referred to as "lacey" or "holey" should be used. Instead of a continuous carbon film, these have a porous nature. This allows the researcher to locate a region of sample that either has adhered to the inside edge of one of the holes within the film or completely suspends across a gap in the film.[10] This results in the electron beam passing through the TEM column, interacting with the sample, and transmitting through to the image capture end without interacting with the sample support in any way. This maximizes the resolution and minimizes the contribution of any nonsample material during elemental analysis.

9.2.2 Transmission Electron Microscopy sample preparation

Sample preparation is a highly varied process, as many different sample types go through vastly different preparation processes prior to imaging and will not be individually covered here. The main consideration for choosing what process to use is what your sample is made of and what you want to learn about it. Whatever your material, it must be able to be prepared in such a way as to survive the very harsh conditions of the sample chamber. The chamber is usually pumped to a very low pressure of around 10^{-4} Pa or lower in HRTEM, to sustain the applied voltage between the cathode and ground without creating an arc through the sample and to minimize the interactions with the electron beam by various gasses in the column. The sample must also be able to withstand the electron bombardment without absorbing to much energy and simply burning up in the beam.

This means biological samples such as cells need to go through very careful processing, usually dehydration, embedding in resin, and then sectioning with an ultramicrotome into sections usually around 60 nm thick. In Cry-oEM, the sample is very precisely frozen using liquid ethane before being imaged. This allows the sample to be viewed in a more natural state and without the conformational artifacts that may otherwise be caused by standard preparation techniques of samples that are in a naturally hydrated state. Liquid sample holders also exist that enable the observation of specimens while under flow or in a static liquid environment. Known as in situ TEM, these accessories allow the examination of a sample in a nonstatic environment. This allows researchers to observe chemical interactions with a sample or the growth modes of nanoparticles in real time.[11,12] The ability to alter a nanoparticle's environment and observe the sample's response directly using the powerful analysis capabilities of a TEM enables a far more rapid research process than producing many samples with slight variations and examining them one by one on a traditional system. These liquid sample holders are especially valuable for investigating real-time

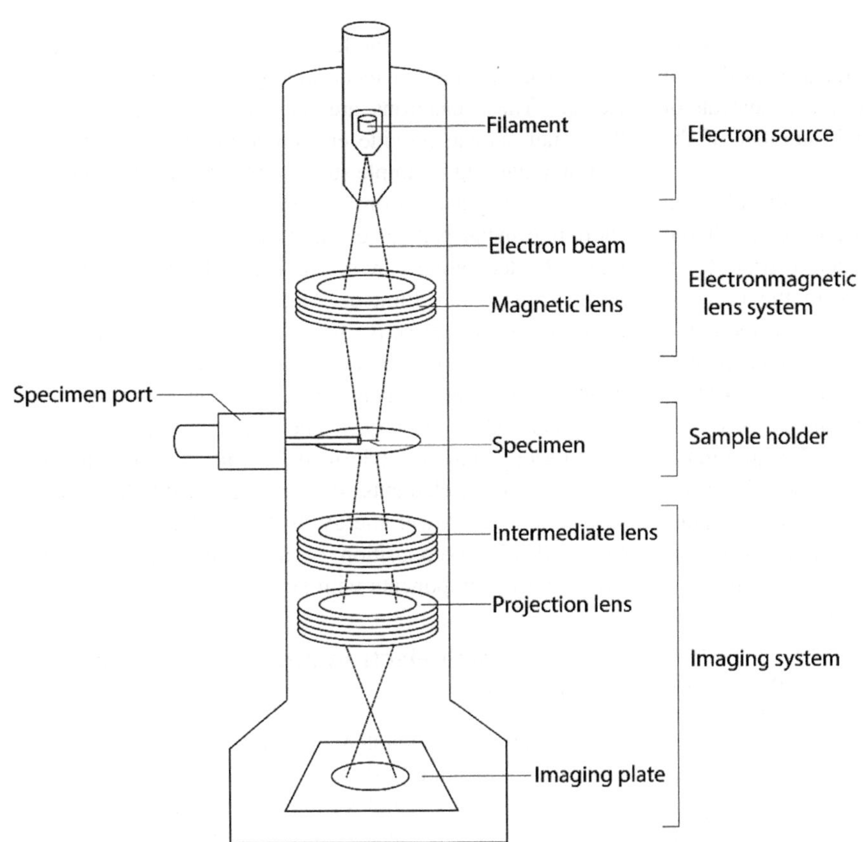

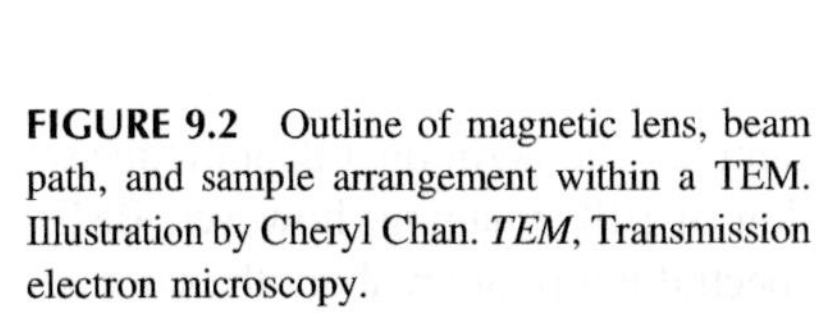

FIGURE 9.2 Outline of magnetic lens, beam path, and sample arrangement within a TEM. Illustration by Cheryl Chan. *TEM*, Transmission electron microscopy.

electrochemical interactions, but they are highly specialized, and currently, few facilities currently own these accessories.

Simple ceramic or metallic samples can be easily prepared for TEM examination provided their particle size is low enough for the beam to penetrate, or the materials density is low enough for the beam to pass through rather than simply casting a black shadow. Users must be aware that the typical drying process to prepare particle samples will result in any salts or residues in the particle suspension solvent also depositing on the sample grid, potentially making the sample difficult to image. For the best results, wash samples in a pure solvent, preferably MilliQ water or an alcohol, prior to depositing on the grid to minimize the artifacts caused by salts or other residues. Any residual moisture will outgas into the sample chamber causing contamination, or adsorb the energy from the electron beam and cause localized burning and damage to the carbon film, potentially ruining the sample. Ensuring all residual moisture has been removed from the sample prior to imaging is critical. It can be good practice to have your sample sit under a heat lamp for several minutes or stored in a desiccator to ensure it is free of moisture.

Less dense nanoparticles such as liposomes or polymeric particles provide much less contrast and may require staining with metals, such as uranium, to be viewed clearly. Any kind of capsule structures, such as liposomes, tend to suffer from the drying process and collapse on themselves, making imaging many intact liposomes challenging. Unless these types of samples are viewed using CryoEM techniques, users must understand that the sample preparation will induce structural artifacts. Readers are highly encouraged to read a comprehensive guide on sample preparation techniques such as that written by Ayache et al.[10] and speak to experts to determine sample limitations and potential preparation routes.

9.2.3 Scanning electron microscopy

SEM uses a fundamentally different process to form an image than that of TEM. Instead of transmitting the electron beam through a thin sample, the beam rasters across the sample surface and collects electrons after they have interacted with the sample and builds an image pixel by pixel. SEM is able to retain the 3D topography of the sample due to having a much wider depth of field than TEM. The highest resolution images are built by collecting secondary electrons (SEs) that are emitted from very near the surface of the sample producing images with a maximum resolution of around 1 nm. Back-scattered electrons (BSEs) are produced by elastic scattering of electrons from deeper within the sample. The additional depth reduces the maximum resolution of BSE imaging; however, BSEs carry a great deal of spectral information about the sample given that their rate of interaction is directly linked to the atomic number of the elements present within the sample.

Characteristic X-rays are produced when the electron beam interacts with an inner shell electron kicking it out and allowing an electron from a higher shell to drop down and fill the vacancy releasing the X-ray in the process. These X-rays can provide detailed information about the elemental makeup of the sample and are interrogated through energy-dispersive X-ray spectroscopy (EDX). While EDX is a powerful technique, it is generally used for elemental and spatial analysis across samples forming maps of elemental distribution on a sample. The resolution limit of SEM renders the use of EDX for analysis of nanoparticles limited in scope. Nanoparticle samples with applications that are highly dependent on the elemental ratios of specific components such as photocatalysts or biosensors often use EDX to determine their elemental configuration.[13,14] While some samples may lend themselves toward EDX analysis, the resolution of SEM instruments tends to limit their applications; there certainly are samples or experiments that EDX can be applied to, but EDX will not be discussed in detail in this chapter. Researchers wishing to apply this technique are encouraged to seek a grounding on the topic from Refs. 9,15 (Fig. 9.3).

Another beam interaction process may also occur where instead of the excess energy producing an X-ray, it can be directly transferred to another electron in one of the outermost shells causing that electron to gain enough energy to be ejected. These electrons are named Auger electrons, and their analysis can provide elemental and protonation information regarding a sample surface. Due to the relatively low energy of Auger electrons (50 eV to 3 keV) and relatively short free mean path of electrons undergoing this process, while the technique can reveal detailed information, it is intrinsically depth limited. Auger electron spectroscopy, therefore, is more effective when applied to thin films or the surface of nanostructures and is of limited use when investigating many nanoparticle samples. It can, however, be of use when other techniques such as X-ray photoelectron spectroscopy may struggle to determine the difference between spectra of elements, such as Ag and Pd, due to mass similarities. The lower energy of Auger electrons can more easily identify composition of a sample containing high atomic mass components with similar masses.[16]

9.2.4 Scanning electron microscopy sample preparation

SEM samples are mounted on small metal stubs, usually aluminum, often adhered to the surface using conductive carbon tape. Larger samples can be loaded into the chamber; however, great care must be taken with "lumpy" or topographically complex samples, as the SEM pole piece must be in very close proximity (around 5 mm) to the surface and it can be easy to bump and cause significant damage when imaging.

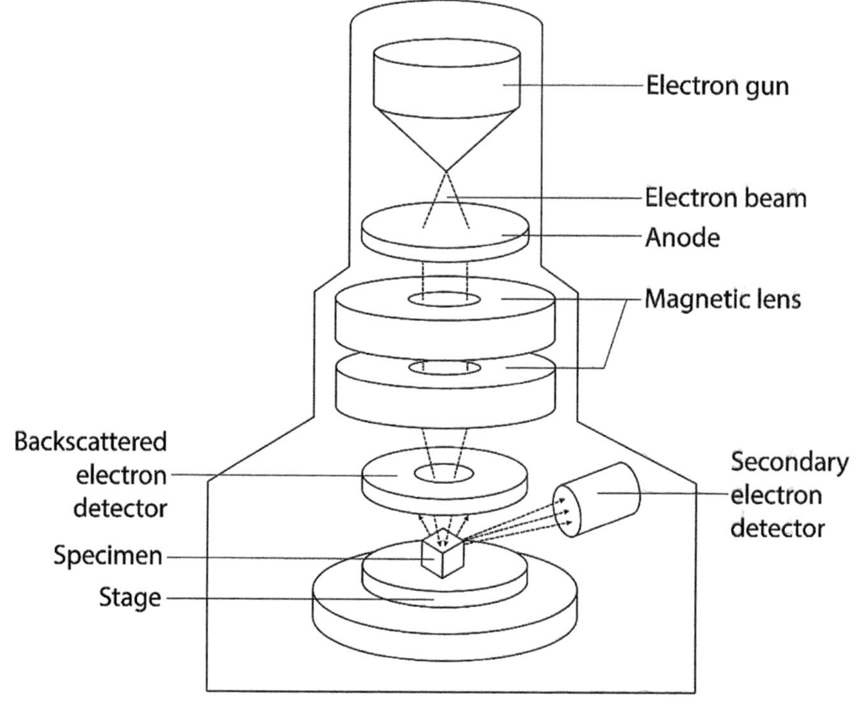

FIGURE 9.3 Outline of magnetic lens, beam path, and sample arrangement within an SEM. Illustration by Cheryl Chan. *SEM*, Scanning electron microscopy.

The primary concern with SEM samples is conductivity; for artifact-free images to be collected, the sample must be adequately conductive and grounded to the sample stub to avoid surface charging caused by the bombardment of electron from the beam building up on the surface of the sample until discharge, making the image seem to pulse. If the sample you wish to examine is not naturally conductive and reducing the accelerating voltage is not sufficient, it should be coated with a thin layer of a conductive material via a radio frequency sputtering technique. Only a few angstroms of conductive material are required, and a carefully coated sample can still maintain its surface morphology, but care should be taken to be selective in the choice of conductive coating if elemental analysis is required. Platinum, carbon, and gold are the standard conductive layers deposited.[7]

Should elemental analysis be required, choosing a conductive coating that will be easy to isolate from sample signal (i.e., platinum if no platinum is present within the sample) is required. Magnetic samples, such as iron oxide nanoparticles, are to be avoided due to the magnetic lenses of the SEM potentially causing the particles to lift from the sample stud and contaminate the walls and sensitive instrumentation of the sample chamber. Care should always be taken to avoid contamination of the sample chamber due to breakdown of the sample under the imaging conditions or magnetic attraction to internal components. The cleaning process required to remove contaminants from the sample chamber is laborious and requires significant instrument downtime.

9.2.5 Environmental scanning electron microscopy

Environmental scanning electron microscopy is a variant of SEM specifically designed to operate at higher pressures so as to enable the analysis of more hydrated or softer samples such as polymers that would not survive the conditions of a normal SEM. An ESEM can operate at pressures above 500 Pa compared with down to 10^{-4} Pa in conventional SEM instruments. This allows samples to be imaged without having to coat them in conductive layers and retains moisture so that samples can be observed in their hydrated state. This reduces the risk of contaminating the chamber and detectors from sample components outgassing or breaking down in the low vacuum of the SEM chamber. ESEM instruments are often completely separate instruments from standard SEM systems; however, some traditional SEM systems are able to operate in an ESEM mode. ESEMs may be useful for examining polymer-based particles or for examining harder metallic particles contained within a biological environment. Methods similar to immunohistochemistry can be applied to a sample using gold nanoparticles instead of optical labels. This can enable the visualization of features such as EGFR expression on the surface of a cell.[17]

9.2.6 Considerations

EM is an incredibly powerful tool to interrogate nanoparticles, but great care must be taken to ensure accurate information is being produced. Sample preparation is of critical importance to ensure no artifacts such as charging or burning alter the perceived morphology. Appropriate imaging modes must be selected for that specific sample and the desired analysis. It must also be understood that the image is being produced by collecting electrons that are undergoing different types of interaction with the surface of the sample. For SEM, understanding the electron interaction volume (Fig. 9.1) is of great importance when asserting exactly where a signal is coming from. Given the beam interaction physics, the interrogated volume is always larger than the beam spot size, and the signal will always be exponentially weighted toward the surface of the sample. For deeper investigation, ion beams can be used to accurately etch layers off the surface and allow for depth profiling of the sample. One critical strength of TEM is the extreme resolution; however, this greatly limits the field of view, and in doing so can give the researcher a false idea of the totality of the sample. Care must be taken not to attribute structural or elemental properties observed in a few sample locations to the whole sample. Wide field images showing the observational trend should always be collected to provide context rather than relying on the images of one or two highly characterized particles out of the hundreds of thousands present in the sample.

9.3 Elemental analysis

Variations of each of the elemental analysis techniques can be applied with an SEM or TEM with certain trade-offs or advantages to using one system or another. Electron energy loss spectroscopy (EELS) and EDX have overlapping function, but in general, EDX is better for heavier elements, whereas EELS can provide much better information on lighter elements. Both techniques can be used to produce elemental surface maps of samples, but EDX is often the more commonly used due to its versatility, simplicity, and availability. However, due to the energy resolution of these techniques, EELS is capable to determine the difference in the oxidation state of an element, whereas EDX is not. The choice of which technique to use will depend on many factors relevant to the sample and desired information. For these reasons, it is common to use more than one technique to investigate a sample, and the limiting factor becomes which techniques the researcher has access to.

9.3.1 Electron diffraction

Electron diffraction is performed on a TEM by using the magnetic lenses of the beam column to focus the beam down to a point that can be aimed at a single particle or edge of a larger crystal. The result is a black image with points of light where the crystal structure is causing the beam to scatter. With the main beam blocked in the center of the image, these points of light or rings in the case of an amorphous or polycrystalline material can be used to calculate information on the crystal structure of the sample. Crystal structure can be of great importance when producing core shell nanoparticles or developing materials with drug release or adsorption properties. This technique is routinely performed on TEM instruments; however, for further understanding, the reader is directed toward work by Zuo et al. who describes the methodology in significant detail.[18]

While electron diffraction can be used to study the crystal structure of specific particles within a sample, X-ray diffraction (XRD) will provide similar information and may be easier to access for many researchers. XRD will require significantly more sample for analysis, up to 0.2 cm^2, but is nondestructive. Should only a small amount of sample be available, general area diffraction systems (GADDS) can provide similar data with less sample. Due to the ability to do both imaging and crystallographic analysis on a minute sample of a nanoparticle material, electron diffraction is often the choice for particle analysis unless the researcher has access to XRD instrumentation and is producing the larger quantities of material required. XRD will provide the average crystal structure of a very large number of particles, potentially making it more of an accurate representation yet may miss the spatially relevant detail provided by performing electron diffraction on a single particle in TEM.

9.3.2 Electron energy loss spectroscopy

EELS relies on bombardment of the sample with an electron beam with a very well-defined range of kinetic energy. A subset of these electrons will undergo inelastic scattering, and their energy loss will be proportional to both the element that the beam interacts with and what type of interaction occurred, i.e., Cherenkov radiation, phonon or plasmon excitations, intra- or interband transitions, and inner shell ionizations, which are especially effective at determining the elemental makeup of a sample.

The EELS spectral window can be generally split between the low loss region <50eV loss and the high loss region >50eV. The high loss region includes spectral information from inner shell ionizations, which provide excellent chemical information on the species present within the sample. The low loss spectral window can reveal dielectric properties and band structures due to both the zero loss and plasmon peaks occurring in these energy ranges.

EELS is an effective technique to produce chemistry and element-based maps of nanoparticles or thin films. When used in a TEM, EELS is also able to provide thickness measurements of samples coregistered with TEM imagery making bias in elemental distribution within a nanoparticle clearly visible and quantifiable. This is especially useful with core shell nanoparticles or semiconductor particles. The reader is encouraged to seek further information on the capabilities of EELS from Ergeton et al.[19]

9.3.3 Inductively coupled plasma mass spectrometry

An inductively coupled plasma mass spectrometer (ICP-MS) is a mass spectrometer that uses a high-temperature plasma source to convert a sample into ions. The elemental makeup of the sample can then be determined by separating all the ions by their mass-to-charge ratio. Elemental analysis techniques such as this are useful when a researcher wants to understand the elemental ratios present within a complex nanoparticle consisting of more than one element such as a CdSe quantum dot. Less commonly, ICP-MS or related elemental analysis techniques can provide biodistribution or specific tissue loading for a nanoparticle.[20] However, these experiments are significantly more complex and may have higher error for reasons that we will discuss further on.

ICP-MS is part of a family of elemental analysis techniques that range in cost, detection range, elemental specificity, sample size, and ability to automate. This includes techniques such as inductively coupled plasma atomic emission spectroscopy (ICP-AES), which is also referred to as inductively coupled plasma optical emission spectroscopy (ICP-OES), or flame-based techniques such as flame atomic absorption spectroscopy (FAAS) also known by the name atomic absorption spectroscopy (AAS). Many of these related techniques could likely supply the elemental information sought by nanoparticle researchers. However, in this chapter, we will discuss the most commonly used and accessible technique to keep focus. Further reading on elemental analysis techniques related to ICP-MS can be found by Lindon et al.[21] and Gauglitz et al.[22]

ICP-MS can be used to simultaneously detect multiple elements within a given sample. This contrasts with techniques such as AAS that must sequentially identify sample components. A wide range of elements can be analyzed this way but not all. Typically, from atomic mass 7 up to 250 can be analyzed; however, some omissions occur due to the introduction of argon to form the plasma. For example, to accurately determine Fe content, an additional reaction chamber must be present, or a high-resolution system (HR-ICP-MS) is needed to resolve the Fe peak away from the ArO peak. In this case, the additional slits are used to reduce overall sensitivity and trade spectral resolution for detection limits.

ICP-MS typically uses a nebulizer to aerosolize liquid samples, or a laser to aerosolize solid samples. The aerosol is introduced to the argon plasma, where it first becomes a gas, and is then converted into ions as it travels through the plasma. The center of the ion stream is sampled using two metal disks with 1 mm diameter holes separated by a vacuum. These metal disks are called the sample cone and skimmer cone, and they funnel the sample into the mass spectrometer component of the instrument. Plasma is generated by applying oscillating electric and magnetic fields to argon gas using a radio frequency load coil. The argon is ionized by introducing a spark from a Tesla unit, and these colliding ions create plasma, at about 6000–10,000°K. Plasma ionization is superior to flame ionization because it prevents oxidization. Argon plasma forms mostly positive ions, which makes the detection of negatively ionizing elements more difficult, such as iodine and bromine.

Most ICP-MS systems use a quadrupole mass spectrometer. Alternating DC voltages and AC RF fields are applied to four rods, each 1 cm in diameter and 15–20 cm in length. This creates a mass-to-charge ratio filter, which only allows one type of ion to pass through at any time, effectively sorting the ions by isotope. Due to the atomization and excitation potential of plasma, up to 60 elements can be analyzed simultaneously, which is a drastic improvement over flame-based elemental analysis. Further reading on specific applications of ICP-MS can be found in *Practical Guide to ICP-MS* by Robert Thomas.[23]

9.3.4 Inductively coupled plasma mass spectrometry sample preparation

Taking a gold nanoparticle as a simple example of a nanoparticle for ICP-MS analysis, the sample preparation for ICP-MS or other related techniques would generally be performed as follows. The particle sample would be digested in acid so that the Au present in the nanoparticles is converted to Au^{3+} in solution. Many metals can simply be digested using hydrochloric acid; however, all samples must be diluted such that the acid content is less than 2% and 0.2% dissolved solids before running through the system to avoid damage. This dilution may present difficulty if the sample mass is quite small, as it may decrease the analyte concentration below the minimum detection limits of the specific element. This is mostly problematic when dealing with the detection of nanoparticles within tissues for biodistribution studies as the particle number of particles per gram of tissue may already be exceptionally low. This additional dilution may result in a false negative for an organ, making claims of "no uptake" or "complete clearance" using only ICP-MS questionable without very robust experimental procedures and/or secondary tissue analysis techniques such as EM. Microwave digestion is sometimes implemented to aid digestion of metal nanoparticles in tissue samples using less acid volume to reduce the required dilution volume, and in the case of Au, nitric acid is also added given the reluctance of Au to dissolve in HCl alone.

9.4 Particle counting

Counting particles is not as easy as it sounds. Specifically, being able to state how many particles you have of, one kind or another per milliliter can be difficult because of the nature of the particle population and the way that population is interrogated. There are methods of calculating total particle concentration using UV–visible spectroscopy for some materials such as gold; however, these techniques tend to rely heavily on assumptions that breakdown as polydispersity increases, yielding false information, which in turn can reduce the validity of experimental results. To count and characterize a particle sample properly, researchers must choose the correct technique for their material and fully understand the limitations of that technique in giving them a true picture of their sample.

There are three primary modes of interrogating a population of particles in solution: using a light source and its interaction with the sample to extrapolate different information from the scattering e.g., dynamic light scattering (DLS); tracking the Brownian motion of individual nanoparticles as they flutter in a known volume of thermally controlled medium to extrapolate size, NTA; and passing the sample through a tiny pore in a membrane or microfluidic structure and detecting changes in voltage between the inner and outer fluid reservoir, a process called Coulter counting, sometimes referred to as tunable resistive pulse sensing (TRPS).

DLS determines information about the Brownian motion of the particle in a solvent of known viscosity, thereby inferring its hydrodynamic size because the larger the particle, the slower its Brownian fluctuations will be. DLS has been a standard technique to determine size for many years. Samples that fit well for DLS measurement have low polydispersity and little variation of scattering cross section such as metal nanoparticles or micelles.

The first consideration is the polydispersity of the sample. Often, it is best to build an understanding of the sample through techniques such as TEM, so you can properly choose the counting technique that will provide the best information. If you find your sample is polydisperse, you may need to build a model that takes this variability into account when interpreting data or select a method that is less vulnerable to the effects of polydispersity. It should be understood that all methods that measure particles within a liquid will provide a hydrodynamic radius. Hydrodynamic radius is the radius of a sphere that would diffuse in the solvent at the same rate as the measured particle. This is slightly larger than the "physical" particle, as it includes the distance of charge projection into the surrounding solvent. A 1–5 nm increase in particle size under DLS compared with TEM is in the realm of acceptability, but it will heavily depend on the zeta potential. A hydrodynamic radius may be more informative for many biological applications, as it is the apparent size or diameter of effect of the particle. All counting techniques likely require dilution of the sample to a specific range; DLS is less restrictive. A bottle of PBS buffer that has sat with the lid open for a lunch break will be contaminated with dust particles ranging in size but will now be counted along with your sample should you use it for dilution. Fresh buffer and high-quality filtration is required before undertaking particle counting experiments; however, even the cleanest solvents contain a particle background that should at least be known and controlled for.

9.4.1 Nanoparticle tracking analysis

NTA analysis, such as TRPS or Coulter counting techniques, is able to provide both size and concentration of nanoparticles per milliliter with great accuracy and only a few caveats. Samples with broader polydispersity or an unknown particle population are excellent for NTA analysis, this being the instrument's main strength. A sample containing a wide population of particles can be equally as accurately measured as a highly monodisperse sample. NTA records the size of all particles within the sample down to 1 nm accuracy, and the presence of a 300 nm population does not interfere with the ability to measure a subpopulation of 50-nm particles unlike DLS.[24] NTA primarily uses the scattering of a particle to determine its location in real time. Using high-speed video recording, the movements of the particle are tracked and measured. With a known temperature and solvent viscosity, the Brownian motion of the particle is used to calculate the hydrodynamic radius of a sphere that would diffuse at the same rate as the particle being tracked.

NTA analysis is excellent for polydisperse particles because using the video tracking of individual particles to build a data set by interrogating every single particle moving through the light path means there are fewer generalizations. By analyzing a few thousand particles directly, a more accurate histogram representing the particle distribution can be produced. Concentration is calculated simply by knowing the optical volume being collected and the flow rate of the sample.

There are two primary ways through which NTA instruments are set up, but the data collection and analysis are essentially the same. Flow cell systems use a thermally controlled fluidic channel to pass sample through a laser path with a collection objective directly above to collect the scattered light. Cuvette-based systems are simpler; instead of flowing sample past the data collection point, the objective focuses on a single volume within the sample, and data are collected for a period before the sample is agitated and fresh sample is brought to the sample volume. Both techniques make multiple video recordings of the particle tracks during the data collection period and then average out the results obtained (Fig. 9.4). Longer acquisition periods and multiple acquisitions decrease the error with flow style systems, whereas cuvette-based instruments benefit more from increasing the number of total acquisitions.

Flow cell style instruments should be considered destructive, as collecting the sample after analysis can lead to contamination, usually around 300 μL of sample is consumed, whereas cuvette style instruments allow easy contamination-free recovery of the sample. However, given the instruments require the samples to be very dilute means little sample volume is needed. To produce quality data, the concentration should typically be between 10^6 and 10^9 particle/mL; any higher or lower will result in poor data. The instrument will often inform you if the particle density is too high or low. This means that samples must be accurately diluted and the final concentration back calculated to your stock solution.

Because NTA analysis needs to be able to individually track nanoparticles, the particles must scatter the particular wavelength of laser light being used by the instrument. Some instruments exist that simultaneously use multiple laser wavelengths to ensure the entire population is being accurately represented. Multiwavelength instruments are typically more expensive but are the most proficient at measuring highly polydisperse particle samples. Other instruments provide options on which wavelength to include with the instrument based on the sample type expected to most commonly be

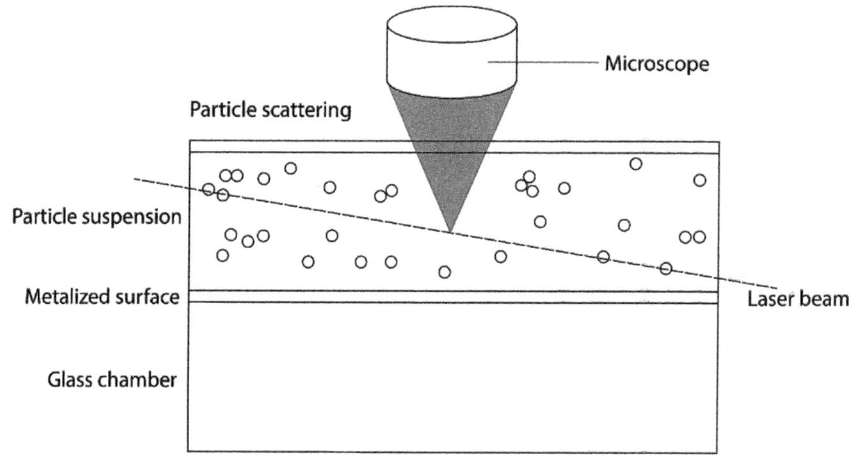

FIGURE 9.4 Side cut of fluidic channel style NTA particle counting system. Illustration by Cheryl Chan. *NTA*, Nanoparticle tracking analysis.

measured within that lab. While detecting the scattered light position and ignoring the intensity removes the need to include a scattering coefficient, it does mean the particles need to scatter enough so as to be individually visualized and tracked. This means that NTA is excellent for particle analysis down to about 20 nm, but below that scattering is too weak even for highly scattering gold particles. DLS is the best option if your particles are below this limit; however, concentration information is no longer possible to measure.

9.4.2 Considerations

NTA analysis provides highly detailed size distribution and concentration data, but care must be taken to ensure that the data are being collected and interpreted correctly. Misalignments of the optical mount or incorrect camera settings can alter the counting quality. In microfluidic variants of NTA systems, trapped bubbles can be a significant problem, and care must always be taken to avoid bubbles, making their way into the fluidic channel. Flow cell style instruments can be delicate given the mating surface of the fluidic cell and the optical surface need to be seated and unseated after every data collection session. Careful handling and maintenance of both the fluidic cell and optical surface is required to ensure quality data are collected.

9.4.3 Coulter counting

Named for its inventor, Wallace H. Coulter, the Coulter principle states that a particle transiting a small pore can be detected and measured by the momentary change in impedance between the opposite sides of the pore if an electric current is flowing through the same pore (Fig. 9.5). The change in impedance is caused by displacement of electrolyte by the particle and is therefore proportional to the volume of the particle. In this regard, all Coulter counting–based instruments, some which now called the principle "tunable resistive pulse sensing" (TRPS), use an electrolyte cell divided by a single pore of a known size.

Coulter counting was initially applied in the clinic measuring complete blood counts, differentiating between white and red blood cells rapidly and with little sample volume requirement. Recently, this technique has been applied to counting nanosized particles with little change required in the overall design of the system except for significantly reducing the size of the pore and dealing with surface tension.[25] On the nanoscale, surface tension can become difficult to overcome especially in cartridge-based systems that include a filtration mechanism. In these cases, surfactants may need to be used to ensure complete wetting of the filtration system and transit pore. Researchers should be aware of the effects of both the electrolyte, typically phosphate buffer, and any surfactant may have on their sample, and care must be taken to avoid the introduction of any contamination that may affect the collected data.

Coulter counting–based systems benefit from measuring individual particles and building a data set one particle at a time. This means there is less chance for assumptions or missed populations of particles within the sample such as in the case with DLS. However, the difficulty of physically constricting the sample through a submicron-sized pore brings with it challenges such as sample clogging, which some designs deal with by making the prefiltration and measurement pore a single use cartridge or using a polymer-based pore that can be deformed. For all Coulter counting–based instruments, dilute samples are required so as not to overwhelm the measurement. Concentrations in the range of 10^5–10^{11} particles/mL can be measured, which is a slightly wider window than NTA.

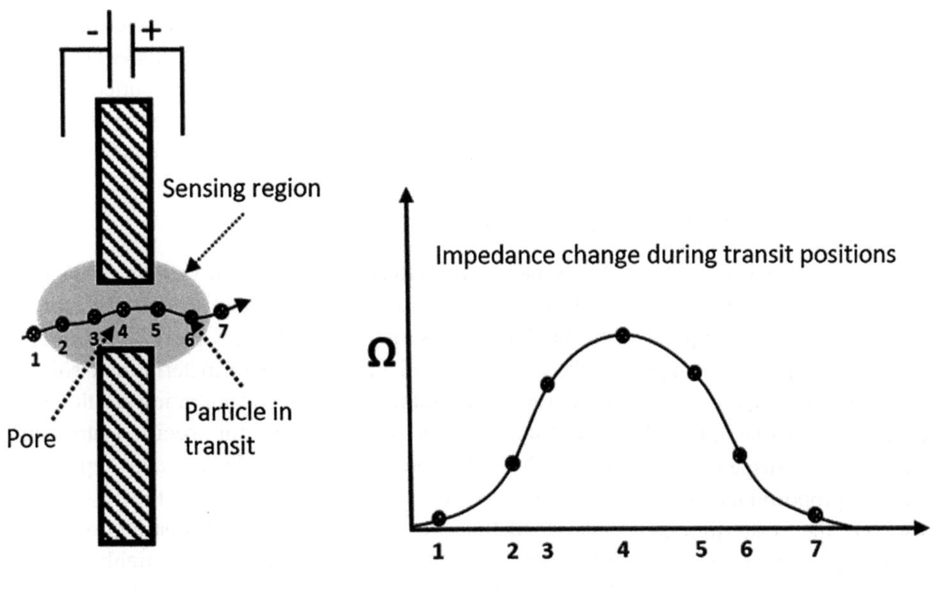

FIGURE 9.5 Coulter counting principle: (Left) Particle passing through the sensing pore. (Right) Change in impedance during particle track depicted on left panel. Illustration by Cheryl Chan.

9.4.4 Considerations

Given that the measured signal is proportional to the electrolyte displacement, porous particles will not displace the same amount of electrolyte, leading to an artificially small diameter reading. It is recommended that a secondary method is first used to correlate the apparent particle size of a porous sample with a more absolute measurement such as that can be provided by TEM. Measurement artifacts may occur such as coincident readings that are difficult to determine if it is a single larger particle or two particles transiting in close proximity. This is easily reduced by decreasing the overall particle concentration; however, the type of pore used may also induce false or difficult to determine signals. Aperture-based pores are far more susceptible to the uneven distribution of charge and liquid flow through the pore causing inconsistent measurements such as "shoulders" on the recorded impedance. Signal processing can be applied to tease out the correct signals in these cases.

9.4.5 Dynamic light scattering

DLS has become a core method of sizing particles in solution due to both the ease of measurement and the relative abundance of benchtop instruments available. DLS has excellent dynamic range and is likely the best technique for measuring particle sizes below 20 nm; however, the technique struggles with polydisperse samples. Unless there is a significant size difference between several monodisperse populations approximately 100 nm, the technique will often fail to differentiate between them and will bias toward the sample with the higher scattering coefficient, i.e., the larger component. DLS is best used to confirm the size and polydispersity of a sample that a researcher is already familiar with. It will quickly and easily indicate deviation from expected quality standards, which is why it is a mainstay technique in pharmaceutical development. Polydisperse samples may be better addressed using other techniques such as NTA or Coulter counting/TRPS-based analysis, as the particles are addressed on a more individual basis and combined to produce a data set rather than inferring the result from the behaviors of a whole population that may not scatter evenly. This section will only cover practical considerations and caveats for using DLS to analyze nanoparticles; a deeper technical understanding of DLS can be found in the works by Schärtl et al.[26] and Robert Pecora[27].

The method uses the variability in scattering conditions based on particle sizes and the proportional Brownian motion to determine the size of particles with some basic information about the sample such as the refractive index of both the sample and solvent. Nanoparticles suspended in solution scatter incident light at a rate proportional to the sixth power of their radius; however, the scattering intensity of some materials such as gold can cause data interpretation problems if the sample is not monodisperse.

When reading DLS data, there are several important values. Polydispersity index (PDI) is a measure of the size distribution within the sample and calculated via a two-parameter fit to the correlation data. The value is dimensionless, but set so that only exceptionally monodisperse samples, like bead standards, reach a value close to 0.05; most samples will fall in the range of 0.05–0.7. Any value higher than 0.7 indicates that the sample is likely too polydisperse for DLS and that your sample is changing during the measurement or improperly prepared. The correlation curve and its Y-intercept value provide the best indication of the validity of the sample data. The correlation curve should be smooth, and the Y-intercept, which depicts the signal to noise ratio within the data, should be greater than 0.6 with anything above 0.9 being of exceptional quality.[28] Selecting an appropriate correlation function fit for your data can significantly change the outcome of your data analysis, and choices should be made based on prior knowledge of your sample. The cumulant model is the simplest method and fits a single exponential decay function, and is particularly robust as it is minimally affected by noise in the signal.[29] However, this means it is less capable when examining polydisperse samples. The CONTIN method uses inverse Laplace transforms and multiple exponentials to fit the correlation curve and is far more capable with polydisperse or multimodal samples.[30]

Sample concentration is an important factor; DLS has a wider dynamic range of acceptable sample concentrations than either NTA or Coulter/TRPS-based methods. Those methods also require lower concentrations of particles due to needing to make measurements on an individual basis. If concentrations are too high, they struggle to differentiate the signal and data quality suffers. The limitations for DLS come from higher or lower concentrations altering the way in which light is scattering from the sample. High concentrations can cause multiple scattering, which decreases the intensity of the scattered light as it undergoes sequential scattering events before being detected, thus reducing the reported particle radius. Lower concentrations simply decrease the amount of scattered light and decrease the signal-to-noise ratio.

9.4.6 Considerations

Many factors can affect the quality and validity of the data collected via DLS, and it is important to create a reliable protocol for measuring your specific particle type. This includes entering all the appropriate material and solvent properties and finding a reliable concentration for the laser power and detector sensitivity of your specific instrument. Once these parameters are established and repeatable measurements are routine, DLS provides the fastest and easiest method to measure size and distribution in a monodisperse nanoparticle sample. DLS is highly susceptible to hiding populations of particles or producing a size value incompatible with EM measurements due to the large number of assumptions used to calculate the properties of the sample. Polydisperse samples, or samples with large changes in scattering coefficient, or samples undergoing flocculation due to dilution can significantly alter the obtained results. Careful attention must be given to the PDI and correlation curve to determine the validity of a sample measurement. Soft samples like micelles or liposomes are more difficult to confirm the results orthogonally; however, hard metallic particles should be examined under EM to ensure DLS results truly reflect the sample.

An example of the same sample made from two distinct particle populations mixed together at equivalent concentrations and examined under NTA and DLS is shown below (Fig. 9.6). The sample, made by mixing smaller gold nanoparticles and larger silica nanoparticles, can be identified as two distinct populations under NTA. However, DLS is unable to determine the two populations from each other due to its lower resolution. In this case, the NTA data are a more accurate representation of the size distribution of the particles within the sample, and the subpopulations would have been overlooked with DLS. Using DLS for sizing analysis is perfectly acceptable if your sample is well known and characterized orthogonally using electron microscopy or a technique like NTA or Coulter counting. DLS provides many indications that some component of your sample is not fitting the usual pattern; however, this data are often not as obvious unless the researcher is looking for it. The particle size distribution is calculated as a single curve to best fit the data collected, whereas the NTA data represent many individual measurements with far less regard for fitting an expectation.

Some instruments are available with the ability to measure the sample from multiple angles, which greatly increases the robustness of the correlograms. A single-angle DLS requires that samples differ in size by a factor of 3 to be accurately separated from each other. Multiangle instruments are able to reduce the required size differential between populations for differentiation from 3:1 to 2:1.[31] Many instruments are also able to perform zeta potential analysis, making the benchtop DLS instrument a common sight in nanoparticle labs around the world. Additional understanding of the physical principles of DLS can be found in laser light scattering by Johnson and Gabriel.[32]

9.5 Zeta potential

Zeta potential is a measurement of the electrical potential between the outer region of the particles charge cloud and the solvent it is suspended (Fig. 9.5). However, it should not be confused with, or equated to, the electric surface potential or the Stern potential. These are separate definitions of electrical properties that have specifically defined locations of measurement within the electrical double layer system. For a more complete understanding of colloidal stability and the specific variables that interact to balance a stable colloidal system, the reader should examine DLVO theory (named for its contributors Derjaguin, Landau, Verwey, and Overbeek) and the formation mechanics of the electrical double layer.[33,34] These topics will outline the reason why certain chemistries are used to infer advantageous charge properties for specific applications. An excellent and detailed discussion on zeta potential and its effects on colloidal systems can be found in Ref. [35].

Zeta potential measurement is carried out by applying an electric field to the sample. The degree to which the particles alter their movement proportional to the externally applied field is referred to as the electrophoretic mobility (μ_e). Once measured, the zeta potential can be calculated using the Henry equation.

$$\mu_e = \frac{2\varepsilon z f(k\alpha)}{\eta} \tag{9.2}$$

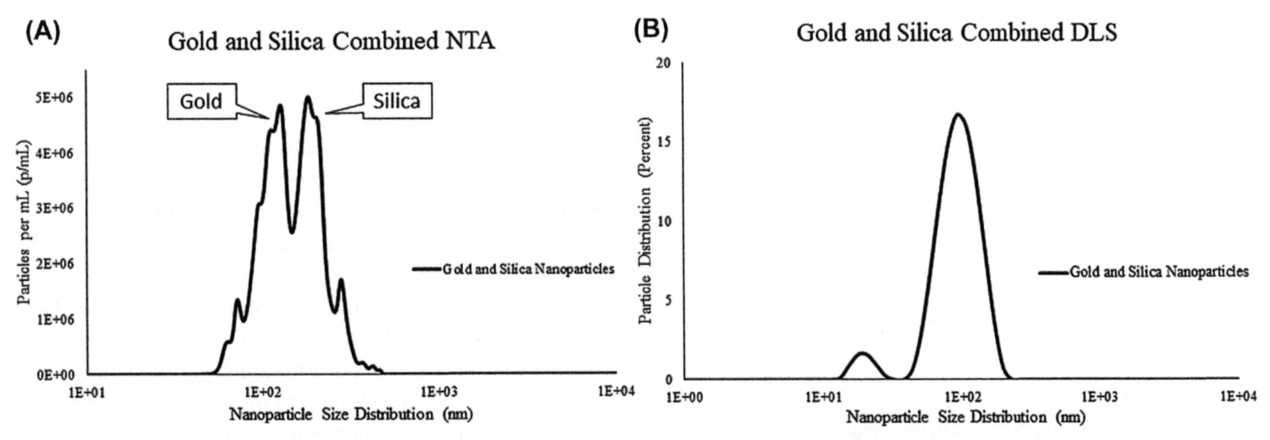

FIGURE 9.6 Comparison of NTA and DLS data collected for the same mixed sample of gold and silica nanoparticles of different sizes: (A) NTA data, (B) DLS data. *NTA*, nanoparticle tracking analysis; *DLS*, dynamic light scattering.

where z is the zeta potential, μ_e the electrophoretic mobility, ε is the dielectric constant, η the viscosity, and $f(k\alpha)$ the Henry function. Within the Henry function, k is the Debye parameter thickness of the electrical double layer and α is the radius of the particle. Typically, 1 or 1.5 is used as an approximation of Henry's function.

The relationship between zeta potential and colloidal stability is often the most broadly discussed. However, the relationship is not as clear cut as it is often portrayed. Often, a zeta potential of 0 mV may be claimed to result in unstable particle suspensions, whereas a zeta potential of ±40 mV provides stability. However, in practice, we find a deeper understanding of DLVO theory provides better predictions than a direct relationship between increased zeta potential and colloidal stability. This is because zeta potential measurements give no information regarding the attractive van der Waals forces at play in the colloidal system. Many particles can form stable colloids at very low zeta potentials, e.g., silica beads, if their Hamaker constant is low.[36] With low attractive van der Waals forces, a significantly lower repulsive zeta potential is required to maintain colloidal stability (e.g., 10−15 mV). Keeping the zeta potential close to zero while maintaining colloidal stability also reduces the risk of large changes in behavior as the particles begin to interact with complex fluids. In this regard, zeta potential remains a critical factor to determine colloidal stability, but there is no set value at which all colloids will aggregate or remain stable. So long as the repulsive forces overcome the attractive van der Waals component stability can be maintained (Fig. 9.7).

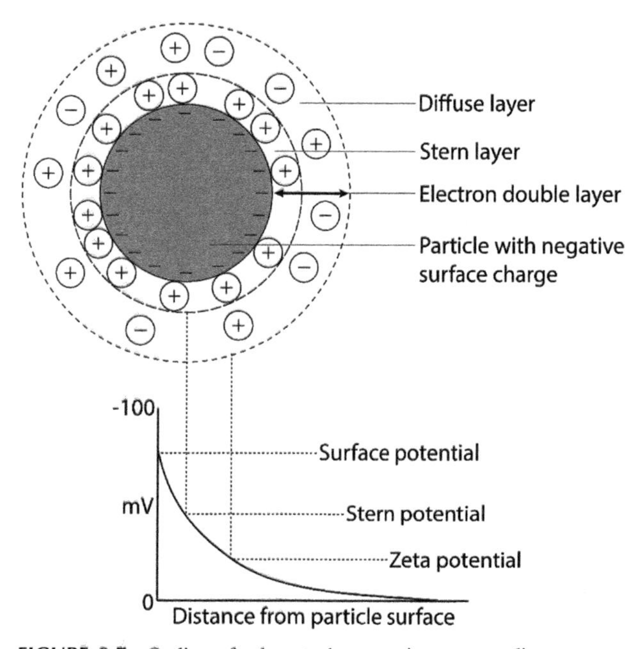

FIGURE 9.7 Outline of relevant charge regions surrounding a nanoparticle. Illustration by Cheryl Chan.

While stability in solution may be of great importance, by its nature, the zeta potential will change when it is introduced to a new environment. Therefore, the particle may have perfect stability while stored in solution but its application environment (such as the bloodstream, cytoplasm, or any complex biological fluid) will likely change the zeta potential and may lead to undesired behavior such as flocculation. This will also alter its ability to cross membranes, adsorb analytes, bind to targets, avoid or seek immune cells, and generally dictate the formation of the inevitable protein corona.

The protein corona is a critical consideration when intending to apply nanoparticles in biological environments. In brief, it refers to the principle that whenever you introduce a nanoparticle into a complex biological solution, it is rapidly coated with proteins and other charged components from its environment. These form two primary layers on the surface of the particle, a "hard corona" where the proteins have high binding affinity and long residence times and the "soft corona" where proteins have weak affinity and short residence times. Zeta potential and crystallographic structure play a strong role in determining which serum proteins bind and ultimately form the interaction surface for the particle. The degree to which the particle interacts with serum proteins may have a larger effect on the function of the particle than any engineered surface moiety on the particle. Zeta potential, therefore, becomes an important engineering consideration when designing a nanoparticle for a specific application.

A particle with a surface charge in excess of ±80 mV will be considered a significant energy gradient, and while it may increase uptake or binding efficiency in vitro, the high charge *may* cause unwanted interactions with components of complex biological fluids and decrease the interaction with a desired target. Given the specific nature of most nanoparticle applications, an appropriate zeta potential must be chosen and implemented. This general description of the role of zeta potential serves only as an umbrella discussion to highlight considerations and general principles. It is highly recommended that the readers seek literature directly related to their field of interest when determining the desired zeta potential for their particles.

Zeta potential measurements are generally carried out on bulk populations of particles, giving an average value for a population. Similar to size or shape variability, a wide variance of zeta potential across a population can hide data or misrepresent the true nature of a particle sample. Again, care while producing the particles and careful zeta potential measurement will give a much clearer picture of the effect of zeta potential on the application. Zeta potential measurement can be carried out on single particles; however, these measurements are limited to instruments that measure particles individually rather than across the whole population. This means some instruments based on the Coulter principle or TRPS can perform this measurement but not those based on DLS techniques.

9.6 Brunauer-Emmet-Teller

Measurements of specific surface area and pore sizes of a particle sample can be critical in developing catalytic materials or potential nanocarriers for drug or other biological payloads. The Brunauer-Emmet-Teller (BET) theory (named for its creators) uses the behavior of gases as they adsorb onto the surface of a material to determine the material's specific surface area and average pore volume.[37] The theory is an extension to the Langmuir theory and assumes gas molecules adsorb onto the surface of the material and form infinitely thick stacks of monolayers of absorbed gases that only interact with their adjacent layers. The absorption process is driven by van der Waals forces between the gas and the material surface and is monitored by a continuous gas flow procedure or a volumetric analysis.

BET analysis can be a useful tool to determine how a nanomaterial will perform with other materials, given many of the properties of these materials are surface area limited. Typically, the measurements are carried out under liquid nitrogen on powder samples. This technique works best with solid particles such as metals that will not alter morphology while undergoing the drying/freezing process of the measurement cycle. The accuracy of this technique is heavily related to the mass of material being measured; the more the sample mass, the greater the accuracy. Sample masses of less than 0.1 g are considered poor quality, and masses of 0.2 g and up are typically considered enough mass for a measurement with acceptable error. For some nanoparticle samples, this mass of material can be difficult to produce; however, this is a nondestructive technique so sample is not lost after measurement.

9.7 Concluding remarks

Characterizing nanoparticles can be a difficult process due to many factors affecting the outcome of experiments, especially when interacting with biological systems. Each variable may have a significant effect and should be characterized independently to form a more comprehensive understanding of the sample. Not only does a single particle have multiple properties that may be relevant, but each of those properties will vary across the population. You have to accept that the best path is to be thorough in your choice of characterization techniques, while accepting that there are no absolutes. The best that can be done is to know your population variables and control for them with strong experimental design.

We have come a long way from squinting down an optical microscope trying to discern detail from the realm of the submicron. Advancements in electron microscopy and chemical analysis have enabled researchers to quantify crystal structure, surface chemistry, protein structure, elemental configuration, and interaction kinetics among a myriad of other parameters. We now have a huge array of tools at our disposal to examine and aid in the design of nanoparticle systems, CryoEm, and in situ TEM being the greatest shifts in the way we see the nanoscale world from the last decade. We are learning at an exponentially growing rate, yet our limited knowledge, especially in regard to biology, reminds us that new ways of examining biological interactions are needed. Advancements in imaging technologies such as magnetic particle imaging, multiphoton microscopy, photo and radio frequency acoustics are providing a window into the interactions and trafficking of nanoparticles in living biological systems. Coupled with greater design accuracy and more robust characterization techniques nanoparticles will continue to find greater applications in biological research and the clinic.

References

1. Nikoobakht B, El-Sayed MA. Preparation and growth mechanism of gold nanorods (NRs) using seed-mediated growth method. *Chem Mater* 2003;**15**(10):1957–62.
2. Xie X, et al. The effect of shape on cellular uptake of gold nanoparticles in the forms of stars, rods, and triangles. *Sci Rep* 2017;**7**(1):3827.
3. Fromen CA, et al. Nanoparticle surface charge impacts distribution, uptake and lymph node trafficking by pulmonary antigen-presenting cells. *Nanomedicine* 2016;**12**(3):677–87.
4. Abbe E. Ueber einen neuen Beleuchtungsapparat am Mikroskop. *Arch Mikrosk Anat* 1873;**9**(1):469–80.
5. Kuo J. *Electron microscopy: methods and protocols*. 2014.
6. Oho E. Digital image processing technology for scanning electron microscopy. In: Hawkes PW, editor. *Advances in imaging and electron physics*. Elsevier; 1998. p. 77–140.
7. Echlin P. *Handbook of sample preparation for scanning electron microscopy and X-ray microanalysis*. US: Springer; 2011.
8. Scarff CA, et al. Variations on negative stain electron microscopy methods: tools for tackling challenging systems. *J Vis Exp* 2018;(132):57199.
9. Lyman CE, et al. *Scanning electron microscopy, X-ray microanalysis, and analytical electron microscopy: a laboratory workbook*. US: Springer; 2012.
10. Ayache J, et al. *Sample preparation handbook for transmission electron microscopy: methodology*. New York: Springer; 2010.
11. Evans JE, et al. Controlled growth of nanoparticles from solution with in situ liquid transmission electron microscopy. *Nano Lett* 2011;**11**(7):2809–13.
12. Taheri ML, et al. Current status and future directions for in situ transmission electron microscopy. *Ultramicroscopy* 2016;**170**:86–95.
13. Sobana N, Muruganadham M, Swaminathan M. Nano-Ag particles doped TiO_2 for efficient photodegradation of direct azo dyes. *J Mol Catal A Chem* 2006;**258**(1):124–32.
14. Baby TT, Ramaprabhu S. SiO_2 coated Fe_3O_4 magnetic nanoparticle dispersed multiwalled carbon nanotubes based amperometric glucose biosensor. *Talanta* 2010;**80**(5):2016–22.

15. Goldstein JI, et al. *Scanning electron microscopy and X-ray microanalysis*. New York: Springer; 2017.
16. Sutter E, et al. In situ liquid-cell electron microscopy of silver–palladium galvanic replacement reactions on silver nanoparticles. *Nat Commun* 2014;**5**:4946.
17. Peckys DB, et al. Epidermal growth factor receptor subunit locations determined in hydrated cells with environmental scanning electron microscopy. *Sci Rep* 2013;**3**:2626.
18. Zuo JM, Spence JCH. *Advanced transmission electron microscopy: imaging and diffraction in nanoscience*. New York: Springer; 2018.
19. Egerton RF. *Electron energy-loss spectroscopy in the electron microscope*. US: Springer; 2013.
20. Sancey L, et al. Long-term in vivo clearance of gadolinium-based AGuIX nanoparticles and their biocompatibility after systemic injection. *ACS Nano* 2015;**9**(3):2477–88.
21. Lindon JC. *Encyclopedia of spectroscopy and spectrometry*. Elsevier Science; 2010.
22. Gauglitz G, Moore DS. *Handbook of spectroscopy*. Wiley; 2014.
23. Thomas R. *Practical guide to ICP-MS: a tutorial for beginners*. 3rd ed. Taylor & Francis; 2013.
24. Filipe V, Hawe A, Jiskoot W. Critical evaluation of Nanoparticle Tracking Analysis (NTA) by NanoSight for the measurement of nanoparticles and protein aggregates. *Pharm Res* 2010;**27**(5):796–810.
25. Henriquez RR, et al. The resurgence of Coulter counting for analyzing nanoscale objects. *Analyst* 2004;**129**(6):478–82.
26. Schärtl W. *Light scattering from polymer solutions and nanoparticle dispersions*. Berlin Heidelberg: Springer; 2007.
27. Pecora R. *Dynamic light scattering: applications of photon correlation spectroscopy*. US: Springer; 2013.
28. Stetefeld J, McKenna SA, Patel TR. Dynamic light scattering: a practical guide and applications in biomedical sciences. *Biophysical reviews* 2016;**8**(4):409–27.
29. Koppel DE. Analysis of macromolecular Polydispersity in intensity correlation spectroscopy: the method of cumulants. *J Chem Phys* 1972;**57**(11):4814–20.
30. Provencher SW. CONTIN: a general purpose constrained regularization program for inverting noisy linear algebraic and integral equations. *Comput Phys Commun* 1982;**27**(3):229–42.
31. Malvern Panalytical. Improved component resolution with Multi-Angle DLS (MADLS). September 27 2018 August, 30, 2019]; Available from: https://www.malvernpanalytical.com/en/learn/knowledge-center.
32. Johnson CS, Gabriel DA. *Laser light scattering*. Dover Publications; 1994.
33. Derjaguin B, Landau L. Theory of the stability of strongly charged lyophobic sols and of the adhesion of strongly charged particles in solutions of electrolytes. *Prog Surf Sci* 1993;**43**(1):30–59.
34. Verwey EJW. Theory of the stability of lyophobic colloids. *J Phys Colloid Chem* 1947;**51**(3):631–6.
35. Bhattacharjee S. DLS and zeta potential – what they are and what they are not? *J Control Release* 2016;**235**:337–51.
36. Hamaker HC. The London—van der Waals attraction between spherical particles. *Physica* 1937;**4**(10):1058–72.
37. Brunauer S, Emmett PH, Teller E. Adsorption of gases in multimolecular layers. *J Am Chem Soc* 1938;**60**(2):309–19.

Chapter 10

Liposomal delivery system

Yuan Zhang[1] and Leaf Huang[2]

[1]*Department of Biomedical and Pharmaceutical Sciences, College of Pharmacy, University of Rhode Island, Kingston, RI, United States;* [2]*Division of Pharmacoengineering and Molecular Pharmaceutics and Center for Nanotechnology in Drug Delivery, Eshelman School of Pharmacy, University of North Carolina at Chapel Hill, Chapel Hill, NC, United States*

Liposomes are one of the most promising vectors for efficient drug and gene delivery. Liposomes could efficiently encapsulate a wide range of molecules for medical applications. Many liposomal formulations are under clinical investigations or have been approved for clinical use. This book chapter will discuss the design and fabrication of a variety of liposomal delivery systems including stimuli-responsive liposomes and active targeting liposomes, as well as their in vivo delivery hurdles and the strategies to overcome the in vivo barriers to achieve efficient drug and gene delivery, such as overcoming the polyethylene glycol (PEG) dilemma and the surveillance of the reticuloendothelial system (RES) as well as promoting endosomal escape.[1]

10.1 Liposomes

Liposomes are biocompatible phospholipid vesicles composing of at least one concentric lipid bilayers enclosing a central aqueous compartment.[2] Based on lamellarity, liposomes are divided into unilamellar liposome vesicles containing a single lipid bilayer and multilamellar liposome vesicles (MLVs) composed of multiple liposomal membranes.[3] Based on the liposome size, unilamellar vesicles are divided into giant unilamellar vesicles (GUVs) (1 μm and larger), large unilamellar vesicles (LUVs) (100 −400 nm), and small unilamellar vesicles (SUVs) (20 −100 nm).[4] Liposomal systems can entrap both lipophilic and hydrophilic compounds, which enable the efficient encapsulation of diverse drugs and their combination. The lipid composition of liposomes allows for improved endocytosis and tissue compatibility.[5] Liposomes as a nanocarrier have the potential to increase the drug concentration accumulated in target cells, therefore increasing the therapeutic index of drugs.[6] In addition, liposomes reduce drug toxicity and improve drug stability.[7] Additionally, the surface charge of liposomes can impact their in vivo behavior. For instance, positively charged liposomes with a high proportion of cationic lipid can increase cytotoxicity in culture and impair colloidal stability.[1,8]

There are several types of liposomal delivery systems. Conventional liposomes consist of a lipid bilayer containing phospholipids (cationic, anionic, or neutral lipids) and cholesterol. The inclusion of cholesterol can increase liposome stability and lipid flexibility, and minimize phospholipid exchange with other physiological components.[9] Conventional liposomes reduced the in vivo toxicity of encapsulated compounds, but often display short circulating half-life and rapid elimination from the bloodstream which compromises their therapeutic efficacy. The fast clearance is due to the opsonization by plasma components and phagocytosis by the RES, mainly in the liver and spleen.[1] To minimize liposome elimination in blood, PEG was modified on the surface of conventional liposomes, creating PEGylated liposomes, also known as stealth liposomes.[10] The modification with PEG, also called PEGylation, prevents opsonin binding from physiological fluids such as plasma and helps liposomes circumvent the surveillance of RES, providing a prolonged half-life in blood circulation.[11,12] The steric barrier of PEG improves the liposome stability and reduces side effects.[13] Considering the physiological characteristics of tumor tissues, PEGylated liposomes can passively target and accumulate to tumors through the enhanced permeability and retention (EPR) effect, with particle sizes typically in the range of 100−200 nm in diameter.[14] (Fig. 10.1). The EPR effect refers to the increased permeability of the vasculature that supplies pathological tissues including tumors and inflammatory conditions, and the lack of effective lymphatic drainage in tumor tissues.[2] The EPR effect enhances the extravasation and accumulation of macromolecules and

Nanoparticles for Biomedical Applications. https://doi.org/10.1016/B978-0-12-816662-8.00010-2

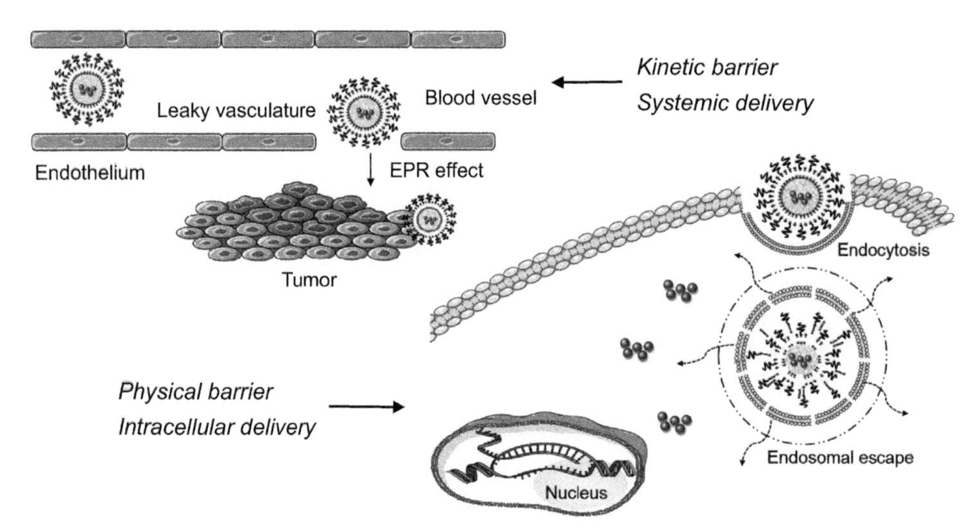

FIGURE 10.1 Schematic illustration of liposome systemic delivery and its intracellular delivery. *EPR*, Enhanced permeability and retention.

nanoparticles in solid tumor tissues by passive targeting. In order to promote the site-specific drug delivery to tumors and other tissues, PEGylated liposomes can be functionalized with various targeting ligands, such as antibodies, peptides/proteins, and small molecules. These targeting ligands can specifically bind to certain receptors/antigens overexpressing on target cells with high affinity, which facilitates receptor-mediated endocytosis.

10.2 Methods of preparation

There are several methods of liposome preparation, including the mechanical dispersion method, solvent dispersion method, and detergent removal method.[15] The solvent dispersion method is commonly known as ethanol injection, and detergent removal methods involve using detergents such as cholate, alkylglycoside, and Triton X-100. The resulting liposomes can be mechanically downsized by sonication or by membrane extrusion cycles through a polycarbonate filter.[16,17]

The microfluidic method is a recently developed approach for liposome preparation. Microfluidics devices generate and control fluid flow in channels with cross-sectional dimensions in the range of 5−500 μm, leading to the formation of lipid vesicles by self-assembly.[18] Lipids in alcohol solution flow in the central channel. The lipid stream is mixed with and sheathed by aqueous buffers flowing from one or two additional channels within the device. The aqueous buffers contain molecules that will be encapsulated in lipid vesicles. Due to the well-defined flow rate and channel architectures, the microfluidic method has potential to achieve superior control over the final physical properties of lipid vesicles, such as liposome size, size distribution, lamellarity, and homogeneity. The microfluidic device with higher channel aspect ratio results in more uniform liposomes and higher production rates.[19]

Liposome's behavior and function are strongly dependent on its properties such as size, shape, and surface charge which can be measured by dynamic light scattering (DLS).[18] Cholesterol is often added to the formulation to stabilize the phospholipid bilayer and control the stiffness of the liposome.[20] The encapsulation efficiency (EE) of the drug within liposomes is calculated by: EE = Amount of drug encapsulated/total amount of drug used for nanoparticle production. The EE and the interaction between drug and lipids depend on the chemical structures of the loaded drug, lipids, and the fabrication method of liposomes.[21]

Liposomes tend to form aggregates or experience drug leakage in aqueous formulation during storage, which limits their clinical application. Lyophilization, also called freeze-drying, can be employed to prolong the shelf life of liposomes without compromising their biological functions.[22] The phospholipid has an intrinsic rotational freedom, which may cause leakage of the liposome contents.[23] To prevent the lipid membrane damage by ice crystal formation during the freeze-drying process, lyoprotectants such as monosaccharides and disaccharides are added before freezing the liposome solution. Lyoprotectants also prevent the leakage of encapsulated drugs from liposomes.[24]

10.3 Barriers and strategies of liposome drug delivery

10.3.1 Reticuloendothelial system and opsonization

The reticuloendothelial system (RES), also known as the mononuclear phagocytic system (MPS), is part of the immune system and its main function includes phagocytosis of foreign particles and abnormal cells.[25,26] MPS cells originate from precursor cells in the bone marrow.[27] Major organs associated with the MPS include the liver, kidney, spleen, and lymph nodes. The liver has the largest capacity for retaining liposomes through phagocytosis by macrophages and kupffer cells.[2] Conventional liposomes face biological challenges, such as MPS clearance. They interact with and bind to plasma proteins via opsonization,[2] promoting phagocytic clearance. To overcome RES through steric stabilization, the surface of liposomes is often modified with amphiphilic polymers such as PEG. After intravenous (IV) administration, small PEGylated stealth liposomes can effectively avoid RES surveillance, leading to prolonged circulation half-life. Liposomes with ~100 nm in diameter are optimal for intratumoral drug delivery.[23] Liposomes can improve the intracellular uptake and effectively deliver therapeutic agents to the target site.

10.3.2 Intracellular trafficking and endosomal escape

The plasma membrane is a significant barrier for cellular entry as depicted in Fig. 10.1. Since both liposomes and cell membranes are composed of phospholipid bilayers, liposomes can bypass drug transporters by membrane fusion or endocytosis.[28,29] For efficient cell-specific uptake, active targeting liposomes are synthesized, and they could efficiently enter the target cells by receptor-mediated endocytosis. Inside the cell, through endocytotic pathways, nanoparticles are entrapped in endosomes and lysosomes where acidic enzymes degrade the nanoparticles and their loaded cargos. Escaping from the endosome to the cytosol is essential for nanoparticles to exert their biological functions intracellularly. A number of mechanisms proposed for endosomal escape are described below.

10.3.2.1 Ion-pair formation (inverted hexagonal phase)

Cationic lipids have been widely used for the fabrication of liposomes for drug and gene delivery. The electrostatic interaction between cationic lipids on liposomes and ionic lipids on the endosome membrane can promote the formation of the inverted hexagonal (H_{II}) phase which is an intermediate structure when two lipid bilayers fuse together.[30–33] Cationic lipids with bulky acyl or alkyl chains are prone to form H_{II} phase and confer improved fusogenicity comparing to lipids with saturated phospholipid tails, which are correlated with the extent of unsaturation of the hydrophobic tail in cationic lipids.[31,34–36] The lipid fusion and ion-pair formation between the liposomal and endosomal membranes destabilize the endosome membrane and further promote de-assembly of the entrapped liposomes, which results in the release of cargos encapsulated within liposomes from the endosome to cytoplasm. The incorporation of fusogenic lipids into liposomes can promote endosomal escape by increasing the lipids' interaction between the liposomal and endosomal membranes.[35–38]

10.3.2.2 pH-buffering effect (proton sponge effect)

The amine groups and histidine structures on lipids or lipoplexes show different pKa values and confer a buffering effect. They are prone to be protonated in acidic endosomes, causing an influx of protons. To balance the ionic concentrations and osmotic pressure, an extensive inflow of chloride ions and water into the endosomal compartment occurs, which subsequently results in the swelling and rupture of the endosomal membrane, releasing the entrapped cargos from the endosome to the cytoplasm.[28] Biomaterials with amine groups and histidine structures have been widely incorporated into liposomes, leading to the disruption of endosomes, and allow the entrapped cargos to be biofunctional intracellularly.[39–42] In addition to the pH-buffering effect of biomaterials, Jun Li et al. designed a lipid calcium phosphate (LCP) nanoparticle containing a drug-loaded calcium phosphate (CaP) microprecipitate coating with an asymmetrical lipid bilayer.[43] The CaP core in an LCP dissolves in acidic endosomes, resulting in the de-assembly of the LCP. The increased ionic concentrations result in an inflow of water into the endosomal compartment, causing endosome swelling. The increased osmotic pressure could disrupt the endosomes, releasing entrapped cargos to the cytoplasm.[44]

10.3.2.3 Fusogenic peptides and proteins

Some peptides, known as cell-penetrating peptides (CPPs), are able to translocate across biological membranes. CPPs can be modified or incorporated in liposomes to promote endosomal escape.[45] Some hydrophobic proteins could destabilize membranes by creating channels and facilitate ion flow across biological membranes.[46] For example, peptides derived from the endodomain of the HIV gp41 envelope glycoprotein and influenza-derived fusogenic peptide dilNF-7 were reported to promote the intracellular trafficking and endosomal release of the entrapped cargos.[47–49]

10.3.3 PEG dilemma and environment-responsive liposomes

The prolonged circulation half-life provided by PEGylation enhances the intratumoral drug delivery through the EPR effect. However, PEGylation inhibits the cellular uptake of liposomes and their interaction with target cells due to the steric hindrance property of the PEG layer. This issue associated with PEGylation is called the "PEG dilemma." Employing strategies to promote PEG shedding from PEGylated liposomes can overcome the issue of the PEG dilemma. To this end, cleavable PEG is designed by covalently conjugating pH or redox sensitive linkers as well as designing specific enzyme and reductase recognition sites on the PEG chains,[50,51] as listed below.

10.3.3.1 pH-responsive liposomes

One of the common ways to overcome the PEG dilemma is to design pH-sensitive detachable linkers on the PEG chains before coating the functional PEG on the liposome surface. The acidic tumor microenvironment can trigger the PEG cleavage and PEG shedding off the liposome surface, which promotes cellular uptake. In the cytosol, pH-sensitive liposomes undergo destabilization at acidic endolysosomal compartments,[52,53] which disrupts endosomes/lysosomes and releases the encapsulated drugs to the cytosol to deliver therapeutic activities. This strategy improved the intracellular drug release and the pharmacological effects of the encapsulated drugs including chemotherapeutic drugs, proteins, and gene molecules.[54] Guan et al. used a PEG aldehyde derivative to react with the amino group of polyethylenimine (PEI)/DNA by the Schiff base reaction. The Schiff base bond is unstable and cleaved off in the acidic environment of the tumor, which allows the particles to effectively uptake inside tumor cells, enhancing the therapeutic efficacy of loaded drugs.[55] Hama et al. developed charge-invertible nanoparticles modified with an acidic pH-sensitive peptide comprised of histidine and glutamic acid residues, resulting in an overall negative charge on the particle surface to avoid enzymatic degradation in systemic circulation. Once they reach the tumor site, the peptide residues get protonated and the charge changes from negative to positive in response to the acidic pH in the intratumoral environment, which facilitates cellular uptake by tumor cells.[56] Other pH-sensitive liposomes can shed off PEG by breaking hydrazone bonds[57] or vinyl ether bonds in acidic tumor tissues,[51,58] promoting cellular uptake of liposomes.

10.3.3.2 Redox-responsive liposomes

The glutathione (GSH) concentration in tumor cells is much higher than extracellular compartments. Concentrations of GSH in blood and extracellular matrices are 2–20 μM; while concentrations of GSH within cancer cells are 2–10 mM which is 100- to 500-fold higher than normal tissues.[59,60] Liposomes responsive to GSH have improved intracellular release of the encapsulated drugs within cancer cells. The commonly used reducible linkers include disulfide bonds, thioether bonds, and diselenide bonds, and triggering the cleavage of disulfide bonds is the most common strategy.[60,61] The great difference in GSH levels between cancer cells and normal tissues serves as an external stimulus for intracellular drug release within cancer cells after cellular uptake of liposomes.

10.3.3.3 Enzyme-responsive liposomes

The drug release of enzyme-sensitive liposomes is triggered by extracellular or intracellular enzymes in the target tissue, and the amount of released drug is often proportional to the concentration of the enzyme at the target site.[62] Yu et al. engineered a nanoparticle that has a targeting middle layer and hydrophobic innermost core encapsulating camptothecin (CPT) by mixing a matrix metalloproteinase MMP2- and MMP9-sensitive copolymers and folate receptor–targeted copolymers. The PEG layer could detach from the particle surface by the extracellular MMP2 and MMP9 in tumors. The folate ligand was then exposed on the particle surface, which improves the cellular internalization of CPT via folate receptor–mediated endocytosis. This nanoparticle increased the CPT accumulation in the tumor site and suppressed the tumor growth.[63] To promote cellular uptake and endosomal escape, Hatakeyama and coworkers designed a multifunctional envelope-type nanodevice (MEND) for nucleic acid delivery.[64–67] A fusogenic PEG-peptide-DOPE (PPD) construct and a pH-sensitive fusogenic GALA peptide were incorporated in the lipid layer.[65] The peptide sequence in the PPD construct can be cleaved by matrix metalloproteinases in the tumor extracellular matrix, enhancing the intracellular delivery to tumor cells, and the GALA peptide could further promote endosomal escape.[64,65]

10.3.3.4 Thermosensitive liposomes

Tumor tissues have relatively higher temperature than the normal body. Thermosensitive liposomes are stable at body temperature (37°C), and they are often used to treat cancers upon the temperature elevation at the disease site.[68] In combination with radiofrequency ablation (RFA), the thermosensitive liposomal formulation ThermoDox (Celsion, Lawrenceville, NJ, USA) rapidly changes structure when heated to 40–45°C, creating openings in the liposome, followed by releasing doxorubicin directly into the targeted tumor and around the tumor margin. ThermoDox contains MSPC phospholipid (1-myristoyl-2-stearoyl-sn-glycero-3-phosphocholine) with a transition temperature of 40°C.[69] This treatment (the OPTIMA Study) is currently in Phase III clinical trials for primary liver cancer.

10.4 Targeting ligands and coupling strategies

Due to the steric hindrance and biologically inert properties, PEGylated liposomes have limited binding affinity to cells, which compromises their cellular uptake and intracellular delivery. The tissue distribution and cell-type-specific uptake of PEGylated liposomes can be modulated by conjugating appropriate targeting ligands on the surface of nanoparticles. Targeting ligands can be monoclonal antibodies, proteins, peptides, aptamers, and small molecules, binding to proteins or receptors overexpressing on the cell surface. The efficiency of cellular uptake depends on the expression level of the corresponding proteins or receptors. For brain delivery nanoparticles, some biologically active ligands are anchored on the liposome surface, which lead to the absorptive-mediated or receptor-mediated transcytosis through the brain endothelial cells and facilitates the liposome transport across the blood–brain barrier (BBB).[70,71] The BBB prevents blood from flowing in the cerebral parenchyma, which limits the transport of therapeutic agents into the brain.[72] The surface of PEGylated liposomes is conjugated with specific monoclonal antibody (mAb) targeting a receptor of brain endothelial cells on the BBB, known as Trojan horse liposomes (THLs) or immunoliposomes.[73,74]

Different ligand's density on the liposome surface results in different binding affinity to the target cells. Optimizing and tailoring the ligand density can ensure the best targeting efficiency and cellular internalization, as well as prevent stability issues such as aggregation which may be caused by increasing the ligand density beyond an optimal level.[68,75]

Liposomes are functionalized with various targeting ligands mainly through the following reactions: (1) formation of amide bond by reacting carboxyl and amino groups; (2) formation of disulfide bond by oxidation of thiol groups; and (3) formation of thioether bond by reacting maleimide and thiol groups.[68] Some typical ligand-conjugated liposomes are described below.

10.4.1 Antibody-conjugated liposomes

Antibodies or their fragments such as fragment antigen-binding (Fab') and single-chain variable fragment (scFv) can be conjugated to the liposome's surface to generate immunoliposomes through the covalent coupling to the modified PEG termini distal.[76] The Fc region of mAbs is prone to bind to Fc receptors on macrophages and other cells, which results in the uptake of mAb-modified nanoparticles by phagocytes and their fast clearance from circulation. To prevent the Fc receptor–mediated phagocytosis of immunoliposomes, the Fc portion of mAbs can be enzymatically cleaved and the Fab portion is isolated for surface modification on liposomes. The disulfide bond in the hinge region on Fab portion is reduced to expose the free thiol group before coupling on the liposome surface through thiol–maleimide conjugation chemistry.[77]

10.4.2 Peptide-conjugated liposomes

Peptides can be conjugated to liposomes through a variety of covalent linkages, such as maleimide linkage, peptide bond, sulfanyl bond, disulfide bond, and thioester linkage.[68,78] Two categories of peptides can be used for surface functionalization of liposomes, including nonspecific CPPs and receptor-specific cell-targeting peptide.[79] The peptide-targeted liposomes demonstrated enhanced cellular uptake in target cells and superior therapeutic efficacy compared to nontargeted liposomes.[80–82] It is reported that a 4% CPP to lipid ratio displayed the optimal cellular internalization efficiency of the liposomes.[83]

10.4.3 Aptamer-conjugated liposomes

Aptamers are short single-stranded RNA or DNA oligonucleotides capable of targeting certain receptors. Aptamers are evolved from systemic evolution of a ligand by exponential enrichment (SELEX) technology, and the resulting aptamers have high binding affinity to target molecules.[84–86] Anti-PSMA (prostate-specific membrane antigen) aptamer–modified liposomes were developed to enhance binding to prostate cancer cells overexpressing PSMA, leading to the reduction in tumor size compared to nontargeted liposomes.[87–89]

10.4.4 Small molecule–conjugated liposomes

Small molecules with high binding affinity to cell surface receptors can be functionalized to the surface of liposomes to improve their tissue-/cell-targeting specificity. The folate-directed liposomes have been formulated to deliver a variety of therapeutics for cancer treatment, since many cancer cells overexpress folate receptors.[90–96] Anisamide is a small molecule ligand that has a high binding affinity to sigma receptors overexpressing in many cancer cell lines. A portion of DSPE-PEG in PEGylated liposomes was replaced by DSPE-PEG-anisamide to specifically target to sigma receptors on cancer cells, for enhanced antitumor efficacy of many therapeutic cargos.[43,97–99]

10.5 Conclusion

The use of liposomes as nanocarriers to assist drug and gene delivery has a great impact on biomedical research and drug development. A wide range of therapeutic compounds can be efficiently loaded in liposomes, with improved targeting efficiency, pharmacokinetic profile, and biodistribution of the loaded compounds as well as reduced side effects. Liposomes can be synthesized by a variety of biocompatible and biodegradable lipids and functionalized with different kinds of targeting molecules to direct the tissue targeting and intracellular delivery. In addition, many cationic lipids, polymers, or peptides can be incorporated in the liposomal bilayers to enhance the endosomal escape capability, which allows the release of the entrapped drug molecules into the cytoplasm to deliver their therapeutic activities. In order to enhance the intracellular uptake of liposomes while rendering them prolonged circulation half-life, PEGylated liposomes in response to intracellular or extracellular stimuli are created by incorporating cleavable PEGylated lipids. The advance of liposomal technology is expected to address many translational limitations and clinical development in the drug discovery process.

References

1. Zhang Y, Satterlee A, Huang L. In vivo gene delivery by nonviral vectors: overcoming hurdles? *Mol Ther* 2012;**20**:1298–304.
2. Sercombe L, et al. Advances and challenges of liposome assisted drug delivery. *Front Pharmacol* 2015;**6**:286.
3. Zylberberg C, Matosevic S. Pharmaceutical liposomal drug delivery: a review of new delivery systems and a look at the regulatory landscape. *Drug Deliv* 2016;**23**:3319–29.
4. Martins S, Sarmento B, Ferreira DC, Souto EB. Lipid-based colloidal carriers for peptide and protein delivery–liposomes versus lipid nanoparticles. *Int J Nanomed* 2007;**2**:595–607.
5. Malam Y, Loizidou M, Seifalian AM. Liposomes and nanoparticles: nanosized vehicles for drug delivery in cancer. *Trends Pharmacol Sci* 2009;**30**:592–9.
6. Chang HI, Yeh MK. Clinical development of liposome-based drugs: formulation, characterization, and therapeutic efficacy. *Int J Nanomed* 2012;**7**:49–60.
7. Li J, et al. Photoinduced PEG deshielding from ROS-sensitive linkage-bridged block copolymer-based nanocarriers for on-demand drug delivery. *Biomaterials* 2018;**170**:147–55.
8. Miller CR, Bondurant B, McLean SD, McGovern KA, O'Brien DF. Liposome-cell interactions in vitro: effect of liposome surface charge on the binding and endocytosis of conventional and sterically stabilized liposomes. *Biochemistry* 1998;**37**:12875–83.
9. Willis M, Forssen E. Ligand-targeted liposomes. *Adv Drug Deliv Rev* 1998;**29**:249–71.
10. Klibanov AL, Maruyama K, Beckerleg AM, Torchilin VP, Huang L. Activity of amphipathic poly(ethylene glycol) 5000 to prolong the circulation time of liposomes depends on the liposome size and is unfavorable for immunoliposome binding to target. *Biochim Biophys Acta* 1991;**1062**:142–8.
11. Hatakeyama H, Akita H, Harashima H. The polyethyleneglycol dilemma: advantage and disadvantage of PEGylation of liposomes for systemic genes and nucleic acids delivery to tumors. *Biol Pharm Bull* 2013;**36**:892–9.
12. Schnyder A, Huwyler J. Drug transport to brain with targeted liposomes. *NeuroRx* 2005;**2**:99–107.
13. Allen TM. Long-circulating (sterically stabilized) liposomes for targeted drug delivery. *Trends Pharmacol Sci* 1994;**15**:215–20.
14. Bozzuto G, Molinari A. Liposomes as nanomedical devices. *Int J Nanomed* 2015;**10**:975–99.
15. Enoch HG, Strittmatter P. Formation and properties of 1000-A-diameter, single-bilayer phospholipid vesicles. *Proc Natl Acad Sci USA* 1979;**76**:145–9.
16. Ming-Ren Toh GNCC. Liposomes as sterile preparations and limitations of sterilisation techniques in liposomal manufacturing. *Asian J Pharm Sci* 2013;**8**:88–95.
17. Akbarzadeh A, et al. Liposome: classification, preparation, and applications. *Nanoscale Res Lett* 2013;**8**:102.
18. Patil YP, Jadhav S. Novel methods for liposome preparation. *Chem Phys Lipids* 2014;**177**:8–18.
19. Hood RR, DeVoe DL. High-throughput continuous flow production of nanoscale liposomes by microfluidic vertical flow focusing. *Small* 2015;**11**:5790–9.
20. Briuglia ML, Rotella C, McFarlane A, Lamprou DA. Influence of cholesterol on liposome stability and on in vitro drug release. *Drug Deliv Transl Res* 2015;**5**:231–42.
21. Kumari A, Yadav SK, Yadav SC. Biodegradable polymeric nanoparticles based drug delivery systems. *Colloids Surfaces B Biointerfaces* 2010;**75**:1–18.
22. Li B, et al. Lyophilization of cationic lipid-protamine-DNA (LPD) complexes. *J Pharm Sci* 2000;**89**:355–64.
23. Pattni BS, Chupin VV, Torchilin VP. New developments in liposomal drug delivery. *Chem Rev* 2015;**115**:10938–66.
24. Yoshimoto M. Stabilization of enzymes through encapsulation in liposomes. *Methods Mol Biol* 2017;**1504**:9–18.
25. Baas J, Senninger N, Elser H. [The reticuloendothelial system. An overview of function, pathology and recent methods of measurement]. *Z Gastroenterol* 1994;**32**:117–23.
26. Pascal M, Lavoie OL. Mononuclear phagocyte system- overview of the mononuclear phagocyte system. *Fetal Neonatal Physiol* 2017.
27. Albegger KW. Sturcture and function of the mononuclear phagocytic system (MPS) in chronic rhinosinusitis. A light and electron microscopic investigation (author's transl). *Arch Oto-Rhino-Laryngol* 1976;**214**:27–48.
28. Varkouhi AK, Scholte M, Storm G, Haisma HJ. Endosomal escape pathways for delivery of biologicals. *J Control Release* 2011;**151**:220–8.
29. Pollock S, et al. Uptake and trafficking of liposomes to the endoplasmic reticulum. *FASEB J* 2010;**24**:1866–78.
30. Xu Y, Szoka Jr FC. Mechanism of DNA release from cationic liposome/DNA complexes used in cell transfection. *Biochemistry* 1996;**35**:5616–23.
31. Hafez IM, Maurer N, Cullis PR. On the mechanism whereby cationic lipids promote intracellular delivery of polynucleic acids. *Gene Ther* 2001;**8**:1188–96.
32. Hafez IM, Cullis PR. Roles of lipid polymorphism in intracellular delivery. *Adv Drug Deliv Rev* 2001;**47**:139–48.
33. Ewert KK, Ahmad A, Evans HM, Safinya CR. Cationic lipid-DNA complexes for non-viral gene therapy: relating supramolecular structures to cellular pathways. *Expert Opin Biol Ther* 2005;**5**:33–53.
34. Tseng YC, Mozumdar S, Huang L. Lipid-based systemic delivery of siRNA. *Adv Drug Deliv Rev* 2009;**61**:721–31.
35. Heyes J, Palmer L, Bremner K, MacLachlan I. Cationic lipid saturation influences intracellular delivery of encapsulated nucleic acids. *J Control Release* 2005;**107**:276–87.
36. Dominska M, Dykxhoorn DM. Breaking down the barriers: siRNA delivery and endosome escape. *J Cell Sci* 2010;**123**:1183–9.
37. Farhood H, Serbina N, Huang L. The role of dioleoyl phosphatidylethanolamine in cationic liposome mediated gene transfer. *Biochim Biophys Acta* 1995;**1235**:289–95.
38. Litzinger DC, Huang L. Phosphatidylethanolamine liposomes: drug delivery, gene transfer and immunodiagnostic applications. *Biochim Biophys Acta* 1992;**1113**:201–27.
39. Miller DK, Griffiths E, Lenard J, Firestone RA. Cell killing by lysosomotropic detergents. *J Cell Biol* 1983;**97**:1841–51.

40. Pack DW, Putnam D, Langer R. Design of imidazole-containing endosomolytic biopolymers for gene delivery. *Biotechnol Bioeng* 2000;**67**:217–23.
41. Moreira C, et al. Improving chitosan-mediated gene transfer by the introduction of intracellular buffering moieties into the chitosan backbone. *Acta Biomater* 2009;**5**:2995–3006.
42. Lin C, Engbersen JF. Effect of chemical functionalities in poly(amido amine)s for non-viral gene transfection. *J Control Release* 2008;**132**:267–72.
43. Li J, Yang Y, Huang L. Calcium phosphate nanoparticles with an asymmetric lipid bilayer coating for siRNA delivery to the tumor. *J Control Release* 2012;**158**:108–14.
44. Li J, Chen YC, Tseng YC, Mozumdar S, Huang L. Biodegradable calcium phosphate nanoparticle with lipid coating for systemic siRNA delivery. *J Control Release* 2010;**142**:416–21.
45. Endoh T, Ohtsuki T. Cellular siRNA delivery using cell-penetrating peptides modified for endosomal escape. *Adv Drug Deliv Rev* 2009;**61**:704–9.
46. Gonzalez ME, Carrasco L. Viroporins. *FEBS Lett* 2003;**552**:28–34.
47. Costin JM, Rausch JM, Garry RF, Wimley WC. Viroporin potential of the lentivirus lytic peptide (LLP) domains of the HIV-1 gp41 protein. *Virol J* 2007;**4**:123.
48. Kwon EJ, Bergen JM, Pun SH. Application of an HIV gp41-derived peptide for enhanced intracellular trafficking of synthetic gene and siRNA delivery vehicles. *Bioconjug Chem* 2008;**19**:920–7.
49. Oliveira S, van Rooy I, Kranenburg O, Storm G, Schiffelers RM. Fusogenic peptides enhance endosomal escape improving siRNA-induced silencing of oncogenes. *Int J Pharm* 2007;**331**:211–4.
50. Xing H, et al. Multimodal detection of a small molecule target using stimuli-responsive liposome triggered by aptamer-enzyme conjugate. *Anal Chem* 2016;**88**:1506–10.
51. Fang Y, et al. Cleavable PEGylation: a strategy for overcoming the "PEG dilemma" in efficient drug delivery. *Drug Deliv* 2017;**24**:22–32.
52. Xu H, Paxton JW, Wu Z. Development of long-circulating pH-sensitive liposomes to circumvent gemcitabine resistance in pancreatic cancer cells. *Pharm Res* 2016;**33**:1628–37.
53. Xu H, et al. Design and evaluation of pH-sensitive liposomes constructed by poly(2-ethyl-2-oxazoline)-cholesterol hemisuccinate for doxorubicin delivery. *Eur J Pharm Biopharm* 2015;**91**:66–74.
54. Paliwal SR, Paliwal R, Vyas SP. A review of mechanistic insight and application of pH-sensitive liposomes in drug delivery. *Drug Deliv* 2015;**22**:231–42.
55. Guan X, et al. A pH-responsive detachable PEG shielding strategy for gene delivery system in cancer therapy. *Biomacromolecules* 2017;**18**:1342–9.
56. Hama S, et al. Overcoming the polyethylene glycol dilemma via pathological environment-sensitive change of the surface property of nanoparticles for cellular entry. *J Control Release* 2015;**206**:67–74.
57. Kanamala M, Palmer BD, Ghandehari H, Wilson WR, Wu Z. PEG-Benzaldehyde-Hydrazone-Lipid based PEG-sheddable pH-sensitive liposomes: abilities for endosomal escape and long circulation. *Pharm Res* 2018;**35**:154.
58. Zununi Vahed S, Salehi R, Davaran S, Sharifi S. Liposome-based drug co-delivery systems in cancer cells. *Mater Sci Eng C Mater Biol Appl* 2017;**71**:1327–41.
59. Torchilin VP. Multifunctional, stimuli-sensitive nanoparticulate systems for drug delivery. *Nat Rev Drug Discov* 2014;**13**:813–27.
60. Liu D, Yang F, Xiong F, Gu N. The smart drug delivery system and its clinical potential. *Theranostics* 2016;**6**:1306–23.
61. Zhou L, Wang H, Li Y. Stimuli-responsive nanomedicines for overcoming cancer multidrug resistance. *Theranostics* 2018;**8**:1059–74.
62. Fouladi F, Steffen KJ, Mallik S. Enzyme-responsive liposomes for the delivery of anticancer drugs. *Bioconjug Chem* 2017;**28**:857–68.
63. Yu H, et al. Enzyme sensitive, surface engineered nanoparticles for enhanced delivery of camptothecin. *J Control Release* 2015;**216**:111–20.
64. Hatakeyama H, et al. Development of a novel systemic gene delivery system for cancer therapy with a tumor-specific cleavable PEG-lipid. *Gene Ther* 2007;**14**:68–77.
65. Hatakeyama H, et al. A pH-sensitive fusogenic peptide facilitates endosomal escape and greatly enhances the gene silencing of siRNA-containing nanoparticles in vitro and in vivo. *J Control Release* 2009;**139**:127–32.
66. Kogure K, Akita H, Harashima H. Multifunctional envelope-type nano device for non-viral gene delivery: concept and application of programmed packaging. *J Control Release* 2007;**122**:246–51.
67. Kogure K, et al. Development of a non-viral multifunctional envelope-type nano device by a novel lipid film hydration method. *J Control Release* 2004;**98**:317–23.
68. Riaz MK, et al. Surface functionalization and targeting strategies of liposomes in solid tumor therapy: a review. *Int J Mol Sci* 2018;**19**.
69. Needham D, Park JY, Wright AM, Tong J. Materials characterization of the low temperature sensitive liposome (LTSL): effects of the lipid composition (lysolipid and DSPE-PEG2000) on the thermal transition and release of doxorubicin. *Faraday Discuss* 2013;**161**:515–34. discussion 563-589.
70. Wu D, Yang J, Pardridge WM. Drug targeting of a peptide radiopharmaceutical through the primate blood-brain barrier in vivo with a monoclonal antibody to the human insulin receptor. *J Clin Investig* 1997;**100**:1804–12.
71. Vieira DB, Gamarra LF. Getting into the brain: liposome-based strategies for effective drug delivery across the blood-brain barrier. *Int J Nanomed* 2016;**11**:5381–414.
72. Lai F, Fadda AM, Sinico C. Liposomes for brain delivery. *Expert Opin Drug Deliv* 2013;**10**:1003–22.
73. Pardridge WM. Preparation of Trojan horse liposomes (THLs) for gene transfer across the blood-brain barrier. *Cold Spring Harb Protoc* 2010;**2010**. pdb prot5407.
74. Pardridge WM. Blood-brain barrier delivery of protein and non-viral gene therapeutics with molecular Trojan horses. *J Control Release* 2007;**122**:345–8.
75. Feng L, Mumper RJ. A critical review of lipid-based nanoparticles for taxane delivery. *Cancer Lett* 2013;**334**:157–75.
76. Cheng WW, Allen TM. The use of single chain Fv as targeting agents for immunoliposomes: an update on immunoliposomal drugs for cancer treatment. *Expert Opin Drug Deliv* 2010;**7**:461–78.
77. Zhang Y, Li N, Suh H, Irvine DJ. Nanoparticle anchoring targets immune agonists to tumors enabling anti-cancer immunity without systemic toxicity. *Nat Commun* 2018;**9**(6).
78. Koren E, Torchilin VP. Cell-penetrating peptides: breaking through to the other side. *Trends Mol Med* 2012;**18**:385–93.
79. Dissanayake S, Denny WA, Gamage S, Sarojini V. Recent developments in anticancer drug delivery using cell penetrating and tumor targeting peptides. *J Control Release* 2017;**250**:62–76.

80. Chen Z, Deng J, Zhao Y, Tao T. Cyclic RGD peptide-modified liposomal drug delivery system: enhanced cellular uptake in vitro and improved pharmacokinetics in rats. *Int J Nanomed* 2012;**7**:3803–11.
81. Zhang X, et al. Liposomes equipped with cell penetrating peptide BR2 enhances chemotherapeutic effects of cantharidin against hepatocellular carcinoma. *Drug Deliv* 2017;**24**:986–98.
82. Wu H, Yao L, Mei J, Li F. Development of synthetic of peptide-functionalized liposome for enhanced targeted ovarian carcinoma therapy. *Int J Clin Exp Pathol* 2015;**8**:207–16.
83. Ding Y, et al. An efficient PEGylated liposomal nanocarrier containing cell-penetrating peptide and pH-sensitive hydrazone bond for enhancing tumor-targeted drug delivery. *Int J Nanomed* 2015;**10**:6199–214.
84. Darmostuk M, Rimpelova S, Gbelcova H, Ruml T. Current approaches in SELEX: an update to aptamer selection technology. *Biotechnol Adv* 2015;**33**:1141–61.
85. Moosavian SA, Abnous K, Badiee A, Jaafari MR. Improvement in the drug delivery and anti-tumor efficacy of PEGylated liposomal doxorubicin by targeting RNA aptamers in mice bearing breast tumor model. *Colloids Surfaces B Biointerfaces* 2016;**139**:228–36.
86. Powell D, et al. Aptamer-functionalized hybrid nanoparticle for the treatment of breast cancer. *Eur J Pharm Biopharm* 2017;**114**:108–18.
87. Baek SE, et al. RNA aptamer-conjugated liposome as an efficient anticancer drug delivery vehicle targeting cancer cells in vivo. *J Control Release* 2014;**196**:234–42.
88. Catuogno S, Esposito CL, de Franciscis V. Aptamer-mediated targeted delivery of therapeutics: an update. *Pharmaceuticals* 2016;**9**.
89. Stuart CH, et al. Prostate-specific membrane antigen-targeted liposomes specifically deliver the Zn(2+) chelator TPEN inducing oxidative stress in prostate cancer cells. *Nanomedicine* 2016;**11**:1207–22.
90. Sriraman SK, Salzano G, Sarisozen C, Torchilin V. Anti-cancer activity of doxorubicin-loaded liposomes co-modified with transferrin and folic acid. *Eur J Pharm Biopharm* 2016;**105**:40–9.
91. Moghimipour E, et al. Folic acid-modified liposomal drug delivery strategy for tumor targeting of 5-fluorouracil. *Eur J Pharm Sci* 2018;**114**:166–74.
92. Chaudhury A, Das S. Folate receptor targeted liposomes encapsulating anti-cancer drugs. *Curr Pharmaceut Biotechnol* 2015;**16**:333–43.
93. Gupta Y, Jain A, Jain P, Jain SK. Design and development of folate appended liposomes for enhanced delivery of 5-FU to tumor cells. *J Drug Target* 2007;**15**:231–40.
94. Yamada A, et al. Design of folate-linked liposomal doxorubicin to its antitumor effect in mice. *Clin Cancer Res* 2008;**14**:8161–8.
95. Lohade AA, et al. A novel folate-targeted nanoliposomal system of doxorubicin for cancer targeting. *AAPS PharmSciTech* 2016;**17**:1298–311.
96. Lee RJ, Low PS. Delivery of liposomes into cultured KB cells via folate receptor-mediated endocytosis. *J Biol Chem* 1994;**269**:3198–204.
97. Zhang Y, Kim WY, Huang L. Systemic delivery of gemcitabine triphosphate via LCP nanoparticles for NSCLC and pancreatic cancer therapy. *Biomaterials* 2013;**34**:3447–58.
98. Chen Y, Bathula SR, Yang Q, Huang L. Targeted nanoparticles deliver siRNA to melanoma. *J Investig Dermatol* 2010;**130**:2790–8.
99. Li SD, Chen YC, Hackett MJ, Huang L. Tumor-targeted delivery of siRNA by self-assembled nanoparticles. *Mol Ther* 2008;**16**:163–9.

Chapter 11

Virus like particles: fundamental concepts, biological interactions, and clinical applications

Candace Benjamin*, Olivia Brohlin*, Arezoo Shahrivarkevishahi and Jeremiah J. Gassensmith

Department of Chemistry and Biochemistry, University of Texas at Dallas, Richardson, Texas, United States

11.1 Introduction

Nanotechnology has offered hopes for the delivery of new technologies in medicine and drug delivery, yet a growing number of voices have begun to express skepticism[1] that these long sought advances may have been over promised.[2] Specifically, issues with targeting and delivering payloads have been called out as being difficult obstacles that still need to be overcome.[3] The reasons for these shortcomings are multiple and linked to issues with biocompatibility,[4] bioaccumulation,[5] and pharmacokinetics,[6,7] all of which can be addressed through clever materials chemistry and bioengineering. The present and persistent issue in nanotech, we must remember, is the "tech" and not the "nano." Nature has very effectively employed nanoscale delivery vehicles for highly selective and targeted gene delivery in the form of viruses. Indeed, their efficacy in delivering sickness to people has created some skepticism to their use, but recent efforts to chemically and biologically engineer "virus-like particles" (VLPs) that take structural cues from these natural nanoparticles have begun to yield important new medicines. For instance, one oncolytic viral nanoparticle[8,9] has made it to the clinic[10–12] and is saving lives,[10,13–15] but many more are in the FDA's approval pipeline and even more are active targets of research for delivery, imaging, stimulation, and biosensing applications.

Viral capsids are extremely useful for these applications as they are easy to produce and straightforward to employ. This is simply owing to the biological nature of the VLP, which imbues five major aspects that define the capsids' value in these fields: (1) ease of production, (2) ability to self-assemble, (3) facile modification, (4) biocompatibility, and (5) immunogenicity. To date, more than 30 different VLPs have been generated[71] through the removal and replacement of the natural viral genome with a modified set of genetic material. These "stripped down" versions spontaneously assemble in noninfectious[72,73] analogs of their viral parents that lack an ability to self-proliferate while preserving many of the other native viral traits. VLPs, typically 15–400 nm,[74] can be replicated and purified from many heterologous expression systems such as bacteria, plants, and yeast[75] to produce ready-to-use nanoparticles for further modification. These methods of replication allow for the scalable production of uniform VLPs with a narrow size distribution, which is crucial for medical applications. These characteristics permit more precise loading of cargos inside of the carrier and regularly spaced functional handles, most commonly lysines, tyrosines, glutamates, aspartates, and cysteines for the development of a multifunctional nanocarrier (Table 11.1). Multiple conjugates can also be attached as a cargo to VLPs, thanks to the multivalency of these subunits that make up the virus including bimodal imaging agents,[76] targeted biosensors,[77,78] and shielded drug carriers.[79,80] Biodistribution studies have been performed using a few of the icosahedral VLPs, which show the particles mostly accumulate in the liver and spleen[81,82] and are usually cleared within 24 h.[83] These carriers can be further modified to help determine their in vivo fate by installing moieties designed to alter the surface charge of the particle[84,85] or stealth capability[86–88]

* These authors contributed equally to this manuscript.

Nanoparticles for Biomedical Applications. https://doi.org/10.1016/B978-0-12-816662-8.00011-4

TABLE 11.1 Examples of bioconjugation reactions on popular virus-like particles.

	Residue	Chemical reaction	Incorporated material
MS2			
	Y85	Diazotization	Diazonium salt,[16] FAM-SE,[17] [^{18}F]-benzaldehyde,[18] Gd(III) complex[19]
		Potassium ferricyanide–mediated oxidative coupling	Gold NPs[20]
	T19pAF	$NaIO_4$-mediated oxidative coupling	AF 488,[21] DNA,[21] DNA aptamers,[22] fibrin,[23] peptides,[24] PEG,[25] porphyrin[26]
		Photolysis/coupling with aniline groups	DNA[27]
	N87C	Thiol-maleimide	AF 488,[22] AF 680,[23] DOTA,[25] AF 350,[26] Oregon Green 488,[26] Gd(III) complex,[28] Taxol[29]
	K106, K113, N-terminus	Isothiocyanate coupling	PEG[17] TREN-bis-HOPO-TAM ligand[19]
TMV			
	Y139	Diazotization and oximation	Diazonium salts and alkoxyamines[30]
		Iodogen method	$Na^{125}I$[31]
		Diazotization/CuAAC	Gd(DOTA),[32,33] Tn antigen,[34] pyrene PEG,[35] RGD peptide,[36] β-cyclodextrin,[37] oligoaniline[38]
	E97, E106	Amide formation/CuAAC	PEG[32]
		Amide formation	Amines[30]
	S123C	Maleimide coupling/CuAAC	Maleimide derivatives of alkynes followed by azido bearing Tn antigen,[34] maleimide derivatives of thiol-reactive chromophores[39,40]
	PAG (S123C mutant)	Potassium ferricyanide–mediated oxidative coupling	*o*-aminophenols or o-catechols[41]

Qβ			
	K2, K13, K16, N-terminus	Acylation/CuAAC	Tn antigen,[42] bovine serum albumin,[43] fluorescein,[43] triple-sulfated ligand,[44] AF 488,[45] AF 568,[46] human holo-transferrin,[46] poly(2-oxazoline),[47] PEG-C_{60},[48] oligomannosides,[49] LacNAc,[50] BPC sialic acid,[50] Gd(DOTA)[51]
	M16HPG	CuAAC	Oligomannosides[49]
	T93AHA	CuAAC	RGD-PEG,[52] biotin[52]
P22			
	S39C	EDC/NHS	Mn porphyrin[53]
		ATRP	AEMA[54]
	K118C	ATRP	THMMA[54]
		Thiol-maleimide	Bortezomib[55]
		CUAAC	DTPA-Gd[56]
	T183C, M338C, C-terminus	Thiol	MIANS,[57] HIV-TAT CPP,[58] mCherry[59]
CPMV			
	K34, K38, K82, K99, K199	CUAAC	Peptides,[60,61] folic acid,[62] fluorescein-PEG,[63,64] transferrin,[63] GD-DOTA[65]
		EDC/NHS	OG 488,[61] AF 568,[61] AF 555,[61] AF647,[66,67] PEG,[66,67] ferrocene,[68] peptides[69]
	R82C, A141/163C	Thiol-maleimide	Proteins[70]

AEMA, Aminoethyl methacrylate; *AF*, Alexa Fluor; *CuAAC*, copper-catalyzed azide alkyne 1,3-dipolar cycloaddition; *MIANS*, 2-(4′-maleimidylanilino) naphthalene-6-sulfonic acid; *PEG*, Poly(ethylene glycol); *RGD*, arginyl-glycyl-aspartyl; *THMMA*, tris(hydroxymethyl)methylacrylamide.

as a means of controlling uptake. This ability to further functionalize VLPs allows researchers to go one step further than simply improving capsid stability through the use of groups like polyethylene glycol (PEG); it allows the design of smarter delivery vessels that can be targeted to specific cell types[89,90] or introduce stimuli responsive release.[91,92] Recently, more focus has been placed on understanding the immunogenicity[42,93–95] of these particles and employing them to treat aggressive diseases.[14,15] Their application as vaccines is plausible considering their small size and ability to illicit an immune response via their repetitive epitope display[95] that also shows promise as an innate adjuvant. With these characteristics in mind, this chapter highlights the advantages VLPs offer to biomedical applications. Each of the aforementioned characteristics affords VLPs the ability to overcome limitations associated with current state-of-the-art technologies. Because most research has been focused on developing VLPs for imaging, sensing, and drug delivery applications, overviews of these areas will be presented to demonstrate the characteristics of VLPs that provide specific advantages over traditional systems. It is worth mentioning that VLPs are relatively easy for the nonbiologist to produce and require only a small investment in equipment. A number of detailed protocols, including video protocols, exist and are worth reviewing.[96–99]

11.2 Imaging applications

VLPs are biocompatible macromolecules that bring many advantages to imaging applications. The monodisperse and multivalent coat proteins that make up the VLP contain repeating functional handles from lysine, cysteine, aspartate, glutamate, and tyrosine residues that can be used in bioconjugation reactions to attach imaging agents to the virus.[100] The monodispersity of the coat proteins allows for uniformly spaced attachment of many imaging agents to each VLP for improved resolution.[101] Furthermore, the multivalency of the coat proteins allows for the utilization of a second functional handle that can be used to attach a targeting ligand orthogonally for improved localization of the imaging agent in a desired region of the body.[80] In certain contexts, these attributes make VLPs attractive alternatives to hard nanoparticles, which tend to bioaccumulate and have limited surface chemistry for functionalization.[102] They also offer atomistically precise surfaces for functionalization in contrast to polymeric systems, which are polydisperse and have spatially disordered functional handles. The proteinaceous makeup of the VLP can help make conjugated synthetic and inorganic imaging agents more biocompatible improving the ability of these agents to translate into *in vitro* and *in vivo* studies.[103] Additionally, VLPs come in different shapes and sizes that can be selected for longer retention times which allow for higher accumulation in the desired area and can extend imaging time.[103] For instance, isotropic VLPs can endure longer circulation times, whereas anisotropic VLPs can avoid phagocytosis by macrophages. Additionally, larger VLPs have been shown to accumulate in tumors because of the enhanced permeation and retention (EPR) effect. These characteristics make VLPs good candidates for next-generation imaging applications.

In this section, we will highlight VLP-based imaging platforms focusing on fluorescence and magnetic resonance imaging (MRI). These two areas of imaging specifically have drawn the interest of many research groups who work with VLPs. Through their work, they have been able to increase the brightness and localization of fluorescent probes as well as increase the relaxivity rates of commonly used lanthanide-based contrast agents. A few examples of these advances in imaging technology are discussed in the following section.

11.2.1 Fluorescent and optical probes

One of the earliest applications of VLPs in biotechnology was to use them as fluorescent nanoparticles for cell imaging. By attaching fluorescent dyes to the multivalent surface of a VLP, the local density of the small molecule fluorophores creates brighter imaging agents for higher-resolution imaging.[100] Furthermore, by reacting at specific sites on the protein that are physically separated in space, collisional quenching between adjacent fluorophores can be avoided, thereby improving the brightness of the nanoparticle. Small molecules can be conjugated to VLPs through a variety of high-yielding bioconjugation reactions.[100] For instance, EDC/NHS chemistry can be used to attach small molecules to lysine residues, diazonium coupling for tyrosine residues, carbodiimide chemistry for glutamate residues, and maleimides for cysteine residues.[104] More recently, "rebridging reactions" on VLPs have made the disulfide bridge an amenable functional handle.[105]

Some of the first work done on creating fluorescent VLPs for *in vitro* imaging applications came out of the Manchester group. Lewis et al. attached[106] 120 Alexa Fluor 555 molecules to each CPMV (cowpea mosaic virus) without any self-quenching of the fluorophores. This conjugate was determined to be much brighter compared with conventional imaging agents made from polystyrene nanospheres carrying the same dye—demonstrating a practical benefit over polymeric systems. Because the multivalency of the VLP coat proteins allow for the attachment of a dye to one functional handle and a targeting ligand to another,[107] it is possible to make bright targeted probes using two-relatively straightforward chemical reactions. For example, Carrico et al. demonstrated[108] that

M13 phage could be modified with both Alexa Fluor 488 and antibody fragments to epidermal growth factor receptor (EGFR) or human epidermal growth factor receptor 2 (HER2) to target imaging of breast cancer cells for diagnostic applications (Fig. 11.1). *In vitro* studies demonstrated the selective uptake of the targeted VLPs in cells expressing EGFR or HER2 by flow cytometry as well as localized fluorescence of the VLP conjugate in these cells by confocal microscopy. This works provides a very strong example of how targeted VLPs can be used in high-resolution fluorescence imaging.

VLPs come in different shapes, sizes, and charges that can be selected for and employed as a targeting function for the imaging agent. For instance, positively charged VLPs encourage cell uptake;[69] larger VLPs are more likely to accumulate in tumors due to the EPR effect,[109] and elongated VLPs avoid phagocytosis by macrophages.[110] Bruckman et al. utilized[32] the elongated rod shape of the plant viral nanoparticle, tobacco mosaic virus (TMV), to target vascular cell adhesion molecule (VCAM)-1 for imaging of atherosclerosis. The elongated shape (300×18 nm) of the VLP enhances the ability of the nanoparticle to bind to the flat walls of the arteries displaying VCAM-1.

As this technology matures, new chemistries are demanded to increase the number of fluorophores and conjugate handles for targeting ligands to help increase the scope and utility of VLPs. For instance, recent work from Chen et al. established[105] a high-yielding method to conjugate a variety of dibromomaleimide handles to the disulfide bonds that bridge the pores of the VLP Qβ. Disulfides are typically structurally vital to protein tertiary structure, but Chen's approach effectively retained the covalent bond character. Furthermore, the resulting five-membered ring that bridges the disulfide is itself fluorescent. The resulting dithiomaleimide cores are modestly bright yellow fluorophores, which allow the conjugates to be imaged *in vitro* (Fig. 11.2) while concurrently allowing for additional functional handles or PEG chains.

In conclusion, the conjugation of fluorescent dyes to the VLP capsid can improve the resolution of fluorescent imaging due to the high loading capabilities and monodisperse display of the dye on the VLP. Similarly, the same characteristics of the VLP capsid can be exploited to obtain high contrast MRI. In the next section, we will discuss some of the advantages VLPs offer for MRI contrast agents.

11.2.1.1 Contrast agents

Contrast-enhanced MRI is an imaging technique that uses contrast agents to greatly exacerbate the relaxation of water molecules compared with their environment making them appear either very bright (T_1 contrast) or very dark (T_2 contrast). Paramagnetic contrast agents, such as gadolinium (Gd^{3+}) ions, are commonly used to increase contrast (T_1) by altering relaxation times.[111] How well a given contrast agent works is related to a number of physical phenomena, one of which can be altered by simply attaching the small molecule to something very large. Large macromolecules, like VLPs, have slow rotational dynamics in solution compared with small molecules.[112–114] Quite generally, though exceptions exist, there is an inverse relationship between the rate of rotational dynamics (rotational correlation time) and the relaxation rate (relaxivities) denoted as r_n n = 1, 2 for T_1 or T_2 of a contrast agent. Consequently, one way to improve the overall ability of a given small molecule contrast agent is to stick it onto something very big. One of the first examples of VLPs used to augment T_1 contrast was done by Qazi et al., who attached an impressive 1900 chelated Gd^{3+} ions to P22 to achieve high relaxivity values, specifically $r_{1,\text{ionic}} = 21.7$ mM/s and $r_{1,\text{particle}} = 41{,}300$ mM/s at 298 K, 0.65 T (28 MHz).[56] This improves the localization density of the contrast agents and lowers the threshold detection limit of imaging agents used in MRI.[115]

Additionally, the large size of VLPs can be harnessed to slow the tumbling rate of contrast agents to improve MRI resolution. Prasuhn et al. conjugated[51] 223 Gd(DOTA) molecules to the exterior surface of CPMV and 153 to the exterior surface of Qβ. This resulted in a doubling of the relaxivity of Gd as compared with the FDA-approved Magnevist MRI contrast agent. The improved relaxivity is attributed to the limited rotational movement and diffusion associated with large VLPs. Similarly, Liepold et al. utilized[111] the large size of the 28 nm cowpea chlorotic mottle virus (CCMV) to conjugate up to 360 Gd(DOTA) to the exterior lysines on each capsid for a slowed tumbling rate and improved r_1 and r_2 relaxivities as compared with free gadolinium ions (Fig. 11.3).

Another method to improve the effectiveness of contrast agents is to incur rigidity within the chelated Gd^{3+}. This can be achieved by conjugating Gd(DOTA) to a functional handle on a VLP. Bruckman et al. found[33] that Gd(DOTA) conjugated to the tyrosine residues on the surface of TMV-improved relaxation threefold compared with free Gd(DOTA) and twofold when conjugated to the glutamate residues on the interior surface (Fig. 11.4). According to the authors, conjugation to the tyrosine residues offered higher rigidity compared with the more flexible carboxylic acids from the glutamate residues, which correspondingly enhanced the Gd(DOTA) relaxivity, though an alternative explanation might also include the slower water diffusion through the internal pore of TMV.

The multivalent functional handles on the VLP also allow for the conjugation of a targeting ligand for localization of the contrast agents in a specified region of the body. Hu et al. created[116] a TMV bimodal imaging agent that targeted prostate cancer cells. To do so, Cy7.5 and Dy(DOTA) were conjugated to the interior glutamate

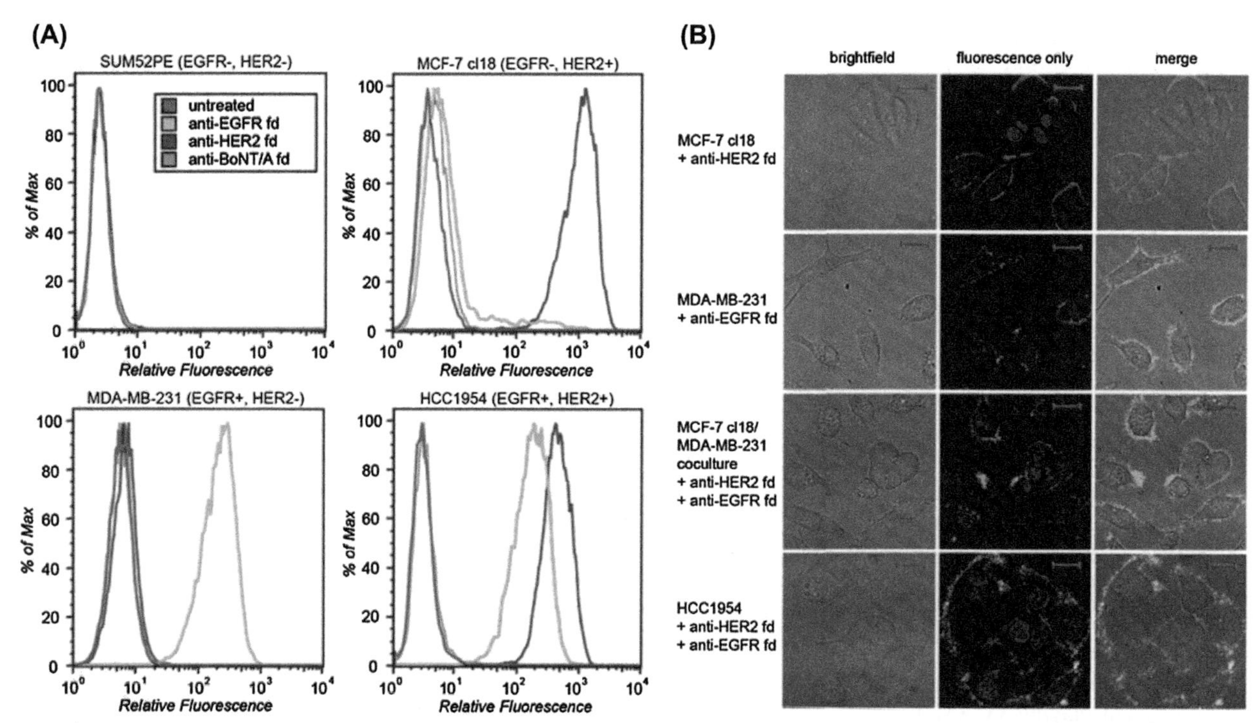

FIGURE 11.1 The N-terminus of phages was conjugated to fluorophores. The phage-displayed antibodies targeted breast cancer cells by recognizing epidermal growth factor receptor (EGFR) or human epidermal growth factor receptor 2 (HER2). It is shown in (A) that the phage–fluorophore conjugate was able to specifically recognize the EGFR and HER2 epitopes as determined by flow cytometry. It is shown in (B) that the phage–fluorophore conjugate targets breast cancer cells with the EGFR or HER2 for visualization by confocal microscopy. *Reproduced with permission from Carrico ZM, Farkas ME, Zhou Y, Hsiao SC, Marks JD, Chokhawala H, Clark DS, Francis MB, N-Terminal labeling of filamentous phage to create cancer marker imaging agents.* ACS Nano *2012;**6**(8):6675–6680.*

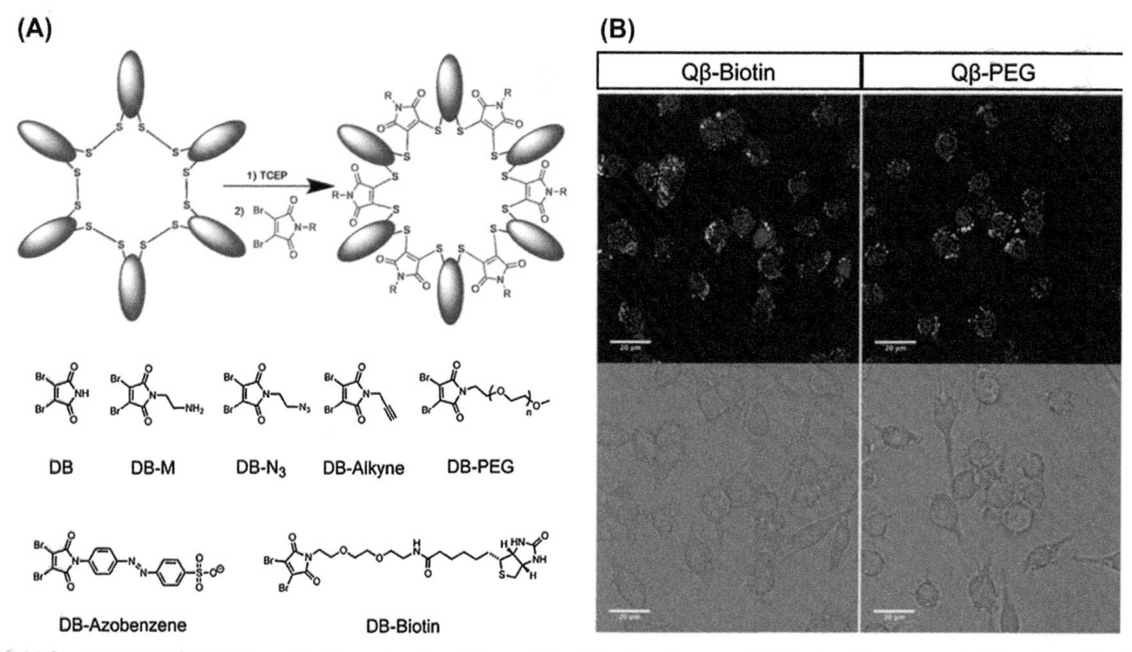

FIGURE 11.2 (A) Synthesis of Qβ–maleimide conjugates with a variety of functional groups. (B) *In vitro* fluorescence imaging by confocal microscopy of biologically relevant Qβ conjugates. The yellow fluorescence is from the five-membered dithio-maleimide rings created in the bioconjugation reaction. *Reproduced with permission from Chen Z, Boyd SD, Calvo JS, Murray KW, Mejia GL, Benjamin CE, Welch RP, Winkler DD, Meloni G, D'Arcy S, Gassensmith JJ. Fluorescent functionalization across quaternary structure in a virus-like particle.* Bioconjug Chem *2017;**28**(9):2277–2283.*

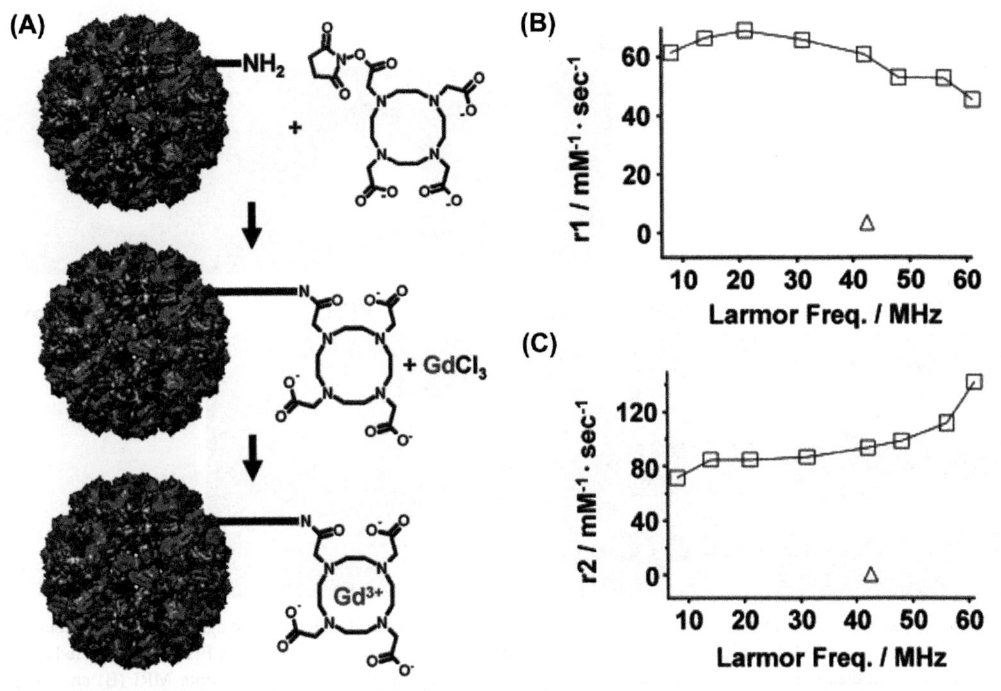

FIGURE 11.3 The relaxivities of “free” gadolinium ions ($GdCl_3$) are compared with gadolinium ions conjugated to the VLP cowpea chlorotic mottle virus. (A) shows the attachment of Gd. The triangles represent the free Gd, and the squares represent the conjugated Gd. (B) shows the r_1 values, and (C) shows the r_2 values. It is clear from both (B) and (C) that the conjugated gadolinium ions have higher relaxivities suggesting that the slowed tumbling rate improves the efficacy of the contrast agent. *Reproduced with permission from Liepold L, Anderson S, Willits D, Oltrogge L, Frank JA, Douglas T, Young M. Viral capsids as MRI contrast agents.* Magn Reson Med *2007;**58(5)**:871–879.*

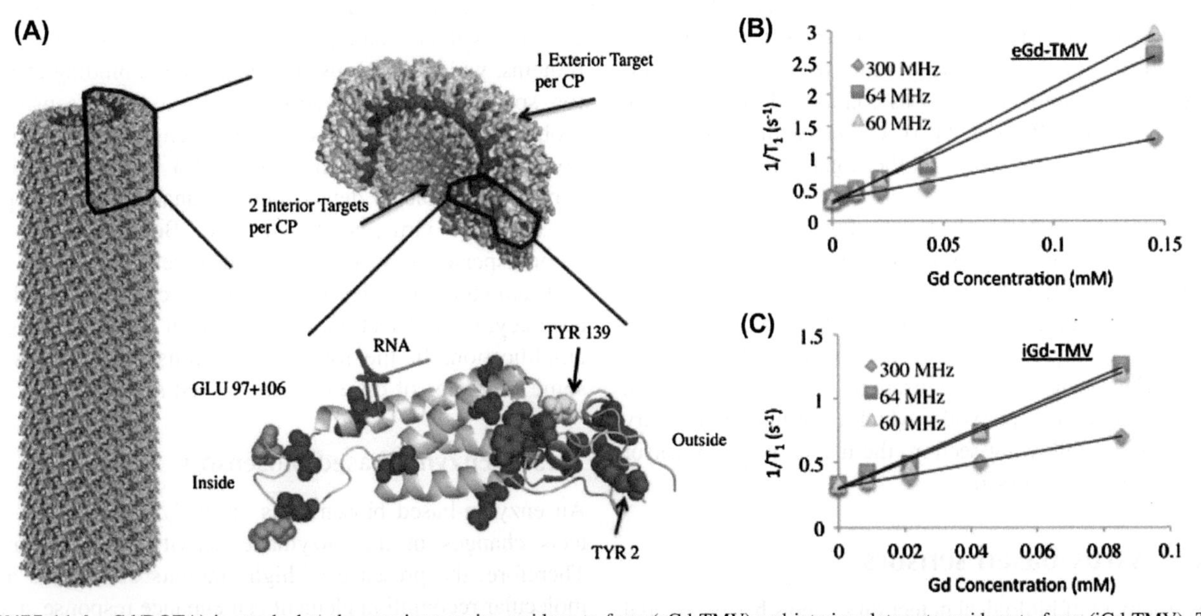

FIGURE 11.4 Gd(DOTA) is attached to the exterior tyrosine residues to form (eGd-TMV) and interior glutamate residues to form (iGd-TMV). The attachment sites are highlighted in (A). At 60 MHz, the slope of eGd-TMV shown in plot (B) gives an r_1 value of 18.4 mM/s which is threefold higher than free Gd(DOTA) (4.9 mM/s at 60 MHz). At 60 MHz, the slope of iGd-TMV shown in plot (C) gives an r_1 value of 10.7 mM/s which is twofold higher than free Gd(DOTA). These plots suggest incurred rigidity of the Gd(DOTA) after conjugation to the VLP with the highest rigidity and relaxation values when conjugated to the exterior tyrosine residues. *Reproduced with permission from Bruckman MA, Hern S, Jiang K, Flask CA, Yu X, Steinmetz NF. Tobacco mosaic virus rods and spheres as supramolecular high-relaxivity MRI contrast agents.* J Mater Chem B *2013;**1(10)**:1482–1490.*

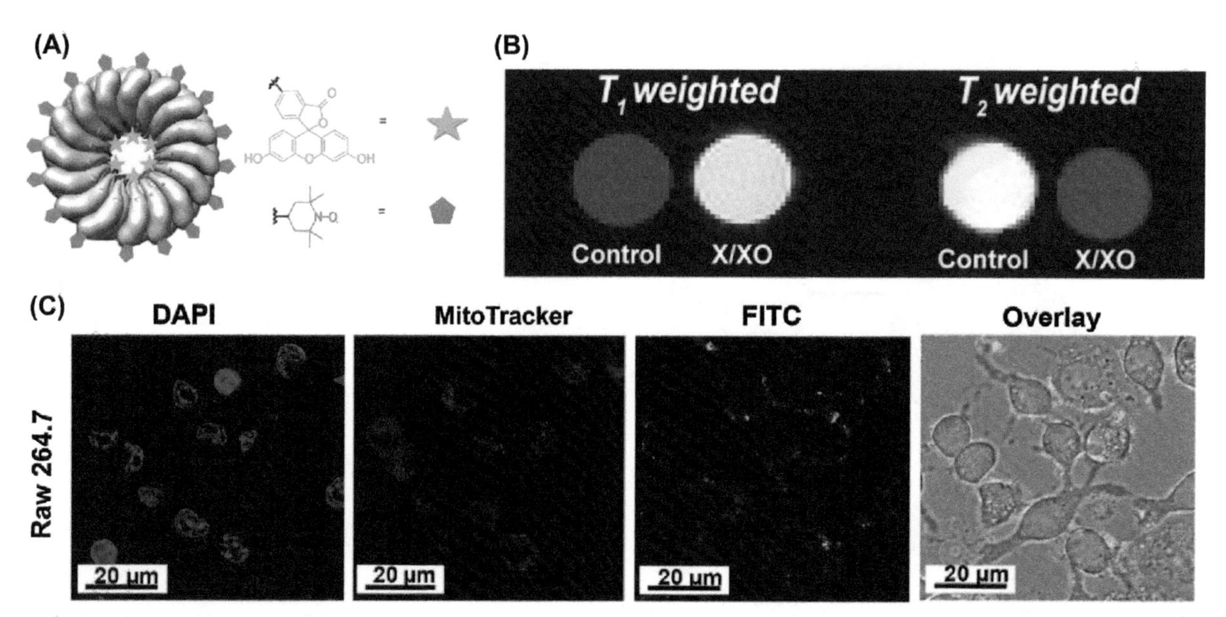

FIGURE 11.5 The virus-like particle tobacco mosaic virus (TMV) is shown to work as both an MRI contrast agent and a fluorescent probe. (A) TEMPO is conjugated to the exterior surface of TMV and works as a contrast agent for MRI imaging (orange pentagon). FITC is conjugated to the interior surface of the TMV and is used for fluorescent imaging (green star). Together the TMV conjugate can be used in both MRI (B) and fluorescence imaging (C) applications. *Reproduced with permission from Dharmarwardana M, Martins AF, Chen Z, Palacios PM, Nowak CM, Welch RP, Li S, Luzuriaga MA, Bleris L, Pierce BS, Sherry AD, Gassensmith JJ. Nitroxyl modified tobacco mosaic virus as a Metal-free high-relaxivity MRI and EPR active superoxide sensor.* Mol Pharm *2018;**15**(8):2973–2983.*

residues of TMV for NIR imaging and MRI. PEG and DGEA were conjugated to the tyrosines on the exterior surface for a biocompatible probe that specifically images prostate cancer.

Another bimodal imaging agent using TMV was designed by Dharmarwardana et al. in which FITC was conjugated[76] to the exterior tyrosine residues for fluorescence imaging and TEMPO was conjugated to the interior glutamates for MRI (Fig. 11.5). Uniquely, this MRI probe is also a superoxide sensor as the organic radical contrast agent, TEMPO, is reduced in *in vitro* and *in vivo* environments into an MRI silent state, but upon oxidation by superoxide, it functions as a "turn on" MRI sensor. This allows the sensor to "turn on" in T_1 and T_2 weighted imaging. The reduced state is MRI inactive, showing up as dark (T_1) or light (T_2), while the oxidized state is MRI active. This sensor can be used to show areas of high concentrations of superoxide, which exist in certain injury states. In the following section, the use of VLPs in sensor applications is discussed.

11.3 Virus-based sensors

Development of biological detection systems has received a considerable amount of attention in the biomedical field owing to its vital importance in clinical diagnosis and treatment. However, many available biosensors such as enzyme, cell-based, electrochemical, and color-based sensors suffer from limited sensitivity, selectivity, reliability, simplicity, and stability to detect and identify biological targets with high levels of certainty.[116–118] Accordingly, there is a pressing need for the invention of advanced biorecognition probes to overcome these challenges. VLPs have been employed as a sensing platform, thanks to their ease of synthetic and genetic modification to their coat proteins, which can be used to enhance the binding affinity for specific targets to solve selectivity and sensitivity problems. Moreover, by strategically engineering or functionalizing the multivalent surface of a viral capsid, these particles are able to detect multiple analytes such as proteins, DNA, virus, antibodies, etc. Because VLPs are monodisperse, they allow the attachment of precise and high amounts of target analytes to the capsid giving high accuracy, rapid detection, and significant response to signal amplification. In the following sections, we will review some examples of different virus-based sensors.

11.3.1 Enzyme-based biosensors

An enzyme-based biosensor is an analytical tool that detects changes in the enzymatic activity of a substrate. Therefore, the presence of high amounts of enzyme as a molecular recognition element can enhance response signal toward the target molecule, resulting in a highly sensitive sensor with a short detection time. Moreover, using highly specific enzymes toward the desired target allows for enhanced selectivity of the sensor. At present, there are several examples of selective and sensitive enzyme

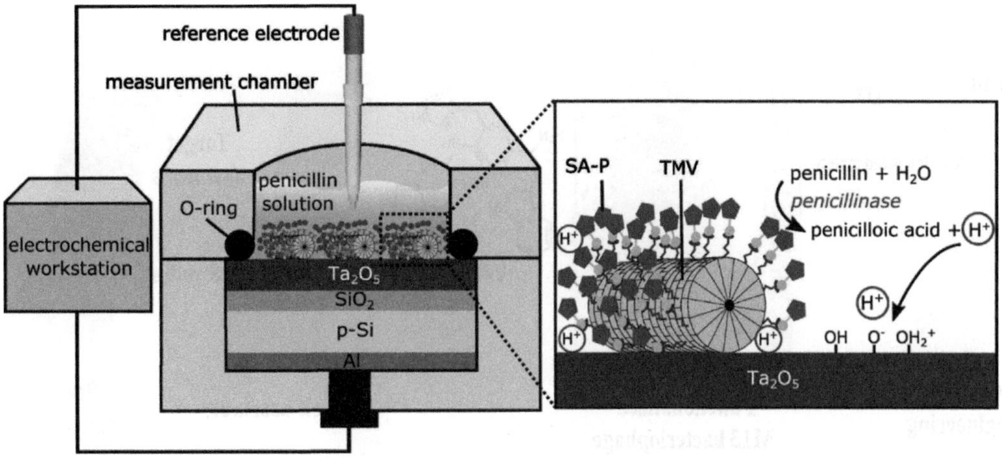

FIGURE 11.6 Schematic structure of modified tobacco mosaic virus (TMV) and penicillin biosensor. TMV modified with biotin groups to conjugated penicillinase–streptavidin (SA-P). The sensor is built up by immobilization of functionalized TMV on a pH-sensitive Ta_2O_5 gate EIS. The probe can detect hydrolysis of penicillin through monitoring the changes in hydrogen ion concentration (pH) near the surface of Ta_2O_5. The result is a change in the surface charge of Ta_2O_5 gate and the depletion capacitance in the silicon, which leads to changes in the overall capacitance of the EIS biosensor. *Reproduced with permission Poghossian A, Jablonski M, Koch C, Bronder TS, Rolka D, Wege C, Schoning MJ. Field-effect biosensor using virus particles as scaffolds for enzyme immobilization.* Biosens Bioelectron *2018:**110**, 168–174.*

biosensors, such as the glucose biosensor that generally uses glucose oxidase (GO) to catalyze oxidation of β-D-glucose.[119] Although these sensors are selective, they suffer from instability, high detection limits, and high production costs.[120] These limitations result from poorly absorbed enzymes, environmental changes (pH and temperature), low enzyme activity, and low signal detection.

To address these problems, there are several reports on integration of available probes with VLPs.[121–124] A recent example is coupling,[125] the enzyme modified TMV to a Pt sensor chip for amperometric detection of glucose. For this purpose, a streptavidin-conjugated glucose oxidase ([SA]-GOD) complex was immobilized on the surface of biotinylated TMV through bioaffinity binding. The functionalized TMV was loaded on the Pt electrode which caused a significant increase in enzyme density on the surface of the sensor chip. The result is higher glucose signal, lower detection limit, and high enzyme activity.

Additionally, VLPs can be used as a specific sensing platform for β-galactosidase. Nanduri et al. has shown that[77] the filamentous bacteriophage 1G40 has high binding affinity to galactosidase which can be used for sensitive and specific detection of this enzyme. They immobilized IG40 on a gold surface of SPR SPREETATM sensor chip and compared the sensor performance with an F8-5 as a control phage (nonspecific to β-gal). Their data showed a 10-fold enhancement in detection response compared with control phage.

Additionally, the surface of VLPs exposes thousands of identical binding sites that permit the attachment of a large number of enzymes to the viral capsid in a spatially controlled manner. Conjugated enzymes maintain their structure and catalytic activity, both of which are required for a sensitive enzyme-based probe. One example of the conjugation of enzymes to a VLP for the development of a probe was shown by Poghossian et al. In this study, they demonstrated[124] the strong immobilization of penicillinase enzyme on TMV via biotin and streptavidin–penicillinase binding affinity. The modified TMV was loaded on Al-p-Si-SiO_2-Ta_2O_5 as an electrolyte insulator semiconductor to build a highly sensitive and stable biosensor (Fig. 11.6). The modified sensor is able to detect penicillin concentrations in the range of 0.1–10 mM with a 50 μM lower detection limit.

VLPs have great potential for successful integration with other sensors owing to their desirable properties such as coupling biological elements like enzymes, high thermal and chemical stability, and lack of toxicity. This will help with the emergence of novel sensors with promoted performance like the analyte detection over low concentration range, high specificity, and stability.

In addition to use of VLPs in developing the enzyme-based sensors, they can be applied as a color-based probes and use different optical techniques (fluorescence spectrometry, UV/Vis, chemiluminescence) for biomolecular interaction analysis and specific detection and identification of a variety of biological analytes. In the following section, we will show the examples of VLPs as a colorimetric sensor.

11.3.2 Colorimetric biosensors

Colorimetric biosensors produce human and machine-readable color changes in response to biological analytes. General drawbacks of these sensors tend to be poor selectivity and relatively low sensitivity, which limit their clinical applications; therefore, there is a need for new

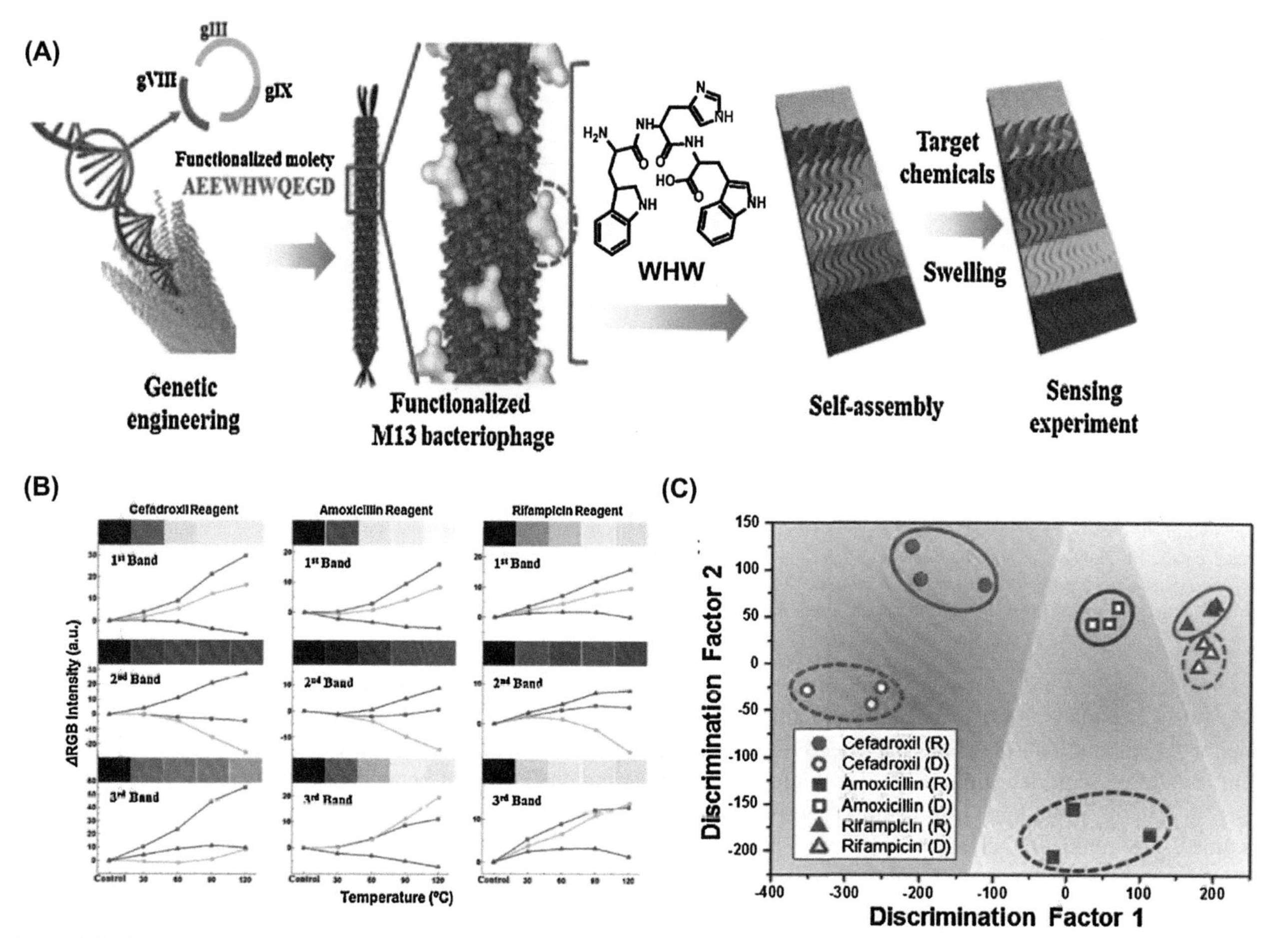

FIGURE 11.7 Schematic illustration of colorimetric sensor composed of filamentous M13 modified with WHW peptide. (A) The self-assembly properties of M13 has been used to make liquid crystalline thin films by the pulling technique. (B) The RGB signal intensity was changed in the presence of different antibiotics at different temperatures owing to changes in the M13-based bundle nanostructure. (C) Principal component analysis (PCA) was used to show discrimination ability of the sensor for different antibiotics (cephalosporin, penicillin, and rifampin). *Modified with permission from Moon JS, Park M, Kim WG, Kim C, Hwang J, Seol D, Kim CS, Sohn JR, Chung H, Oh JW, M-13 bacteriophage based structural color sensor for detecting antibiotics.* Sens Actuators B Chem *2017:***240***, 757–762.*

architectures to enhance sensitivity toward bioanalytes. VLPs can be engineered chemically and genetically to promote intrinsic affinity toward a specific analyte. For example, Oh and coworkers introduced[78] a selective and stable colorimetric probe for the detection of different types of antibiotics by using the self-assembly properties of a genetically engineered nonlytic M13 VLP. In this study, an M13 was functionalized with the WHW peptide to have 1000 copies of tryptophan (W) histidine (H) tryptophan (W) sequences which can act as a receptor for antibiotics. Target binding causes the quasi-ordered bundles of phage matrices to swell or shrink, which induces a change in the optical scattering properties on the chip surface following interaction with different target antibiotics (Fig. 11.7). This scattering of light results in an apparent color, even though no chromophores are present.

For early disease diagnostics, there is critical need for tools to sense and measure different biological molecules, proteins, and biomarkers on cancerous cells. To date, several colorimetric sensors such as enzyme-linked immunosorbent assay (ELISA) and cell-based ELISA (CELISA) have emerged for this purpose; however, because of the limited number of attached enzymes and high dissociation constant between antibody and antigen, their detection limit is in the nanomolar range.[126,127] Recently, VLPs have offered several improved colorimetric sensing systems with higher response signals.[128–131] For example, Brasino et al. improved[127] ELISA sensing performance by dually decorating a filamentous bacteriophage Fd with antibodies for specific antigen detection and horseradish peroxidase to generate an amplified colorimetric signal. In another work, Wang et al. successfully designed[131] a "CELISA" using a modified TMV to detect folate receptors overexpressed on cancer cells. For this purpose, the exterior surface of TMV was modified with platinum nanoparticles as a peroxidase surrogate and folic acid as a cancer cell targeting mechanism. When the modified TMV binds to cancer cells that overexpress folic

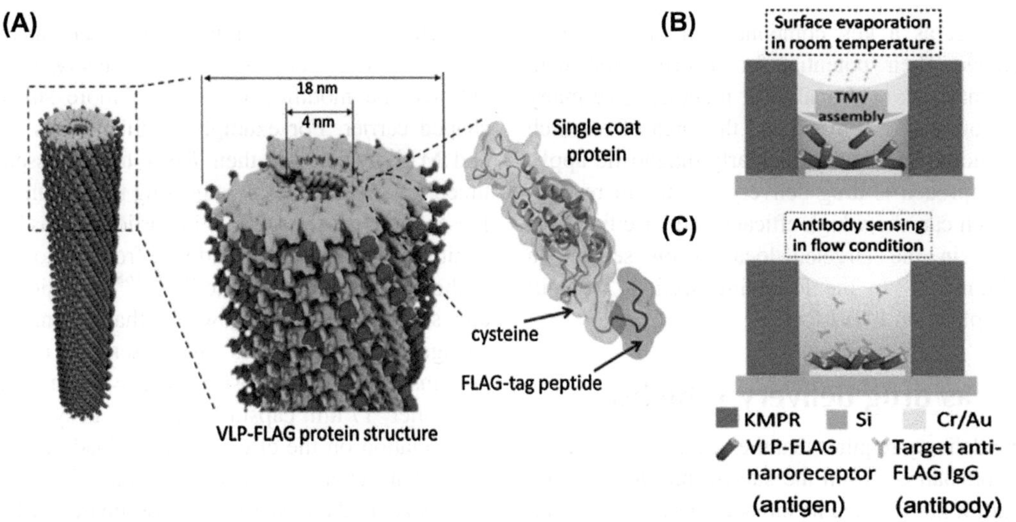

FIGURE 11.8 A) Three-dimensional schematic of modified tobacco mosaic virus (TMV) expressing cysteine residues and receptor peptide FLAG-tag. (B) Surface functionalization of TMV-FLAG. (C) Antibody detection in the sensor system. *Reproduced with permission from Zang F, Gerasopoulos K, Brown AD, Culver JN, Ghodssi R. Capillary Microfluidics-Assembled virus-like particle bionanoreceptor Interfaces for label-free biosensing.* ACS Appl Mater Interfaces *2017;**9**(10):8471–8479.*

acid receptors, superoxide is supplemented to provide a colorimetric indicator of which cells are cancerous. Consequently, modification of VLPs has afforded a new color biosensing system that could be used for biomedical applications and diagnostics assays. Another example is an M13 bacteriophage–DNA conjugated system that has been developed[130] by Domaille et al. for protein detection. In this study, acyl hydrazone linkages were utilized for DNA sequence incorporation, which led to a strong and detectable change in absorption signal (410 nm) on interaction with IgG as a model protein. Thus, by using the phage as a sensing platform, they created a rapid and extremely sensitive tool for protein detection in the range of 0–1000 fmol.

11.3.3 Electrochemical biosensors

Electrochemical biosensors are involved in the generation or consumption of electrons over an interaction between biochemical receptors and an electrochemical transduction element. Although these sensors are usually selective and sensitive toward target biomolecules, they suffer from narrow temperature ranges, limited half-life, and high background signal. In recent decades, VLPs have received much attention for their thermal stability and robustness. Combining VLPs as a sensing receptor with analytical methods such as electrochemical methods can be a reliable way to simultaneously increase electrochemical sensor performance and improve sensor stability. For instance, Ghodssi and coworkers developed[132] a novel electrochemical biosensor for schizophrenia analysis. In this study, they modified the surface of electrode with TMV, nickel, and gold following introduction of ssDNA for Neuregulin-1 gene detection. The modified probe showed a high surface area with strong current change on DNA hybridization, which lead to an 8-fold increase in signal and 9.5-fold enhancement in biosensing performance.[132]

Coating VLPs on the surface of electrodes is a way to increase the electrode surface area, thus allowing for a higher electrochemical signal, decreased signal to noise ratio, and greater sensitivity. For example, a new impedance sensor was developed[133] by Zang et al. that applied FLAG-tag–modified TMV on an electrode surface by capillary action and surface evaporation for label-free antibody detection. Thus, owing to the high surface to volume ratio of TMV nanotubes and several hundred available binding sites on its surface, a high peptide density could anchor to the electrode, which maximized antibody detection (Fig. 11.8).[129]

Additionally, VLPs can be used as a sensing platform for biomarker and cancer cell detection. One example is the immobilization of a filamentous M13 phage on the surface of a modified Si_3N_4 chip by reacting the N terminal domain of the phage coat protein with an aldehyde group on the chip surface to make a light addressable potentiometric sensor (LAPS). Jia et al. showed[134] the sensor is able to detect human phosphatase of regenerating liver-3(hPRL-3) at concentrations of 0.04–400 nM and mammary adenocarcinoma cell (MDAMB231) at concentrations of 0–105 cells/mL through specific binding to the phage, which had been evolved via phage display, and subsequent change of the output voltage of LAPS. Therefore, integration of bionanoreceptors with conventional electrochemical methods can be an effective strategy for improving sensor performance.

VLPs can act as a key component in different biosensing systems. Their potential for incorporation with different nanomaterials and analytical methods give many opportunities for scientists to expand this area of research and progress biomedical and particularly diagnostic applications. One approach is drug delivery by stimuli responsive VLPs which can show high efficacy and specificity for cargo delivery in the targeted location on sensing a particular stimulus.[135] In the following section, we will discuss this application of VLPs.[131]

11.4 VLPs as drug delivery vehicles

Effective drug delivery requires that the desired cargo passes several transport barriers from the site of introduction into the patient until it has reached its intended destination while avoiding off-target effects. Unfortunately, there are many barriers to successful delivery. The reticuloendothelial system hampers dosage efficacy especially if the materials have long circulation times which subsequently leads to faster clearance from the body. Additionally, cellularly targeted drugs need to permeate the membrane and avoid or survive endosomal trafficking before it releases its cargo.[136] Several nanoscale platforms are being investigated for drug delivery as nanoparticle based therapeutics as a result of their small size[137] and favorable pharmacokinetics,[7,138] which offer solutions to many of the problems associated with conventional drug administration. Despite growing interest in their use and development, the number of FDA approved nanoparticle drugs is limited, and more than half of the formulations currently undergoing trial are liposomal.[139] These systems have been shown to suffer from rapid and dose-dependent clearance from the body[140–144] and conflicting results on the efficacy of attaching targeting ligands.[145,146] VLPs, on the other hand, are capable of accomplishing this task by carrying a diverse set of therapeutic cargos ranging from nucleic acids,[130,147–151] genes,[152,153] aptamers,[154,155] therapeutic drugs,[156–162] larger proteins,[163,164] to dendrimers,[165,166] while still being amenable to further functionalization—some have even been cleared for use by the FDA.[75] This paves a path for drug delivery to make further advancements through the utilization of a robust and tunable carrier to circumvent the issues plaguing current delivery methods.

11.4.1 Cargo loading

As discussed in previous sections, VLP geometries can play an important role in targeting and cell specificity. Because the shape of nanoparticles is known to alter their pharmacokinetics, the VLP geometry makes for a uniquely tunable parameter for drug delivery. For instance, small icosahedral nanoparticles diffuse well into tissues but have smaller cargo capacities while their larger, filamentous counterparts are better suited for aligning with vessel walls, though they do not infiltrate cells as well. Fortunately, many viral capsids can be modified to create a more suitably sized or shaped carrier. For example, rodlike VLPs such as TMV and M13, which use their RNA to self-assemble, can be tuned to specific sizes by adjusting the length of their RNA. Icosahedral viruses, CCMV in particular, has been shown to exhibit an increase in capsid size from 27 to 30 nm linearly as the pH is varied from 5 to 7.[167,168] Asensio et al. has gone one step further and shown[169] that a single amino acid change—S37P—changes the assembly of MS2 capsid proteins from 27 nm capsid with $T = 3$ symmetry to a much a smaller 17 nm capsid with $T = 1$ symmetry. Further investigation on the effects of drug loading was performed by Cadena et al. to elucidate[170] the effects of increasing cargo size on the formation of icosahedral VLPs. They have found that varying lengths of RNA from 140 to 12,000 nt can be completely encapsulated while causing a change in capsid size. For shorter strands, the RNA is packaged into 24 and 26 nm capsids, while a single stand of RNA greater that 4500 nt is packaged by two or more 26–30 nm capsids showing that just changing the length of the structural RNA, various lengths, and sizes of VLPs can be achieved to predetermine the cargo capacity for delivery applications. Utilizing VLPs allows for increased and precise drug loading, which remediates issues with low and inaccurate dosing. Rurup et al. have demonstrated[171] a method of predicting the loading of VLPs using teal fluorescent proteins (TFPs) and CCMV where more than 10 3 nm TFPs can be loaded inside of the 18 nm cavity of the viral capsid (Fig. 11.9). Through the use of homo-FRET, they have determined that tethering the TLPs to the capsid proteins yields more predictive and controlled loading behavior increasing the number of fluorescent proteins from 6—in the coiled coil system—to 20 dimeric units when directly bound to the CPs. This information lays some of the ground work for further progress in the use of VLPs as a drug carrier.

11.4.2 Drug delivery

Encapsulating therapeutics within a nanoparticle offers protection from rapid clearance from the body and the harsh cellular environments that would normally degrade free small molecules before reaching their target destination. The ease of functionalization of VLPs allows for the design of smarter drug delivery vehicles including stimuli responsive release. For example, work by Chen et al. utilizes[91] VLP Qβ, first functionalized with an azide linker on the surface exposed to NH_2, handles via EDC coupling followed by a CUAAC reaction to attach the photocleavable Dox group. The as-synthesized VLP encountered solubility issues so to remedy this, they further functionalized the surface by adding a second functional group—PEG 1K or 2K through dibromomaleimide

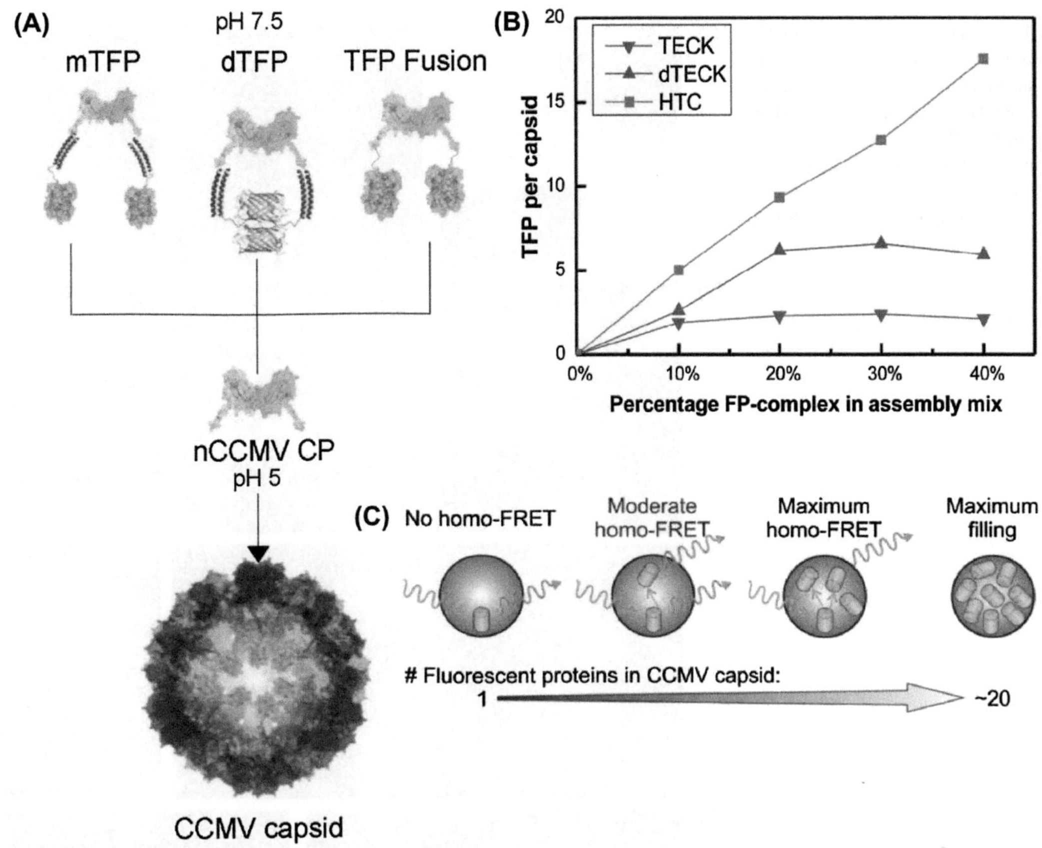

FIGURE 11.9 (A) Schematic representation of the different design principles described in this work for the rational loading of CCMV. The first approach utilizes leucine zipper like E-coils tethered to monomeric TFP (mTFP) or dimeric TFP (dTFP), which form electrostatic interactions at pH 7.5 with the complementary K-coil tethered to CCMV. The formed complex is referred to as TECK and dTECK, respectively. The second approach utilizes a genetically engineered TFP peptide linker-CCMV fusion protein, when complexed, referred to as HTC. In all cases, lowering the pH to 5.0 promotes the encapsulation of TFP cargo inside CCMV. (B) Typical capsid TFP loading as a function of percentage of complex (TECK, dTECK, or HTC) in assembly. (C) Schematic explaining how homo-FRET works. *Reproduced with permission from Rurup WF, Verbij F, Koay MST, Blum C, Subramaniam V, Cornelissen JJLM. Predicting the loading of virus-like particles with fluorescent proteins.* Biomacromolecules *2014;**15**(2):558–563.*

chemistry. The final VLP is a soluble, low toxicity carrier that shows cytotoxicity on stimulation with UV light which cleaves the linker, activating Dox release in the cells. The Steinmetz group has also done[160] extensive work showing that the conjugation of molecules such as Dox can be attached and successfully delivered to cells. They have made use of the VNP CPMV decorated with covalently bound Dox on the exterior surface demonstrating that the functionalized particle in low doses is more cytotoxic than free Doxorubicin and exhibits a time-delayed release. This work has also determined that the CPMV-Dox particles get trafficked to endosomal compartments, as seen in Fig. 11.10 in HeLa cells, where the proteinaceous carrier is degraded, and the drug molecules are released into the cellular environment.

11.4.3 Targeting

The addition of a targeting functionality offers several advantages over nontargeted drugs. Mainly they consist of reducing the side effects associated with damage to healthy tissues and enhancement of uptake into afflicted cells. Targeting can be approached in either a passive or active manner depending on the nature of the particle in use and the functionalities incorporated into its design. Passive targeting includes (1) the EPR effect, (2) approaches relying on the tumor microenvironment, and (3) intratumoral delivery.[89] The EPR effect is a phenomenon where increased permeability of the tumor vasculature is combined with poor lymphatic drainage, which makes it difficult for high molecular weight carriers to be removed from the tumor environment. EPR coupled with release based on the tumor microenvironment or an external stimulus offers some solution to healthy tissue damage and has been demonstrated across nanomedicine to be effective.[79]

Many of these functionalities are applicable to VLPs that can be further modified to increase targeting specificity. Active targeting of a drug delivery system allows for the preferential accumulation into specific cells that can be selected for by a variety of tumor markers, such as small

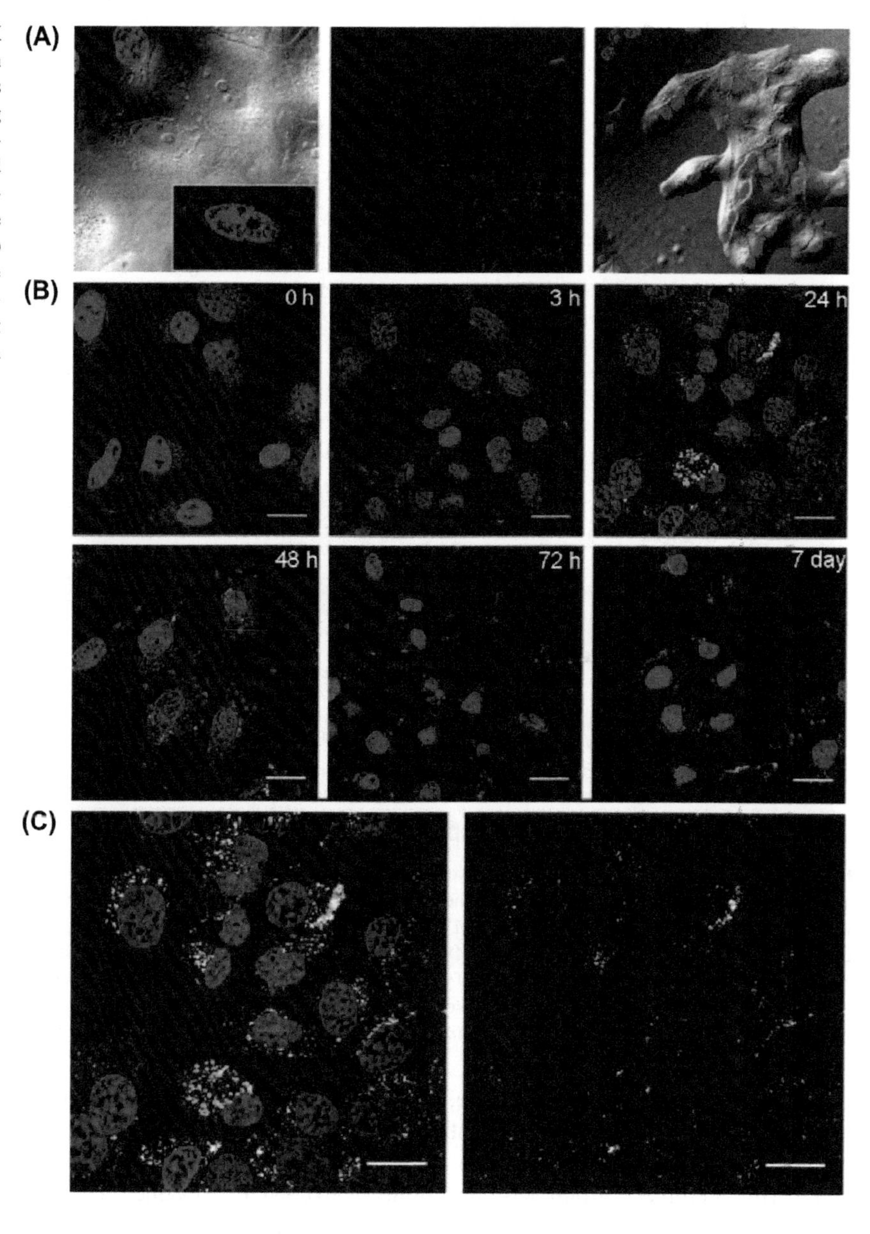

FIGURE 11.10 (A) Imaging of CPMV-DOX in HeLa 3 h postincubation. CPMV is shown in red, nuclei are shown in blue, and DIC overlay is shown in gray. (B) Time course study showing cellular uptake of CPMV using confocal scanning microscopy; CPMV was immunostained (pseudocolored in green). Endolysosomes pseudocolored in red. Nuclei are shown in blue. Scale bar is 50 μm. (C) Colocalization analysis (white) of CPMV and Lamp-1 staining. Scale bars are 50 μm. *Reproduced with permission from Aljabali AA, Shukla S, Lomonossoff GP, Steinmetz NF, Evans DJ. CPMV-DOX delivers.* Mol Pharm *2013;**10**(1):3–10.*

peptides and antigens as well as cell surface receptors[45] and biomarkers. These moieties have been used throughout the literature to up the chances of delivery to maligned cells—sparing the healthy ones. In an effort to increase specificity in delivery, targeting molecules have been employed such as folic acid or small peptides like cyclic RGD. For instance, Stephanopoulos et al. has constructed[172] an MS2 capsid where they have attached aptamers specific to Jurkat leukemia T cells onto engineered *p*-aminophenylalanine (paF) groups followed by the conjugation of porphyrins on onto the interior cysteines that generate reactive oxygen when irradiated with blue light (Fig. 11.11). Approximately 20 aptamers were attached per capsid increasing the targeting specificity of the VLP. This dual-modal delivery system was shown to localize only in the Jurkat cells when cocultured with other cells and successfully and selectively initiated apoptosis through photoredox ROS generation.

11.5 Vaccines

Vaccines are continually used as a method of disease treatment and prevention since their inception by making use of inactivated native viral proteins to bolster our immune systems against foreign bodies. VLPs—lacking their viral genome—produce similar immune responses to those of native, infectious diseases. The highly organized structure of the VLP surface presents several repeating amino

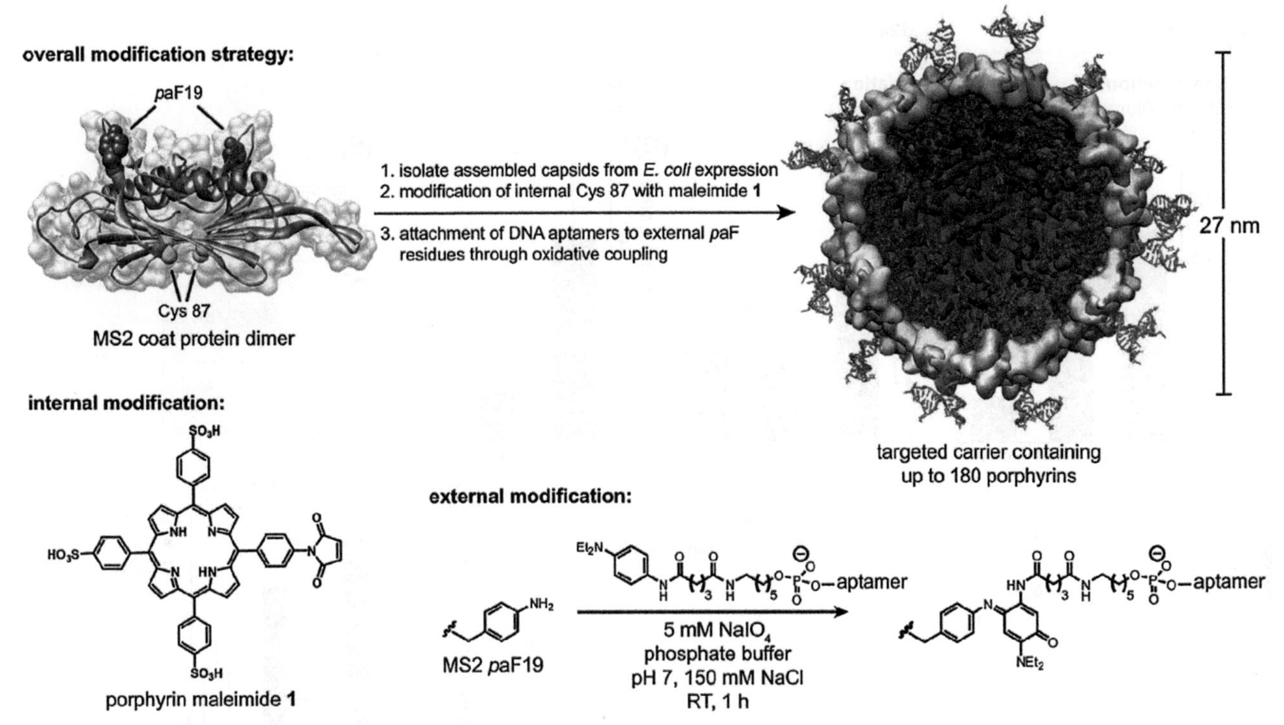

FIGURE 11.11 Construction of a multivalent cell-targeted photodynamic therapy vehicle using recombinant bacteriophage MS2. Cysteine residues on the capsid interior were modified using porphyrin maleimide 1 (rendered in purple), enabling the generation of singlet oxygen on illumination at 415 nm. Exterior *p*-aminophenylalanine (*pa*F) residues were coupled to phenylene diamine–modified DNA aptamers to bind tyrosine kinase 7 receptors. *Reproduced with permission from Stephanopoulos N, Tong, GJ, Hsiao SC, Francis MB. Dual-surface modified virus capsids for targeted delivery of photodynamic agents to cancer cells.* ACS Nano *2010;4(10):6014–6020.*

acid sequences which can cross-link B-cell receptors which, in turn, quickens the activation of antibody responses.[93] In addition, the encapsulated genome itself is capable of activating toll-like receptors and further eliciting an immune response with the added benefit of including a customized genetic cargo. Several VLP-based vaccines, such as human papilloma virus (HPV) and hepatitis B, are already on the market, but many more are under development.[173] The Bachmann group has conducted extensive work utilizing the Qβ VLP to study its immunogenicity showing that the particle alone can transport a therapeutic while behaving as an adjuvant all in one by developing vaccines for influenza,[174] respiratory allergies,[175] and smoking cessation,[176] reporting as much as 100% antibody response to the injection in clinical trials. They have even gone one step further as to show the efficacy of modifying the surface of the VLP Qβ with Fel d1 (Fig. 11.12), a cat allergen to induce a protective immune response without the additional threat of inducing anaphylaxis in mice.[94] In this study, to determine whether Qβ–Fel d1 inhibited mast cell degeneration (which signals immune-stimulated destruction of invasive materials) in an antigen specific manner, BALB/c mice were vaccinated subcutaneously with Qβ or Qβ–Fel d1. When challenged 2 weeks later, mice treated with Qβ–Fel d1 hardly showed an immune response after inoculation of free Fel d1 indicating successful immune memory without adverse effects. This is an important step forward in the medical field as they have shown that VLP-based vaccines may be used as a safe, effective, and customizable method to produce vaccines.

Virus-based vaccines share some of the same problems encountered with any vaccine. Even with efficient immune responses, they rely on the longevity of the host response. In addition, use of VLPs has shown more promise than many other subunit vaccines because they are conformationally the most similar to the native virus yet are safer as they lack genetic material and thus cannot reproduce. The use of other virus-based particles such as HPV and influenza virus has sparked an interest in the further development of VLPs particularly in increasing the efficacy in these particles.

11.6 Conclusion

VLPs offer many advantages to biological applications. In this chapter, we have discussed some of the important characteristics of VLPs that can be harnessed to advance biomedical fields such as imaging, sensing, and drug delivery. There are still some issues in using VLPs in biomedical applications, in particular they are immunogenic, which means repeated exposure will change the

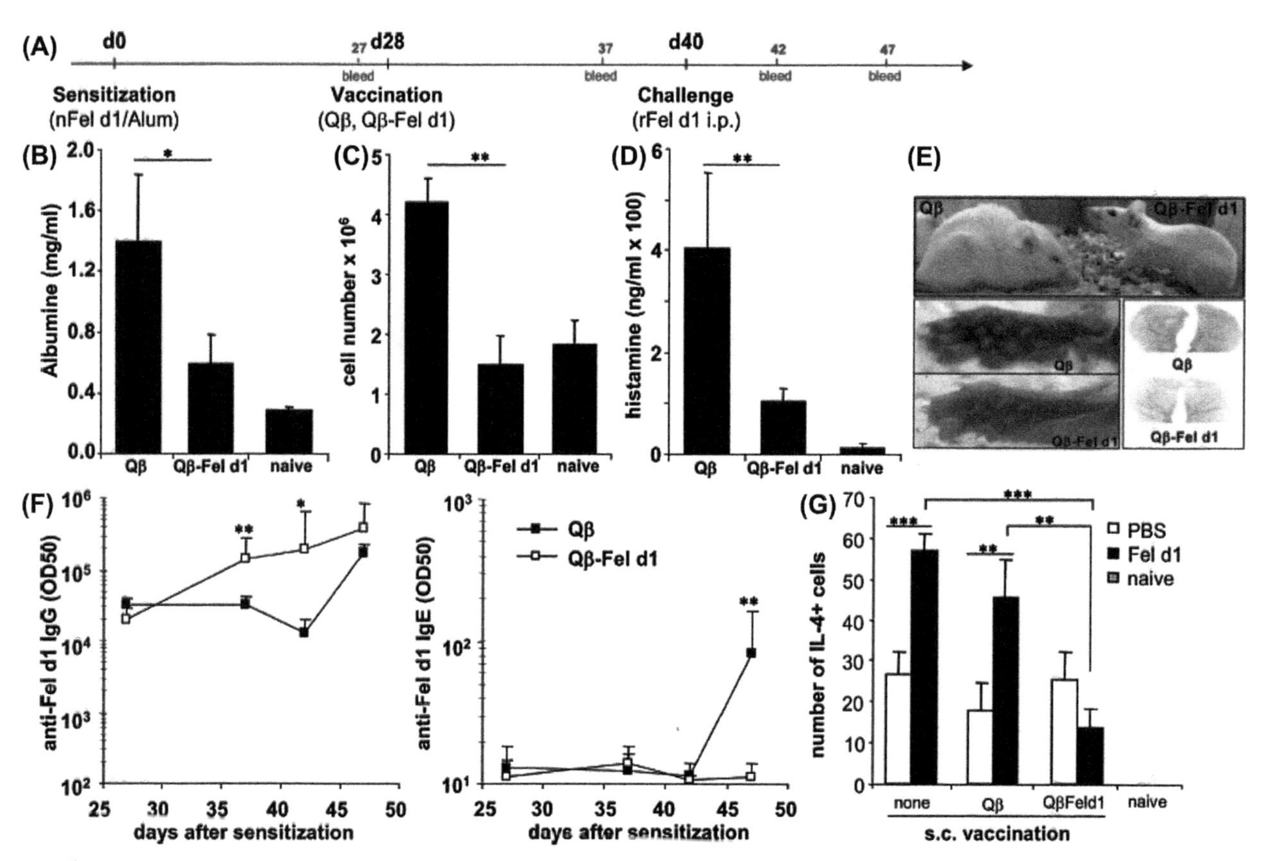

FIGURE 11.12 (A) Schematic outline of the experiment. (B–D) Mast cell activation determined by measurement of peritoneal albumin concentrations (B), peritoneal cell influx (C), and serum histamine levels (D) on antigen challenge. (E) Pictures of representative animals of each experimental group, 40 min after intraperitoneal injection–free Fel d1 challenge. Qβ control animals displayed typical signs of an anaphylactic reaction. (F) Fel d1-specific IgG (left) and Fel d1-specific IgE (right) titers. (G) ELISPOT assays were performed 1 wk after Fel d1 challenge to determine the numbers of IL-4 producing cells per 2 × 105 spleen which are indicative of helper T-cells. *, $P < .05$; **, $P < .005$; ***, $P < .0005$. *Reproduced with permission from Engeroff P, Caviezel F, Storni F, Thoms F, Vogel M, Bachmann MF. Allergens displayed on virus-like particles are highly immunogenic but fail to activate human mast cells.* Allergy *2018;73(2):341–349.*

pharmacokinetics in individual patients. This drawback is not unique to VLPs and is an issue for polymers as well.[177,178] In context of cost, they will be more expensive than synthetic nanomaterials, though they are expressed in *Escherichia coli* in high yields, which would make their eventual scale up in a process setting relatively practical. In imaging applications, the large size of VLPs is helpful in attaching a substantial amount of dye or contrast agent, and monodisperse subunits reduce self-quenching for high-resolution imaging. The functionalizability of VLPs owed to their multivalent subunits can also be used to increase bioprobe sensitivity while maintaining stability of the conjugate. Lastly, the biocompatibility and encapsulating ability of VLPs for drug delivery helps encourage the accumulation of drugs in a specified region with reduced clearance. Because VLPs are relatively new nanocarriers, the extent of the benefits they offer for biomedical applications has yet to be realized.

References

1. Chopra KL. Nanotechnology: hope or hype? *Curr Sci* 2012;**102**(10):1364–6.
2. Mack J. Nanotechnology: what's in it for biotech? *Biotechnol Healthc* 2005;**2**(6):29–36.
3. Wilhelm S, Tavares AJ, Dai Q, Ohta S, Audet J, Dvorak HF, Chan WCW. Analysis of nanoparticle delivery to tumours. *Nature Rev Mater* 2016;**1**:16014.
4. Kohane DS, Langer R. Biocompatibility and drug delivery systems. *Chem Sci* 2010;**1**(4):441–6.
5. Wilson N. Nanoparticles: environmental problems or problem solvers? *Bioscience* 2018;**68**(4):241–6.
6. Hong H, Chen F, Cai W. Pharmacokinetic issues of imaging with nanoparticles: focusing on carbon nanotubes and quantum dots. *Mol Imaging Biol* 2013;**15**(5):507–20.
7. Hoshyar N, Gray S, Han H, Bao G. The effect of nanoparticle size on in vivo pharmacokinetics and cellular interaction. *Nanomedicine* 2016;**11**(6):673–92.

8. NCI FDA Approves Talimogene Laherparepvec to Treat Metastatic Melanoma. https://www.cancer.gov/news-events/cancer-currents-blog/2015/t-vec-melanoma.
9. NCI Talimogene Laherparepvec. https://www.cancer.gov/about-cancer/treatment/drugs/talimogenelaherparepvec.
10. Lang FF, Conrad C, Gomez-Manzano C, Tufaro F, Sawaya R, Weinberg J, Prabhu S, Fuller G, Aldape K, Fueyo J. Nt-18: phase I clinical trial of oncolytic virus delta-24-Rgd (Dnx-2401) with biological endpoints: implications for viro-immunotherapy. *Neuro Oncol* 2014;**16**(Suppl. 5). v162-v162.
11. NCI Oncolytic Virus Therapy: Using Tumor-Targeting Viruses to Treat Cancer. https://www.cancer.gov/news-events/cancer-currents-blog/2018/oncolytic-viruses-to-treat-cancer.
12. Chesney J, Puzanov I, Collichio F, Singh P, Milhem MM, Glaspy J, Hamid O, Ross M, Friedlander P, Garbe C, Logan TF, Hauschild A, Lebbe C, Chen L, Kim JJ, Gansert J, Andtbacka RHI, Kaufman HL. Randomized, open-label phase II study evaluating the efficacy and safety of Talimogene Laherparepvec in combination with Ipilimumab versus Ipilimumab alone in patients with advanced, unresectable melanoma. *J Clin Oncol* 2018;**36**(17):1658−67.
13. Kelly E, Russell SJ. History of oncolytic viruses: genesis to genetic engineering. *Mol Ther* 2007;**15**(4):651−9.
14. Samson A, Scott KJ, Taggart D, West EJ, Wilson E, Nuovo GJ, Thomson S, Corns R, Mathew RK, Fuller MJ, Kottke TJ, Thompson JM, Ilett EJ, Cockle JV, van Hille P, Sivakumar G, Polson ES, Turnbull SJ, Appleton ES, Migneco G, Rose AS, Coffey MC, Beirne DA, Collinson FJ, Ralph C, Alan Anthoney D, Twelves CJ, Furness AJ, Quezada SA, Wurdak H, Errington-Mais F, Pandha H, Harrington KJ, Selby PJ, Vile RG, Griffin SD, Stead LF, Short SC, Melcher AA. Intravenous delivery of oncolytic reovirus to brain tumor patients immunologically primes for subsequent checkpoint blockade. *Sci Transl Med* 2018;**10**(422).
15. Bourgeois-Daigneault MC, Roy DG, Aitken AS, El Sayes N, Martin NT, Varette O, Falls T, St-Germain LE, Pelin A, Lichty BD, Stojdl DF, Ungerechts G, Diallo JS, Bell JC. Neoadjuvant oncolytic virotherapy before surgery sensitizes triple-negative breast cancer to immune checkpoint therapy. *Sci Transl Med* 2018;**10**(422).
16. Hooker JM, Kovacs EW, Francis MB. Interior surface modification of bacteriophage MS2. *J Am Chem Soc* 2004;**126**(12):3718−9.
17. Kovacs EW, Hooker JM, Romanini DW, Holder PG, Berry KE, Francis MB. Dual-surface-modified bacteriophage MS2 as an ideal scaffold for a viral capsid-based drug delivery system. *Bioconjug Chem* 2007;**18**(4):1140−7.
18. Hooker JM, O'Neil JP, Romanini DW, Taylor SE, Francis MB. Genome-free viral capsids as carriers for positron emission tomography radiolabels. *Mol Imaging Biol* 2008;**10**(4):182−91.
19. Datta A, Hooker JM, Botta M, Francis MB, Aime S, Raymond KN. High relaxivity gadolinium hydroxypyridonate-viral capsid conjugates: nanosized MRI contrast agents. *J Am Chem Soc* 2008;**130**(8):2546−52.
20. Capehart SL, ElSohly AM, Obermeyer AC, Francis MB. Bioconjugation of gold nanoparticles through the oxidative coupling of ortho-aminophenols and anilines. *Bioconjug Chem* 2014;**25**(10):1888−92.
21. Capehart SL, Coyle MP, Glasgow JE, Francis MB. Controlled integration of gold nanoparticles and organic fluorophores using synthetically modified MS2 viral capsids. *J Am Chem Soc* 2013;**135**(8):3011−6.
22. Tong GJ, Hsiao SC, Carrico ZM, Francis MB. Viral capsid DNA aptamer conjugates as multivalent cell-targeting vehicles. *J Am Chem Soc* 2009;**131**(31):11174−8.
23. Obermeyer AC, Capehart SL, Jarman JB, Francis MB. Multivalent viral capsids with internal cargo for fibrin imaging. *PLoS One* 2014;**9**(6):e100678.
24. Carrico ZM, Romanini DW, Mehl RA, Francis MB. Oxidative coupling of peptides to a virus capsid containing unnatural amino acids. *Chem Commun* 2008;(10):1205−7.
25. Farkas ME, Aanei IL, Behrens CR, Tong GJ, Murphy ST, O'Neil JP, Francis MB. PET Imaging and biodistribution of chemically modified bacteriophage MS2. *Mol Pharm* 2013;**10**(1):69−76.
26. Stephanopoulos N, Carrico ZM, Francis MB. Nanoscale integration of sensitizing chromophores and porphyrins with bacteriophage MS2. *Angew Chem Int Ed Engl* 2009;**48**(50):9498−502.
27. El Muslemany KM, Twite AA, ElSohly AM, Obermeyer AC, Mathies RA, Francis MB. Photoactivated bioconjugation between ortho-azidophenols and anilines: a facile approach to biomolecular photopatterning. *J Am Chem Soc* 2014;**136**(36):12600−6.
28. Garimella PD, Datta A, Romanini DW, Raymond KN, Francis MB. Multivalent, high-relaxivity MRI contrast agents using rigid cysteine-reactive gadolinium complexes. *J Am Chem Soc* 2011;**133**(37):14704−9.
29. Wu W, Hsiao SC, Carrico ZM, Francis MB. Genome-free viral capsids as multivalent carriers for taxol delivery. *Angew Chem* 2009;**48**(50):9493−7.
30. Schlick TL, Ding Z, Kovacs EW, Francis MB. Dual-surface modification of the tobacco mosaic virus. *J Am Chem Soc* 2005;**127**(11):3718−23.
31. Wu M, Shi J, Fan D, Zhou Q, Wang F, Niu Z, Huang Y. Biobehavior in normal and tumor-bearing mice of tobacco mosaic virus. *Biomacromolecules* 2013;**14**(11):4032−7.
32. Bruckman MA, Jiang K, Simpson EJ, Randolph LN, Luyt LG, Yu X, Steinmetz NF. Dual-modal magnetic resonance and fluorescence imaging of atherosclerotic plaques in vivo using VCAM-1 targeted tobacco mosaic virus. *Nano Lett* 2014;**14**(3):1551−8.
33. Bruckman MA, Hern S, Jiang K, Flask CA, Yu X, Steinmetz NF. Tobacco mosaic virus rods and spheres as supramolecular high-relaxivity MRI contrast agents. *J Mater Chem B* 2013;**1**(10):1482−90.
34. Yin Z, Nguyen HG, Chowdhury S, Bentley P, Bruckman MA, Miermont A, Gildersleeve JC, Wang Q, Huang X. Tobacco mosaic virus as a new carrier for tumor associated carbohydrate antigens. *Bioconjug Chem* 2012;**23**(8):1694−703.
35. Hu J, Wang P, Zhao X, Lv L, Yang S, Song B, Wang Q. Charge-transfer interactions for the fabrication of multifunctional viral nanoparticles. *Chem Commun* 2014;**50**(91):14125−8.
36. Sitasuwan P, Lee LA, Li K, Nguyen HG, Wang Q. RGD-conjugated rod-like viral nanoparticles on 2D scaffold improve bone differentiation of mesenchymal stem cells. *Front Chem* 2014;**2**. 31-31.
37. Chen L, Zhao X, Lin Y, Huang Y, Wang Q. A supramolecular strategy to assemble multifunctional viral nanoparticles. *Chem Commun* 2013;**49**(83):9678−80.
38. Bruckman MA, Liu J, Koley G, Li Y, Benicewicz B, Niu Z, Wang Q. Tobacco mosaic virus based thin film sensor for detection of volatile organic compounds. *J Mater Chem* 2010;**20**(27):5715−9.
39. Miller RA, Presley AD, Francis MB. Self-assembling light-harvesting systems from synthetically modified tobacco mosaic virus coat proteins. *J Am Chem Soc* 2007;**129**(11):3104−9.

40. Miller RA, Stephanopoulos N, McFarland JM, Rosko AS, Geissler PL, Francis MB. Impact of assembly state on the defect tolerance of TMV-based light harvesting arrays. *J Am Chem Soc* 2010;**132**(17):6068–74.
41. Obermeyer AC, Jarman JB, Francis MB. N-terminal modification of proteins with o-aminophenols. *J Am Chem Soc* 2014;**136**(27):9572–9.
42. Yin Z, Comellas-Aragones M, Chowdhury S, Bentley P, Kaczanowska K, BenMohamed L, Gildersleeve JC, Finn MG, Huang X. Boosting immunity to small tumor-associated carbohydrates with bacteriophage Qβ capsids. *ACS Chem Biol* 2013;**8**(6):1253–62.
43. Hong V, Presolski SI, Ma C, Finn MG. Analysis and optimization of copper-catalyzed azide–alkyne cycloaddition for bioconjugation. *Angew Chem Int Ed* 2009;**48**(52):9879–83.
44. Mead G, Hiley M, Ng T, Fihn C, Hong K, Groner M, Miner W, Drugan D, Hollingsworth W, Udit AK. Directed polyvalent display of sulfated ligands on virus nanoparticles elicits heparin-like anticoagulant activity. *Bioconjug Chem* 2014;**25**(8):1444–52.
45. Pokorski JK, Hovlid ML, Finn MG. Cell targeting with hybrid Qβ virus-like particles displaying epidermal growth factor. *Chembiochem* 2011;**12**(16):2441–7.
46. Banerjee D, Liu AP, Voss NR, Schmid SL, Finn MG. Multivalent display and receptor-mediated endocytosis of transferrin on virus-like particles. *Chembiochem* 2010;**11**(9):1273–9.
47. Manzenrieder F, Luxenhofer R, Retzlaff M, Jordan R, Finn MG. Stabilization of virus-like particles with poly(2-oxazoline)s. *Angew Chem* 2011;**50**(11):2601–5.
48. Steinmetz NF, Hong V, Spoerke ED, Lu P, Breitenkamp K, Finn MG, Manchester M. Buckyballs meet viral nanoparticles: candidates for biomedicine. *J Am Chem Soc* 2009;**131**(47):17093–5.
49. Astronomo RD, Kaltgrad E, Udit AK, Wang SK, Doores KJ, Huang CY, Pantophlet R, Paulson JC, Wong CH, Finn MG, Burton DR. Defining criteria for oligomannose immunogens for HIV using icosahedral virus capsid scaffolds. *Chem Biol* 2010;**17**(4):357–70.
50. Kaltgrad E, O'Reilly MK, Liao L, Han S, Paulson JC, Finn MG. On-virus construction of polyvalent glycan ligands for cell-surface receptors. *J Am Chem Soc* 2008;**130**(14):4578–9.
51. Prasuhn JDE, Yeh RM, Obenaus A, Manchester M, Finn MG. Viral MRI contrast agents: coordination of Gd by native virions and attachment of Gd complexes by azide–alkyne cycloaddition. *Chem Commun* 2007;(12):1269–71.
52. Hovlid ML, Lau JL, Breitenkamp K, Higginson CJ, Laufer B, Manchester M, Finn MG. Encapsidated atom-transfer radical polymerization in Qbeta virus-like nanoparticles. *ACS Nano* 2014;**8**(8):8003–14.
53. Qazi S, Uchida M, Usselman R, Shearer R, Edwards E, Douglas T. Manganese(III) porphyrins complexed with P22 virus-like particles as T1-enhanced contrast agents for magnetic resonance imaging. *J Biol Inorg Chem* 2014;**19**(2):237–46.
54. Lucon J, Edwards E, Qazi S, Uchida M, Douglas T. Atom transfer radical polymerization on the interior of the P22 capsid and incorporation of photocatalytic monomer crosslinks. *Eur Polym J* 2013;**49**(10):2976–85.
55. Min J, Moon H, Yang HJ, Shin H-H, Hong SY, Kang S. Development of P22 viral capsid nanocomposites as anti-cancer drug, bortezomib (BTZ), delivery nanoplatforms. *Macromol Biosci* 2014;**14**(4):557–64.
56. Qazi S, Liepold LO, Abedin MJ, Johnson B, Prevelige P, Frank JA, Douglas T. P22 viral capsids as nanocomposite high-relaxivity MRI contrast agents. *Mol Pharm* 2013;**10**(1):11–7.
57. Kang S, Lander GC, Johnson JE, Prevelige PE. Development of bacteriophage P22 as a platform for molecular display: genetic and chemical modifications of the procapsid exterior surface. *Chembiochem* 2008;**9**(4):514–8.
58. Anand P, O'Neil A, Lin E, Douglas T, Holford M. Tailored delivery of analgesic ziconotide across a blood brain barrier model using viral nanocontainers. *Sci Rep* 2015;**5**:12497.
59. Servid A, Jordan P, O'Neil A, Prevelige P, Douglas T. Location of the bacteriophage P22 coat protein C-terminus provides opportunities for the design of capsid-based materials. *Biomacromolecules* 2013;**14**(9):2989–95.
60. Brunel FM, Lewis JD, Destito G, Steinmetz NF, Manchester M, Stuhlmann H, Dawson PE. Hydrazone ligation strategy to assemble multifunctional viral nanoparticles for cell imaging and tumor targeting. *Nano Lett* 2010;**10**(3):1093–7.
61. Hovlid ML, Steinmetz NF, Laufer B, Lau JL, Kuzelka J, Wang Q, Hyypiä T, Nemerow GR, Kessler H, Manchester M, Finn MG. Guiding plant virus particles to integrin-displaying cells. *Nanoscale* 2012;**4**(12):3698–705.
62. Destito G, Yeh R, Rae CS, Finn MG, Manchester M. Folic acid-mediated targeting of cowpea mosaic virus particles to tumor cells. *Chem Bio* 2007;**14**(10):1152–62.
63. Sen Gupta S, Kuzelka J, Singh P, Lewis WG, Manchester M, Finn MG. Accelerated bioorthogonal conjugation: a practical method for the ligation of diverse functional molecules to a polyvalent virus scaffold. *Bioconjug Chem* 2005;**16**(6):1572–9.
64. Comellas-Aragonès M, de la Escosura A, Dirks AJ, van der Ham A, Fusté-Cuñé A, Cornelissen JJLM, Nolte RJM. Controlled integration of polymers into viral capsids. *Biomacromolecules* 2009;**10**(11):3141–7.
65. Singh P, Prasuhn D, Yeh RM, Destito G, Rae CS, Osborn K, Finn MG, Manchester M. Bio-distribution, toxicity and pathology of cowpea mosaic virus nanoparticles in vivo. *J Control Release* 2007;**120**(1–2):41–50.
66. Steinmetz NF, Manchester M. PEGylated viral nanoparticles for biomedicine: the impact of PEG chain length on VNP cell interactions in vitro and ex vivo. *Biomacromolecules* 2009;**10**(4):784–92.
67. Shukla S, Ablack AL, Wen AM, Lee KL, Lewis JD, Steinmetz NF. Increased tumor homing and tissue penetration of the filamentous plant viral nanoparticle Potato virus X. *Mol Pharm* 2013;**10**(1):33–42.
68. Steinmetz NF, Lomonossoff GP, Evans DJ. Decoration of cowpea mosaic virus with multiple, redox-active, organometallic complexes. *Small* 2006;**2**(4):530–3.
69. Wu Z, Chen K, Yildiz I, Dirksen A, Fischer R, Dawson PE, Steinmetz NF. Development of viral nanoparticles for efficient intracellular delivery. *Nanoscale* 2012;**4**(11):3567–76.
70. Chatterji A, Ochoa W, Shamieh L, Salakian SP, Wong SM, Clinton G, Ghosh P, Lin T, Johnson JE. Chemical conjugation of heterologous proteins on the surface of Cowpea mosaic virus. *Bioconjug Chem* 2004;**15**(4):807–13.

71. Noad R, Roy P. Virus-like particles as immunogens. *Trends Microbiol* 2003;**11**(9):438–44.
72. Akahata W, Yang Z-Y, Andersen H, Sun S, Holdaway HA, Kong W-P, Lewis MG, Higgs S, Rossmann MG, Rao S, Nabel GJ. A virus-like particle vaccine for epidemic Chikungunya virus protects nonhuman primates against infection. *Nat Med* 2010;**16**(3):334–8.
73. Naskalska A, Pyrc K. Virus like particles as immunogens and universal nanocarriers. *Pol J Microbiol* 2015;**64**(1):3–13.
74. Roldao A, Mellado MC, Castilho LR, Carrondo MJ, Alves PM. Virus-like particles in vaccine development. *Expert Rev Vaccines* 2010;**9**(10):1149–76.
75. Kushnir N, Streatfield SJ, Yusibov V. Virus-like particles as a highly efficient vaccine platform: diversity of targets and production systems and advances in clinical development. *Vaccine* 2012;**31**(1):58–83.
76. Dharmarwardana M, Martins AF, Chen Z, Palacios PM, Nowak CM, Welch RP, Li S, Luzuriaga MA, Bleris L, Pierce BS, Sherry AD, Gassensmith JJ. Nitroxyl modified tobacco mosaic virus as a metal-free high-relaxivity MRI and EPR active superoxide sensor. *Mol Pharm* 2018;**15**(8):2973–83.
77. Nanduri V, Balasubramanian S, Sista S, Vodyanoy VJ, Simonian AL. Highly sensitive phage-based biosensor for the detection of β-galactosidase. *Anal Chim Acta* 2007;**589**(2):166–72.
78. Moon J-S, Park M, Kim W-G, Kim C, Hwang J, Seol D, Kim C-S, Sohn J-R, Chung H, Oh J-W. M-13 bacteriophage based structural color sensor for detecting antibiotics. *Sens Actuators B Chem* 2017;**240**:757–62.
79. Molino NM, Wang S-W. Caged protein nanoparticles for drug delivery. *Curr Opin Biotechnol* 2014;**28**:75–82.
80. Schwarz B, Douglas T. Development of virus-like particles for diagnostic and prophylactic biomedical applications. *Wiley Interdiscip Rev Nanomed Nanobiotechnol* 2015;**7**(5):722–35.
81. Lee KL, Shukla S, Wu M, Ayat NR, El Sanadi CE, Wen AM, Edelbrock JF, Pokorski JK, Commandeur U, Dubyak GR, Steinmetz NF. Stealth filaments: polymer chain length and conformation affect the in vivo fate of PEGylated potato virus X. *Acta Biomaterialia* 2015;**19**:166–79.
82. Aanei IL, ElSohly AM, Farkas ME, Netirojjanakul C, Regan M, Taylor Murphy S, O'Neil JP, Seo Y, Francis MB. Biodistribution of antibody-MS2 viral capsid conjugates in breast cancer models. *Mol Pharm* 2016;**13**(11):3764–72.
83. Prasuhn Jr DE, Singh P, Strable E, Brown S, Manchester M, Finn MG. Plasma clearance of bacteriophage Qbeta particles as a function of surface charge. *J Am Chem Soc* 2008;**130**(4):1328–34.
84. Agrawal A, Manchester M. Differential uptake of chemically modified cowpea mosaic virus nanoparticles in macrophage subpopulations present in inflammatory and tumor microenvironments. *Biomacromolecules* 2012;**13**(10):3320–6.
85. Lee H, Benjamin CE, Nowak CM, Tuong LH, Welch RP, Chen Z, Dharmarwardana M, Murray KW, Bleris L, D'Arcy S, Gassensmith JJ. Regulating the uptake of viral nanoparticles in macrophage and cancer cells via a pH switch. *Mol Pharm* 2018;**15**(8):2984–90.
86. Mishra P, Nayak B, Dey RK. PEGylation in anti-cancer therapy: an overview. *Asian J Pharm Sci* 2016;**11**(3):337–48.
87. Cho J, Lim SI, Yang BS, Hahn YS, Kwon I. Generation of therapeutic protein variants with the human serum albumin binding capacity via site-specific fatty acid conjugation. *Sci Rep* 2017;**7**(1):18041.
88. Gulati NM, Pitek AS, Czapar AE, Stewart PL, Steinmetz NF. The in vivo fates of plant viral nanoparticles camouflaged using self-proteins: overcoming immune recognition. *J Mater Chem B* 2018;**6**(15):2204–16.
89. Minko T, Dharap SS, Pakunlu RI, Wang Y. Molecular targeting of drug delivery systems to cancer. *Curr Drug Targets* 2004;**5**(4):389–406.
90. Rohovie MJ, Nagasawa M, Swartz JR. Virus-like particles: next-generation nanoparticles for targeted therapeutic delivery. *Bioeng Transl Med* 2017;**2**(1):43–57.
91. Chen Z, Li N, Chen L, Lee J, Gassensmith JJ. Dual functionalized bacteriophage Qbeta as a photocaged drug carrier. *Small* 2016;**12**(33):4563–71.
92. Pokorski JK, Steinmetz NF. The art of engineering viral nanoparticles. *Mol Pharm* 2011;**8**(1):29–43.
93. Kundig TM, Klimek L, Schendzielorz P, Renner WA, Senti G, Bachmann MF. Is the allergen really needed in allergy immunotherapy? *Current Treat Options Allergy* 2015;**2**(1):72–82.
94. Engeroff P, Caviezel F, Storni F, Thoms F, Vogel M, Bachmann MF. Allergens displayed on virus-like particles are highly immunogenic but fail to activate human mast cells. *Allergy* 2018;**73**(2):341–9.
95. Grgacic EV, Anderson DA. Virus-like particles: passport to immune recognition. *Methods* 2006;**40**(1):60–5.
96. Chen Z, Detvo ST, Pham E, Gassensmith JJ. Making conjugation-induced fluorescent PEGylated virus-like particles by dibromomaleimide-disulfide chemistry. *J Vis Exp* 2018;**135**:e57712.
97. van Zyl AR, Hitzeroth II . Purification of virus-like particles (VLPs) from plants. *Methods Mol Biol* 2016;**1404**:569–79.
98. Zeltins A. Construction and characterization of virus-like particles: a review. *Mol Biotechnol* 2013;**53**(1):92–107.
99. Fuenmayor J, Gòdia F, Cervera L. Production of virus-like particles for vaccines. *New Biotechnol* 2017;**39**:174–80.
100. Chen Z, Li N, Li S, Dharmarwardana M, Schlimme A, Gassensmith JJ. Viral chemistry: the chemical functionalization of viral architectures to create new technology. *Wiley Interdiscip Rev Nanomed Nanobiotechnol* 2016;**8**(4):512–34.
101. Li K, Nguyen HG, Lu X, Wang Q. Viruses and their potential in bioimaging and biosensing applications. *Analyst* 2010;**135**(1):21–7.
102. Tagit O, de Ruiter MV, Brasch M, Ma Y, Cornelissen JJLM. Quantum dot encapsulation in virus-like particles with tuneable structural properties and low toxicity. *RSC Adv* 2017;**7**(60):38110–8.
103. Yildiz I, Shukla S, Steinmetz NF. Applications of viral nanoparticles in medicine. *Curr Opin Biotechnol* 2011;**22**(6):901–8.
104. Robertson KL, Liu JL. Engineered viral nanoparticles for flow cytometry and fluorescence microscopy applications. *Wiley Interdiscip Rev Nanomed Nanobiotechnol* 2012;**4**(5):511–24.
105. Chen Z, Boyd SD, Calvo JS, Murray KW, Mejia GL, Benjamin CE, Welch RP, Winkler DD, Meloni G, D'Arcy S, Gassensmith JJ. Fluorescent functionalization across quaternary structure in a virus-like particle. *Bioconjug Chem* 2017;**28**(9):2277–83.
106. Lewis JD, Destito G, Zijlstra A, Gonzalez MJ, Quigley JP, Manchester M, Stuhlmann H. Viral nanoparticles as tools for intravital vascular imaging. *Nat Med* 2006;**12**(3):354–60.

107. Steinmetz NF, Ablack AL, Hickey JL, Ablack J, Manocha B, Mymryk JS, Luyt LG, Lewis JD. Intravital imaging of human prostate cancer using viral nanoparticles targeted to gastrin-releasing peptide receptors. *Small* 2011;**7**(12):1664–72.
108. Carrico ZM, Farkas ME, Zhou Y, Hsiao SC, Marks JD, Chokhawala H, Clark DS, Francis MB. N-Terminal labeling of filamentous phage to create cancer marker imaging agents. *ACS Nano* 2012;**6**(8):6675–80.
109. Wen AM, Rambhia PH, French RH, Steinmetz NF. Design rules for nanomedical engineering: from physical virology to the applications of virus-based materials in medicine. *J Biol Phys* 2013;**39**(2):301–25.
110. Bruckman MA, Randolph LN, VanMeter A, Hern S, Shoffstall AJ, Taurog RE, Steinmetz NF. Biodistribution, pharmacokinetics, and blood compatibility of native and PEGylated tobacco mosaic virus nano-rods and -spheres in mice. *Virology* 2014;**449**:163–73.
111. Liepold L, Anderson S, Willits D, Oltrogge L, Frank JA, Douglas T, Young M. Viral capsids as MRI contrast agents. *Magn Reson Med* 2007;**58**(5):871–9.
112. Sowers MA, McCombs JR, Wang Y, Paletta JT, Morton SW, Dreaden EC, Boska MD, Ottaviani MF, Hammond PT, Rajca A, Johnson JA. Redox-responsive branched-bottlebrush polymers for in vivo MRI and fluorescence imaging. *Nat Commun* 2014;**5**. 5460-5460.
113. Merbach, A.; Helm, L.; Tóth, É., 2013; p 0.
114. Nguyen HVT, Chen Q, Paletta JT, Harvey P, Jiang Y, Zhang H, Boska MD, Ottaviani MF, Jasanoff A, Rajca A, Johnson JA. Nitroxide-based macromolecular contrast agents with unprecedented transverse relaxivity and stability for magnetic resonance imaging of tumors. *ACS Central Science* 2017;**3**(7):800–11.
115. Meldrum T, Seim KL, Bajaj VS, Palaniappan KK, Wu W, Francis MB, Wemmer DE, Pines A. A xenon-based molecular sensor assembled on an MS2 viral capsid scaffold. *J Am Chem Soc* 2010;**132**(17):5936–7.
116. Xiao L, Zhu A, Xu Q, Chen Y, Xu J, Weng J. Colorimetric biosensor for detection of cancer biomarker by Au nanoparticle-decorated Bi2Se3 nanosheets. *ACS Appl Mater Interfaces* 2017;**9**(8):6931–40.
117. Wang P, Xu G, Qin L, Li Y, Li R. Cell-based biosensors and its application in biomedicine. *Sens Actuators B Chem* 2005;**108**(1–2):576–84.
118. Kara P, de la Escosura-Muniz A, Maltez-da Costa M, Guix M, Ozsoz M, Merkoci A. Aptamers based electrochemical biosensor for protein detection using carbon nanotubes platforms. *Biosens Bioelectron* 2010;**26**(4):1715–8.
119. Yoo EH, Lee SY. Glucose biosensors: an overview of use in clinical practice. *Sensors* 2010;**10**(5):4558–76.
120. Mao C, Liu A, Cao B. Virus-based chemical and biological sensing. *Angew Chem* 2009;**48**(37):6790–810.
121. Tscherne DM, Manicassamy B, Garcia-Sastre A. An enzymatic virus-like particle assay for sensitive detection of virus entry. *J Virol Methods* 2010;**163**(2):336–43.
122. Koch C, Wabbel K, Eber FJ, Krolla-Sidenstein P, Azucena C, Gliemann H, Eiben S, Geiger F, Wege C. Modified TMV particles as beneficial scaffolds to present sensor enzymes. *Front Plant Sci* 2015;**6**(1137).
123. Jablonski M, Koch C, Bronder TS, Poghossian A, Wege C, Schöning MJ. Field-effect biosensors modified with tobacco mosaic virus nanotubes as enzyme nanocarrier. *Proceedings* 2017;**1**(4).
124. Poghossian A, Jablonski M, Koch C, Bronder TS, Rolka D, Wege C, Schoning MJ. Field-effect biosensor using virus particles as scaffolds for enzyme immobilization. *Biosens Bioelectron* 2018;**110**:168–74.
125. Bäcker M, Koch C, Eiben S, Geiger F, Eber F, Gliemann H, Poghossian A, Wege C, Schöning MJ. Tobacco mosaic virus as enzyme nanocarrier for electrochemical biosensors. *Sens Actuators B Chem* 2017;**238**:716–22.
126. Kim D, Daniel WL, Mirkin CA. Microarray-based multiplexed scanometric immunoassay for protein cancer markers using gold nanoparticle probes. *Anal Chem* 2009;**81**(21):9183–7.
127. Brasino M, Lee JH, Cha JN. Creating highly amplified enzyme-linked immunosorbent assay signals from genetically engineered bacteriophage. *Anal Biochem* 2015;**470**:7–13.
128. Lee JH, Cha JN. Amplified protein detection through visible plasmon shifts in gold nanocrystal solutions from bacteriophage platforms. *Anal Chem* 2011;**83**(9):3516–9.
129. Lee JH, Xu PF, Domaille DW, Choi C, Jin S, Cha JN. M13 bacteriophage as materials for amplified surface enhanced Raman scattering protein sensing. *Adv Funct Mater* 2013;**24**(14):2079–84.
130. Domaille DW, Lee JH, Cha JN. High density DNA loading on the M13 bacteriophage provides access to colorimetric and fluorescent protein microarray biosensors. *Chem Commun (Camb)* 2013;**49**(17):1759–61.
131. Guo J, Zhao X, Hu J, Lin Y, Wang Q. Tobacco mosaic virus with peroxidase-like activity for cancer cell detection through colorimetric assay. *Mol Pharm* 2018;**15**(8):2946–53.
132. Ben-Yoav H, Brown A, Pomerantseva E, L Kelly D, N Culver J, Ghodssi R. Tobacco mosaaic virus biotemplated electrochemical biosensor. 2012.
133. Zang F, Gerasopoulos K, Brown AD, Culver JN, Ghodssi R. Capillary microfluidics-assembled virus-like particle bionanoreceptor interfaces for label-free biosensing. *ACS Appl Mater Interfaces* 2017;**9**(10):8471–9.
134. Jia Y, Qin M, Zhang H, Niu W, Li X, Wang L, Li X, Bai Y, Cao Y, Feng X. Label-free biosensor: a novel phage-modified Light Addressable Potentiometric Sensor system for cancer cell monitoring. *Biosens Bioelectron* 2007;**22**(12):3261–6.
135. Brun MJ, Gomez EJ, Suh J. Stimulus-responsive viral vectors for controlled delivery of therapeutics. *J Control Release* 2017;**267**:80–9.
136. Hubbell JA, Chilkoti A. Nanomaterials for drug delivery. *Science* 2012;**337**(6092):303–5.
137. Suri SS, Fenniri H, Singh B. Nanotechnology-based drug delivery systems. *J Occup Med Toxicol* 2007;**2**:16.
138. Li SD, Huang L. Pharmacokinetics and biodistribution of nanoparticles. *Mol Pharm* 2008;**5**(4):496–504.
139. Ventola CL. Progress in nanomedicine: approved and investigational nanodrugs. *PT* 2017;**42**(12):742–55.
140. Moghimi SM, Szebeni J. Stealth liposomes and long circulating nanoparticles: critical issues in pharmacokinetics, opsonization and protein-binding properties. *Prog Lipid Res* 2003;**42**(6):463–78.
141. Ishida T, Masuda K, Ichikawa T, Ichihara M, Irimura K, Kiwada H. Accelerated clearance of a second injection of PEGylated liposomes in mice. *Int J Pharm* 2003;**255**(1):167–74.

142. Ishida T, Ichihara M, Wang X, Kiwada H. Spleen plays an important role in the induction of accelerated blood clearance of PEGylated liposomes. *J Control Release* 2006;**115**(3):243–50.
143. Ishida T, Harada M, Wang XY, Ichihara M, Irimura K, Kiwada H. Accelerated blood clearance of PEGylated liposomes following preceding liposome injection: effects of lipid dose and PEG surface-density and chain length of the first-dose liposomes. *J Control Release* 2005;**105**(3):305–17.
144. Gabizon A, Tzemach D, Mak L, Bronstein M, Horowitz AT. Dose dependency of pharmacokinetics and therapeutic efficacy of pegylated liposomal doxorubicin (DOXIL) in murine models. *J Drug Target* 2002;**10**(7):539–48.
145. Allen TM, Cullis PR. Liposomal drug delivery systems: from concept to clinical applications. *Adv Drug Deliv Rev* 2013;**65**(1):36–48.
146. Sercombe L, Veerati T, Moheimani F, Wu SY, Sood AK, Hua S. Advances and challenges of liposome assisted drug delivery. *Front Pharmacol* 2015;**6**. 286-286.
147. Pan Y, Zhang Y, Jia T, Zhang K, Li J, Wang L. Development of a microRNA delivery system based on bacteriophage MS2 virus-like particles. *FEBS J* 2012;**279**(7):1198–208.
148. Prel A, Caval V, Gayon R, Ravassard P, Duthoit C, Payen E, Maouche-Chretien L, Creneguy A, Nguyen TH, Martin N, Piver E, Sevrain R, Lamouroux L, Leboulch P, Deschaseaux F, Bouille P, Sensebe L, Pages JC. Highly efficient in vitro and in vivo delivery of functional RNAs using new versatile MS2-chimeric retrovirus-like particles. *Mol Ther Methods Clin Dev* 2015;**2** (2329-0501 (Print)).
149. Lam P, Steinmetz NF. Plant viral and bacteriophage delivery of nucleic acid therapeutics. *Wiley Interdiscip Rev Nanomed Nanobiotechnol* 2018;**10**(1):e1487.
150. Yao Y, Jia T, Pan Y, Gou H, Li Y, Sun Y, Zhang R, Zhang K, Lin G, Xie J, Li J, Wang L. Using a novel microRNA delivery system to inhibit osteoclastogenesis. *Int J Mol Sci* 2015;**16**(4):8337–50.
151. Kwak M, Minten IJ, Anaya D-M, Musser AJ, Brasch M, Nolte RJM, Müllen K, Cornelissen JJLM, Herrmann A. Virus-like particles templated by DNA micelles: a general method for loading virus nanocarriers. *J Am Chem Soc* 2010;**132**(23):7834–5.
152. Touze A, Coursaget P. In vitro gene transfer using human papillomavirus-like particles. *Nucleic Acids Res* 1998;**26**(5):1317–23.
153. Xu, Y. F.; Zhang YQ - Xu, X. M.; Xu Xm Fau - Song, G. X.; Song, G. X., Papillomavirus virus-like particles as vehicles for the delivery of epitopes or genes. Arch Virol (0304-8608 [Print]).
154. Lau JL, Baksh MM, Fiedler JD, Brown SD, Kussrow A, Bornhop DJ, Ordoukhanian P, Finn MG. Evolution and protein packaging of small-molecule RNA aptamers. *ACS Nano* 2011;**5**(10):7722–9.
155. Fiedler JD, Brown SD, Lau JL, Finn MG. RNA-directed packaging of enzymes within virus-like particles. *Angew Chem* 2010;**49**(50):9648–51.
156. Benjamin CE, Chen Z, Kang P, Wilson BA, Li N, Nielsen SO, Qin Z, Gassensmith JJ. Site-selective nucleation and size control of gold nanoparticle photothermal antennae on the pore structures of a virus. *J Am Chem Soc* 2018;**140**(49):17226–33.
157. Franke CE, Czapar AE, Patel RB, Steinmetz NF. Tobacco mosaic virus-delivered cisplatin restores efficacy in platinum-resistant ovarian cancer cells. *Mol Pharm* 2018;**15**(8):2922–31.
158. Zeng Q, Wen H, Wen Q, Chen X, Wang Y, Xuan W, Liang J, Wan S. Cucumber mosaic virus as drug delivery vehicle for doxorubicin. *Biomaterials* 2013;**34**(19):4632–42.
159. Pitek AS, Wang Y, Gulati S, Gao H, Stewart PL, Simon DI, Steinmetz NF. Elongated plant virus-based nanoparticles for enhanced delivery of thrombolytic therapies. *Mol Pharm* 2017;**14**(11):3815–23.
160. Aljabali AA, Shukla S, Lomonossoff GP, Steinmetz NF, Evans DJ. CPMV-DOX delivers. *Mol Pharm* 2013;**10**(1):3–10.
161. Vernekar AA, Berger G, Czapar AE, Veliz FA, Wang DI, Steinmetz NF, Lippard SJ. Speciation of phenanthriplatin and its analogs in the core of tobacco mosaic virus. *J Am Chem Soc* 2018;**140**(12):4279–87.
162. Masarapu H, Patel BK, Chariou PL, Hu H, Gulati NM, Carpenter BL, Ghiladi RA, Shukla S, Steinmetz NF. Physalis mottle virus-like particles as nanocarriers for imaging reagents and drugs. *Biomacromolecules* 2017;**18**(12):4141–53.
163. Kaczmarczyk SJ, Sitaraman K, Young HA, Hughes SH, Chatterjee DK. Protein delivery using engineered virus-like particles. *Proc Natl Acad Sci USA* 2011;**108**(41):16998–7003.
164. Minten IJ, Hendriks LJA, Nolte RJM, Cornelissen JJLM. Controlled encapsulation of multiple proteins in virus capsids. *J Am Chem Soc* 2009;**131**(49):17771–3.
165. Setaro F, Brasch M, Hahn U, Koay MST, Cornelissen JJLM, de la Escosura A, Torres T. Generation-dependent templated self-assembly of biohybrid protein nanoparticles around photosensitizer dendrimers. *Nano Lett* 2015;**15**(2):1245–51.
166. Madaan K, Kumar S, Poonia N, Lather V, Pandita D. Dendrimers in drug delivery and targeting: drug-dendrimer interactions and toxicity issues. *J Pharm BioAllied Sci* 2014;**6**(3):139–50.
167. Miao Y, Johnson JE, Ortoleva PJ. All-atom multiscale simulation of cowpea chlorotic mottle virus capsid swelling. *J Phys Chem B* 2010;**114**(34):11181–95.
168. Wilts BD, Schaap IAT, Schmidt CF. Swelling and softening of the cowpea chlorotic mottle virus in response to pH shifts. *Biophys J* 2015;**108**(10):2541–9.
169. Asensio MA, Morella NM, Jakobson CM, Hartman EC, Glasgow JE, Sankaran B, Zwart PH, Tullman-Ercek D. A selection for assembly reveals that a single amino acid mutant of the bacteriophage MS2 coat protein forms a smaller virus-like particle. *Nano Lett* 2016;**16**(9):5944–50.
170. Cadena-Nava RD, Comas-Garcia M, Garmann RF, Rao AL, Knobler CM, Gelbart WM. Self-assembly of viral capsid protein and RNA molecules of different sizes: requirement for a specific high protein/RNA mass ratio. *J Virol* 2012;**86**(6):3318–26.
171. Rurup WF, Verbij F, Koay MST, Blum C, Subramaniam V, Cornelissen JJLM. Predicting the loading of virus-like particles with fluorescent proteins. *Biomacromolecules* 2014;**15**(2):558–63.
172. Stephanopoulos N, Tong GJ, Hsiao SC, Francis MB. Dual-surface modified virus capsids for targeted delivery of photodynamic agents to cancer cells. *ACS Nano* 2010;**4**(10):6014–20.
173. Zhang X, Xin L, Li S, Fang M, Zhang J, Xia N, Zhao Q. Lessons learned from successful human vaccines: delineating key epitopes by dissecting the capsid proteins. *Hum Vaccines Immunother* 2015;**11**(5):1277–92.
174. Jegerlehner A, Zabel F, Langer A, Dietmeier K, Jennings GT, Saudan P, Bachmann MF. Bacterially produced recombinant influenza vaccines based on virus-like particles. *PLoS One* 2013;**8**(11):e78947.

175. Storni T, Ruedl C, Schwarz K, Schwendener RA, Renner WA, Bachmann MF. Nonmethylated CG motifs packaged into virus-like particles induce protective cytotoxic T cell responses in the absence of systemic side effects. *J Immunol* 2004;**172**(3):1777–85.

176. Cornuz J, Zwahlen S, Jungi WF, Osterwalder J, Klingler K, van Melle G, Bangala Y, Guessous I, Müller P, Willers J, Maurer P, Bachmann MF, Cerny T. A vaccine against nicotine for smoking cessation: a randomized controlled trial. *PLoS One* 2008;**3**(6):e2547.

177. Watanabe T, Watanabe S, Neumann G, Kida H, Kawaoka Y. Immunogenicity and protective efficacy of replication-incompetent influenza virus-like particles. *J Virol* 2002;**76**(2):767.

178. Li B, Yuan Z, Hung H-C, Ma J, Jain P, Tsao C, Xie J, Zhang P, Lin X, Wu K, Jiang S. Revealing the immunogenic risk of polymers. *Angew Chem Int Ed* 2018;**57**(42):13873–6.

Chapter 12

Engineering gold nanoparticles for photothermal therapy, surgery, and imaging

Jillian Stabile[1,a], Daniel Najafali[1,a], Yahya Cheema[1], Collin T. Inglut[1], Barry J. Liang[1], Swapna Vaja[1], Aaron J. Sorrin[1] and Huang-Chiao Huang[1,2]

[1]*Fischell Department of Bioengineering, University of Maryland, College Park, MD, United States;* [2]*Marlene and Stewart Greenebaum Cancer Center, University of Maryland School of Medicine, Baltimore, MD, United States*

12.1 Introduction—The evolution of gold nanomedicine

The applications of nanotechnology have expanded over the past 4 decades to address the clinical challenges associated with various diseases.[1,2] In its early stages, nanotechnology's role in medicine was overlooked, with efforts instead being focused on studying nanoscale particles from a strictly materials science perspective.[1–7] Over time, it became apparent that the benefits of nanotechnology could be applied to healthcare, initiating a new field of scientific inquiry: nanomedicine.[3–7]

Nanomedicine employs autonomous nanoscale materials toward sites of disease for effective therapy.[6] In 2018, roughly 1,735,350 individuals in the United States were diagnosed with cancer and an estimated 609,640 will die from the disease (cancer.gov). With such a high rate of mortality, theranostic multifunctional nanomaterials have emerged as a promising modality that offers simultaneous diagnosis and treatment.[8] Nanoparticles show promising medical success, adding to the repertoire of cancer treatments, and their capabilities have been extensively explored in drug delivery, bioimaging, and phototherapy. Specifically, gold nanoparticles (GNPs) offer superior chemical, optical, electronic, and physical properties compared to other nanoparticles. Among the list of important properties are strong absorption and accumulation rates, greater biocompatibility compared to other metals, and simplistic surface chemistry that aids molecular attachments.[1,2,6,9]

The surface of GNPs can be decorated and coated with reactive functional groups such as thiol, amine, and phosphate-containing groups, which make functionalizing GNPs with DNA, proteins, and small molecules possible (Fig. 12.1).[1,2,6,9] Modifying the surface chemistry of gold hinders its ability to form aggregates and influences the stability, efficacy, and toxicity of the gold particles.[1,2,6,9] GNPs can be fabricated in a variety of different geometries, including nanospheres, nanorods, nanoshells, nanocages,

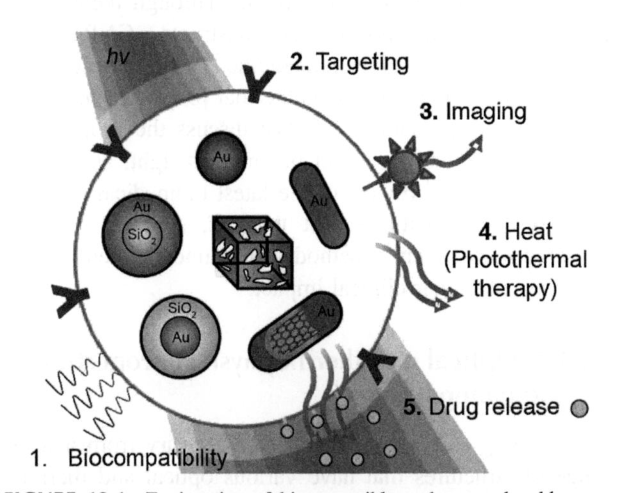

FIGURE 12.1 Engineering of biocompatible and targeted gold nanoparticles (GNPs) for biomedical applications. (1–2) The surface of GNPs can be easily modified with stabilizers and targeting moieties to improve stability and selectivity. (3) Absorption and scattering properties of GNPs can be tuned for biomedical imaging. (4–5) Upon light illumination (hv), the heat generated from the GNPs can be used for photothermal therapy (PTT) and facilitate drug release, allowing for an interactive combination therapy.

a These authors contributed equally to this work.

Nanoparticles for Biomedical Applications. https://doi.org/10.1016/B978-0-12-816662-8.00012-6

nanorings, nanodisks, triangular prisms, and triangular platelets. These structures have a profound effect on the absorption of light via the surface plasmon resonance (SPR) of the GNPs.[10] This phenomenon, responsible for improving the scattering and absorption characteristics of GNPs, is influenced by the size and shape of the nanoparticle. The tunable optical properties of gold are taken advantage of by designing gold-based particles that absorb light in the near-infrared range (NIR; 700–1000 nm).[1,2,6,9] Exposure to light in the NIR range allows for the absorbed light to be converted into energy in the form of heat that can damage cancer cells through localized hyperthermia or be used to release the encapsulated drug.[10] NIR light can be confined to target sites via optical fibers and balloons, minimizing damage to the surrounding normal tissue and allowing for complementary combination therapies to be developed and employed.

Many cancer treatments employ engineered cocktails in conjunction with chemotherapeutic approaches to target proliferating cancer cells. This approach creates systemic toxicities, and the abnormal tumor microenvironment (e.g., extracellular matrix) reduces the concentration of drug that reaches its destination. Synergistic administration of photothermal therapy (PTT) along with chemotherapy to cancer cells provides a method to simultaneously administer the chemotherapeutic drug and induce hyperthermia in cells of interest.[11] Manipulation of the surface chemistry surrounding GNPs via temperature control makes this possible. Overcoming cancer cell resistance to hyperthermia can be circumnavigated using this approach while increasing intracellular drug concentration by permeabilization of the cell membrane. Through their incorporation into theranostic nanoconstructs, GNPs have advanced the field of nanomedicine. Here, we introduce their unique optical and photothermal properties based on their distinct size and shape. We discuss the property of localized SPR and its effect on incident light, as well as provide a detailed review of the latest biomedical applications of GNPs with respect to PTT, surgery, imaging techniques, delivery methods, immunotherapeutic approaches, and their clinical impact.

12.1.1 Optical and thermophysical properties of gold nanoparticles

The makeup and composition of GNPs vary from a wide range of structures that have various optical and thermophysical properties (Table 12.1). These structures include gold nanospheres, gold nanorods (GNRs), gold nanoshells, gold nanocages, gold nanorings, gold nanodisks, gold triangular nanoprisms, and gold triangular platelets. The element gold is used and often combined with a surfactant-containing solvent for the formulation of GNPs, as surfactants may help to stabilize the GNPs and allow for the mean free path and thermal diffusivity of the GNPs to better resemble that of cellular tissue. This allows the GNPs to travel to the desired target in a more efficient manner.[6] A key optical property of GNPs is the localized SPR, which is a resonance that is generated by light when it comes into contact with conductive nanoparticles that are smaller than the incident wavelength of light. This allows for an electric field of incident light to excite electrons of a conduction band on the particle, resulting in localized plasmon oscillations with a resonant frequency that can be change based on the composition, size, geometry, environment, and the amount of nanoparticles encountered.[12] Furthermore, the scattering and absorption properties of GNPs are dependent on the structure and size of the nanoparticles, the amount of light exciting the particle, and the dielectric constant of the surrounding environment or medium.[13] Optical properties of GNPs are determined by the structure and size of the particle. Through modifying the shape and composition of GNPs, the nanoparticles can be tuned to certain wavelengths of incident light.[6] Studies have shown that by manipulating these factors in gold nanoshells and GNRs, the GNPs were tuned to the NIR regime, which aided in identifying where the GNPs could efficiently work inside cellular tissue.[6] It was also discovered that GNRs have a larger peak in the NIR regime along their longitudinal face, whereas the smaller peak in the spectrum was found along the transverse direction.[6]

12.1.2 Classes of gold nanoparticles

12.1.2.1 Gold nanospheres

Gold nanospheres are often colloidal in nature, as they are commonly synthesized through a citrate reduction of gold salt ($HAuCl_4$) in water.[14] As one of the most widely studied nanoparticle systems, gold colloids have been evaluated with regards to a temperature-dependence.[15] Studies have examined gold clusters and determined that the spectrum decreases in intensity and broadens when increasing the temperature from 1.5 to 300 K. It has been shown that the electron–phonon interaction is compensated as temperature decreases by contractions within the thermal lattice of the nanoparticles.[15] By controlling the ratio of the gold and the remainder of the solution, as well as controlling the temperature in which the solution is synthesized, the size of the nanospheres can be manipulated to become larger or smaller in diameter with typical sizes ranging from 2 to 100 nm. The addition of various ligands, copolymers, and reducing agents is often incorporated into gold nanosphere synthesis protocols.[2] Specifically, in the presence of a system consisting of GNPs created using Turkevich et al.'s methodology, the reduction of $HAuCl_4$ with hydroxylamine hydrochloride promotes the formation of larger particles.[16,17] In slightly acidic conditions, the nanoparticles'

TABLE 12.1 Characteristic properties of gold nanoparticles (GNPs). Outline of the characteristics of various GNP structures.

Particle	Sketch	Size	λ_{SPR} (nm)	C_{abs} (nm^2)	η_{abs}	C_{abs}/C_{ext}
Au sphere		$r = 20$ nm	528	2827	2.3	0.94
Si core/Au shell		$r_1 = 60$ nm $r_2 = 75$ nm	800	45,769	2.6	0.53
Au_2S core/Au shell		$r_1 = 21$ nm $r_2 = 25$ nm	~780	2750	1.4	>0.9
Au rod[a]		$L_1 = 13$ nm $L_2 = 49$ nm	797	5674	13.8	0.93
Au cage[b]		$L = 36.7$ nm $t = 3.3$ nm	800	7260	5.4	0.90

Note: The terms in the table are surface plasmon resonance wavelength (λ_{SPR}), absorption cross-section (C_{abs}), absorption efficiency ($\eta_{abs} = C_{abs}/A$), and the ratio of absorption over extinction (C_{abs}/C_{ext})
[a]*L_1 and L_2 are the width and length of the rod. Effective radius (sphere with the same volume $r_{eff} = 11.43$ nm) is used to calculate the geometric cross-section.*
[b]*L is the outer length of the cubic and t is the thickness of the cage. The geometric cross-section used is L^2.*
Reprinted from Royal Society of Chemistry, Zhenpeng Qin and John C. Bischof, Thermophysical and biological responses of gold nanoparticle laser heating, 2011, with permission from Elsevier.

size increases as the reducing agent, hydroxylamine hydrochloride, is nonnucleating.[16,17] As for the properties of gold nanospheres, both the composition and structure reveal that for a nanosphere with a radius of 20 nm, there is a localized SPR wavelength of 528 nm, an absorption cross-section of 2827 nm^2, an absorption efficiency of 2.3, and a ratio of absorbance over extinction of 0.94.[6] The degree to which particles are scattered is determined by comparing the ratio of absorption over extinction. Significant scattering is indicated with a lower ratio, while a larger ratio indicates less scattering of the particles. As the scattering increases, so does the size of the GNPs.[6] These properties show the efficiency at which gold nanospheres absorb light and the value of the electron resonance that is produced when gold nanospheres come in contact with light. In addition, the red shift of the wavelength is seen as a function of size with relation to the GNPs.[6]

12.1.2.2 Gold nanorods

GNRs differ from gold nanospheres in that there are many ways to synthesize them, which have been introduced and implemented by experts in the field. For example, Burdick et al. edited the already existing template method, which was developed by Martin et al.,[18] and consisted of electrochemical and electroless accumulation of gold within the nanopores of particularly porous polycarbonate template membranes. The modified method consisted of preparing the nanorods in a multilayer fashion, with alternating layers of gold and the particularly dissolvable metal, silver. By preparing the nanorods in this manner, there is a significantly higher yield of nanorods compared to traditional template methods that only use one layer of gold, while decreasing the cost of material and preparation time.[19] Another method of GNR synthesis, which was developed by Yu et al.[20] and Chang et al.,[21] is called electrochemical synthesis. This method involves reducing gold anions at the cathode surface or within a specialized cylindrical template comprised of cetyltrimethylammonium bromide (CTAB). One of the most widely used methods for the preparation of GNRs is the seed-mediated growth method which was originally developed by Murphy et al.,[22] as well as Jana et al.[23] This method, which was later edited by Nikoobakht et al.,[24] is a multistep process that first calls for the formation of gold seeds by reducing $HAuCl_4$ with a strong reducing agent (the method calls for sodium borohydride) within the presence of CTAB. Following this step, the gold seeds are placed into a growth solution of $HAuCl_4$ with a weak reducing agent (the method calls for ascorbic acid), as well as a CTAB surfactant. According to Nikoobakht et al.,[25] the CTAB acts to form a bilayer on the surface of the nanorods, which then in turn allows for the appropriate separation of the nanorods from each other, as the cationic head groups of the CTAB surfactant repel each other. However, due to the cytotoxicity of the CTAB surfactant, other strategies and reagents are being pursued in order to complete this nanorod formation process. As for the properties of GNRs, for a nanorod of width 13 nm and length 49 nm, there is a localized SPR value of 797 nm, an absorption cross-section of 5674 nm^2, an absorption efficiency of 13.8, and a ratio of absorbance over extinction of 0.93.[6] The aspect ratio of the rods themselves affects these properties as well, as there are variations in the values when the aspect ratio differs among various nanorods. These properties display the efficiency at which the GNRs absorb light and the value of electron resonance that is produced when they come into contact with light. The absorption efficiency acts as the most comprehensive way to compare light absorption between GNPs. With an efficiency of 13.8, the GNR has the highest absorption efficiency of all the GNPs.[6]

12.1.2.3 Gold nanoshells

Hollow gold nanoshells (HGNs) can be fabricated with a silica coating using the Stöber process.[26] Initially, a microemulsion was produced consisting of 2-propanol and millipore water. Under continuous stirring, ammonia and tetraethyl orthosilicate (TEOS) were added to the system. The resulting silica-coated HGNs generated with the aforementioned Stöber method range from 50–2000 nm in diameter.[27,28] Modulating the specific concentration of reactants, catalysts, and reaction temperature influences the size of the HGNs produced. Increasing the concentration of ammonia and water led to larger particles.[28] Moreover, the initial concentration of TEOS used in the formulation was inversely proportional to the resulting size of the particles.[28] Gold nanoshells are often found to have a composite gold metallic shell and a silica dielectric core. Oldenburg and Halas et al. developed the most well-known method for preparing this shell and core structure, as monodispersed silica cores were prepared through basic reduction of TEOS in ethanol (Stöber method) followed by a surface animation.[29] This animation allows for the negatively charged gold colloid to be absorbed on the silica surface and generate nucleation sites, allowing for the reduction of additional gold ions. Due to this structure of gold nanoshells, they possess a single localized SPR band in the NIR region which can be manipulated based on the thickness of the gold shell. According to the method, by reducing thickness by about 15 nm, there is a shift in the absorption peak read of about 300 nm in the positive direction due to the increased coupling between plasmons. The scattering and absorbing optical properties of the gold nanoshells are dependent on the size of the silica core found within the shell. Often, silica cores that are smaller in size tend to display a higher absorption of energy, while silica cores that are larger in size are more effective at scattering incident light energy.[2] As for the properties of gold nanoshells, for a nanoshell with a silica core of radius 60 nm and a gold shell of radius 75 nm, there is a localized SPR value of 800 nm, an absorption cross-section of 45,769 nm^2, an absorption efficiency of 2.6, and a ratio of absorbance over extinction of 0.53.[6] The thickness of the shells themselves affects these properties as well, as these values represent a shell with thickness of 15 nm. These properties illustrate the efficiency at which the gold nanoshells absorb light and the value of electron resonance as a result.

12.1.2.4 Gold nanocages

Gold nanocages can be formed through a galvanic replacement reaction between silver nanocubes and a $HAuCl_4$ solution, via a method developed by Skrabalak et al.[30] Once the reaction concludes, gold atoms are inserted and silver atoms are removed from the silver nanocubes, and thus a gold and silver alloy shell is formed around the semihollow silver nanocubes. Varying degrees of the galvanic replacement reaction allow for pores to form in the wall of the nanocages and the cube-like structure of the nanocage to form. In terms of optical properties, the hollow and porous nature of the gold nanocage possesses a single localized SPR band around 800 nm.[2]

12.1.2.5 Gold nanodisks, nanorings, triangular nanoprisms, and triangular platelets

Colloidal gold nanorings have been fabricated using a galvanic replacement reaction of cobalt nanoparticles in $HAuCl_4$ solution with a polyvinylpyrrolidone stabilizing agent. Aizpurua et al. introduced a method to form gold nanorings which was later modified to form gold nanodisks, where colloidal polystyrene particles were electrostatically placed onto a soda-glass substrate, which was then followed by a thin gold-film coating.[31] An argon beam was then used to create nanorings around the polystyrene particles by removing unwanted gold atoms. Finally, ultraviolet (UV)-ozone treatment was employed in order to remove any remaining polystyrene particles, thus leaving fully formed gold nanorings in place. To create nanodisks using a similar technique, Tseng et al. edited this sequence of steps and used a silica-deposited sapphire substrate for the electrostatic placement of the colloidal polystyrene particles, replaced the original argon beam with trifluoromethane, and followed this with an ozone treatment.[32] Triangular nanoparticles have been explored and synthesized on soft templates via a seed-mediated growth process in the presence of micelles of CTAB.[33] The SPR band of these particles can be regulated and shifted from 560 to 420 nm by modifying the shape through further aging the particles at high temperatures.[33] Shankar et al. demonstrated that reacting aqueous chloroaurate ions ($AuCl_4^-$) with lemongrass extract yields a high percentage of single-crystalline gold nanotriangles.[34] Gold layers may be employed to protect silver triangular nanoparticles, such as those synthesized by Tsai and colleagues.[35] Gold-coated triangular platelets on the nanometer scale were prepared using a wet chemical method consisting of silver nitrate mixed with trisodium citrate combined with a reducing solution.[35] Centrifuging separated large triangles from smaller spherical particles, and the colloid of triangular platelets were subjected to gold coating.[35] The gold coating protected the silver core, and its presence allowed for future attachment of functional molecules.

12.1.3 Biological applications of GNPs via laser heating

Biological applications that take advantage of GNPs within tissues and the cellular environment via laser irradiation are becoming widely used modalities and targeted therapies. Heat generated by GNPs in response to laser light activation can have a variety of effects depending on the applied temperature.[36] Temperature control is dependent on the energy input driving the heating or cooling of the system as a whole. With high-energy laser pulses, there can be a large temperature increase of near 1000 degrees in just a few seconds.[36] Many biomedical applications and their outcomes are driven by this tunable capability.[37] The wide range of applications involving the laser heating of GNPs span both microscopic and macroscopic levels.

Limitations with implementing laser thermolysis for cancer therapy include a lack of therapeutic efficacy and failure to accurately target malignant tissues. A study conducted by Lopotkho et al. aimed to selectively maximize the damage to human leukemia cells while sparing healthy cells through a two-stage method: delivery of the nanoparticles to the target cells and laser irradiation of the sample. The selective cell killing method is accomplished by laser-activated nanothermolysis and employs vapor microbubbles produced by pulses from a laser around superheated clusters of GNPs.[38] The group used 30 nm spherical GNPs and a wavelength of 532 nm in conjunction with a laser pulse duration of 10 s achieving 0.1%−1.5% of tumor cell and 77%−84% of bone marrow cell survival.[38] With a fluence of 0.6 J/cm^2, larger clusters of GNPs effectively targeted cancerous cells inducing microbubbles, while cells with smaller clusters avoided damage.

Approaches such as laser-activated nanothermolysis and modalities that are focused on applying heat to GNPs have expanded the inventory of cancer therapies. Efforts have focused on damaging target cells while preserving healthy ones through minimally invasive therapeutic approaches. Light activation of GNPs is a promising avenue that has taken advantage of specific geometries that offer optimal characteristics based on different formulations. Here we explore the various methods that take advantage of GNPs and exploit their properties.

12.1.3.1 Applications of laser heating GNPs at the nanoscale level

12.1.3.1.1 Nanoscale membrane and DNA melting

GNPs possess the ability to target the lipids that compose biological membranes. The cellular membrane is mostly hydrophobic and impermeable to substances that are hydrophilic in nature. Urban et al. successfully displayed that GNPs can be used as sources of heat on the phospholipid membrane by illuminating them at their plasmon resonances. More specifically, the GNPs induced and characterized the gel—fluid phase transition of the membrane simultaneously in defined regions within the membrane.[39] Manipulating the membrane to achieve a fluid phase is made possible by increasing the temperature past the melting temperature value (T_m) where intermolecular interactions between phospholipids are reduced. A gel phase is achieved by decreasing the temperature below the T_m value, allowing van der Waals forces between acyl chains to dominate. Control of the phospholipid membrane's viscosity was enhanced by the GNPs as they were positioned at specific locations along the membrane.

DNA assembly to GNPs provides a strategy that makes it possible to tailor the optical, electronic, and structural properties of colloidal gold aggregates through the specificity of DNA interactions that serve to mitigate the interactions between particles.[40] In Mirkin et al.'s strategy, colloidal GNPs are aggregated together both rationally and reversibly by attaching to the surfaces of two batches of 13 nm gold particles' noncomplementary DNA oligonucleotides containing thiol groups at their ends.[40] This aforementioned assembly process can be reversed by employing thermal denaturation.[40] Sharp melting transitions are observed as a result of the nanoparticle size, the surface density of the oligonucleotide on the nanoparticles, the dielectric constant of the surrounding medium, and the position of the nanoparticles with respect to each other.[41] The T_m of the DNA-linked nanoparticle structures increases with increasing salt concentration and also increases as interparticle distance is increased for the DNA-linked nanoparticle aggregates as a result of less electrostatic repulsion.[41] The sharpness of the melting profile relies heavily on nanoparticles size, with 50 nm gold particles displaying a transition of a single degree. The melting of DNA is also influenced by the salt concentration surrounding the molecule, due to DNA being highly negatively charged and the local salt concentration changing once double helices dissociate into single strands.[41]

Heating GNPs provides a mechanism to manipulate macromolecules of a similar size such as DNA. The size of an average GNP ranges from 10 to 200 nm in diameter.[42] Macromolecules of a similar size interact with GNPs through attractive and repulsive forces.[43] Manipulating the amount of heat generated via laser energy makes controlling and reversing heating of macromolecules possible. By utilizing 300 ns laser pulses, Stehr et al. rapidly heated DNA-bound GNPs that were aggregated together and demonstrated that double-stranded DNA melts on a microsecond time scale subsequently leading to the disintegration of those aggregates on a millisecond time scale.[44] GNPs absorb light very efficiently and when irradiated by short laser pulses, they are able to convert the absorbed light energy into thermal energy.[44] This thermal energy generated by laser pulses of 10^6 kW/mm^2 can break the thiol bond of DNA-functionalized nanoparticles.[44]

12.1.3.1.2 Drug release from gold nanoparticles

Applying a pulsed laser creates high temperatures within the local environment surrounding the GNPs. This temperature change nearby the GNPs can be strong enough to break bonds between the particles and ligands attached to the GNPs.[45] In a similar fashion, Jain et al. examined the effects of femtosecond laser heating on GNPs attached to DNA ligands via thiol groups and found that at a wavelength of 400 nm, desorption of thiolated DNA strands from the nanoparticles takes place breaking the gold–sulfur bond.[43] In an effort to study the mechanism behind laser-triggered release as a drug delivery strategy, Xiong et al. loaded hollow gold nanoconstructs with cisplatin and triggered their release using a 15 ns pulsed laser at a repetition rate of 10 Hz.[46] Their system manifested two release mechanisms, one of which resulted in sustained release in the presence of chloride ions. The chloride ions facilitated an ion-exchange process that resulted in the long-term release of Pt(II). Rapid release was achieved once NIR laser irradiation enabled oxidative desorption cleaving gold–sulfur bonds releasing soluble Pt(II). Gold platforms such as nanocages can also be taken advantage of as nanocarriers by exposing the particles to the NIR laser.[47] Yavuz et al. prepared two "smart" polymers, pNIPAAm and pNIPAAm-*co*-pAAm, using atom transfer radical polymerization and attached them to the gold nanostructures via gold–thiolate linkages.[47] These interactions were subsequently broken via NIR laser light, and their system was used to evaluate the release profile of doxorubicin for cancer therapy. Specifically, SK-BR-3 breast cancer cells in the presence of gold nanocages loaded with doxorubicin were irradiated with a Ti:sapphire laser at 20 mW/cm^2 for 2 and 5 mins. The greater the duration of irradiation, the greater the amount of doxorubicin released and as a result, the lower the resulting viability of the cancer cells.

12.1.3.1.3 Selective protein denaturation, interdigitation, and conformational alteration

High temperatures, as a result of laser irradiation, have a wide variety of impacts on the local environment of the particles and on GNPs overall. One remarkable effect in particular is the ability for selective protein denaturation. This occurs in part due to techniques of administering laser pulses. Rather than a continuous stream, pulses allow for photoacoustic effects to occur resulting in thermal expansion of the nanoparticle itself.[48] Photoacoustic effects are sound waves that develop from a material absorbing light. Selective denaturation and inactivation can be very desirable when trying to control cellular behavior. GNPs allow for a higher absorption level compared to dyes and can be of great use for denaturation.[49] In the 1980s, Daniel G. Jay of Harvard Medical School performed a study called chromophore laser-assisted inactivation (CALI).[50] This study showed that once a protein binds to a specific antibody that is conjugated with malachite green, it can be inactivated by laser irradiation at 5 mins of 80 mW of power.[50] This irradiation endured pulses at a frequency of 10 Hz with an average peak power of 0.8 mW. Pulses were used because continuous irradiation would become stagnant after a steady state is reached. The inactivation of the malachite green dye is selective in that the dye is able to absorb the light, but the cellular components are unaffected. The denaturation and inactivation of GNPs can prove to be more efficient than using a dye because GNPs can be targeted to nearly all proteins.[50]

12.1.3.2 Applications of GNP laser heating at the microscale level

12.1.3.2.1 Transmembrane drug delivery

The cell membrane serves as a difficult barrier to overcome when trying to deliver drugs or gene therapies into the cell. Transmembrane drug delivery is especially desirable with respect to cancer treatment, as the need to administer drugs is crucial to the therapeutic efficacy of the treatment. It is possible to penetrate the cell membrane with high intensity light and direct focus on the desired site. Unfortunately, the process speed is limited because only one cell can be targeted at a time. GNPs can be of great use for breaking through the cell membrane and require only pulses of light rather than high intensity focus. In theory, this process will allow for more cells to be affected at one time rather than individual cells.[6,51]

12.1.3.2.2 Liposomal and endosomal release

Endosomal encapsulation is another major barrier to successful drug uptake in cells. GNPs offer a great way of overcoming this barrier. Irradiating HGNs with the NIR pulsed laser can create almost complete liposomal release.[52] With respect to the endosomal release, it was shown that siRNA could be released from the endosome into the cytoplasm with NIR laser pulses, blocking mRNA for green fluorescent protein (GFP) expression. The mechanism of escape is due to the bubbles created during the heating of the GNPs which damage the endosomal and liposomal membranes while maintaining the structure of the cell membrane.[6]

12.1.3.3 Applications of GNP laser heating at the macroscale level

12.1.3.3.1 Photothermal therapy

PTT is a cancer treatment modality that leverages heat generated from the absorbed light of the plasmonic nanoparticles for the thermal ablation of cancer cells.[53,54] When plasmonic nanoparticles are exposed to light at a resonance wavelength, they experience SPRs, which are synchronized oscillations of the valence electrons.[55] The resulting synchronized oscillations can either absorb or scatter the exposed light. In the case of light absorption, the absorbed light is converted to heat, which is exploited for hyperthermia treatment in PTT. Cancerous cells are more sensitive to hyperthermia compared to normal cells because of the chaotic vascular structure that hinders the heat dissipation.[56] PTT typically begins with systematic administration of the plasmonic nanoparticles for passive tumor localization. The tumor is then subjected to spatially and temporally controlled light irradiation, and the light absorbed by the nanoparticles is converted into heat, raising the local environmental temperature in the range of 41−47°C in order to induce apoptosis via DNA damage, protein denaturation, and cell membrane disruption.[57]

Gold-based nanoparticles have emerged as a leading nanoplatform due to their chemical and tunable optical properties.[1] The surface of GNPs can be modified and decorated with targeting modalities or therapeutic compounds via facile gold−thiol chemistry, which improves stability, functionality, and biocompatibility.[58,59] For example, light activation of intratumorally or intravenously injected PEGylated GNRs resulted in pronounced PTT effects, leading to significant tumor volume reductions in squamous cell carcinoma xenograft animal models (Fig. 12.2).[60] In addition to simple surface functionalization, the optical properties of GNPs can be precisely controlled by adjusting their size and structure in order to maximize their light absorption for high photothermal conversion.[61,62] Spatiotemporal distribution of the converted energy has been modeled and characterized by Huang et al. on a monolayer of cells.[63] Due to these unique properties, GNP-based PTT has been studied in vitro, in vivo, and even in clinical trials for head−neck and prostate cancer.[64]

Although there are many advantages to using GNP-based PTT, its therapeutic effect is confined within the area of light irradiation; as a result, the nonirradiated cancer cells and metastatic lesions are unaffected. Currently, researchers are developing strategies to combine PTT with a secondary therapy such as chemotherapy, immunotherapy, or photodynamic therapy (PDT) to improve treatment outcomes.

12.1.3.3.2 Photothermal enhancement of chemotherapy

Chemotherapy is one of the most common types of cancer treatments. The complex tumor microenvironment and cancer survival pathways limit chemotherapeutic delivery and efficacy. PTT has been explored extensively to improve chemotherapeutic outcomes. One of the distinct characteristics of PTT is localized hyperthermia. Raeesi et al. have demonstrated that PTT-induced local hyperthermia can permeabilize the interstitial matrices of tumors by denaturing the dense collagen matrix within the interstitial space between tumor cells and blood vessels.[65] Others have demonstrated an increase in intracellular drug concentration due to an increase in membrane permeability when the therapeutic is administered after initial PTT hyperthermia priming.[66,67]

In addition to increasing tumoral and cell membrane permeability, PTT has been established to have a synergistic effect with chemotherapeutics, particularly DNA-damaging agents. This results in a temperature-dependent DNA repair process.[68,69] Mendes et al. demonstrated that GNP-induced PTT potentiates the therapeutic efficacy of doxorubicin, a topoisomerase I and II inhibitor and DNA intercalating agent, compared to doxorubicin or PTT alone.[67] Van der Heigden et al. showed similar findings where PTT-induced hyperthermia enhanced cytotoxicity of mitomycin-C, E09, epirubicin, and gemcitabine in transitional cell carcinoma.[70]

Aside from the synergistic effect of PTT and chemotherapy, PTT has also been demonstrated to reduce off-target toxicity by selectively releasing the drug at the tumor site upon light irradiation. Currently, there are four common photothermal-triggered drug delivery strategies.[45] First, therapeutics can be embedded within a thermoresponsive polymeric matrix that surrounds the GNP.[71−73] Light-induced localized heating of the GNPs will degrade the polymeric matrix to release the drug. Second, the therapeutic and GNP can be coencapsulated within a thermoresponsive liposome for localized delivery via bursting of the liposome upon light irradiation.[74] Third, therapeutics can be covalently linked to the GNP via a thermoresponsive Diels−Alder adduct and released via a temperature dependent retro−Diels−Alder reaction.[75] Lastly, therapeutics can be noncovalently embedded within a mesoporous silica matrix that surrounds the GNP.[76,77] Drug release occurs when the silica matrix collapses in response to heating of the GNP.

The effects of PTT can be potentiated by the coadministration of a chemotherapeutic. Suboptimal PTT administration can lead to thermotolerance in cancer cells via the heat shock pathway (e.g., release of heat shock proteins). One strategy to overcome such a challenge is the coadministration of heat shock protein inhibitors and PTT. Huang et al. have demonstrated that simultaneous administration of PTT and the chemotherapeutic drug 17-(allylamino)-17-demethoxygeldanamycin (17-AAG), an inhibitor of heat shock protein 90, can improve the hyperthermic effect of PTT, using a biocompatible and degradable matrix (Fig. 12.3).[11] In addition to the ability of PTT to induce localized hyperthermia, rationally

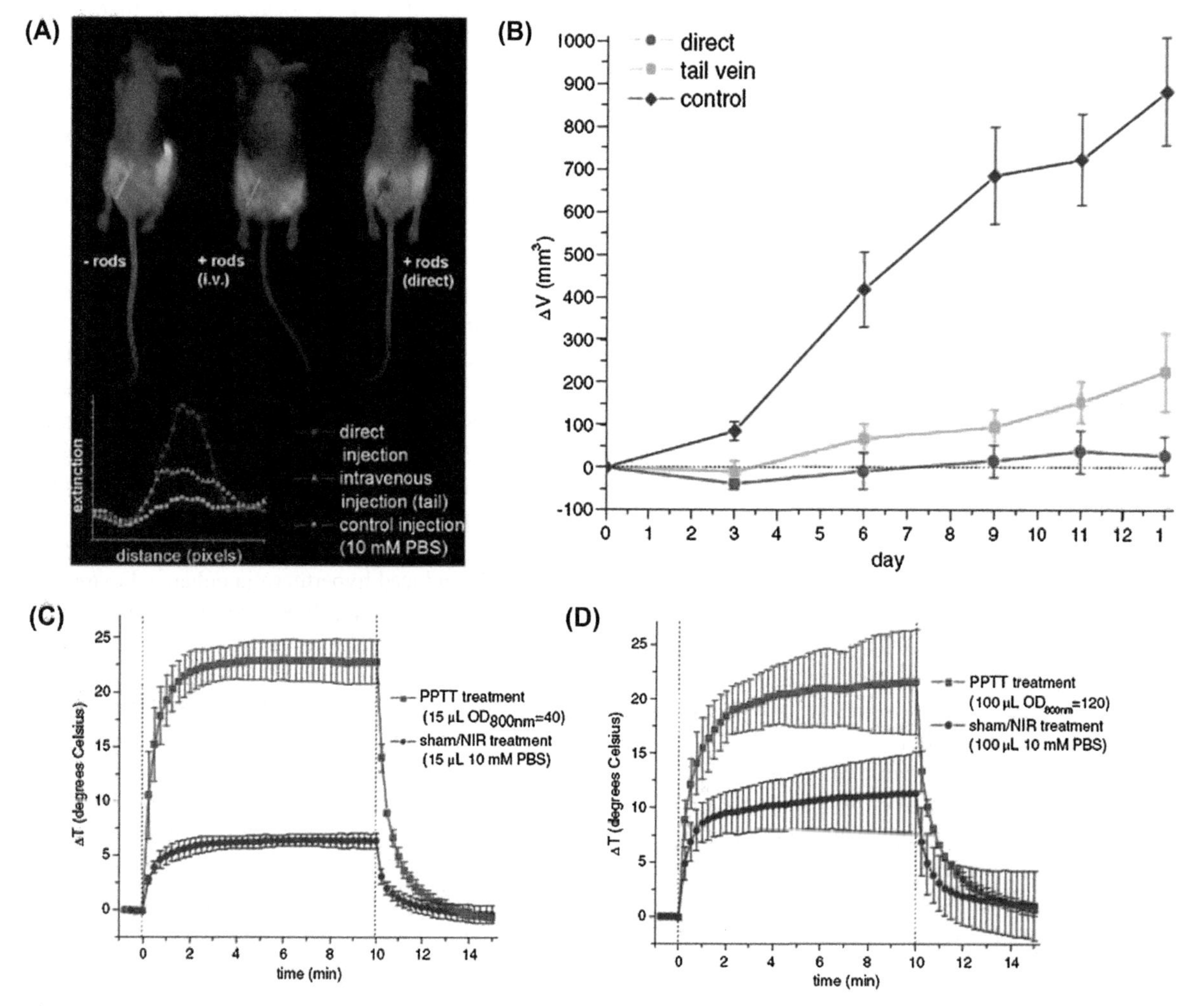

FIGURE 12.2 (A) *In vivo* imaging and (B) PTT using PEGylated gold nanorods (GNRs). (C–D) Tumor temperature was monitored during PTT with (red) or without (blue) PEGylated GNRs.[60] *Reprinted from Dickerson, E.B., et al., Gold nanorod assisted near-infrared plasmonic photothermal therapy (PPTT) of squamous cell carcinoma in mice. Cancer Lett, 2008. 269(1): p. 57–66, Copyright (2008), with permission from Elsevier.*

designed combinations of PTT and chemotherapy hold significant promise for the treatment of cancer.

12.1.3.3.3 Photothermal enhancement of immunotherapy

The use of immunotherapy as a cancer treatment has gained great interest and momentum in recent years due to its unique strategy to combat cancerous cells. Immunotherapy leverages the host's immune system to recognize and destroy cancer cells. However, due to the ever-evolving nature of cancer cells, they have adapted immune-suppressive mechanisms in the tumor environment such as inhibiting maturation of dendritic cells, which capture antigens and present them to cytotoxic T cells for activation, by secreting immune-suppressive cytokines.[78] One of the ways to overcome such a challenge is through the use of PTT to elicit an immunostimulatory response in the tumor microenvironment.[79] Bear et al. have demonstrated that GNP-induced PTT promotes the secretion of proinflammatory cytokines to induce maturation of dendritic cells for activation of antitumor $CD8^+$ cytotoxic T cells.[79]

The use of checkpoint blockade inhibitors in immunotherapy has shown great promise in cancer therapy.[80] Two of the proteins that serve as immune checkpoints are cytotoxic T lymphocyte–associated antigen (CTLA-4) and programmed death-ligand 1 (PD-L1); both serve as inhibitory proteins that regulate T cell activation.[81,82] Many have explored combination treatments of PTT and checkpoint blockade immunotherapy. Wang et al. demonstrated carbon-nanotube-based PTT potentiates anti-CTLA-4 therapy to increase dendritic cell maturation. This leads to higher T cell activation to kill cancer cells and suppress metastasis.[83] Ge et al. improved anti-PD-L1 therapy by adding an imiquimod (R837), a toll-like receptor 7 agonist, within poly(ethylene glycol)-block-poly(lactic-co-glycolic acid) copolymer-encapsulated Fe_3O_4 superparticles.[84]

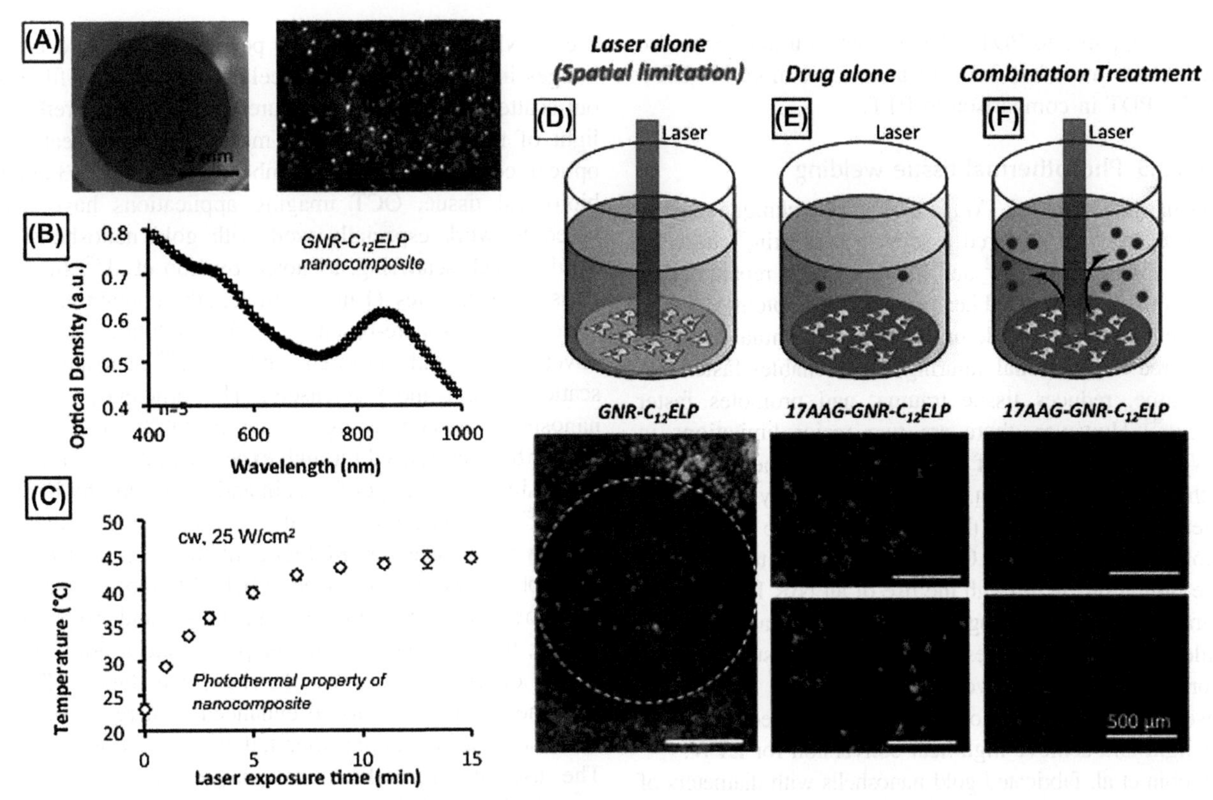

FIGURE 12.3 Gold nanorod-elastin-like polypeptide (GNR-ELP) nanocomposite for combination cancer treatment. Heat generated by the GNR upon laser treatment can induce cell death known as hyperthermia; on the other hand, ELP can act as an encapsulation and release platform for drug molecules. (A) Digital snap shot (left) and scanning electron microscopy image (right) of the GNR-ELP nanocomposite. (B) Absorption spectrum of nanocomposite showing two GNR characteristic peaks. (C) Nanocomposite provides a stable photothermal response up to 43°C upon laser exposure. Human prostate cancer cells were cultured on top of the nanocomposite. (D) The laser was irradiated vertically at the center of the matrix at 25 W/cm^2 for 7 minutes. In the fluorescence image, cells outside the laser path were stained green, indicating living cells. Cells inside the laser path were stained red, indicating cell death. (E) The 17-(allylamino)-17-demethoxygeldanamycin (17-AAG)-loaded nanocomposite can support cell growth with minimal toxicity. (F) Combination treatment. The laser facilitated both the release of 17-AAG and increased the temperature up to 43°C. The fluorescence images indicated both cells inside and outside the laser path are dead and stained red. *Reprinted from Huang, H.-C., et al., Synergistic administration of photothermal therapy and chemotherapy to cancer cells using polypeptide-based degradable plasmonic matrices. Nanomedicine, 2011 6(3): p. 459–473, Copyright (2011), with permission from Elsevier.*

Fe_3O_4-induced PTT ablates the tumor and releases R837 to enhance the antitumor response. The combination of GNP-based PTT and checkpoint blockade immunotherapy has yet to be evaluated; however, given the success of using PTT induced by other plasmonic particles, to potentiate checkpoint blockade immunotherapy, GNP-based PTT should also elicit a similar therapeutic response when combined with checkpoint blockade immunotherapy.

12.1.3.3.4 Photothermal enhancement of photodynamic therapy

Another form of light-activated therapy is PDT, in which red light activates a photosensitizer to produce reactive molecular species (RMS, e.g., singlet oxygen) that damages cells or tissues. This unique photochemistry-based modality does not generate heat and thus is fundamentally and mechanistically distinct from PTT. Unlike chemotherapy, photosensitizers are nontoxic in the absence of light. Upon light irradiation, photons excite electrons within the small molecules to a higher excited state. While the electrons can relax back down to the ground state, some undergo intersystem crossing and begin relaxation from the triplet state. The excess energy released during the relaxation period is utilized for two reactions depending on the type of photosensitizer involved: a type I reaction that produces free radicals and/or a type II reaction that reacts with oxygen in the local environment to generate singlet oxygen.[85] These two reactions can occur simultaneously and are dependent on tissue oxygenation.[86] Light irradiation makes PDT a selective cancer treatment in terms of tumor targeting, unlike chemotherapy. Currently, several groups are working on combining gold-based PTT and PDT for therapeutic treatments.[87–89] Bhana et al. demonstrated that silicon 2,3-naphthalocyanine dihydroxide–loaded GNRs for the combination of PTT and PDT were able to induce 41.1% more cell killing for KB-3-1 cells, head and neck cancer, and 41.6% more cell killing for SK-BR-3 cells, breast cancer, compared to PDT. The combination treatment also killed 23.4% more KB-3-1 cells and 15.6% more SK-BR-3 cells by PDT in comparison to PTT.

12.1.3.3.5 Photothermal tissue welding

Laser tissue welding (LTW) is a surgical technique used to repair a variety of ruptured tissues such as skin,[90] nerve,[91] blood vessel,[91] cornea,[92] and liver.[93] Tissue repair occurs through the light-induced heating of tissue proteins, leading to protein denaturation, deformation, and eventual fusion.[91] Compared to traditional suturing, LTW enables faster surgical time, reduces tissue trauma, and promotes faster healing.[94] However, there are two major limitations in LTW. First, the depth of wound healing depends on the depth of light penetration. Second, LTW may induce peripheral tissue damage as the light path may go through the peripheral healthy tissue. One of the methods to overcome these limitations is through the use of an NIR laser and by leveraging nanotechnology to achieve localized PTT. While NIR light penetrates deeper into the tissue, the light absorption and heat conversion by the tissue is minimal. However, plasmonic nanoparticles can be used to absorb NIR light and achieve high heat conversion for LTW.

Gobin et al. fabricated gold nanoshells with diameters of ~110 nm and a shell thickness of ~10 nm for photothermal-induced LTW.[95] When they combined the gold nanoshells with bovine serum albumin (BSA) solder formulation (35 wt% and 40 wt% BSA) and light irradiation at 20 W/cm^2 for their in vivo studies, they observed that the initial weld strength of 30 kPa for the fused tissue was enough to keep the wound intact for the animal to begin healing. However, the sutured wound had greater strength compared to the welded wound 10 days post operation, suggesting that optimization of this technique is required.

To mimic the wound-healing environment during the cell proliferation stage, Huang et al. engineered gold nanorods-elastin-like polypeptide (GNR-C_{12}ELP) plasmonic nanocomposites for use in LTW (Fig. 12.4).[96] The ex vivo studies in ruptured porcine small intestines demonstrated that the nanocomposites significantly improved the tensile strength, leakage pressure, and bursting pressure of the ruptured tissue. In addition to improving the mechanical properties, nanocomposite-based LTW offers forward-thinking opportunities to incorporate therapeutics to further enhance the healing and repair process.

12.1.4 Applications of gold nanoparticles in biomedical imaging

12.1.4.1 Scattering

12.1.4.1.1 Optical coherence tomography

Optical coherence tomography (OCT) is an imaging technique introduced by Huang et al. in 1991;[97] OCT makes use of NIR and far-IR light to penetrate tissue and create images in real time at the subcellular level. After filtering out scattered light, OCT measures the remaining reflected light of the optical scattering media and thus creates an optical contrast for targets embedded up to 2–3 cm in biological tissue. OCT imaging applications have been noted to work especially well with gold nanoshells for in vivo back scattering, as noted by Loo et al.[98] In comparison to cuvettes (1 mm path length) containing polystyrene microsphere-based scattering solution or saline, cuvettes with gold nanoshell solutions (10^9 nanoshells/mL) scattered light more intensely. The efficiency of gold nanoshells as contrasting agents in OCT imaging has further been correlated through experimental runs in Monte Carlo simulations in porcine skin and rabbit skin by Kirillin et al.[99] and Zaganova et al.[100] Monoclonal epidermal growth factor receptor (EGFR) antibody–conjugated gold nanospheres were synthesized to help differentiate between cells overexpressing EGFR and those underexpressing EGFR; the gold nanospheres helped create a 300% OCT signal difference between the two cell types. Tumor brightness was found to be enhanced as a result of gold nanoshells accumulating after tail vein injection in mice. The use of anti-EGFR functionalized PEGylated gold nanoshells as OCT contrast agents has been observed by Gobin et al.,[101] with improved nanoparticle accumulation in epidermoid tumors in xenograft mouse models. Through the use of antibody-functionalized GNPs, the delivery time of nanoshells to the tumor site was reduced from 6 h to 2 h. Microneedles have been noted as being especially useful for deep penetration of nanospheres, as reported by Kim et al.,[102] as well as creating improved distribution as a result of ultrasonic force generation. In comparison to untreated segments, the mean intensity of OCT images has boosted approximately 177% when employing this newer approach.

12.1.4.1.2 Diffuse reflectance spectroscopy

Diffuse reflectance spectroscopy is a technique used to collect and analyze scattered IR energy, which in turn is used to measure extremely fine particles or course surfaces. Scattering in spectroscopy often relies on well-engineered optical contrast agents, such as gold nanoshells. Efforts to understand the reflectance properties exhibited by gold nanoshells led to a study demonstrating their use as exogenous contrast agents.[103] In comparison to other metal nanoshells, gold nanoshells demonstrate enhanced absorption and scattering behavior due to their strong plasmon resonance in spherical configurations. The peak resonance of gold nanoshells was determined by varying core size and shell thickness across a wide range of light wavelengths from visible light to NIR light. Increasing the core to shell ratio shifts the peak resonance toward the NIR light region

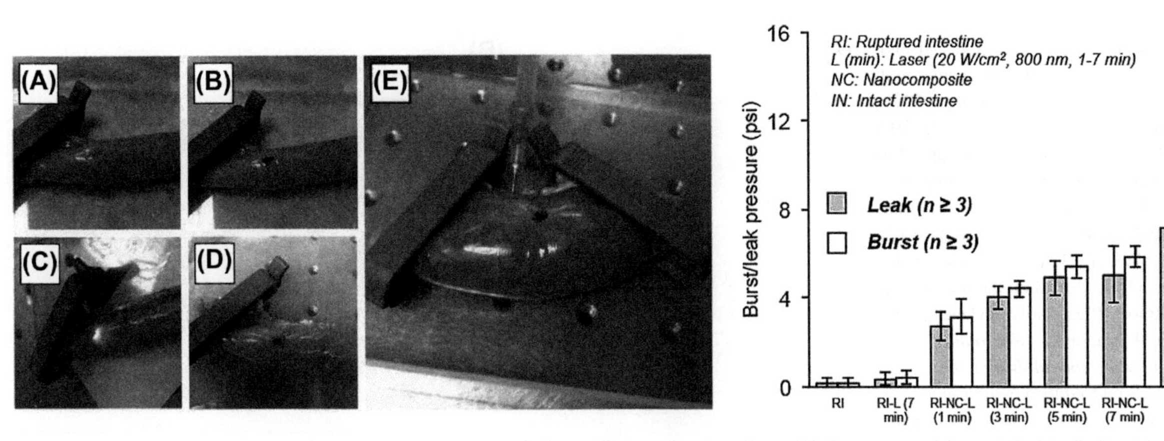

FIGURE 12.4 Nanocomposite-assisted laser tissue welding carried out using porcine intestines. (A) 5 mm cut was first applied to the intestine. (B–D) 2 mg of GNR-C_{12}ELP nanocomposite was then applied to the cut and irradiated with a laser at 20 W/cm^2 for different durations. (E) The leaking and bursting pressures were measured. Ruptured intestine and intact intestine have the lowest and highest bursting/leaking pressures, respectively. The laser application alone did not increase the bursting/leaking pressures. Laser tissue welding (LTW) using nanocomposites enhanced the leaking and bursting pressure of ruptured intestinal tissues from 2% up to 78% and 49% of its original intact form. *Reproduced with permission from Huang, H.C., et al., Laser welding of ruptured intestinal tissue using plasmonic polypeptide nanocomposite solders. ACS Nano, 2013. 7(4): p. 2988–2998, Copyright (2013) with permission from American Chemical Society.*

of values. However, the peak resonance values can be tuned to arrive at the same peak by adjusting the core to shell ratios. It has been noted that regular gold nanoshells demonstrate higher resonance values than colloidal gold particles at NIR wavelengths.

12.1.4.1.3 Surface-enhanced Raman scattering

Surface-enhanced Raman scattering (SERS) is a technique used primarily for bioimaging and bio-diagnosis of cancer cells. Raman spectroscopy measures the inelastic scattering of monochromatic light from different materials. The detection limit is further pushed to singular molecules by enhancing Raman scattering through the adsorption of molecules on a rough metal surface. Laurent et al.[104] reported the Raman imaging and spectra of methylene blue as having a single layer adsorption on gold nanospheres. Huang et al.[105] recognized that the enhanced and polarized Raman spectrum of antibody-conjugated GNRs have been recognized as potential diagnostic signatures for cancer cells. Tumor detection and live animal imaging through SERS GNPs and Raman spectroscopy have also been demonstrated as potentially viable options. Actively targeted SERS nanoparticles were found to possess optical enhancement of Raman spectra up to 10 times more efficiently than nontargeted SERS nanoparticles.[106] A detection limit of 8.125 pM has been demonstrated through multiplexed Raman imaging with four different SERS nanoparticles (all gold core covered with Raman-active material and coated with silica) in mice.[107] According to Bhatia et al.[108] following an injection into athymic mice, SERS-coded polyethylene glycol (PEG)-NRs were able to be detected and provided Raman spectra, with a minimum detection limit between $2x10^{-12}$ M and 4×10^{16} M (Fig. 12.5).

12.1.4.2 Emission

12.1.4.2.1 Fluorescence

GNP fluorescence is a crucial element needed to fully understand imaging techniques often used with GNPs. In a 2008 ACS paper, ensemble fluorescence spectrometry, fluorescence correlation spectroscopy (FCS), and fluorescence microscopy were used to reach several conclusions regarding the fluorescent properties of GNPs. It was noted that an increase in particle size led to a gradual increase in emission intensity, although the emission wavelength remained largely constant at 610 nm. He et al. demonstrated that GNPs have a strong antiphotobleaching effect, which is particularly notable due to their exposure to strong light illumination, a condition that would lead to the bleaching of a large portion of imaging agents.[110] As a result of the antiphotobleaching properties observed in GNPs, it was determined that their use as an imaging agent for cells could be a viable avenue to pursue. Their use as fluorescent probes has also been demonstrated, with GNPs being used as staining agents in cell membranes.[110] These membranes would then be photobleached, and the GNPs, having withstood the power of the illumination and photobleaching, would remain intact and be used as imaging agents. The viability of this technique was proven in practice through the imaging of HeLa cells. It is important to note that the fluorescent properties demonstrated by GNPs change when exposed to fluorophores. Fluorophores have been used in imaging for a long time, serving as optical signal mediators and often playing a crucial role due to

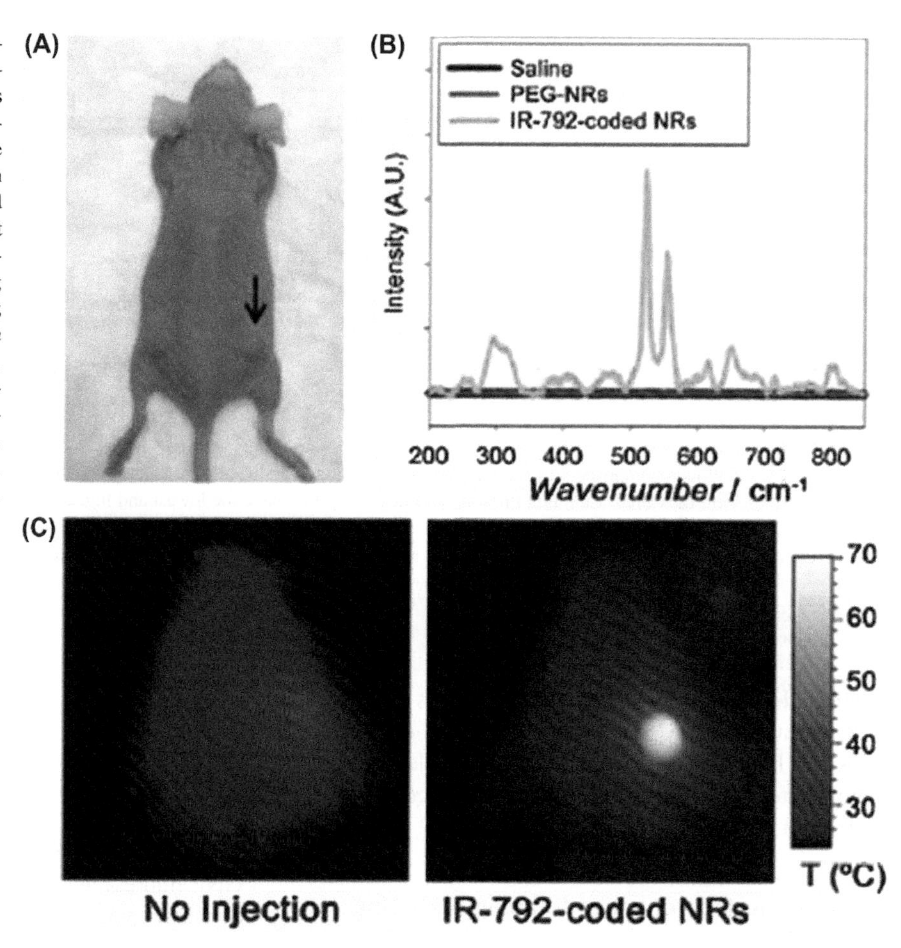

FIGURE 12.5 Raman detection and photothermal heating using Raman-active molecules (IR-792)-loaded PEGylated GNRs (IR-792-coded-GNRs) in mice. (A) IR-792-coded GNRs, PEGylated GNRs, or saline was injected into MDA-MB-435 tumors in mice. (B) Raman spectra of IR-792-coded GNRs and two controls. (C) Light (810 nm, 2 W/cm^2, 3 min) activation of IR-792-coded GNRs for photothermal heating of the tumor. PEG, polyethylene glycol; GNR, gold nanorod. *Reproduced with permission from von Maltzahn, G., et al., SERS-coded gold nanorods as a multifunctional platform for densely multiplexed near-infrared imaging and photothermal heating. Adv Mater, 2009. 21(31): p. 3175-3180, Copyright Wiley-VCH Verlag GmbH & Co. KGaA.*

their sensitivity. In a 2011 article, Kang et al.[43] documented the interactions between Cypate, a fluorophore, and GNPs. The polymer-coated GNPs were exposed to Cypate at approximately 5 nm from the surface, and this resulted in the almost complete fluorescent quenching of Cypate, as well as an approximately 17x image enhancement.

12.1.4.2.2 Two-photon luminescence

Two-photon luminescence (TPL) deals with the two low-energy photonic excitations of electrons from the occupied d band to the unoccupied sp bands of a noble metal atom producing an electron hole in the respective bands. As a result, heat scattering results in some energy loss, with the remainder being projected as a quantifiable luminescent signal because of electron–hole recombination.[111] Gold nanomaterials have been found to possess enhanced luminescent signal properties post resonance coupling due to their surface plasmon characteristics.[112] Imaging of GNR-labeled skin cells in a three-dimensional (3-D) tissue phantom deep down to 75 μm have been found to possess a TPL intensity three times stronger than that of unlabeled cancer cells, as reported by Durr and colleagues.[113] TPL has further been utilized by Park et al.[114] to create multiplexed imaging at an intraorgan level by using GNPs to simultaneously image a cell's nuclei and cytoplasm as well as GNPs within colorectal cancer tumor slices. In addition, Huff et al.[115] have made use of TPL as a mechanism to track the dissemination of GNRs inside oral epithelium-derivate KB cells. When compared to PEGylated GNRs, a higher nonspecific uptake was observed in CTAB-coated GNRs within KB cells. The in vivo TPL imaging of GNRs in mouse earlobe vessels has also come under study.[116] By first injecting picomolar concentrations of GNRs via the tail vein and following with real-time TPL imaging, it was found that the TPL intensities generated through GNRs were approximately three times higher than that of the background intensities.[117]

12.1.4.3 Absorption

12.1.4.3.1 Photoacoustic tomography

Photoacoustic tomography (PAT) deals with the production of acoustic waves produced by a target as a result of irradiation by a short electromagnetic pulse beam. A portion of the short electromagnetic pulse beam is absorbed by the target and creates localized thermal excitation, which in turn creates a buildup of pressure. The difference in pressure between the target and its surroundings eventually produces a detectable ultrasonic wave. The properties of the ultrasonic wave are dependent on the differing thermal and mechanical characteristics of the target of origin. The properties of the wave determine the initial optical absorption and the wave transmission to the transducer. PAT imaging has been demonstrated to offer a spatial resolution around 0.2 mm coupled with a penetration depth of up to 5 cm.[118,119]

PEGylated gold nanospheres have been utilized as a vehicle for PAT imaging of breast tumors in the abdominal wall of a xenograft mouse model.[120] The noninvasive PAT of rat brain vasculature using a maximum of 63% enhancement in optical absorption has been documented.[121] The nanoshells used in the PAT were cleared from the system in 6 hours after three separate, sequential administrations. PEGylated gold nanocages were found to enhance the optical absorption of the cerebral cortex in rats.[122] Penetration depths up to 3 cm were recorded in photoacoustic imaging of sentinel lymph nodes using gold nanocages as contrast agents.[123] Multiwavelength photoacoustic imaging has been documented in subcutaneous gelatin implants in ex vivo mouse tissue through the use of anti-EFGR GNPs targeted toward human epithelial cells.[124] The multiwavelength photoacoustic imaging was further used to distinguish between malignant and benign cells based on their respective absorption patterns. Cancerous cells notably exhibit a characteristic red-shifted peak on the extinction spectra, while benign cells demonstrated a green peak.

12.1.4.3.2 X-ray computed tomography

X-ray computed tomography (CT) imaging is commonly used in clinical settings to produce cross-sectional images of the body by compounding two-dimensional (2-D) slices taken along a single circular axis in the area of interest. CT imaging is well suited for in vivo applications of deep-suited tissues. However, iodine-based agents used in CT imaging have been known to create limitations, and thus, GNPs were introduced as X-ray contrast agents as a potential alternative avenue.[125] In order to test the ability of GNPs as X-ray contrast agents, 2 nm gold nanospheres were injected via the tail vein in mice to create contrast in EMT-6 syngeneic mammary tumors in xenograft mouse models alongside blood vessels. PEGylated GNPs were put into use for in vivo CT imaging of heart vessels,[126] while antibody coated GNRs were used for in vitro cancer targeting and imaging.[127] Both treatments were used to study GNP potential as X-ray contrast agents. Gadolinium chelate–coated GNPs at a 50.7 mM concentration (10 mg of gold/mL) showed an equivalent X-ray absorption as that of 280 mM iodine (35 mg of iodine/mL), as previously established by Alric and colleagues.[128] Bhatia et al. showed that intratumorally injected PEGylated GNRs in MDA-MB-435 human tumor–bearing mice had an X-ray absorption twofold higher than that demonstrated by iodine.[129]

12.1.5 Clinical gold nanomedicine—past, present, and future

Although it is one of the most studied nanotechnology platforms, only one gold nanomedicine has been Food and Drug Administration (FDA) approved for topical applications with five other known technologies within the last decade being translated from animal studies to human clinical trials, summarized in Table 12.2. The review of these technologies will focus on their technical aspects and clinical results. One of the first reported studies of GNPs in modern medicine was carried out by Guy Abraham and Peter Himmel in 1997. Abraham and Himmel demonstrated the use of their 20 nm GNPs for the treatment of rheumatoid arthritis in 10 patients. Daily doses of 30 mg, administered orally for 4 weeks followed by one dose per month for 5 months resulted in no evidence of toxicity and a "rapid and dramatic" decrease in tenderness and swelling of joints.[130] However, no follow-up studies were conducted.

The first gold nanotechnology to complete a phase 1 clinical trial was CYT-6091 (Aurimmune; CytImmune Sciences, Rockville, MD), which was developed to address challenges related to the biodistribution of previous nanomedicines (nonspecific uptake of therapeutics in healthy tissue) and interstitial fluid pressure (which opposes the enhanced permeability and retention [EPR] effect). The 27 nm colloidal gold particle bound with PEG and tumor necrosis factor-α (TNF-α) was used for the treatment of advanced stage solid tumors that were unresponsive to conventional therapies.[131] TNF-α, a cytokine that has shown antitumor effects in animal models, has seen limited clinical use due to dose-limiting toxicities (DLTs), hypotension, thrombocytopenia, and hepatotoxicity, including additional side effects of fever, general malaise, nausea, and vomiting.[132,133] Promising results from the phase 1 clinical trial showed the delivery of TNF-α via CYT-6091 increased the maximum tolerated dose from 225 $\mu g\ m^{-2}$ to 600 $\mu g\ m^{-2}$. Although all patients became febrile, no DLTs were observed at the maximum dose.[131] Since the initial clinical trial, CYT-21000, the second-generation constructs with bound chemotherapeutic paclitaxel analog have been investigated in metastatic thyroid cancer mouse models.[134] Preclinical studies have demonstrated that the delivery of CYT-21000 leads to a greater accumulation of paclitaxel within the tumor, and a 16-fold lower dose compared to free-form paclitaxel to achieve the same decrease in tumor volume.

TABLE 12.2 Summary and timeline of GNPs used in clinical trials.

Name	Description	Size	Disease	Clinical trials	Year Introduced/ Completed
AuroShell	Silica NP with gold shell, coated with PEG	Core = 120 nm Shell = 12 −15 nm	Metastatic Lung tumors, Recurrent tumors of the head and neck prostate	NCT01679470, NCT00848042, NCT02680535	2008/Ongoing
C19-A3 GNP/ EE-ASI	GNP coated with proinsulin peptide	5 nm	Type 1 diabetes	NCT02837094	2016/Ongoing
CYT-6091 (CYT-21000)	GNP coated with TNF-α and PEG (and paclitaxel)	27 nm	Advanced solid tumors, Primary cancer or metastatic cancer	NCT00356980, NCT00436410	2006/Ongoing
NANOM FIM	Silica–gold NP	60/15–70/ 40 nm core/ shell	Atherosclerosis	NCT01270139	2007/2016
NU-0129	Nucleic acids attached to GNP	13 nm	Recurrent glioblastoma or gliosarcoma	NCT03020017, NCT02782026	2017/Ongoing
Sebacia Microparticles	Silica NP with gold shell	Core = 120 nm Shell = 15 nm	Acne vulgaris	NCT02758041, NCT03303170, NCT02217228, NCT02219074, NCT03573115	2011/2018 FDA approval

GNP, gold nanoparticle; NP, nanoparticle; PEG, polyethylene glycol; TNF, tumor necrosis factor.

In order to minimize the side effects involved with conventional therapies and to combat the challenge of healthy tissue damage, AuroShell (Nanospectra Biosciences, Inc., Houston, TX), developed a 120 nm silica nanoparticle containing a 12–15 nm thick gold shell coated with a layer of 5000 molecular weight PEG for photothermal ablation of solid tumors. When activated by NIR light (820 nm, 4 W/cm^2), AuroShell particles can reach temperatures that cause irreversible tissue damage within 6 min, due to their optical absorption peak around ~800 nm.[135,136] In two phase-1 clinical trials, patients diagnosed with tumors of the head and neck received a single intravenous infusion of 24–31 mg/kg nanoshells. Laser energy was then applied 12–14 h post infusion.[137] The initial safety evaluation for the treatment of prostate cancer revealed no significant effect on the patients' chemical balance nor metabolism, with only two causes of adverse effects out of 22 patients.[138] AuroShell particle infusion is currently being tested in an ongoing phase 1 trial for prostate cancer.

Coronary artery disease (atherosclerosis), the most prevalent form of heart disease, killed about 366,000 people in the United States in 2015 (CDC.gov). The first human trial (phase I\II clinical trial) to assess the safety and efficacy of GNP-PTT to eliminate the entire plaque buildup in the artery was Plasmonic Nanophotothermal Therapy of Atherosclerosis (NANOM FIM). This technology utilizes silica GNPs (60/15–70/40 nm core/shell) delivered via a porous bovine scaffold with purified allogeneic stem cells (nanogroup) or targeted microbubbles, compared to stent implantation. Plasmonic PTT using intravascular or transcutaneous NIR laser excitation (821 nm, 35–44 W/cm^2, 7-minute exposure) was conducted 7 days post implantation. Nanoparticle concentrations ranged from 39 to 43 nM (2.23 mg/mL). Results showed an initial 12-month percent atheroma volume reduction of 12.6/44.6% for patients with the nanogroup, while the ferro group witnessed a 13.1/43.2% decrease. Patients within the control group experienced a 20.2%/22.7% reduction. The 12 month follow-up study revealed the major adverse cardiovascular events (MACE)-free survival was 92%, 82%, and 80% for the nano, ferro, and stent group, respectively, while a 5-year follow-up study indicated a cumulative MACE-free survival percentage of 94.3, 91.4, and 90.5, demonstrating a "robust level of safety."[139,140]

A major challenge in glioblastoma (GBM) treatment is the unavoidable recurrence of the cancer caused by resistant cell populations that are not removed during tumor resection nor eradicated during chemoradiotherapy. To overcome this challenge, NU-0129, a 13 nm GNP coated with "densely packed," highly oriented siRNA oligonucleotides, was designed to silence the frequently amplified gene, Bcl2L12, which encodes for proteins that neutralize the effects of caspase-3/caspase-7 and inhibit p53 activity. Preclinical animal trials demonstrated the ability of the nanoparticles to transcytose the blood–brain barrier and transfect cancerous cells, reducing tumor burden.[141,142] NU-0129 is currently under investigation within an early phase 1 clinical trial.

In order to stop white blood cells from damaging the beta cells within the pancreas for patients with type 1 diabetes, the nanomedicine C19-A3 GNP couples the peptide epitope of proinsulin, C19-A3, to 5 nm GNPs, and is administered via microneedles. The vaccine works by exposing the parts of proteins that the immune system targets to the T cells and B cells present in the body, causing them to recognize the body's insulin producing cells. In a phase 1 clinical trial, one participant, who received three doses of 10 μg peptide every 28 days, revealed no systemic reactions nor blood test abnormalities, with potential nanoparticle retention allowing for T cell infiltration and tolerance.[143]

Lastly, the only FDA-approved gold nanotechnology, Sebacia Microparticles, is a 120 nm silica nanoparticle coated with a 15 nm gold shell that is designed for the treatment of acne vulgaris. This nanoparticle has been investigated in multiple clinical trials to evaluate its safety and effectiveness. After being applied topically, the gold-coated silica microparticles localize within sebaceous follicles and cause local thermal damage when activated by NIR (10–50 J/cm^2, 30 ms, 800 nm diode laser pulses). Biodistribution and skin safety studies showed the highest level of gold in any other organ was 40.5 ng/g, a value much lower than the established safety threshold. Clinical trial results indicate a significant reduction in inflammatory lesions 12 weeks post treatment and a 60% reduction at 6 months.[144] Sebacia Microparticles, which has EU approval (CE mark), is sold in select markets and is expected to hit the United States market in 2019.

PTT has become a clinically relevant treatment option for cancer, and these clinical trials have motivated a growing interest in PTT research. While nanotechnology was initially developed to understand biodistribution of existing nanomedicines, GNPs are now being studied for applications of drug delivery and diagnostics due to their novel, tunable properties.

References

1. Huang X, El-Sayed MA. Gold nanoparticles: optical properties and implementations in cancer diagnosis and photothermal therapy. *J Adv Res* 2010;**1**(1):13–28.
2. Huang HCR, Grandhi T, Potta T, Rege K. Gold nanoparticles in cancer imaging and therapeutics. *Nano LIFE* 2010;**01**(03n04): 289–307.
3. Obaid G, et al. Photonanomedicine: a convergence of photodynamic therapy and nanotechnology. *Nanoscale* 2016;**8**(25):12471–503.
4. Shi J, et al. Cancer nanomedicine: progress, challenges and opportunities. *Nat Rev Cancer* 2016;**17**:20.

5. Wang AZ, Langer R, Farokhzad OC. Nanoparticle delivery of cancer drugs. *Annu Rev Med* 2012;**63**(1):185–98.
6. Qin Z, Bischof JC. Thermophysical and biological responses of gold nanoparticle laser heating. *Chem Soc Rev* 2012;**41**(3):1191–217.
7. Huang HC, Hasan T. The "nano" World in photodynamic therapy austin. *J Nanomed Nanotechnol* 2014;**2**(3):1020.
8. Baptista P, et al. Gold nanoparticles for the development of clinical diagnosis methods. *Anal Bioanal Chem* 2008;**391**(3):943–50.
9. Dreaden EC, et al. The golden age: gold nanoparticles for biomedicine. *Chem Soc Rev* 2012;**41**(7):2740–79.
10. Lim E-K, et al. Nanomaterials for theranostics: recent advances and future challenges. *Chem Rev* 2015;**115**(1):327–94.
11. Huang H-C, et al. Synergistic administration of photothermal therapy and chemotherapy to cancer cells using polypeptide-based degradable plasmonic matrices. *Nanomedicine* 2011;**6**(3):459–73.
12. Petryayeva E, Krull UJ. Localized surface plasmon resonance: nanostructures, bioassays and biosensing—a review. *Anal Chim Acta* 2011;**706**(1):8–24.
13. El-Sayed MA. Some interesting properties of metals confined in time and nanometer space of different shapes. *Accounts Chem Res* 2001;**34**(4):257–64.
14. Turkevich J, Stevenson PC, Hillier J. the formation of colloidal gold. *J Phys Chem* 1953;**57**(7):670–3.
15. Robenek H. In: Hayat MA, editor. *Colloidal gold: principles, methods, and applications vols. I and II. III in preparation).* New York: Academic Press, Inc.; 1989. ISBN 0–12–333927–8, Vol. I, 536 pages ISBN 0–12–333928–6, Vol. II, *484 pages.* Scanning, 1990. 12(4): pp. 244–244.
16. Kimling J, et al. Turkevich method for gold nanoparticle synthesis revisited. *J Phys Chem B* 2006;**110**(32):15700–7.
17. Turkevich J, Stevenson PC, Hillier J. A study of the nucleation and growth processes in the synthesis of colloidal gold. *Discuss Faraday Soc* 1951;**11**(0):55–75.
18. Martin CR. Nanomaterials: a membrane-based synthetic approach. *Science* 1994;**266**(5193):1961–6.
19. Jared B, et al. High-throughput templated multisegment synthesis of gold nanowires and nanorods. *Nanotechnology* 2009;**20**(6):065306.
20. Yu, et al. Gold Nanorods: electrochemical synthesis and optical properties. *J Phys Chem B* 1997;**101**(34):6661–4.
21. Chang S-S, et al. The shape transition of gold nanorods. *Langmuir* 1999;**15**(3):701–9.
22. Gole A, Murphy CJ. Seed-mediated synthesis of gold Nanorods: role of the size and nature of the seed. *Chem Mater* 2004;**16**(19):3633–40.
23. Jana NR, et al. Anisotropic chemical reactivity of gold spheroids and nanorods. *Langmuir* 2002;**18**(3):922–7.
24. Nikoobakht B, El-Sayed MA. Evidence for bilayer assembly of cationic surfactants on the surface of gold nanorods. *Langmuir* 2001;**17**(20):6368–74.
25. Nikoobakht B, El-Sayed MA. Preparation and growth mechanism of gold nanorods (NRs) using seed-mediated growth method. *Chem Mater* 2003;**15**(10):1957–62.
26. Liz-Marzán LM, Giersig M, Mulvaney P. Synthesis of nanosized Gold–Silica Core–Shell particles. *Langmuir* 1996;**12**(18):4329–35.
27. Prouzet É, Boissière C. A review on the synthesis, structure and applications in separation processes of mesoporous MSU-X silica obtained with the two-step process. *Compt Rendus Chem* 2005;**8**(3):579–96.
28. Bogush GH, Tracy MA, Zukoski CF. Preparation of monodisperse silica particles: control of size and mass fraction. *J Non-Cryst Solids* 1988;**104**(1):95–106.
29. Westcott SL, et al. Formation and adsorption of clusters of gold nanoparticles onto functionalized silica nanoparticle surfaces. *Langmuir* 1998;**14**(19):5396–401.
30. Skrabalak SE, et al. Facile synthesis of Ag nanocubes and Au nanocages. *Nat Protoc* 2007;**2**:2182.
31. Aizpurua J, et al. Optical properties of gold nanorings. *Phys Rev Lett* 2003;**90**(5):057401.
32. Lee C-K, et al. Characterizing the localized surface plasmon resonance behaviors of Au nanorings and tracking their diffusion in bio-tissue with optical coherence tomography. *Biomed Opt Express* 2010;**1**(4):1060–73.
33. Chen S, Carroll DL. Synthesis and characterization of truncated triangular silver nanoplates. *Nano Lett* 2002;**2**(9):1003–7.
34. Shankar SS, et al. Biological synthesis of triangular gold nanoprisms. *Nat Mater* 2004;**3**(7):482–8.
35. Tsai D-S, Chen C-H, Chou C-C. Preparation and characterization of gold-coated silver triangular platelets in nanometer scale. *Mater Chem Phys* 2005;**90**(2):361–6.
36. Govorov AO, Richardson HH. Generating heat with metal nanoparticles. *Nano Today* 2007;**2**(1):30–8.
37. Sperling RA, et al. Biological applications of gold nanoparticles. *Chem Soc Rev* 2008;**37**(9):1896–908.
38. Lapotko D, et al. Method of laser activated nano-thermolysis for elimination of tumor cells. *Cancer Lett* 2006;**239**(1):36–45.
39. Urban AS, et al. Controlled nanometric phase transitions of phospholipid membranes by plasmonic heating of single gold nanoparticles. *Nano Lett* 2009;**9**(8):2903–8.
40. Mirkin CA, et al. A DNA-based method for rationally assembling nanoparticles into macroscopic materials. *Nature* 1996;**382**(6592): 607–9.
41. Jin R, et al. What controls the melting properties of DNA-linked gold nanoparticle assemblies? *J Am Chem Soc* 2003;**125**(6):1643–54.
42. Link S, El-Sayed MA. Size and temperature dependence of the plasmon absorption of colloidal gold nanoparticles. *J Phys Chem B* 1999;**103**(21):4212–7.
43. Jain PK, Qian W, El-Sayed MA. Ultrafast cooling of photoexcited electrons in gold Nanoparticle–Thiolated DNA conjugates involves the dissociation of the Gold–Thiol bond. *J Am Chem Soc* 2006;**128**(7):2426–33.
44. Stehr J, et al. Gold NanoStoves for microsecond DNA melting analysis. *Nano Lett* 2008;**8**(2):619–23.
45. Guerrero AR, et al. Gold nanoparticles for photothermally controlled drug release. *Nanomedicine* 2014;**9**(13):2023–39.
46. Xiong C, et al. Cisplatin-loaded hollow gold nanoparticles for laser-triggered release. *Cancer Nanotechnol* 2018;**9**(1):6.
47. Yavuz MS, et al. Gold nanocages covered by smart polymers for controlled release with near-infrared light. *Nat Mater* 2009;**8**:935.
48. Pustovalov VK, Smetannikov AS, Zharov VP. Photothermal and accompanied phenomena of selective nanophotothermolysis with gold nanoparticles and laser pulses. *Laser Phys Lett* 2008;**5**(11):775.
49. You C-C, et al. Tunable inhibition and denaturation of α-chymotrypsin with amino acid-functionalized gold nanoparticles. *J Am Chem Soc* 2005;**127**(37):12873–81.

50. Jay DG. Selective destruction of protein function by chromophore-assisted laser inactivation. *Proc Natl Acad Sci USA* 1988;**85**(15):5454–8.
51. Dreaden EC, et al. Size matters: gold nanoparticles in targeted cancer drug delivery. *Ther Deliv* 2012;**3**(4):457–78.
52. Wu G, et al. Remotely triggered liposome release by near-infrared light absorption via hollow gold nanoshells. *J Am Chem Soc* 2008;**130**(26):8175–7.
53. Shanmugam V, Selvakumar S, Yeh CS. Near-infrared light-responsive nanomaterials in cancer therapeutics. *Chem Soc Rev* 2014;**43**(17):6254–87.
54. Alkilany AM, et al. Gold nanorods: their potential for photothermal therapeutics and drug delivery, tempered by the complexity of their biological interactions. *Adv Drug Deliv Rev* 2012;**64**(2):190–9.
55. Kennedy LC, et al. A new era for cancer treatment: gold-nanoparticle-mediated thermal therapies. *Small* 2011;**7**(2):169–83.
56. Song CW. Effect of local hyperthermia on blood flow and microenvironment: a review. *Cancer Res* 1984;**44**(10 Suppl. l):4721s–30s.
57. Riley RS, Day ES. Gold nanoparticle-mediated photothermal therapy: applications and opportunities for multimodal cancer treatment. *Wiley Interdiscip Rev Nanomed Nanobiotechnol* 2017;**9**(4):e1449.
58. DeLong RK, et al. Functionalized gold nanoparticles for the binding, stabilization, and delivery of therapeutic DNA, RNA, and other biological macromolecules. *Nanotechnol Sci Appl* 2010;**3**:53–63.
59. Jazayeri MH, et al. Various methods of gold nanoparticles (GNPs) conjugation to antibodies. *Sensing Bio-Sensing Res* 2016;**9**:17–22.
60. Dickerson EB, et al. Gold nanorod assisted near-infrared plasmonic photothermal therapy (PPTT) of squamous cell carcinoma in mice. *Cancer Lett* 2008;**269**(1):57–66.
61. Cole JR, et al. Photothermal efficiencies of nanoshells and nanorods for clinical therapeutic applications. *J Phys Chem C* 2009;**113**(28):12090–4.
62. Wang Y, et al. Comparison study of gold nanohexapods, nanorods, and nanocages for photothermal cancer treatment. *ACS Nano* 2013;**7**(3):2068–77.
63. Huang HC, Rege K, Heys JJ. Spatiotemporal temperature distribution and cancer cell death in response to extracellular hyperthermia induced by gold nanorods. *ACS Nano* 2010;**4**(5):2892–900.
64. Nanospectra biosciences, I. Pilot study of AuroLase(tm) therapy in refractory and/or recurrent tumors of the head and neck. Available from: https://ClinicalTrials.gov/show/NCT00848042.
65. Raeesi V, Chan WC. Improving nanoparticle diffusion through tumor collagen matrix by photo-thermal gold nanorods. *Nanoscale* 2016;**8**(25):12524–30.
66. Fay BL, Melamed JR, Day ES. Nanoshell-mediated photothermal therapy can enhance chemotherapy in inflammatory breast cancer cells. *Int J Nanomed* 2015;**10**:6931–41.
67. Mendes R, et al. Photothermal enhancement of chemotherapy in breast cancer by visible irradiation of Gold Nanoparticles. *Sci Rep* 2017;**7**(1):10872.
68. Wust P, et al. Hyperthermia in combined treatment of cancer. *Lancet Oncol* 2002;**3**(8):487–97.
69. Schaaf L, et al. Hyperthermia synergizes with chemotherapy by inhibiting PARP1-dependent DNA replication arrest. *Cancer Res* 2016;**76**(10):2868–75.
70. van der Heijden AG, et al. Effect of hyperthermia on the cytotoxicity of 4 chemotherapeutic agents currently used for the treatment of transitional cell carcinoma of the bladder: an in vitro study. *J Urol* 2005;**173**(4):1375–80.
71. Liu J, et al. Gold nanorods coated with a thermo-responsive poly(-ethylene glycol)-b-poly(N-vinylcaprolactam) corona as drug delivery systems for remotely near infrared-triggered release. *Polym Chem* 2014;**5**(3):799–813.
72. Campardelli R, et al. Au–PLA nanocomposites for photothermally controlled drug delivery. *J Mater Chem B* 2014;**2**(4):409–17.
73. Huang J, Jackson KS, Murphy CJ. Polyelectrolyte wrapping layers control rates of photothermal molecular release from gold nanorods. *Nano Lett* 2012;**12**(6):2982–7.
74. Rengan AK, et al. Multifunctional gold coated thermo-sensitive liposomes for multimodal imaging and photo-thermal therapy of breast cancer cells. *Nanoscale* 2014;**6**(2):916–23.
75. Yamashita S, et al. Controlled-release system mediated by a retro Diels-Alder reaction induced by the photothermal effect of gold nanorods. *Langmuir* 2011;**27**(23):14621–6.
76. Yang J, et al. Spatially confined fabrication of core–shell gold Nanocages@Mesoporous silica for near-infrared controlled photothermal drug release. *Chem Mater* 2013;**25**(15):3030–7.
77. Zhang Z, et al. Mesoporous silica-coated gold nanorods as a light-mediated multifunctional theranostic platform for cancer treatment. *Adv Mater* 2012;**24**(11):1418–23.
78. Munn DH, Bronte V. Immune suppressive mechanisms in the tumor microenvironment. *Curr Opin Immunol* 2016;**39**:1–6.
79. Bear AS, et al. Elimination of metastatic melanoma using gold nanoshell-enabled photothermal therapy and adoptive T cell transfer. *PLoS One* 2013;**8**(7):e69073.
80. Ribas A, Wolchok JD. Cancer immunotherapy using checkpoint blockade. *Science* 2018;**359**(6382):1350–5.
81. Swaika A, Hammond WA, Joseph RW. Current state of anti-PD-L1 and anti-PD-1 agents in cancer therapy. *Mol Immunol* 2015;**67**(2):4–17. Part A.
82. Callahan MK, Wolchok JD, Allison JP. Anti-CTLA-4 antibody therapy: immune monitoring during clinical development of a novel immunotherapy. *Semin Oncol* 2010;**37**(5):473–84.
83. Wang C, et al. Immunological responses triggered by photothermal therapy with carbon nanotubes in combination with anti-CTLA-4 therapy to inhibit cancer metastasis. *Adv Mater* 2014;**26**(48):8154–62.
84. Bakhtiari ABS, et al. An efficient method based on the photothermal effect for the release of molecules from metal nanoparticle surfaces. *Angew Chem Int Ed* 2009;**48**(23):4166–9.
85. Castano AP, Demidova TN, Hamblin MR. Mechanisms in photodynamic therapy: part one—-photosensitizers, photochemistry and cellular localization. *Photodiagn Photodyn Ther* 2004;**1**(4):279–93.
86. Ding H, et al. Photoactivation switch from type II to type I reactions by electron-rich micelles for improved photodynamic therapy of cancer cells under hypoxia. *J Control Release* 2011;**156**(3):276–80.
87. Bhana S, et al. Photosensitizer-loaded gold nanorods for near infrared photodynamic and photothermal cancer therapy. *J Colloid Interface Sci* 2016;**469**:8–16.
88. Wei X, et al. Combined photodynamic and photothermal therapy using cross-linked polyphosphazene nanospheres decorated with gold nanoparticles. *ACS Applied Nano Materials* 2018;**1**(7):3663–72.
89. Ge R, et al. Photothermal-activatable Fe_3O_4 superparticle nanodrug carriers with PD-L1 immune checkpoint blockade for anti-metastatic cancer immunotherapy. *ACS Appl Mater Interfaces* 2018;**10**(24): 20342–55.

90. Yang P, et al. Light-activated sutureless closure of wounds in thin skin. *Lasers Surg Med* 2012;**44**(2):163–7.
91. Wolf-de Jonge IC, Beek JF, Balm R. 25 years of laser assisted vascular anastomosis (LAVA): what have we learned? *Eur J Vasc Endovasc Surg* 2004;**27**(5):466–76.
92. Matteini P, et al. Microscopic characterization of collagen modifications induced by low-temperature diode-laser welding of corneal tissue. *Lasers Surg Med* 2007;**39**(7):597–604.
93. Wadia Y, Xie H, Kajitani M. Liver repair and hemorrhage control by using laser soldering of liquid albumin in a porcine model. *Lasers Surg Med* 2000;**27**(4):319–28.
94. McNally KM, et al. Photothermal effects of laser tissue soldering. *Phys Med Biol* 1999;**44**(4):983–1002. discussion 2 pages follow.
95. Gobin AM, et al. Near infrared laser-tissue welding using nanoshells as an exogenous absorber. *Lasers Surg Med* 2005;**37**(2):123–9.
96. Huang HC, et al. Laser welding of ruptured intestinal tissue using plasmonic polypeptide nanocomposite solders. *ACS Nano* 2013;**7**(4):2988–98.
97. Huang D, et al. Optical coherence tomography. *Science* 1991;**254**(5035):1178–81.
98. Loo C, et al. Nanoshell-enabled photonics-based imaging and therapy of cancer. *Technol Cancer Res Treat* 2004;**3**(1):33–40.
99. Kirillin MY, et al. *Contrasting Properties of Gold Nanoshells and Titanium dioxide Nanoparticles for Optical Coherence Tomography Imaging of Skin: Monte Carlo Simulations and in vivo Study*. SPIE; 2009.
100. Zagaynova EV, et al. Contrasting properties of gold nanoparticles for optical coherence tomography: phantom, in vivo studies and Monte Carlo simulation. *Phys Med Biol* 2008;**53**(18): 4995–5009.
101. Gobin AM, et al. Near-infrared resonant nanoshells for combined optical imaging and photothermal cancer therapy. *Nano Lett* 2007;**7**(7):1929–34.
102. Kim CS, et al. Enhanced detection of early-stage oral cancer in vivo by optical coherence tomography using multimodal delivery of gold nanoparticles. *J Biomed Opt* 2009;**14**(3):034008.
103. Lin AWH, et al. Reflectance spectroscopy of gold nanoshells: computational predictions and experimental measurements. *J Nanoparticle Res* 2006;**8**(5):681–92.
104. Laurent G, et al. Imaging surface plasmon of gold nanoparticle arrays by far-field Raman scattering. *Nano Lett* 2005;**5**(2):253–8.
105. Huang X, et al. Cancer cells assemble and align gold nanorods conjugated to antibodies to produce highly enhanced, sharp, and polarized surface Raman spectra: a potential cancer diagnostic marker. *Nano Lett* 2007;**7**(6):1591–7.
106. Qian X, et al. In vivo tumor targeting and spectroscopic detection with surface-enhanced Raman nanoparticle tags. *Nat Biotechnol* 2008;**26**(1):83–90.
107. Keren S, et al. Noninvasive molecular imaging of small living subjects using Raman spectroscopy. *Proc Natl Acad Sci USA* 2008;**105**(15):5844–9.
108. von Maltzahn G, et al. SERS-coded gold nanorods as a multifunctional platform for densely multiplexed near-infrared imaging and photothermal heating. *Adv Mater* 2009;**21**(31):3175–80.
109. He H, Xie C, Ren J. Nonbleaching fluorescence of gold nanoparticles and its applications in cancer cell imaging. *Anal Chem* 2008;**80**(15):5951–7.
111. Boyd GT, Yu ZH, Shen YR. Photoinduced luminescence from the noble metals and its enhancement on roughened surfaces. *Phys Rev B* 1986;**33**(12):7923–36.
112. Bouhelier A, et al. Surface plasmon characteristics of tunable photoluminescence in single gold nanorods. *Phys Rev Lett* 2005;**95**(26):267405.
113. Durr NJ, et al. Two-photon luminescence imaging of cancer cells using molecularly targeted gold nanorods. *Nano Lett* 2007;**7**(4):941–5.
114. Park J, et al. Intra-organ biodistribution of gold nanoparticles using intrinsic two-photon induced photoluminescence. *Lasers Surg Med* 2010;**42**(7):630–9.
115. Huff TB, et al. Controlling the cellular uptake of gold nanorods. *Langmuir* 2007;**23**(4):1596–9.
116. Wang H, et al. In vitro and in vivo two-photon luminescence imaging of single gold nanorods. *Proc Natl Acad Sci U S A* 2005;**102**(44):15752–6.
117. Zhang G, et al. Influence of anchoring ligands and particle size on the colloidal stability and in vivo biodistribution of polyethylene glycol-coated gold nanoparticles in tumor-xenografted mice. *Biomaterials* 2009;**30**(10):1928–36.
118. Wang X, et al. Noninvasive laser-induced photoacoustic tomography for structural and functional in vivo imaging of the brain. *Nat Biotechnol* 2003;**21**(7):803–6.
119. Ku G, Wang LV. Deeply penetrating photoacoustic tomography in biological tissues enhanced with an optical contrast agent. *Opt Lett* 2005;**30**(5):507–9.
120. Zhang Q, et al. Gold nanoparticles as a contrast agent for in vivo tumor imaging with photoacoustic tomography. *Nanotechnology* 2009;**20**(39):395102.
121. Wang Y, et al. Photoacoustic tomography of a nanoshell contrast agent in the in vivo rat brain. *Nano Lett* 2004;**4**(9):1689–92.
122. Yang X, et al. Photoacoustic tomography of a rat cerebral cortex in vivo with Au nanocages as an optical contrast agent. *Nano Lett* 2007;**7**(12):3798–802.
123. Song KH, et al. Near-infrared gold nanocages as a new class of tracers for photoacoustic sentinel lymph node mapping on a rat model. *Nano Lett* 2009;**9**(1):183–8.
124. Mallidi S, et al. Multiwavelength photoacoustic imaging and plasmon resonance coupling of gold nanoparticles for selective detection of cancer. *Nano Lett* 2009;**9**(8):2825–31.
125. Hainfeld JF, et al. Gold nanoparticles: a new X-ray contrast agent. *Br J Radiol* 2006;**79**(939):248–53.
126. Kim D, et al. Antibiofouling polymer-coated gold nanoparticles as a contrast agent for in vivo X-ray computed tomography imaging. *J Am Chem Soc* 2007;**129**(24):7661–5.
127. Popovtzer R, et al. Targeted gold nanoparticles enable molecular CT imaging of cancer. *Nano Lett* 2008;**8**(12):4593–6.
128. Alric C, et al. Gadolinium chelate coated gold nanoparticles as contrast agents for both X-ray computed tomography and magnetic resonance imaging. *J Am Chem Soc* 2008;**130**(18): 5908–15.
129. von Maltzahn G, et al. Computationally guided photothermal tumor therapy using long-circulating gold nanorod antennas. *Cancer Res* 2009;**69**(9):3892–900.
130. Abraham GE, Himmel PB. Management of rheumatoid arthritis: rationale for the. *J Nutr Environ Med* 1997;**7**(4):295.

131. Libutti SK, et al. Phase I and pharmacokinetic studies of CYT-6091, a novel PEGylated colloidal gold-rhTNF nanomedicine. *Clin Cancer Res* 2010;**16**(24):6139–49.
132. Taguchi T. Phase I study of recombinant human tumor necrosis factor (rHu-TNF:PT-050). *Cancer Detect Prev* 1988;**12**(1–6):561–72.
133. Kimura K, et al. Phase I study of recombinant human tumor necrosis factor. *Cancer Chemother Pharmacol* 1987;**20**(3):223–9.
Nilubol N, et al. Novel dual-action targeted nanomedicine in mice with metastatic thyroid cancer and pancreatic neuroendocrine tumors. *JNCI, J Natl Cancer Inst* 2018;**110**(9):1019–29.
135. Hirsch LR, et al. Nanoshell-mediated near-infrared thermal therapy of tumors under magnetic resonance guidance. *Proc Natl Acad Sci USA* 2003;**100**(23):13549–54.
136. James WD, et al. Application of INAA to the build-up and clearance of gold nanoshells in clinical studies in mice. *J. Radioanal. Nucl. Chem.* 2007;**271**(2):455–9.
137. Gad SC, et al. Evaluation of the toxicity of intravenous delivery of auroshell particles (gold-silica nanoshells). *Int J Toxicol* 2012;**31**(6):584–94.
138. Stern JM, et al. Initial evaluation of the safety of nanoshell-directed photothermal therapy in the treatment of prostate disease 2016;**35**(1):38–46.
139. Kharlamov AN, et al. Silica–gold nanoparticles for atheroprotective management of plaques: results of the NANOM-FIM trial. *Nanoscale* 2015;**7**(17):8003–15.
140. Kharlamov AN, et al. Plasmonic photothermal therapy of atherosclerosis with nanoparticles: long-term outcomes and safety in. *NANOM-FIM trial* 2017;**13**(4):345–63.
141. Jensen SA, et al. Spherical nucleic acid nanoparticle conjugates as an RNAi-based therapy for glioblastoma. *Sci Transl Med* 2013;**5**(209). p. 209ra152-209ra152.
142. Rosi NL, et al. Oligonucleotide-modified gold nanoparticles for intracellular gene regulation. *Science* 2006;**312**(5776):1027–30.
143. *Case reports* 2018;**35**(S1):13–5.
144. Paithankar DY, et al. Acne treatment based on selective photothermolysis of sebaceous follicles with topically delivered light-absorbing gold microparticles. *J Investig Dermatol* 2015;**135**(7):1727–34.

Chapter 13

Magnetic nanoparticles

Shehaab Savliwala[1], Andreina Chiu-Lam[1], Mythreyi Unni[1], Angelie Rivera-Rodriguez[2], Eric Fuller[2], Kacoli Sen[1], Marcus Threadcraft[3] and Carlos Rinaldi[1,2]

[1]*Department of Chemical Engineering, University of Florida, Gainesville, FL, United States;* [2]*J. Crayton Pruitt Family Department of Biomedical Engineering, University of Florida, Gainesville, FL, United States;* [3]*College of Medicine, University of Florida, Gainesville, FL, United States*

13.1 Introduction

Magnetic nanoparticles (MNPs) are of interest in numerous biomedical applications due to the intrinsic biocompatibility of some of their phases and their interaction with externally applied magnetic fields. MNPs can distort the magnetic field in their surroundings, forming the basis for enhanced contrast in magnetic resonance imaging (MRI). In other applications, applied magnetic fields can induce magnetic forces and torques on their magnetic dipoles, resulting in particle translation, rotation, and even energy dissipation in the form of heat. These phenomena give rise to applications in biomarker/cell separation, magnetically targeted drug delivery, magnetomechanical actuation of cell surface receptors, magnetic hyperthermia and triggered drug release, and biomedical imaging. In the past decade, there has been a tremendous amount of research on the synthesis, characterization, and postsynthesis application-specific modification of magnetic iron oxide and substituted ferrite nanoparticles, leading to many emerging applications in a wide array of fields. For a general review of the applications of MNPs, there are several review articles published in the past few years that serve as an excellent starting point.[1–6]

In this chapter, we will focus on the applications of MNPs specific to the biomedical setting. The chapter is organized as follows. We start by introducing the chemical and physical properties of iron oxide and ferrite nanoparticles commonly used for biomedical applications. Then, we describe the most important and widely reported magnetic properties of these particles, followed by the most common methods of synthesis. Next, we summarize applications of these particles that have achieved clinical translation, including use as MRI contrast agents, magnetic hyperthermia, and in sentinel lymph node (SLN) mapping. Finally, we summarize a few emerging applications that rely on the response of MNPs to alternating magnetic fields (AMFs).

13.2 Magnetite, maghemite, and substituted ferrites

13.2.1 Magnetic nanoparticles and biomedicine

MNPs can be made from a variety of materials and compositions, with varying magnetic and physical properties relevant to intended applications. However, in the biomedical arena, one must consider their potential biocompatibility/toxicity and long-term in vivo fate and clearance. These considerations restrict the nanoparticle compositions and formulations that can be used safely without introducing harm or side effects to living tissue,[7,8] making a specific subset of ferrite nanoparticles ($M_xFe_{3-x}O_4$, where M can be Fe, Mn, Ni, or Zn) excellent candidates for biomedical applications.[9–12]

One reason for the reduced concern with biocompatibility of iron oxide MNPs is that the healthy human body already has mechanisms for handling, storage, and use of iron.[13] As an essential nutrient, iron is required to sustain human health and survival. Iron is both an antioxidant and pro-oxidant that participates in the transport and storage of oxygen throughout the body, DNA synthesis, energy production, and metabolism and detoxification. In fact, the average human body contains about 4 g of iron (as well as much smaller amounts of the other metals mentioned above) in the form of two extremely important molecules, ferritin and hemoglobin.[14]

Ferritin is an intracellular protein found in the cytoplasm of every cell type[15], its primary function being the capture, storage, and controlled release of iron. A ferritin molecule weighs 474 kDa, consisting of 24 ferritin subunits (19 kDa, 21 kDa) bound to form a hollow globular protein 8–12 nm in diameter.[15,16] Free iron ions can be toxic to cells by acting as catalysts in the formation of reactive oxygen species via the Fenton reaction.[17] A single ferritin

Nanoparticles for Biomedical Applications. https://doi.org/10.1016/B978-0-12-816662-8.00013-8

complex can capture and store roughly 4500 Fe^{3+} ions in the form of phosphate and hydroxide salts of iron, ensuring that the iron is stored in a soluble and nontoxic form, and preventing accumulation of free iron ions inside cells.[16] In its role as a carrier and transport molecule, ferritin is released into the serum/plasma, and iron can be released from ferritin when required by the process of ferritin degradation, which occurs in lysosomes.[18]

Hemoglobin is an iron-containing protein found in the blood of all vertebrates, as well as some invertebrates.[19] In vertebrates, its primary function is oxygen transport through the blood, which it does by providing four iron binding sites[20] for molecular oxygen per 64 kDa (four subunits, each 16 kDa) globular complex. Hemoglobin is also involved in vital transport processes of other gases in the body, such as CO_2 and nitric oxide.[21,22] Additionally, hemoglobin is found in several other cell types in the body, where it is reported to play a role as an antioxidant and regulator of iron metabolism.[23]

Another compelling reason for the preference for ferrite MNPs over others for biomedical applications is that there has been extensive testing regarding the safety of these nanoparticles in laboratory, preclinical, and clinical settings. In fact, several formulations of iron oxide have been approved by regulatory agencies in both the United States and Europe for clinical stage investigation and use, notable examples being for the treatment of pancreatic and brain tumors,[24–30] their use in imaging and diagnostic settings via MRI, and their application for SLN mapping.[31–33] These applications are discussed further below.

13.2.2 Phases of iron oxide

There are 16 phases of iron oxides commonly found in nature, made up of a mix of iron oxides, hydroxides, and oxide-hydroxides.[34] Not all of these are phases that generally show up in iron oxide/ferrite nanoparticles when synthesized by wet chemical methods, but they can occur when the preparation method is through physical size reduction[35] or gas phase deposition processes.[36] The reason a distinction must be made between different phases of iron oxide is that the physical, chemical, and magnetic properties of the phases are extremely different, and weakly magnetic or nonmagnetic compositions must be identified and avoided when the intended use relies on nanoscale magnetic properties. Similarly, substituted ferrites (those where the divalent iron atom has been substituted by another divalent metal element), while not commonly found in nature, show chemical, physical, and crystallographic properties similar to the iron oxide phase they derive from, yet, their magnetic properties can be tuned by the proper selection of the substituent metal atom(s).[37–41] Table 13.1 lists the names, chemical compositions, type of magnetic response, crystal geometry, and unit cell dimensions[34] of the five iron oxide phases that will be of most relevance to this chapter, namely: magnetite, maghemite, hematite, wüstite, and goethite. For an extensive review into the chemistry of iron oxides, the book by Cornell and Schwertmann is an excellent reference.[34]

Magnetite or maghemite: Magnetite (Fe_3O_4) is the most magnetic naturally occurring mineral and, as such, is a highly desirable crystal phase when preparing MNPs. Magnetite crystals have a face-centered cubic inverse spinel crystal geometry with a unit cell dimension of $a = 0.8396$ nm. The unit cell consists of 32 O^{2-} ions in a cubic close packed arrangement, 8 Fe^{2+} ions occupying half the octahedral sites, and 16 Fe^{3+} atoms occupying the remaining octahedral and tetrahedral sites. Magnetite is a ferrimagnetic material and exhibits superparamagnetism at the nanoscale with a reported upper limit for single domain

TABLE 13.1 Phases of iron oxides encountered in nanoparticle formulations relevant to the biomedical setting.

Phase	Chemical composition	Type of magnetism	Crystal structure
Magnetite	Fe_3O_4	Ferrimagnetic. Exhibits superparamagnetism at the nanoscale.	Cubic. $a = 0.8396$ nm
Maghemite	γ-Fe_2O_3	Ferrimagnetic. Exhibits superparamagnetism at the nanoscale.	Cubic or tetragonal. $a = 0.8374$ nm
Hematite	α-Fe_2O_3	Weakly ferromagnetic or antiferromagnetic.	Rhombohedral Hexagonal. $a = 0.5036$ nm, $c = 1.3749$ nm
Wustite	FeO	Antiferromagnetic.	Cubic. $a = 0.4302$–0.4275 nm
Goethite	α-FeOOH	Antiferromagnetic.	Orthorhombic. $a = 0.9956$ nm, $b = 0.3022$ nm, $c = 0.4608$ nm

Adapted from Cornell RM, Schwertmann U. The iron oxides: structure, properties, reactions, occurrences and uses: Wiley; 2006.

particles of approximately 80–100 nm[42–44] and a high mass saturation magnetization of 92 Am^2/kg at 293 K.[45]

Maghemite is closely related to magnetite in structure, with the main difference being that all the iron exists as Fe^{3+}. Maghemite also exhibits a cubic face-centered inverse spinel geometry and a unit cell dimension of $a = 0.8374$ nm. This makes it extremely hard to distinguish from magnetite, especially for polydisperse nanoparticle populations, by conventional methods of crystal-phase determination for particulates such as X-ray diffraction (XRD), Raman spectroscopy, high-resolution transmission electron microscopy (TEM), and electron diffraction. Maghemite is ferrimagnetic and also exhibits superparamagnetism at the nanoscale for single domain particles but has a lower mass saturation magnetization of 76 Am^2/kg[45], thus making it slightly less desirable than magnetite as the optimal MNP platform for applications. However, magnetite can easily be oxidized to maghemite in an oxygen-rich environment, making the synthesis of phase-pure magnetite challenging and raising concerns that particle properties will change over time. This has prompted some groups to purposefully oxidize magnetite nanoparticles to maghemite prior to use.[46–49] Challenges with synthesis of phase-pure magnetite are discussed further in Section 13.3.

Goethite, Hematite, and Wüstite: Goethite and hematite are two of the most thermodynamically stable phases of iron oxide at room temperature[34] and are often the end result of oxidation or multiple phase transitions from other phases. Both are very weakly antiferromagnetic, and reliable measurements of saturation magnetization are hard to obtain because the materials require very high external fields to saturate. Neither exhibits superparamagnetism at the nanoscale, making them undesirable for most biomedical applications of MNPs. However, they can occur as impurities during synthesis of magnetite and maghemite, and they can be distinguished using XRD as they have different crystal structures compared to magnetite and maghemite.

Wüstite has a composition of $Fe_{1-x}O$, a sodium chloride–type body-centered cubic structure, and usually exists as a metastable compound that is intermediate between magnetite, maghemite, and goethite. Wüstite can be reduced to goethite over time or oxidized to magnetite/maghemite via disproportionation or oxidation.[34] It is weakly antiferromagnetic, does not exhibit superparamagnetism at the nanoscale, and is generally undesirable for use in common biomedical applications of MNPs. However, wüstite has been reported to form in place of magnetite and maghemite when synthesis of nanoparticles is conducted under anoxic conditions, which will be discussed further in Section 13.3.

13.3 Summary of magnetic properties

MNPs are of interest in biomedicine precisely because of their magnetic properties. However, many beginning practitioners in the field lack an understanding of what these properties are and how they are typically measured and reported. Here we provide a brief summary of some of the most important and widely reported magnetic properties and refer the reader to other sources for additional information.[50–52]

13.3.1 Magnetization curves and types of magnetic materials

The magnetic response of materials to an external magnetic field is influenced by the electronic configuration of its constituent elements, the way they combine chemically, and temperature. Some common types of magnetic materials are explained below.

Diamagnets: In a diamagnetic material, all the electron spins in the material are paired, and they exhibit the weakest type of magnetic behavior. An external magnetic field induces a torque on the spin dipoles of these electron pairs, which causes the electron pairs to undergo an angular displacement. The direction of realignment is such that the magnetic moment created acts to oppose the inducing field, resulting in materials with a negative initial susceptibility. The initial susceptibility of a magnetic material, which we address fully in Section 13.2.2, is defined by the slope of the magnetization versus external field data, as seen in Fig. 13.1. Inert gases, most nonmetals, and organic compounds are common diamagnets, and their response is weakly dependent on temperature.

Paramagnets: Paramagnetic materials are those in which individual atoms have uncompensated spins that are

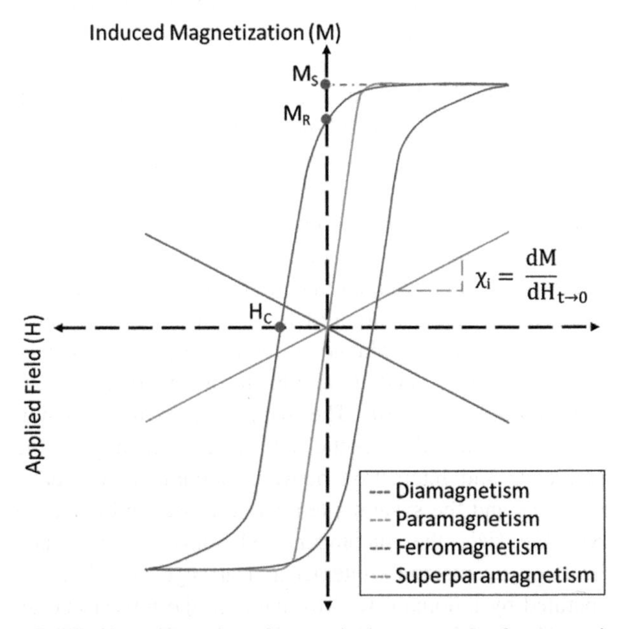

FIGURE 13.1 Illustration of magnetization curves for ferromagnetic, paramagnetic, diamagnetic, and superparamagnetic materials. Here, M_S, M_R, H_C, and χ_i are the saturation magnetization, remanent magnetization, coercive field threshold, and the initial susceptibility of the material.

randomly aligned. In the presence of an external magnetic field, the uncompensated spin moments tend to align in the direction of the field. The degree of alignment of the uncompensated spins with the applied magnetic field therefore depends on the strength of the field (the stronger the field, the greater the degree of alignment up to very high fields) and the temperature (the higher the temperature of the material, the lower the degree of alignment for the same applied field). As shown in Fig. 13.1, they have a positive magnetic susceptibility.

Ferromagnets: The magnetic moments in each domain of a ferromagnet are oriented along an easy axis of magnetization, corresponding to a low-energy state. Uncompensated electrons in individual atoms tend to interact, resulting in coupling of spins in a preferred orientation. In ferromagnets, uncompensated spins in individual atoms of a ferromagnetic material may couple either directly (direct exchange) or through an intermediate anion—usually oxygen (super exchange). Unlike paramagnets, when the applied field is removed, they may retain a component of magnetization in the direction of the applied field causing them to be "permanently" magnetized. In fact, the magnetization is kinetically trapped at experimental time scales. As seen in Fig. 13.1, the response is an open curve and these materials exhibit hysteresis. On removal of the field, the extent to which the material remains magnetized is quantified by the remanent magnetization (M_R), and the field required to demagnetize the material is the coercive field (H_c). Ferromagnetism is mostly seen in metals like iron, nickel, cobalt, and manganese. The field at which the material reaches saturation is a measure of how magnetically "hard" or "soft" it is.

In the case of ferromagnets, the coupling of spins need not always be in the same direction, thereby resulting in materials exhibiting special kinds of ferromagnetism. When uncompensated spins are coupled antiparallel to one other, materials are antiferromagnetic. Due to spin canting or lattice defects, they might possess a net magnetization. Ferromagnets in which the spins of neighboring lattices are antiparallel and of unequal magnitude are called ferrimagnets. The net magnetization of ferrimagnets is greater than for antiferromagnets. Magnetite, commonly found in biological organisms, tends to exhibit ferrimagnetism.

Superparamagnetism: The magnetic response of a material to an external magnetic field depends mainly on the prevalence and interaction between uncompensated electron spins and the system's temperature. Beyond a certain crystallite size, the uncompensated spins in ferro- and ferrimagnetic materials interact and arrange into domains separated by a domain wall to maintain the lowest energy state. Conversely, there is a critical size (80—100 nm for mixed ferrites[44]) below which it is energetically unfavorable for domain walls to form, resulting in single domain nanoparticles.[53] As predicted by Louis Nèel,[54] at a high enough temperature, nanoparticles in the single domain regime do not exhibit hysteresis behavior in an applied magnetic field, while their magnetization (volume density of magnetic dipoles) quickly increases and then saturates as the strength of the applied magnetic field increases. This condition is referred to as superparamagnetism. Small ferromagnetic nanoparticles tend to behave as superparamagnets. The size below which superparamagnetism is predominant depends on the balance between magnetocrystalline anisotropy energy, thermal energy, and the magnetic energy of the applied magnetic field.[55] Analogous to paramagnets, superparamagnets tend to lose their magnetism in the absence of a field and do not exhibit any hysteresis. As illustrated in Fig. 13.1, high initial susceptibility, saturation of magnetization, and negligible coercivity and remanence are hallmarks of superparamagnets.

13.3.2 Commonly reported magnetic properties

Initial susceptibility: At low enough applied magnetic fields, the dependence between the magnetization and applied magnetic field for paramagnetic and superparamagnetic materials is linear, and the slope of this relation is called the initial susceptibility. As such, the initial susceptibility is a measure of how easy it is to align the magnetic dipoles in the material with the field, for situations where the energy associated with the magnetic field is small relative to thermal energy. In a paramagnetic material, the uncompensated electron spins are uncoupled, hence the balance is between the magnetic torque on a single electron spin and the thermal energy. Because the torque on single electrons is very weak, the magnetic energy is much lower than the thermal energy for technically feasible magnetic fields; the ratio of magnetic to thermal energy is always $<<1$ and the initial susceptibility is relatively low (10^{-5} to 10^{-7}). For superparamagnetic nanoparticles, the magnetic torque acts on a collection of coupled electron spins, resulting in a much higher initial susceptibility (10^{-2} to 10^{-3}). For a collection of noninteracting, spherical, monodisperse MNPs the initial susceptibility is given by[55]

$$\chi_i = \frac{\pi}{18} \Phi \mu_o \frac{M_d^2 d^3}{kT} \tag{13.1}$$

where ϕ is the volume fraction of magnetic solids, μ_0 is the initial permeability, M_d is the domain magnetization, k is Boltzmann's constant, T is the absolute temperature, and d is the diameter of the particles.

Magnetic saturation: In the presence of an applied magnetic field, magnetic spins in a superparamagnetic particle tend to align in the direction of the field, resulting in an induced magnetization.[56] At high enough magnetic fields, all the magnetic spins are aligned in the direction of the field, resulting in the maximum induced magnetization, which is often called the saturation magnetization of the sample. Saturation magnetization is often used as a metric to compare magnetic properties across different particles (say, obtained by different methods or with varied sizes and compositions) as it is related to the strength of the nanoparticle's overall dipole moment.

Blocking temperature: Superparamagnetism is largely dependent on system temperature and the size of the particle. Superparamagnetism corresponds to a state where the energy barrier to dipole moment rotation in the crystal is much smaller than the thermal energy and the dipoles can freely rotate to align with an applied magnetic field. The temperature at which thermal energy is low enough to "freeze" the spontaneous alignment of magnetization is called the blocking temperature. Above the blocking temperature a material may act as a superparamagnet, while it may act as a ferromagnet below the blocking temperature. The blocking temperature is often determined using temperature dependence of the magnetization of a sample cooled to cryogenic temperature in zero field, and the value of the blocking temperature determined in this way can be used to estimate the so-called magnetocrystalline anisotropy energy density that characterizes the energy barrier to dipole rotation.[50] However, care must be taken when interpreting such measurements, as the blocking temperature is not an intrinsic property of the sample and depends on the conditions of the measurement.[57]

Brownian and Néel relaxation: For a collection of noninteracting MNPs in suspension, the change in orientation of the particle's magnetic dipoles in response to a time-varying magnetic field may occur by two basic mechanisms (illustrated in Fig. 13.2): (i) physical particle rotation, known as Brownian relaxation and (ii) internal dipole rotation, known as Néel relaxation. When particles relax by the Brownian mechanism, their dipoles are thought to be locked along a given crystal direction, therefore the torque on the magnetic dipole induces rotation of the particle as a whole and against the drag of the surrounding medium. In contrast, when particles relax by the Néel mechanism, their dipoles are thought to either freely rotate between crystal directions or switch between crystal directions that correspond to energy minima and are often called "easy axes." Both mechanisms occur simultaneously albeit with different rates, quantified by their characteristic relaxation times, and the dominant mechanism will be the one with the fastest rate (i.e., shortest relaxation time).

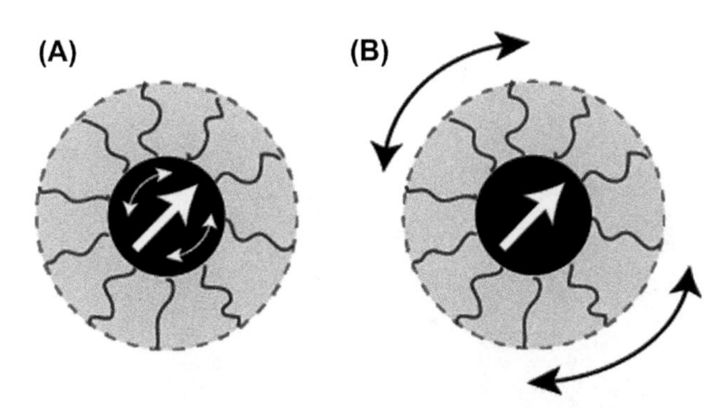

FIGURE 13.2 Illustration of mechanisms by which particles relax in the presence of an alternating magnetic field: (A) Internal dipole rotation or Néel mechanism and (B) physical particle rotation or Brownian mechanism.

Magnetogranulometry and the concept of magnetic diameter: The most commonly used MNPs are ferrites that exhibit a spinel or inverse spinel structure. The distribution of the metal ions relative to the oxygen ions in the crystal lattice results in the formation of dipoles and determines the overall magnetization of the material. Common routes of synthesis often result in particles that have saturation magnetization below the bulk value.[58] This is often attributed to the existence of a "magnetically dead layer" on the surface of the nanoparticles, where spin canting and other phenomena may lead to disorder of the magnetic dipoles.[59,60] Alternatively, the nanoparticle may possess magnetic subdomains that are smaller than the overall physical dimensions of the particles. These cases are illustrated in Fig. 13.3A. In both such cases, there is a mismatch between the magnetic volume of particles that experiences a magnetic force/torque and contributes to the magnetic response, and the actual physical volume of the particles, often determined from TEM. The magnetic volume, or the associated magnetic diameter, is a measure of the ordering and strength of the dipoles in single domain particles. Magnetization measurements as a function of applied magnetic field can be analyzed to obtain the distribution of magnetic diameters in a sample, a technique often called magnetogranulometric analysis.[61] This is often achieved by fitting the Langevin function describing superparamagnetic magnetization, weighted using a lognormal size distribution,[62] to experimental magnetization measurements

$$M(\alpha) = M_S \int_0^\infty n_v(D_m) L(\alpha) dD_m \tag{13.2}$$

$$n_v(D_m) = \frac{1}{\sqrt{2\pi} D_m \ln \sigma} \exp\left[-\frac{\ln^2\left(\frac{D_m}{D_{mv}}\right)}{2\ln^2 \sigma}\right] \tag{13.3}$$

$$L(\alpha) = \coth \alpha - \frac{1}{\alpha}; \quad \alpha = \frac{\pi \mu_0 M_d D_m^3 H}{6 k_B T} \tag{13.4}$$

In Eqs. (13.2)–(13.4), α is the Langevin parameter (the ratio of magnetic to thermal energy), M_s is the saturation magnetization of the sample consisting of a collection of MNPs in a nonmagnetic medium, D_m is the magnetic diameter of the particles, D_{mv} is the volume weighted

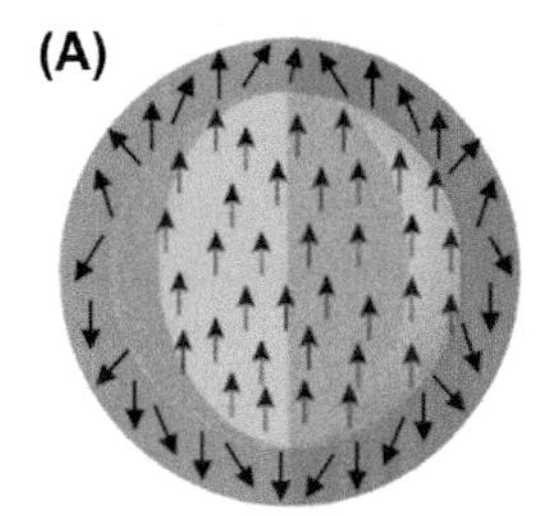

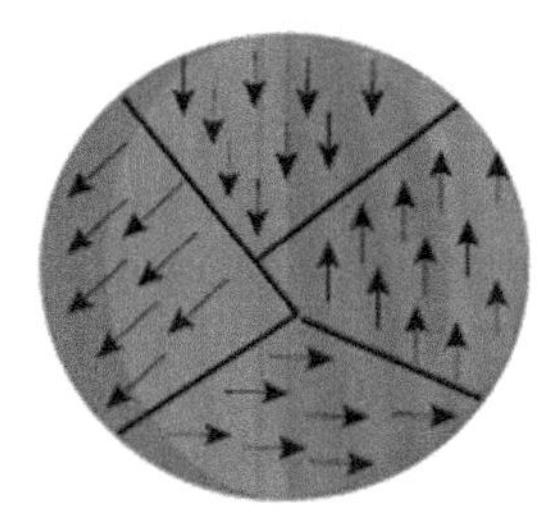
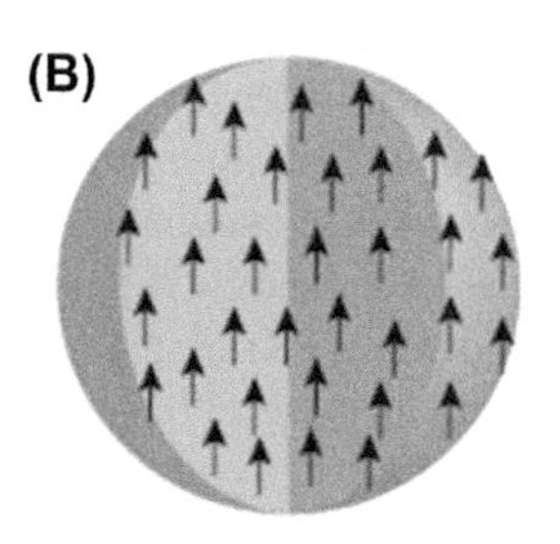

FIGURE 13.3 Schematic of magnetic nanoparticles (MNPs) (A) where the spins are not ordered at the surface or throughput the volume, resulting in an effective magnetic volume that is smaller than the physical volume and (B) where the spins are ordered throughout, and the physical and magnetic volumes are equal.

median magnetic diameter, σ is the geometric standard deviation of the magnetic diameter distribution, and H is the externally applied magnetic field.

MNPs are of interest in several biomedical applications where the response of the nanoparticles' magnetic dipole to an applied time-varying or constant magnetic field plays a key role in performance as discussed in the sections below. Application-relevant properties such as the rate of energy dissipation used in nanoscale thermal cancer therapy[63] and magnetically triggered drug release,[64] the magnetic forces relevant in ferrofluids[1] or magnetic capture,[65] and signal intensity in magnetic particle imaging (MPI)[66] are all expected to scale with the magnitude of the particle's magnetic dipoles, which in turn depend on the magnetic diameter of the particle. Thus, single domain nanoparticle with uniform magnetization and equal physical and magnetic diameters (Fig. 13.3B) are often desirable for such applications.

13.4 Common methods of synthesis

Synthesis methods for MNPs are numerous and fall into one of three categories: solid phase size reduction from bulk materials, gas phase deposition processes, and liquid phase wet chemical syntheses. The main advantage of solid phase syntheses is that they can be easily scaled up to produce large quantities of nanoparticles, but the product is characterized by high polydispersity and is partially amorphous as-synthesized,[35] requiring high-temperature annealing to achieve crystalline particles. Thus, solid phase synthesis is often undesirable for applications that require uniformity in nanoparticle physical and magnetic properties. Gas phase deposition methods, such as chemical vapor deposition, atomic vapor deposition, and spray pyrolysis, are options for manufacturing magnetic nanomaterials with high purity and yield but often result in size polydispersity due to difficulty in controlling gas phase evaporation and particle formation processes.[67] Furthermore, aggregation of nanoparticles formed by gas phase processes is a significant challenge. These drawbacks make use of MNPs obtained by gas phase synthesis challenging for many biomedical applications. Finally, wet chemical synthesis methods can yield MNPs with excellent control over size and shape, excellent crystallinity, and magnetic ordering and can prevent aggregation using surfactant capping agents. As such, wet synthesis methods are the most commonly reported to obtain MNPs for biomedical applications. The two most common wet synthesis methods, coprecipitation and thermal decomposition, are compared below. Fig. 13.4 shows representative TEM images of iron oxide nanoparticles synthesized through each of the methods.

13.4.1 Aqueous Coprecipitation

The coprecipitation synthesis, studied systematically by Massart in 1980,[69,70] offers an easy, inexpensive, low-temperature method of synthesizing iron oxide nanoparticles

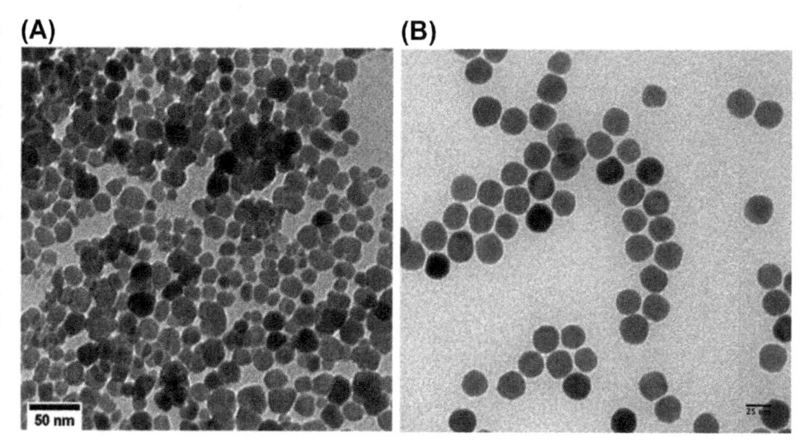

FIGURE 13.4 Representative images of iron oxide nanoparticles synthesized by (A) aqueous coprecipitation and (B) thermal decomposition methods. Coprecipitation is easily scalable at the cost of relatively poor size and shape control of the particles. Conversely, thermal decomposition offers superior size and shape control of particles, at the cost of smaller scale (<1g) yield of nanoparticles. *TEM image in (A) reprinted with permission from Merida F, Chiu-Lam A, Bohorquez A, Maldonado-Camargo L, Perez ME, Pericchi L, Torres-Lugo M, Rinaldi C. Optimization of synthesis and peptization steps to obtain iron oxide nanoparticles with high energy dissipation rates. J Magn Magn Mater. 2015;394:361-371. doi: 10.1016/j.jmmm.2015.06.076. Copyright © 2015 Elsevier (B)V.*

via the use of a basic precipitating agent in a room-temperature to mildly heated (60–80°C) reaction and using close to a stoichiometric mixture of ferrous (Fe^{2+}) and ferric (Fe^{3+}) salts. A common choice for the salts used are ferric and ferrous chloride, and a common precipitating agent used is ammonium hydroxide.[68] The precipitated iron hydroxides are dispersed into aqueous media by vigorous agitation or ultrasonication, sometimes with the addition of a counter-cation to provide electrostatic stability to the suspension.[71] This method is extremely scalable, with syntheses at the scale of a few grams easily achievable in a lab setting. Although skilled execution of this synthesis can yield a much greater degree of size control than either the physical or the gas phase synthesis methods, the method still falls short of achieving a highly monodisperse population, and there is usually very little or no size or shape control.[72] Since the precipitated particles are mostly iron hydroxides, the magnetic properties of the product are subpar as-synthesized. Annealing procedures can be used to oxidize the particles and improve magnetic properties to some extent but involve high-temperature heating for long times.[73] Ultimately, the lack of size and shape control limits the applicability of this synthesis method to cases where a large quantity of moderately MNPs are needed and uniformity of size and magnetic properties is not a principal consideration for application.

13.4.2 Thermal decomposition

Rapidly becoming the method of choice for the synthesis of high-quality, monodisperse, highly crystalline MNPs, the thermal decomposition method is based on the controlled high-temperature decomposition of an organometallic precursor in a high boiling point combination of solvents and surfactant, usually at the reflux temperature of the reaction solvent and under a blanket of inert gas to maintain anoxic conditions as well as alleviate safety concerns associated with flammability of reactant vapors at the high temperatures used. The high degree of size and shape control in this synthesis route is achieved by the temporal separation of the nanoparticle nucleation and growth stages,[74–78] which involves careful selection of reaction process variables such as the choice of solvent (which dictates the reaction temperature) and surfactant, the organometallic precursor used, as well as the concentrations of the precursor and surfactant in the system. The state of the art in size control for this synthesis method is represented by the work of Vreeland et al.[79,80] in an article demonstrating high degree of reproducibility and exquisite control over nanoparticle size in a semibatch synthesis of spherical iron oxide nanoparticles. Nanoparticles from thermal decomposition are coated with an organic surfactant layer as-synthesized and suspend readily after washes in organic solvents, but this means they need to undergo postsynthesis surface chemistry modification for transfer to aqueous media prior to use in biomedical applications. Because of the high degree of crystallinity, size, and shape control, the magnetic properties of the nanoparticles obtained by thermal decomposition are often better than those obtained by other synthesis methods. However, it has recently become clear that the anoxic conditions used prevent the full oxidation of synthesized nanoparticles to the magnetite phase, resulting instead in nanoparticles with multiple magnetic phases and domains, some of them identified to be nonmagnetic phases like wüstite.[81–83] This causes only a fraction of the total nanoparticle volume to contribute to the magnetic properties, resulting in a drop in magnetic properties as compared to bulk magnetite. For an indication of how significant a drop this can cause, in the same work by Vreeland et al.,[79,80] the saturation magnetization of the as-synthesized nanoparticles was at best 74% of the bulk value for magnetite.

13.4.3 Recent advances in thermal decomposition synthesis

As discussed above, while exquisite control over size and shape of iron oxide nanoparticles has been demonstrated, magnetic properties may be subpar due to the lack of sufficiently oxidizing conditions to promote the formation of magnetite, especially for large diameter particles. Since Vreeland's work was published, some investigations into the effect of adding oxidizing species in the synthesis for iron oxide NPs have been conducted. One way to oxidize as-synthesized mixed phase multidomain particles and improve their magnetic properties was demonstrated by Krishnan and collaborators,[84,85] who used a 1% oxygen in argon gas stream blown over or bubbled into the reaction mixture after the nanoparticle growth stage was completed, and aliquots taken over the course of the synthesis and during the extended period of controlled oxygen exposure showed a trend of improving magnetic properties. However, postsynthesis oxidation becomes less effective as the diameter of the particles increased. To overcome this limitation, Unni et al. [86] demonstrated an approach involving the bubbling of molecular oxygen under mass-flow control into a semibatch thermal decomposition synthesis, with measures taken to ensure safe introduction of the oxygen, to promote the formation of phase-pure magnetite in situ. Particles in the size range of 10–25 nm were synthesized with magnetic properties close to the bulk straight out of synthesis and were demonstrated to have excellent agreement between the physical, magnetic, and crystal size.[86] Fig. 13.5, adapted from ref. 76, is a representation of the improvement in magnetic properties and crystal order achieved using the bubbled oxygen approach. In yet another novel approach, Chen et al. demonstrated that the crystal phase of particles in thermal decomposition synthesis could be manipulated by tuning the redox phase activity of the reaction solvent mixture and that single

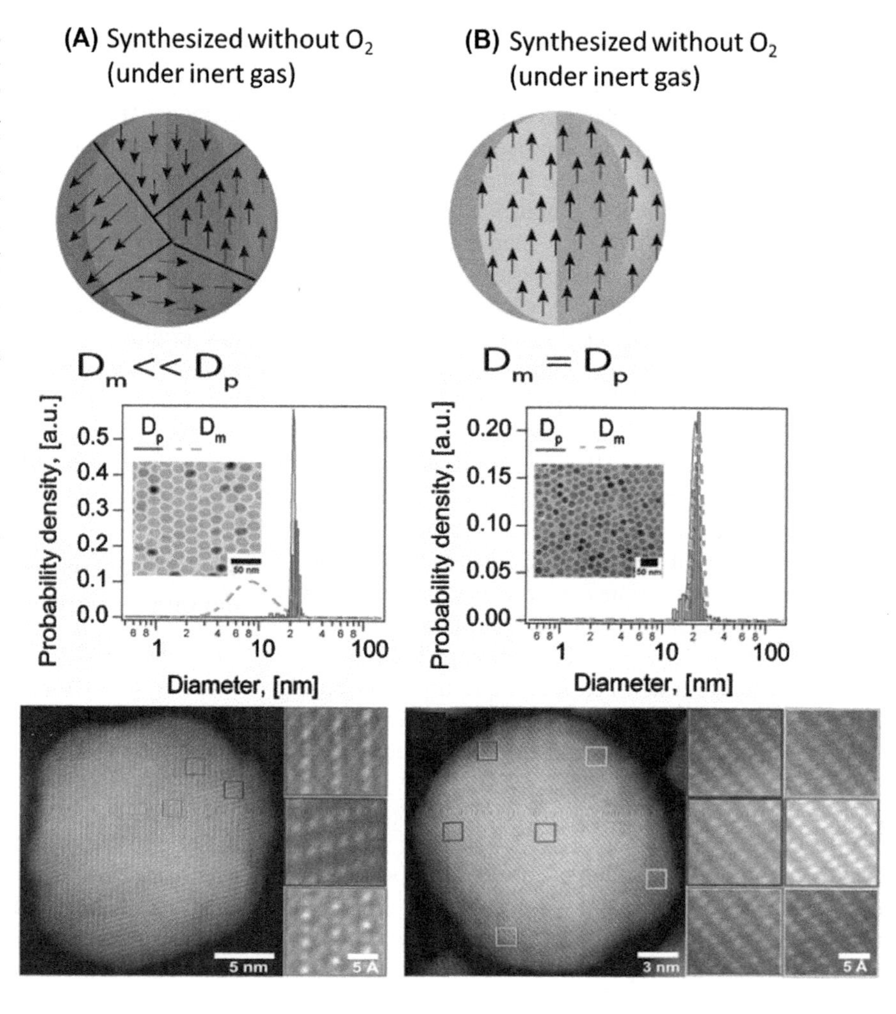

FIGURE 13.5 (A) Iron oxide nanoparticles synthesized by thermal decomposition synthesis under an inert atmosphere are made up of multiple magnetic domains (top left). As a result, they can possess a large "magnetically dead layer," with a smaller mean magnetic diameter and wider distribution of magnetic sizes than the physical size distribution (middle left). High angle annular dark field scanning transmission electron microscopy (TEM) (HAADF-STEM) images of iron oxide nanoparticles synthesized under an inert atmosphere (bottom left) show that there are several different crystal lattice arrangements within the same particle. (B) In contrast, particles synthesized in the presence of oxygen or in an oxidative environment can be controllably synthesized to consist almost entirely of the magnetite phase (top right). The magnetic diameter distribution is comparable to the physical diameter distribution, and particles have a negligible magnetically dead layer (middle right). HAADF-STEM images (bottom right) show that the particles synthesized with oxygen possess the same crystal orientation throughout the particle, indicating phase purity and a single domain. *Adapted with permission from Unni M, Uhl AM, Savliwala S, Savitzky BH, Dhavalikar R, Garraud N, Arnold DP, Kourkoutis LF, Andrew JS, Rinaldi C. Thermal decomposition synthesis of iron oxide nanoparticles with diminished magnetic dead layer by controlled addition of oxygen. ACS Nano. 2017;11(2):2284–2303. Epub 2017/02/09. https://doi.org/10.1021/acsnano.7b00609, Copyright 2017 American Chemical Society.*

domain magnetite could be obtained in oxidizing solvent mixtures.[87] Although additional work is needed, these advances suggest that thermal decomposition methods may yield MNPs with improved magnetic properties suitable for current and emerging applications.

13.5 Clinical applications

Due to their nontoxic and biocompatible nature, superparamagnetic iron oxide nanoparticles (SPIONs) are used as iron supplements in anemic patients.[88,89] They are also being studied for imaging vasculature and tumors,[44,90,91] gene therapy,[92] drug delivery,[92] tracking of labeled cells,[93] thermal ablation of tumors via magnetic heating,[25–27,94] and organ preservation.[89] Within the last decade, the FDA approval of ferumoxytol (Feraheme) to treat patients with iron deficiency and chronic kidney disease highlighted the clinical applicability of SPIONs in therapy.[88] Fishbane et al.[95] reported that patients tolerated up to 510 mg_{Fe}/injection, with subsequent increases in hemoglobin level post injection.[95] Another study reported that in 396 US patients who received a total of 570 IV injections of SPION therapy, no serious adverse events were observed.[96] Minor side effects such as headache, nausea, flushing, muscle pain (myalgias), chest discomfort, and itching (pruritus) requiring modified dosage were noted. However, some severe adverse effects have been noted with the use of SPION therapy. A 1-year retrospective observational study including 8666 US patients noted adverse effects such as hypotension, dyspnea, hypersensitivity and anaphylactoid reactions, and loss of consciousness.[97,98] While the long-term safety of SPION therapy is still under investigation, the clinical use of iron oxide nanoparticles for therapeutic benefit remains promising due to their apparent biocompatibility and the results of safety studies conducted so far. Table 13.2 reports dosage and half-life values of selected iron oxide nanoparticle formulations used in humans as part of various clinical trials.

Concerns about the fate of iron oxide deposited in the body are largely allayed because of intrinsic mechanisms the human body has for the sequestration, storage, and

TABLE 13.2 SPIONs in Clinical Use: Dosing and Blood Half-Lives of nanoparticle formulations after injection in humans.[92]

Core Size/Hydrodynamic Size	Coating	Name	Charge (mV)	Dose (mg_{Fe}/kg BW)	Blood $t_{1/2}$ (h)	Application	References
5/30	Dextran	N/A	Not available	2.6	21–30	MRI of lymph nodes	99
5/30	Dextran	USPIO	Not available	1.7	>24	General MRI evaluation	100
4-6/227	Dextran	Ferumoxides	Not available	0.56–0.84	2	Liver MRI	101
7/30	Carboxy dextran	Ferumoxytol (AMI7228)	Anionic	<4	10–14	MR angiography	102,103
5-7/25	PEG + starch	Clariscan (NC100150)	Anionic	3–4	3–4	MR angiography	104
4/8.6	Citrate coating	VSOP–C184	Not available	0.84–4.2	0.5–1.5	General MRI applications	105

eventual incorporation or removal of iron. However, there is still some concern that usage of SPIONs can cause chronic, iron overloaded states (i.e., transferrin saturation > 75%), resulting in iron deposits in the parenchyma of organs (e.g., liver, heart, and endocrine organs) that express higher levels of transferrin receptors, with possible damage and side effects. However, due to the transient nature of SPION treatment, chronic iron overload is rarely a concern in the clinic. In the setting of acute iron overload (e.g., iron overdoses), toxicity consisting of cellular damage due to free radical formation is observed when more than 60 mg/kg of iron is ingested.[106]

Uncoated iron oxide nanoparticles have been reported to have an LD-50 of 300–600 mg_{Fe} kg^{-1} body weight in rodents.[92,107] SPIONs coated with dextran showed higher LD-50 of 2000–6000 mg_{Fe} kg^{-1} body weight in rodents.[92,107] To date, most preclinical and clinical research studies have been limited to the use of dextran-coated SPIONs or silica-coated SPIONs.[92] While toxicity studies must be conducted to determine the specific LD-50 for SPIONs coated with other polymers or surface modifications, the studies cited above suggest that the iron oxide nanocrystal itself is not likely to be the cause of serious toxicity concerns. Degradation, biotransformation, and excretion of nanoparticles intended for clinical use is an important consideration. For iron oxide nanoparticles coated with dextran, it has been reported that the nanoparticle's iron is incorporated into hemoglobin after intravenous administration in rats, suggesting a pattern of degradation similar to that of ferritin.[108–110] Another study on Feridex particles concluded that biodegradation of iron oxides occurred in the lysosomes of macrophages.[111]

13.5.1 Magnetic resonance imaging

Magnetic resonance imaging (MRI) is a noninvasive imaging technology that produces three-dimensional anatomical images valuable for disease detection, diagnosis, and treatment monitoring. MRI is based on the magnetic response of proton dipoles, usually from water molecules, that are normally randomly oriented within the tissue being examined.[112–114] A powerful and uniform external magnetic field is applied to align the magnetic moments of these protons, producing an equilibrium magnetization along the z-axis (M_z).[112] Next, the equilibrium magnetization is disrupted by the introduction of an external radio frequency (RF) pulse that transfers energy to protons by rotating their magnetic moments off the z-axis, in phase and at an angle called the flip angle.[108,115] The protons return to their resting alignment through various relaxation processes while emitting RF energy.[116] After a certain period, the emitted RF signals are measured, and Fourier transformation is used to convert the signal from each location into grayscale images that represent the distribution of signal intensity levels.[116,117] The transmitted RF pulses can be used in sequence to differentiate particular tissue or abnormalities. Different tissues relax at different rates when the transmitted RF pulse is switched off.[116,117] The time taken for the protons to relax is denoted as T_1 (spin–lattice) or T_2 (spin–spin) relaxation.[115] The first is the time taken for the magnetic vector to return to its resting state, and the second is the time needed for the axial spin to return to its resting state.[112,113] In most tissues, differences between T_1 and T_2 relaxation times are small, and often a contrast agent is employed to enhance contrast between the region of interest and surrounding tissue.[113]

Most T_1 contrast agents are paramagnetic complexes of manganese (Mn^{2+}), iron (Fe^{3+}), or gadolinium (Gd^{3+}).[113] The first generation of T_1 contrast agents (also known as *positive contrast agents*), consisted of high-spin paramagnetic metal ions that produced hyperintense signals by close proximity of the metal ions with the protons of water molecules.[108,113,114] The chemical structures of these T_1 contrast agents are generally characterized by neutral or anionic metal complexes.[113] Several Gd contrast agents have been approved by the US Food and Drug Administration (FDA) and by the European Medicines Agency (EMA) for use in MRI.[113] Due to the intrinsic toxicity of these cations, they need to be complexed with chelates. However, metal chelates cannot be used in renal disease patients.[112,113] Another limitation of T_1 contrast agents is that their efficiency decreases with higher magnetic fields.[113] Hence, there has been interest in the use of SPIONs as T_2 contrast agents. T_2 contrast agents (*negative contrast agents*) produce hypointense signals in T_2 (natural relaxation time) and T_2* (transverse relaxation time) signals.[108,113] This is due to a decrease in the MR signal intensity in the regions where they are delivered, and thus the affected regions appear darker (Fig. 13.6).

Iron oxides have been used as MRI contrast agents for more than 25 years in the form of superparamagnetic nanoparticles. Both magnetite (Fe_3O_4) and maghemite (γ-Fe_2O_3) are often used in biomedical applications due to their stability in physiological conditions, negligible toxicity, and high magnetic moments.[113,116,119] The two iron oxide formulations currently approved for use as MRI T_2 contrast agents are Feridex and Resovist. While Resovist received approval only in Europe and Japan for contrast-enhanced MRI of the liver, Feridex was approved for MRI of the liver in the United States, Europe, and Japan.[119] However, as of today, Feridex has been withdrawn from all markets, and Resovist is only available in Japan. Feridex, also known as ferumoxides, was the first clinically approved contrast agent.[119] The iron oxide nanoparticles in Feridex are made by the coprecipitation method.[120] The core material is a mixture of magnetite and maghemite, coated with dextran. The core and hydrodynamic diameters are ~4.8–5.6 nm and ~80–200 nm, respectively, with an r_2 relaxivity of 90–160 $mmol^{-1}s^{-1}$.[111,121,122] Resovist, also known as Ferucarbotran, is also made by the coprecipitation method[121,123] but is coated with carboxydextran.[113,121,123,124] The core and hydrodynamic diameters are approximately 4.2 and 62 nm, respectively, with r_2 relaxivity of 150–190 $mmol^{-1}s^{-1}$.[113,121,124]

While initially exciting examples of the potential of nanotechnology to impact clinical practice, iron oxide nanoparticle MRI contrast agents did not gain widespread clinical use and were eventually withdrawn. While not enough has been reported on the subject, one can begin to understand this failure by considering how they were used to image cancer lesions in the liver. Because the nanoparticles generate a hypointense (dark) signal and accumulate readily in healthy liver tissue, cancer lesions are highlighted against a dark background (see Fig. 13.6). This mechanism of enhancing contrast requires significant and selective accumulation of the nanoparticles in the tissue surrounding the tumor that is to be highlighted. Alternatively, one could imagine using nanoparticles that would selectively accumulate in the tumor lesion itself, making it appear as a hypointense (dark) region. However, the clinically approved iron oxide nanoparticle MRI contrast agents Feridex and Resovist accumulate primarily in the reticuloendothelial system, resulting in limited clinical utility, and do not have adequate tumor penetration and accumulation profiles. The selective delivery and accumulation of nanoparticles to specific organs or tissues has been an area of intense research for the past 2 decades, with limited success.[125,126] One way to potentially achieve this is through engineering the nanoparticle surface, often by coating with relatively thick polymer layers. However, thick coatings negatively affect contrast efficiency in T_2-weighted MRI by reducing the interaction between the particle's magnetic dipole and water protons.[113] Furthermore, another disadvantage of the negative contrast mechanism of iron oxide T_2 contrast agents is that the resulting dark signal can be hard to distinguish from other

(A)

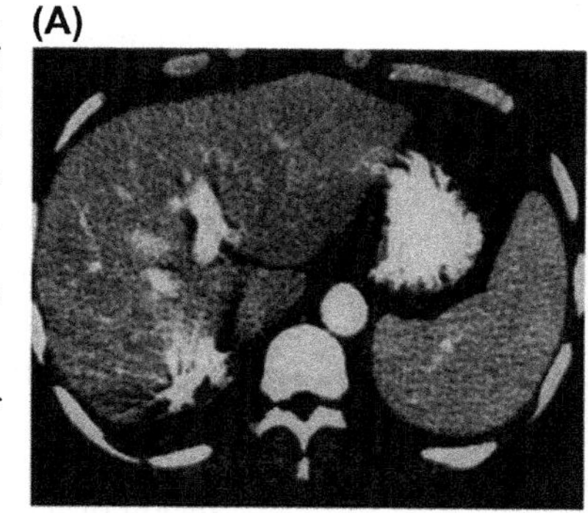

(B)

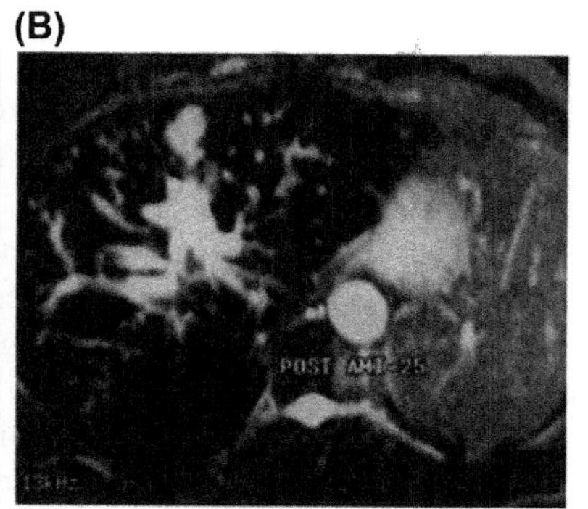

FIGURE 13.6 T2-weighted magnetic resonance images obtained (A) before and (B) after injection of superparamagnetic iron oxide nanoparticles (SPIONs) showing that lesions are more easily detected by contrast-enhanced imaging. *Reprinted with permission from Winter TC, Freeny PC, Nghiem HV, Mack LA, Patten RM, Thomas CR, Elliott S. MR imaging with i.v. superparamagnetic iron oxide: efficacy in the detection of focal hepatic lesions. Am J Roentgenol. 1993;161(6):1191–1198. https://doi.org/10.2214/ajr.161.6.8249724, Copyright 1993 American Journal of Roentgenology.*

anatomical features (normal or pathogenic) or imaging artifacts. This makes T_2-weighted MR images more difficult to interpret, limiting their impact on improved patient outcomes. Additionally, the high susceptibility of T_2 contrast agents induces distortion of the magnetic field in neighboring healthy tissues, called a susceptibility artifact or "blooming effect," resulting in lower resolution compared to T_1 images, and images with no background around the lesions.[113,114,119,127] These limitations suggest that SPIONs are not ideal for clinical MRI contrast in low signal body regions, in organs with intrinsic high magnetic susceptibility (e.g., lungs), or in the presence of hemorrhagic events.[113,127]

Despite the failure of initial clinically approved formulations, demonstration that ultrasmall superparamagnetic iron oxide (USPIO) nanoparticles can serve as T1 (positive) contrast agents has led to renewed interest in developing formulations for MRI contrast applications.[128,129] Furthermore, while the initial formulations eventually failed to gain widespread clinical use, their development and approval studies taught many important lessons that support the study of iron oxide nanoparticles for other applications. Importantly, these studies suggest that iron oxide nanoparticles are not toxic and eventually degrade in vivo, with the iron being incorporated into the body's iron pool.[15,18,95,130–132]

13.5.2 Magnetic fluid hyperthermia

Magnetic fluid hyperthermia (MFH), refers to a therapeutic procedure that uses SPIONs and an AMF to produce energy in the form of heat and elevate tissue temperature to 40–47°C.[133–135] This phenomenon is the result of particle rotation or movement of the magnetic dipole and can be quantified in the form of an energy dissipation rate of SPIONs, commonly quantified as the specific absorption rate (SAR). The fact that energy is only dissipated under high-frequency and moderate amplitude fields that can be constrained to the tumor region make MFH a highly promising form of noninvasive, externally activated cancer thermal treatment. MFH can be applied as an adjunctive therapy or as part of a multimodal oncological strategy with various established cancer treatments to create synergistic effects, such as radiotherapy and chemotherapy.[28,136–138] Magnetic particle heating can be accomplished without any limitations related to tissue penetration, and the AMF can be applied to treat tumors located virtually anywhere in the human body.[139–142] Also, the same particles used for heating can be used for imaging through MRI or MPI (discussed below), enabling theranostic application.[141,143]

Many in vitro and in vivo preclinical studies have demonstrated the potential efficacy of MFH treatment in a wide range of cancers, including breast, prostate, ovarian, melanoma, cervical, and bone cancers, among others.[134,137,144–146] These promising results led to clinical trials in Europe, where MFH is approved for treatment of glioblastoma multiforme (GBM).[27,28,94,147] GBM is the most common and most aggressive primary brain tumor.[148] According to the American Cancer Society, GBM increases in frequency with age and affects more men than women. The GBM 5-year relative survival rates range from 19% for patients who are 20–44 years to 5% for patients who are 55–64 years old. Current treatment options vary depending on factors that include tumor size, position, and whether the cancer has spread to other regions of the brain. Surgery, radiotherapy, chemotherapy, and targeted therapy are commonly employed.[149] Despite this, there is a need to find better treatments that can improve and prolong the quality of life for these patients.

NanoTherm Therapy, developed by MagForce AG, is the first and only nanotechnology-based therapy with European regulatory approval for the treatment of brain tumors through MFH (Fig. 13.7). The therapy is based on injecting iron oxide nanoparticles (NanoTherm) directly into solid tumors and heating them in the AMF using a human-scale applicator (NanoActivator). Depending on treatment duration and temperature achieved within the tumor tissue, cancer cells can be damaged or sensitized for additional MFH, chemotherapy, or radiotherapy treatments.[27]

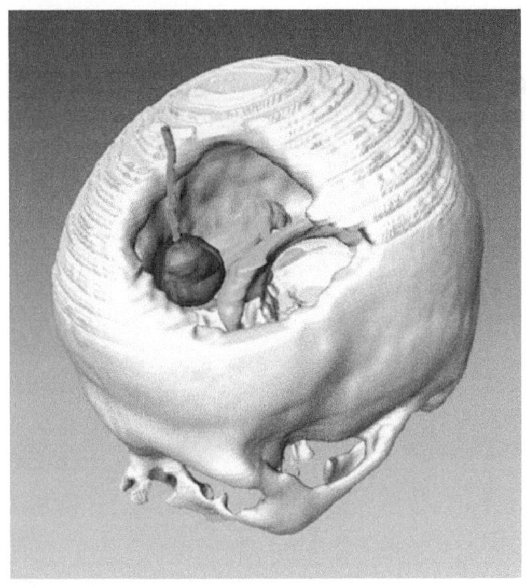

FIGURE 13.7 Three-dimensional reconstruction (MagForce NanoPlan software) of a skull with a frontal glioblastoma multiforme after magnetic resonance imaging and computed tomography. Calculated 42°C treatment isotherm surface (red) enclosing the whole tumor (brown), thermometry catheter (green), and ventricle (light blue). *Reprinted with permission from Maier-Hauff K, Rothe R, Scholz R, Gneveckow U, Wust P, Thiesen B, Feussner A, von Deimling A, Waldoefner N, Felix R, Jordan A. Intracranial thermotherapy using magnetic nanoparticles combined with external beam radiotherapy: results of a feasibility study on patients with glioblastoma multiforme. J Neuro Oncol. 2007;81(1):53-60. https://doi.org/10.1007/s11060-006-9195-0 Copyright Springer Science + Business Media (B)V. 2006.*

Maier-Hauff et al.[28] investigated the clinical outcome effects of intratumoral MFH using MNPs in GBM. In a single-arm clinical study, 66 patients, of which 59 had recurrent GBM, received neuronavigational-controlled intratumoral instillation of a solution of MNPs in a process like a brain needle biopsy. The median amount of magnetic fluid injected was 4.5 mL, corresponding to a dosage of 0.28 mL of magnetic fluid/cm^3 of tumor volume. Following instillation, a closed-end thermometry catheter was placed in the target area. The MFH treatment consisted of six semiweekly sessions of 1 h of AMF application. The NanoTherm therapy was combined with fractionated stereotactic radiotherapy using a median dose of 30 Gy in 5 × 2 Gy/week, performed immediately before or after MFH. The study endpoint was overall survival following diagnosis of first tumor recurrence (OS-2), while the secondary endpoint was overall survival after primary tumor diagnosis (OS-1). The median OS-2 among the 59 patients with recurrent GBM was 13.4 months, while the median OS-1 was 23.2 months and the median time interval between primary diagnosis and tumor recurrence was 8 months. This represents an improvement in overall survival compared with conventional therapies that show an OS-2 of 6.2 months and OD-1 of 14.6 months (Fig. 13.8). With regards to safety, only moderate side effects (e.g., disorientation, sweating, headaches, convulsions, and motor disturbances) were reported following MFH treatment.

Recently, MagForce USA received US Food and Drug Administration (FDA) Investigational Device Exemption (IDE) approval to conduct a clinical trial with NanoTherm therapy as a focal ablation treatment for intermediate-risk prostate cancer.[151] In clinical studies by Johannsen et al.,[25,152,153] the treatment-related morbidity and quality of life (QoL) during NanoTherm therapy in patients with recurrent prostate cancer were investigated. Temperatures of up to 55°C were achieved, and after a median follow-up of 17.5 months, no systemic toxicity was observed, treatment-related morbidity was moderate, and QoL was only temporarily impaired. MagForce is also studying the application of NanoTherm therapy in other cancers, such as esophageal and pancreatic cancer, with results yet to be published.

The nanoparticle formulation used by MagForce consists of aminosilane-coated SPIONs.[154] The particles are made by the coprecipitation method and then coated with aminopropyltriethoxysilane.[154] The particles have a reported core diameter of 12−15 nm, hydrodynamic diameter of 15−17 nm, are highly positive due to the aminosilane coating, and have an SAR of 120−150 W/g Fe. There are several advantages and disadvantages to this platform from the point of view of nanoparticles used and therapy, as summarized in Table 13.3.

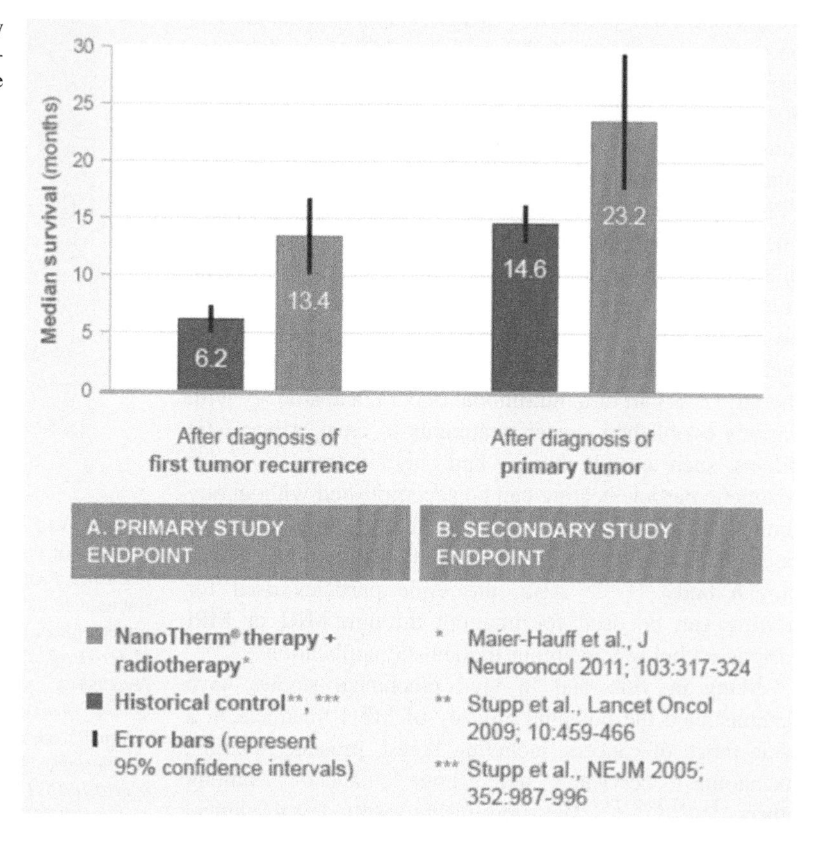

FIGURE 13.8 Survival benefit of NanoTherm therapy in combination with stereotactic radiotherapy in 59 patients with recurrent glioblastoma multiforme (GBM).[150]

TABLE 13.3 Clinical advantages and disadvantages associated with NanoTherm.

Advantages	Disadvantages
• Grams of particles can be produced from a single batch • Highly positive coating leads to high uptake[145] • Positively charged particles aggregate upon injection into the tumor, forming stable deposits allowing for repeated treatments[155]	• Particles are highly polydisperse, resulting in nonuniform heating properties • Due to lack of reproducibility, direct temperature measurements are required initially[27,155] • Aggregation limits ability to uniformly distribute particles intratumorally by interstitial application[94,155] • Invasive localized therapy, not suitable for disseminated tumors [155]

Despite the limitations with the current clinically approved NanoTherm therapy, one must recognize that this is an exciting example of successful translation of nanotechnology to clinical use in a therapeutic setting. For this reason, the use of iron oxide nanoparticles for cancer thermal treatment is still an exciting area of research, especially in combination with other therapies. Much of the research that has followed includes improvement in synthesis and reproducibility of iron oxide nanoparticles,[156,157] improved coating strategies,[156,157] modification with agents to target tumors and cancer cells,[157] and studies of biological effects of iron oxide and MFH treatment.[157,158] This research may one day lead to wider application and improved patient outcomes in the clinic.

13.5.3 Sentinel lymph node imaging

The lymphatic system is an important part of the immune system, consisting of a complex network of vessels and glands throughout the body. Lymph nodes (glands) are small bean-shaped structures which function as nodes to filter lymphatic fluid, removing viruses, bacteria, cancer cells, and waste metabolites. Additionally, antigen presentation and important steps in the communication between cells in the humoral immune system occur in lymph nodes. A SLN is defined as the first lymph node collecting drainage from a primary tumor tissue. In some cases, there may be more than one SLN for a given tumor. SLNs play a critical role since they are the site with maximum probability of spread from the primary tumor. As such, the presence of cancer in SLNs or in nearby lymph nodes (regional lymph nodes) and/or other associated organs helps oncologists determine the stage and extent of spread (metastasis) of the cancer and informs the development of an appropriate treatment regimen. Absence of cancer cells in SLNs indicates that spread has not occurred and could also suggest low metastatic ability of the cancer in the patient. Cancer staging and determining the degree of metastasis in a patient is critical since they are important predictors of recurrence and survival. SLN biopsy involves identification of the draining lymph node (dLN) closest to the cancer, followed by lymphadenectomy for biopsy to determine the presence of cancer cells.

Traditionally, SLN mapping involved injecting visible dyes (e.g., Evans blue) into the lymphatic system, which has limited applicability due to fast clearance, poor tissue contrast, and low penetration depth of light. This was followed by the use of radionucleotide tracers. However, their low spatial resolution, lack of anatomic details in the SLN mapping procedure, and unnecessary exposure to ionizing radiation in patients and healthcare personnel made this approach undesirable. Conventional preoperative and intraoperative SLN detection methods in use today include ultrasound, computed tomography, and MRI.[31] Development of better contrast agents for high soft-tissue contrast and spatial resolution has made MRI a noninvasive imaging modality for SLN mapping in recent times.

In 2001, Torchia and colleagues demonstrated detection of SLNs using ultrasmall superparamagnetic iron oxide (USPIO) (0.2–5 mg of ferumoxtran-10) in anesthetized pigs by interstitial and intradermal injections.[32] The first-generation USPIO nanoparticle, ferumoxtran-10 (Combidex, Advanced Magnetics Incorporated, Cambridge, MA), has a core diameter of 4–6 nm and hydrodynamic diameter of 20–40 nm, with an iron oxide core coated with a layer of dextran. These particles have significant T_1 relaxation effects. The dextran coating allows ferumoxtran to have a long plasma half-life of more than 24h in humans. Because of its long blood half life, ferumoxtran was found to evade the reticuloendothelial system in the body. This made it particularly suitable for sentinel node mapping. MRI images in the study were used to identify SLNs at time points as early as 15 min to as late as 48h post injection.

In another novel approach, Hiraiwa et al. tested a few commercially available thermoresponsive MNPs as MRI contrast agents by subcutaneous injection of these particles into the thoracic wall of rats.[33] This study provided insight on the feasibility of application of commercially available MNPs for SLN mapping. The MNPs evaluated had different thermoresponsive polymer loadings [poly(N-isopropylacrylamide]. Histological studies postMRI suggested the inability of Therma-Max 36 to enter the SLN due to aggregation, while Ferridex, Therma-Max 42, and Therma-Max 55 were able to enter the SLN. Formulations with lower critical solution temperature (LCST) of 36°C (Therma-Max 36) showed inability to accumulate in SLN while the optimal LCST was 42°C (Therma-Max 42) since above those values, the formulations also accumulated in the distal tumors, making them suboptimal for SLN mapping.

Pouw et al. investigated magnetic SLN mapping in *ex-vivo* colorectal cancer tissue (12 patients) as a proof of concept for the application of a handheld magnetic probe based on a vibrating sample magnetometer (Sentimag, Endomagnetics LTD., London, UK) to quantify the amount of SPIONs in lymph nodes.[159] To obtain a comparative estimation of the distribution of SPIONs in the lymph nodes, high-field MRI was also performed. Magtrace, which uses a proprietary nanoformulation in conjunction with the Sentimag magnetic localization systems (Endomagnetics, Inc.), received US FDA approval in July 2018 as a magnetic device system for guiding lymph node biopsies in breast cancer patients undergoing mastectomy.[160] The machine detects injected Resovist particles during SLN biopsy procedures for surgical removal (Fig. 13.9). Resovist, comprised of carboxydextran-coated iron oxide nanoparticle clusters with core and hydrodynamic sizes of roughly 4.2 and 62 nm[124] was found to accumulate in the lymph nodes via a macrophage capture pathway,[111] and approval for clinical use was obtained following a breast cancer clinical trial involving 147 patients comparing classical blue dye and the Sentimag

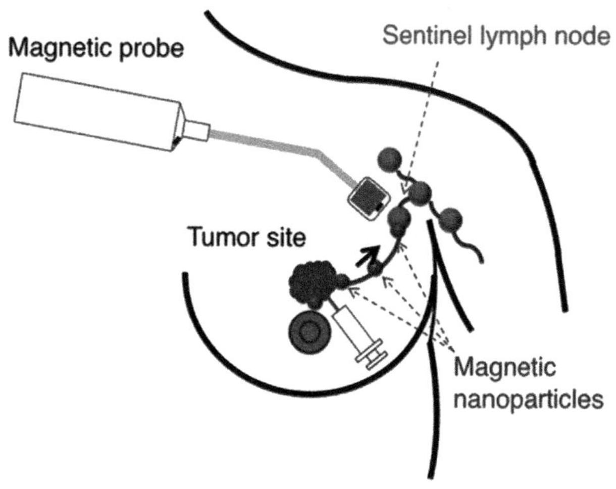

FIGURE 13.9 Schematic illustration describing the principle of magnetic detection of sentinel lymph nodes (SLNs) using a handheld magnetic probe and magnetic nanoparticles (MNPs) for breast cancer patients. MNPs injected accumulate in the SLNs via the axillary lymphatic system which are then detected by a magnetometer. *Reprinted with permission from Sekino M, Kuwahata A, Ookubo T, Shiozawa M, Ohashi K, Kaneko M, Saito I, Inoue Y, Ohsaki H, Takei H, Kusakabe M. Handheld magnetic probe with permanent magnet and Hall sensor for identifying sentinel lymph nodes in breast cancer patients. Sci Rep. 2018;8(1):1195. https://doi.org/10.1038/s41598-018-19480-1. Copyright © 2018, Springer Nature.*

system to identify the SLN. The Sentimag system achieved a higher lymph node detection rate of 94.3%, compared to a 93.5% detection rate obtained using the dye.[160]

With the renewed interest in noninvasive SLN imaging modalities, MNP-based systems are an attractive and viable approach with the potential to emerge as the diagnostic tool of choice. The higher sensitivity for tracers and images with better resolution and no tissue penetration depth limitations offer definite advantages in comparison to conventional diagnostic strategies.

13.6 Emerging applications

13.6.1 Magnetic particle imaging

Magnetic particle imaging (MPI) is a tomographic tracer imaging technology that relies on the nonlinear magnetization of SPIONs in a time-varying magnetic field. The concept was introduced by Gleich and Weizenecker in 2005[161] and has since attracted much attention as a novel imaging modality with several potential clinical applications. MPI is a safer alternative to other tracer modalities such as positron emission tomography and single-photon emission computed tomography because no ionizing radiation is needed for MPI and biocompatible iron oxide nanoparticles are used as tracers. The strength of the signal in MPI is linearly proportional to the concentration of SPIONs, providing quantitative information of tracer distribution. Due to the high sensitivity and quantitative nature of MPI, there are various potential clinical applications under development, including blood pool imaging, traumatic brain injury imaging, stem cell tracking, and monitoring accumulation of particles in tumors and the lymphatic system.[132,159,160,162–165]

Image formation: MPI images are generated in an MPI scanner. Several small animal preclinical scanners are in use, while scanners large enough for imaging humans are under development. The key principles in signal generation in MPI are illustrated in Fig. 13.10. The MPI signal is derived from the nonlinear response of the MNPs in the so-called field-free region (FFR).[139] Everywhere else, the response of the nanoparticles is prevented due to the action of a nonuniform constant bias magnetic field (the selection field). The bias magnetic field can be generated using combinations of opposing permanent magnets and electromagnets and can have field free line and field free point configurations. In most MPI scanners, the FFR is moved electronically or mechanically during imaging. Another solenoid coil is used to generate an AMF, referred to as the drive field. The drive field is superimposed on the bias field. Particles that are in the FFR respond to the drive field, but those which are far away from the FFR and saturated by the bias field do not. The particles in the FFR give a periodic magnetization response which induces a voltage in a

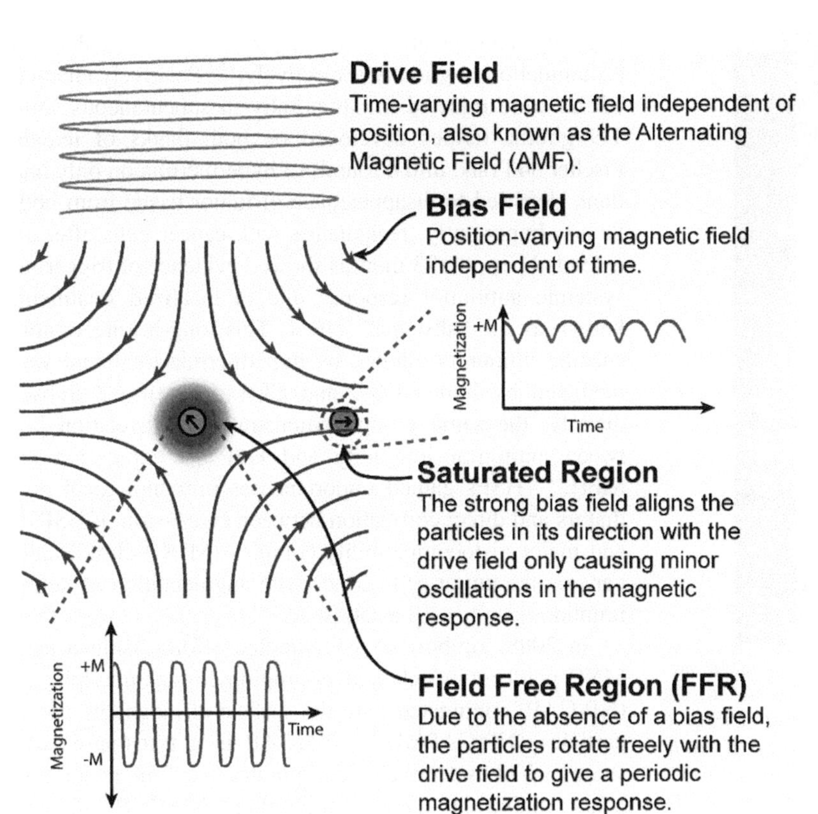

FIGURE 13.10 Key principles of signal generation in magnetic particle imaging.

receive coil. The signal can then be reconstructed using harmonic space reconstruction or x-space reconstruction. Both approaches have been used in various MPI applications.[161,166,167]

Magnetic particle imaging is distinct from magnetic resonance imaging (MRI): Although the hardware and imaging concepts may appear similar, the physics of magnetic particle imaging (MPI) is different from that of MRI.[168] This can lead to some confusion, and it is therefore important to point out the differences. Those familiar with magnetic field gradients, transmit and receiver coils, pulse sequences, relaxation effects, and the reciprocity principle from MRI will understand similar concepts in MPI. However, while MRI generates a signal from tissue, the signal from MPI arises solely from the magnetic nanoparticle (MNP) tracers. There is no background signal arising from anatomy in MPI. As such, MPI is classified as a "molecular imaging" technique.

Sample applications of MPI. Gastrointestinal (GI) bleeding causes many hospitalizations per year, and imaging plays a vital role in locating the source of the bleed. The robust contrast, sensitivity, safety, and ability to image anywhere in the body make MPI a promising tool for imaging GI bleeding. Fig. 13.11 illustrates imaging of blood pooling in vivo.[164]The ability to image blood pooling could also be useful for traumatic brain injury, allowing clinicians to see the extent of internal bleeding and the rate at which this responds to treatment.[163] MPI also has the potential to improve preclinical and clinical research by enabling stem cell tracking and imaging nanoparticle accumulation in tumors. Stem cell therapy is an active area of research with promise for regenerative medicine. No satisfactory method exists as of now to confirm the accuracy of stem cell targeting and long-term viability in these organs.[168] Application of MPI for SLN mapping was reported in female C57B6 mice by Finas et al. in a breast cancer model.[162]

13.6.2 Magnetic fluid hyperthermia to induce antitumor immune response

The primary reason for death in most cancer patients is due to metastasis.[169–171] Treatment regimens for metastatic disease involve the use of systemic nontargeted chemotherapeutics, leading to significant side effects and morbidity. The recent success of anticancer immunotherapies has given hope that the immune system can be primed to actively pursue and eradicate metastatic disease. Immunotherapy is based on the premise of priming the patient's immune system to recognize and differentiate between self "normal" and self "tumor" tissue and preferentially attack the tumor tissue. Interestingly, there is evidence in the literature that thermal therapy using MNPs, MFH, may give rise to antitumor immune response, suggesting the potential of MFH for cancer immunotherapy.

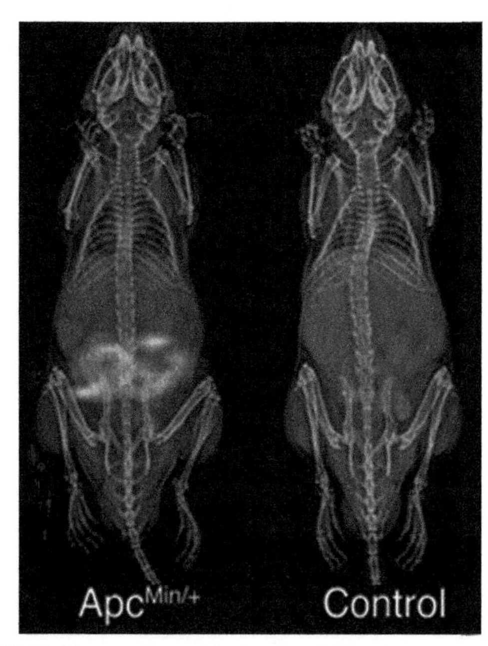

FIGURE 13.11 agnetic particle imaging (MPI) of mouse model predisposed to GI polyp development ($Apc^{Min/+}$) shows GI bleeding via MPI. *Reprinted with permission from Yu EY, Chandrasekharan P, Berzon R, Tay ZW, Zhou XY, Khandhar AP, Ferguson RM, Kemp SJ, Zheng B, Goodwill PW, Wendland MF, Krishnan KM, Behr S, Carter J, Conolly SM. Magnetic particle imaging for highly sensitive, quantitative, and safe in vivo gut bleed detection in a murine model. ACS Nano. 2017,11(12):12067-12076. Epub 2017/11/23. https://doi.org/10.1021/acsnano.7b04844. Copyright © 2017 American Chemical Society.*

Some of the major contributors on the topic of antitumor effects caused by MFH are the groups led by Kobayashi, Honda, Jimbow, and Fiering. The strategy involves utilization of an AMF to heat MNPs or magnetoliposomes introduced in vivo, either directly in the tumor or via intravenous systemic administration.[172] MFH can differentially heat tumor tissue to a desired temperature, resulting in direct damage to the tumor without damaging surrounding normal tissue using tumor targeting MNPs[173] or using spatially localized AMFs.[166]

One of the earliest reports of antitumor immunity induction by MFH was by Kobayashi's group in 1998 and involved the use of magnetic cationic liposomes.[174] At that point, the role of immunostimulatory heat shock protein (HSP) in inducing the T cell responses was already proposed and established in contexts other than MNP-based hyperthermia.[175–177] Even though they were unable to demonstrate a direct correlation between HSP and anticancer immunity, their work showed for the first time that MFH-elicited T cell–based cancer regression. Kobayashi's group moved away from dextran nanoparticles[178] and aminosilane-coated particles[179] being reported by contemporaries to antibody-conjugated magnetoliposomes (AMLs) and magnetic cationic liposomes (MCLs) as heating mediators for hyperthermia to achieve active targeting and positive surface charge–based enhanced accumulation in glioma, respectively.[180] Positively charged MCLs were injected intratumorally in subcutaneous solid T-9 glioma tissues developed on both flanks of female Fischer 344 rats. Initial rounds of hyperthermia on only one flank (left) led to disappearance of tumor tissue from both flanks. Importantly, rechallenge with cancer cells after an extended period of 3 months showed evidence of triggering systemic antitumor response due to localized treatment, known as the "abscopal" effect. This long-lasting tumor-specific immunity elicited by hyperthermia treatment was mediated by both CD8+ and CD4+ T cells.[174] Subsequently, the same group demonstrated a correlation between antitumor immunity and HSP 70 expression by MFH.[181] HSPs gained importance as immunological mediators and direct correlation between expression of HSP70 and major histocompatibility complex (MHC) class I antigens on the tumor cell surface with augmentation of tumor immunogenicity was established.[182]

In 2008, Jimbow et al. rekindled efforts using a new MNP platform which had N-propionylcysteaminylphenol (NPrCAP) conjugated onto the surface of magnetite nanoparticles (NPrCAP/M).[183] NPrCAP is a tyrosinase substrate, which selectively incorporates itself in melanoma cells, inhibiting their proliferation. NPrCAP allowed localized delivery of magnetite particles in melanoma cells and inhibited their proliferation by free radical generation. In the presence of the AMF using the NPrCAP/M nanoformulation, hyperthermic temperatures of 43°C were achieved which led to heat shock protein (HSP70)/melanoma peptide complex production and localized necrotic degradation of melanoma cells. Melanoma-derived heat shock protein 70 (HSP70)–peptide complexes (PCs) were shown to stimulate an antitumor response against tumor cells.[184]

Fiering and collaborators showed that controlled MFH at 43°C for 30 min in B16 primary tumors had the potential to activate dendritic cells (DCs) as well as dLN-based CD8(+) T cells. This study evaluated the abscopal effect, with rechallenge using B16 cells 1 week post initial hyperthermia treatment resulting in no tumor formation on both the primary tumor side and the contralateral side in a CD8(+) T cell–dependent manner.[185] The CD8(+) T cell–dependent resistance imparted was primary tumor specific and observable only at a narrow temperature range around 43°C. Subsequently, Fiering and collaborators demonstrated the role of immunosuppressive peritoneal phagocytes as a delivery vehicle for nanoparticles injected intraperitoneally due to their enhanced recruitment and association with SPIONs for local targeted SPION-mediated hyperthermia.[186] More recent studies by Fiering and collaborators involved spontaneous canine tumor occurrences receiving singular or combination therapy regimens of hypofractionated radiation, MFH, and intratumoral injection of virus-like nanoparticles (VLP-modified version of the cowpea mosaic virus).[187] Animals either received all three therapeutic modalities or dual therapeutic regimens of radiation and hyperthermia or radiation and VLP or single therapeutic regimen of MFH over a period of 14 days. The results described in the study suggest that both hypofractionated radiation and MFH trigger effective immune responses which can be potentiated by VLP treatment and the underlying molecular triggers which augment the immune response are HSP70/90, calreticulin, and CD-47.

The studies conducted so far suggest that cancer cells subjected to mild hyperthermia (<43°C) release immunostimulatory HSPs. These HSPs cause antigen presenting cells (APCs) to cross-present cancer antigen to prime T cells (CD4+/CD8+), resulting in an antitumor immune response. These observations motivate future studies to further understand the mechanisms of priming of the immune system by MFH, with the goal of achieving improved efficacy against reoccurring or metastatic cancer.

13.6.3 Magnetically triggered drug release

Because nanoparticles accumulate in various organs and tissues in addition to the intended target site, there has been significant interest in developing nanoparticle drug carriers that release their drug cargo in response to an externally applied stimulus.[188–193] Magnetism is one of the many mechanisms for achieving "triggered" release, with light, ultrasound, and temperature being other prominent examples. The use of magnetism can be advantageous because triggered drug release can be combined with imaging modalities such as MRI or MPI, or with other treatment options such as MFH. Additionally, magnetic triggering does not suffer from tissue penetration depth limitations, and MNPs can be tailored and functionalized in many ways.[194] Various platforms have been used to achieve magnetically triggered release, including liposomes, polymeric nanoparticles, core-shell nanoparticles, and hydrogels. Each of these platforms has distinct drug release mechanisms in the AMF, which will be described below. While a significant amount of in vitro work has been done, challenges including low tumor accumulation of particles and marginal differences between passive (diffusion driven) and triggered release have severely limited the number of in vivo studies performed.[188]

Liposomes have been a popular candidate for drug delivery in general due to their biocompatibility. Doxil, a liposomal form of the chemotherapeutic drug doxorubicin, is currently clinically used and reduces the cardiotoxicity of doxorubicin.[195] Several other liposomal nanomedicines have been used clinically, but in general, they do not show improvements in overall survival compared to administering the free drug.[196] For this reason, methods of triggering drug release in liposomes have been researched, such as creating magnetoliposomes that can release drug in response to an AMF (see Fig. 13.12). In an AMF, the MNPs release heat, which raises the temperature of the liposomal membrane above its transition temperature, allowing the drug to then diffuse out of the liposome.[192,197,198] Liposomes are advantageous because of their biocompatibility and well-studied properties, but their disadvantages can include low drug loading and premature drug release.

Polymeric nanoparticles and hydrogels have also been used for magnetically triggered release.[199–202] The mechanism of release is similar to that used for liposomes—heat generated via MNPs in an AMF is used to actuate a transition in the polymer or hydrogel that allows increased drug release. Additionally, drug cargo can be loaded onto the particle via thermally labile bonds which break in the presence of an AMF.[203–205] The main challenge with using these carriers lies in achieving a method of limiting the passive, diffusion-driven release at body temperature to near zero while maintaining significant release in the AMF.

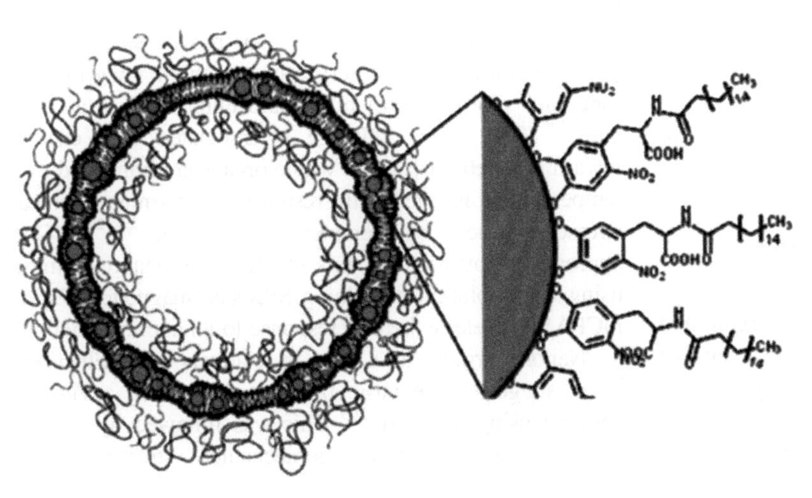

FIGURE 13.12 Sample magnetoliposome. Magnetic nanoparticles (MNPs, orange) inside the lipid bilayer make the liposome responsive to magnetic fields. In an alternating magnetic field (AMF), heat generated from MNPs can raise the liposomal membrane above its transition temperature and cause drug release.

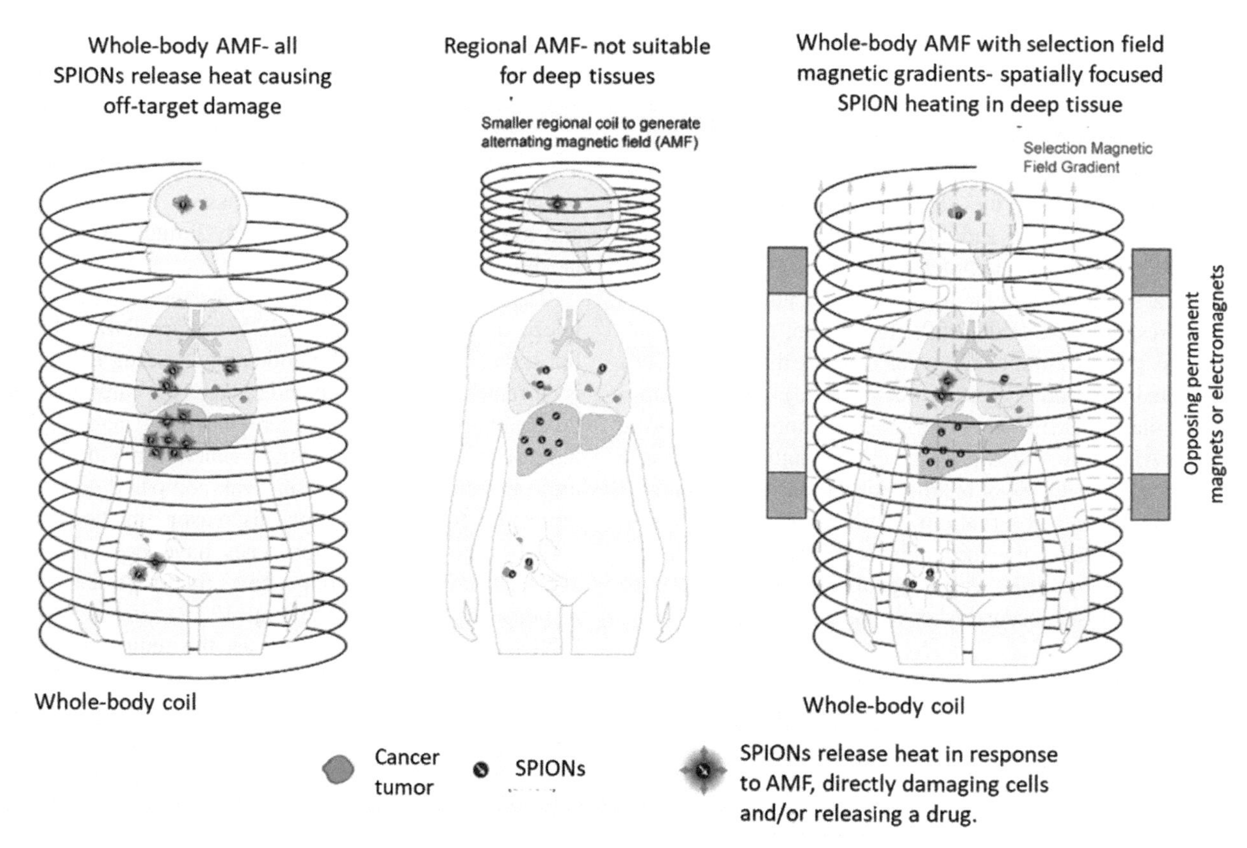

FIGURE 13.13 Image-guided drug delivery with magnetic particle imaging (MPI). Selection field gradients with superposed alternating magnetic fields (AMFs) can be used to image and/or heat magnetic nanoparticles (MNPs). This approach could enable clinicians to see where the drug and MNP are located and then actuate heat and drug release in desired regions only.

Fig. 13.13 illustrates the concept of MPI guided and externally triggered drug delivery via localized particle heating,[141,166] which could be possible through combination of triggered release of drug from MNPs and imaging through MPI. In this approach, nanoparticle drug carriers would be administered to patients, then imaged via MPI to determine the location of the particles and heated via an AMF to achieve localized drug release. The AMF strengths used for imaging with MPI are much weaker than those used to actuate heat and drug release, therefore particles could be imaged without significant heating. Given the many potential platforms for magnetically triggered release and the developing technology for MPI, the outlook for magnetically triggered drug release is promising.

13.6.4 Nanorewarming of cryopreserved tissues and organs

The lack of technologies to preserve vascularized organs and tissues is a major challenge in addressing the needs of transplant patients. Extending the window between procurement and transplantation beyond the current preservation time frame (3–24 h depending on the organ/tissue) would enable comprehensive testing of the organ/tissue, in-depth donor-to-recipient matching, and facilitate treatment planning.[206] Cryopreservation by vitrification has great potential in extending tissue shelf-life.[206] This approach allows storage of biologics at cryogenic temperature using highly concentrated solutions of cryoprotective agents (CPAs).[207] CPAs allow the liquid to transition to a glassy state when cooling, which suppresses crystallization and prevents the harmful effects of ice formation within the tissue.[207] Although vitrifying small tissues has proven successful, it has been difficult to preserve the structural integrity and functional physiology of bulk multicellular tissues and organs.[208] The main challenge is associated with current rewarming methods, where whole organs are immersed in a temperature-controlled bath, resulting in thermomechanical stresses caused by temperature gradients.[206,207] One approach to overcoming this challenge is nanorewarming using CPA solution containing SPIONs (magnetic CPA or mCPA) that release heat in response to an applied AMF.[206]

Nanorewarming as a field is relatively new. Etheridge et al. suggested the basic principle of heating a vitrified solution using an AMF.[209] This was followed by a theoretical evaluation of thermomechanical stresses during nanorewarming.[210] More recent studies evaluated nanorewarming for cryopreservation of cells and tissues. Wang et al. performed nanorewarming for cryopreservation of human umbilical cord mesenchymal stem cells (hUCM-MSC).[211] The authors demonstrated that using mCPA improved the viability of vitrified cells after rewarming with AMF.[211] Particles used in the experiments were made through the coprecipitation method. The authors do not mention if the particles were coated nor was particle stability in the CPA solution studied. Particles made by the coprecipitation method without any coating are highly susceptible to aggregation and precipitation in solution other than water.[211] Highly negative particles also lead to rapid nonspecific internalization, as observed in their uptake studies.

Manuchehrabadi et al. demonstrated scale-up of nanorewarming to porcine arteries of 1 cm^2.[212] They found that convective warming of large samples (>3 mL) caused a decrease in viability. However, with nanorewarming viability was only slightly lower than for fresh samples.[212] The rate at which the sample is rewarmed had a significant effect on viability. This study showed great promise in using mCPA for rewarming large samples without loss in viability. The authors utilized coprecipitation particles purchased from Ferrotec, Inc.,[212] and formed a mesoporous silica shell around the particles. They noticed the particles were only stable for a few hours and further coated the particles with polyethylene glycol.[212] Although stability analysis was performed, this was limited to only 1 day.

While still at a nascent stage, nanorewarming appears highly promising for organ banking. Studies thus far have been performed using nanoparticles made by the coprecipitation method. The advantage of this method of synthesis is the ease to produce large quantities of nanoparticles. However, the main disadvantages include polydispersity and poor reproducibility in warming rates. Physicochemical and magnetic characterization of mCPAs reported in prior studies is limited, which makes critical evaluation of improvements in formulations impossible. More importantly, the SPIONs used were not optimized for heat dissipation which is their primary function. Studies on particle stability in mCPA solution before and after vitrification are limited as well. Although this may not be as important for past studies, which were focused on immersion of very thin samples, this will be important when moving to whole tissue/organ perfusion, as aggregation and precipitation will limit uniform spread of the particles and change the heat dissipation rate.

13.7 Concluding Remarks

MNPs, specifically superparamagnetic iron oxide crystals, have been an area of active research for biomedical application for several decades. The successful clinical translation of these nanoparticles for application in MR contrast imaging, cancer treatment through hyperthermia, and SLN mapping stand as clear examples of the promise of nanotechnology to transform clinical practice and result in improved patient care. Furthermore, advances in iron oxide nanoparticle synthesis and modification over the past decade, emerging understanding of the potential immunomodulatory role of nanoscale heat, and new technologies such as MPI and nanorewarming suggest that MNPs still have much to offer to clinicians and patients.

References

1. Torres-Diaz I, Rinaldi C. Recent progress in ferrofluids research: novel applications of magnetically controllable and tunable fluids. *Soft Matter* 2014;**10**(43):8584–602. https://doi.org/10.1039/c4sm01308e. PubMed PMID: WOS:000343992100001.
2. Wu W, Wu ZH, Yu T, Jiang CZ, Kim WS. Recent progress on magnetic iron oxide nanoparticles: synthesis, surface functional strategies and biomedical applications. *Sci Technol Adv Mater* 2015;**16**(2). https://doi.org/10.1088/1468-6996/16/2/023501. PubMed PMID: WOS:000353641100003.
3. Weissleder R, Nahrendorf M, Pittet MJ. Imaging macrophages with nanoparticles. *Nat Mater* 2014;**13**(2):125–38. https://doi.org/10.1038/nmat3780. PubMed PMID: WOS:000330182700018.
4. Wu LH, Mendoza-Garcia A, Li Q, Sun SH. Organic phase syntheses of magnetic nanoparticles and their applications. *Chem Rev* 2016;**116**(18):10473–512. https://doi.org/10.1021/acs.chemrev.5b00687. PubMed PMID: WOS:000384518600004.
5. Kozissnik B, Dobson J. Biomedical applications of mesoscale magnetic particles. *MRS Bull* 2013;**38**(11):927–32. https://doi.org/10.1557/mrs.2013.257. PubMed PMID: WOS:000330345500019.
6. Ling D, Lee N, Hyeon T. Chemical synthesis and assembly of uniformly sized iron oxide nanoparticles for medical applications. *Acc Chem Res* 2015;**48**(5):1276–85. https://doi.org/10.1021/acs.accounts.5b00038. PubMed PMID: WOS:000355055700008.
7. Lewinski N, Colvin V, Drezek R. Cytotoxicity of nanoparticles. *Small* 2008;**4**(1):26–49. https://doi.org/10.1002/smll.200700595.
8. Kong B, Seog JH, Graham LM, Lee SB. Experimental considerations on the cytotoxicity of nanoparticles. *Nanomedicine* 2011;**6**(5):929–41. https://doi.org/10.2217/nnm.11.77. PubMed PMID: PMC3196306.
9. Umut E. *Surface modification of nanoparticles used in biomedical applications*. 2013.
10. Srinivasan SY, Paknikar KM, Bodas D, Gajbhiye V. Applications of cobalt ferrite nanoparticles in biomedical nanotechnology. *Nanomedicine* 2018;**13**(10):1221–38. https://doi.org/10.2217/nnm-2017-0379.
11. Sharifi I, Shokrollahi H, Amiri S. Ferrite-based magnetic nanofluids used in hyperthermia applications. *J Magn Magn Mater* 2012;**324**(6):903–15. https://doi.org/10.1016/j.jmmm.2011.10.017. PubMed PMID: WOS:000298864100002.
12. Xu C, Sun S. New forms of superparamagnetic nanoparticles for biomedical applications. *Adv Drug Deliv Rev* 2013;**65**(5):732–43. https://doi.org/10.1016/j.addr.2012.10.008.
13. Hentze MW, Muckenthaler MU, Andrews NC. Balancing acts: molecular control of mammalian iron metabolism. *Cell* 2004;**117**(3):285–97. https://doi.org/10.1016/s0092-8674(04)00343-5. PubMed PMID: WOS:000221176400004.
14. Gropper SAS, Smith JL. *Advanced nutrition and human metabolism*. Belmont, CA: Wadsworth/Cengage Learning; 2013.

15. Theil EC. Ferritin – structure, gene-regulation, and cellular function IN animals, plants, and microorganisms. *Annu Rev Biochem* 1987;**56**:289–315. https://doi.org/10.1146/annurev.biochem.56.1.289. PubMed PMID: WOS:A1987H963200011.
16. Andrews SC, Arosio P, Bottke W, Briat JF, Vondarl M, Harrison PM, Laulhere JP, Levi S, Lobreaux S, Yewdall SJ. Structure, function, and evolution of ferritins. *J Inorg Biochem* 1992;**47**(3–4):161–74. https://doi.org/10.1016/0162-0134(92)84062-r. PubMed PMID: WOS:A1992JG96200003.
17. Orino K, Lehman L, Tsuji Y, Ayaki H, Torti SV, Torti FM. Ferritin and the response to oxidative stress. *Biochem J* 2001;**357**(Pt 1):241–7. PubMed PMID: PMC1221947.
18. Zhang YH, Mikhael M, Xu DX, Li YY, Shan SL, Ning B, Li W, Nie GJ, Zhao YL, Ponka P. Lysosomal proteolysis is the primary degradation pathway for cytosolic ferritin and cytosolic ferritin degradation is necessary for iron exit. *Antioxid Redox Signal* 2010;**13**(7):999–1009. https://doi.org/10.1089/ars.2010.3129. PubMed PMID: WOS:000281100300005.
19. Maton A. *Human biology and health*. Englewood Cliffs, N.J.: Prentice Hall; 1993.
20. Costanzo LS. *Physiology*. Lippincott Williams & Wilkins; 2007.
21. Hsia CCW. Respiratory function of hemoglobin. *N Engl J Med* 1998;**338**(4):239–48. https://doi.org/10.1056/NEJM199801223380407.
22. Patton KT, Thibodeau GA. *Anatomy & physiology*. Elsevier; 2018.
23. Biagioli M, Pinto M, Cesselli D, Zaninello M, Lazarevic D, Roncaglia P, Simone R, Vlachouli C, Plessy C, Bertin N, Beltrami A, Kobayashi K, Gallo V, Santoro C, Ferrer I, Rivella S, Beltrami CA, Carninci P, Raviola E, Gustincich S. Unexpected expression of alpha- and beta-globin in mesencephalic dopaminergic neurons and glial cells. *Proc Natl Acad Sci USA* 2009;**106**(36):15454–9. https://doi.org/10.1073/pnas.0813216106. PubMed PMID: WOS:000269632400067.
24. Johannsen M, Thiesen B, Jordan A, Taymoorian K, Gneveckow U, Waldofner N, Scholz R, Koch M, Lein M, Jung K, Loening SA. Magnetic fluid hyperthermia (MFH) reduces prostate cancer growth in the orthotopic dunning R3327 rat model. *Prostate* 2005;**64**(3):283–92. https://doi.org/10.1002/pros.20213. PubMed PMID: WOS:000230371000008.
25. Johannsen M, Gneveckow U, Taymoorian K, Thiesen B, Waldoefner N, Scholz R, Jung K, Jordan A, Wust P, Loening SA. Morbidity and quality of life during thermotherapy using magnetic nanoparticles in locally recurrent prostate cancer: results of a prospective phase I trial. *Int J Hyperth* 2007;**23**(3):315–23. https://doi.org/10.1080/02656730601175479. PubMed PMID: WOS:000247379300008.
26. Jordan A, Maier-Hauff K, Wust R, Rau B, Johannsen M. Thermotherapy using magnetic nanoparticles. *Der Onkologe* 2007;**13**(10):896. https://doi.org/10.1007/s00761-007-1263-3. PubMed PMID: WOS:000254519600002.
27. Maier-Hauff K, Rothe R, Scholz R, Gneveckow U, Wust P, Thiesen B, Feussner A, von Deimling A, Waldoefner N, Felix R, Jordan A. Intracranial thermotherapy using magnetic nanoparticles combined with external beam radiotherapy: results of a feasibility study on patients with glioblastoma multiforme. *J Neuro Oncol* 2007;**81**(1):53–60. https://doi.org/10.1007/s11060-006-9195-0. PubMed PMID: WOS:000242970100007.
28. Maier-Hauff K, Ulrich F, Nestler D, Niehoff H, Wust P, Thiesen B, Orawa H, Budach V, Jordan A. Efficacy and safety of intratumoral thermotherapy using magnetic iron-oxide nanoparticles combined with external beam radiotherapy on patients with recurrent glioblastoma multiforme. *J Neuro Oncol* 2011;**103**(2):317–24. https://doi.org/10.1007/s11060-010-0389-0. PubMed PMID: WOS:000290773100015.
29. Akiyama S, Kawasaki S, Kodera Y, Hibi K, Kato S, Ito K, Nakao A. A new method of thermo-chemotherapy using a stent for patients with esophageal cancer. *Surg Today* 2006;**36**(1):19–24. https://doi.org/10.1007/s00595-005-3089-1. PubMed PMID: WOS:000234207500004.
30. Deger S, Taymoorian K, Boehmer D, Schink T, Roigas J, Wille AH, Budach V, Wernecke K-D, Loening SA. Thermoradiotherapy using interstitial self-regulating thermoseeds: an intermediate analysis of a phase II trial. *Eur Urol* 2004;**45**(5):574–80. https://doi.org/10.1016/j.eururo.2003.11.012.
31. Zhou Z, Chen H, Lipowska M, Wang L, Yu Q, Yang X, Tiwari D, Yang L, Mao H. A dual-modal magnetic nanoparticle probe for preoperative and intraoperative mapping of sentinel lymph nodes by magnetic resonance and near infrared fluorescence imaging. *J Biomater Appl* 2013;**28**(1):100–11. https://doi.org/10.1177/0885328212437883.
32. Torchia MG, Nason R, Danzinger R, Lewis JM, Thliveris JA. Interstitial MR lymphangiography for the detection of sentinel lymph nodes. *J Surg Oncol* 2001;**78**(3):151–6. discussion 7. PubMed PMID: 11745796.
33. Hiraiwa K, Ueda M, Takeuchi H, Oyama T, Irino T, Yoshikawa T, Kondo A, Kitagawa Y. Sentinel node mapping with thermoresponsive magnetic nanoparticles in rats. *J Surg Res* 2012;**174**(1):48–55. https://doi.org/10.1016/j.jss.2010.11.884.
34. Cornell RM, Schwertmann U. *The iron oxides: structure, properties, reactions, occurrences and uses*. Wiley; 2006.
35. Leslie-Pelecky DL, Rieke RD. Magnetic properties of nanostructured materials. *Chem Mater* 1996;**8**(8):1770–83. https://doi.org/10.1021/cm960077f.
36. Strobel R, Pratsinis SE. Direct synthesis of maghemite, magnetite and wustite nanoparticles by flame spray pyrolysis. *Adv Powder Technol* 2009;**20**(2):190–4. https://doi.org/10.1016/j.apt.2008.08.002.
37. Lee JH, Jang JT, Choi JS, Moon SH, Noh SH, Kim JW, Kim JG, Kim IS, Park KI, Cheon J. Exchange-coupled magnetic nanoparticles for efficient heat induction. *Nat Nanotechnol* 2011;**6**(7):418–22. https://doi.org/10.1038/nnano.2011.95. PubMed PMID: WOS:000292463000010.
38. Im GH, Kim SM, Lee D-G, Lee WJ, Lee JH, Lee IS. Fe_3O_4/MnO hybrid nanocrystals as a dual contrast agent for both T1- and T2-weighted liver MRI. *Biomaterials* 2013;**34**(8):2069–76. https://doi.org/10.1016/j.biomaterials.2012.11.054.
39. Angelakeris M, Li ZA, Hilgendorff M, Simeonidis K, Sakellari D, Filippousi M, Tian H, Van Tendeloo G, Spasova M, Acet M, Farle M. Enhanced biomedical heat-triggered carriers via nanomagnetism tuning in ferrite-based nanoparticles. *J Magn Magn Mater* 2015;**381**:179–87. https://doi.org/10.1016/j.jmmm.2014.12.069. PubMed PMID: WOS:000349361100027.
40. Muscas G, Singh G, Glomm WR, Mathieu R, Kumar PA, Concas G, Agostinelli E, Peddis D. Tuning the size and shape of oxide nanoparticles by controlling oxygen content in the reaction environment:

morphological analysis by aspect maps. *Chem Mater* 2015;**27**(6):1982–90. https://doi.org/10.1021/cm5038815. PubMed PMID: WOS:000351971600011.

41. Singh P, Mott DM, Maenosono S. Gold/Wustite core-shell nanoparticles: suppression of iron oxidation through the electron-transfer phenomenon. *ChemPhysChem* 2013;**14**(14):3278–83. https://doi.org/10.1002/cphc.201300471. PubMed PMID: WOS:000325157100022.
42. Butler RF, Banerjee SK. Single-domain grain-size limits for metallic iron. *J Geophys Res* 1975;**80**(2):252–9. https://doi.org/10.1029/JB080i002p00252. PubMed PMID: WOS:A1975V323500005.
43. Butler RF, Banerjee SK. Theoretical single-domain grain-size range IN magnetite and titanomagnetite. *J Geophys Res* 1975;**80**(29):4049–58. https://doi.org/10.1029/JB080i029p04049. PubMed PMID: WOS:A1975AV27400005.
44. Krishnan KM. Biomedical nanomagnetics: a spin through possibilities in imaging, diagnostics, and therapy. *IEEE Trans Magn* 2010;**46**(7):2523–58. https://doi.org/10.1109/tmag.2010.2046907. PubMed PMID: WOS:000281747800001.
45. Cullity BD, Graham CD. *Introduction to magnetic materials*. Wiley; 2011.
46. Schwaminger SP, Bauer D, Fraga-Garcia P, Wagner FE, Berensmeier S. Oxidation of magnetite nanoparticles: impact on surface and crystal properties. *CrystEngComm* 2017;**19**(2):246–55. https://doi.org/10.1039/c6ce02421a. PubMed PMID: WOS:000395439000007.
47. Rebodos RL, Vikesland PJ. Effects of oxidation on the magnetization of nanoparticulate magnetite. *Langmuir* 2010;**26**(22):16745–53. https://doi.org/10.1021/la102461z. PubMed PMID: WOS:000283837800021.
48. Frison R, Cernuto G, Cervellino A, Zaharko O, Colonna GM, Guagliardi A, Masciocchi N. Magnetite–maghemite nanoparticles in the 5–15 nm range: correlating the core–shell composition and the surface structure to the magnetic properties. A total scattering study. *Chem Mater* 2013;**25**(23):4820–7. https://doi.org/10.1021/cm403360f.
49. Santoyo Salazar J, Perez L, de Abril O, Truong Phuoc L, Ihiawakrim D, Vazquez M, Greneche J-M, Begin-Colin S, Pourroy G. Magnetic iron oxide nanoparticles in 10–40 nm range: composition in terms of magnetite/maghemite ratio and effect on the magnetic properties. *Chem Mater* 2011;**23**(6):1379–86. https://doi.org/10.1021/cm103188a.
50. Maldonado-Camargo L, Unni M, Rinaldi C. Magnetic characterization of iron oxide nanoparticles for biomedical applications. In: Petrosko SH, Day ES, editors. *Biomedical nanotechnology: methods and protocols*. New York, NY: Springer New York; 2017. p. 47–71.
51. Spaldin NA. *Magnetic materials: fundamentals and applications*. 2 ed. Cambridge: Cambridge University Press; 2010.
52. Callister WD, Rethwisch DG. *Materials science and engineering: an introduction*. 2014.
53. Kittel C. Physical theory of ferromagnetic domains. *Rev Mod Phys* 1949;**21**(4):541–83. https://doi.org/10.1103/RevModPhys.21.541.
54. Neel L. Thermoremanent magnetization of fine powders. *Rev Mod Phys* 1953;**25**(1):293–6. https://doi.org/10.1103/RevModPhys.25.293. PubMed PMID: WOS:A1953UK67700055.
55. Rosensweig RE. *Ferrohydrodynamics*. Dover Publications; 2013.
56. Jiles D. *Introduction to magnetism and magnetic materials*. Boca Raton, FL: CRC Press; 2015.
57. Livesey KL, Ruta S, Anderson NR, Baldomir D, Chantrell RW, Serantes D. Beyond the blocking model to fit nanoparticle ZFC/FC magnetisation curves. *Sci Rep* 2018;**8**(1):11166. https://doi.org/10.1038/s41598-018-29501-8.
58. Luigjes B, Woudenberg SMC, de Groot R, Meeldijk JD, Galvis HMT, de Jong KP, Philipse AP, Erne BH. Diverging geometric and magnetic size distributions of iron oxide nanocrystals. *J Phys Chem C* 2011;**115**(30):14598–605. https://doi.org/10.1021/jp203373f. PubMed PMID: WOS:000293192100020.
59. Lieberma L, Clinton J, Edwards DM, Mathon J. Dead layers in ferromagnetic transition metals. *Phys Rev Lett* 1970;**25**(4):232–&. https://doi.org/10.1103/PhysRevLett.25.232. PubMed PMID: WOS:A1970G854900012.
60. Morales MP, Veintemillas-Verdaguer S, Montero MI, Serna CJ, Roig A, Casas L, Martinez B, Sandiumenge F. Surface and internal spin canting in gamma-Fe_2O_3 nanoparticles. *Chem Mater* 1999;**11**(11):3058–64. https://doi.org/10.1021/cm991018f. PubMed PMID: WOS:000083776000012.
61. Pshenichnikov AF, Mekhonoshin VV, Lebedev AV. Magneto-granulometric analysis of concentrated ferrocolloids. *J Magn Magn Mater* 1996;**161**:94–102. https://doi.org/10.1016/s0304-8853(96)00067-4. PubMed PMID: WOS:A1996VR56200014.
62. Chantrell RW, Popplewell J, Charles SW. Measurements of particle-size distribution parameters in ferrofluids. *IEEE Trans Magn* 1978;**14**(5):975–7. https://doi.org/10.1109/Tmag.1978.1059918. PubMed PMID: WOS:A1978FQ11200210.
63. Creixell M, Bohorquez AC, Torres-Lugo M, Rinaldi C. EGFR-targeted magnetic nanoparticle heaters kill cancer cells without a perceptible temperature rise. *ACS Nano* 2011;**5**(9):7124–9. https://doi.org/10.1021/nn201822b. PubMed PMID: WOS:000295187400041.
64. Bonini M, Berti D, Baglioni P. Nanostructures for magnetically triggered release of drugs and biomolecules. *Curr Opin Colloid Interface Sci* 2013;**18**(5):459–67. https://doi.org/10.1016/j.cocis.2013.07.007. PubMed PMID: WOS:000324356400009.
65. Wang Y, Jia HZ, Han K, Zhuo RX, Zhang XZ. Theranostic magnetic nanoparticles for efficient capture and in situ chemotherapy of circulating tumor cells. *J Mater Chem B* 2013;**1**(27):3344–52. https://doi.org/10.1039/c3tb20509f. PubMed PMID: WOS:000320664200002.
66. Ferguson RM, Khandhar AP, Kemp SJ, Arami H, Saritas EU, Croft LR, Konkle J, Goodwill PW, Halkola A, Rahmer J, Borgert J, Conolly SM, Krishnan KM. Magnetic particle imaging with tailored iron oxide nanoparticle tracers. *IEEE Trans Med Imaging* 2015;**34**(5):1077–84. https://doi.org/10.1109/tmi.2014.2375065. PubMed PMID: WOS:000353899600006.
67. Kang YC, Park SB, Kang YW. Preparation OF high-surface-area nanophase particles BY low-pressure spray-pyrolysis. *Nanostructured Mater* 1995;**5**(7–8):777–91. https://doi.org/10.1016/0965-9773(95)00289-q. PubMed PMID: WOS:A1995TD69200004.
68. Merida F, Chiu-Lam A, Bohorquez A, Maldonado-Camargo L, Perez ME, Pericchi L, Torres-Lugo M, Rinaldi C. Optimization of synthesis and peptization steps to obtain iron oxide nanoparticles with high energy dissipation rates. *J Magn Magn Mater* 2015;**394**:361–71. https://doi.org/10.1016/j.jmmm.2015.06.076. PubMed PMID: WOS:000360025800055.
69. Massart R. Preparation of aqueous ferrofluids without using surfactant – behavior as a function of the PH and the counterions.

Comptes Rendus Hebd Seances Acad Sci Ser A C 1980;**291**(1):1–3. PubMed PMID: WOS:A1980KF42700001.
70. Massart R. Preparation OF aqueous magnetic liquids IN alkaline and acidic media. *IEEE Trans Magn* 1981;**17**(2):1247–8. https://doi.org/10.1109/tmag.1981.1061188. PubMed PMID: WOS:A1981LK31900013.
71. Duarte W, Meguekam A, Colas M, Vardelle M, Rossignol S. Effects of the counter-cation nature and preparation method on the structure of $La_2Zr_2O_7$. *J Mater Sci* 2015;**50**(1):463–75. https://doi.org/10.1007/s10853-014-8606-4. PubMed PMID: WOS:000345077000048.
72. Laurent S, Forge D, Port M, Roch A, Robic C, Vander Elst L, Muller RN. Magnetic iron oxide nanoparticles: synthesis, stabilization, vectorization, physicochemical characterizations, and biological applications. *Chem Rev* 2008;**108**(6):2064–110. https://doi.org/10.1021/cr068445e.
73. Ferreira TAS, Waerenborgh JC, Mendonca M, Nunes MR, Costa FM. Structural and morphological characterization of $FeCo_2O_4$ and $CoFe_2O_4$ spinels prepared by a coprecipitation method. *Solid State Sci* 2003;**5**(2):383–92. https://doi.org/10.1016/s1293-2558(03)00011-6. PubMed PMID: WOS:000182558600017.
74. Park J, An KJ, Hwang YS, Park JG, Noh HJ, Kim JY, Park JH, Hwang NM, Hyeon T. Ultra-large-scale syntheses of monodisperse nanocrystals. *Nat Mater* 2004;**3**(12):891–5. https://doi.org/10.1038/nmat1251. PubMed PMID: WOS:000225453200022.
75. Park J, Joo J, Kwon SG, Jang Y, Hyeon T. Synthesis of monodisperse spherical nanocrystals. *Angew Chem Int Ed* 2007;**46**(25):4630–60. https://doi.org/10.1002/anie.200603148. PubMed PMID: WOS:000247558200003.
76. Murray CB, Norris DJ, Bawendi MG. Synthesis and characterization of nearly monodisperse CDE (E = S, SE, TE) semiconductor nanocrystallites. *J Am Chem Soc* 1993;**115**(19):8706–15. https://doi.org/10.1021/ja00072a025. PubMed PMID: WOS:A1993LZ13300025.
77. Kwon SG, Piao Y, Park J, Angappane S, Jo Y, Hwang NM, Park JG, Hyeon T. Kinetics of monodisperse iron oxide nanocrystal formation by "heating-up" process. *J Am Chem Soc* 2007;**129**(41):12571–84. https://doi.org/10.1021/ja074633q. PubMed PMID: WOS:000250105500056.
78. Lamer VK, Dinegar RH. Theory, production and mechanism of formation of monodispersed hydrosols. *J Am Chem Soc* 1950;**72**(11):4847–54. https://doi.org/10.1021/ja01167a001. PubMed PMID: WOS:A1950UB71500001.
79. Vreeland E. *Development of novel synthetic methods for size-tunable synthesis of superparamagnetic iron oxide nanoparticles*. Albuquerque, New Mexico: University of New Mexico; 2014.
80. Vreeland EC, Watt J, Schober GB, Hance BG, Austin MJ, Price AD, Fellows BD, Monson TC, Hudak NS, Maldonado-Camargo L, Bohorquez AC, Rinaldi C, Huber DL. Enhanced nanoparticle size control by extending LaMer's mechanism. *Chem Mater* 2015;**27**(17):6059–66. https://doi.org/10.1021/acs.chemmater.5b02510. PubMed PMID: WOS:000361086100030.
81. Chalasani R, Vasudevan S. Form, content, and magnetism in iron oxide nanocrystals. *J Phys Chem C* 2011;**115**(37):18088–93. https://doi.org/10.1021/jp204697f. PubMed PMID: WOS:000294875200008.
82. Pichon BP, Gerber O, Lefevre C, Florea I, Fleutot S, Baaziz W, Pauly M, Ohlmann M, Ulhaq C, Ersen O, Pierron-Bohnes V, Panissod P, Drillon M, Begin-Colin S. Microstructural and magnetic investigations of wustite-spinel core-shell cubic-shaped nanoparticles. *Chem Mater* 2011;**23**(11):2886–900. https://doi.org/10.1021/cm2003319. PubMed PMID: WOS:000291294100027.
83. Casula MF, Jun YW, Zaziski DJ, Chan EM, Corrias A, Alivisatos AP. The concept of delayed nucleation in nanocrystal growth demonstrated for the case of iron oxide nanodisks. *J Am Chem Soc* 2006;**128**(5):1675–82. https://doi.org/10.1021/ja056139x. PubMed PMID: WOS:000235224700062.
84. Hufschmid R, Arami H, Ferguson RM, Gonzales M, Teeman E, Brush LN, Browning ND, Krishnan KM. Synthesis of phase-pure and monodisperse iron oxide nanoparticles by thermal decomposition. *Nanoscale* 2015;**7**(25):11142–54. https://doi.org/10.1039/c5nr01651g. PubMed PMID: WOS:000356515900035.
85. Kemp SJ, Ferguson RM, Khandhar AP, Krishnan KM. Monodisperse magnetite nanoparticles with nearly ideal saturation magnetization. *RSC Adv* 2016;**6**(81):77452–64. https://doi.org/10.1039/C6RA12072E.
86. Unni M, Uhl AM, Savliwala S, Savitzky BH, Dhavalikar R, Garraud N, Arnold DP, Kourkoutis LF, Andrew JS, Rinaldi C. Thermal decomposition synthesis of iron oxide nanoparticles with diminished magnetic dead layer by controlled addition of oxygen. Epub 2017/02/09 *ACS Nano* 2017;**11**(2):2284–303. https://doi.org/10.1021/acsnano.7b00609. PubMed PMID: 28178419; PMCID: PMC6004320.
87. Chen R, Christiansen MG, Sourakov A, Mohr A, Matsumoto Y, Okada S, Jasanoff A, Anikeeva P. High-performance ferrite nanoparticles through nonaqueous redox phase tuning. *Nano Lett* 2016;**16**(2):1345–51. https://doi.org/10.1021/acs.nanolett.5b04761. PubMed PMID: WOS:000370215200077.
88. Lu M, Cohen MH, Rieves D, Pazdur R. FDA report: ferumoxytol for intravenous iron therapy in adult patients with chronic kidney disease. Epub 2010/03/05 *Am J Hematol* 2010;**85**(5):315–9. https://doi.org/10.1002/ajh.21656. PubMed PMID: 20201089.
89. Anselmo AC, Mitragotri S. Nanoparticles in the clinic. Epub 2016/06/03 *Bioeng Transl Med* 2016;**1**(1):10–29. https://doi.org/10.1002/btm2.10003. PubMed PMID: 29313004; PMCID: PMC5689513.
90. Rosen JE, Chan L, Shieh DB, Gu FX. Iron oxide nanoparticles for targeted cancer imaging and diagnostics. Epub 2011/09/21 *Nanomedicine* 2012;**8**(3):275–90. https://doi.org/10.1016/j.nano.2011.08.017. PubMed PMID: 21930108.
91. McAteer MA, Akhtar AM, von Zur Muhlen C, Choudhury RP. An approach to molecular imaging of atherosclerosis, thrombosis, and vascular inflammation using microparticles of iron oxide. Epub 2009/11/04 *Atherosclerosis* 2010;**209**(1):18–27. https://doi.org/10.1016/j.atherosclerosis.2009.10.009. PubMed PMID: 19883911; PMCID: PMC2839076.
92. Arami H, Khandhar A, Liggitt D, Krishnan KM. In vivo delivery, pharmacokinetics, biodistribution and toxicity of iron oxide nanoparticles. Epub 2015/09/22 *Chem Soc Rev* 2015;**44**(23):8576–607. https://doi.org/10.1039/c5cs00541h. PubMed PMID: 26390044; PMCID: PMC4648695.
93. Berman SC, Galpoththawela C, Gilad AA, Bulte JW, Walczak P. Long-term MR cell tracking of neural stem cells grafted in immunocompetent versus immunodeficient mice reveals distinct differences in contrast between live and dead cells. Epub 2010/10/12 *Magn Reson Med* 2011;**65**(2):564–74. https://doi.org/10.1002/mrm.22613. PubMed PMID: 20928883; PMCID: PMC3031985.

94. van Landeghem FK, Maier-Hauff K, Jordan A, Hoffmann KT, Gneveckow U, Scholz R, Thiesen B, Bruck W, von Deimling A. Post-mortem studies in glioblastoma patients treated with thermotherapy using magnetic nanoparticles. Epub 2008/10/14 *Biomaterials* 2009;**30**(1):52–7. https://doi.org/10.1016/j.biomaterials.2008.09.044. PubMed PMID: 18848723.
95. Fishbane S, Bolton WK, Winkelmayer WC, Strauss W, Li Z, Pereira BJ. Factors affecting response and tolerability to ferumoxytol in nondialysis chronic kidney disease patients. *Clin Nephrol* 2012;**78**(3):181–8. Epub 2012/08/10. PubMed PMID: 22874106.
96. Auerbach M, Pappadakis JA, Bahrain H, Auerbach SA, Ballard H, Dahl NV. Safety and efficacy of rapidly administered (one hour) one gram of low molecular weight iron dextran (INFeD) for the treatment of iron deficient anemia. Epub 2011/09/17 *Am J Hematol* 2011;**86**(10):860–2. https://doi.org/10.1002/ajh.22153. PubMed PMID: 21922526.
97. McCormack PL. Ferumoxytol: in iron deficiency anaemia in adults with chronic kidney disease. Epub 2012/09/22 *Drugs* 2012;**72**(15):2013–22. https://doi.org/10.2165/11209880-000000000-00000. PubMed PMID: 22994536.
98. Schiller B, Bhat P, Sharma A. Safety and effectiveness of ferumoxytol in hemodialysis patients at 3 dialysis chains in the United States over a 12-month period. Epub 2013/12/10 *Clin Ther* 2014;**36**(1):70–83. https://doi.org/10.1016/j.clinthera.2013.09.028. PubMed PMID: 24315802.
99. Sigal R, Vogl T, Casselman J, Moulin G, Veillon F, Hermans R, Dubrulle F, Viala J, Bosq J, Mack M, Depondt M, Mattelaer C, Petit P, Champsaur P, Riehm S, Dadashitazehozi Y, de Jaegere T, Marchal G, Chevalier D, Lemaitre L, Kubiak C, Helmberger R, Halimi P. Lymph node metastases from head and neck squamous cell carcinoma: MR imaging with ultrasmall superparamagnetic iron oxide particles (Sinerem MR) – results of a phase-III multicenter clinical trial. Epub 2002/04/27 *Eur Radiol* 2002;**12**(5):1104–13. https://doi.org/10.1007/s003300101130. PubMed PMID: 11976854.
100. McLachlan SJ, Morris MR, Lucas MA, Fisco RA, Eakins MN, Fowler DR, Scheetz RB, Olukotun AY. Phase I clinical evaluation of a new iron oxide MR contrast agent. *J Magn Reson Imaging* 1994;**4**(3):301–7. Epub 1994/05/01. PubMed PMID: 8061425.
101. Clement O, Siauve N, Cuenod CA, Frija G. Liver imaging with ferumoxides (Feridex): fundamentals, controversies, and practical aspects. *Top Magn Reson Imaging* 1998;**9**(3):167–82. Epub 1998/06/11. PubMed PMID: 9621405.
102. Simon GH, von Vopelius-Feldt J, Fu Y, Schlegel J, Pinotek G, Wendland MF, Chen MH, Daldrup-Link HE. Ultrasmall supraparamagnetic iron oxide-enhanced magnetic resonance imaging of antigen-induced arthritis: a comparative study between SHU 555 C, ferumoxtran-10, and ferumoxytol. *Investig Radiol* 2006;**41**(1):45–51. Epub 2005/12/16. PubMed PMID: 16355039.
103. Li W, Tutton S, Vu AT, Pierchala L, Li BS, Lewis JM, Prasad PV, Edelman RR. First-pass contrast-enhanced magnetic resonance angiography in humans using ferumoxytol, a novel ultrasmall superparamagnetic iron oxide (USPIO)-based blood pool agent. Epub 2004/12/22 *J Magn Reson Imaging* 2005;**21**(1):46–52. https://doi.org/10.1002/jmri.20235. PubMed PMID: 15611942.
104. Weishaupt D, Hilfiker PR, Schmidt M, Debatin JF. Pulmonary hemorrhage: imaging with a new magnetic resonance blood pool agent in conjunction with breathheld three-dimensional magnetic resonance angiography. *Cardiovasc Interv Radiol* 1999;**22**(4):321–5. Epub 1999/07/23. PubMed PMID: 10415223.
105. Taupitz M, Wagner S, Schnorr J, Kravec I, Pilgrimm H, Bergmann-Fritsch H, Hamm B. Phase I clinical evaluation of citrate-coated monocrystalline very small superparamagnetic iron oxide particles as a new contrast medium for magnetic resonance imaging. *Investig Radiol* 2004;**39**(7):394–405. Epub 2004/06/15. PubMed PMID: 15194910.
106. Mills KC, Curry SC. Acute iron poisoning. *Emerg Med Clin N Am* 1994;**12**(2):397–413. Epub 1994/05/01. PubMed PMID: 8187690.
107. Wada S, Yue L, Tazawa K, Furuta I, Nagae H, Takemori S, Minamimura T. New local hyperthermia using dextran magnetite complex (DM) for oral cavity: experimental study in normal hamster tongue. *Oral Dis* 2001;**7**(3):192–5. Epub 2001/08/10. PubMed PMID: 11495196.
108. Weissleder R, Reimer P. Superparamagnetic iron oxide for MRI. *Eur Radiol* 1993;**3**:198–212.
109. Cook JD, Hershko C, Finch CA. Storage iron kinetics. I. Measurement of the cellular distribution of 59 Fe in rat liver. *J Lab Clin Med* 1972;**80**(5):613–23. PubMed PMID: 5081660.
110. Hershko C, Cook JD, Finch DA. Storage iron kinetics. 3. Study of desferrioxamine action by selective radioiron labels of RE and parenchymal cells. *J Lab Clin Med* 1973;**81**(6):876–86. PubMed PMID: 4196982.
111. Weissleder R, Stark DD, Engelstad BL, Bacon BR, Compton CC, White DL, Jacobs P, Lewis J. Superparamagnetic iron oxide: pharmacokinetics and toxicity. *Am J Roentgenol* 1988:167–73.
112. Stephen ZR, Kievit FM, Zhang M. Magnetite nanoparticles for medical MR imaging. *Mater Today* 2011;**14**(7–8):330–8. https://doi.org/10.1016/s1369-7021(11)70163-8.
113. Estelrich J, Sanchez-Martin MJ, Busquets MA. Nanoparticles in magnetic resonance imaging: from simple to dual contrast agents. Epub 2015/04/03 *Int J Nanomed* 2015;**10**:1727–41. https://doi.org/10.2147/IJN.S76501. PubMed PMID: 25834422; PMCID: PMC4358688.
114. Bunnemain B. Superparamagnetic agents in Magnetic Resonance Imaging: physicochemical characteristics and clinical applications a review. *J Drug Target* 1998;**6**(3):167–74. Epub 2009.
115. Berger A. *Magnetic resonance imaging*. 2002.
116. Yadollahpour A, Hosseini SA, Rashidi S, Farhadi F. Applications of magnetic nanoparticles as contrast agents in MRI: recent advances and clinical challenges. *Int J Pharm Res Allied Sci* 2016;**5**(2):251–7.
117. Gallagher TA, Nemeth AJ, Hacein-Bey L. An introduction to the Fourier transform: relationship to MRI. Epub 2008/04/24 *AJR Am J Roentgenol* 2008;**190**(5):1396–405. https://doi.org/10.2214/AJR.07.2874. PubMed PMID: 18430861.
118. Winter TC, Freeny PC, Nghiem HV, Mack LA, Patten RM, Thomas CR, Elliott S. MR imaging with i.v. superparamagnetic iron oxide: efficacy in the detection of focal hepatic lesions. *Am J Roentgenol* 1993;**161**(6):1191–8. https://doi.org/10.2214/ajr.161.6.8249724.
119. Wang YX. Current status of superparamagnetic iron oxide contrast agents for liver magnetic resonance imaging. Epub 2015/12/31 *World J Gastroenterol* 2015;**21**(47):13400–2. https://doi.org/10.3748/wjg.v21.i47.13400. PubMed PMID: 26715826; PMCID: PMC4679775.

120. Josephson EVG.L, inventor; Advanced Magnetics Incorporated, assignee. Biologically degradable superparamagnetic particles for use as nuclear magnetic resonance imaging agents. USA patent 4,770,183. 1986 Sep. 13, 1988.
121. Wang YX, Hussain SM, Krestin GP. Superparamagnetic iron oxide contrast agents: physicochemical characteristics and applications in MR imaging. *Eur Radiol* 2001;**11**(11):2319–31. https://doi.org/10.1007/s003300100908. PubMed PMID: 11702180.
122. Reimer P, Tombach B. Hepatic MRI with SPIO: detection and characterization of focal liver lesions. *Eur Radiol* 1998;**8**(7):1198–204. https://doi.org/10.1007/s003300050535. PubMed PMID: WOS:000076035200020.
123. Hamm B, Staks T, Taupitz M, SHU 555A. A new superparamagnetic iron oxide contrast agent for magnetic resonance imaging. *Investig Radiol* 1994;**29**(Suppl. 2):S87–9. PubMed PMID: 7928280.
124. Reimer P, Balzer T. Ferucarbotran (Resovist): a new clinically approved RES-specific contrast agent for contrast-enhanced MRI of the liver: properties, clinical development, and applications. Epub 2003/05/24 *Eur Radiol* 2003;**13**(6):1266–76. https://doi.org/10.1007/s00330-002-1721-7. PubMed PMID: 12764641.
125. Barua S, Mitragotri S. Challenges associated with penetration of nanoparticles across cell and tissue barriers: a review of current status and future prospects. *Nano Today* 2014;**9**(2):223–43. https://doi.org/10.1016/j.nantod.2014.04.008.
126. Bae YH, Park K. Targeted drug delivery to tumors: myths, reality and possibility. Epub 2011/06/06 *J Control Release* 2011;**153**(3):198–205. https://doi.org/10.1016/j.jconrel.2011.06.001. PubMed PMID: 21663778.
127. Krupa K, Bekiesinska-Figatowska M. Artifacts in magnetic resonance imaging. Epub 2015/03/10 *Pol J Radiol* 2015;**80**:93–106. https://doi.org/10.12659/PJR.892628. PubMed PMID: 25745524; PMCID: PMC4340093.
128. Wei H, Bruns OT, Kaul MG, Hansen EC, Barch M, Wisniowska A, Chen O, Chen Y, Li N, Okada S, Cordero JM, Heine M, Farrar CT, Montana DM, Adam G, Ittrich H, Jasanoff A, Nielsen P, Bawendi MG. Exceedingly small iron oxide nanoparticles as positive MRI contrast agents. *Proc Natl Acad Sci USA* 2017;**114**(9):2325–30. https://doi.org/10.1073/pnas.1620145114. PubMed PMID: WOS:000395101200066.
129. Shen Z, Wu A, Chen X. Iron oxide nanoparticle based contrast agents for magnetic resonance imaging. *Mol Pharm* 2017;**14**(5):1352–64. https://doi.org/10.1021/acs.molpharmaceut.6b00839.
130. Bourquin J, Milosevic A, Hauser D, Lehner R, Blank F, Petri-Fink A, Rothen-Rutishauser B. Biodistribution, clearance, and long-term fate of clinically relevant nanomaterials. *Adv Mater* 2018;**30**(19):1704307. https://doi.org/10.1002/adma.201704307.
131. Lartigue L, Alloyeau D, Kolosnjaj-Tabi J, Javed Y, Guardia P, Riedinger A, Péchoux C, Pellegrino T, Wilhelm C, Gazeau F. Biodegradation of iron oxide nanocubes: high-resolution in situ monitoring. *ACS Nano* 2013;**7**(5):3939–52. https://doi.org/10.1021/nn305719y.
132. Keselman P, Yu EY, Zhou XY, Goodwill PW, Chandrasekharan P, Ferguson RM, Khandhar AP, Kemp SJ, Krishnan KM, Zheng B, Conolly SM. Tracking short-term biodistribution and long-term clearance of SPIO tracers in magnetic particle imaging. Epub 2017/02/09 *Phys Med Biol* 2017;**62**(9):3440–53. https://doi.org/10.1088/1361-6560/aa5f48. PubMed PMID: 28177301; PMCID: PMC5739049.
133. Jordan A, Wust P, Fahling H, John W, Hinz A, Felix R. Inductive heating of ferrimagnetic particles and magnetic fluids - physical evaluation of their potential for hyperthermia. *Int J Hyperth* 1993;**9**(1):51–68. https://doi.org/10.3109/02656739309061478. PubMed PMID: WOS:A1993KG76800005.
134. Jordan A, Scholz R, Wust P, Fahling H, Krause J, Wlodarczyk W, Sander B, Vogl T, Felix R. Effects of magnetic fluid hyperthermia (MFH) on C_3H mammary carcinoma in vivo. Epub 1998/01/09 *Int J Hyperth* 1997;**13**(6):587–605. https://doi.org/10.3109/02656739709023559. PubMed PMID: 9421741.
135. Jordan A, Wust P, Scholz R, Tesche B, Fähling H, Mitrovics T, Vogl T, Cervós-navarro J, Felix R. Cellular uptake of magnetic fluid particles and their effects on human adenocarcinoma cells exposed to AC magnetic fields in vitro. *Int J Hyperth* 1996;**12**(6):705–22. https://doi.org/10.3109/02656739609027678.
136. Thiesen B, Jordan A. Clinical applications of magnetic nanoparticles for hyperthermia. *Int J Hyperth* 2008;**24**(6):467–74. https://doi.org/10.1080/02656730802104757.
137. Jordan A, Scholz R, Maier-Hauff K, van Landeghem FK, Waldoefner N, Teichgraeber U, Pinkernelle J, Bruhn H, Neumann F, Thiesen B, von Deimling A, Felix R. The effect of thermotherapy using magnetic nanoparticles on rat malignant glioma. Epub 2005/11/30 *J Neuro Oncol* 2006;**78**(1):7–14. https://doi.org/10.1007/s11060-005-9059-z. PubMed PMID: 16314937.
138. Johannsen M, Thiesen B, Gneveckow U, Taymoorian K, Waldofner N, Scholz R, Deger S, Jung K, Loening SA, Jordan A. Thermotherapy using magnetic nanoparticles combined with external radiation in an orthotopic rat model of prostate cancer. Epub 2005/08/23 *Prostate* 2006;**66**(1):97–104. https://doi.org/10.1002/pros.20324. PubMed PMID: 16114060.
139. Dhavalikar R, Rinaldi C. Theoretical predictions for spatially-focused heating of magnetic nanoparticles guided by magnetic particle imaging field gradients. *J Magn Magn Mater* 2016;**419**:267–73. https://doi.org/10.1016/j.jmmm.2016.06.038.
140. Giustini AJ, Petryk AA, Cassim SM, Tate JA, Baker I, Hoopes PJ. Magnetic nanoparticle hyperthermia in cancer treatment. Epub 2010/03/01 *Nano Life* 2010;**1**(1n02). https://doi.org/10.1142/S1793984410000067. PubMed PMID: 24348868; PMCID: PMC3859910.
141. Hensley D, Tay ZW, Dhavalikar R, Zheng B, Goodwill P, Rinaldi C, Conolly S. Combining magnetic particle imaging and magnetic fluid hyperthermia in a theranostic platform. *Phys Med Biol* 2017;**62**(9):3483–500. https://doi.org/10.1088/1361-6560/aa5601.
142. Jordan A, Scholz R, Maier-Hauff K, Johannsen M, Wust P, Nadobny J, Schirra H, Schmidt H, Deger S, Loening S, Lanksch W, Felix R. Presentation of a new magnetic field therapy system for the treatment of human solid tumors with magnetic fluid hyperthermia. *J Magn Magn Mater* 2001;**225**(1–2):118–26. https://doi.org/10.1016/S0304-8853(00)01239-7.
143. Thomas R, Park IK, Jeong YY. Magnetic iron oxide nanoparticles for multimodal imaging and therapy of cancer. Epub 2013/08/06 *Int J Mol Sci* 2013;**14**(8):15910–30. https://doi.org/10.3390/ijms140815910. PubMed PMID: 23912234; PMCID: PMC3759893.
144. Asin L, Stepien G, Moros M, Fratila RM, JMdl F. Magnetic nanoparticles for cancer treatment using magnetic hyperthermia. In:

Clinical applications of magnetic nanoparticles. CRC Press; 2018. p. 305–17.

145. Jordan A, Scholz R, Wust P, Schirra H, Schiestel T, Schmidt H, Felix R. Endocytosis of dextran and silan-coated magnetite nanoparticles and the effect of intracellular hyperthermia on human mammary carcinoma cells in vitro. *J Magn Magn Mater* 1999:185–96.
146. Rivera-Rodriguez A, Chiu-Lam A, Morozov VM, Ishov AM, Rinaldi C. Magnetic nanoparticle hyperthermia potentiates paclitaxel activity in sensitive and resistant breast cancer cells. Epub 2018/09/11 *Int J Nanomed* 2018;**13**:4771–9. https://doi.org/10.2147/IJN.S171130. PubMed PMID: 30197514; PMCID: PMC6112810.
147. Wankhede M, Bouras A, Kaluzova M, Hadjipanayis CG. Magnetic nanoparticles: an emerging technology for malignant brain tumor imaging and therapy. Epub 2012/03/07 *Expert Rev Clin Pharmacol* 2012;**5**(2):173–86. https://doi.org/10.1586/ecp.12.1. PubMed PMID: 22390560; PMCID: PMC3461264.
148. Borasi G, Nahum A. A new Glioblastoma treatment, potentially highly effective, combining focused ultrasound generated hyperthermia and radiations. *JSM Brain Science* 2017;**2**(1).
149. Davis ME. Glioblastoma: overview of disease and treatment. Epub 2016/09/27 *Clin J Oncol Nurs* 2016;**20**(5 Suppl. l):S2–8. https://doi.org/10.1188/16.CJON.S1.2-8. PubMed PMID: 27668386; PMCID: PMC5123811.
150. AG M. NanoTherm® therapy information for the treatment of brain tumors mag force 2007–2018. Available from: https://www.magforce.com/en/patienten/beschreibung-der-therapie.html.
151. AG M. *MagForce receives FDA investigational device exemption approval to conduct a clinical trial with NanoTherm® therapy as focal ablation treatment for intermediate risk prostate cancer*. 2018. Available from: https://www.magforce.com/uploads/media/180210_eCN_IDE_Approval.pdf.
152. Johannsen M, Gneveckow U, Eckelt L, Feussner A, Waldofner N, Scholz R, Deger S, Wust P, Loening SA, Jordan A. Clinical hyperthermia of prostate cancer using magnetic nanoparticles: presentation of a new interstitial technique. *Int J Hyperth* 2005;**21**(7):637–47. https://doi.org/10.1080/02656730500158360.
153. Johannsen M, Gneveckow U, Thiesen B, Taymoorian K, Cho CH, Waldofner N, Scholz R, Jordan A, Loening SA, Wust P. Thermotherapy of prostate cancer using magnetic nanoparticles: feasibility, imaging, and three-dimensional temperature distribution. Epub 2006/11/28 *Eur Urol* 2007;**52**(6):1653–61. https://doi.org/10.1016/j.eururo.2006.11.023. PubMed PMID: 17125906.
154. Lesniak C, Schiestel T, Nass R, Schmidt H. *Process for preparing agglomerate-free nanoscalar iron-oxide particles with a hydrolysis resistant coating*. United States; 2001.
155. Jordan A. Hyperthermia classic commentary: 'Inductive heating of ferrimagnetic particles and magnetic fluids: physical evaluation of their potential for hyperthermia. Epub 2009/10/24 *Int J Hyperth* 2009;**25**(7):512–6. https://doi.org/10.3109/02656730903183445. PubMed PMID: 19848613.
156. Grüttner C, Müller K, Teller J, Westphal F. Synthesis and functionalisation of magnetic nanoparticles for hyperthermia applications. *Int J Hyperth* 2013;**29**(8):777–89. https://doi.org/10.3109/02656736.2013.835876. PubMed PMID: 91929214.
157. Arias LS, Pessan JP, Vieira APM, Lima TMT, Delbem ACB, Monteiro DR. Iron oxide nanoparticles for biomedical applications: a perspective on synthesis, drugs, antimicrobial activity, and toxicity. *Antibiotics* 2018;**7**(2):46. https://doi.org/10.3390/antibiotics7020046. PubMed PMID: 29890753.
158. Valdiglesias V, Kilic G, Costa C, Fernandez-Bertolez N, Pasaro E, Teixeira JP, Laffon B. Effects of iron oxide nanoparticles: cytotoxicity, genotoxicity, developmental toxicity, and neurotoxicity. *Environ Mol Mutagen* 2015;**56**(2):125–48. https://doi.org/10.1002/em.21909. PubMed PMID: WOS:000350356800005.
159. Pouw JJ, Fratila RM, Velders AH, ten Haken B, Pankhurst QA, Klaase JM. Ex vivo magnetic sentinel lymph node detection in colorectal cancer with a SPIO tracer 2012;**140**:181–5. https://doi.org/10.1007/978-3-642-24133-8_29.
160. Sekino M, Kuwahata A, Ookubo T, Shiozawa M, Ohashi K, Kaneko M, Saito I, Inoue Y, Ohsaki H, Takei H, Kusakabe M. Handheld magnetic probe with permanent magnet and Hall sensor for identifying sentinel lymph nodes in breast cancer patients. *Sci Rep* 2018;**8**(1):1195. https://doi.org/10.1038/s41598-018-19480-1.
161. Gleich B, Weizenecker J. Tomographic imaging using the nonlinear response of magnetic particles. *Nature* 2005;**435**:1214. https://doi.org/10.1038/nature03808.
162. Finas D, Baumann K, Heinrich K, Ruhland B, Sydow L, Gräfe K, Sattel T, Lüdtke-Buzug K, Buzug T. Distribution of superparamagnetic nanoparticles in lymphatic tissue for sentinel lymph node detection in breast cancer by magnetic particle imaging 2012;**140**:187–91. https://doi.org/10.1007/978-3-642-24133-8_30.
163. Orendorff R, Peck AJ, Zheng B, Shirazi SN, Matthew Ferguson R, Khandhar AP, Kemp SJ, Goodwill P, Krishnan KM, Brooks GA, Kaufer D, Conolly S. First in vivo traumatic brain injury imaging via magnetic particle imaging. Epub 2017/04/06 *Phys Med Biol* 2017;**62**(9):3501–9. https://doi.org/10.1088/1361-6560/aa52ad. PubMed PMID: 28378708; PMCID: PMC5736300.
164. Yu EY, Chandrasekharan P, Berzon R, Tay ZW, Zhou XY, Khandhar AP, Ferguson RM, Kemp SJ, Zheng B, Goodwill PW, Wendland MF, Krishnan KM, Behr S, Carter J, Conolly SM. Magnetic particle imaging for highly sensitive, quantitative, and safe in vivo gut bleed detection in a murine model. Epub 2017/11/23 *ACS Nano* 2017;**11**(12):12067–76. https://doi.org/10.1021/acsnano.7b04844. PubMed PMID: 29165995; PMCID: PMC5752588.
165. Nejadnik H, Pandit P, Lenkov O, Lahiji AP, Yerneni K, Daldrup-Link HE. Ferumoxytol can Be used for quantitative magnetic particle imaging of transplanted stem cells. Epub 2018/09/09 *Mol Imaging Biol* 2018. https://doi.org/10.1007/s11307-018-1276-x. PubMed PMID: 30194566.
166. Tay ZW, Chandrasekharan P, Chiu-Lam A, Hensley DW, Dhavalikar R, Zhou XY, Yu EY, Goodwill PW, Zheng B, Rinaldi C, Conolly SM. Magnetic particle imaging-guided heating in vivo using gradient fields for arbitrary localization of magnetic hyperthermia therapy. *ACS Nano* 2018;**12**(4):3699–713. https://doi.org/10.1021/acsnano.8b00893.
167. Panagiotopoulos N, Duschka RL, Ahlborg M, Bringout G, Debbeler C, Graeser M, Kaethner C, Ludtke-Buzug K, Medimagh H, Stelzner J, Buzug TM, Barkhausen J, Vogt FM, Haegele J. Magnetic particle imaging: current developments and future directions. *Int J Nanomed* 2015;**10**:18. https://doi.org/10.2147/ijn.s70488. PubMed PMID: WOS:000353281900001.
168. Saritas EU, Goodwill PW, Croft LR, Konkle JJ, Lu K, Zheng B, Conolly SM. Magnetic particle imaging (MPI) for NMR and MRI

researchers. *J Magn Reson* 2013;**229**:116–26. https://doi.org/10.1016/j.jmr.2012.11.029.

169. Geiger TR, Peeper DS. Metastasis mechanisms. *Biochim Biophys Acta Rev Canc* 2009;**1796**(2):293–308. https://doi.org/10.1016/j.bbcan.2009.07.006. PubMed PMID: WOS:000270767600019.
170. Massague J, Obenauf AC. Metastatic colonization by circulating tumour cells. *Nature* 2016;**529**(7586):298–306. https://doi.org/10.1038/nature17038. PubMed PMID: WOS:000368354800031.
171. Chaffer CL, Weinberg RA. A perspective on cancer cell metastasis. *Science* 2011;**331**(6024):1559–64. https://doi.org/10.1126/science.1203543. PubMed PMID: WOS:000288754500044.
172. Toraya-Brown S, Fiering S. Local tumour hyperthermia as immunotherapy for metastatic cancer. *Int J Hyperth* 2014;**30**(8):531–9. https://doi.org/10.3109/02656736.2014.968640.
173. Kobayashi T, Ito A, Honda H. *Magnetic nanoparticle-mediated hyperthermia and induction of anti-tumor immune responses*. 2016. p. 137–50. https://doi.org/10.1007/978-981-10-0719-4_13.
174. Yanase M, Shinkai M, Honda H, Wakabayashi T, Yoshida J, Kobayashi T. Antitumor immunity induction by intracellular hyperthermia using magnetite cationic liposomes. *Jpn J Cancer Res* 1998;**89**(7):775–82. https://doi.org/10.1111/j.1349-7006.1998.tb03283.x.
175. Mukasa Y, Kobayashi M, Nomoto K. Gamma delta T cells in infection-induced and autoimmune-induced testicular inflammation. *Immunology* 1998;**95**(3):395–401. https://doi.org/10.1046/j.1365-2567.1998.00585.x.
176. Srivastava PK, Menoret A, Basu S, Binder RJ, McQuade KL. Heat shock proteins come of age: primitive functions acquire new roles in an adaptive world. *Immunity* 1998;**8**(6):657–65. https://doi.org/10.1016/s1074-7613(00)80570-1.
177. Udono H, Srivastava PK. Comparison of tumor-specific immunogenicities of stress-induced proteins gp96, hsp90, and hsp70. *J Immunol* 1994;**152**(11):5398–403. PubMed PMID: 8189059.
178. Mitsumori M, Hiraoka M, Shibata T, Okuno Y, Masunaga S, Koishi M, Okajima K, Nagata Y, Nishimura Y, Abe M, Ohura K, Hasegawa M, Nagae H, Ebisawa Y. Development of intra-arterial hyperthermia using a dextran-magnetite complex. *Int J Hyperth* 2009;**10**(6):785–93. https://doi.org/10.3109/02656739409012371.
179. Jordan A, Wust P, Fähling H, John W, Hinz A, Felix R. Inductive heating of ferrimagnetic particles and magnetic fluids: physical evaluation of their potential for hyperthermia. *Int J Hyperth* 2009;**25**(7):499–511. https://doi.org/10.3109/02656730903287790.
180. Kobayashi T. Cancer hyperthermia using magnetic nanoparticles. *Biotechnol J* 2011;**6**(11):1342–7. PubMed PMID: WOS:000297559600006.
181. Ito A, Shinkai M, Honda H, Yoshikawa K, Saga S, Wakabayashi T, Yoshida J, Kobayashi T. Heat shock protein 70 expression induces antitumor immunity during intracellular hyperthermia using magnetite nanoparticles. *Cancer Immunol Immunother* 2003;**52**(2):80–8. https://doi.org/10.1007/s00262-002-0335-x. PubMed PMID: WOS:000181664000002.
182. Ito A, Honda H, Kobayashi T. Cancer immunotherapy based on intracellular hyperthermia using magnetite nanoparticles: a novel concept of "heat-controlled necrosis" with heat shock protein expression. *Cancer Immunol Immunother* 2005;**55**(3):320–8. https://doi.org/10.1007/s00262-005-0049-y.
183. Jimbow K, Takada T, Sato M, Sato A, Kamiya T, Ono I, Yamashita T, Tamura Y, Sato S, Miyamoto A, Ito A, Honda H, Wakamatsu K, Ito S. Melanin biology and translational research strategy; melanogenesis and nanomedicine as the basis for melanoma-targeted DDS and chemothermoimmunotherapy. *Pigm Cell Melanoma R* 2008;**21**(2):243–4. PubMed PMID: WOS:000255061700022.
184. Gao Y, Gao W, Chen X, Cha N, Wang X, Jia X, Wang B, Ren M, Ren J. Enhancing the treatment effect on melanoma by heat shock protein 70-peptide complexes purified from human melanoma cell lines. *Oncol Rep* 2016;**36**(3):1243–50. https://doi.org/10.3892/or.2016.4947. PubMed PMID: 27431432; PMCID: 4968617.
185. Toraya-Brown S, Sheen MR, Zhang P, Chen L, Baird JR, Demidenko E, Turk MJ, Hoopes PJ, Conejo-Garcia JR, Fiering S. Local hyperthermia treatment of tumors induces CD8+ T cell-mediated resistance against distal and secondary tumors. *Nanomed Nanotechnol Biol Med* 2014;**10**(6):1273–85. https://doi.org/10.1016/j.nano.2014.01.011.
186. Toraya-Brown S, Sheen MR, Baird JR, Barry S, Demidenko E, Turk MJ, Hoopes PJ, Conejo-Garcia JR, Fiering S. Phagocytes mediate targeting of iron oxide nanoparticles to tumors for cancer therapy. *Integr Biol* 2013;**5**(1):159–71. https://doi.org/10.1039/c2ib20180a.
187. Ryan TP, Hoopes PJ, Moodie KL, Petryk AA, Petryk JD, Sechrist S, Gladstone DJ, Steinmetz NF, Veliz FA, Bursey AA, Wagner RJ, Rajan A, Dugat D, Crary-Burney M, Fiering SN. Hypo-fractionated radiation, magnetic nanoparticle hyperthermia and a viral immunotherapy treatment of spontaneous canine cancer 2017;**10066**:1006605. https://doi.org/10.1117/12.2256213.
188. Wang Y, Kohane DS. External triggering and triggered targeting strategies for drug delivery. *Nature* 2017;**2**:17020. https://doi.org/10.1038/natrevmats.2017.20.
189. Brazel CS. Magnetothermally-responsive nanomaterials: combining magnetic nanostructures and thermally-sensitive polymers for triggered drug release. *Pharm Res* 2009;**26**(3):644–56. https://doi.org/10.1007/s11095-008-9773-2. PubMed PMID: WOS:000263116600018.
190. Rwei AY, Wang W, Kohane DS. Photoresponsive nanoparticles for drug delivery. *Nano Today* 2015;**10**(4):451–67. https://doi.org/10.1016/j.nantod.2015.06.004.
191. Jhaveri A, Deshpande P, Torchilin V. Stimuli-sensitive nanopreparations for combination cancer therapy. *J Control Release* 2014;**190**:352–70. https://doi.org/10.1016/j.jconrel.2014.05.002. PubMed PMID: WOS:000345910900020.
192. Amstad E, Kohlbrecher J, Muller E, Schweizer T, Textor M, Reimhult E. Triggered release from liposomes through magnetic actuation of iron oxide nanoparticle containing membranes. Epub 2011/03/01 *Nano Lett* 2011;**11**(4):1664–70. https://doi.org/10.1021/nl2001499. PubMed PMID: 21351741.
193. Amstad E, Reimhult E. Nanoparticle actuated hollow drug delivery vehicles. *Nanomedicine* 2012;**7**(1):145–64. https://doi.org/10.2217/nnm.11.167. PubMed PMID: WOS:000300212600023.
194. Estelrich J, Escribano E, Queralt J, Busquets M. Iron oxide nanoparticles for magnetically-guided and magnetically-responsive drug delivery. *Int J Mol Sci* 2015;**16**(4):8070. https://doi.org/10.3390/ijms16048070. PubMed PMID:.
195. Barenholz Y. Doxil(R)–the first FDA-approved nano-drug: lessons learned. Epub 2012/04/10 *J Control Release* 2012;**160**(2):117–34. https://doi.org/10.1016/j.jconrel.2012.03.020. PubMed PMID: 22484195.

196. Petersen GH, Alzghari SK, Chee W, Sankari SS, La-Beck NM. Meta-analysis of clinical and preclinical studies comparing the anticancer efficacy of liposomal versus conventional non-liposomal doxorubicin. *J Control Release* 2016;**232**:255–64. https://doi.org/10.1016/j.jconrel.2016.04.028.
197. Chen Y, Chen Y, Xiao D, Bose A, Deng R, Bothun GD. Low-dose chemotherapy of hepatocellular carcinoma through triggered-release from bilayer-decorated magnetoliposomes. Epub 2014/02/20 *Colloids Surfaces B Biointerfaces* 2014;**116**:452–8. https://doi.org/10.1016/j.colsurfb.2014.01.022. PubMed PMID: 24549047; PMCID: PMC3995871.
198. Soenen SJ, Hodenius M, De Cuyper M. Magnetoliposomes: versatile innovative nanocolloids for use in biotechnology and biomedicine. Epub 2009/02/06 *Nanomedicine* 2009;**4**(2):177–91. https://doi.org/10.2217/17435889.4.2.177. PubMed PMID: 19193184.
199. Kim DH, Vitol EA, Liu J, Balasubramanian S, Gosztola DJ, Cohen EE, Novosad V, Rozhkova EA. Stimuli-responsive magnetic nanomicelles as multifunctional heat and cargo delivery vehicles. Epub 2013/01/29 *Langmuir* 2013;**29**(24):7425–32. https://doi.org/10.1021/la3044158. PubMed PMID: 23351096.
200. Oliveira H, Pérez-Andrés E, Thevenot J, Sandre O, Berra E, Lecommandoux S. Magnetic field triggered drug release from polymersomes for cancer therapeutics. *J Control Release* 2013;**169**(3):165–70. https://doi.org/10.1016/j.jconrel.2013.01.013.
201. Qu Y, Li J, Ren J, Leng J, Lin C, Shi D. Enhanced synergism of thermo-chemotherapy by combining highly efficient magnetic hyperthermia with magnetothermally-facilitated drug release. *Nanoscale* 2014;**6**(21):12408–13. https://doi.org/10.1039/C4NR03384A.
202. Shirakura T, Kelson TJ, Ray A, Malyarenko AE, Kopelman R. Hydrogel nanoparticles with thermally controlled drug release. Epub 2014/11/25 *ACS Macro Letters* 2014;**3**(7):602–6. https://doi.org/10.1021/mz500231e. PubMed PMID: 25419487; PMCID: PMC4235390.
203. N'Guyen TT, Duong HT, Basuki J, Montembault V, Pascual S, Guibert C, Fresnais J, Boyer C, Whittaker MR, Davis TP, Fontaine L. Functional iron oxide magnetic nanoparticles with hyperthermia-induced drug release ability by using a combination of orthogonal click reactions. Epub 2013/11/21 *Angew Chem* 2013;**52**(52):14152–6. https://doi.org/10.1002/anie.201306724. PubMed PMID: 24255024.
204. Riedinger A, Guardia P, Curcio A, Garcia MA, Cingolani R, Manna L, Pellegrino T. Subnanometer local temperature probing and remotely controlled drug release based on azo-functionalized iron oxide nanoparticles. Epub 2013/05/11 *Nano Lett* 2013;**13**(6):2399–406. https://doi.org/10.1021/nl400188q. PubMed PMID: 23659603.
205. Yoo D, Jeong H, Noh SH, Lee JH, Cheon J. Magnetically triggered dual functional nanoparticles for resistance-free apoptotic hyperthermia. Epub 2013/11/28 *Angew Chem* 2013;**52**(49):13047–51. https://doi.org/10.1002/anie.201306557. PubMed PMID: 24281889.
206. Lewis JK, Bischof JC, Braslavsky I, Brockbank KG, Fahy GM, Fuller BJ, Rabin Y, Tocchio A, Woods EJ, Wowk BG, Acker JP, Giwa S. The Grand Challenges of Organ Banking: proceedings from the first global summit on complex tissue cryopreservation. *Cryobiology* 2016;**72**(2):169–82. https://doi.org/10.1016/j.cryobiol.2015.12.001. PubMed PMID: 26687388.
207. Fahy GM, Wowk B. Principles of cryopreservation by vitrification. *Methods Mol Biol* 2015;**1257**:21–82. https://doi.org/10.1007/978-1-4939-2193-5_2. PubMed PMID: 25428002.
208. Taylor M, Song Y, Brockbank K. Vitrification in tissue preservation: new developments. *Life in the Frozen State* 2004;**22**:616–55. https://doi.org/10.1201/9780203647073.
209. Etheridge ML, Xu Y, Rott L, Choi J, Glasmacher B, Bischof JC. RF heating of magnetic nanoparticles improves the thawing of cryopreserved biomaterials. *Technology* 2014;**02**(03):229–42. https://doi.org/10.1142/s2339547814500204.
210. Eisenberg DP, Bischof JC, Rabin Y. Thermomechanical stress in cryopreservation via vitrification with nanoparticle heating as a stress-moderating effect. *J Biomech Eng-T Asme.* 2016;**138**(1). Artn 011010 10.1115/1.4032053. PubMed PMID: WOS:000366758400010.
211. Wang JY, Zhao G, Zhang ZL, Xu XL, He XM. Magnetic induction heating of superparamagnetic nanoparticles during rewarming augments the recovery of hUCM-MSCs cryopreserved by vitrification. *Acta Biomater* 2016;**33**:264–74. https://doi.org/10.1016/j.actbio.2016.01.026. PubMed PMID: WOS:000372688700026.
212. Manuchehrabadi N, Gao Z, Zhang JJ, Ring HL, Shao Q, Liu F, McDermott M, Fok A, Rabin Y, Brockbank KGM, Garwood M, Haynes CL, Bischof JC. Improved tissue cryopreservation using inductive heating of magnetic nanoparticles. *Sci Transl Med* 2017;**9**(379). ARTN eaah4586 10.1126/scitranslmed.aah4586. PubMed PMID: WOS:000395754100003.

Chapter 14

Carbon nanomaterials: fundamental concepts, biological interactions, and clinical applications

Edward Kai-Hua Chow[1,2], Mengjie Gu[1,2] and Jingru Xu[1,2]

[1]Department of Pharmacology, National University of Singapore, Singapore; [2]Cancer Science Institute of Singapore, National University of Singapore, Singapore

14.1 Introduction

There was a burst in the research of various nanomaterials, thanks to the enormous advancements of nanotechnology during the past decades.[1] Among all the advanced materials, carbon nanomaterials represent a class of low-dimensional materials with increasing interest. These low-dimensional carbon nanomaterials possess a variety of unusual physical, chemical, optical, magnetic, and electrical properties.[1] Because of their unique properties, carbon nanomaterials have been widely explored in the fields of electronics, photonics, renewable energy, as well as biomedicine. We will focus on their biomedical applications in this chapter.

Typically, nanomaterials refer to the particles whose size ranges from 1 nm to 1 μm. One striking advantage of nanomaterials is that they utilize the enhanced permeability and retention effect (EPR effect for short), which describes the enhanced permeability of nanoparticles into tumor blood vessels due to the larger epithelial junctions (40−1000 nm in tumor vessel compared with 8 nm in normal blood vessel) as well as the enhanced retention due to the deficient lymphatic drainage in tumor sites.[2−5] The EPR effect helps nanoparticles to passively target tumors while minimizing the side effects against normal tissues, which makes them an ideal delivery platform to load and deliver molecules, such as chemotherapy drugs (which will be discussed in detail in Section 3.1), to specific targets.

Among all the nanomaterials, carbon nanomaterials exhibit large diversity in terms of structures. According to the number of dimensions, carbon nanomaterials can be categorized into zero-dimensional (0D) materials, such as fullerenes and carbon dots; one-dimensional (1D) materials, such as carbon nanotubes (CNTs); two-dimensional (2D) layered materials, such as graphene; and three-dimensional (3D) structures, such as nanodiamonds (NDs) (Fig. 14.1). They display different properties in terms of shape, functional groups, as well as atomic hybridization (sp, sp^2 or sp^3).[1] In addition, the diversities of different carbon nanomaterials result in distinct physicochemical properties such as electrochemical and redox potential and therefore further influence their biological behaviors.[6−9] Herein, we will mainly highlight three classes of carbon nanomaterials, namely, fullerenes, CNTs, and NDs.

14.1.1 Fullerenes

Fullerenes are among one of the most rapidly studied carbon nanomaterials, while the most investigated fullerene is Buckminsterfullerene (C_{60}), which contains 60 carbon atoms and is a truncated icosahedron with 20 hexagons and 12 pentagons, resembling a football in shape.[10] The diameter of a C_{60} fullerene molecule is approximately 1 nm.[11] The synthesis of fullerenes mainly includes two approaches, namely top-down method (by laser- or heat-induced evaporation of graphite)[1,11,12] and bottom-up method (direct chemical synthesis from smaller aromatic precursors).[13] Importantly, their ultrasmall size, uniform dispersity, as well as tunable chemical modifications, receive increasing interest in the fields of biomedical research, highlighting in therapeutics, diagnostics, and bioimaging.[1,14]

Considering previous publications on fullerenes, this chapter will discuss the most recent developments, mainly

Nanoparticles for Biomedical Applications. https://doi.org/10.1016/B978-0-12-816662-8.00014-X

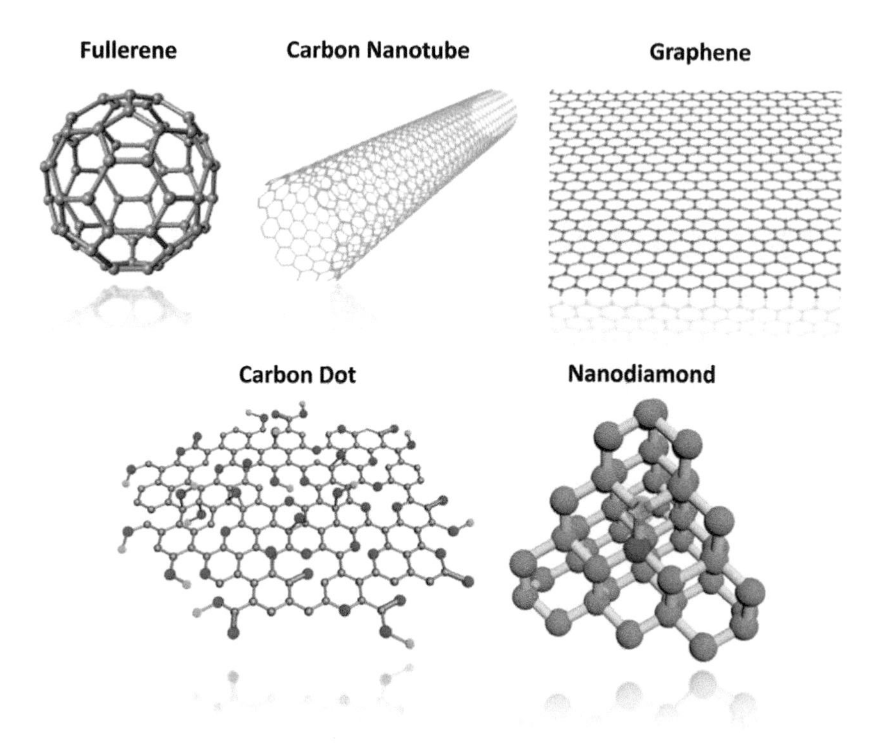

FIGURE 14.1 The structures of carbon nanomaterials.[1] *Reprinted (adapted) with permission from Hong G., Diao S., Antaris A.L., Dai H., Carbon nanomaterials for biological imaging and nanomedicinal therapy.* Chem Rev *2015;**115**(19):10816–906. Copyright [2015] American Chemical Society.*

focusing on their significant role in promoting novel delivery platforms of biomolecules and theranostic tools.[15]

14.1.2 Carbon nanotubes

CNTs are well-ordered, one-dimensional macromolecules, composed of single or multiple coaxial tubes of graphitic sheets. They can be mainly classified into two types: single-walled carbon nanotubes (SWCNTs), which were constructed by a single graphitic layer, and multiwalled carbon nanotubes (MWCNTs), which were constructed by multiple coaxial graphitic layers. There are three main techniques used for CNTs production: the carbon arc-discharge method,[16] the laser-ablation method,[17] and the chemical vapor deposition (CVD) method.[18]

CNTs become an appealing candidate for biomedical research because of their unique chemical, structural, mechanical, optical, and electrical properties. The high aspect ratio and multifunctional surface chemistry of CNTs lead to valid drug delivery capacity. Also, SWCNTs have unique optical properties because of the existence of the bandgap in semiconducting SWCNTs, based on which SWCNTs have been applied in photothermal and photodynamic therapy.[19–21] Meanwhile, the outstanding flexibility as well as strength under mechanical duress and biocompatibility have made CNTs promising materials for tissue engineering.[22–25] Hydrophobic CNTs can be modified to impart water solubility, and the solubilized CNTs have lower toxicity and better biocompatibility than the unmodified CNTs.

14.1.3 Nanodiamonds

NDs represent another unique class of carbon nanomaterials, specifically in the emerging field for novel delivery systems with the ability of protecting, loading, delivering, and unloading their payloads to the specific sites of action. Essentially, NDs are carbon particles with diameter of 2–8 nm. The geometric structure of a single ND particle is a faceted truncated octahedral architecture.[26] They are mainly composed of carbon sp^3 hybridization in the core, with sp^2 hybridization and disorder/defect carbons on the surface.[27,28] NDs can be classified into different categories according to their synthesis methods. Among them, detonation NDs (DNDs) and high-pressure high-temperature (HPHT) NDs are the most widely utilized in biomedical applications. As the name implies, detonation NDs are generally synthesized by decomposing high-explosive mixtures using negative oxygen balance in a nonoxidizing medium (usually an inert gas or water/ice coolant).[28,29] The resulting product, detonation soot, is a mixture of diamond particles and other carbon allotropes as well as impurities. Therefore, further purification process needs to be conducted. The composition of the surface chemistry is a result of the synthesis route for ND. As a result of a purification process using oxygenating acids that remove the residual noncarbon impurities and nondiamond carbon, NDs have a high amount of oxygen species at the surface (mainly carboxyl groups), thus forming high surface potentials and stable aqueous dispersions.[10]

There are several distinct advantages of NDs over other carbon nanomaterials. Above all, they can be versatilely surface modified with a variety of functional groups, such as carboxyl group, amino group, and hydroxyl group, without many alterations to its diamond core. Additionally, NDs possess strong electrostatic fields on each of its facets, attracting surrounded water molecules and creating a hydration shell at the ND–solvent interface, which mediates their binding with ions and water molecules. This reversible and potent drug binding capacity results in sustained release as drug molecules are exchanged on the surface of NDs.[26] In one study, Wang et al. reported that ND–epirubicin complexes formulated by physical adsorption had sustained release under physiological condition (pH = 7), whereas negligible premature drug release in blood was observed in mice,[30] indicating these complexes were lack of systemic toxicity. Most importantly, unlike other carbon nanomaterials (e.g., fullerenes, CNTs), NDs were reported to possess higher biocompatibility.[31–33] After intravenous administration of NDs at high dosages, no change of serum indicators of liver and systemic toxicity was observed in mice, rats, and nonhuman primates.[26,34] This superiority is probably caused by NDs'capability of whole-body clearance. Rapid clearance of NDs was observed from the lung, followed by more gradual clearance from the spleen, liver, and kidney over 10-day period.[26] On the contrary, long-term retention of CNTs in the lung might cause fibrosis and has potential chronic pulmonary toxicity.[35]

Due to the aforementioned advantageous properties such as small size, large surface area,unique optical properties, and superior mechanical properties, carbon nanomaterials stand out among all nanomaterials. Furthermore, the preparation process of carbon nanomaterials (e.g., ND–drug complexes) is usually facile and readily reproducible, making them more suitable than other nanomaterials for scale-up production and further translation to the clinic. In this chapter, we will cover the most recent progress in the applications of therapy, bioimaging, diagnosis, and tissue engineering and repair using carbon nanomaterials, specifically fullerenes, CNTs, and NDs. We will also try to provide some insights with regard to the future directions and major challenges for furthering their clinical applications.

14.2 Surface functionalization

From the perspective of clinical applications, the most vital consideration of using these exogenous nanoparticles is biocompatibility. Biological interactions with biomacromolecules (such as proteins, lipids, and polysaccharide) not only influence their accumulation in living tissues and organs, elimination pathways, but also determine their eventual fate in organisms. The successful translation of nanomaterials is based on a comprehensive understanding of their biological interactions.[27]

To solve the water solubility issue of carbon nanomaterials, as well as to impede their toxicity, multiple methods have been proposed.[36,37] Desirable solubility under physiological solutions (for example, in phosphate buffer saline (PBS) or in cell culture medium) provides opportunities for carbon nanomaterials to load a broad range of therapeutic molecules such as peptides, proteins, nucleic acids, and so forth.[15] To obtain the purpose of sustained release or stimuli-dependent release of cargo, carbon nanomaterials can be functionalized in a controllable way for further interaction with therapeutic molecules, that is, stimuli-responsive delivery system (or so-called "smart" drug delivery system).[38,39]

Because of their hydrophobic properties, fullerenes show a poor aqueous solubility, therefore limiting their biomedical applications.[40,41] Interestingly, chemical modification with hydroxyl, carboxyl, or amino groups through covalent reactions has been demonstrated to enhance the aqueous solubility of fullerene derivatives, leading to higher biocompatibility.[42] On the other hand, fullerene derivatives can also be linked with a variety of other functional groups such as pyrrolidinium and peptides.[43–45] Moreover, the tunable surface modifications of fullerenes have endowed their capability of bioconjugation with targeting molecules to selectively target to specific biomarkers.[1,46]

Also, the hydrophobicity of CNTs limits their biomedical applications. Luckily, there are several ways, either noncovalently or covalently functionalized to improve water solubility. The noncovalent functionalization, including π-πstaking and hydrophobic interactions, can minimize the structural damage and intrinsic properties disturbance to the carbon nanomaterial. In terms of SWCNT, the noncovalent functionalization maintains the properties and electronic of SWCNTs, especially the NIR-II fluorescence emission.

Kinds of small molecule surfactants, such as sodium dodecyl sulfate (SDS), sodium deoxycholate, sodium taurodeoxycholate, and cetylpyridinium chloride, have been used to disperse and solubilize pristine SWCNTs.[47,48] The surfactant molecules spontaneously form columnar micelles in water when the concentration of surfactants reaches the critical micelle concentration (CMC). SWCNTs are encapsulated through hydrophobic interactions in the hydrophobic core of micelles; meanwhile, the hydrophilic shell of micelles provides solvation in an aqueous environment. However, it is reported that the micelle-stabilized SWCNTs have toxicity to cells because of the existence of the surfactants, even at a low concentration.[49]

However, it is difficult for noncovalently functionalized CNTs to be further modified. Covalent functionalization can not only improve the solubility of CNTs, but also introduce functional motifs for further conjugation. One popular approach for the covalent functionalization of CNTs is through controlled oxidation using certain oxidizing agents. With many carboxylic acid groups on the open ends, CNTs can further react with other functional groups, such as poly-(propionylethylenimine-co-ethylenimine) (PPEI-EI), ligands with amine groups, and thiolated RGD peptide.[50–52]

Similarly, the dispersity and stability under physiological environment still remain as a predominant hurdle for ND application. There also have been numerous studies on functionalizing ND with various biocompatible macromolecules such as polyethylene glycol (PEG),[53–55] chitosan,[56] amino acid,[57,58]polyethylenimine (PEI),[59] and so on.[60] Among them, PEG is the most successfully integrated with different nanoparticles (such as liposomes, gold nanoparticles, and quantum dots[61–64]) to increase their solubility, stability, and permeability, meanwhile avoid quick recognition and elimination by the immune system, therefore prolonging the circulation time of certain nanoparticles[53,61,62].

Facile surface functionalization of carbon nanomaterials further increases their adaptability toward delivering a variety of therapeutics and imaging reagents, consequently widening their range for clinical applications.[65] We will highlight their significant importance in promoting new delivery platforms for biomolecules in the following sections.[15]

14.3 Biological interactions

Owing to a wide scope of biomedical applications of carbon nanomaterials, there is an urgent need to elucidate their toxicological and pharmacological profiles. Although comprehensive in vivo studies using different animal models (e.g., mouse, rat, and nonhuman primate) have shown that carbon nanomaterials such as NDs do not cause toxic effects,[15,66] there are still gaps we need to fill. For instance, fullerenes were reported to inhibit vascular endothelial growth factor (VEGF).[65,67] Additionally, cellular toxicity caused by the generation of reactive oxygen species (ROS) was also reported in several studies.[68–70] Moreover, the heavy metal residues resulted from using metallic catalysts during the synthesis procedure further influence cellular processes, which has been reported for CNTs.[71,72] NDs were shown to increase intracellular oxidative stress within the endothelial cells and thus activate key signaling pathways.[65] As such, careful considerations of accumulation, degradation, and/or excretion in the organism must be made.

One major and inevitable concern when applying in vivo (especially via intravenous administration and exposure to blood circulatory system) is the interactions between plasma proteins and carbon nanomaterials, which has drawn increasing attention in recent years.[73–75] On one hand, this nanomaterial–protein binding is usually influenced by the surface properties of the nanomaterial.[76–78] Due to the inherent strong electrostatic properties, the resulting electronic interactions with proteins may lead to an alteration of protein conformation and even trigger immune response.[79] Studies have also demonstrated the oxygenated functional group density of the nanomaterials, particularly the amount of their C–O and C=O bonds, might have strong influence on these electronic interactions.[80] To some extent, the dimensionality and surface area of nanomaterials also played a vital role.[80] On the other hand, avoiding quick recognition and blood clearance by the reticuloendothelial system (RES) so as to improve biodistribution is also a key issue for nanoparticles.[81,82]To reduce rapid clearance, the desirable size for nanoparticles appears to be 5–30 nm.[81] Ideally, neutral surface charge and nonspherical shape can also reduce their reactivity and protein adsorption trend.[83,84] Moreover, the strategy of using stealth coating (e.g., PEGylation) has shown particular potential in enhancing the half-life of nanoparticles.[85,86]

Among all the biocompatibility assessments of nanomaterials, their potential effects on the immune system are of key importance.[27,87] Some studies have indicated functionalized carbon nanomaterials might act as immune stimulatory agents since they were involved in interacting with immune cells (e.g., macrophages and dendritic cells) and activating immune-related pathways in monocytes.[27,87–92] Another reason for the underlying toxicity of carbon nanomaterials might be caused by their hydrophobic character, which enables them to penetrate through cell membranes,[93] namely, cellular uptake. Taking NDs as an example, it has been revealed that they could efficiently deliver a payload into cells via endocytosis pathway, particularly clathrin-mediatedendocytosis and macropinocytosis.[30,94] This enhanced cellular uptake of the payload leads to enhanced retention as well as improved therapeutic efficiency.

Although the enhanced cellular retention might serve as an advantage for drug delivery systems that are designed to stay within the target organ or tissue, their possible accumulation in other organs should also be considered, specifically the liver. The liver is the primary organ responsible for the accumulation of multiple substances due to its function of breaking down or modifying toxins,[95] which makes the liver quite susceptible to the damages caused by nanoparticles, further triggering oxidative stress and inflammation.[96] However, studies have confirmed no toxic effect to the liver and no harmful systemic side effects after long-term expose using a rat model.[66] There is no doubt that further studies regarding the potential applicability of carbon nanomaterials need to be conducted.

Luckily, more recent studies have suggested surface modification strategies to improve the biocompatibility of carbon nanomaterials.[27] Besides biocompatibility, biodegradation is another vital issue that needs to be carefully considered. Several studies have reported that biodegradation of carbon nanomaterials can be easily tuned by chemical functionalization.[97–100] Specifically, enzymatic degradation provides such an approach to alleviate their accumulation issue. In one study, Star and coworkers found that carboxylated SWCNTs could be degraded by horseradish peroxidase (HRP) in the presence of low concentrations of H_2O_2.[101,102] Nearly all the nanotubes were found degraded within 10 days. In another similar study, SWCNTs were demonstrated to be biodegradable in fluids mimicking the phagolysosome milieu (phagolysosomal simulating fluid), which was medium designed to simulate the acidic oxidizing environment inside the late-stage endosomes and phagolysosomes of macrophages.[103]

14.4 Therapeutic applications

Thanks to their desirable size range, considerably high surface area, tunable surface chemistry, as well as the potential for controlled release, novel functionalized carbon nanomaterials possess satisfactory drug loading capacity, high biocompatibility, as well as remarkably pharmaceutical efficiency. Additionally, carbon nanomaterials can be functionalized with a wide spectrum of therapeutics, including chemotherapy drugs, bioactive peptides, proteins, and nucleic acids.[15]

14.4.1 Applications in chemotherapy drugs

Cancer is a heterogeneous disease, and different patient populations might have dramatically different responses toward the same therapeutic combination.[65] Notably, thanks to the EPR effect, delivery using carbon nanomaterials could achieve similar efficacy at lower dosage compared with conventional chemotherapy drugs, thus reducing the associated side effects induced by chemotherapy drugs.

One predominant application of carbon nanomaterials is overcoming drugefflux–based chemoresistance. Among which, a common mechanism of drug resistance is induced by ABC transporter (ATP-binding cassette transporter), since multiple ABC transporters are able to efflux drug molecules, particularly anthracyclines.[104–106] There have been diverse studies with regard to ND-anthracycline complexes, which not only increased the antitumor efficacy but also reduced the toxic side effects caused by anthracyclines.[26,30,107–109] In this case, compared with the drug alone, NDs sequestered the drug molecules for a longer time, which decreased the efficacy during the very first period. However, these ND–drug complexes possessed a delayed but time-controlled/sustained drug release, which in turn prolonged the overall efficacy during the treatment.[104] Besides solid tumors, ND-based delivery has also been used to combat chemoresistant leukemia and was demonstrated with enhanced efficacy compared with daunorubicin alone, by overcoming efflux mechanisms.[108] Interestingly, NDs were reported to have antiangiogenic junctions, resulting in tumor growth inhibition,[6,110] which makes ND itself a promising anticancer agent.

Thanks to the optimal sizes and hydrophobic surface properties, functionalized fullerenes also serve as favorable nanocarriers for chemotherapy drugs. One major advantage of fullerenes is their ability to easily cross cell membranes.[15,42] Some clinically used chemotherapy drugs (e.g., paclitaxel, doxorubicin) were conjugated on the surface of C_{60},[111,112] and the resultant conjugates displayed satisfactory release profiles and antitumor activities. Likewise, a water-soluble and biocompatible fluorescent fullerene (C_{60}-TEG–COOH)–coated mesoporous silica nanoparticle (named MSN) was designed in one study.[113] This smart delivery system showed a pH-sensitive release profile; meanwhile the loading of doxorubicin was associated with high toxicity in HeLa cells, demonstrating their reserved killing capability toward cancer cells.[15,113]

CNTs have been considered as a promising drug delivery system owing to their unique structures and functional surface groups. Various molecules can be conjugated to the modified CNTs with available functional groups. Otherwise, hydrophobic drugs can be adsorbed to the CNTs through $\pi-\pi$ stacking or hydrophobic interactions. Paclitaxel (PTX) was successfully covalently linked to SWCNTs, and SWCNT-PTX showed high water solubility as well as the long blood circulation time, meanwhile exhibited similar toxicity as Taxol, the clinical drug formulation of PTX. Furthermore, the in vivo cancer treatment shows the significant inhibition of tumor growth and low side effects.[114] Another commonly used drug in chemotherapy, doxorubicin (DOX), was loaded onto CNTs through $\pi-\pi$ stacking with high drug loading capacity (up to 4g DOX every 1g of SWCNTs).[115] With PEG coating, the blood circulation time of the CNTs-DOX has been prolonged In the meantime, the CNTs-DOX were sensitive to acidic environments while stable at neutral pH, which was a desirable property for in vivo drug delivery. Accordingly, an in vivo study showed that the CNTs-DOX achieved enhanced treatment efficacy and low toxicity compared with the free DOX and DOXIL.

14.4.2 Other applications besides cancer

Although carbon nanomaterials–based drug delivery platform has received most attention in cancer treatment, there are also various studies exploring these versatile nanomaterials for treating other kinds of diseases. Among which, one aspect is antibacterial drugs. Developing novel antibacterial materials is of vital importance owing to the increasing prevalence of resistant bacteria strains.[10] Ideally, all carbon nanomaterials are capable of showing antibacterial properties because of their inherent antibacterial properties.[10,69] Direct contact of bacteria with carbon nanomaterials was reported to affect their cellular membrane integrity, metabolic processes, and morphology.[116] For example, SWCNTs could cause severe membrane damage and subsequent cell death.[117] One possible hypothesis was that formation of cell-CNTs aggregates caused damage of cell wall of bacteria and then release of their DNA content.[118] For fullerene, the antibacterial effect was probably caused by inhibiting energy metabolism after internalization into the bacteria.[116] Lyon et al.[119] in their study demonstrated that fractions of nC_{60} containing smaller fullerene aggregates showed greater antibacterial activity. Wehling et al. found that the antibacterial activity of NDs depends on surface chemistry to a great extent.[120] Likewise, taking advantage of the strong interactions between fullerene derivatives and cell membranes, Pantarotto et al. found that they demonstrate substantiated antimicrobial activities against the gram-positive bacterium, *Staphylococcus aureus*, and lysed erythrocytes.[44]

Of note, carbon nanomaterials are commonly used as a delivery platform of antiinflammation drugs as well. In one study, taking advantage of NDs' rich surface chemistry, octadecylamine-modified ND (termed ND-ODA) was designed as a platform to deliver dexamethasone, an antiinflammation drug.[121] The ability of ND-ODA to promote antiinflammatory and prophagocytic behavior in macrophages suggested its promising role as an antiinflammatory therapeutic carrier to directly target macrophages.

Waterinsolubility has always been a dominant challenge for biomedically active molecules. A lot of compounds that possess remarkable therapeutic properties have poor water solubility, therefore limiting further potential biomedical applications. Chen et al. reported in their studies that NDs were able to load poorly water-soluble compounds (Purvalanol A, 4-hydroxytamoxifen, and dexamethasone were used in their studies) to enhance their dispersibility in water.[122] Meanwhile, biological activity of these drugs was preserved, indicating the broad feasibility of NDs in delivering poorly water-soluble molecules to achieve novel treatment routes.

The high surface areas and aspect ratios make CNTs the ideal platform for drug delivery. In addition, the needle-like shape of CNTs can improve the transmembrane penetration of the drug molecule.[123] Thus, there are kinds of investigations on CNTs as drug delivery agents for treatment of inflammation (dexamethasone[124]), infection (amphotericin B,[125]pazufloxacin mesylate[126]), and hypertension (diltiazem hydrochloride,[127] metoprolol tartrate[128]), demonstrating superior effect and low toxicity. In terms of brain diseases, for example, Alzheimer disease (AD), CNTs can effectively deliver acetylcholine (Ach) into the brain. Free Ach cannot directly enter into the brain because of its poor lipophilicity and strong polarity. However, the defects of Ach can be overcome by using CNTs as a delivery system due to its lipophilicity.[129] In this study, mice were administered by gastrogavage with SWCNTs–Ach mixture. Once inside the brain, they enter the lysosomes of neurons and release the Ach because of the low pH condition.

14.4.3 Applications in proteins and peptides

Protein-based drugs hold great potential as therapeutic agents, which include monoclonal antibodies, hormones, cytokines, and therapeutic peptides. However, the instability of protein-based drugs under physiological conditions limits their further applications.[130–132] That is, when administrated in vivo, nonspecific proteases in the blood circulation can rapidly degrade proteins before they reach the target sites. Therefore, the requirement of increasing the stability of proteins by proficient delivery systems is of crucial importance to achieve enhanced efficacy.

A broad spectrum of methods have been utilized to improve the stability and therapeutic efficacy of proteins using carbon nanomaterials–mediated delivery systems either through noncovalent binding or covalent conjugation.[57,94,133–135] In one study, bovine insulin was loaded onto NDs via physical adsorption, and this ND–insulin complex presented pH-dependent desorption under alkaline conditions.[133]In vitro assays revealed that the loaded insulin remained inactive under neutral pH and only desorbed under alkaline medium. Another study focused on NDs' capability of delivering antibodies (Abs).[136] NDs were shown to bind readily with the Abs, and the resultant ND-Ab complexes were demonstrated to be stable in water with no Ab release even after 10 days. These ND-Ab complexes were triggered to release when exposed to physiological conditions, whereas the functionality of Abs was preserved during the adsorption/desorption process. CNTs were also used to noncovalently and nonspecifically bind with various types of proteins ($\leq$80 kD). After uptake by cell lines, the protein–nanotube conjugates were released from the endosome, entering into the cytoplasm to perform biological functions.[137]

14.4.4 Applications in gene delivery

Gene therapy has attracted increasing attention because of its capability of actively controlling the expression of certain proteins that play vital roles in disease progressions, by introducing foreign genetic materials into host cells. However, genetic molecules such as DNA, plasmid DNA, mRNA, siRNA, and shRNA are unstable in a biological environment, which has been an unneglectable obstacle for further translation. Therefore, developing vehicles that can enhance nucleic acid stability as well as targeting specificity is a key determinant to pave their way to clinical applications.[138] Additionally, considering the high potential of immune response and carcinogenicity risks brought by viral vectors, researchers have shifted their efforts toward-nonviral vectors, in particular, nanocarriers.[138–141]

Efficient delivery of nucleic acids into cells and release of the nucleic acids are of significant importance for successful transfection.[142] Considerable efforts have been made to develop carbon nanomaterials suitable for gene delivery. Notably, NDs and their complexes with PEI possess significantly low toxicity and excellent biocompatibility,[59,143] while maintaining high transfection efficiency when delivering plasmid DNA, siRNA, as well as miRNA,[59,143,144] usually via electrostatic interactions between nucleic acids and PEI-modified NDs. Furthermore, in addition to electrostatic attachment, covalent linkage approach is utilized in ND-based gene delivery as well.[145] In one study regarding siRNA delivery, compared with lipofectamine, which serves as a commercial gold standard for transfection, ND-PEI complexes were demonstrated to exhibit enhanced transfection efficiency under biological conditions, signifying the translational promise of this biocompatible siRNA delivery strategy.[143]

Likewise, studies have also been conducted to prepare various complexes for gene delivery based on fullerenes.[15,146–149] For instance, Maeda-Mamiya et al. developed the cationic tetraaminofullerene with a high hydrophilicity to deliver plasmid DNA in their study.[150] Their results suggested that delivery of the insulin 2 gene increased the plasma insulin level in female C57/BL6 mice, meanwhile decreased the blood glucose concentration. Their study indicates the potential therapeutic application of fullerene derivatives as gene delivery nanocarriers. Additionally, no acute toxicity of the fullerene complexes was observed after administration.

CNTs show promise as an effective tool in gene delivery as well. The first type of nucleic acid transfected successfully in vitro by CNTs was plasmid DNA. In addition, CNTs have been utilized to deliver different kinds of plasmid DNA since then, green fluorescent protein (GFP) gene,[151–154] for example. However, there is very limited in vivo study with regard to plasmid DNA delivered by CNTs. The study by Kam, et al.[155] showed that the conjugates of SWCNTs and siRNA with cleavable bonds can efficiently transport siRNA into cells and downregulate the targeted protein. After this pioneering study, more and more investigations on CNTs as an ideal platform for siRNA delivery have been reported both in vitro and in vivo.[156–161] It has been shown that CNTs are suitable for transfecting difficult cell types, such us skeletal muscle cells, primary cardiomyocytes, and T cells.[157,162,163]

14.4.5 Applications in photothermal therapy

Having fluorescence with the emission wavelengths from visible to near infrared (NIR) allows some carbon nanomaterials to be used for bioimaging and treatment simultaneously. When the photosensitizers accumulate in specific tissues, the electromagnetic radiation can be used to heat the tissues, which leads to photocoagulation and cell death.[164] CNTs with some surface modification can escape from the immune system. Additionally, CNTs have strong absorbance in the NIR region, which has better tissue penetration compared with the visible region. These superiorities make CNTs an ideal photothermal agent.

Single-walled CNTs (SWCNTs) are the first carbon nanomaterial developed for photothermal therapy.[165] Once delivered into cells by CNTs, endosomal disruption was triggered by NIR laser pulses, and then the loaded oligonucleotides could be transferred to the nucleus. Meanwhile, continuous NIR radiation resulted in cell death. In this study, the SWCNTs played two roles at the same time: molecular cargo and photosensitizer. Both the intratumoral injection and intravenous injection can be applied to transport SWCNTs into the tumor.[20,166]

14.4.6 Applications in photodynamic therapy

Photoexcitation capability is another unique photochemical property of fullerene. Upon photoexcitation, ground-state, singlet C_{60} can absorb photon energy, followed by being excited to the triplet C_{60}. This transfers its stored energy to their surrounding oxygen molecules and then turns them into ROS (such as singlet oxygen and oxygen-free radicals) through both energy transfer and electron transfer.[15,167–169] These ROS are highly active in DNA cleavage and thus can be cytotoxic. Therefore, C_{60} molecules can be used as photosensitizers in photodynamic therapy.[170]

CNTs can be used as a platform to deliver the photosensitizers for PDT, and there are a few studies that used CNTs themselves as a photosensitizer.[21,171] In the work of Shi et al.,[172] hyaluronic acid–modified CNTs (HA-CNTs) with high solubility in water were linked with HMME, a PDT agent, by $\pi-\pi$ stacking interaction. The resultant HMME-HA-CNTs, possessing photodynamic and photothermal properties simultaneously, showed tumor growth suppression both in vivo and in vitro.

14.5 Applications in bioimaging

14.5.1 Applications in optical imaging

Carbon nanomaterials have drawn a lot of attention for bioimaging applications because of their unique optical properties.[1] For instance, SWCNTs have the intrinsic fluorescence emission at long wavelengths (1000–1700 nm), which allows them for deep-tissue fluorescence imaging due to the reduced scattering of photons.[173–175] In another example, NDs were shown to have remarkably long fluorescence lifetime, making them suitable for distinguishing the NDs-labeled fluorescence from tissue autofluorescence.[176] In addition, based on the intrinsic photoluminescence of fullerenes (C_{60}), they are also utilized in fluorescence imaging.[177–180]

Indeed, some NDs, especially those synthesized using the HTHP method, are capable of emitting fluorescent signals.[181–183] This self-fluorescent of NDs is mainly due to the impurity of nitrogen and its incorporation into the diamond crystal vacancy during the production of NDs.[184,185] The vacancies in the diamond core occupied by nitrogen atoms form different color centers based on the structure of the nitrogenvacancy (NV) defect, making the ND self-fluorescent under red or near-infrared wavelengths.[186] Linking or adsorbing various fluorophores onto NDs provides another way to produce fluorescent NDs (FNDs). FNDs serve as a powerful sensor by monitoring surface changes within the bonding environment. Importantly, FNDs combine the advantages of quantum dots with biocompatibility and rich surface chemistry, making them well suited as in vivo imaging tools.[28] Moreover, because of their negligible photobleaching and toxicity, FNDs are broadly used to track their fate after administering in vivo. Studies also suggested that FNDs represented an excellent nanocarrier for intracellular transport and long-term imaging applications.[134,187]

Nowadays, CNTs have been widely used as imaging agents both in vitro and in vivo. Some studies used CNTs as molecular transporters to deliver organic fluorophores into cells for fluorescent imaging.[188] However, Cherukuri et al.[189] detected the intrinsic fluorescence of SWCNTs, and the intracellular distribution of SWCNTs in macrophages was successfully imaged. This investigation provides a new method for SWCNTs to be used in bioimaging directly through its intrinsic fluorescence. Welsher et al.[173] used SWCNTs as fluorescent imaging agents in the low albedo NIR IIregion for videorate in vivo imaging of mice via intravenous injection and studied the pathway of SWCNTs through mouse anatomy. As useful fluorophores, the SWCNTs are bright enough to be imaged inside mice at high frame rates.

Another important bioimaging method of CNTs is Raman imaging. Raman scattering is the inelastic scattering process of a photon that can gain or lose energy. Based on this, researchers can gain information about materials from Raman spectroscopy. SWCNTs exhibit Raman peak at the graphitic band, which can be easily differentiated from the autofluorescence background. With the large Raman scattering cross sections, SWCNTs can be used as the Raman labels and probes for biomedical imaging. Strano et al.[190] first reported that DNA-functionalized SWCNTs showed continuous Raman scattering and variational fluorescence spectra in mammalian cells. Moreover, the Raman signals could be seen inside cells during the experiment. Raman spectroscopy was also used to measure the blood circulation of SWCNTs by intravenous injection as well as to detect the distribution in different organs and tissues of mice ex vivo.[191] Moreover, Raman imaging of CNTs was also used in vivo in several investigations.[192–194]

14.5.2 Applications in nonoptical imaging

Carbon nanomaterials are ideal for photoacoustic imaging for the reason that they are good light absorbers in the entire visible and near-infrared window. Meanwhile, they can convert incoming photons to heat more efficiently thanks to their low fluorescence quantum yields. The first and most broadly applied carbon nanomaterial in the photoacoustic imaging field is SWCNTs. There are several reports on photoacoustic imaging using SWCNTs in vivo.[52,192] One interesting work developed a two-color photoacoustic imaging platform by adding magnetic nanoparticles with photoacoustic response to gold-plated CNTs where the absorption maxima of the two materials were at different wavelengths.[195] This two-color photoacoustic imaging nanoparticle system was more specific in detecting tumor cells since tumor cells are heterogeneous, expressing different biomarkers. Overall, SWCNTs are recognized as good contrast agents for thermoacoustic imaging as well as photothermal imaging.

14.5.3 Applications in clinically relevant imaging modalities

Nowadays, computed tomography (CT), magnetic resonance imaging (MRI), and positron emission tomography (PET) are among the most prevalently applied in the clinical setting. Among them, MRI has become an increasingly popular tool for clinical diagnosis due to the lack of ionizing radiation.[196] In most cases, to improve the resolution and quality of MR images, contrast agents will be used. Generally speaking, MRI contrast agents contain a paramagnetic metal ion, such as ferrum (or iron, Fe), gadolinium (Gd), and manganese (Mn). By applying contrast agents, the image contrast between normal tissues and diseased tissues can be significantly enhanced.[197] However, conventional contrast agents are usually small molecules, and many reports have showed that Gd-based contrast agents had the potential of causing nephrogenic systemic fibrosis (NSF), especially for those patients with end-stage renal diseases.[198,199] Therefore, developing novel MRI contrast agents with improved tissue specificity and safety is essential.

On NDs, facet-specific electrostatics have played a vital role in coordinating water molecules close to the ND surface, which could be utilized to prepare ND–metal conjugates, resulting in increased interactions between water molecules and metal ions, as well as improving the per ion relaxivity.[65] For instance, Hou et al. developed a dual-mode contrast agent ND–Mn (ND–manganese conjugates), which enhanced both T_1 (longitudinal relaxation time)- and T_2 (transverse relaxation time)-weighted MR imaging.[200] Promisingly, demonstrated using an orthotopic liver cancer mouse model, these ND–Mn complexes displayed enhanced contrast imaging while reducing the concentration of toxic-free Mn^{2+} ions in the blood circulation.

Functionalized fullerenes have also been widely utilized for MRI diagnosis. Metallofullerene represents a promising family of MRI contrast agents. Of note, because of their unique structures and novel electronic properties, electron could transfer from the encaged metal atoms to the fullerene cages.[201,202] The closed network of carbon atoms has the advantages of preventing any leakage of the metal atoms from the fullerene cage, meanwhile retaining all of the metal's physical properties.[203] Several studies have indicated that such Gd-containing endohedral fullerenes possessed a higher signal enhancement at lower doses, as well as higher relaxivity, compared with the commercial Gd-DTPA (gadopentetate dimeglumine).[204–206]

As a delivery platform, CNTs can also be used to load MRI contrast agents, Gd^{3+}, for example.[207] However, with the metal impurities at the ends as residual catalysts, CNTs themselves can perform as MRI agents. SWCNTs were prepared at high pressure (30–50 atm) with $Fe(CO)_5$ as the iron-containing catalyst precursor, resulting in iron oxide nanoparticles linked to the end of the SWCNTs. This procedure is called the HiPco process. Based on this, the multifunctionality of SWCNTs/iron oxide nanoparticles were reported and engulfed by macrophage cells, which were imaged using MRI and NIR mapping.[208]

14.6 Applications in biosensing/diagnosis and theranostics

Carbon nanomaterials have emerged as an excellent biosensing platform due to their diverse and robust intrinsic optic and electronic properties.[209] Additionally, their high surface area renders simultaneous detection events. Integrated smart release delivery and sensor devices based on ND–peptide complexes have been proposed using stimuli-responsive systems in one study.[135] One peptide that can be specifically cleaved by MMP-9 (matrix metalloproteinase-9), an endopeptidase, whose expression level has been shown to be indicative of cancer metastasis, was covalentlyconjugated onto NDs. Moreover, the MMP-9-specific substrate peptide was labeled with fluorescent dye, so that the protease activity of MMP-9 cleaving the peptide can be accurately monitored and correlated to MMP-9 expression. Importantly, the resultant ND–peptide complexes also possessed an enhanced capability of protecting the peptide from nonspecific serum protease cleavage. This quantitative stimuli-responsive output function, combined with enhanced peptide stability, provided strong evidence for developing carbon nanomaterials-mediated biosensor for metastasis site detection.

Thanks to the remarkable progress made so far, multifunctional or multimodal nanomaterial-based delivery systems are made possible. One major strategy incorporating therapeutic functionality and imaging capability in one system is termed theranostics. Particularly, the unique physicochemical properties of carbon nanomaterials make them quite promising in meeting these demands.[82] Carbon nanomaterials–based electrochemical sensors represent a novel class of biosensors where their increased conductivity and surface area are readily explored. Petrakova et al. fabricated a FNDs-based platform that combined nucleic acids delivery and label-free intracellular tracking.[142] The sensing function was achieved by utilizing NV color centers, which provide stable nonblinking luminescence. The molecular events such as binding and release of DNA from FNDs surface will lead to changes in the electrical charge, thus monitoring nucleic acid transfection, and the payload release inside cells can be achieved. This creative device innovates the strategies for nucleic acid delivery and imaging simultaneously, meanwhile avoids affecting cellular processing of the nucleic acids.

CNTs were used in constructing enzyme biosensors because of their high aspect ratio, which contributes to the biomolecular conjugation. One of the important applications of currently used biosensors is glucose detection. The SWCNTs field-effect transistor biosensors are able to detect glucose by catalyzing glucose to gluconic acid and hydrogen peroxide under aerobic conditions.[210] The other widely used CNT biosensors are DNA biosensors. Single-strand DNA (ssDNA) can strongly bind to CNTs, whereas double-strand DNA (dsDNA) cannot bind to CNTs; based on this, CNT–DNA complexes have been built to target different molecules. It was reported that SWCNT-FET-based electronic DNA sensors can be easily integrated with high-density sensor arrays in "system-on-a-chip" for microanalysis devices.[211] In general, SWCNT acts as a transducer in the sensors that can translate and amplify DNA hybridization on Au into the electrical signal. The SWCNT DNA sensors are easier to be developed compared with optical and other electrochemical methods.

14.7 Applications in tissue engineering and repair

In addition to the aforementioned features of carbon nanomaterials, SWCNTs with pristine carbon networks and extended structures have superior mechanical properties that are successfully used for enhancing the strengths of tissue scaffolds.[1,24,212–215] The shape and structure of CNTs provides a particular strength toward applications in regenerative medicine, which leads to stem cell differentiation and even stem cell banking.[65]

There are several different cells that have been reported to successfully grow on the scaffolds of CNTs. As a scaffold for the growth of artificial bone material, hydroxyapatite (HA), chemically modified SWCNTs with negative charges were able to attract calcium cations and result in nucleation and initiating the crystallization of HA.[213] The growth direction of HA can be controlled by using different functionalized SWCNTs. For neural tissue engineering applications, MWCNTs-coated nanofibers can enhance the electrical properties of the scaffolds so as to improve the neurite outgrowth of rat dorsal root ganglia (DRG) neurons and focal adhesion kinase (FAK) expression of PC-12 cells.[216] Another example of CNTs scaffolds' application is in cardiac tissue growth. It was reported that CNT-incorporated photocross-linkable gelatin methacrylate (GelMA) showed outstanding mechanical integrity and electrophysiological functions, meanwhile reducing the electrical impedance, indicating promise as cardiac scaffolds.[217] There is also interesting work on controlling stem cell behaviors by using a polypyrrole (Ppy) array.[218] The Ppy array can switch between highly adhesive hydrophobic CNTs and poorly adhesive hydrophilic nanotips via an electrochemical oxidation or reduction, and it provided dynamic attachment and detachment stimuli on cell surfaces. The cytoskeleton can detect the stimuli via anchor points at focal adhesions and transduce the stimuli into nuclear signals, so as to guide mesenchymal stem cell osteogenic fate.

Besides CNTs, NDs have also been developed as nanocomposite hydrogels for tissue engineering, specifically stem cell–guided bone regeneration.[219,220] A hydrogel using photocross-linkable gelatin methacrylamide (GelMA) and NDs as a 3D scaffold was synthesized. The incorporation of NDs increased the network stiffness, which in turn enhanced the traction forces generated by human adipose stem cells (hASCs). Furthermore, dexamethasone (Dex) was adsorbed onto NDs to form complexes, which promoted the osteogenic differentiation of hASCs. The ND–Dex complexes were demonstrated to modulate gene expression in hASCs, focal adhesion surface area, as well as their focal adhesion number, confirming that the bioactivity of Dex was retained after complexation with NDs.

Interestingly, NDs have also been utilized for root canal therapy (RCT), which is already under clinical investigation (clinicaltrials.gov identifer: NCT02698163; NCT03376984.).[65,221,222] In one study, NDs were embedded with gutta percha, an inert thermoplastic polymer that is composed of the gutta percha latex, zinc oxide, a radiopacifier to allow for X-ray imaging to monitor treatment progress, and a plasticizer.[221,223] Notably, this thermoplastic material was the current standard material for RCT obturation to address reinfection and bone loss following RCT. Sustained apical wound healing with no reinfection or pain issues were reported during the interventional treatment. This study illustrated a foundation for the continued clinical translation of nanomaterials for a broad spectrum of applications.

14.8 Summary: future directions and main hurdles

The aforementioned studies serve as the foundation for further exploring carbon nanomaterials for clinical indications. Several carbon nanomedicines have been translated to the clinic with more under clinical trials, which are summarized in Table 14.1.[28,82,224–226]

Despite all the achievements obtained so far, there is still a long way to go due to the complexity of the clinical setting. First of all, there are some other major concerns regarding carbon nanomaterials, for example, poor water solubility, low biodegradability, as well as undesirable biosafety issues.[15,230–232] Even though preclinical and early clinical studies have proved their safety, more extensive clinical studies are required.[65] Second, taking the undesirable efficacy of nanomedicines in cancer treatment as an example, the major limitations are caused by the heterogeneity of tumor tissues. Since solid tumors have irregular vasculature, even after successful administration, nanoparticles are usually moved away from the center of the tumor mass by the high interstitial pressure.[233] Nevertheless, opportunities still exist to solve these issues. For instance, tumor retention of nanoparticles could be enhanced by increasing tumor permeability with some molecules, such as NO (nitric oxide)—releasing agents and ACE (angiotensin-convertingenzyme) inhibitors.[233] Filling such a gap between the lab and the clinic is key toward successfully applying nanomedicines in the future.[82]

Herein, we have comprehensively discussed the potential clinical applications of carbon nanomaterials. Besides nanotechnology, the next generation of nanomedicine development might rely on more advanced approaches, such as combination therapies, artificial intelligence (AI), as well as precision and personalized medicine (PPM), which will surely catalyze their development. The versatility of carbon nanomaterials will definitely make contributions to developing a truly personalized medical future

TABLE 14.1 Summary of the current clinical applications of carbon nanomaterials.

Type of carbon nanomaterial	Applications	Translational status	Disease/animal models	Key details of study	References
Nanodiamond	Tissue engineering and repair	Clinical trials	Dental pulp diseases Dental pulp necrosis Nerve root pain necrosis	Nanodiamond-modified gutta percha (NDGP) composite for nonsurgical root canal therapy (RCT) filler material (NCT02698163)	222
	Tissue engineering and repair	Clinical trials	Dental pulp diseases Dental pulp necrosis Nerve root pain necrosis	NDGP composite biomaterials for RCT (NCT03376984)	222 221
	Drug delivery	Preclinical	Both murine liver tumor and mammary carcinoma models	ND loaded with DOX can prolong the drug retention and increase the apoptotic response of tumor and animal survival.	26
Nanotube	Biological imaging	Clinical trials	Breast neoplasms	Comparison of stationary breast tomosynthesis and 2-D digital mammography in patients with known breast lesions (NCT01773850)	227
	Biological imaging	Clinical trials	Dental caries	Conventional bite wing radiography versus stationary intraoral tomosynthesis (NCT02873585)	
	Biosensors	Clinical trials	Tuberculosis	Noninvasive TB triage and patient mapping platform using breath via low-cost titanium dioxide nanotube sensor (NCT02681445)	
	Biosensors	Clinical trials	Stomach diseases	Diagnosis of gastric lesions with Nanose	228,229
	Biosensors	Clinical trials	Parkinson's disease Parkinsonism	Using nanotechnology to detect biomarkers of Parkinson's disease from exhaled breath (NCT01246336)	
	Drug delivery	Preclinical	Murine 4T1 breast-cancer model	SWCNTs-paclitaxel conjugate have higher tumor suppression efficacy than the clinical drug formulation Taxol in vivo	114
	Gene delivery	Preclinical	Human lung carcinoma xenograft model	MWCNTs loaded with siRNA can effectively inhibit the tumor growth and significantly increase survival compared with bare siRNA or siRNA delivered by cationic liposome in vivo	161

and, in turn, improvement in healthcare.[65] Combined with AI and PPM, carbon nanomaterials have potential to launch a new biomedical era.

References

[1] Hong G, Diao S, Antaris AL, Dai H. Carbon nanomaterials for biological imaging and nanomedicinal therapy. *Chem Rev* 2015;**115**(19):10816–906. https://doi.org/10.1021/acs.chemrev.5b00008.

[2] Chow EK-H, Ho D. Cancer nanomedicine: from drug delivery to imaging. *Sci Transl Med* 2013;**5**(216). https://doi.org/10.1126/scitranslmed.3005872. 216rv4-216rv4.

[3] Maeda H, Wu J, Sawa T, Matsumura Y, Hori K. Tumor vascular permeability and the EPR effect in macromolecular therapeutics: a review. *J Control Release* 2000;**65**(1–2):271–84. https://doi.org/10.1016/s0168-3659(99)00248-5.

[4] Jain RK, Reviews M. Transport of molecules across tumor vasculature. *Cancer Metast Rev* 1987;**6**(4):559–93. https://doi.org/10.1007/bf00047468.

[5] Maeda H, Nakamura H, Fang J. The EPR effect for macromolecular drug delivery to solid tumors: improvement of tumor uptake, lowering of systemic toxicity, and distinct tumor imaging in vivo. *Adv Drug Deliv Rev* 2013;**65**(1):71–9. https://doi.org/10.1016/j.addr.2012.10.002.

[6] Strojny B, Kurantowicz N, Sawosz E, Grodzik M, Jaworski S, Kutwin M, Wierzbicki M, Hotowy A, Lipińska L, Chwalibog A. Long term influence of carbon nanoparticles on health and liver status in rats. *PLoS ONE* 2015;**10**(12):e0144821. https://doi.org/10.1371/journal.pone.0144821.

[7] Kulakova II. Surface chemistry of nanodiamonds. *Phys Solid State* 2004;**46**(4):636–43. https://doi.org/10.1134/1.1711440.

[8] Kurantowicz N, Sawosz E, Jaworski S, Kutwin M, Strojny B, Wierzbicki M, Szeliga J, Hotowy A, Lipińska L, Koziński RJ. Interaction of graphene family materials with *Listeria monocytogenes* and *Salmonella enterica*. *Nanoscale Res Lett* 2015;**10**(1):23. https://doi.org/10.1186/s11671-015-0749-y.

[9] Wierzbicki M, Sawosz E, Grodzik M, Prasek M, Jaworski S, Chwalibog A. Comparison of anti-angiogenic properties of pristine carbon nanoparticles. *Nanoscale Res Lett* 2013;**8**(1):195. https://doi.org/10.1186/1556-276x-8-195.

[10] Maas M. Carbon nanomaterials as antibacterial colloids. *Materials* 2016;**9**(8):617. https://doi.org/10.3390/ma9080617.

[11] Kroto HW, Heath JR, O'Brien SC, Curl RF, Smalley RE. C60: buckminsterfullerene. *Nature* 1985;**318**(6042):162. https://doi.org/10.1038/318162a0.

[12] Krätschmer W, Lamb LD, Fostiropoulos K, Huffman DR. Solid C60: a new form of carbon. *Nature* 1990;**347**(6291):354. https://doi.org/10.1038/347354a0.

[13] Scott LT, Boorum MM, McMahon BJ, Hagen S, Mack J, Blank J, Wegner H, de Meijere AJS. A rational chemical synthesis of C60. *Science* 2002;**295**(5559):1500–3. https://doi.org/10.1126/science.1068427.

[14] Cha C, Shin SR, Annabi N, Dokmeci MR, Khademhosseini A. Carbon-based nanomaterials: multifunctional materials for biomedical engineering. *ACS Nano* 2013;**7**(4):2891–7. https://doi.org/10.1021/nn401196a.

[15] Mohajeri M, Behnam B, Sahebkar A. Biomedical applications of carbon nanomaterials: drug and gene delivery potentials. *J Cell Physiol* 2019;**234**(1):298–319. https://doi.org/10.1002/jcp.26899.

[16] Iijima S. Helical microtubules of graphitic carbon. *Nature* 1991;**354**(6348):56. https://doi.org/10.1038/354056a0.

[17] Thess A, Lee R, Nikolaev P, Dai H, Petit P, Robert J, Xu C, Lee YH, Kim SG, Rinzler AG, Colbert DT, Scuseria GE, Tomanek D, Fischer JE, Smalley RE. Crystalline ropes of metallic carbon nanotubes. *Science* 1996;**273**(5274):483–7. https://doi.org/10.1126/science.273.5274.483.

[18] José-Yacamán M, Miki-Yoshida M, Rendon L, Santiesteban JJ. Catalytic growth of carbon microtubules with fullerene structure. *Appl Phy Lett* 1993;**62**(6):657–9.

[19] Sun X, Zaric S, Daranciang D, Welsher K, Lu Y, Li X, Dai H. Optical properties of ultrashort semiconducting single-walled carbon nanotube capsules down to sub-10 nm. *J Am Chem Soc* 2008;**130**(20):6551–5. https://doi.org/10.1021/ja8006929.

[20] Robinson JT, Welsher K, Tabakman SM, Sherlock SP, Wang H, Luong R, Dai H. High performance in vivo near-IR (>1 μm) imaging and photothermal cancer therapy with carbon nanotubes. *Nano Res* 2010;**3**(11):779–93. https://doi.org/10.1007/s12274-010-0045-1.

[21] Murakami T, Nakatsuji H, Inada M, Matoba Y, Umeyama T, Tsujimoto M, Isoda S, Hashida M, Imahori H. Photodynamic and photothermal effects of semiconducting and metallic-enriched single-walled carbon nanotubes. *J Am Chem Soc.* 2012;**134**(43):17862–5. https://doi.org/10.1021/ja3079972.

[22] Iijima S, Brabec C, Maiti A, Bernholc J. Structural flexibility of carbon nanotubes. *J Chem Phys* 1996;**104**(5):2089–92. https://doi.org/10.1063/1.470966.

[23] Wei H, Wei Y, Wu Y, Liu L, Fan S, Jiang K. High-strength composite yarns derived from oxygen plasma modified super-aligned carbon nanotube arrays. *Nano Res* 2013;**6**(3):208–15. https://doi.org/10.1007/s12274-013-0297-7.

[24] Correa-Duarte MA, Wagner N, Rojas-Chapana J, Morsczeck C, Thie M, Giersig M. Fabrication and biocompatibility of carbon nanotube-based 3D networks as scaffolds for cell seeding and growth. *Nano Lett* 2004;**4**(11):2233–6. https://doi.org/10.1021/nl048574f.

[25] Shi X, Sitharaman B, Pham QP, Liang F, Wu K, Edward Billups W, Wilson LJ, Mikos AG. Fabrication of porous ultra-short single-walled carbon nanotube nanocomposite scaffolds for bone tissue engineering. *Biomaterials* 2007;**28**(28):4078–90. https://doi.org/10.1016/j.biomaterials.2007.05.033.

[26] Chow EK, Zhang X-Q, Chen M, Lam R, Robinson E, Huang H, Schaffer D, Osawa E, Goga A, Ho DJ. Nanodiamond therapeutic delivery agents mediate enhanced chemoresistant tumor treatment. *Sci Transl Med* 2011;**3**(73). https://doi.org/10.1126/scitranslmed.3001713. 73ra21-73ra21.

[27] Bhattacharya K, Mukherjee SP, Gallud A, Burkert SC, Bistarelli S, Bellucci S, Bottini M, Star A, Fadeel B. Biological interactions of carbon-based nanomaterials: from coronation to degradation. *Biol Med* 2016;**12**(2):333–51. https://doi.org/10.1016/j.nano.2015.11.011.

[28] Mochalin VN, Shenderova O, Ho D, Gogotsi Y. The properties and applications of nanodiamonds. *Nature Nanotech* 2012;**7**(1):11. https://doi.org/10.1038/nnano.2011.209.

[29] Dolmatov VY. Detonation-synthesis nanodiamonds: synthesis, structure, properties and applications. *Russian Chem Rev* 2007;**76**(4):339–60. https://doi.org/10.1070/rc2007v076n04abeh003643.

[30] Wang X, Low XC, Hou W, Abdullah LN, Toh TB, Mohd Abdul Rashid M, Ho D, Chow EK-H. Epirubicin-adsorbed nanodiamonds kill chemoresistant hepatic cancer stem cells. *ACS Nano* 2014;**8**(12):12151–66. https://doi.org/10.1021/nn503491e.

[31] Schrand AM, Huang H, Carlson C, Schlager JJ, Ōsawa E, Hussain SM, Dai L. Are diamond nanoparticles cytotoxic? *J Phys Chem B* 2007;**111**(1):2–7. https://doi.org/10.1021/jp066387v.

[32] Schrand AM, Hens SAC, Shenderova OA. Nanodiamond particles: properties and perspectives for bioapplications. *Crit Rev Solid State Mater Sci* 2009;**34**(1–2):18–74. https://doi.org/10.1080/10408430902831987.

[33] Manna SK, Sarkar S, Barr J, Wise K, Barrera EV, Jejelowo O, Rice-Ficht AC, Ramesh GT. Single-walled carbon nanotube induces oxidative stress and activates nuclear transcription factor-κB in human keratinocytes. *Nano Lett* 2005;**5**(9):1676–84. https://doi.org/10.1021/nl0507966.

[34] Ho D, Wang C-HK, Chow EK-H. Nanodiamonds: the intersection of nanotechnology, drug development, and personalized medicine. *Sci Adv* 2015;**1**(7):e1500439. https://doi.org/10.1126/sciadv.1500439.

[35] Manke A, Wang L, Rojanasakul Y. Pulmonary toxicity and fibrogenic response of carbon nanotubes. *Toxicol Mech Methods* 2013;**23**(3):196–206. https://doi.org/10.3109/15376516.2012.753967.

[36] Mukherjee A, Majumdar S, Servin AD, Pagano L, Dhankher OP, White JC. Carbon nanomaterials in agriculture: a critical review. *Front Plant Sci* 2016;**7**:172. https://doi.org/10.3389/fpls.2016.00172.

[37] Perepelytsina OM, Yakymchuk OM, Sydorenko MV, Bakalinska ON, Bloisi F, Vicari LR. Functionalization of carbon nanomaterial surface by doxorubicin and antibodies to tumor markers. *Nanoscale Res Lett* 2016;**11**(1):314. https://doi.org/10.1186/s11671-016-1537-z.

[38] Mura S, Nicolas J, Couvreur P. Stimuli-responsive nanocarriers for drug delivery. *Nature Mater* 2013;**12**(11):991. https://doi.org/10.1038/nmat3776.

[39] Gu M, Wang X, Toh TB, Chow EK-H. Applications of stimuli-responsive nanoscale drug delivery systems in translational research. *Drug Discovery Today* 2018;**23**(5):1043–52. https://doi.org/10.1016/j.drudis.2017.11.009.

[40] Durdagi S, Mavromoustakos T, Chronakis N, Papadopoulos MG, chemistry m. Computational design of novel fullerene analogues as potential HIV-1 PR inhibitors: analysis of the binding interactions between fullerene inhibitors and HIV-1 PR residues using 3D QSAR, molecular docking and molecular dynamics simulations. *Bioorg Med Chem* 2008;**16**(23):9957–74. https://doi.org/10.1016/j.bmc.2008.10.039.

[41] Horie M, Fukuhara A, Saito Y, Yoshida Y, Sato H, Ohi H, Obata M, Mikata Y, Yano S, Niki E. Antioxidant action of sugar-pendant C60 fullerenes. *Bio Med Chem Lett* 2009;**19**(20):5902–4. https://doi.org/10.1016/j.bmcl.2009.08.067.

[42] Montellano A, Da Ros T, Bianco A, Prato M. Fullerene C60 as a multifunctional system for drug and gene delivery. *Nanoscale* 2011;**3**(10):4035–41. https://doi.org/10.1039/c1nr10783f.

[43] Mashino T, Nishikawa D, Takahashi K, Usui N, Yamori T, Seki M, Endo T, Mochizuki M. Antibacterial and antiproliferative activity of cationic fullerene derivatives. *Bioorg Med Chem Lett* 2003;**13**(24):4395–7. https://doi.org/10.1016/j.bmcl.2003.09.040.

[44] Pantarotto D, Bianco A, Pellarini F, Tossi A, Giangaspero A, Zelezetsky I, Briand J-P, Prato M. Solid-phase synthesis of fullerene-peptides. *J Am Chem Soc* 2002;**124**(42):12543–9. https://doi.org/10.1021/ja027603q.

[45] Tang YJ, Ashcroft JM, Chen D, Min G, Kim C-H, Murkhejee B, Larabell C, Keasling JD, Chen FF. Charge-associated effects of fullerene derivatives on microbial structural integrity and central metabolism. *Nano Lett* 2007;**7**(3):754–60. https://doi.org/10.1021/nl063020t.

[46] Ashcroft JM, Tsyboulski DA, Hartman KB, Zakharian TY, Marks JW, Weisman RB, Rosenblum MG, Wilson LJ. Fullerene (C60) immunoconjugates: interaction of water-soluble C60 derivatives with the murine anti-gp240 melanoma antibody. *Chem Commun* 2006;(28):3004–6. https://doi.org/10.1039/b601717g.

[47] O'connell MJ, Bachilo SM, Huffman CB, Moore VC, Strano MS, Haroz EH, Rialon KL, Boul PJ, Noon WH, Kittrell CJS. Band gap fluorescence from individual single-walled carbon nanotubes. *Science* 2002;**297**(5581):593–6. https://doi.org/10.1126/science.1072631.

[48] Wenseleers W, Vlasov II, Goovaerts E, Obraztsova ED, Lobach AS, Bouwen A. Efficient isolation and solubilization of pristine single-walled nanotubes in bile salt micelles. *Adv Funct Mater* 2004;**14**(11):1105–12. https://doi.org/10.1002/adfm.200400130.

[49] Dong L, Joseph KL, Witkowski CM, Craig MM. Cytotoxicity of single-walled carbon nanotubes suspended in various surfactants. *Nanotechnol* 2008;**19**(25):255702. https://doi.org/10.1088/0957-4484/19/25/255702.

[50] Riggs JE, Guo Z, Carroll DL, Sun Y-P. Strong luminescence of solubilized carbon nanotubes. *J Am Chem Soc* 2000;**122**(24):5879–80. https://doi.org/10.1021/ja9942282.

[51] Huang W, Taylor S, Fu K, Lin Y, Zhang D, Hanks TW, Rao AM, Sun Y-P. Attaching proteins to carbon nanotubes via diimide-activated amidation. *Nano Lett* 2002;**2**(4):311–4. https://doi.org/10.1021/nl010095i.

[52] De La Zerda A, Zavaleta C, Keren S, Vaithilingam S, Bodapati S, Liu Z, Levi J, Smith BR, Ma T-J, Oralkan O, Cheng Z, Chen X, Dai H, Khuri-Yakub BT, Gambhir SS. Carbon nanotubes as photoacoustic molecular imaging agents in living mice. *Nature Nanotech* 2008;**3**(9):557. https://doi.org/10.1038/nnano.2008.231.

[53] Wang D, Tong Y, Li Y, Tian Z, Cao R, Yang B, Materials R. PEGylated nanodiamond for chemotherapeutic drug delivery. *Diamond Relat Mater* 2013;**36**:26–34. https://doi.org/10.1016/j.diamond.2013.04.002.

[54] Zhang X, Fu C, Feng L, Ji Y, Tao L, Huang Q, Li S, Wei Y. PEGylation and polyPEGylation of nanodiamond. *Polymer* 2012;**53**(15):3178–84. https://doi.org/10.1016/j.polymer.2012.05.029.

[55] Zhao L, Xu Y-H, Akasaka T, Abe S, Komatsu N, Watari F, Chen X. Polyglycerol-coated nanodiamond as a macrophage-evading platform for selective drug delivery in cancer cells. *Biomaterials* 2014;**35**(20):5393–406. https://doi.org/10.1016/j.biomaterials.2014.03.041.

[56] Wang H-D, Yang Q, Niu CH. Functionalization of nanodiamond particles with N,O-carboxymethyl chitosan. *Diamond Relat Mater*

2010;**19**(5–6):441–4. https://doi.org/10.1016/j.diamond.2010.01.032.

[57] Huang L-CL, Chang H-C. Adsorption and immobilization of cytochromecon nanodiamonds. *Langmuir* 2004;**20**(14):5879–84. https://doi.org/10.1021/la0495736.

[58] Kaur R, Chitanda JM, Michel D, Maley J, Borondics F, Yang P, Verrall RE, Badea IJI. Lysine-functionalized nanodiamonds: synthesis, physiochemical characterization, and nucleic acid binding studies. *Int J Nanomedicine* 2012;**7**:3851.

[59] Zhang X-Q, Chen M, Lam R, Xu X, Osawa E, Ho D. Polymer-functionalized nanodiamond platforms as vehicles for gene delivery. *ACS Nano* 2009;**3**(9):2609–16. https://doi.org/10.1021/nn900865g.

[60] Schüll C, Frey H. Grafting of hyperbranched polymers: from unusual complex polymer topologies to multivalent surface functionalization. *Polymer* 2013;**54**(21):5443–55. https://doi.org/10.1016/j.polymer.2013.07.065.

[61] Immordino ML, Dosio F, Cattel L. Stealth liposomes: review of the basic science, rationale, and clinical applications, existing and potential. *Int J Nanomedicine* 2006;**1**(3):297.

[62] Milla P, Dosio F, Cattel L. PEGylation of proteins and liposomes: a powerful and flexible strategy to improve the drug delivery. *Curr Drug Metab* 2012;**13**(1):105–19. https://doi.org/10.2174/138920012798356934.

[63] Bhattacharjee B, Ganguli D, Chaudhuri S. Luminescent CdS nanoparticles embedded in polyethylene glycol (PEG 300) matrix thin film. *J Nanoparticle Res* 2002;**4**(3):225–30. https://doi.org/10.1023/a:1019926512111.

[64] Daou TJ, Li L, Reiss P, Josserand V, Texier I. Effect of Poly(-ethylene glycol) length on the in vivo behavior of coated quantum dots. *Langmuir* 2009;**25**(5):3040–4. https://doi.org/10.1021/la8035083.

[65] Loh KP, Ho D, Chiu GNC, Leong DT, Pastorin G, Chow EK-H. Clinical applications of carbon nanomaterials in diagnostics and therapy. *Adv. Mater.* 2018;**30**(47):1802368. https://doi.org/10.1002/adma.201802368.

[66] Moore L, Yang J, Lan TTH, Osawa E, Lee D-K, Johnson WD, Xi J, Chow EK-H, Ho D. Biocompatibility assessment of detonation nanodiamond in non-human primates and rats using histological, hematologic, and urine analysis. *ACS Nano* 2016;**10**(8):7385–400. https://doi.org/10.1021/acsnano.6b00839.

[67] Murugesan S, Mousa SA, O'Connor LJ, Lincoln DW, Linhardt RJ. Carbon inhibits vascular endothelial growth factor- and fibroblast growth factor-promoted angiogenesis. *FEBS Lett* 2007;**581**(6):1157–60. https://doi.org/10.1016/j.febslet.2007.02.022.

[68] Pulskamp K, Diabate S, Krug H. Carbon nanotubes show no sign of acute toxicity but induce intracellular reactive oxygen species in dependence on contaminants. *Toxicol Lett* 2007;**168**(1):58–74. https://doi.org/10.1016/j.toxlet.2006.11.001.

[69] Jacobsen NR, Pojana G, White P, Møller P, Cohn CA, Smith Korsholm K, Vogel U, Marcomini A, Loft S, Wallin H. Genotoxicity, cytotoxicity, and reactive oxygen species induced by single-walled carbon nanotubes and C60fullerenes in the FE1-MutaMouse lung epithelial cells. *Environ Mol Mutagen* 2008;**49**(6):476–87. https://doi.org/10.1002/em.20406.

[70] Liao K-H, Lin Y-S, Macosko CW, Haynes CL. Cytotoxicity of graphene oxide and graphene in human erythrocytes and skin fibroblasts. *ACS Appl Mater Interfaces* 2011;**3**(7):2607–15. https://doi.org/10.1021/am200428v.

[71] Poland CA, Duffin R, Kinloch I, Maynard A, Wallace WAH, Seaton A, Stone V, Brown S, MacNee W, Donaldson K. Carbon nanotubes introduced into the abdominal cavity of mice show asbestos-like pathogenicity in a pilot study. *Nature Nanotech* 2008;**3**(7):423. https://doi.org/10.1038/nnano.2008.111.

[72] Porter AE, Gass M, Muller K, Skepper JN, Midgley PA, Welland M. Direct imaging of single-walled carbon nanotubes in cells. *Nature Nanotech* 2007;**2**(11):713. https://doi.org/10.1038/nnano.2007.347.

[73] Loh KP, Lim CT. Molecular hemocompatibility of graphene oxide and its implication for antithrombotic applications. *Small* 2015;**11**(38):5105–17.

[74] Loh KP, Lim CT. Molecular interactions of graphene oxide with human blood plasma proteins. *Nanoscale* 2016;**8**(17):9425–41.

[75] Loh KP, Lim CT. Selective concentration-dependent manipulation of intrinsic fluorescence of plasma proteins by graphene oxide nanosheets. *J RSC Adv* 2016;**6**(52):46558–66.

[76] Lundqvist M, Stigler J, Elia G, Lynch I, Cedervall T, Dawson KA. Nanoparticle size and surface properties determine the protein corona with possible implications for biological impacts. *Proc Natl Acad Sci USA* 2008.

[77] Verma A, Stellacci F. Effect of surface properties on nanoparticle-cell interactions. *Small* 2010;**6**(1):12–21. https://doi.org/10.1002/smll.200901158.

[78] Saptarshi SR, Duschl A, Lopata AL. Interaction of nanoparticles with proteins: relation to bio-reactivity of the nanoparticle. *J Nanobiotechnology* 2013;**11**(1):26. https://doi.org/10.1186/1477-3155-11-26.

[79] Mahmoudi M, Lynch I, Ejtehadi MR, Monopoli MP, Bombelli FB, Laurent S. Protein–nanoparticle interactions: opportunities and challenges. *Chem Rev* 2011;**111**(9):5610–37. https://doi.org/10.1021/cr100440g.

[80] Geldert A, Liu Y, Loh KP, Lim CT. Nano-bio interactions between carbon nanomaterials and blood plasma proteins: why oxygen functionality matters. *NPG Asia Mater* 2017;**9**(8):e422.

[81] Duncan R, Gaspar R. Nanomedicine(s) under the microscope. *Mol Pharmaceutics* 2011;**8**(6):2101–41. https://doi.org/10.1021/mp200394t.

[82] Marchesan S, Melchionna M, Prato M. Carbon nanostructures for nanomedicine: opportunities and challenges. *Nanotubes C Nanostructures* 2014;**22**(1–3):190–5. https://doi.org/10.1080/1536383x.2013.798726.

[83] Albanese A, Tang PS, Chan WCW. The effect of nanoparticle size, shape, and surface chemistry on biological systems. *Annu Rev Biomed Eng* 2012;**14**:1–16. https://doi.org/10.1146/annurev-bioeng-071811-150124.

[84] Daum N, Tscheka C, Neumeyer A, Schneider M. Novel approaches for drug delivery systems in nanomedicine: effects of particle design and shape. *Wiley Interdiscip Rev Nanomed Nanobiotechnol* 2012;**4**(1):52–65. https://doi.org/10.1002/wnan.165.

[85] Liu X, Tao H, Yang K, Zhang S, Lee S-T, Liu Z. Optimization of surface chemistry on single-walled carbon nanotubes for in vivo photothermal ablation of tumors. *Biomaterials* 2011;**32**(1):144–51. https://doi.org/10.1016/j.biomaterials.2010.08.096.

[86] Liu Z, Cai W, He L, Nakayama N, Chen K, Sun X, Chen X, Dai H. In vivo biodistribution and highly efficient tumour targeting of

carbon nanotubes in mice. *Nature Nanotech* 2007;**2**(1):47. https://doi.org/10.1038/nnano.2006.170.

[87] Farrera C, Fadeel B. It takes two to tango: understanding the interactions between engineered nanomaterials and the immune system. *Eur J Pharm Biopharm* 2015;**95**:3–12. https://doi.org/10.1016/j.ejpb.2015.03.007.

[88] Boraschi D, Costantino L, Italiani P. Interaction of nanoparticles with immunocompetent cells: nanosafety considerations. *Nanomedicine (Lond)* 2012;**7**(1):121–31. https://doi.org/10.2217/nnm.11.169.

[89] Tkach AV, Shurin GV, Shurin MR, Kisin ER, Murray AR, Young S-H, Star A, Fadeel B, Kagan VE, Shvedova AA. Direct effects of carbon nanotubes on dendritic cells induce immune suppression upon pulmonary exposure. *ACS Nano* 2011;**5**(7):5755–62. https://doi.org/10.1021/nn2014479.

[90] Tkach AV, Yanamala N, Stanley S, Shurin MR, Shurin GV, Kisin ER, Murray AR, Pareso S, Khaliullin T, Kotchey GP, Castranova V, Mathur S, Fadeel B, Star A, Kagan VE, Shvedova AA. Graphene oxide, but not fullerenes, targets immunoproteasomes and suppresses antigen presentation by dendritic cells. *Small* 2013;**9**(9-10):1686–90. https://doi.org/10.1002/smll.201201546.

[91] Shurin MR, Yanamala N, Kisin ER, Tkach AV, Shurin GV, Murray AR, Leonard HD, Reynolds JS, Gutkin DW, Star A, Fadeel B, Savolainen K, Kagan VE, Shvedova AA. Graphene oxide attenuates Th2-type immune responses, but augments airway remodeling and hyperresponsiveness in a murine model of asthma. *ACS Nano* 2014;**8**(6):5585–99. https://doi.org/10.1021/nn406454u.

[92] Pescatori M, Bedognetti D, Venturelli E, Ménard-Moyon C, Bernardini C, Muresu E, Piana A, Maida G, Manetti R, Sgarrella F, Bianco A, Delogu LG. Functionalized carbon nanotubes as immunomodulator systems. *Biomaterials* 2013;**34**(18):4395–403. https://doi.org/10.1016/j.biomaterials.2013.02.052.

[93] Monteiro-Riviere NA, Nemanich RJ, Inman AO, Wang YY, Riviere JE. Multi-walled carbon nanotube interactions with human epidermal keratinocytes. *Toxicol Lett* 2005;**155**(3):377–84. https://doi.org/10.1016/j.toxlet.2004.11.004.

[94] Gu M, Wang X, Toh TB, Hooi L, Tenen DG, Chow EKH. Nanodiamond-based platform for intracellular-specific delivery of therapeutic peptides against hepatocellular carcinoma. *Adv Therap* 2018;**1**(8):1800110. https://doi.org/10.1002/adtp.201800110.

[95] Pessayre D, Fromenty B, Berson A, Robin M-A, Lettéron P, Moreau R, Mansouri A. Central role of mitochondria in drug-induced liver injury. *Drug Metabol Rev* 2012;**44**(1):34–87. https://doi.org/10.3109/03602532.2011.604086.

[96] Buzea C, Pacheco II, Robbie K. Nanomaterials and nanoparticles: sources and toxicity. *Biointerphases* 2007;**2**(4):MR17–71. https://doi.org/10.1116/1.2815690.

[97] Al-Jamal KT, Nunes A, Methven L, Ali-Boucetta H, Li S, Toma FM, Herrero MA, Al-Jamal WT, ten Eikelder HM, Foster JJAC. Degree of chemical functionalization of carbon nanotubes determines tissue distribution and excretion profile. *Angew Chem Int Ed Engl* 2012;**124**(26):6495–9.

[98] Kostarelos K, Bianco A, Prato M. Promises, facts and challenges for carbon nanotubes in imaging and therapeutics. *Nature Nanotech* 2009;**4**(10):627. https://doi.org/10.1038/nnano.2009.241.

[99] Bianco A, Kostarelos K, Prato M. Making carbon nanotubes biocompatible and biodegradable. *Chem Commun* 2011;**47**(37):10182–8. https://doi.org/10.1039/c1cc13011k.

[100] Ali-Boucetta H, Nunes A, Sainz R, Herrero MA, Tian B, Prato M, Bianco A, Kostarelos K. Asbestos-like pathogenicity of long carbon nanotubes alleviated by chemical functionalization. *Angew Chem Int Ed Engl* 2013;**125**(8):2330–4.

[101] Allen BL, Kotchey GP, Chen Y, Yanamala NVK, Klein-Seetharaman J, Kagan VE, Star A. Mechanistic investigations of horseradish peroxidase-catalyzed degradation of single-walled carbon nanotubes. *J Am Chem Soc* 2009;**131**(47):17194–205. https://doi.org/10.1021/ja9083623.

[102] Allen BL, Kichambare PD, Gou P, Vlasova II, Kapralov AA, Konduru N, Kagan VE, Star A. Biodegradation of single-walled carbon nanotubes through enzymatic catalysis. *Nano Lett* 2008;**8**(11):3899–903. https://doi.org/10.1021/nl802315h.

[103] Liu X, Hurt RH, Kane AB. Biodurability of single-walled carbon nanotubes depends on surface functionalization. *Carbon* 2010;**48**(7):1961–9. https://doi.org/10.1016/j.carbon.2010.02.002.

[104] Bianco A, Kostarelos K, Prato M. Opportunities and challenges of carbon-based nanomaterials for cancer therapy. *Expert Opin Drug Deliv* 2008;**5**(3):331–42. https://doi.org/10.1517/17425247.5.3.331.

[105] Choi C-H. ABC transporters as multidrug resistance mechanisms and the development of chemosensitizers for their reversal. *Cancer Cell Int* 2005;**5**(1):30.

[106] Fletcher JI, Haber M, Henderson MJ, Norris MD. ABC transporters in cancer: more than just drug efflux pumps. *Nat Rev Cancer* 2010;**10**(2):147. https://doi.org/10.1038/nrc2789.

[107] Toh T-B, Lee D-K, Hou W, Abdullah LN, Nguyen J, Ho D, Chow EK. Nanodiamond-mitoxantrone complexes enhance drug retention in chemoresistant breast cancer cells. *Mol Pharm* 2014;**11**(8):2683–91. https://doi.org/10.1021/mp5001108.

[108] Man HB, Kim H, Kim H-J, Robinson E, Liu WK, Chow EK-H, Ho D. Synthesis of nanodiamond-daunorubicin conjugates to overcome multidrug chemoresistance in leukemia. *Nanomedicine* 2014;**10**(2):359–69. https://doi.org/10.1016/j.nano.2013.07.014.

[109] Huang H, Pierstorff E, Osawa E, Ho D. Active nanodiamond hydrogels for chemotherapeutic delivery. *Nano Lett* 2007;**7**(11):3305–14. https://doi.org/10.1021/nl071521o.

[110] Grodzik M, Sawosz E, Wierzbicki M, Orlowski P, Hotowy A, Niemiec T, Szmidt M, Mitura K, Chwalibog AJ. Nanoparticles of carbon allotropes inhibit glioblastoma multiforme angiogenesis in ovo. *Int J Nanomedicine* 2011;**6**:3041.

[111] Liu J-H, Cao L, Luo PG, Yang S-T, Lu F, Wang H, Meziani MJ, Haque SA, Liu Y, Lacher S, Sun Y-P. Fullerene-conjugated doxorubicin in cells. *ACS Appl Mater Interfaces* 2010;**2**(5):1384–9. https://doi.org/10.1021/am100037y.

[112] Zakharian TY, Seryshev A, Sitharaman B, Gilbert BE, Knight V, Wilson LJ. A fullerene–paclitaxel chemotherapeutic: synthesis, characterization, and study of biological activity in tissue culture. *J Am Chem Soc* 2005;**127**(36):12508–9. https://doi.org/10.1021/ja0546525.

[113] Tan L, Wu T, Tang Z-W, Xiao J-Y, Zhuo R-X, Shi B, Liu C-J. Water-soluble photoluminescent fullerene capped mesoporous silica for pH-responsive drug delivery and bioimaging. *Nanotechnology* 2016;**27**(31):315104. https://doi.org/10.1088/0957-4484/27/31/315104.

[114] Liu Z, Chen K, Davis C, Sherlock S, Cao Q, Chen X, Dai H. Drug delivery with carbon nanotubes for in vivo cancer treatment. *Cancer Res* 2008;**68**(16):6652–60. https://doi.org/10.1158/0008-5472.can-08-1468.

[115] Liu Z, Fan AC, Rakhra K, Sherlock S, Goodwin A, Chen X, Yang Q, Felsher DW, Dai H. Supramolecular stacking of doxorubicin on carbon nanotubes for in vivo cancer therapy. *Angew Chem Int Ed Engl* 2009;**121**(41):7804–8. https://doi.org/10.1002/ange.200902612.

[116] Maleki Dizaj S, Mennati A, Jafari S, Khezri K, Adibkia K. Antimicrobial activity of carbon-based nanoparticles. *Adv Pharm Bull* 2015;**5**(1):19–23.

[117] Kang S, Pinault M, Pfefferle LD, Elimelech M. Single-walled carbon nanotubes exhibit strong antimicrobial activity. *Langmuir* 2007;**23**(17):8670–3. https://doi.org/10.1021/la701067r.

[118] Arias LR, Yang L. Inactivation of bacterial pathogens by carbon nanotubes in suspensions. *Langmuir* 2009;**25**(5):3003–12. https://doi.org/10.1021/la802769m.

[119] Lyon DY, Adams LK, Falkner JC, Alvarez PJJ. Antibacterial activity of fullerene water suspensions: effects of preparation method and particle size. *Environ Sci Technol* 2006;**40**(14):4360–6. https://doi.org/10.1021/es0603655.

[120] Wehling J, Dringen R, Zare RN, Maas M, Rezwan K. Bactericidal activity of partially oxidized nanodiamonds. *ACS Nano* 2014;**8**(6):6475–83. https://doi.org/10.1021/nn502230m.

[121] Pentecost AE, Witherel CE, Gogotsi Y, Spiller KL. Anti-inflammatory effects of octadecylamine-functionalized nanodiamond on primary human macrophages. *Biomater Sci* 2017;**5**(10):2131–43. https://doi.org/10.1039/c7bm00294g.

[122] Chen M, Pierstorff ED, Lam R, Li S-Y, Huang H, Osawa E, Ho D. Nanodiamond-mediated delivery of water-insoluble therapeutics. *ACS Nano* 2009;**3**(7):2016–22. https://doi.org/10.1021/nn900480m.

[123] Wong BS, Yoong SL, Jagusiak A, Panczyk T, Ho HK, Ang WH, Pastorin G. Carbon nanotubes for delivery of small molecule drugs. *Adv Drug Deliv Rev* 2013;**65**(15):1964–2015. https://doi.org/10.1016/j.addr.2013.08.005.

[124] Murakami T, Ajima K, Miyawaki J, Yudasaka M, Iijima S, Shiba K. Drug-loaded carbon nanohorns: adsorption and release of dexamethasone in vitro. *Mol Pharm* 2004;**1**(6):399–405. https://doi.org/10.1021/mp049928e.

[125] Rosen Y, Mattix B, Rao A, Alexis F, Disease RH, editors. *Carbon nanotubes and infectious diseases*; 2011. p. 249–67.

[126] Jiang L, Liu T, He H, Pham-Huy LA, Li L, Pham-Huy C, Xiao D. Adsorption behavior of pazufloxacin mesilate on amino-functionalized carbon nanotubes. *J Nanosci Nanotechnol* 2012;**12**(9):7271–9. https://doi.org/10.1166/jnn.2012.6562.

[127] Bhunia T, Giri A, Nasim T, Chattopadhyay D, Bandyopadhyay A. A transdermal diltiazem hydrochloride delivery device using multi-walled carbon nanotube/poly(vinyl alcohol) composites. *Carbon* 2013;**52**:305–15. https://doi.org/10.1016/j.carbon.2012.09.032.

[128] Garala K, Patel J, Patel A, Dharamsi A. Enhanced encapsulation of metoprolol tartrate with carbon nanotubes as adsorbent. *Appl Nanosci* 2011;**1**(4):219–30. https://doi.org/10.1007/s13204-011-0030-3.

[129] Yang Z, Zhang Y, Yang Y, Sun L, Han D, Li H, Wang C. Pharmacological and toxicological target organelles and safe use of single-walled carbon nanotubes as drug carriers in treating Alzheimer disease. *Nanomedicine* 2010;**6**(3):427–41. https://doi.org/10.1016/j.nano.2009.11.007.

[130] Palm C, Jayamanne M, Kjellander M, Hällbrink M. Peptide degradation is a critical determinant for cell-penetrating peptide uptake. *Biochim Biophys Acta* 2007;**1768**(7):1769–76. https://doi.org/10.1016/j.bbamem.2007.03.029.

[131] Johnson-Léger C, Power CA, Shomade G, Shaw JP, Proudfoot AE. Protein therapeutics - lessons learned and a view of the future. *Expert Opin Biol Ther* 2006;**6**(1):1–7. https://doi.org/10.1517/14712598.6.1.1.

[132] Lu Y, Yang J, Sega E. Issues related to targeted delivery of proteins and peptides. *AAPS J* 2006;**8**(3):E466–78. https://doi.org/10.1208/aapsj080355.

[133] Shimkunas RA, Robinson E, Lam R, Lu S, Xu X, Zhang X-Q, Huang H, Osawa E, Ho D. Nanodiamond-insulin complexes as pH-dependent protein delivery vehicles. *Biomaterials* 2009;**30**(29):5720–8. https://doi.org/10.1016/j.biomaterials.2009.07.004.

[134] Kuo Y, Hsu T-Y, Wu Y-C, Chang H-C. Fluorescent nanodiamond as a probe for the intercellular transport of proteins in vivo. *Biomaterials* 2013;**34**(33):8352–60. https://doi.org/10.1016/j.biomaterials.2013.07.043.

[135] Wang X, Gu M, Toh TB, Abdullah NLB, Chow EK-H. Stimuli-responsive nanodiamond-based biosensor for enhanced metastatic tumor site detection. *SLAS Technol* 2018;**23**(1):44–56. https://doi.org/10.1177/2472630317735497.

[136] Smith AH, Robinson EM, Zhang X-Q, Chow EK, Lin Y, Osawa E, Xi J, Ho D. Triggered release of therapeutic antibodies from nanodiamond complexes. *Nanoscale* 2011;**3**(7):2844–8. https://doi.org/10.1039/c1nr10278h.

[137] Kam NW, Dai H. Carbon nanotubes as intracellular protein transporters: generality and biological functionality. *J Am Chem Soc* 2005;**127**(16):6021–6. https://doi.org/10.1021/ja050062v.

[138] Yin H, Kanasty RL, Eltoukhy AA, Vegas AJ, Dorkin JR, Anderson DG. Non-viral vectors for gene-based therapy. *Nat Rev Genet* 2014;**15**(8):541. https://doi.org/10.1038/nrg3763.

[139] Nayak S, Herzog RW. Progress and prospects: immune responses to viral vectors. *Gene Ther* 2010;**17**(3):295. https://doi.org/10.1038/gt.2009.148.

[140] Ramamoorth M, Narvekar A. Non viral vectors in gene therapy- an overview. *J Clin Diagn Res* 2015;**9**(1):GE01–6. https://doi.org/10.7860/JCDR/2015/10443.5394.

[141] Riley M, Vermerris W. Recent advances in nanomaterials for gene delivery-a review. *Nanomaterials* 2017;**7**(5):94. https://doi.org/10.3390/nano7050094.

[142] Petrakova V, Benson V, Buncek M, Fiserova A, Ledvina M, Stursa J, Cigler P, Nesladek M. Imaging of transfection and intracellular release of intact, non-labeled DNA using fluorescent nanodiamonds. *Nanoscale* 2016;**8**(23):12002–12. https://doi.org/10.1039/c6nr00610h.

[143] Chen M, Zhang X-Q, Man HB, Lam R, Chow EK, Ho D. Nanodiamond vectors functionalized with polyethylenimine for siRNA delivery. *J Phys Chem Lett* 2010;**1**(21):3167–71. https://doi.org/10.1021/jz1013278.

[144] Alhaddad A, Adam M-P, Botsoa J, Dantelle G, Perruchas S, Gacoin T, Mansuy C, Lavielle S, Malvy C, Treussart F, Bertrand J-R. Nanodiamond as a vector for siRNA delivery to Ewing sarcoma

cells. *Small* 2011;**7**(21):3087–95. https://doi.org/10.1002/smll.201101193.

[145] Ushizawa K, Sato Y, Mitsumori T, Machinami T, Ueda T, Ando T. Covalent immobilization of DNA on diamond and its verification by diffuse reflectance infrared spectroscopy. *Chem Phys Lett* 2002;**351**(1–2):105–8. https://doi.org/10.1016/s0009-2614(01)01362-8.

[146] Isobe H, Nakanishi W, Tomita N, Jinno S, Okayama H, Nakamura E. Gene delivery by aminofullerenes: structural requirements for efficient transfection. *Chem Asian J* 2006;**1**(1-2):167–75. https://doi.org/10.1002/asia.200600051.

[147] Klumpp C, Lacerda L, Chaloin O, Ros TD, Kostarelos K, Prato M, Bianco A. Multifunctionalised cationic fullerene adducts for gene transfer: design, synthesis and DNA complexation. *Chem Commun* 2007;(36):3762–4. https://doi.org/10.1039/b708435h.

[148] Shin SR, Jin KS, Lee CK, Kim SI, Spinks GM, So I, Jeon J-H, Kang TM, Mun JY, Han S-S, Ree M, Kim SJ. Fullerene attachment enhances performance of a DNA nanomachine. *Adv Mater* 2009;**21**(19):1907–10. https://doi.org/10.1002/adma.200803429.

[149] Sitharaman B, Zakharian TY, Saraf A, Misra P, Ashcroft J, Pan S, Pham QP, Mikos AG, Wilson LJ, Engler DA. Water-soluble fullerene (C60) derivatives as nonviral gene-delivery vectors. *Mol Pharm* 2008;**5**(4):567–78. https://doi.org/10.1021/mp700106w.

[150] Maeda-Mamiya R, Noiri E, Isobe H, Nakanishi W, Okamoto K, Doi K, Sugaya T, Izumi T, Homma T, Nakamura E. In vivo gene delivery by cationic tetraamino fullerene. *Proc Natl Acad Sci USA* 2010;**107**(12):5339–44. https://doi.org/10.1073/pnas.0909223107.

[151] Gao L, Nie L, Wang T, Qin Y, Guo Z, Yang D, Yan X. Carbon nanotube delivery of the GFP gene into mammalian cells. *ChemBioChem* 2006;**7**(2):239–42. https://doi.org/10.1002/cbic.200500227.

[152] Qin W, Yang K, Tang H, Tan L, Xie Q, Ma M, Zhang Y, Yao S, Biointerfaces SB. Improved GFP gene transfection mediated by polyamidoamine dendrimer-functionalized multi-walled carbon nanotubes with high biocompatibility. *Colloids Surf B: Biointerfaces* 2011;**84**(1):206–13. https://doi.org/10.1016/j.colsurfb.2011.01.001.

[153] Hao Y, Xu P, He C, Yang X, Huang M, Xing J, Chen J. Impact of carbondiimide crosslinker used for magnetic carbon nanotube mediated GFP plasmid delivery. *Nanotechnology* 2011;**22**(28):285103. https://doi.org/10.1088/0957-4484/22/28/285103.

[154] Inoue Y, Fujimoto H, Ogino T, Iwata H. Site-specific gene transfer with high efficiency onto a carbon nanotube-loaded electrode. *J R Soc Interface* 2008;**5**(25):909–18. https://doi.org/10.1098/rsif.2007.1295.

[155] Kam NWS, Liu Z, Dai H. Functionalization of carbon nanotubes via cleavable disulfide bonds for efficient intracellular delivery of siRNA and potent gene silencing. *J Am Chem Soc* 2005;**127**(36):12492–3. https://doi.org/10.1021/ja053962k.

[156] Wang X, Ren J, Qu X. Targeted RNA interference of cyclin A2 mediated by functionalized single-walled carbon nanotubes induces proliferation arrest and apoptosis in chronic myelogenous leukemia K562 cells. *ChemMedChem* 2008;**3**(6):940–5. https://doi.org/10.1002/cmdc.200700329.

[157] Krajcik R, Jung A, Hirsch A, Neuhuber W, Zolk O. Functionalization of carbon nanotubes enables non-covalent binding and intracellular delivery of small interfering RNA for efficient knock-down of genes. *Biochem Biophys Res Commun* 2008;**369**(2):595–602. https://doi.org/10.1016/j.bbrc.2008.02.072.

[158] Ladeira MS, Andrade VA, Gomes ERM, Aguiar CJ, Moraes ER, Soares JS, Silva EE, Lacerda RG, Ladeira LO, Jorio A, Lima P, Fatima Leite M, Resende RR, Guatimosim S. Highly efficient siRNA delivery system into human and murine cells using single-wall carbon nanotubes. *Nanotechnology* 2010;**21**(38):385101. https://doi.org/10.1088/0957-4484/21/38/385101.

[159] Bartholomeusz G, Cherukuri P, Kingston J, Cognet L, Lemos R, Leeuw TK, Gumbiner-Russo L, Weisman RB, Powis G. In vivo therapeutic silencing of hypoxia-inducible factor 1 alpha (HIF-1α) using single-walled carbon nanotubes noncovalently coated with siRNA. *Nano Res* 2009;**2**(4):279–91. https://doi.org/10.1007/s12274-009-9026-7.

[160] Al-Jamal KT, Gherardini L, Bardi G, Nunes A, Guo C, Bussy C, Herrero MA, Bianco A, Prato M, Kostarelos K, Pizzorusso T. Functional motor recovery from brain ischemic insult by carbon nanotube-mediated siRNA silencing. *Proc Natl Acad Sci USA* 2011;**108**(27):10952–7. https://doi.org/10.1073/pnas.1100930108.

[161] Podesta JE, Al-Jamal KT, Herrero MA, Tian B, Ali-Boucetta H, Hegde V, Bianco A, Prato M, Kostarelos KJS. Antitumor activity and prolonged survival by carbon-nanotube-mediated therapeutic siRNA silencing in a human lung xenograft model. *Small* 2009;**5**(10):1176–85. https://doi.org/10.1002/smll.200990047.

[162] Lanner JT, Bruton JD, Assefaw-Redda Y, Andronache Z, Zhang S-J, Severa D, Zhang Z-B, Melzer W, Zhang S-L, Katz A, Westerblad H. Knockdown of TRPC3 with siRNA coupled to carbon nanotubes results in decreased insulin-mediated glucose uptake in adult skeletal muscle cells. *FASEB J* 2009;**23**(6):1728–38. https://doi.org/10.1096/fj.08-116814.

[163] Liu Z, Winters M, Holodniy M, Dai H. siRNA delivery into human T cells and primary cells with carbon-nanotube transporters. *Angew Chem Int Ed Engl* 2007;**119**(12):2069–73. https://doi.org/10.1002/ange.200604295.

[164] O'Neal DP, Hirsch LR, Halas NJ, Payne JD, West JL. Photo-thermal tumor ablation in mice using near infrared-absorbing nanoparticles. *Cancer Lett* 2004;**209**(2):171–6. https://doi.org/10.1016/j.canlet.2004.02.004.

[165] Kam NWS, O'Connell M, Wisdom JA, Dai H. Carbon nanotubes as multifunctional biological transporters and near-infrared agents for selective cancer cell destruction. *Proc Natl Acad Sci USA* 2005;**102**(33):11600–5.

[166] Moon HK, Lee SH, Choi HC. In vivo near-infrared mediated tumor destruction by photothermal effect of carbon nanotubes. *ACS Nano* 2009;**3**(11):3707–13. https://doi.org/10.1021/nn900904h.

[167] Yamakoshi Y, Umezawa N, Ryu A, Arakane K, Miyata N, Goda Y, Masumizu T, Nagano T. Active oxygen species generated from photoexcited fullerene (C60) as potential medicines: O2-versus 1O2. *J Am Chem Soc* 2003;**125**(42):12803–9. https://doi.org/10.1021/ja0355574.

[168] Iwamoto Y, Yamakoshi Y. A highly water-soluble C60-NVP copolymer: a potential material for photodynamic therapy. *Chem Commun* 2006;(46):4805–7. https://doi.org/10.1039/b614305a.

[169] Markovic Z, Trajkovic V. Biomedical potential of the reactive oxygen species generation and quenching by fullerenes (C60). *Biomaterials* 2008;**29**(26):3561–73. https://doi.org/10.1016/j.biomaterials.2008.05.005.

[170] Sharma SK, Chiang LY, Hamblin MR. Photodynamic therapy with fullerenesin vivo: reality or a dream? *Nanomedicine* 2011;**6**(10):1813–25. https://doi.org/10.2217/nnm.11.144.

[171] Wang L, Shi J, Liu R, Liu Y, Zhang J, Yu X, Gao J, Zhang C, Zhang Z. Photodynamic effect of functionalized single-walled carbon nanotubes: a potential sensitizer for photodynamic therapy. *Nanoscale* 2014;**6**(9):4642–51. https://doi.org/10.1039/c3nr06835h.

[172] Shi J, Ma R, Lei Wang L, Zhang J, Liu RRuiyuan, Liu Y, Yu X, Gao J, Li L, Hou L, Zhang Z. The application of hyaluronic acid-derivatized carbon nanotubes in hematoporphyrin monomethyl ether-based photodynamic therapy for in vivo and in vitro cancer treatment. *Int J Nanomedicine* 2013;**8**:2361. https://doi.org/10.2147/ijn.s45407.

[173] Welsher K, Sherlock SP, Dai H. Deep-tissue anatomical imaging of mice using carbon nanotube fluorophores in the second near-infrared window. *Proc Natl Acad Sci USA* 2011;**108**(22):8943–8. https://doi.org/10.1073/pnas.1014501108.

[174] Hong G, Lee JC, Robinson JT, Raaz U, Xie L, Huang NF, Cooke JP, Dai H. Multifunctional in vivo vascular imaging using near-infrared II fluorescence. *Nat Med* 2012;**18**(12):1841. https://doi.org/10.1038/nm.2995.

[175] Hong G, Diao S, Chang J, Antaris AL, Chen C, Zhang B, Zhao S, Atochin DN, Huang PL, Andreasson KI, Kuo CJ, Dai H. Through-skull fluorescence imaging of the brain in a new near-infrared window. *Nature Photon* 2014;**8**(9):723. https://doi.org/10.1038/nphoton.2014.166.

[176] Wu T-J, Tzeng Y-K, Chang W-W, Cheng C-A, Kuo Y, Chien C-H, Chang H-C, Yu J. Tracking the engraftment and regenerative capabilities of transplanted lung stem cells using fluorescent nanodiamonds. *Nature Nanotech* 2013;**8**(9):682. https://doi.org/10.1038/nnano.2013.147.

[177] Jeong J, Jung J, Choi M, Kim JW, Chung SJ, Lim S, Lee H, Chung BH. Color-tunable photoluminescent fullerene nanoparticles. *Adv Mater* 2012;**24**(15):1999–2003. https://doi.org/10.1002/adma.201104772.

[178] Levi N, Hantgan RR, Lively MO, Carroll DL, Prasad GL. C 60-Fullerenes: detection of intracellular photoluminescence and lack of cytotoxic effects. *J Nanobiotechnol* 2006;**4**(1):14. https://doi.org/10.1186/1477-3155-4-14.

[179] Jeong J, Cho M, Lim YT, Song NW, Chung BH. Synthesis and characterization of a photoluminescent nanoparticle based on fullerene-silica hybridization. *Angewandte Chemie Int Ed* 2009;**48**(29):5296–9. https://doi.org/10.1002/anie.200901750.

[180] Lin S, Jones DX, Mount AS, Ke PC. *Fluorescence of water-soluble fullerenes in biological systems*. NSTI--Nanotech; 2007. p. 238–41.

[181] Boudou J-P, Curmi PA, Jelezko F, Wrachtrup J, Aubert P, Sennour M, Balasubramanian G, Reuter R, Thorel A, Gaffet E. High yield fabrication of fluorescent nanodiamonds. *Nanotechnology* 2009;**20**(23):235602. https://doi.org/10.1088/0957-4484/20/23/235602.

[182] Chang Y-R, Lee H-Y, Chen K, Chang C-C, Tsai D-S, Fu C-C, Lim T-S, Tzeng Y-K, Fang C-Y, Han C-C, Chang H-C, Fann W. Mass production and dynamic imaging of fluorescent nanodiamonds. *Nature Nanotech* 2008;**3**(5):284. https://doi.org/10.1038/nnano.2008.99.

[183] Yu S-J, Kang M-W, Chang H-C, Chen K-M, Yu Y-C. Bright fluorescent nanodiamonds: no photobleaching and low cytotoxicity. *J Am Chem Soc* 2005;**127**(50):17604–5. https://doi.org/10.1021/ja0567081.

[184] Rondin L, Dantelle G, Slablab A, Grosshans F, Treussart F, Bergonzo P, Perruchas S, Gacoin T, Chaigneau M, Chang H-C. Surface-induced charge state conversion of nitrogen-vacancy defects in nanodiamonds. *Mater Sci* 2010;**82**(11):115449. https://doi.org/10.1103/physrevb.82.115449.

[185] Doherty MW, Manson NB, Delaney P, Jelezko F, Wrachtrup J, Hollenberg LCL. The nitrogen-vacancy colour centre in diamond. *Phys Rep* 2013;**528**(1):1–45. https://doi.org/10.1016/j.physrep.2013.02.001.

[186] Holt KB. Diamond at the nanoscale: applications of diamond nanoparticles from cellular biomarkers to quantum computing. *Philos Trans A Math Phys Eng Sci* 2007;**365**(1861):2845–61. https://doi.org/10.1098/rsta.2007.0005.

[187] Vaijayanthimala V, Cheng P-Y, Yeh S-H, Liu K-K, Hsiao C-H, Chao J-I, Chang H-C. The long-term stability and biocompatibility of fluorescent nanodiamond as an in vivo contrast agent. *Biomaterials* 2012;**33**(31):7794–802. https://doi.org/10.1016/j.biomaterials.2012.06.084.

[188] Shi Kam NW, Jessop TC, Wender PA, Dai H. Nanotube molecular transporters: internalization of carbon nanotube–protein conjugates into mammalian cells. *J Am Chem Soc* 2004;**126**(22):6850–1. https://doi.org/10.1021/ja0486059.

[189] Cherukuri P, Bachilo SM, Litovsky SH, Weisman RB. Near-infrared fluorescence microscopy of single-walled carbon nanotubes in phagocytic cells. *J Am Chem Soc* 2004;**126**(48):15638–9. https://doi.org/10.1021/ja0466311.

[190] Heller DA, Baik S, Eurell TE, Strano MS. Single-walled carbon nanotube spectroscopy in live cells: towards long term labels and optical sensors. *Adv Mater* 2005;**17**(23):2793–9. https://doi.org/10.1002/adma.200500477.

[191] Liu Z, Davis C, Cai W, He L, Chen X, Dai H. Circulation and long-term fate of functionalized, biocompatible single-walled carbon nanotubes in mice probed by Raman spectroscopy. *Proc Natl Acad Sci USA* 2008;**105**(5):1410–5. https://doi.org/10.1073/pnas.0707654105.

[192] Wang C, Ma X, Ye S, Cheng L, Yang K, Guo L, Li C, Li Y, Liu Z. Protamine functionalized single-walled carbon nanotubes for stem cell labeling and in vivo Raman/Magnetic resonance/photoacoustic triple-modal imaging. *Adv Funct Mater* 2012;**22**(11):2363–75. https://doi.org/10.1002/adfm.201200133.

[193] Keren S, Zavaleta C, Cheng Z, de La Zerda A, Gheysens O, Gambhir SS. Noninvasive molecular imaging of small living subjects using Raman spectroscopy. *Proc Natl Acad Sci USA* 2008;**105**(15):5844–9. https://doi.org/10.1073/pnas.0710575105.

[194] Zavaleta C, De La Zerda A, Liu Z, Keren S, Cheng Z, Schipper M, Chen X, Dai H, Gambhir SS. Noninvasive Raman spectroscopy in living mice for evaluation of tumor targeting with carbon nanotubes. *Nano Lett* 2008;**8**(9):2800–5. https://doi.org/10.1021/nl801362a.

[195] Galanzha EI, Shashkov EV, Kelly T, Kim J-W, Yang L, Zharov VP. In vivo magnetic enrichment and multiplex photoacoustic detection of circulating tumour cells. *Nature Nanotech* 2009;**4**(12):855. https://doi.org/10.1038/nnano.2009.333.

[196] Martins MBAF, Corvo ML, Marcelino P, Marinho HS, Feio G, Carvalho A. New long circulating magnetoliposomes as contrast agents for detection of ischemia-reperfusion injuries by MRI. *Nanomedicine* 2014;**10**(1):207–14. https://doi.org/10.1016/j.nano.2013.06.008.

[197] Caravan P, Ellison JJ, McMurry TJ, Lauffer RB. Gadolinium(III) chelates as MRI contrast agents: structure, dynamics, and applications. *Chem Rev* 1999;**99**(9):2293–352. https://doi.org/10.1021/cr980440x.

[198] Perazella M. Gadolinium-contrast toxicity in patients with kidney disease: nephrotoxicity and nephrogenic systemic fibrosis. *Curr Drug Saf* 2008;**3**(1):67–75. https://doi.org/10.2174/157488608783333989.

[199] Perazella MA. Current status of gadolinium toxicity in patients with kidney disease. *Clin J Am Soc Nephrol* 2009;**4**(2):461–9. https://doi.org/10.2215/cjn.06011108.

[200] Hou W, Toh TB, Abdullah LN, Yvonne TWZ, Lee KJ, Guenther I, Chow EK-H. Nanodiamond–manganese dual mode MRI contrast agents for enhanced liver tumor detection. *Nanomed Nanotechnol* 2017;**13**(3):783–93. https://doi.org/10.1016/j.nano.2016.12.013.

[201] Chen Z, Ma L, Liu Y, Chen C. Applications of functionalized fullerenes in tumor theranostics. *Theranostics* 2012;**2**(3):238. https://doi.org/10.7150/thno.3509.

[202] Kato H, Kanazawa Y, Okumura M, Taninaka A, Yokawa T, Shinohara H. Lanthanoid endohedral metallofullerenols for MRI contrast agents. *J Am Chem Soc* 2003;**125**(14):4391–7. https://doi.org/10.1021/ja027555+.

[203] Ghiassi KB, Olmstead MM, Balch AL. Gadolinium-containing endohedral fullerenes: structures and function as magnetic resonance imaging (MRI) agents. *Dalton Trans* 2014;**43**(20):7346–58. https://doi.org/10.1039/c3dt53517g.

[204] Mikawa M, Kato H, Okumura M, Narazaki M, Kanazawa Y, Miwa N, Shinohara H. Paramagnetic water-soluble metallofullerenes having the highest relaxivity for MRI contrast agents. *Bioconjugate Chem* 2001;**12**(4):510–4. https://doi.org/10.1021/bc000136m.

[205] Fatouros PP, Corwin FD, Chen Z-J, Broaddus WC, Tatum JL, Kettenmann B, Ge Z, Gibson HW, Russ JL, Leonard AP, Duchamp JC, Dorn HC. In vitro and in vivo imaging studies of a new endohedral metallofullerene nanoparticle. *Radiology* 2006;**240**(3):756–64. https://doi.org/10.1148/radiol.2403051341.

[206] Zhang J, Fatouros PP, Shu C, Reid J, Owens LS, Cai T, Gibson HW, Long GL, Corwin FD, Chen Z-J, Dorn HC. High relaxivity trimetallic nitride (Gd3N) metallofullerene MRI contrast agents with optimized functionality. *Bioconjugate Chem* 2010;**21**(4):610–5. https://doi.org/10.1021/bc900375n.

[207] Richard C, Doan B-T, Beloeil J-C, Bessodes M, Tóth É, Scherman D. Noncovalent functionalization of carbon nanotubes with amphiphilic Gd^{3+} chelates: toward powerful T1and T2 MRI contrast agents. *Nano Lett* 2008;**8**(1):232–6. https://doi.org/10.1021/nl072509z.

[208] Choi JH, Nguyen FT, Barone PW, Heller DA, Moll AE, Patel D, Boppart SA, Strano MS. Multimodal biomedical imaging with asymmetric single-walled carbon nanotube/iron oxide nanoparticle complexes. *Nano Lett* 2007;**7**(4):861–7. https://doi.org/10.1021/nl062306v.

[209] Liu H, Zhang L, Yan M, Yu J. Carbon nanostructures in biology and medicine. *J Mater Chem B* 2017;**5**(32):6437–50. https://doi.org/10.1039/c7tb00891k.

[210] Pourasl AH, Ahmadi M, Rahmani M, Chin H, Lim C, Ismail R, Tan ML. Analytical modeling of glucose biosensors based on carbon nanotubes. *Nanoscale Res Lett* 2014;**9**(1):33. https://doi.org/10.1186/1556-276x-9-33.

[211] Tang X, Bansaruntip S, Nakayama N, Yenilmez E, Chang Y-l, Wang Q. Carbon nanotube DNA sensor and sensing mechanism. *Nano Lett* 2006;**6**(8):1632–6. https://doi.org/10.1021/nl060613v.

[212] Shin SR, Bae H, Cha JM, Mun JY, Chen Y-C, Tekin H, Shin H, Farshchi S, Dokmeci MR, Tang S, Khademhosseini A. Carbon nanotube reinforced hybrid microgels as scaffold materials for cell encapsulation. *ACS Nano* 2011;**6**(1):362–72. https://doi.org/10.1021/nn203711s.

[213] Zhao B, Hu H, Mandal SK, Haddon RC. A bone mimic based on the self-assembly of hydroxyapatite on chemically functionalized single-walled carbon nanotubes. *Chem Mater* 2005;**17**(12):3235–41. https://doi.org/10.1021/cm0500399.

[214] Li N, Zhang Q, Gao S, Song Q, Huang R, Wang L, Liu L, Dai J, Tang M, Cheng GJ. Three-dimensional graphene foam as a biocompatible and conductive scaffold for neural stem cells. *Sci Rep* 2013;**3**:1604. https://doi.org/10.1038/srep01604.

[215] Nayak TR, Andersen H, Makam VS, Khaw C, Bae S, Xu X, Ee P-LR, Ahn J-H, Hong BH, Pastorin G, Özyilmaz B. Graphene for controlled and accelerated osteogenic differentiation of human mesenchymal stem cells. *ACS Nano* 2011;**5**(6):4670–8. https://doi.org/10.1021/nn200500h.

[216] Jin G-Z, Kim M, Shin US, Kim H-W. Neurite outgrowth of dorsal root ganglia neurons is enhanced on aligned nanofibrous biopolymer scaffold with carbon nanotube coating. *Neurosci Lett* 2011;**501**(1):10–4. https://doi.org/10.1016/j.neulet.2011.06.023.

[217] Shin SR, Jung SM, Zalabany M, Kim K, Zorlutuna P, Kim Sb, Nikkhah M, Khabiry M, Azize M, Kong J, Wan K-t, Palacios T, Dokmeci MR, Bae H, Tang X, Khademhosseini A. Carbon-nanotube-embedded hydrogel sheets for engineering cardiac constructs and bioactuators. *ACS Nano* 2013;**7**(3):2369–80. https://doi.org/10.1021/nn305559j.

[218] Wei Y, Mo X, Zhang P, Li Y, Liao J, Li Y, Zhang J, Ning C, Wang S, Deng X, Jiang L. Directing stem cell differentiation via electrochemical reversible switching between nanotubes and nanotips of polypyrrole array. *ACS Nano* 2017;**11**(6):5915–24. https://doi.org/10.1021/acsnano.7b01661.

[219] Pacelli S, Maloney R, Chakravarti AR, Whitlow J, Basu S, Modaresi S, Gehrke S, Paul A. Controlling adult stem cell behavior using nanodiamond-reinforced hydrogel: implication in bone regeneration therapy. *Sci Rep* 2017;**7**(1):6577. https://doi.org/10.1038/s41598-017-06028-y.

[220] Whitlow J, Pacelli S, Paul A. Multifunctional nanodiamonds in regenerative medicine: recent advances and future directions. *J Control Release* 2017;**261**:62–86. https://doi.org/10.1016/j.jconrel.2017.05.033.

[221] Lee D-K, Kee T, Liang Z, Hsiou D, Miya D, Wu B, Osawa E, Chow EK-H, Sung EC, Kang MK. Clinical validation of a nanodiamond-embedded thermoplastic biomaterial. *Proc Natl Acad Sci USA* 2017. 201711924.

[222] Lee D-K, Kim SV, Limansubroto AN, Yen A, Soundia A, Wang C-Y, Shi W, Hong C, Tetradis S, Kim Y, Park N-H, Kang MK, Ho D. Nanodiamond-gutta percha composite biomaterials for root canal therapy. *ACS Nano* 2015;**9**(11):11490–501. https://doi.org/10.1021/acsnano.5b05718.

[223] Friedman CM, Sandrik JL, Heuer MA, Rapp GW. Composition and mechanical properties of gutta-percha endodontic points. *J Dent Res* 1975;**54**(5):921–5. https://doi.org/10.1177/00220345750540052901.

[224] Liu Z, Tabakman S, Welsher K, Dai H. Carbon nanotubes in biology and medicine: in vitro and in vivo detection, imaging and drug delivery. *Nano Res* 2009;**2**(2):85–120. https://doi.org/10.1007/s12274-009-9009-8.

[225] Tran PA, Zhang L, Webster TJ. Carbon nanofibers and carbon nanotubes in regenerative medicine. *Adv Drug Deliv Rev* 2009;**61**(12):1097–114. https://doi.org/10.1016/j.addr.2009.07.010.

[226] Morales-Narváez E, Merkoçi A. Graphene oxide as an optical biosensing platform. *Adv Mater* 2012;**24**(25):3298–308.

[227] Lee Y, Kuzmiak C. Comparison of stationary breast tomosynthesis and 2-D digital mammography in patients with known breast lesions. *Acad Radiol* 2017.

[228] Xu Z-q, Broza YY, Ionsecu R, Tisch U, Ding L, Liu H, Song Q, Pan Y-y, Xiong F-x, Gu K-s, Sun G-p, Chen Z-d, Leja M, Haick H. A nanomaterial-based breath test for distinguishing gastric cancer from benign gastric conditions. *Br J Cancer* 2013;**108**(4):941. https://doi.org/10.1038/bjc.2013.44.

[229] Amal H, Leja M, Funka K, Skapars R, Sivins A, Ancans G, Liepniece-Karele I, Kikuste I, Lasina I, Haick H. Detection of precancerous gastric lesions and gastric cancer through exhaled breath. *Gut* 2016;**65**(3):400–7. https://doi.org/10.1136/gutjnl-2014-308536.

[230] Al-Jumaili A, Alancherry S, Bazaka K, Jacob M. Review on the antimicrobial properties of carbon nanostructures. *Materials* 2017;**10**(9):1066. https://doi.org/10.3390/ma10091066.

[231] Hou J, Wan B, Yang Y, Ren X-M, Guo L-H, Liu J-F. Biodegradation of single-walled carbon nanotubes in macrophages through respiratory burst modulation. *Int J Mol Sci* 2016;**17**(3):409. https://doi.org/10.3390/ijms17030409.

[232] Notarianni M, Liu J, Vernon K, Motta N. Synthesis and applications of carbon nanomaterials for energy generation and storage. *Beilstein J Nanotechnol* 2016;**7**(1):149–96. https://doi.org/10.3762/bjnano.7.17.

[233] Moghimi SM, Hunter AC, Andresen TL. Factors controlling nanoparticle pharmacokinetics: an integrated analysis and perspective. *Annu Rev Pharmacol Toxicol* 2012;**52**:481–503. https://doi.org/10.1146/annurev-pharmtox-010611-134623.

Chapter 15

Quantum Dots

Tyler Maxwell[1,2], Maria Gabriela Nogueira Campos[2,3], Stephen Smith[1,2], Mitsushita Doomra[2,4], Zon Thwin[1,2] and Swadeshmukul Santra[1,2,4,5]

[1]*Department of Chemistry, University of Central Florida, Orlando, FL, United States;* [2]*NanoScience Technology Center, University of Central Florida, Orlando, FL, United States;* [3]*Institute of Science and Technology, Federal University of Alfenas, Poços de Caldas, Minas Gerais, Brazil;* [4]*Burnett School of Biomedical Science, University of Central Florida, Orlando, FL, United States;* [5]*Department of Materials Science and Engineering, University of Central Florida, Orlando, FL, United States*

15.1 Introduction to quantum dots

Quantum dots (QDs) are ultrasmall size semiconductor nanocrystals made up of 100–10,000 atoms,[1] within the size range of 1.5–10 nm. QDs exhibit size unique optical properties due to changes in band gap energy caused by quantum confinement effects. On absorption of light, electrons are promoted from the valence band (lower electronic energy state) to the conduction band (upper electronic energy state), producing an electron–hole pair, called an "exciton." When the electron and hole recombine, energy is released in the form of a photon (radiative recombination). In bulk materials, the exciton can spread out over the delocalized lattice. However, when the particle size falls under the Bohr radius, the energy required to create an exciton increases. This effect is termed "quantum confinement," and it is typically observed in ultrasmall size, crystalline, semiconductor materials. Smaller QDs possess larger band gap energy thereby emitting photons of higher energy (blue shifted) and vice versa. Tunability of optical properties of QDs is shown in Fig. 15.1. QDs have been synthesized with emissions ranging from near ultraviolet[2] to infrared.[3]

QDs were first described by Ekimov and Onushenko in 1981.[4] In 1982, Efros and Efros[5] postulated that quantum size effects cause the change in optical and optoelectronic properties of nanoparticles. In 1984, Louis Brus pioneered the field of colloidal semiconductor nanocrystals[6] for which he was awarded the Kavli Prize in Nanotechnology in 2008. QDs were first introduced as biological probes in 1988.[7] Their broad absorption spectrum, narrow tunable emission, and increased photostability compared with organic dyes made them attractive materials for bioimaging.

QDs are synthesized from group II–VI (CdSe, CdS, ZnO, ZnS), III–V (GaN, GaP, InP), and IV–VI (PbSe, PbS) elements in the periodic table due to their semiconductor properties. Impurities can be purposely doped into the crystal lattice to alter their optical properties. Transition metal dopants, such as Mn^{2+}, Cu^{2+}, Fe^{2+}, Cr^{2+}, and Co^{2+}, are widely studied to modulate QD's magnetic and optical properties.[9] Advantages of doping can include improved quantum yield (QY)[10] and longer excited state lifetime.[11] High QY gives better limits of detection of QDs for imaging. Longer excited state lifetimes in doped QDs are beneficial for eliminating background fluorescence in biological systems.

QDs have a high surface-to-volume ratio, which means a large percentage of the atoms are located on the particle surface. For example, a 5 nm diameter particle would have ~20% of its atoms on the surface, whereas a 20 nm particle would have ~5% surface atoms.[12] The surface dangling bonds or defects can serve as a nonradiative recombination centers and reduce QY. This is due to entrapment of excited state electrons and holes which migrated to the nonpassivated QD surface. Nonradiative recombination can be minimized by passivating the QD surface with an inorganic shell layer having a wide band gap (such as ZnS or ZnSe) to produce a core/shell (C–S) QD structure. In C–S QDs, excitons are more effectively confined within the core, thereby improving QY.[13,14] However, mismatches in the lattice spacing of the core with shell material can result in an unstable structure. QDs have been designed with multiple shell layers such as CdSe/CdS/ZnS to minimize the lattice mismatch.[15]

15.2 Quantum dot synthesis

One of the most commonly studied techniques to produce highly fluorescent QDs is known as the hot injection synthesis. In hot injection synthesis,[16] a metal precursor, such as cadmium oleate or CdO, is dissolved in a

Nanoparticles for Biomedical Applications. https://doi.org/10.1016/B978-0-12-816662-8.00015-1

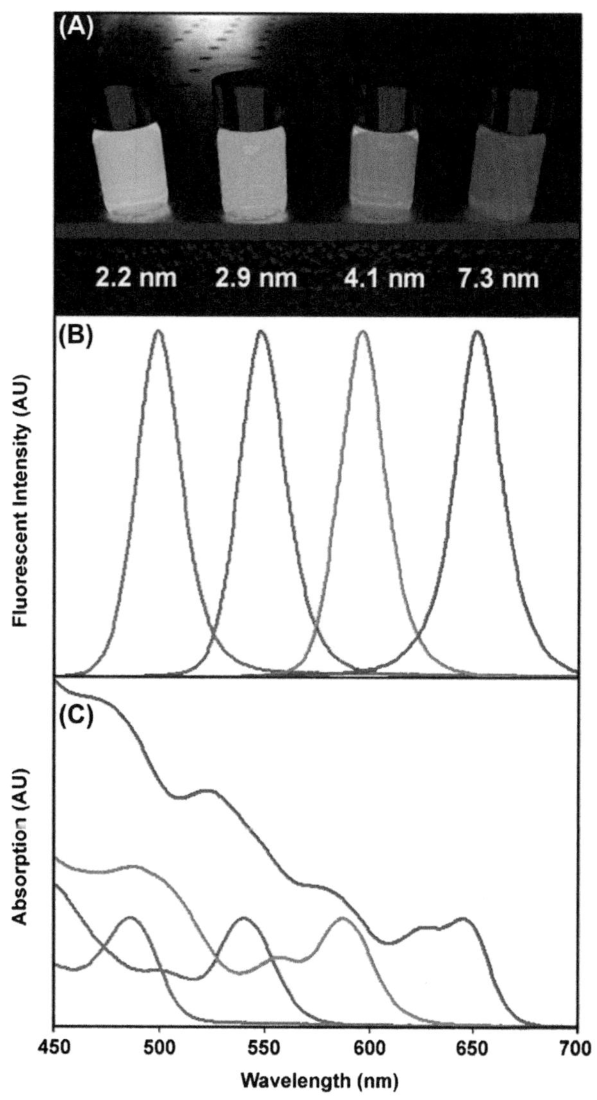

FIGURE 15.1 (A) Image of different sized CdSe quantum dots (QDs) excited by an ultraviolet lamp demonstrating the quantum confinement effect. (B) Fluorescence emission spectra of the same QD samples. (C) Absorption spectra of the QD samples. *From Smith, AM, et al., Bioconjugated quantum dots for in vivo molecular and cellular imaging.* Adv Drug Deliv Rev *2008;**60**(11):1226–1240.*

coordinating organic solvent such as trioctyl phosphine oxide (TOPO) or trioctyl phosphine. Coordinating solvents are used to control the QD nucleation and growth as they bind to the surface of the nucleating particles. An organic solution containing an anion source (for example, Se^{-2} or S^{-2}) is then injected, followed by heating for a set amount of time, with a longer growth time resulting in larger QDs (Fig. 15.2). QD growth is halted by injection of cold acetone or methanol to precipitate the QDs. Because the reagents are air sensitive, the whole reaction is performed under argon flow. QDs produced by this method are more fluorescent than those synthesized by other techniques due to the reduction and passivation of surface defects by the thick layer of organic coating on the surface of the QD. A limitation of this synthesis technique is the requirement of expensive high-purity organic solvents and stringent synthesis steps such as precise heating and argon flow settings and recovery of QDs through purification process. QDs produced by this method also tend to have larger hydrodynamic diameters from the thick hydrophobic coatings imparted by the coordinating solvent.

Water-in-oil (W/O) microemulsion (also known as reverse micelle) method is an alternative QD synthesis method.[18] A reverse microemulsion is the dispersion of water in oil in which a surfactant is added to create extremely small water droplets. W/O microemulsion parameters such as water-to-surfactant molar ratio are varied to control the water droplet size.[19] The size of the water droplet has an effect on the particle size. Usually, particle size increases with the increase of water droplet size but other factors such as reaction time, intermicellular exchange rate, and concentration of reagents also play a role.[20,21] For QD microemulsion synthesis, water-soluble salts are dissolved in two separate microemulsions, one for the anion and one for the cation. The ions are not soluble in the bulk oil phase and are therefore confined to the dispersed water droplets. QD crystals are produced when the two microemulsion are slowly mixed together at room temperature (Fig. 15.3A). During mixing, water droplets undergo collision and coalescence processes, resulting in the formation of QDs within the water droplet. The W/O microemulsion synthesis requires large amounts of high purity oil and surfactant, making it expensive and not environmentally friendly.

Sol–gel is another process for making metal oxide or metal sulfide–based QDs at room temperature. This method involves the formation of a colloidal solution called a "sol" from a metal precursor dispersed in a solvent, followed by formation of a continuous network or "gel" (Fig. 15.3B). A stabilizing agent such as glutathione (GSH), mercaptopropionic acid (MPA), or mercaptoundecanoic acid is incorporated in the reaction mix to control the growth of QD.[22] Inexpensive solvents such as ethanol[23] or water can be used for this method, making it cost-effective. Another advantage of using sol–gel synthesis is that less waste is produced making it more environmentally friendly than hot injection or microemulsion methods. Major drawbacks for this method include broad size distribution and high level of surface defects.

Pyrolysis and hydrothermal processes can be used to prepare inorganic or carbon QDs (CQDs). These methods are one-pot synthesis procedures where the reactant precursors are dissolved in water and heated at high temperature (and high pressure for hydrothermal process). This heating partially decomposes chemicals and facilitates collisions, which cause QD formation (Fig. 15.3C). To

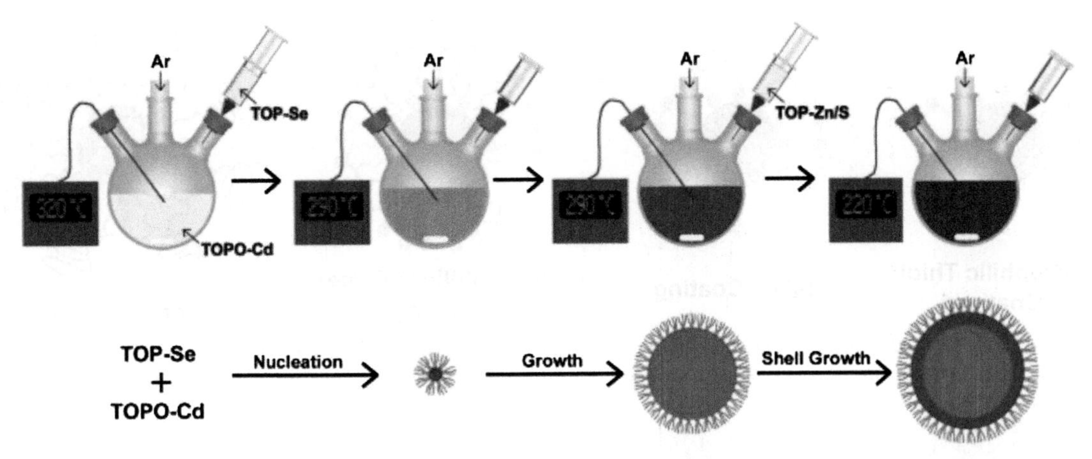

FIGURE 15.2 Hot injection synthesis of CdSe/ZnS quantum dots. *TOPO*, Trioctyl phosphine oxide; *TOP*, Trioctyl phosphine. *From Bailey, RE, A.M. Smith, and S. Nie, Quantum dots in biology and medicine.* Physica E (Amsterdam, Neth.), *2004;**25**(1):1–12.*

prepare CQDs, organic precursors such as ammonium citrate,[24,25] glucose,[26] chitosan,[27] or other carbon sources are used. Nitric acid is commonly added during synthesis to increase water dispersibility by oxidizing surface groups of the CQDs to carboxyl groups. These methods are scalable, low-cost, and environmentally friendly.[28] However, the effect of the heat source on particle formation is still poorly understood.[29]

15.3 Quantum dot surface modification and bioconjugation

After synthesis, many QDs have a hydrophobic coating which must be replaced or further modified to give them aqueous dispersibility. A few common strategies for this include coating with hydrophilic thiols, silica, amphiphilic polymers, and polyethylene glycol (PEG) (Fig. 15.4).

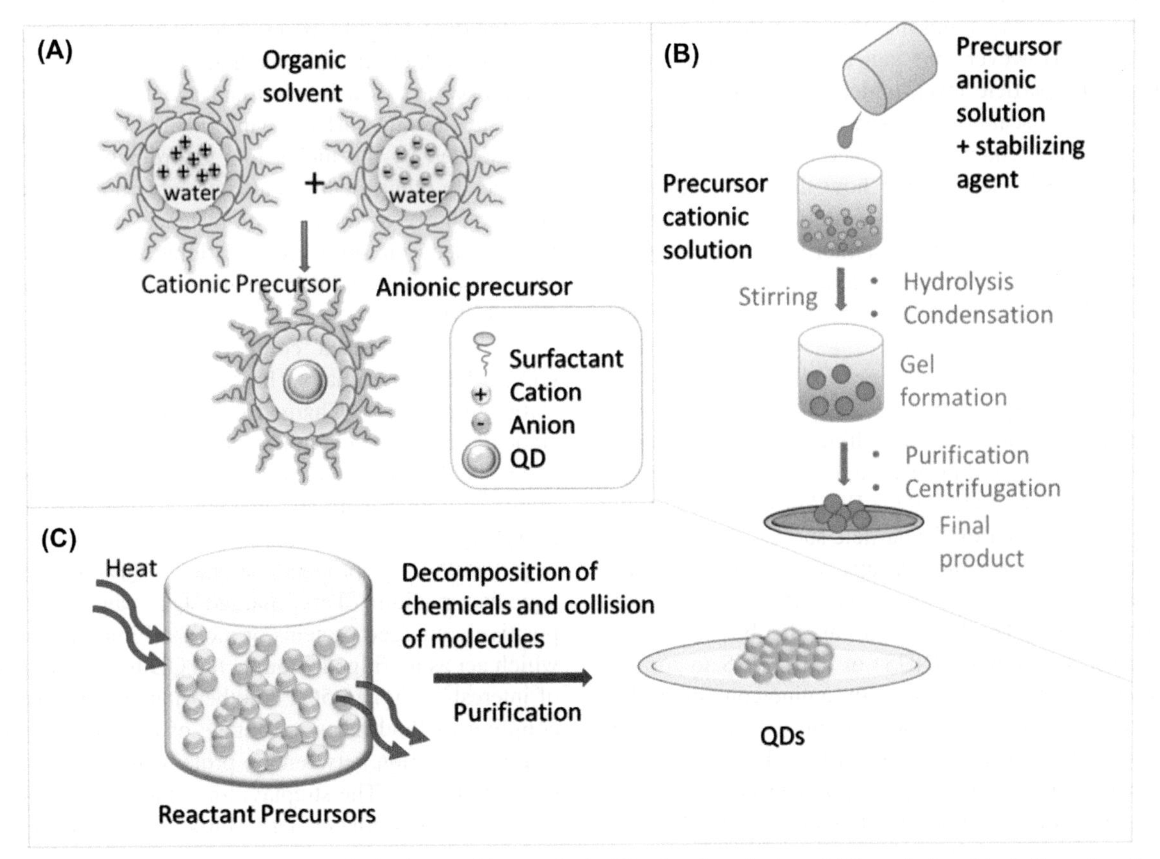

FIGURE 15.3 Schematic representation of (A) microemulsion synthesis, (B) sol–gel synthesis, and (C) pyrolysis and hydrothermal syntheses.

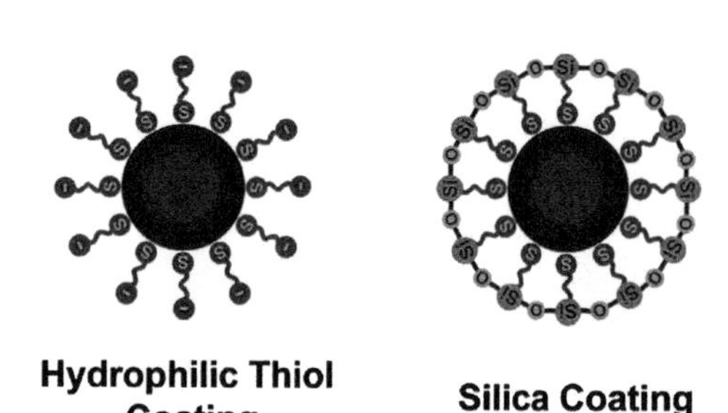

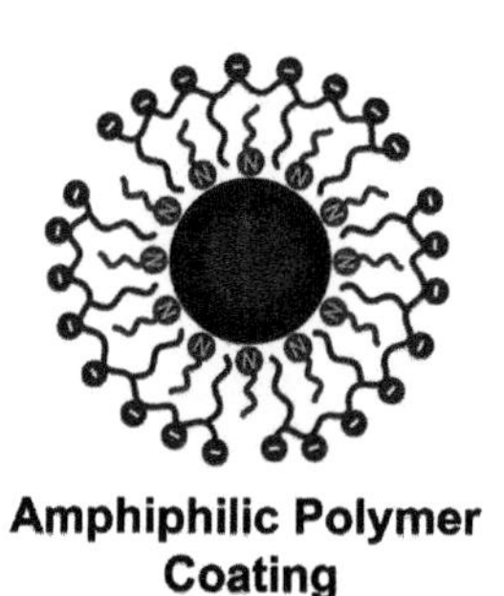

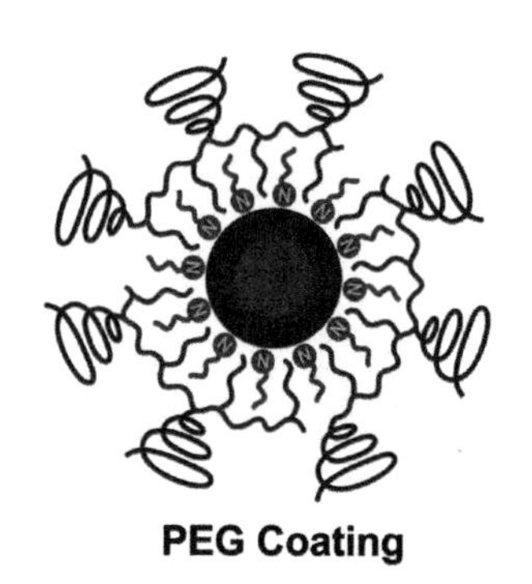

FIGURE 15.4 Types of coating materials used to functionalize quantum dot surface for future conjugation. PEG, polyethylene glycol. *Modified from Smith AM, et al., Bioconjugated quantum dots for in vivo molecular and cellular imaging.* Adv Drug Deliv Rev, *2008;60(11):1226–1240.*

Thiol groups can bind with both sulfur and metal atoms, such as zinc and cadmium on the QD surface. Small molecule coating agents containing thiol and carboxyl groups are the most commonly used surface capping for QDs. Thiols bind to the QD surface, while the carboxyl groups are exposed to the solvent. At neutral pH, most carboxyl groups remain deprotonated, producing a negatively charged QD surface. Therefore, QDs in aqueous solution are stabilized via electrostatic repulsion. Zeta potential (ζ) is a measurement of overall particle surface charge (positive or negative). If the ζ value is more than ± 20 mV, one can expect stable colloidal solution (no settlement over days) and therefore minimal aggregation of particles. However, one can still expect some aggregation at the particle level, which can be detected using sensitive light scattering–based measurements such as dynamic light scattering. Surface chemistry plays an important role in determining how the QD will interact with a biological system. For example, heavy-metal ion toxicity of QD can be masked either by the shell layer or by ligand capping with biomolecules. Conjugation with biomolecules can not only provide colloidal stability but also improve biocompatibility.[8]

One of the most common methods for attaching biomolecules to QD surface is EDC (1-ethyl-3-(3-dimethylaminopropyl) carbodiimide hydrochloride) covalent coupling. In this method, carboxyl-modified QDs are activated with water-soluble EDC in buffer to generate a reactive EDC ester on the particle surface. This ester can then react with the amine groups on the biomolecule to form a stable amide (peptide) bond between the QD and the biomolecule. The EDC ester can also be reacted with N-hydroxy succinimide (NHS) or sulfo-NHS to form an NHS ester before reacting with amine-containing biomolecules in a two-step conjugation. The advantage of using the two-step conjugation is that the NHS ester is more stable and gives higher yields than the initial EDC ester.[30] In addition, the negatively charged sulfo-NHS can help maintain repulsive forces between particles, which increase their stability during conjugation.

Sulfhydryl cross-linkers, such as maleimides and pyridyl disulfides, can also be used for biomolecule conjugation. The maleimide–thiol reaction is selective to thiol groups which are present on naturally occurring cysteine residues (Fig. 15.5A). The availability of cysteine residue on the protein can be a limiting factor for this conjugation strategy. Thiol groups can also be purposely introduced into a protein's chain by the reaction of primary amine groups with sulfhydryl reagents (i.e., Traut's reagent).

Histidine tagging is another method for conjugating proteins a QD. In this method, nickel–nitrilotriacetate complexes act as a bifunctional agent, which covalently binds to the QD surface, while histidine-tagged proteins are chelated by the nickel ion. Coordination of histidine residues to other metals is also possible due to histidine's strong affinity to metals. For instance, zinc ions on the QD surface can serve as a histidine chelator for direct attachment of the biomolecule to the QD surface[31] (Fig. 15.5B).

Noncovalent-based conjugation of biomolecules to QD surface is primarily based on Coulombic (electrostatic) interactions. Charged QD surfaces can be electrostatically assembled with oppositely charged ligands to create stable conjugates. Usually, QDs are surface-modified with negatively charged molecules such as N-acetyl cysteine (NAC) that minimizes particle–particle aggregation and produces a stable QD dispersion in aqueous medium. This charged QD can interact with positively charged proteins or modified immunoglobulins, which act as a bridge to couple the QD to the biomolecule of interest[32] (Fig. 15.5C). Another noncovalent-based QD coupling method takes advantage of the specific biomolecular interaction between the protein streptavidin and the biotin molecule. The streptavidin–biotin system is one of the strongest noncovalent biological protein–ligand

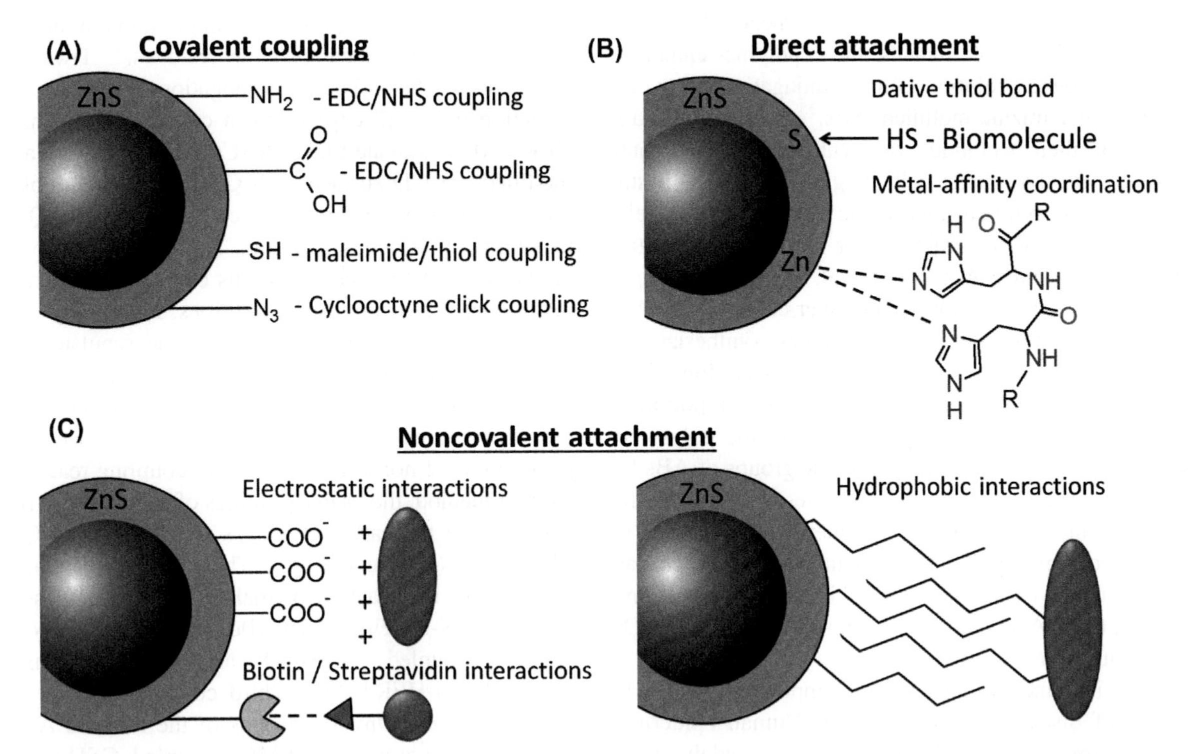

FIGURE 15.5 Schematic representation of different methods of conjugating biomolecules to quantum dots (QDs). (A) Covalent attachment of biomolecules through the amine, thiol, or carboxyl groups displayed on the QD surface. (B) Direct attachment (zero-length coupling) of biomolecules to atoms on the QD surface, by either dative thiol bonding or metal affinity–driven coordination. (C) Electrostatic (noncovalent) interactions between QD surfaces and oppositely charged proteins or other biomolecules. *Modified from Sapsford KE, et al., Biosensing with luminescent semiconductor quantum dots.* Sensors *2006;6(8):925–953.*

interactions known to date and is a widely used tool for bioconjugation.

15.4 Quantum dot–based antibody probes

Antibodies (ABs) or immunoglobulins are glycoproteins mainly produced by plasma cells. ABs are "Y"-shaped proteins composed of four polypeptide chains: two light chains and two heavy chains. Both heavy and light chains are composed of antigen recognition domains. AB fragments (nanobodies), such as the heavy chain and single variable domain, can also be used as therapeutics, for site recognition and/or target detection due to their high specificity to the antigen. These properties make ABs suitable for several biological applications, such as immunoassays for diagnoses of diseases, bioimaging, biosensing, and for detection of toxins, biomarkers, and other molecules of interest.

To prepare AB-based probes, a reporting molecule (fluorophore) is attached to the AB. Organic dyes have been used for this purpose, but QDs have been proposed as alternatives due to their attractive photophysical properties. The use of QDs in probes for biological and clinical applications has been considered advantageous because of their interesting optical properties, small size, and versatility.[34] Detection probes, immunoprobes, biosensors, and drug-delivery systems are some of the several applications of QDs in the biomedical area. Moreover, conjugation of QDs with ABs has recently captured interest due to the potential for targeted delivery, disease diagnosis, and monitoring therapy.

15.4.1 Antibody conjugation

Selection of bioconjugate chemistry has impact on the stability and functional activity of the QD-AB probe. Recognition sites of ABs need to be preserved during conjugation to maintain the specificity of binding to the target molecules, such as antigens. Molecular conformation is an important parameter that affects the specificity of the reaction between antigen and AB, as well as the success of conjugation between QD and ABs. Direct attachment of AB to QD surface using "zero-length" coupling chemistry (such as cyanogen bromide based) increases the chances of blocking the antigen-binding site, thus compromising AB performance.

Han et al. synthesized norbornene-QD/tetrazine-AB conjugates for in vivo cytometric imaging in mice.[35] Norbornene, which is an uncharged bridging cycling hydrocarbon, was incorporated to the QD to avoid nonspecific binding to cells or biomolecules due to surface charge. The authors reported passivation of the norbornene-QD surface with PEG-polyimidazole ligands; the copolymer enhanced the QY in aqueous solution before conjugation by cycloaddition with tetrazine-modified ABs.[35] Some of the advantages of their technique on synthesizing conjugates suitable for in vivo single cell imaging include high stability and QYs, minimal nonspecific interaction with cells and serum, and narrow emission for multiplex cytometric imaging.[35] Fernandez-Arguelles et al. reported a simple bioconjugation of amphiphilic polymer-coated QD with ABs for immunoassays.[36] The authors synthesized a polymer based on poly(maleic anhydride) functional groups to improve stability and brightness of polymer-coated QD. Then, the carboxylic groups of the polymeric coating were cross-linked with the amine groups of ABs by water-soluble EDC chemistry.[36] The results showed the ability of a highly fluorescent, polymer-coated QD-AB to selectively recognize an antigen/toxin. This approach can be used to develop multiplexed immunoassays using several types of ABs conjugated with different sized QDs that emit at different wavelengths.[36]

Sensitivity and selectivity are important for early detection of diseases, such as cancer. Human epidermal growth factor receptor 2 (HER2) is a widely used biomarker for the detection of several types of cancer, including lung and breast cancers. Several studies reported the conjugation of anti-HER2 ABs to QDs for cancer diagnostics. Rakovich et al. prepared highly sensitive, ultrasmall, and bright nanoprobes for detection of HER2 biomarker in lung and breast cancer cells by conjugating maleimide-activated QDs with single-domain antibodies (SDABs) through their cysteine residues.[37] Tiwari et al. also studied the effect of conjugation chemistry on the detection of HER2 expression in cancer cells, using anti-HER2 AB conjugated to CdSe/CdZnS QD.[38] The authors modified the QD surface with GSH, a natural thiol compound that is present in most cells, to improve QD dispersibility in aqueous medium. The thiol group of GSH binds to the QD surface, while its carboxyl group remains deprotonated at neutral pH conditions. Negatively charged QDs remain stable through electrostatic repulsion. Three different coupling agents were tested, and the resulting probes were evaluated in their ability to stain HER2 in breast cancer cells (Fig. 15.6). The first and second conjugations were nonselective covalent coupling reactions. In the first method, the primary amines of anti-HER2 AB were reacted with the carboxyl groups of GSH-coated QD via EDC/sulfo-NHS coupling. The second conjugation occurred by the reaction of maleimide groups of succinimidyl 4-(N-maleimidomethyl)cyclohexane-1-carboxylate (SMCC)−coupled GSH-QD and the iminothiolane-modified anti-HER2 ABs. Third conjugation was specifically between sulfhydryl groups of the reduced ABs and the maleimide groups of SMCC-coupled GSH-QD. The specific conjugation of the QD with the thiol group of ABs resulted in a more stable conjugate with proper orientation. A desired orientation is one in which the active site of the AB is pointed out and away from the QD, so it is accessible to the antigen. If the antigen-binding site is coupled to the QD, it may become inaccessible due to steric effects.

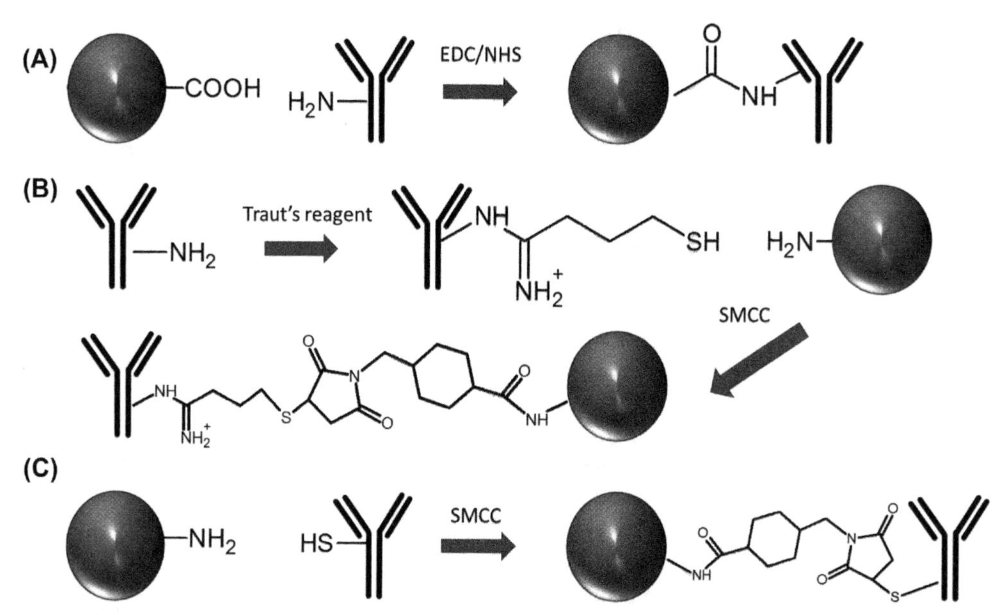

FIGURE 15.6 Schematic representation for the coupling reactions between glutathione-quantum dots and anti−human epidermal growth factor receptor 2 antibodies. (A) EDC/sulfo-N-hydroxy succinimide, (B) iminothiolate/sulfo-SMCC, and (C) sulfo-SMCC coupling. *Modified from Tiwari DK, et al., Synthesis and characterization of anti-HER2 antibody conjugated CdSe/CdZnS quantum dots for fluorescence imaging of breast cancer cells. Sensors 2009;9(11):9332−9354.*

Orientation of the AB is controlled through the functional groups used for attachment to the QD. HER2 may contain many amine groups near its binding site and thus when these groups are coupled to the QD, the antigen binding is compromised. With the AB coupled via thiol groups, the probe demonstrated superior detection of HER2 expression in cancer cells.[38] Therefore, conjugation chemistry plays an important role in the specificity and sensitivity of AB-QD conjugates.

15.4.2 Compact quantum dot—antibody probe design

Direct conjugation of an AB to a QD surface produces a compact probe. Wu et al. used the direct conjugation approach to immobilize anti-HER2 ABs to the ZnS QD surface. Histidine-modified ADAPTs (albumin-binding, domain-derived affinity proteins) were self-assembled on Zn on the QD surface. This method allows for a very close proximity between the QD and AB by self-assembly of ADAPTs on the QD surface, resulting in smaller conjugates.[39]

Liu et al. studied the conjugation of biotin-coated QD with single-domain AB-rhizavidin (RZ) fusions. RZ is a protein with affinity for biotin, as well as streptavidin. Fusion of SDABs with biotin-affinity proteins is another strategy for direct conjugation of ABs to biotin-coated QDs. The authors reported that RZ-SDABs conjugate structure is smaller than the streptavidin one, because RZ is organized as a homodimer. Streptavidin is a larger quaternary protein (tetramer). The advantages of using RZ-SDABs fusion include oriented binding to biotin-coated QD and efficient packing. This improves the active surface without compromising antigen recognition.[40]

Goldman et al. reported the conjugation of QD with immunoglobulin G (IgG) using another type of engineered adaptor protein. The authors added a positively charged leucine zipper to the C-terminus of a two-domain recombinant protein. The leucine zipper is a heptad repetition of leucine residues that facilitates protein—protein interactions by forming parallel helix—helix association. These residues were introduced into the IgG by genetic fusion for further conjugation with the DHLA-coated QD by electrostatic interaction between surficial negative charges of QD and positive charges of the leucine zipper attached to the IgG.[32] According to the authors, synthesis of QD-IgG is simple, reproducible, and readily formed. They also claimed QD-IgG conjugates can be used for several immunoassays due to their optical properties, such as resistance to photobleaching and wide emission wavelengths.[32]

15.4.3 Factors controlling antibody loading to quantum dot surface

The number of ABs attached to the surface of a QD will depend on the QD surface functionalization, bioconjugation chemistry, orientation of ABs, and size of the QD-AB conjugate.

Recently, Umakoshi et al. reported for the first time the visualization of QD-AB conjugation using high-speed atomic force microscopy.[41] They were also able to count the number of ABs bound to a QD (Fig. 15.7), which in the past was only possible by indirect methods or estimative calculations.[42] Conjugation was achieved by reacting a maleimide-functionalized QD with thiol groups of ABs. To expose thiol groups before conjugation, the AB molecules were treated using a reducing agent tris(2-carboxyetheyl)phosphine (TCEP). This methodology leads to small size structures and well-oriented QD-AB conjugation. The authors observed ABs split in two steps, as well as the formation of an intermediate state for conjugation with QD.[41]

Pathak et al. reported the use of quantitative electrophoresis experiments to derive the number of IgG ABs conjugated to the QD.[42] The authors used both covalent (maleimide based) and noncovalent (streptavidin—biotin based) coupling methods to prepare QD-IgG.[42] Interestingly, the authors found very low number of ABs per QD, and the results were much lower for covalent conjugation. It was suggested that orientation of the AB molecule plays an important role in bioconjugation. Moreover, covalent conjugation using maleimide chemistry requires pretreatment of ABs to expose bioavailable thiol groups, which may compromise the AB functionality. However, IgG attachment to the QD surface using streptavidin—biotin interaction increased the yield of functional ABs.[42]

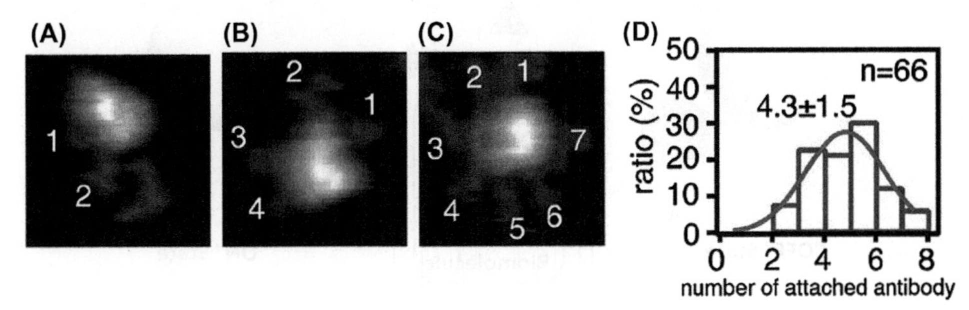

FIGURE 15.7 High-speed AFM analysis of the number of attached antibodies (ABs) on quantum dots (QDs). (A)–(C) H-S AFM images of QD-ABs conjugates. (D) Histogram for the number of attached ABs on QDs. *Modified from Umakoshi T., et al., Quantum-dot antibody conjugation visualized at the single-molecule scale with high-speed atomic force microscopy.* Colloids Surfaces B Biointerfaces *2018;167:267–274.*

QD-AB conjugates have some advantages for in vivo cell-labeling studies, such as broad absorption, narrow emission, and large multiphoton cross sections. Long-term, deep tissue tracking and sensing experiments may benefit from the use of near-infrared (NIR)–emitting QDs.[35] Organic NIR dyes have limited QY and photostability compared with QDs.[43] Controlling AB orientation on the QD surface remains a challenge because the surface properties of QDs vary based on their preparation. The size of QD-AB probes may also impact their usefulness as larger probes may not be able to reach desired target due to steric effects. On the other hand, for ex vivo assays, where size of probe is not a concern, QD-ABs conjugates can be designed using different types of ABs for simultaneous detection of biomarkers for a number of diseases, and/or for more accurate/sensitive detection of diseases at early stage.

15.5 Quantum dot biosensors

Biosensors are systems engineered to produce a distinguishable signal in response to a specific analyte in a complex biological matrix. Fluorescence probes are useful tools for biosensing due to their fast response times and in situ nondestructive sample analysis. There has been extensive research using fluorescent dyes and nanomaterials as biosensors, but more sensitive biosensing probes are still needed to help understand complex biological interactions. QDs have been employed to improve the sensitivity and selectivity of the detection of biomolecules. QDs offer advantages over other nanomaterials, in that their emission can be tuned to allow better spectral overlap with quencher molecules for improved sensitivity. Improved photostability over organic dyes and proteins is another attractive QD property because it facilitates long-term biosensing or tracking applications.

QD biosensors have been developed to sense various biologically relevant stimuli, such as pH changes,[44–54] reactive oxygen species (ROS),[55–59] metal ions,[60–64] and biomolecules.[33,61,65–71] Typically, QD biosensors are designed with a fluorescence quencher bound to the QD in a way that the analyte of interest can remove or change the quencher so that the QD fluorescence is restored. When the quencher is bound to the QD, it exhibits low fluorescence intensity or "OFF" state. When the quencher is removed, the system is shifted to a high fluorescence or "ON" state (Fig. 15.8). This "OFF/ON" design is advantageous over "always ON" probes because these probes have higher signal-to-noise ratio, lower detection limit, and are capable of real-time detection in living organisms.[72,73]

15.5.1 Quantum dot pH sensors

Many diseases such as cancer and Alzheimer's can cause unidirectional changes in pH to more acidic levels of the cellular environment and/or organelles. Change in pH is observed in inflamed tissue (e.g., cancer tissue) due to increased rates of glycolysis of those cells.[74,75] As this pH change is universal trend for these diseases, sensing pH changes at the cellular level has been studied for diagnostic purposes.

QD-based pH sensors can be synthesized by attachment of a ligand with pH-dependent redox properties to the QD to control the fluorescence. Mattoussi et al. accomplished this by binding dopamine (neurotransmitter) to the surface of CdSe/ZnS QDs. Dopamine isothiocyanate was attached to amine-terminated PEG on the QD surface. Dopamine exists in its reduced catechol form at low pH and oxidized quinone at high pH. The quinone state can accept electrons from the excited QD to quench the QD's fluorescence. The authors show the QD-dopamine probe was sensitive to pH changes between 4 and 10 (Fig. 15.9). The QD probe was injected into COS-1 (fibroblast) cells to test intracellular pH-sensing capabilities. An increase in fluorescence over time was observed as the pH of the endosomes decreased.[46,47]

Ratiometric fluorescence sensors combine an analyte-sensitive fluorophore and an analyte-insensitive fluorophore

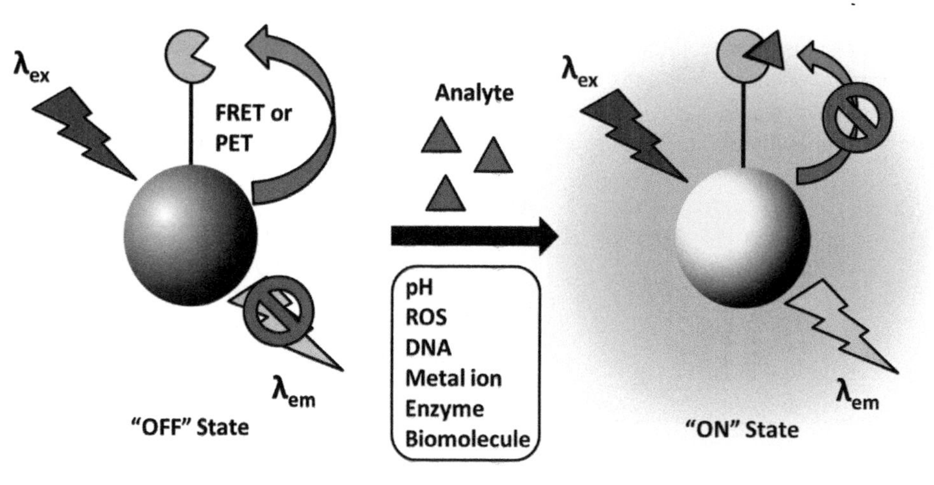

FIGURE 15.8 Scheme showing the design of quantum dot–based biosensors.

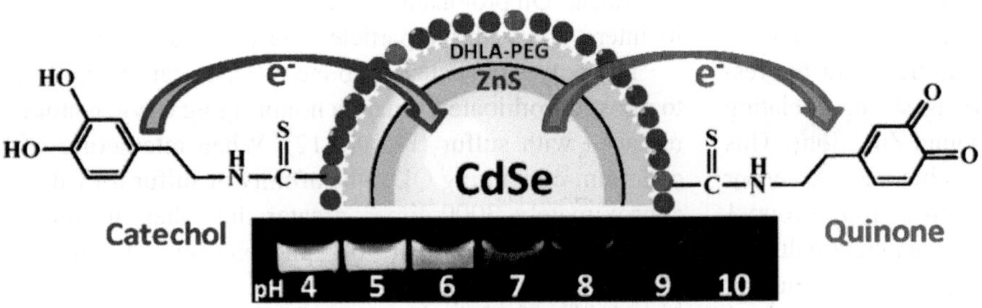

FIGURE 15.9 Schematic design of pH-responsive quantum dot–dopamine probe (top) and a photograph of probe fluorescence emission in the pH range of 4–10 (bottom). *From Ji X, et al., On the pH-dependent quenching of quantum dot photoluminescence by redox active dopamine.* J Am Chem Soc *2012;134(13):6006–6017.*

(usually the QD) to obtain information on the analyte. Information is obtained based on the fluorescence intensity ratio of the two fluorophores. Ratiometric sensors have advantages over redox-based sensors, in that they provide probes with a self-calibration ability to improve their sensitivity and selectivity. The concentration of the probe can be calculated from the insensitive fluorophore, and the pH-sensitive fluorophore would report on pH change. For sensing pH in the range from 6 to 8, Miyazaki et al. attached fluorescein isothiocyanate (FITC) to GSH-capped CdTe/ZnS QDs.[76] The QY of fluorescein is pH sensitive, it decreases as the carboxyl groups (pKa 6.4) are protonated.

Sensing pH in the endosome and lysosome compartments requires probes to have a working pH range between 4 and 6. Todd et al. designed an acid reactive probe by attaching a thiol-modified dye (2-(dimethylamino) ethyl) aminonaphthalimide to CdSe/ZnS QDs. The tertiary amine group on the dye shifts the fluorescence spectra when protonated. Energy transfer from the dye to QD occurs at acidic pH enhancing QD fluorescence.[51]

In conclusion, QD pH sensors have been synthesized with the capability of measuring physiologically relevant pHs at the cellular level such as those in the endosome. Because of their good photostability, these QDs may be useful for longer duration studies. Currently, cell membrane permeable pH-reactive dyes are the most effective at quantifying intercellular pH as they can easily penetrate into cell. Transport of QDs to areas outside the endosome is still a challenge limiting their usefulness.

15.5.2 Quantum dot metal ion sensors

The sensing of metal ions is vital to understanding many different diseases and metabolic processes. To obtain subcellular information on metal ions, it is necessary to use either metal ion selective electrodes or dyes. Electrodes are limited by their large size which results in poor spatial resolution. Optical-based probes are well suited for subcellular visualization of metal ions with fluorescent detection being the most utilized. Organic dyes modified with metal-binding groups are widely available to report on intracellular metal ion concentrations. QDs with metal-binding ligands can be used in place of these organic dyes resulting in probes that are more photostable. Cyclic ethers (crown ethers) and azamacrocycles (aza-crown) have been attached to QDs to create metal ion sensors. These cyclic compounds are electron rich and thus quench the QD fluorescence through electron transfer (Fig. 15.10). When the crown ether is bound to a metal cation, its ability to quench the QD is reduced.[77]

A zinc ion sensor was synthesized by Hall et al. by linking an azamacrocycle (cyclam or cyclen) to MPA-capped CdSe/ZnS QDs by carbodiimide coupling. Cyclam was able to quench the QD fluorescence through electron transfer. When bound to a Zn^{2+} ion, cyclam's

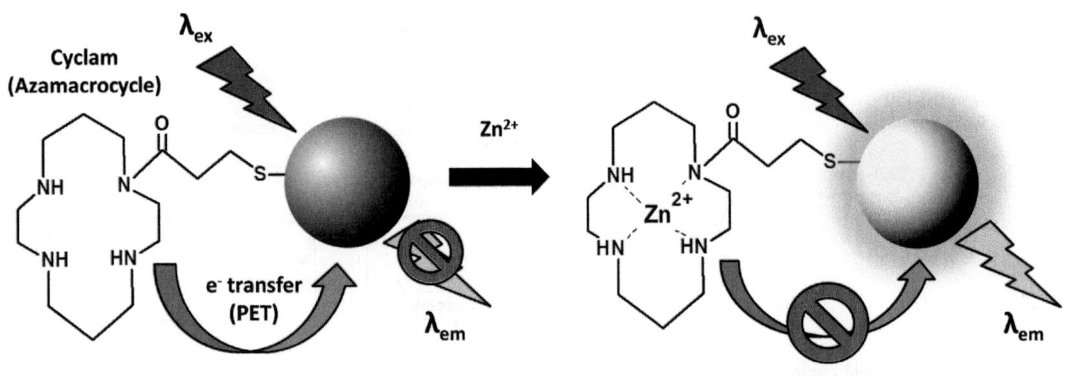

FIGURE 15.10 Mechanism of quantum dot zinc ion sensor. *Based on Ruedas-Rama MJ, Hall EAH. Azamacrocycle activated quantum dot for zinc ion detection.* Anal Chem (Washington, DC, U S)*, 2008;**80**(21):8260–8268.*

molecular orbitals were no longer available for electron transfer. The authors showed that QD fluorescence intensity responded linearly to Zn^{2+} ion concentration, and fluorescence was again quenched after applying strong chelating agent (EDTA) which would remove bound Zn^{2+} ions. This shows that the Zn^{2+} binding was reversible and the sensor can be reused. There was little interference from Group 1 and 2 metals (Na, K, Ca, Mg); however, copper, cobalt, and iron all bind very strongly to the ZnS shell causing interference.[64]

15.6 Quantum dot—DNA probes

In clinical diagnostics, the ability to rapidly detect or sequence low concentrations of DNA is critical for the early diagnosis of many diseases such as cancer. QD biosensors have reported improved detection limits compared with traditional molecular assays. These low limits are achieved due to the QDs' very high QY and their capacity to immobilize multiple recognition biomolecules. The hybridization of a single target DNA molecule at the surface is capable of recruiting multiple reporter probe molecules. QD-DNA/RNA constructs have been demonstrated to successfully monitor the delivery of therapeutic agents like small interfering RNA (siRNA) to cells.[78–80]

15.6.1 Quantum Dot–DNA noncovalent conjugation strategies

The method of conjugation of the nucleic acid to the QD is important to consider when developing biosensors. Strategies for conjugating DNA to QDs via noncovalent coupling may be categorized into two groups: affinity and biological interactions.

Imidazoles carry high affinity toward the surface of QDs and can be employed for anchoring groups onto the QD surface. To utilize this affinity in conjugation strategies, DNA may be tagged with polyhistidine peptides (Fig. 15.11).[81,82] However, the affinity of the imidazole functional group toward the particle surface is pH dependent. On protonation ($pH < 6$) of the imidazole group, its interaction with the particle's surface is destabilized.

The polyphosphate backbone of DNA can be modified to phosphorothioates, where a nonbridging oxygen atom is replaced with sulfur (Fig. 15.12). When interacting with cadmium-containing QDs, the affinity of sulfur for Cd^{+2} is approximately 3000 times greater than that of oxygen. Successful conjugation of phosphorothioate-modified DNA molecules to many types of QDs has been reported.[83–85] However, the conjugated DNA will no longer hybridize complementary DNA due to conformational distortion.[83] To overcome this limitation, a DNA overhang with a phosphodiester backbone which contains the target sequence may be added to the phosphorothioate-modified DNA to preserve functionality in biosensing applications.[86]

Phospholipids self-assemble on the surface of the QDs, allowing polar groups to promote water solubility of the QDs. The resulting lipid encapsulated QDs may be optimized to display functional groups capable of conjugating DNA by controlling the composition of encapsulating phospholipids used (Fig. 15.13).[87,88] This conjugation strategy requires the QD to possess a hydrophobic shell (e.g., QD coated with TOPO). These hydrophobic QDs may then be encapsulated by an amphiphilic compound such as 1,2-dioleoyl-sn-glycero-3-phosphocholine (DOPC). Lipid-conjugated oligonucleotides are then added to amphiphilic DOPC–coated QD. Oligonucleotides are thus immobilized onto QDs through hydrophobic–hydrophobic interaction, forming a stable conjugate.[89] This method does suffer from a lack of control regarding loading efficiency. In addition, these phospholipid formulations are generally poor at delivering cargo to the cytoplasm and crossing the cellular lipid bilayer.[90–92]

The negatively charged phosphate backbone of DNA may also adsorb QDs with positively charged surfaces by electrostatic interactions. QDs with positively charged coatings can be loaded with DNA by simply mixing the two together. However, interactions of the DNA with the QD in this manner may distort the conformation of the

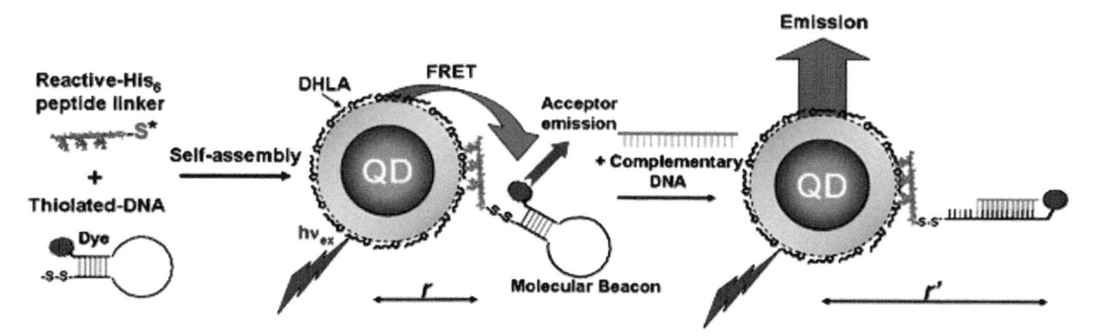

FIGURE 15.11 Imidazole-mediated conjugation. *From Medintz IL, et al., A reactive peptidic linker for self-assembling hybrid quantum Dot–DNA bioconjugates.* Nano Lett *2007;7(6):1741–1748.*

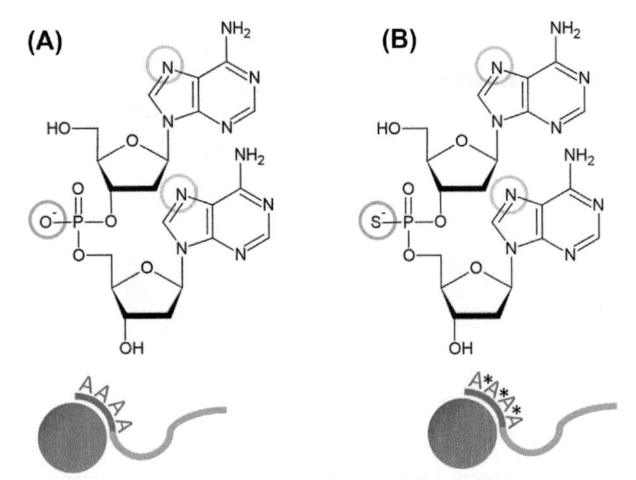

FIGURE 15.12 Phosphorothioate DNA conjugation. Unmodified DNA (A) will coordinate to the particle's surface via N7 position interactions of adenine (circled in yellow) and nonbridging oxygen (circled in blue). Phosphorothioate DNA (B) produces stronger complexes by coordinating on the particle's surface via the higher-affinity sulfur (circled in blue) interactions. *From Zhou W, et al., Tandem phosphorothioate Modifications for DNA adsorption Strength and polarity control on gold nanoparticles.* ACS Appl Mater Interfaces *2014;**6**(17):14795–14800.*

DNA and are pH dependent.[93] DNA attached electrostatically is also subject to premature release by displacement by biomolecules.

QDs functionalized with streptavidin can bind biotinylated DNA. This strategy has been widely used and offers a simple "mix and shake" route for conjugation.[94] However, with an additional layer of protein, the resulting QD-conjugate size may exceed the desired range for many biological applications. D'Agata et al. reported a hydrodynamic diameter of 31.1 nm when 19 nm particles were functionalized with streptavidin[95]. On binding of biotinylated DNA in the study, the hydrodynamic diameter further increased to 40 nm. In addition, the quantity of DNA molecules loaded per QD in this method is not homogenous.[96]

15.6.2 Quantum Dot–DNA covalent conjugation strategies

Covalent conjugation strategies are also used to functionalize QDs with DNA. Covalent conjugation not only increases the QD-DNA stability but also provides flexibility for controlling the orientation of DNA on the particle surface. Limitations of covalent binding of DNA include tedious sample preparation and purification processes that often involve multiple steps. Carboxyl-modified QDs can be linked to amine-functionalized DNA via carbodiimide coupling chemistry which forms a stable amide bond between the QD and DNA. The conjugation strategy generally results in minimal size increase of the QDs. However, when the surface carboxyl groups esterify with EDC-NHS, colloidal stability of the particle can be compromised.[97]

Covalent conjugation of DNA to QDs may also be accomplished using commercially available bifunctional linking reagents. The linker sulfosuccinimidyl-4-(N-maleimido-methyl) cyclohexane-1-carboxylate (sSMCC) is well-suited use for this purpose. After labeling DNA molecules with amine groups, reaction with terminal NHS groups of sSMCC produces DNA-maleimide (Fig. 15.14). Polymer coatings on the QDs may be reduced with TCEP to produce free thiol groups at the particle's surface. The thiol displaying QDs and DNA-maleimide are then reacted to produce DNA-conjugated QDs[98]

Copper-free click chemistry can be used to conjugate azide functionalized biomolecules to ligands with alkyne moieties via cycloaddition. Originally, the reaction employed copper ions as catalysts, but copper is known to quench QD photoluminescence.[99] Recently, copper-free alternatives have been demonstrated to successfully conjugate the DNA while preserving high QYs.[100] Zhang et al. reported DHLA-PEG-N_3-coated QDs added to cyclooctyne-functionalized DNA resulted in nearly two-third of the DNA to be successfully conjugated. The loading efficiency in conjunction with the commercial availability of these linkers makes this conjugation

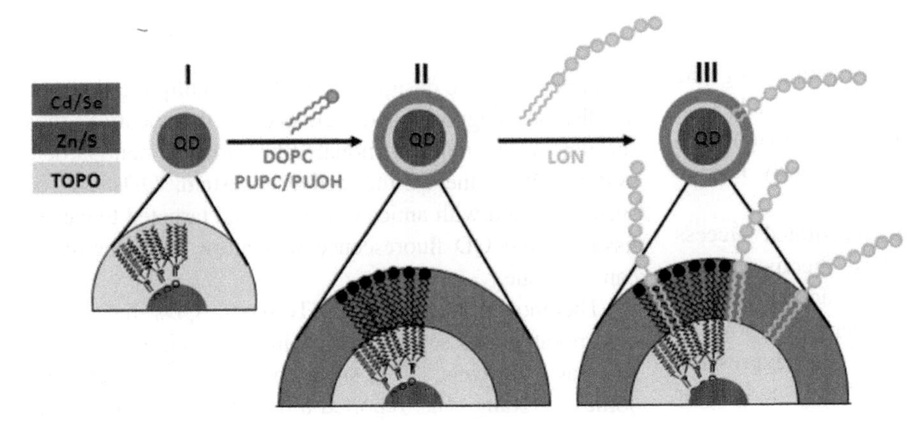

FIGURE 15.13 Lipid oligonucleotide conjugation. Lipid oligonucleotide conjugates formed from 1,2-dioleoyl-sn-glycero-3-phosphocholine (DOPC), palmitic uridine phosphocholine (PUPC), and palmitic uridine (PUOH). *From Aimé A, et al., Quantum dot lipid oligonucleotide bioconjugates: toward a new anti-micro RNA nanoplatform.* Bioconjug Chem *2013;**24**(8):1345–1355.*

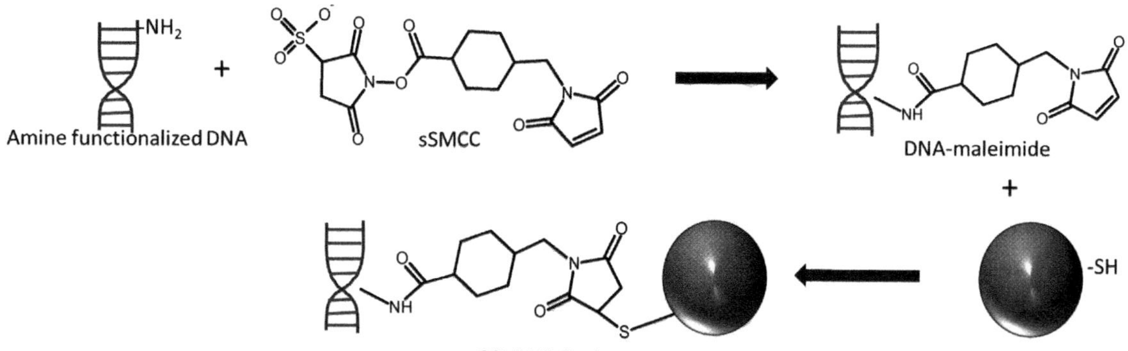

FIGURE 15.14 Amine to thiol-reactive linker (sulfo-SMCC)–mediated conjugation.

strategy one of the most popular for producing QD-DNA conjugates.

15.6.3 Quantum Dot–DNA sensor applications

QD-DNA conjugates employing FRET-based biosensing have been reported to detect single point mutations in clinical samples with lower detection limits than molecular beacon probes.[101] The system reported by Zhang et al. labeled reporter probes with a fluorescent dye and the capture probes with biotin. In the presence of target DNA, these probes form a sandwiched hybrid (Fig. 15.15). When streptavidin-functionalized QDs are introduced, the sandwiched hybrid forms an FRET donor–acceptor nanostructure via interactions between the biotinylated capture probe and the streptavidin-functionalized QD. Now in proximity with the QD, and on selective excitation of the QD, the dye labeled reporter probe generates fluorescence signal through FRET from excited QD to dye. Displaying multiple biotin–binding sites, the QD can act as a concentrator to amplify signals by confining multiple dye molecules on a single probe.

Utilizing QDs in lieu of traditional fluorophores offers comparatively higher signal-to-noise ratios. Capable of detecting target nucleic acid molecules at concentrations less than 1 femtomol,[102] the utility of QD-FRET–based biosensors in molecular diagnostics is clear. The primary limitation of these biosensors exists in controlling the number of DNA molecules associated with each QD. Future success of these sensors in molecular diagnostics depends on the ability to produce homogenously labeled conjugates.[98]

QD-DNA conjugates have also demonstrated success in delivering therapeutics to cells. These therapeutic applications are the regulation of gene expression or delivery of gene therapies. One of the earliest demonstrations of using QD-DNA conjugates to regulate gene expression was reported in 2006.[80,103] Plasmid DNA, coded for enhanced green fluorescent protein (EGFP) expression, was covalently attached to QDs using amine–thiol reactive linkers. After cellular internalization, delivery of the plasmid to the nucleus was tracked by monitoring the QD fluorescence signal over time. Simultaneous time-dependent monitoring of the GFP signal allows confirmation of successful delivery and expression of the plasmid in the nucleus.

Successful siRNA-mediated gene silencing has been reported using QD-siRNA conjugates. Derfus et al. produced QDs with targeting F3 peptides and siRNA against EGFP covalently attached using thiol–amine reactive linkers.[78] The ability of these siRNA delivery vehicles to escape the endosome is a limiting factor for their usefulness. To promote endosomal escape, cationic liposomes were incubated with cells having already internalized the QD-siRNA conjugates. These liposomes were internalized by new endosomes, which then fused with the QD-siRNA–containing endosomes. The acidic environment induced osmotic lysis, resulting in release of the trapped QD-siRNA conjugates. On endosomal escape, mRNA homologous to the siRNA was degraded and EGFP knockdown was observed. Other genes have been silenced successfully with similar design strategies.[78–80]

15.7 Quantum dot drug delivery systems for cancer therapy

Quantum Dots are designed to perform multiple tasks such as disease diagnosis and delivery of therapeutics, thus serving as a multifunctional (theranostic) nanoparticle system. As a therapeutic delivery system, QDs can be surface loaded with anticancer drugs and targeted to cancer tissue, while QD fluorescence will allow for imaging of cancer tissue.

Theranostic CdSe and CdTe-based QDs have been incorporated into several composite drug delivery systems such as hydrogels,[104,105] silica, polymers,[106,107] or liposomes.[108] Kang et al. reported a multifunctional system in

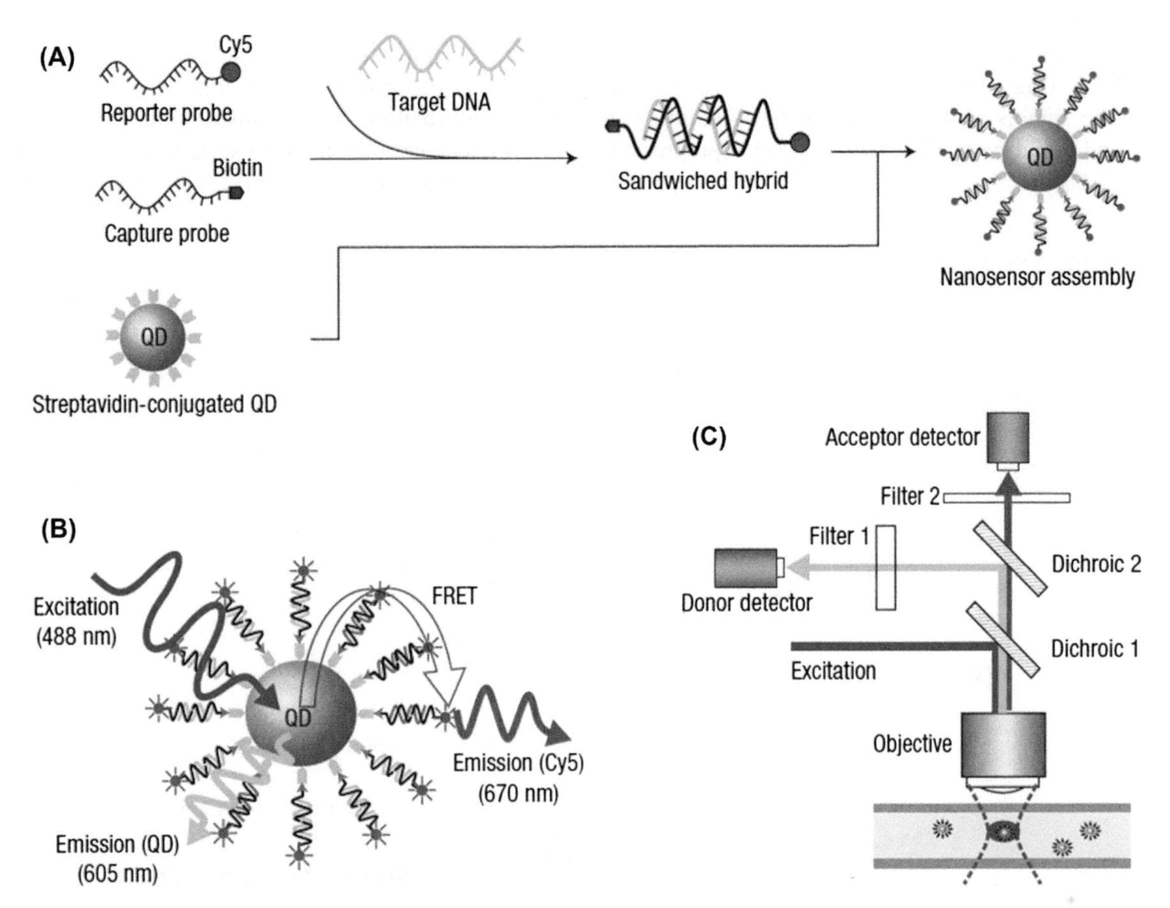

FIGURE 15.15 (A) Scheme showing the formation of the nanosensor by the sandwiching of the target DNA between the capture probe and reporter probe. (B) Florescence emission of the dye-labeled (Cy5) reporter probe by FRET from the QD to Cy5. As FRET is distance dependent unbound reporter probes do not participate in FRET with QD and are not fluorescent (C) Confocal microscopy experimental setup utilizing a continuous-flow of nanosensor to minimize photobleaching. *From Zhang CY, et al., Single-quantum-dot-based DNA nanosensor.* Nat Mater *2005;4(11):826–831.*

which core/shell CdSe/ZnS QDs and paclitaxel (PTX, anticancer drug) were encapsulated in lipid micelles consisting of phosphatidylethanolamine (DSPE) and maleimide-functionalized PEG (Fig. 15.16). The micelle was targeted to cancer cells with antiepidermal growth factor receptor (EGFR, receptor commonly overexpressed in cancer) ABs.[109] The AB was thiolated with Traut's reagent and then reacted with maleimide-functionalized PEG. In the low pH environment of tumor tissue, the micelle structure was destabilized via protonation of amine groups on the phospholipid. This response gives the micelle an activatable release mechanism where the drug would be released when the micelle encounters the low pH environment of tumor tissue. *In vivo* fluorescence imaging results confirmed successful entry and delivery of QD micelles into tumor tissue, LS174T-xenograft BALB/c mice after 24 h. The QD signal remained elevated in tumor tissue with the EGFR-targeted treatment as opposed to nontargeted micelles. It was also observed that the targeted micelles were more effective in reducing tumor growth than nontargeted micelles and free PTX.

While many studies have shown Cd-based QDs when properly coated are nontoxic, over time they do carry some risk of toxicity due to heavy metal ion leakage from the core.[110] Thus, non–heavy metal-containing QDs have been explored as nontoxic alternatives to Cd-containing QDs. InP QDs have been shown to be less toxic than Cd-containing QDs.[111,112] InP QDs can also be tailored to have emissions in the NIR range. Wang et al. encapsulated InP/ZnS QDs and aminoflavone (AF, anticancer compound) in a micelle composed of PEG-PLA block copolymer.[113] First, the InP/ZnS QDs were coated with mercaptoacetic acid through ligand exchange, then carbodiimide coupling (DMF/DMAP) was used to link hydroxyl groups on the polymer (PLA-PEG-maleimide and PLA-PEG-OCH_3) to carboxyl groups on the QD. An anti- (EGFR) nanobody, 7D12 Nb, was employed for targeting and was attached to the micelle by maleimide–thiol reaction (Fig. 15.17A). It was shown that the nanobody increased micelle uptake on EGFR-overexpressing cells and improved its cytotoxic effect in vitro. Both targeted and nontargeted QD micelles inhibited tumor growth in vivo with the targeted treatment performing significantly better at reducing tumor volume (Fig. 15.17B). The presence of the QD allowed the tumors to be imaged by NIR fluorescence in vivo and could be used to monitor tumor progression (Fig. 15.17C).

Nanocarriers that incorporate multiple modes of imaging, i.e., fluorescence and magnetic resonance imaging (MRI) or positron emission tomography, can provide more information on biodistribution and biological fate of the particles than those with only a single modality. Iron oxide NPs (IONP, a T2 contrast agent) or

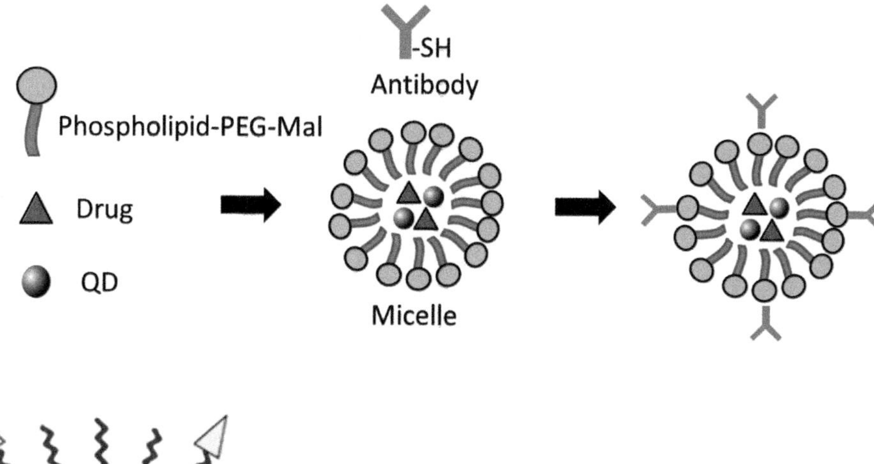

FIGURE 15.16 Synthesis of paclitaxel (PTX) and quantum dot (QD)–loaded lipid micelles. *Based on Kang SJ, et al., Anti-EGFR lipid micellar nanoparticles co-encapsulating quantum dots and paclitaxel for tumor-targeted theranosis.* Nanoscale *2018;**10**(41):19338–19350.*

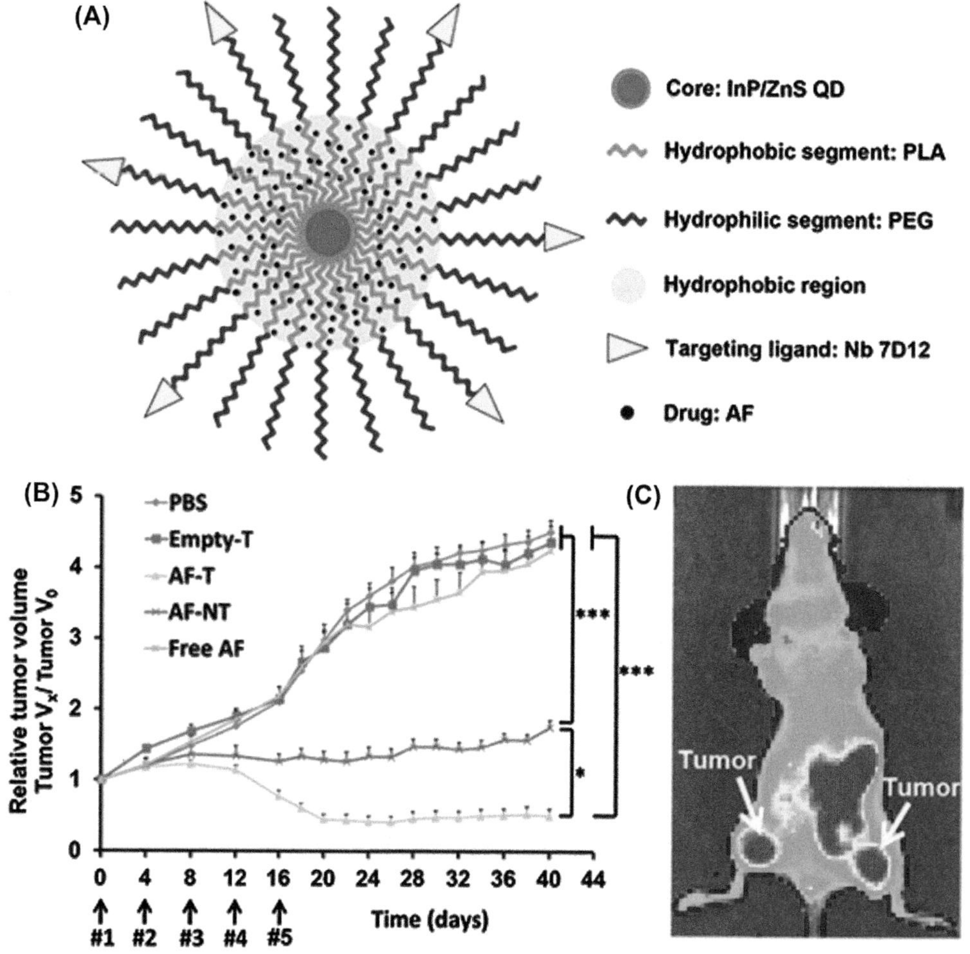

FIGURE 15.17 (A) Design of InP/ZnS quantum dot (QD) micelle drug delivery system. (B) Normalized tumor volumes plotted over time of targeted (T) or nontargeted (NT) QD micelles with anticancer drug (AF). near-infrared imaging of mouse and tumor after injection with targeted QD micelle. *Modified from Wang Y, et al., Quantum-dot-based theranostic micelles conjugated with an anti-EGFR nanobody for triple-negative breast cancer therapy.* ACS Appl Mater Interfaces *2017;**9**(36):30297–30305.*

gadolinium ions (Gd^{3+}, a T1 contrast agent) can be linked to QDs to provide contrast enhancement for MRI imaging capabilities. QD drug delivery platforms incorporating this can be imaged through both MRI and QD fluorescence. MRI is advantageous as it is more tissue penetrating than fluorescence, which makes it better for in vivo imaging, whereas fluorescence is better for in vitro cellular imaging or histological studies. Ye et al. used a biodegradable polymer, poly(lactic-co-glycolic acid) (PLGA), to link ZnS:Mn QDs to IONPs and busulfan (cancer therapeutic) in an oil-in-water emulsion (Fig. 15.18 top).[114] First, oleate-stabilized IONPs were mixed with a solution of decanethiol-capped ZnS:Mn QDs in dichloromethane (DCM). PLGA (15 kDa MW) was then added to the particles in DCM which was mixed with an aqueous solution (1:20 oil/water ratio) of poly lactic acid (PLA) under sonication to form an emulsion. The oil was then evaporated, and the particles were purified by dialysis. The QD-IONP system could be tracked by fluorescence in vitro. Darker contrast appeared in the liver (7 minutes post injection), confirming accumulation of these particles in the animal model (Fig. 15.18 bottom).

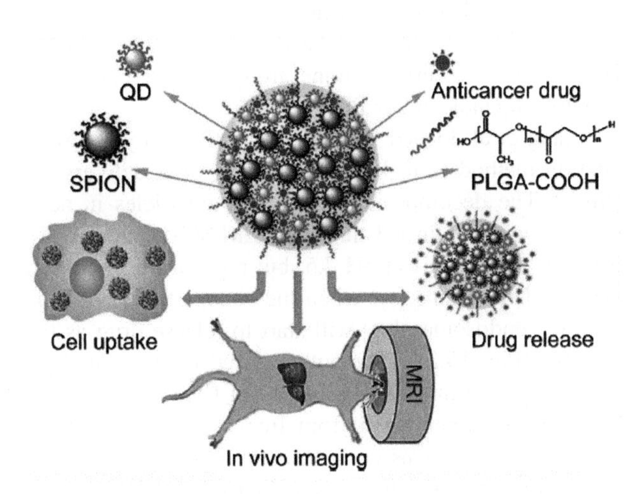

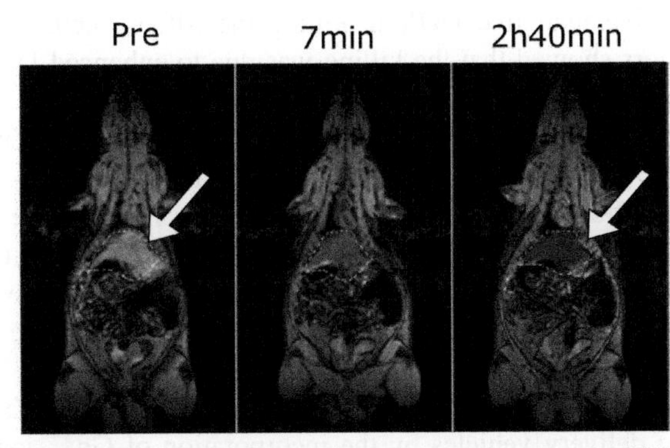

FIGURE 15.18 Scheme showing the applications of quantum dot (QD)–iron oxide nanoparticles and T_2*-weighted in vivo MR images of a rat before, 7min after, and 2h 40 min after injection of QD-IONPs. *Modified from Ye F, et al., Biodegradable polymeric vesicles containing magnetic nanoparticles, quantum dots and anticancer drugs for drug delivery and imaging.* Biomaterials *2014;**35**(12):3885–3894.*

15.7.1 Activatable quantum dot drug delivery systems

Drug delivery systems that incorporate stimuli responsive or "activatable" QDs, where QD fluorescence is altered by a stimulus such as the presence of a biomolecule or change in pH, can provide additional information on the drug delivery event. Activatable drug release can help maximize the bioavailability of a therapeutic by minimizing premature drug release.

Multimodal activatable QDs have been synthesized by Santra et al. with folic acid (FA) acting as a targeting ligand and quencher for QD fluorescence.[115] First, a microemulsion was used to synthesize CdS:Mn/ZnS QDs. FA was bound to NAC using EDC chemistry. The FA-NAC was attached to the QD via a disulfide bond. FA was able to quench QD fluorescence emission by transferring electrons to the excited QD. The QD fluorescence can be restored ("OFF" to "ON") by cleaving the disulfide bond connecting FA to the QD. When the QD comes in contact with GSH (antioxidant), it is able to reductively cleave the disulfide bond (Fig. 15.19).[116–118] An anticancer drug (SF-1-046, STAT3 inhibitor) is also released on activation because it too is attached to the QD via disulfide bond. With this design, the QD releases the drug after interacting with GSH, and it is also able to report on the drug delivery event through increased fluorescence. Utilizing GSH as an activator for NP drug delivery systems is attractive as some cancer types have high concentrations of GSH in their cytosol.[119] This QD was attached to an IONP to give the ability of MRI imaging.

Zinc oxide (ZnO) is generally regarded as safe (GRAS) by the United States Food and Drug Administration and is used in many foods and cosmetics. ZnO QDs can be synthesized in large-scale economically when compared with other nanomaterials.[120] For these reasons, ZnO QDs have great potential for use in commercial biomedical applications. The increased solubility of ZnO QDs in slightly acidic environment (pH 5.0) can be exploited for use in activatable drug delivery. One of the hallmarks of cancers is decreased pH of the tumor microenvironment. This acidic environment can be used to activate or dissolve ZnO-based drug carriers, thereby releasing the bound drug where it can kill the cancer. On dissolution in microenvironment, released zinc ions have also been demonstrated to induce cytotoxic effect. Studies have shown ZnO QDs themselves can be cytotoxic to some cultured malignant cells.[121,122] The release of zinc ions from ZnO QDs has been proposed to be used as a mechanism of killing for cancer treatment.[123] High concentrations of free zinc ions can bind to DNA changing its conformation and potentially disrupting

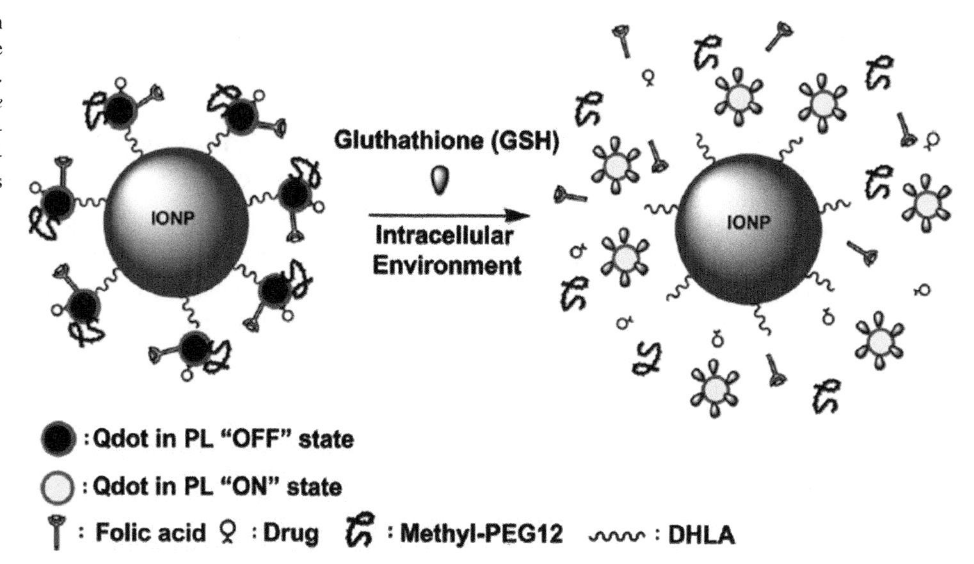

FIGURE 15.19 Scheme of an activatable quantum dot–iron oxide nanoparticle drug delivery platform. *From Mitra RN, et al., An activatable multimodal/multifunctional nanoprobe for direct imaging of intracellular drug delivery.* Biomaterials *2012;**33**(5):1500–1508.*

its transcription.[124,125] ZnO QDs have also been shown to generate damaging ROS as well as cause cell membrane damage (Fig. 15.20). These intrinsic properties of ZnO QDs have the potential to work synergistically to enhance the activity of bound therapeutics.[122] ROS generation can make the cancer cells more sensitive to chemotherapy, and membrane disruption could enhance the bioavailability of therapeutics.[126]

One of the most widely used methods of preparing ZnO-drug conjugates exploits the high reactivity of surface Zn to bind to functional groups such as ketone and alcohols.[127,128] This method involves the simple mixing of ZnO QDs with the drug and does not involve any complex cross-linking reagents. Drugs attached in this way are rapidly released when the ZnO QD dissolves, providing an activatable release mechanism. ZnO QD-drug conjugates have been synthesized with doxorubicin (DOX),[129–139] tangeretin140, paclitaxel,[141] and others[122,142] to make pH-responsive drug delivery vehicles. A protective shell of silica (SiO_2) is commonly added to the ZnO QDs before drug loading. This shell increases the stability of the QDs and can also provide functional groups (such as amine) for further derivatization. Amine-derivatized silane, (3-aminopropyl)triethoxysilane (APTES), is often used to provide reactive surface amine groups for the coupling of targeting ligands and/or PEG.

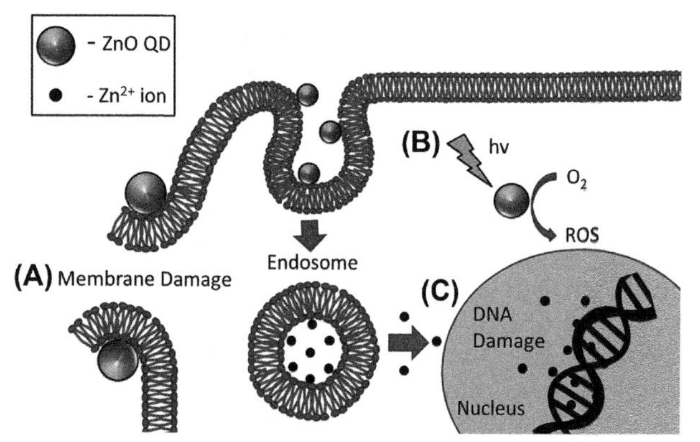

FIGURE 15.20 Scheme showing the different modes of action ZnO quantum dots can take to damage cells: (A) membrane damage, (B) reactive oxygen species (ROS) production, and (C) Zn^{2+} ion release.

Liang et al. loaded ZnO QDs with DOX by a coprecipitation method to make an activatable drug delivery system.[132] The decomposition of the nanoparticles in acidic solution was confirmed through TEM/SEM analysis. The particles were stable at pH 7.5, but rapidly decomposed at pH 5.0. This means that when the nanoparticles are in the acidified endosome, they will start to release drug as they dissolve (Fig. 15.21). The authors used flow cytometry to show increased intracellular uptake of DOX from the ZnO QD-DOX treatment than from free DOX. The increased delivery of DOX was confirmed through MTT (cell proliferation) assay which showed ZnO QD-DOX was more effective than free DOX at killing the MCF-7 cells. The authors showed that the killing was due to enhanced DOX delivery because the ZnO particles themselves had no toxicity on MCF-7 cells at the concentrations tested. ZnO QD-DOX was also effective at killing resistant MCF-7R cells where free DOX had no effect. This may be due to the high localized concentration of DOX delivered by the QDs. Zhu et al. built on this system by showing the synergistic anticancer activity of ZnO QDs with DOX due to ROS generation from the ZnO.[138]

Multimodal imaging capability can be extended to ZnO drug delivery vehicles by the incorporation of Gd^{3+} ions. Polymer-coated ZnO QDs were synthesized with excess carboxyl groups, and they were mixed with Gd^{3+} and DOX to create a fluorescence (600–700 nm) and MRI trackable pH-responsive drug delivery vehicle.[133] The authors

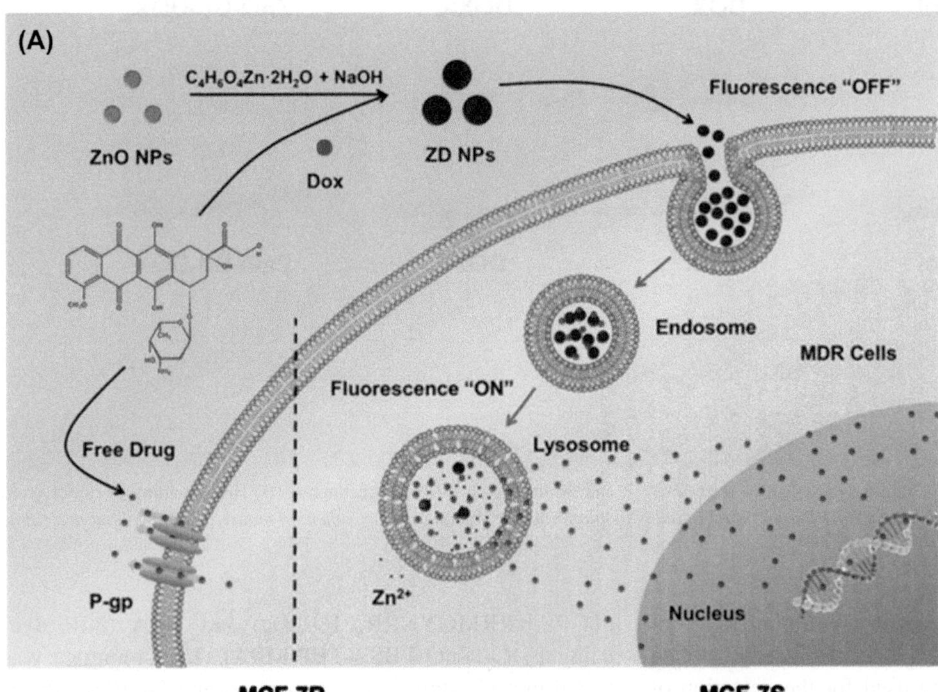

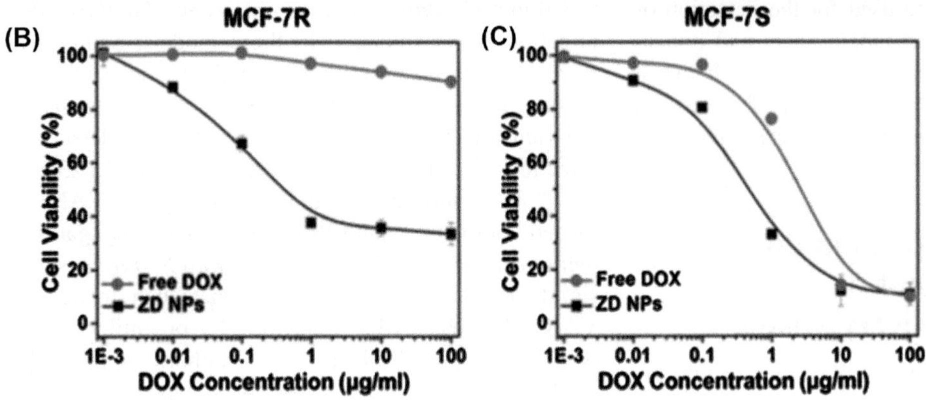

FIGURE 15.21 (A) Scheme showing the pH-induced delivery of doxorubicin (DOX) by ZnO QDs compared to free DOX. In vitro cytotoxicity of free DOX and DOX loaded ZnO QDs (ZD NPs) on (B) drug resistant cells (MCF-7R) and (C) drug sensitive cells (MCF-7S). *Modified from Liu J, et al., Zinc oxide nanoparticles as adjuvant to facilitate doxorubicin intracellular accumulation and visualize pH-responsive release for overcoming drug resistance. Mol Pharm 2016;**13**(5):1723–1730.*

reported significant antitumor activity of the particles on BxPC-3 tumor-bearing nude mice. Fig. 15.22A shows an increase in tumor size for the control, whereas no change in tumor size was observed for DOX, Doxil, or ZnO-Gd-DOX QD treatments. Hematoxylin and eosin (H&E) staining of the tumor showed that QD-DOX treatment damaged the tumor cells more severely than DOX or Doxil treatments, making it a more effective treatment (Fig. 15.22B).

15.8 Imaging of bacteria using fluorescent quantum dots

The photoluminescent properties of QDs can be employed to detect bacteria both *in vitro* and *in vivo*. Detection of bacteria is important to identify contaminated food or water and to diagnose infections. For bacterial detection, QDs are generally conjugated to a molecule such as an AB or sugar moiety in order to provide bacterial recognition. Many different kinds of QDs have been used for bacterial detection such as CdSe/ZnS,[143] CdSe,[144] CQDs,[145] and ZnO.[146]

It is possible to reliably detect low levels of bacterial cells in a sample using QDs due to their high QY in comparison with organic dyes. Hahn et al. used biotinylated anti-*Escherichia coli* O157:H7 ABs that specifically bind to the outer membrane of *E. coli* O157:H7 cells. Bacterial cells were then labeled with streptavidin-conjugated CdSe/ZnS QDs. The authors showed that streptavidin-QD labeling showed around two orders of magnitude more sensitive detection of bacterial cells than streptavidin-FITC (organic dye). The QDs were even capable of detecting a single pathogenic cell.[143]

QDs can also be used for the quantification of bacteria. CdSe-thioglycolic acid (TGA) QDs were coupled to *Salmonella typhimurium* membrane proteins using EDC coupling chemistry. QD fluorescence intensity responded

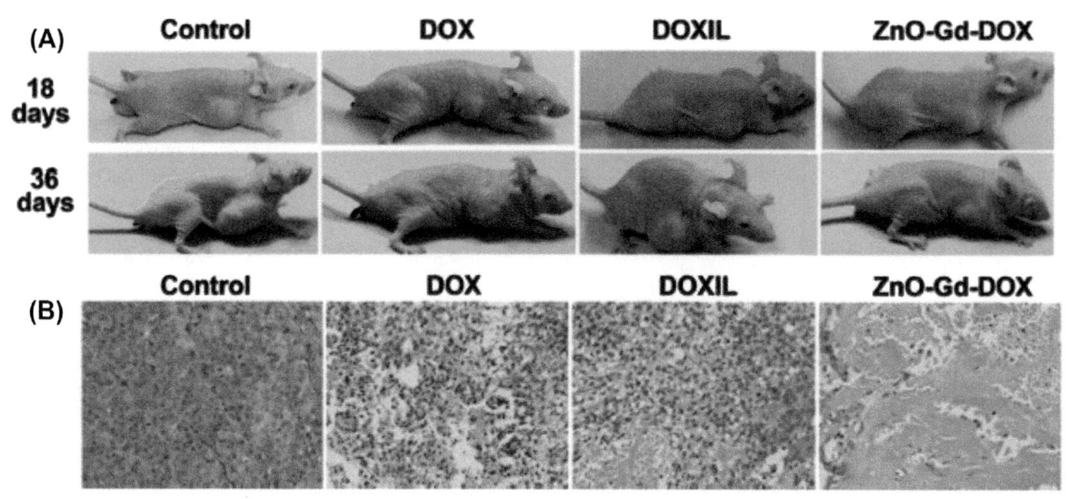

FIGURE 15.22 (A) Images of BxPC-3 tumor-bearing nude mice after 18 and 36 days with different treatments. (B) H&E staining of tumor cross sections after 36 days treatment. *Modified from Ye DX, et al., ZnO-based Nanoplatforms for labeling and treatment of mouse tumors without detectable toxic Side effects.* ACS Nano *2016;**10**(4):4294–4300.*

linearly to bacterial counts over a concentration range of 10^2–10^6 CFU/mL of bacteria.[144] Lai et al. demonstrated that mannose CQDs can also be used for the detection of bacteria in samples of tap water, apple juice, and human urine. The authors employed specific interaction between mannose and *E. coli* bacterial protein FimH for the bacterial labeling and showed that this QD probe has the potential to be used in clinical applications.[145]

15.9 Application of quantum dots as an antimicrobial agent or antimicrobial delivery system

Several studies have demonstrated applications of QDs as antibacterial agents such as CdTe,[147,148] ZnSe/ZnS,[149] and ZnO.[150,151] Chen et al. also examined ZnO QDs as an antimicrobial delivery system.[146] Although ROS generation is shown to play a role in antibacterial mechanisms of QDs, the comprehensive understanding of interactions between QDs and bacteria remains unclear.[147,148,151]

It has been also reported that certain QDs when conjugated to antibiotics are able to enhance the efficacy of the antibiotic. The antibiotic ceftriaxone (Rocephin) when conjugated to CdTe QDs demonstrated a synergistic effect of killing *E. coli*.[152] Using EDC coupling chemistry, Jijie et al. conjugated ampicillin (-carboxyl) to amine-functionalized CQDs. The conjugate was significantly more effective in killing *E. coli* than ampicillin alone. Authors suggested that the increased efficacy was likely due to the cooperative antibacterial activity of QD-ampicillin as compared with free antibiotic.[153]

For diagnostic applications, Chen et al. synthesized ZnO QDs coated with BSA and then functionalized with a cationic antimicrobial peptide (PEP) $UBI_{29\text{-}41}$ (TGRAKRRMQYNRR, 1693Da) and MPA (NIR dye) using EDC (ZnO@BSA-PEP-MPA). The conjugate was tested in both *Staphylococcus aureus* and *Bacillus subtilis* infection mouse models. In these models, *S. aureus* or *B. subtilis* suspensions were injected into the right axillary fossa, followed by exposure to the QD conjugates through tail-vein injection. QD fluorescence allowed detection of infection site after 6 h of treatment (Fig. 15.23B and C).[146] In a subsequent study, vancomycin (VAN) was loaded onto the ZnO-PEP-MPA QD conjugates for theranostic activity. Mice infected with *S. aureus* showed significant reduction in skin lesions when treated with VAN@ZnO-PEP-MPA than the QD or antibiotic alone (Fig. 15.23D).[146] Thus, the authors suggest that ZnO@BSA-PEP-MPA serves as a nanocarrier for the targeted delivery of VAN.

15.10 Conclusions and perspective

QD composition along with a number of physical and chemical properties is important to consider when selecting them for biomedical applications. Other than QD composition, particle size, surface charge, surface chemistry, and targeting ligands must be carefully selected to make them suitable for use in biological systems. Selection of appropriate coupling chemistry for bioconjugation is important for efficient loading, stability, and orientation of target molecules such as ABs, proteins, antibiotics, and anticancer drugs onto the QD surface.

For biomedical applications, QDs offer many advantages over traditional organic fluorescent dyes for sensitive imaging, target detection, targeted delivery of therapeutics, as well as monitoring of therapy due to their high QY, photostability, long lifetime, and large Stokes' shift

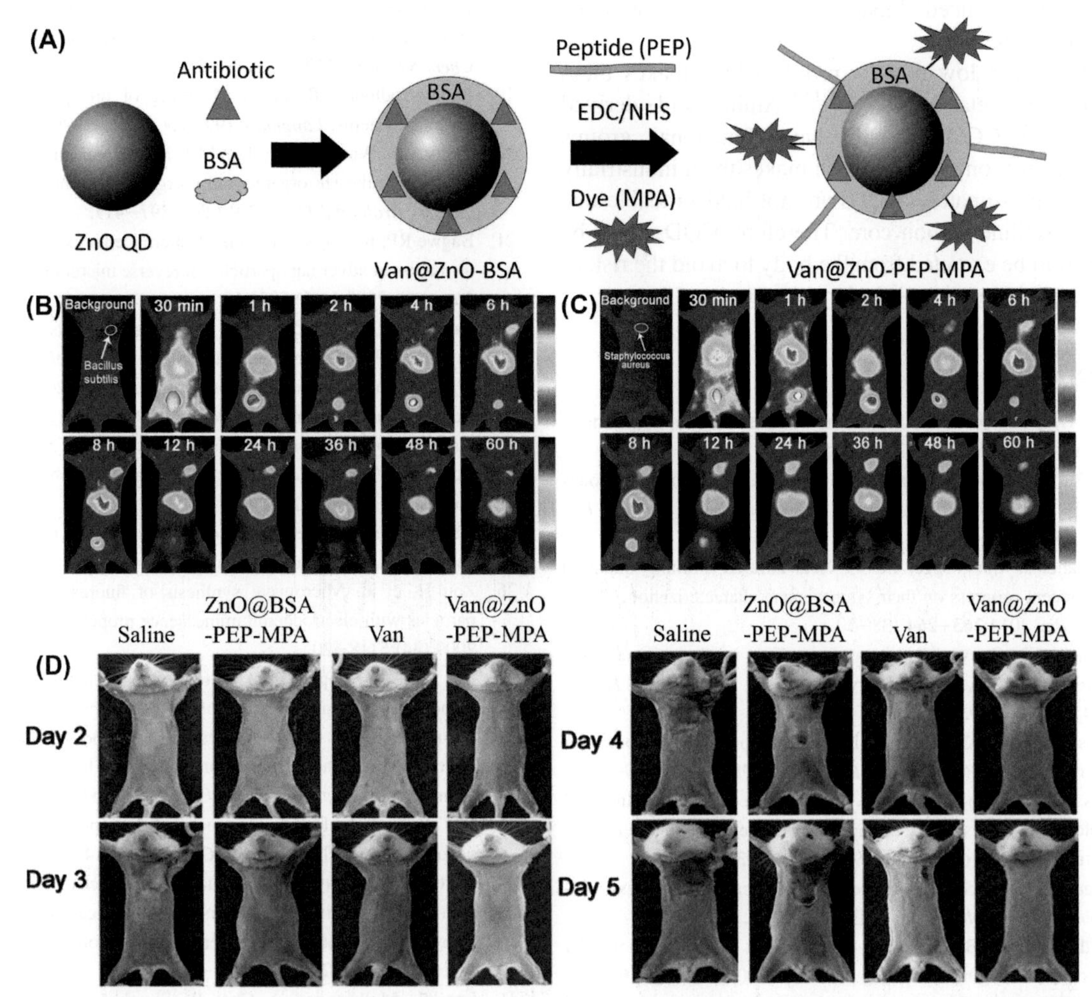

FIGURE 15.23 Figure shows *in vivo* detection and treatment of bacterial infection by ZnO QD conjugate. Synthesis of antibiotic-ZnO QD complex (A), *in vivo* detection of *Bacillus subtilis* (B) and *Staphylococcus aureus* (C) site of infection by ZnO QD conjugate are shown. (D) Reduction of skin lesion in *S. aureus* infection mouse model on treatment with antibiotic–QD complex compared with QD conjugate or antibiotic alone. *Modified from Chen H, et al., Versatile antimicrobial peptide-based ZnO quantum dots for in vivo bacteria diagnosis and treatment with high specificity.* Biomaterials *2015;**53**:532–544.*

(separation of excitation and emission wavelengths). Because of large surface-to-volume ratio, QDs serve as an excellent nanoscale payload carrier for therapeutic cargoes.

Several reports have shown that the capability of QDs to improve the bioavailability therapeutics at the target site as well synergistic effect on therapeutic efficacy. Many of these applications rely on careful control of physiochemical properties of surface-modified QD that allows for recognition of cell-specific surface receptor proteins.

For successful clinical applications of QD nanotechnology as a drug delivery system, there are many questions that must be answered. Despite careful QD surface engineering, only small fractions of them are able to reach the target site.[154] This demands further advancement in QD design that will avoid their premature removal from the circulatory system by the reticuloendothelial system followed by their excretion through liver or kidney. In general, particles that have extended circulation times can draw additional benefit from the EPR effect which helps increase accumulation at the tumor site.[155] The incorporation of PEG to the surface of NP systems can help to minimize nonspecific interactions and serum protein adsorption that promote circulatory clearance via opsonisation.[156] Detailed study of QD interactions with biological systems leading to their uptake, mobility, clearance, and degradation will allow for gaining new knowledge based on which more efficient QD systems can be developed.

QD toxicity and accumulation in off-target tissue also must be addressed.[157] QDs containing heavy-metals, despite their biocompatible coating, may not be suitable for in vivo applications due to high risk of toxic metal ion release. However, ex vivo use of QDs for diagnostic purposes could be feasible. ZnO-based QDs are attractive as they can be eventually degraded to Zn^{2+} ions, entering to the metabolic pool. Ultrasmall size QDs (<10 nm size) coated with PEGylated silica (SiO_2)[158] will have the advantage of reduced bioaccumulation and could be excreted from the body.

CQDs have a low toxicity profile which makes them attractive over metal-based QDs.[159] Amino acid–derived as-synthesized CQDs usually have functional groups available for bioconjugation which makes them industrially attractive. Unfortunately, CQDs are not biodegradable due to their crystalline carbon core. Therefore, CQDs must be engineered to be excreted from the body to avoid the risk of tissue accumulation, in particular the nontarget tissue.

References

1. Bera D, et al. Quantum dots and their multimodal applications: a review. *Materials* 2010;**3**:2260–345.
2. Kwak J, et al. High-power genuine ultraviolet light-emitting diodes based on colloidal nanocrystal quantum dots. *Nano Lett* 2015;**15**(6):3793–9.
3. Pichaandi J, van Veggel FCJM. Near-infrared emitting quantum dots: recent progress on their synthesis and characterization. *Coord Chem Rev* 2014;**263–264**:138–50.
4. Ekimov AI, O AA. Quantum size effect in three-dimensional microscopic semiconductor crystals. *JETP Lett (Engl Transl)* 1981;**34**(6):345–9.
5. Efros AL, Efros AL. Interband light absorption in a semiconductor sphere. *Fiz Tekh Poluprovodn (Leningrad)* 1982;**16**(7):1209–14.
6. Brus LE. Electron-electron and electron-hole interactions in small semiconductor crystallites: the size dependence of the lowest excited electronic state. *J Chem Phys* 1984;**80**(9):4403–9.
7. Lippa A. *Fluorescence immunoassay involving energy transfer between two fluorophores.* USA: Ethigen Corp.; 1987. p. 27.
8. Smith AM, et al. Bioconjugated quantum dots for in vivo molecular and cellular imaging. *Adv Drug Deliv Rev* 2008;**60**(11):1226–40.
9. Wu P, Yan X-P. Doped quantum dots for chemo/biosensing and bioimaging. *Chem Soc Rev* 2013;**42**(12):5489–521.
10. Sun L-W, et al. Lanthanum-doped ZnO quantum dots with greatly enhanced fluorescent quantum yield. *J Mater Chem* 2012;**22**(17):8221–7.
11. Bol AA, Meijerink A. Long-lived Mn2+ emission in nanocrystalline ZnS:Mn2+. *Phys Rev B* 1998;**58**(24):R15997–6000.
12. Neus GB, et al. *The reactivity of colloidal inorganic nanoparticles.* 2012.
13. Lee W, et al. An effective oxidation approach for luminescence enhancement in CdS quantum dots by H_2O_2. *Nanoscale Res Lett* 2012;**7**(1):672.
14. Vela J, et al. Effect of shell thickness and composition on blinking suppression and the blinking mechanism in 'giant' CdSe/CdS nanocrystal quantum dots. *J Biophot* 2010;**3**(10–11):706–17.
15. Talapin DV, et al. CdSe/CdS/ZnS and CdSe/ZnSe/ZnS Core--Shell–Shell nanocrystals. *J Phys Chem B* 2004;**108**(49):18826–31.
16. Murray CB, Norris DJ, Bawendi MG. Synthesis and characterization of nearly monodisperse CdE (E = sulfur, selenium, tellurium) semiconductor nanocrystallites. *J Am Chem Soc* 1993;**115**(19):8706–15.
17. Bailey RE, Smith AM, Nie S. Quantum dots in biology and medicine. *Physica E* 2004;**25**(1):1–12.
18. Kortan AR, et al. Nucleation and growth of CdSe on ZnS quantum crystallite seeds, and vice versa, in inverse micelle media. *J Am Chem Soc* 1990;**112**(4):1327–32.
19. Bandyopadhyaya R, et al. Modeling of precipitation in reverse micellar systems. *Langmuir* 1997;**13**(14):3610–20.
20. Malik MA, Wani MY, Hashim MA. Microemulsion method: a novel route to synthesize organic and inorganic nanomaterials: 1st Nano Update. *Arabian J Chem* 2012;**5**(4):397–417.
21. Bagwe RP, Khilar KC. Effects of intermicellar exchange rate on the formation of silver nanoparticles in reverse microemulsions of AOT. *Langmuir* 2000;**16**(3):905–10.
22. Samanta A, Deng Z, Liu Y. Aqueous synthesis of glutathione-capped CdTe/CdS/ZnS and CdTe/CdSe/ZnS core/shell/shell nanocrystal heterostructures. *Langmuir* 2012;**28**(21):8205–15.
23. Bera D, et al. Photoluminescence of ZnO quantum dots produced by a sol-gel process. *Opt Mater* 2008;**30**(8):1233–9.
24. Bourlinos AB, et al. Surface functionalized carbogenic quantum dots. *Small* 2008;**4**(4):455–8.
25. Yang Z, et al. Nitrogen-doped, carbon-rich, highly photoluminescent carbon dots from ammonium citrate. *Nanoscale* 2014;**6**(3):1890–5.
26. Zhu H, et al. Microwave synthesis of fluorescent carbon nanoparticles with electrochemiluminescence properties. *Chem Commun* 2009;(34):5118–20.
27. Liu X, et al. Simple approach to synthesize amino-functionalized carbon dots by carbonization of chitosan. *Sci Rep* 2016;**6**:31100.
28. Chiu S-H, et al. Rapid fabrication of carbon quantum dots as multifunctional nanovehicles for dual-modal targeted imaging and chemotherapy. *Acta Biomater* 2016;**46**:151–64.
29. Zhu Y-J, Chen F. Microwave-assisted preparation of inorganic nanostructures in liquid phase. *Chem Rev* 2014;**114**(12):6462–555.
30. Staros JV. N-hydroxysulfosuccinimide active esters: bis(N-hydroxysulfosuccinimide) esters of two dicarboxylic acids are hydrophilic, membrane-impermeant, protein cross-linkers. *Biochemistry* 1982;**21**(17):3950–5.
31. Lao UL, Mulchandani A, Chen W. Simple conjugation and purification of quantum dot-antibody complexes using a thermally responsive elastin-protein L scaffold as immunofluorescent agents. *J Am Chem Soc* 2006;**128**(46):14756–7.
32. Goldman ER, et al. Conjugation of luminescent quantum dots with antibodies using an engineered adaptor protein to provide new reagents for fluoroimmunoassays. *Anal Chem* 2002;**74**(4):841–7.
33. Sapsford KE, et al. Biosensing with luminescent semiconductor quantum dots. *Sensors* 2006;**6**(8):925–53.
34. Medintz IL, et al. Quantum dot bioconjugates for imaging, labelling and sensing. *Nat Mater* 2005;**4**(6):435–46.
35. Han HS, et al. Quantum dot/antibody conjugates for in vivo cytometric imaging in mice. *Proc Natl Acad Sci USA* 2015;**112**(5):1350–5.
36. Fernandez-Arguelles MT, et al. Simple bio-conjugation of polymer-coated quantum dots with antibodies for fluorescence-based immunoassays. *Analyst* 2008;**133**(4):444–7.
37. Rakovich TY, et al. Highly sensitive single domain antibody-quantum dot conjugates for detection of HER2 biomarker in lung and breast cancer cells. *ACS Nano* 2014;**8**(6):5682–95.
38. Tiwari DK, et al. Synthesis and characterization of anti-HER2 antibody conjugated CdSe/CdZnS quantum dots for fluorescence imaging of breast cancer cells. *Sensors* 2009;**9**(11):9332–54.

39. Wu YT, et al. Quantum dot-based FRET immunoassay for HER2 using ultrasmall affinity proteins. *Small* 2018;**14**(35).
40. Liu JL, et al. Conjugation of biotin-coated luminescent quantum dots with single domain antibody-rhizavidin fusions. *Biotechnol Rep* 2016;**10**:56–65.
41. Umakoshi T, et al. Quantum-dot antibody conjugation visualized at the single-molecule scale with high-speed atomic force microscopy. *Colloids Surf., B* 2018;**167**:267–74.
42. Pathak S, Davidson MC, Silva GA. Characterization of the functional binding properties of antibody conjugated quantum dots. *Nano Lett* 2007;**7**(7):1839–45.
43. Resch-Genger U, et al. Quantum dots versus organic dyes as fluorescent labels. *Nat Methods* 2008;**5**:763.
44. Liu Y-S, et al. pH-sensitive photoluminescence of CdSe/ZnSe/ZnS quantum dots in human ovarian cancer cells. *J Phys Chem C* 2007;**111**(7):2872–8.
45. Huang X, Li W, He W. pH tunable turn on and turn off quantum dots conjugated with poly(2-dialkylamino)ethyl methacrylate). *Adv Mater Res* 2014:998–9 (Advances in Applied Sciences, Engineering and Technology II): pp. 75–78, 5 pp.
46. Medintz IL, et al. Quantum-dot/dopamine bioconjugates function as redox coupled assemblies for in vitro and intracellular pH sensing. *Nat Mater* 2010;**9**:676.
47. Ji X, et al. On the pH-dependent quenching of quantum dot photoluminescence by redox active dopamine. *J Am Chem Soc* 2012;**134**(13):6006–17.
48. Maria Jose R-R, Elizabeth AHH. pH sensitive quantum dot–anthraquinone nanoconjugates. *Nanotechnology* 2014;**25**(19):195501.
49. Snee PT, et al. A ratiometric CdSe/ZnS nanocrystal pH sensor. *J Am Chem Soc* 2006;**128**(41):13320–1.
50. Kurabayashi T, et al. CdSe/ZnS quantum dots conjugated with a fluorescein derivative: a FRET-based pH sensor for physiological alkaline conditions. *Anal Sci* 2014;**30**(5):545–50.
51. Ast S, Rutledge PJ, Todd MH. pH-Responsive quantum dots (RQDs) that combine a fluorescent nanoparticle with a pH-sensitive dye. *Phys Chem Chem Phys* 2014;**16**(46):25255–7.
52. Paek K, et al. Fluorescent and pH-responsive diblock copolymer-coated core-shell CdSe/ZnS particles for a color-displaying, ratiometric pH sensor. *Chem Commun* 2011;**47**(37):10272–4.
53. Dennis AM, et al. Quantum dot-fluorescent protein FRET probes for sensing intracellular pH. *ACS Nano* 2012;**6**(4):2917–24.
54. Pratiwi FW, et al. Construction of single fluorophore ratiometric pH sensors using dual-emission Mn2+-doped quantum dots. *Biosens Bioelectron* 2016;**84**:133–40.
55. Yuan J, Guo W, Wang E. Utilizing a CdTe quantum dots-enzyme hybrid system for the determination of both phenolic compounds and hydrogen peroxide. *Anal Chem* 2008;**80**(4):1141–5.
56. Bhattacharya S, et al. Detection of reactive oxygen species by a carbon-dot-ascorbic acid hydrogel. *Anal Chem* 2017;**89**(1):830–6.
57. Huang XY, et al. Quantum dot-based FRET for sensitive determination of hydrogen peroxide and glucose using tyramide reaction. *Talanta* 2013;**106**:79–84.
58. Adegoke O, Khene S, Nyokong T. Fluorescence "switch on" of conjugates of CdTe@ZnS quantum dots with Al, Ni and Zn tetraamino-phthalocyanines by hydrogen peroxide: characterization and applications as luminescent nanosensors. *J Fluoresc* 2013;**23**(5):963–74.
59. Liu R, et al. Design of a new near-infrared ratiometric fluorescent nanoprobe for real-time imaging of superoxide anions and hydroxyl radicals in live cells and in situ tracing of the inflammation process in vivo. *Anal Chem* 2018;**90**(7):4452–60.
60. Wang J, et al. Diethyldithiocarbamate functionalized CdSe/CdS quantum dots as a fluorescent probe for copper ion detection. *Spectrochim Acta A Mol Biomol Spectrosc* 2011;**81**(1):178–83.
61. Liao S, et al. Novel S, N-doped carbon quantum dot-based "off-on" fluorescent sensor for silver ion and cysteine. *Talanta* 2018;**180**:300–8.
62. Ma Q, et al. A novel carboxymethyl chitosan-quantum dot-based intracellular probe for Zn^{2+} ion sensing in prostate cancer cells. *Acta Biomater* 2014;**10**(2):868–74.
63. Ren H-B, et al. Silica-coated S2–enriched manganese-doped ZnS quantum dots as a photoluminescence probe for imaging intracellular Zn^{2+} ions. *Anal Chem* 2011;**83**(21):8239–44.
64. Ruedas-Rama MJ, Hall EAH. Azamacrocycle activated quantum dot for zinc ion detection. *Anal Chem* 2008;**80**(21):8260–8.
65. Wang G, Li Z, Ma N. Next-generation DNA-functionalized quantum dots as biological sensors. *ACS Chem Biol* 2018;**13**(7):1705–13.
66. Ebrahim S, et al. CdTe quantum dots as a novel biosensor for *Serratia marcescens* and Lipopolysaccharide. *Spectrochim Acta, Part A* 2015;**150**:212–9.
67. Zhu G, Yang K, Zhang C-y. A single quantum dot-based biosensor for telomerase assay. *Chem Commun* 2015;**51**(31):6808–11.
68. Wu P, et al. Analyte-activable probe for protease based on cytochrome C-capped Mn: ZnS quantum dots. *Anal Chem* 2014;**86**(20):10078–83.
69. Zhou Z-M, Yu Y, Zhao Y-D. A new strategy for the detection of adenosine triphosphate by aptamer/quantum dot biosensor based on chemiluminescence resonance energy transfer. *Analyst* 2012;**137**(18):4262–6.
70. Yang C, et al. Quantum-dot-based biosensor for simultaneous detection of biomarker and therapeutic drug: first steps toward an assay for quantitative pharmacology. *Analyst* 2012;**137**(5):1205–9.
71. Geissler D, et al. Quantum dot biosensors for ultrasensitive multiplexed diagnostics. *Angew Chem Int Ed* 2010;**49**(8):1396–401. S1396/1-S1396/9.
72. Stanisavljevic M, et al. Quantum dots-fluorescence resonance energy transfer-based nanosensors and their application. *Biosens Bioelectron* 2015;**74**:562–74.
73. Bakalova R, Zhelev Z, Ohba H. Quantum dots open new trends in biosensor evolution. *Sens Lett* 2006;**4**(4):452–4.
74. Yamagata M, et al. The contribution of lactic acid to acidification of tumors: studies of variant cells lacking lactate dehydrogenase. *Br J Canc* 1998;**77**(11):1726–31.
75. Jaehde E, et al. pH in human tumor xenografts and transplanted rat tumors: effect of insulin, inorganic phosphate, and m-iodobenzylguanidine. *Cancer Res* 1992;**52**(22):6209–15.
76. Jin T, et al. A quantum dot-based ratiometric pH sensor. *Chem Commun* 2010;**46**(14):2408–10.
77. Castanho MARB, Prieto MJE. Fluorescence quenching data interpretation in biological systems: the use of microscopic models for data analysis and interpretation of complex systems. *Biochim Biophys Acta Biomembr* 1998;**1373**(1):1–16.
78. Derfus AM, et al. Targeted quantum dot conjugates for siRNA delivery. *Bioconjug Chem* 2007;**18**(5):1391–6.

79. Elbakry A, et al. Layer-by-Layer assembled gold nanoparticles for siRNA delivery. *Nano Lett* 2009;**9**(5):2059–64.
80. Qi L, Gao X. Quantum Dot–Amphipol nanocomplex for intracellular delivery and real-time imaging of siRNA. *ACS Nano* 2008;**2**(7):1403–10.
81. Sapsford KE, et al. Kinetics of metal-affinity driven self-assembly between proteins or peptides and CdSe–ZnS quantum dots. *J Phys Chem C* 2007;**111**(31):11528–38.
82. Medintz IL, et al. A reactive peptidic linker for self-assembling hybrid quantum Dot–DNA bioconjugates. *Nano Lett* 2007;**7**(6):1741–8.
83. Zhou W, et al. Tandem phosphorothioate Modifications for DNA adsorption Strength and polarity control on gold nanoparticles. *ACS Appl Mater Interfaces* 2014;**6**(17):14795–800.
84. Liu C, et al. Aptamer-functionalized CdTe:Zn^{2+} quantum dots for the detection of tomato systemin. *Analytical Methods* 2015;**7**(18):7748–52.
85. Jiang G, et al. Cascaded FRET in conjugated polymer/quantum dot/dye-labeled DNA complexes for DNA hybridization detection. *ACS Nano* 2009;**3**(12):4127–31.
86. Farlow J, et al. Formation of targeted monovalent quantum dots by steric exclusion. *Nat Methods* 2013;**10**:1203.
87. Carion O, et al. Synthesis, encapsulation, purification and coupling of single quantum dots in phospholipid micelles for their use in cellular and in vivo imaging. *Nat Protoc* 2007;**2**:2383.
88. Dubertret B, et al. In vivo imaging of quantum dots encapsulated in phospholipid micelles. *Science* 2002;**298**(5599):1759.
89. Aimé A, et al. Quantum dot lipid oligonucleotide bioconjugates: toward a new anti-micro RNA Nanoplatform. *Bioconjug Chem* 2013;**24**(8):1345–55.
90. Van Lehn RC, et al. Lipid tail protrusions mediate the insertion of nanoparticles into model cell membranes. *Nat Commun* 2014;**5**:4482.
91. Chen AA, et al. Quantum dots to monitor RNAi delivery and improve gene silencing. *Nucleic Acids Res* 2005;**33**(22). p. e190-e190.
92. Nel AE, et al. Understanding biophysicochemical interactions at the nano–bio interface. *Nat Mater* 2009;**8**:543.
93. Algar WR, Krull UJ. Adsorption and hybridization of oligonucleotides on mercaptoacetic acid-capped CdSe/ZnS quantum dots and quantum Dot–Oligonucleotide conjugates. *Langmuir* 2006;**22**(26):11346–52.
94. Chen Y, et al. Manganese oxide-based multifunctionalized mesoporous silica nanoparticles for pH-responsive MRI, ultrasonography and circumvention of MDR in cancer cells. *Biomaterials* 2012;**33**(29):7126–37.
95. D'Agata R, Palladino P, Spoto G. Streptavidin-coated gold nanoparticles: critical role of oligonucleotides on stability and fractal aggregation. *Beilstein J Nanotechnol* 2017;**8**:1–11.
96. Zhang Y, et al. Mapping DNA quantity into electrophoretic mobility through quantum dot nanotethers for high-resolution genetic and epigenetic analysis. *ACS Nano* 2012;**6**(1):858–64.
97. Smith AM, et al. A systematic examination of surface coatings on the optical and chemical properties of semiconductor quantum dots. *Phys Chem Chem Phys* 2006;**8**(33):3895–903.
98. Banerjee A, et al. Quantum dots–DNA bioconjugates: synthesis to applications. *Interface Focus* 2016;**6**(6).
99. Beaune G, et al. Luminescence of polyethylene glycol coated CdSeTe/ZnS and InP/ZnS nanoparticles in the presence of copper cations. *ChemPhysChem* 2011;**12**(12):2247–54.
100. Zhang H, et al. Robust and specific ratiometric biosensing using a copper-free clicked quantum dot–DNA aptamer sensor. *Nanoscale* 2013;**5**(21):10307–15.
101. Zhang CY, et al. Single-quantum-dot-based DNA nanosensor. *Nat Mater* 2005;**4**(11):826–31.
102. Liang R-Q, et al. An oligonucleotide microarray for microRNA expression analysis based on labeling RNA with quantum dot and nanogold probe. *Nucleic Acids Res* 2005;**33**(2). p. e17-e17.
103. Srinivasan C, et al. Labeling and intracellular tracking of functionally active plasmid DNA with semiconductor quantum dots. *Mol Ther* 2006;**14**(2):192–201.
104. Wu W, et al. In-situ immobilization of quantum dots in polysaccharide-based nanogels for integration of optical pH-sensing, tumor cell imaging, and drug delivery. *Biomaterials* 2010;**31**(11):3023–31.
105. Li Z, et al. Quantum dots loaded nanogels for low cytotoxicity, pH-sensitive fluorescence, cell imaging and drug delivery. *Carbohydr Polym* 2015;**121**:477–85.
106. Huang H-K, et al. A novel cancer nanotheranostics system based on quantum dots encapsulated by a polymer-prodrug with controlled release behaviour. *Aust J Chem* 2017;**70**(12):1302–11.
107. Glueckert R, et al. Nanoparticle mediated drug delivery of rolipram to tyrosine kinase B positive cells in the inner ear with targeting peptides and agonistic antibodies. *Front Aging Neurosci* 2015;**7**:1–18.
108. Olerile LD, et al. Near-infrared mediated quantum dots and paclitaxel co-loaded nanostructured lipid carriers for cancer theragnostic. *Colloids Surf B Biointerfaces* 2017;**150**:121–30.
109. Kang SJ, et al. Anti-EGFR lipid micellar nanoparticles co-encapsulating quantum dots and paclitaxel for tumor-targeted theranosis. *Nanoscale* 2018;**10**(41):19338–50.
110. Derfus AM, Chan WCW, Bhatia SN. Probing the cytotoxicity of semiconductor quantum dots. *Nano Letters* 2004;**4**(1):11–8.
111. Chibli H, et al. Cytotoxicity of InP/ZnS quantum dots related to reactive oxygen species generation. *Nanoscale* 2011;**3**(6):2552–9.
112. Brunetti V, et al. InP/ZnS as a safer alternative to CdSe/ZnS core/shell quantum dots: in vitro and in vivo toxicity assessment. *Nanoscale* 2013;**5**(1):307–17.
113. Wang Y, et al. Quantum-dot-based theranostic micelles conjugated with an anti-EGFR nanobody for triple-negative breast cancer therapy. *ACS Appl Mater Interfaces* 2017;**9**(36):30297–305.
114. Ye F, et al. Biodegradable polymeric vesicles containing magnetic nanoparticles, quantum dots and anticancer drugs for drug delivery and imaging. *Biomaterials* 2014;**35**(12):3885–94.
115. Mitra RN, et al. An activatable multimodal/multifunctional nanoprobe for direct imaging of intracellular drug delivery. *Biomaterials* 2012;**33**(5):1500–8.
116. Maxwell T, et al. Non-cytotoxic quantum dot-chitosan nanogel biosensing probe for potential cancer targeting agent. *Nanomaterials* 2015;**5**(4):2359–79.
117. Li Q-L, et al. pH and glutathione dual-responsive dynamic cross-linked supramolecular network on mesoporous silica nanoparticles for controlled anticancer drug release. *ACS Appl Mater Interfaces* 2015;**7**(51):28656–64.
118. Banerjee S, et al. Quantum dot-based OFF/ON probe for detection of glutathione. *J Phys Chem C* 2009;**113**(22):9659–63.
119. Calvert P, et al. Clinical studies of reversal of drug resistance based on glutathione. *Chem Biol Interact* 1998;**111–112**:213–24.

120. Liu K-K, et al. Large-scale synthesis of ZnO nanoparticles and their application as phosphors in light-emitting devices. *Opt Mater Express* 2017;**7**(7):2682–90.
121. Ostrovsky S, et al. Selective cytotoxic effect of ZnO nanoparticles on glioma cells. *Nano Res* 2009;**2**(11):882–90.
122. Guo D, et al. Synergistic cytotoxic effect of different sized ZnO nanoparticles and daunorubicin against leukemia cancer cells under UV irradiation. *J Photochem Photobiol B* 2008;**93**(3):119–26.
123. Cory H, et al. Preferential killing of cancer cells and activated human T cells using ZnO nanoparticles. *Nanotechnology* 2008;**19**(29):295103.
124. Langlais M, Tajmir-Riahi HA, Savoie R. Raman spectroscopic study of the effects of Ca^{2+}, Mg^{2+}, Zn^{2+}, and Cd^{2+} ions on calf thymus DNA: binding sites and conformational changes. *Biopolymers* 1990;**30**(7–8):743–52.
125. Martínez-Balbás MA, Jiménez-García E, Azorín F. Zinc(II) ions selectively interact with DNA sequences present at the TFIIIA binding site of the Xenopus 5S-RNA gene. *Nucleic Acids Res* 1995;**23**(13):2464–71.
126. Chakraborty P, et al. Sensitization of cancer cells to cyclophosphamide therapy by an organoselenium compound through ROS-mediated apoptosis. *Biomed Pharmacother* 2016;**84**:1992–9.
127. Abraham SA, et al. Formation of transition metal-doxorubicin complexes inside liposomes. *Biochim Biophys Acta Biomembr* 2002;**1565**(1):41–54.
128. Fiallo MML, et al. How Fe^{3+} binds anthracycline antitumour compounds. The myth and the reality of a chemical sphinx. *J Inorg Biochem* 1999;**75**(2):105–15.
129. Barick KC, Nigam S, Bahadur D. Nanoscale assembly of mesoporous ZnO: a potential drug carrier. *J Mater Chem* 2010;**20**(31):6446–52.
130. Muhammad F, et al. Acid degradable ZnO quantum dots as a platform for targeted delivery of an anticancer drug. *J Mater Chem* 2011;**21**(35):13406–12.
131. Zhang ZY, et al. Biodegradable ZnO@polymer core–shell nanocarriers: pH-triggered release of doxorubicin In Vitro. *Angew Chem Int Ed* 2013;**52**(15):4127–31.
132. Liu J, et al. Zinc oxide nanoparticles as adjuvant to facilitate doxorubicin intracellular accumulation and visualize pH-responsive release for overcoming drug resistance. *Mol Pharm* 2016;**13**(5):1723–30.
133. Ye D-X, et al. ZnO-based Nanoplatforms for labeling and treatment of mouse tumors without detectable toxic Side effects. *ACS Nano* 2016;**10**(4):4294–300.
134. Zhang J, et al. Dextran microgels loaded with ZnO QDs: pH-triggered degradation under acidic conditions. *J Appl Polym Sci* 2018;**135**(6):n/a.
135. Cai X, et al. pH-sensitive ZnO quantum dots-doxorubicin nanoparticles for lung cancer targeted drug delivery. *ACS Appl Mater Interfaces* 2016;**8**(34):22442–50.
136. Muhammad F, et al. pH-Triggered controlled drug release from mesoporous silica nanoparticles via intracelluar dissolution of ZnO nanolids. *J Am Chem Soc* 2011;**133**(23):8778–81.
137. Kim S, Lee SY, Cho H-J. Doxorubicin-wrapped zinc oxide nanoclusters for the therapy of colorectal adenocarcinoma. *Nanomaterials* 2017;**7**(11):354/1–354/13.
138. Wang J, et al. Exploration of zinc oxide nanoparticles as a multitarget and multifunctional anticancer nanomedicine. *ACS Appl Mater Interfaces* 2017;**9**(46):39971–84.
139. Cai X, et al. pH-responsive ZnO nanocluster for lung cancer chemotherapy. *ACS Appl Mater Interfaces* 2017;**9**(7):5739–47.
140. Roshini A, et al. pH-sensitive tangeretin-ZnO quantum dots exert apoptotic and anti-metastatic effects in metastatic lung cancer cell line. *Mater Sci Eng C* 2018;**92**:477–88.
141. Puvvada N, et al. Novel ZnO hollow-nanocarriers containing paclitaxel targeting folate-receptors in a malignant pH-microenvironment for effective monitoring and promoting breast tumor regression. *Sci Rep* 2015;**5**:11760.
142. Tripathy N, et al. Enhanced anticancer potency using an acid-responsive ZnO-incorporated liposomal drug-delivery system. *Nanoscale* 2015;**7**(9):4088–96.
143. Hahn MA, Tabb JS, Krauss TD. Detection of single bacterial pathogens with semiconductor quantum dots. *Anal Chem* 2005;**77**(15):4861–9.
144. Crespo RF, Perez OJP, Ramirez C. Total count of *Salmonella typhimurium* coupled on water soluble CdSe quantum dots by fluorescence detection. *J Electron Mater* 2018;**47**(8):4379–84.
145. Lai IP-J, et al. Solid-state synthesis of self-functional carbon quantum dots for detection of bacteria and tumor cells. *Sens Actuators B Chem* 2016;**228**:465–70.
146. Chen H, et al. Versatile antimicrobial peptide-based ZnO quantum dots for in vivo bacteria diagnosis and treatment with high specificity. *Biomaterials* 2015;**53**:532–44.
147. Lu Z, et al. Mechanism of antimicrobial activity of CdTe quantum dots. *Langmuir* 2008;**24**(10):5445–52.
148. Dumas E-M, et al. Toxicity of CdTe quantum dots in bacterial strains. *IEEE Trans Nanobioscience* 2009;**8**(1):58–64.
149. Mir IA, et al. Antimicrobial and biocompatibility of highly fluorescent ZnSe core and ZnSe@ ZnS core-shell quantum dots. *J Nanoparticle Res* 2018;**20**(7):174.
150. Jin T, et al. Antimicrobial efficacy of zinc oxide quantum dots against *Listeria monocytogenes*, *Salmonella enteritidis*, and *Escherichia coli* O157: h7. *J Food Sci* 2009;**74**(1):M46–52.
151. Dutta RK, et al. Studies on antibacterial activity of ZnO nanoparticles by ROS induced lipid peroxidation. *Colloids Surfaces B Biointerfaces* 2012;**94**:143–50.
152. Luo Z, et al. Cooperative antimicrobial activity of CdTe quantum dots with rocephin and fluorescence monitoring for *Escherichia coli*. *J Colloid Interface Sci* 2011;**362**(1):100–6.
153. Jijie R, et al. Enhanced antibacterial activity of carbon dots functionalized with ampicillin combined with visible light triggered photodynamic effects. *Colloids Surfaces B Biointerfaces* 2018;**170**(1):347–54.
154. Dai Q, et al. Quantifying the ligand-coated nanoparticle delivery to cancer cells in solid tumors. *ACS Nano* 2018;**12**(8):8423–35.
155. Greish K, et al. Macromolecular therapeutics. *Clin Pharmacokinet* 2003;**42**(13):1089–105.
156. Salmaso S, Caliceti P. Stealth properties to improve therapeutic efficacy of drug nanocarriers. *J Drug Delivery* 2013;**2013**:19.
157. Park K. Facing the truth about nanotechnology in drug delivery. *ACS Nano* 2013;**7**(9):7442–7.
158. Chen F, et al. Ultrasmall targeted nanoparticles with engineered antibody fragments for imaging detection of HER2-overexpressing breast cancer. *Nat Commun* 2018;**9**(1):4141.
159. Kang Y-F, et al. Carbon quantum dots for zebrafish fluorescence imaging. *Sci Rep* 2015;**5**:11835.

Chapter 16

Mesoporous silica nanoparticles: synthesis, properties, and biomedical applications

Marco A. Downing and Piyush K. Jain

Department of Chemical Engineering, Herbert Wertheim College of Engineering, University of Florida

16.1 What are silica nanoparticles?

The Food and Drug Administration (FDA) defines nanoparticles as particles less than 1000 nm. In contrast to the FDA, the medical field commonly defines nanoparticles as less than 500 nm, as nanoparticles that are less than 500 nm can be endocytosed by cells. However, particles between 500 and 1000 nm can be used for medical applications, as they can possess useful bulk properties such as optical or magnetic properties despite not being able to enter cells. Nanoparticles' role in medicine has mainly focused on drug delivery, as many types of nanoparticles can act as stable vectors in vivo while transporting less stable therapeutic drugs. Nanoparticles are chemical delivery vectors, opposed to the biological viral vectors, such as adenovirus, lentivirus, or adeno-associated virus. However, new research on modular nanoparticles that contain both biological components such as peptides or lipids and traditional chemical components such as silica or iron oxide show promise as a future sector of drug delivery. This chapter will focus on a type of nanoparticle that is particularly promising for medical applications: silica nanoparticles.

Silica nanoparticles, also known as nanosilica, make up a major section of nanoparticle research with an emphasis on biomedical applications due to their low toxicity and stability in the body. Silica nanoparticles are often referred to as mesoporous silica nanoparticles (MSNs) due to their unique property of being mesoporous or containing pores between 2 and 50 nm in diameter. MSNs have a structure of $(SiO_2)_n$ and can be made in a variety of ways resulting in vastly different properties. MSN synthesis only requires four main components: a silica precursor such as silane, a catalyst, solvents, and a surfactant.[1–3] However, even though synthesis only requires these four components, MSNs with different properties such as diameter, pore size, surface area, and shape can be achieved.[4]

There are three unique properties that make the mesoporous nature of MSNs ideal for biomedical application, see Fig. 16.1.

First, their porosity makes MSNs effective carriers of small molecules and proteins for easy drug delivery. Second, their structure also provides MSNs with a half-life long enough to be stable in blood serum while also degrading by physiological systems at longer residence

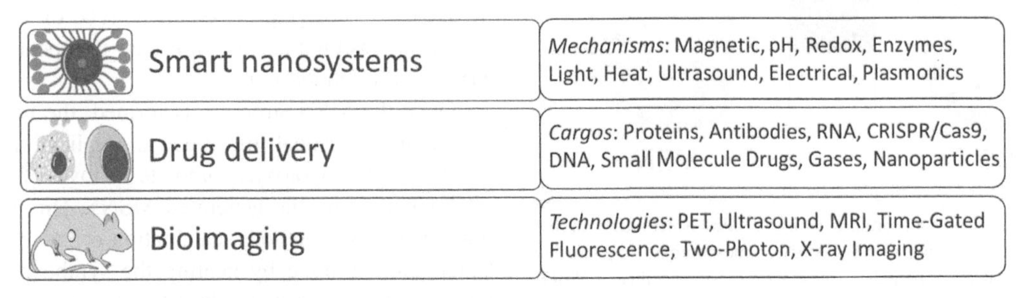

FIGURE 16.1 Biomedical systems design and applications using silica. *Credit: Original figure.*

Nanoparticles for Biomedical Applications. https://doi.org/10.1016/B978-0-12-816662-8.00016-3

times. This is important, as any nanoparticle used in medical applications must not build up in the body. Finally, MSN formulation provides consistent and predictable particle sizes with tunable features such as diameter, shape, porosity, and both core and surface features. This tunability allows a wide variety of MSNs to exist and is a broad area of research, as different structures will be ideal for different medical applications, whether that is targeting different tissues or carrying different cargo.

Recently, new areas of research in silica nanoparticles have arisen with developments in mesoporous organosilica nanoparticles (MONs) and periodic mesoporous organosilica (PMO) nanoparticles. Changing the silica precursor to include an organic R group has created these novel nanoparticles. This leads to a particle structure of $(SiO_{1.5}$-R-$SiO_{1.5})_n$ and can have significantly more complex internal chemistry, depending on the chosen functional R group.[5–17] MONs and PMOs have potential for unique medical applications but will have a larger barrier to pass clinical trials. Toxicological studies on MSNs translate to other MSNs but do not translate over to MONs or PMOs. Additional toxicological testing would be required for each R group configuration of MON/PMO, adding an additional challenge to their medical use. For further reading on MONs and PMOs, refer to these excellent review articles[1,18–21] which go into much more detail on these novel systems (Fig. 16.2).

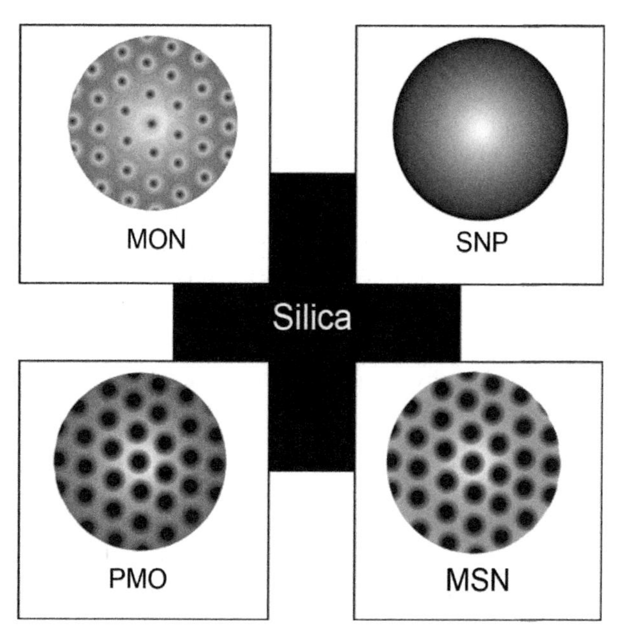

FIGURE 16.2 Silica nanoparticles variants: silica nanoparticle (SNP), mesoporous silica nanoparticle (MSN), mesoporous organosilica nanoparticle (MON), periodic mesoporous organosilica (PMO). *Credit: Original figure.*

16.2 How are silica nanoparticles made?

Silica nanoparticle production usually occurs under the sol–gel process, a soft chemistry process occurring at ambient temperature in either acidic or basic conditions. The process starts with a precursor, some type of silane such as tetraethyl orthosilicate (TEOS) $Si(OEt)_4$ or tetramethyl orthosilicate (TMOS) $Si(OMe)_4$ in an aqueous solution. The reaction occurs through a hydrolysis and condensation reaction in the presence of either an acid or base catalyst such as HCl or NH_3.[22–28]

As the reaction occurs, the precursors form a crystalline nanostructure as shown in Fig. 16.3. The choice of an acid or a base as the catalyst determines whether the hydrolysis or the condensation step is faster. In the case of an acid-catalyzed reaction, hydrolysis is much faster than condensation, leading to many small silica particles forming. These smaller particles tend to form a gel-like structure. Conversely, the base-catalyzed reaction has a faster condensation step than the hydrolysis step, which forms larger silica nanoparticles. If only these three ingredients are used, the silica particles made are nonporous and tend to form either gel networks (acid-catalyzed) or solid spheres (base-catalyzed) (Fig. 16.4).

MSN production is both simple and complicated; while requiring only four key components, the tuning of the process can give a wide variety of results. The addition of a surfactant to the solution allows the formation of MSNs. The generation of mesopores within the silica nanoparticles is due to the surfactant acting as a template for the growth of the silica structures. The choice of surfactant is important for determining the mesopore structure. A common surfactant used is cetyltrimethylammonium bromide, as it can form micelles in aqueous solutions when above a critical micellar concentration. A micelle is formed when the hydrophilic portion of the surfactant orients itself toward the aqueous solution, making the hydrophobic region orient inward. The hydrophobic regions then aggregate forming a sphere-like micelle (Fig. 16.5).

As you increase the concentration of surfactant, these micelles change shape, going from spheres to cylinders to hexagonal channels. If larger pores are needed, the addition of a hydrophobic swelling agent as the fifth component can be used. By changing the quantity, type of surfactant, and by adding swelling agent,[31] it is easy to repeatedly generate MSNs with defined porosity.

Once the MSN structure is formed, the removal of the surfactant is critical for medical applications. As most surfactants are cytotoxic, complete removal of surfactants is vital for utilizing the generated MSNs. This is commonly done using two methods: calcination or solvent extraction. Calcination is done by heating the synthesized MSNs to temperatures as hot as 800°C. These extremely high

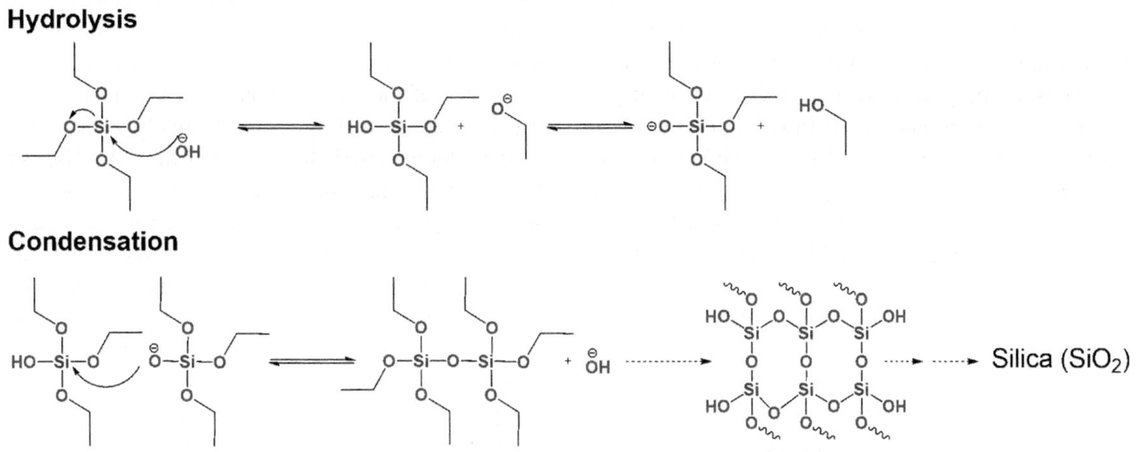

FIGURE 16.3 Hydrolysis and condensation reactions of silanes. *Credit: Ref. 29.*

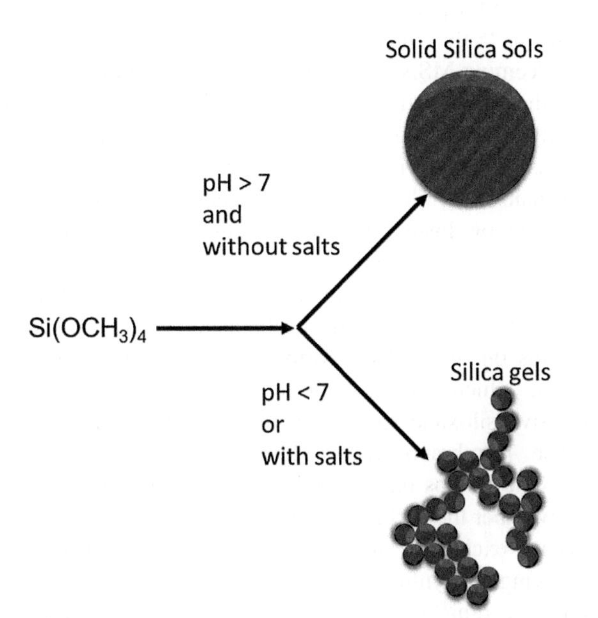

FIGURE 16.4 Silica synthesis pathways under acidic(gels) and basic conditions(sols). *Credit: Original Figure.*

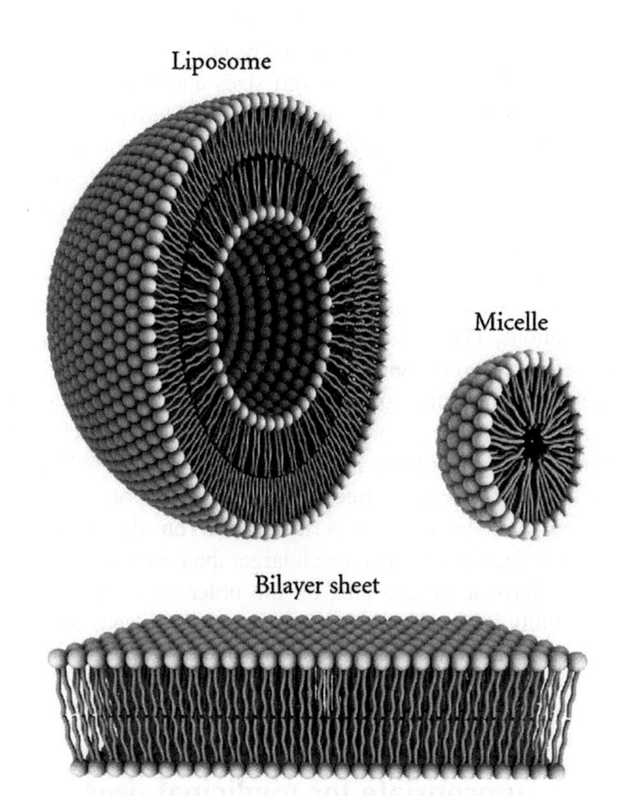

FIGURE 16.5 Variations in micelle shape formation which lead to an array of silica pore sizes. *Credit: Ref. 30.*

temperatures are required to bring the solution above the decomposition point for the surfactant in solution. The downsides of calcination are the high temperature, energy requirement, and the surface modifications that occur. At high temperatures, the Si—OH bonds on the surface of the MSNs react together to form Si—O—Si bonds. This constricts the surface and pores, changing the pore size and making the particle more hydrophobic. Solvent extraction can also be used depending on the surfactant and whether the reaction occurred at acidic or basic conditions. An example of solvent extraction is using ammonium nitrate to extract the nanoparticles. The advantage of solvent extraction is the significantly lower temperature and energy requirement. The main downside to solvent extraction is the potential need for more costly separation processes downstream due to additional solvents being used. Regardless of which method is used, complete removal of the surfactant must be confirmed before use of the MSN.

Further modification of the MSNs can be done to functionalize the core, the surface, or both the core and the surface. Surface modifications can be through either chemical reactions or various coatings. Different surface chemistry reactions are possible on MSNs, depending on whether the surface groups are silanol (Si—OH) or siloxane (Si—O—Si). Adding functional groups to the surface of

MSNs has been used for controlling the rate of drug release, determining the location of drug release, and reducing the toxicity of MSNs. Common coatings for MSNs have been different types of polymers such as polyethylene glycol (PEG),[32] polyethyleneimine (PEI)-PEG copolymer,[33] or poly (N-isopropylacrylamide).[34] Core modifications are commonly used for hybrid nanoparticles. For example, MSN-coated iron oxide (Fe_3O_4) nanoparticles can be used to impart magnetic properties to MSN particles.[35] Other metal cores such as gold-core MSNs[36–41] and silver-core MSNs[34] have been made, with more hybrids being published every year.

The variety of MSNs leads to vastly different property ranges for size, pore shape, pore volume, surface area, etc. Common MSNs for biomedical applications can have diameters ranging from 300 nm to less than 10 nm.[25] Particles can be made as a monopore (hollow silica nanoparticle with only one pore) with a diameter less than 10 nm[42] allowing for very specific cargo sizes and pore diameters ranging from 30 nm to as small as 2 nm.[43] Pores have been generated with a variety of shapes such as hexagonal,[44] cubic,[45] concentric,[46] foam-like,[46] radial wrinkle-like,[47] worm-like,[48,49] hierarchical dual,[50] and triple porosity[51] (Fig. 16.6).

The hierarchical porosity structures can be formed through stepwise synthesis using different surfactant concentrations. The variation in the pore types allows for vastly different cargo-carrying capabilities. Most MSNs have a well-defined ability to carry cargo with a pore volume of 1 cm^3/g; however, they can have a pronounced capacity for carrying cargo with the largest pore volume reported being as high as 4.5 cm^3/g. Because of the large pore volume, MSNs also have large surface areas on the order of 1000 m^2/g, making them much larger than nonporous silica which have a surface area on the order of 10 m^2/g. The variability in the physical properties of MSNs leads them to have a wide variety of medical applications.

16.3 Why are silica nanoparticles appropriate for medicinal use?

Silica nanoparticles have great potential for medicinal use due to their biocompatibility, lack of toxicity, and biodegradability. MSNs have well-understood biocompatibility in the human body with numerous studies having been performed. While some nanoparticles have issues with acute toxicity, MSNs have been found to have dose-dependent toxicity.[1] The therapeutic dose for MSN delivery is well below the toxic dose, making MSNs an excellent option for medical applications. A big part of MSNs' biocompatibility comes from the generation of a protein corona on the surface of MSN particles.[51,53–57] A protein corona is a dynamic coating of proteins that binds to the outside of the MSN particles, masking it as it travels through the body. This protein corona can be utilized to improve MSN toxicity and stability by adjusting the surface chemistry of the MSNs. Finally, a key factor for medical use is whether a drug can effectively clear the body or whether there is toxic buildup over time. MSNs, as they are fundamentally just SiO_2, are biodegradable for longer time spans in the body. This biodegradability is due to a hydrolysis reaction in the body that occurs on the surfaces of MSNs, breaking apart the silica nanoparticles into silicic acid. This reaction prevents the toxic buildup of MSNs in the body. MSNs are readily available for medical use as they have excellent compatibility with the human body compared with other potential nanoparticle vectors.

Silica has been recognized as safe for use by the FDA due to their known biocompatibility, making them very attractive for pharmaceutical use. The FDA has recognized silica as "safe" for over 50 years, which makes the hurdle for deeming MSN-based drugs as "safe" mainly dependent on the modifications and cargo of choice. Silica nanoparticles, without modifications, have two primary mechanisms for toxicity in the human body.[46] The first mechanism is due to surface silanol groups becoming reactive on losing their hydrogens. The reactive Si–O- group causes membranolysis by reacting with the tetraalkylammonium-containing phospholipids[58] on the cell membrane. The second mechanism is due to siloxane groups on the surface, forming three-membered siloxane rings, which are unstable and, hence, reactive. These reactive siloxane rings, like the silanol groups, can also cause membranolysis.[59] The presence of silanols and siloxane groups on the surface of the MSNs is dependent on whether the surfactant was removed through calcination or ion-exchange during MSN synthesis. This makes knowing the synthesis route of your MSNs important when understanding potential toxicity of your MSNs. It is important to note that both mechanisms are dependent on the surface chemistry of MSNs. Targeting surface modifications will have an acute effect on toxicity and is important when designing new MSNs for drug treatment. Regardless of whether the surface is primarily silanols or siloxanes, the potential for toxicity at higher dosages is present. Luckily, these mechanisms are not readily seen in MSNs at the dosages used for therapeutics.[60] Therapeutic in vivo particle dosages have been shown to typically be anywhere from 1 to 50 mg/kg[61] with 80 mg/kg being shown to be well tolerated.[62] This is significantly less than the LD_{50} for MSNs which has been proposed to be around 1000 mg/kg.[62] The high LD_{50} for MSNs suggests that regardless of what mechanisms there are for MSN toxicity, they do not pose major issues for biocompatibility at therapeutic dosages. Targeting the primary cause of toxicity, the surface of MSNs, should be the focus of increasing biocompatibility.

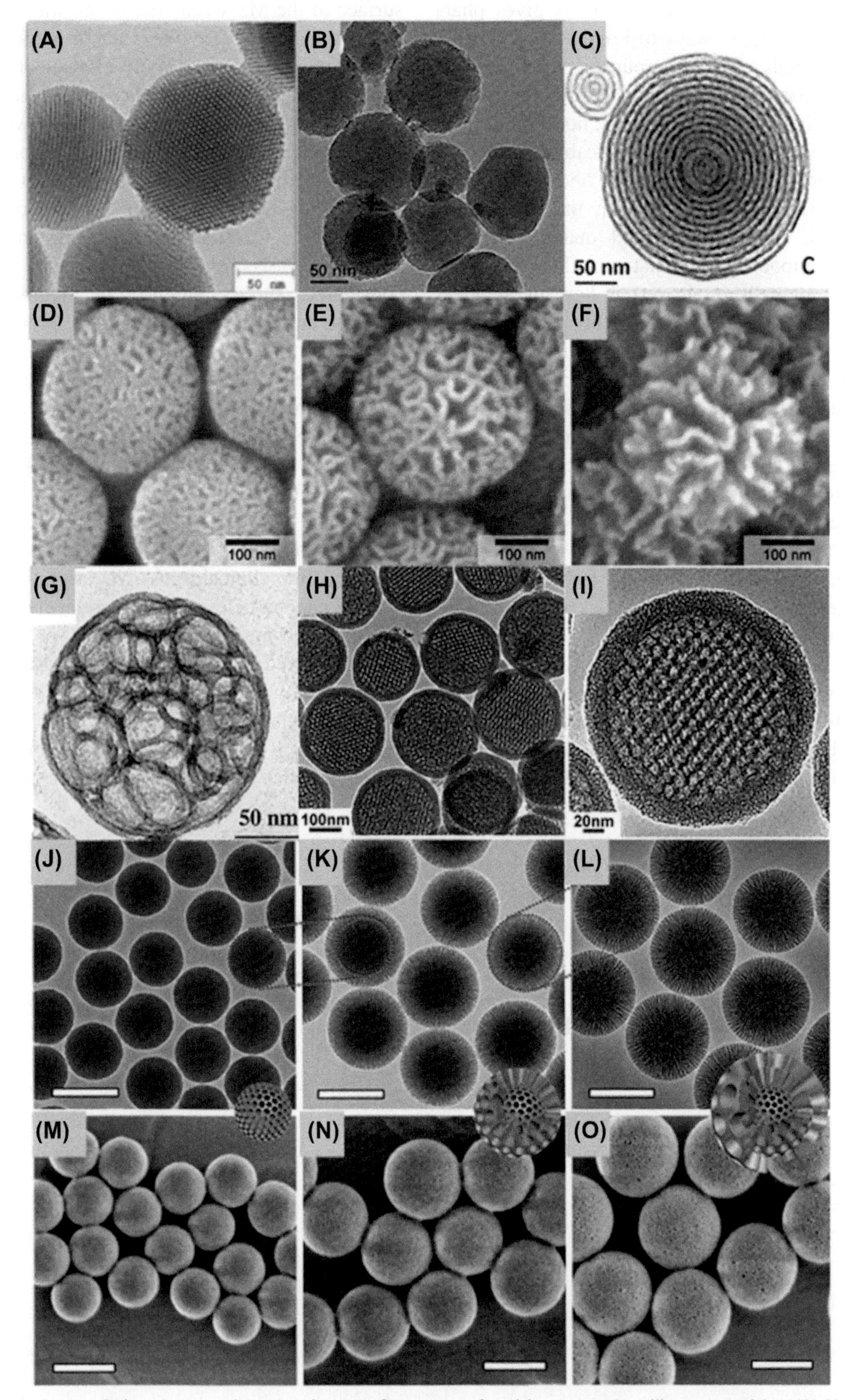

FIGURE 16.6 Typical transmission electron microscopy images of pore types found in mesoporous silica nanoparticles. (A) Hexagonal, (B) cubic, (C) concentric, (D–F) radial wrinkle-like, (G) foam-like, (H–I) hierarchical dual, (J–O) triple porosity. *Credit: Refs. 1,44–49,52.*

Surface chemistry and biology of MSNs gives pharmaceutical chemists unique ways to improve the medical applicability of MSNs. Surface groups are the primary reactive species that can cause toxicity due to MSNs. Through surface chemistry modifications, not only can the toxicity be changed but the medical applicability of MSNs can also be improved. Modification of the surface can change the biodistribution of MSNs in the body. Biodistribution is the understanding and quantification of where a target compound accumulates in the body. Targeting of tissues or cells of interest is key for an ideal biodistribution, which will be effective for medical treatment. Through improving the specificity of nanoparticle delivery to the cells of interest, the therapeutic dose is effectively reduced because less dosage is wasted. For MSNs, this has primarily been done with surface modifications allowing for targeting specific tissues or diseases. For example, treatment of MSN's surface with PEI-PEG copolymer increased the percentage of MSNs that arrived in the target tumor cells from less than 1%–10%.[33] This increase in specificity would allow for lower magnitude dosages to achieve the same results.

MSNs are unique, in that their surface modifications can be done not just chemically but also biologically due to the presence of a protein corona. The protein corona is formed through proteins adsorbing onto the mesoporous surface, creating a shell around the nanoparticles.[63,64] This is important because the nature of proteins that attach to the surface of the MSN can change the way the body interacts with the MSN. Effectively, the presence of the protein corona reduces the hemolytic effect of the surface of the MSN[65,66] and effects cellular internalization.[67] This can potentially mask surface modifications, which is important to remember during MSN design. The protein corona can also allow for particles to pass through the blood–brain barrier[68] or to be taken up by monocytes or macrophages.[69,70] Considering the protein corona while designing MSNs for drug delivery is key; if it is not considered, surface engineering modifications may not have the desired expectations.[71] The protein corona can be controlled indirectly by changing surface charge, pore size, pore shape, and hydrophobicity/hydrophilicity. As the protein coronas are dynamic in vivo, it can be hard to pretreat MSNs with proteins before use. However, further research in binding proteins to the MSNs could allow that to be a useful option for improving specificity and reducing toxicity.

Degradability of silica in the body promotes a fast track of MSNs into clinical trials. The largest barrier for clinical trials of nanoparticles is the requirement of particles to clear the body and not accumulate. Thus, proving that any particles delivered to the body will not have long-term effects due to accumulation is vital (Fig. 16.7).

Silica nanoparticles have great promise for degrading in the body, as it is the third most abundant trace element in the body. Silica nanoparticles have one of highest potentials

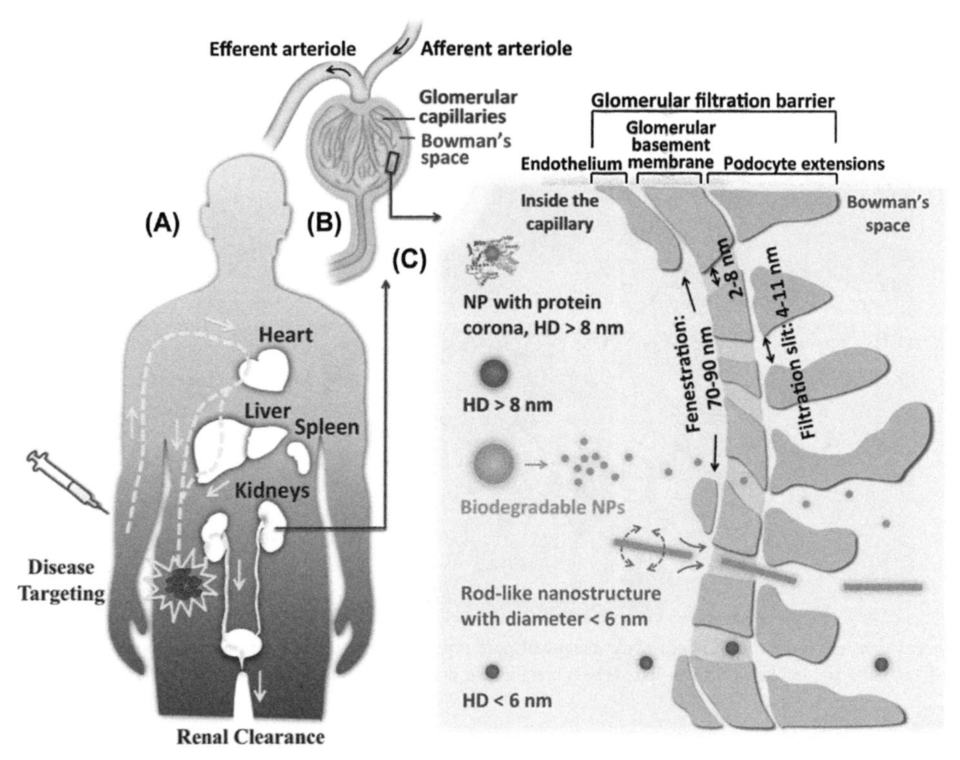

FIGURE 16.7 Degradation pathways of nanoparticles in vivo. *Credit: Refs. 18,72.*

for medical applications, being readily degraded in the body through a three-step reaction mechanism.[73] The MSN's surface first goes through a hydration step where water adsorbs onto the surface. Next, a hydrolysis reaction occurs as water reacts with the siloxane groups converting them to silanol groups. The silanol groups can then participate in an ion-exchange reaction, which causes the Si to leave the nanostructure in the form of silicic acid. Silicic acid is considered nontoxic[18,74] and clears the body through the urine.[75] This dissolution of Si from the nanostructure has been shown to follow this dissolution reaction rate, via Ehrlich, Demadis et al.[76]:

$$R_{diss} = k_1\left[SiOH_2^+\right]^m + k_2[SiOH]^m + k_3[SiO^-]^p. \quad [16.1]$$

The dissolution rate and order of reaction is determined by which form of silanols are present on the surface of the nanoparticles, with m and p being the reaction orders. The pH of the system will determine whether the surface silanols are protonated, neutral or deprotonated effecting the overall rate of dissolution. Because the reactions occur primarily on surfaces, pore size and, by extension, surface area are important for degradation times. As the porosity increases, the rate at which the particle degrades in the body increases. Once silica degrades, it can be used in the body, and excess silicic acid or poly-silicic acid nanoparticles (less than 6 nm) can be excreted through the kidneys into the urine.[77,78] The clearance time of MSNs can vary widely due to differences in surface coatings, morphology, thermal oxidation, and surface functionalization. This variance in clearance times mimics the variability in MSNs and is something that should be considered when designing new MSNs. Anything that limits or halts clearance of the MSNs will have the potential of introducing long-term toxicity and buildup.

16.4 What kinds of cargo can MSNs deliver?

For any kind of medical use, silica nanoparticles are simply delivery vectors that can be tailored for a specific cargo of choice. Silica nanoparticles have the capability of carrying cargo in their mesoporous structure, ranging from small molecules to large proteins. This is primarily due to the tunability of the pore sizes and shape, allowing for accommodation of small (1 nm size pores)[42] to large (50 nm size pores) molecules or proteins.[79] Cargo can be loaded to MSNs without any kind of additional surface treatment. Specifically, MSNs can deliver two types of cargos: noncovalently loaded hydrophobic cargos and noncovalently loaded hydrophilic cargos. However, without surface treatment, MSNs have the issue of leaking cargo during delivery. One solution to this problem is the surface engineering of "pore-gates" or molecules that act as a way of sealing the MSNs pores on the surface, preventing leakage. This is key for avoiding side effects and loss of efficiency, due to leakage, to nontarget tissues and cells.

Scientists have created a myriad of "pore-gates" that can have a variety of drug-release "triggers." Often the type of "pore-gates" used act as cleavable molecular bridges, or nanovalves, that perform conformational changes. These bridges can be activated in a variety of ways—some under the control of the drug administrator, and some dependent on tissue/cell location. Many mechanisms have advantages and disadvantages due to their respective technologies. Thus, it is important to always consider the unique qualities of the disease or tissues of interest before selecting a drug-release method (Fig. 16.8).

One common release mechanism is pH-dependent drug release. This works as MSNs are brought into the cell through endocytosis. During this process, the endosome carrying the MSN will continually drop in pH. If the cleavable group reacts at a pH between physiological pH (<7.4), but higher than lysosomal pH ($4.5 >$), then drug release can be triggered during the endosome to lysosome transition. This drop in pH can either cleave the molecular bridges or change their orientation on the surface of the MSN, releasing the cargo from the MSN. However, it is important to consider the cargo, as many things can be degraded at such a low pH. Endosomal escape is imperative for release of cargo from the endosome/lysosome into the cell. One example of pH changing the surface conformation is rotaxane, which gradually changes its conformation as the pH drops below 5.[81] Dissolvable coatings have also been used on MSNs such as a calcium phosphate.[82]

Like pH-based groups, redox-based groups have also been used. Targeting compounds upregulated in specific tissues or diseases that act as reducing agents allows for targeted delivery. For example, glutathione, a reducing agent, has a much higher intra- rather than extracellular concentration. One group took advantage of this property to trigger the redox reaction of disulfide groups of a nanocap formed from β-cyclodextrin with disulfide connecting groups. They showed that the extracellular concentration was not high enough to trigger the redox reaction and that leakage did not occur.[83]

Functional groups that are cleavable by specific enzymes have also been created. Specificity can be increased if the tissue of interest is the only tissue expressing a certain enzyme. For example, a group has used a molecular α-cyclodextrin with adamantane as "stoppers" to close the pores of silica nanoparticles, which can then be opened with the enzyme porcine liver esterase.[84] A medical application of this has been performed with anticancer drug delivery, specifically targeting colon cancer. Drug delivery was limited to the colon by utilizing a polysaccharide coating, guar gum, which can only be cleaved by enzymes present in the colon. This is often very important as drugs

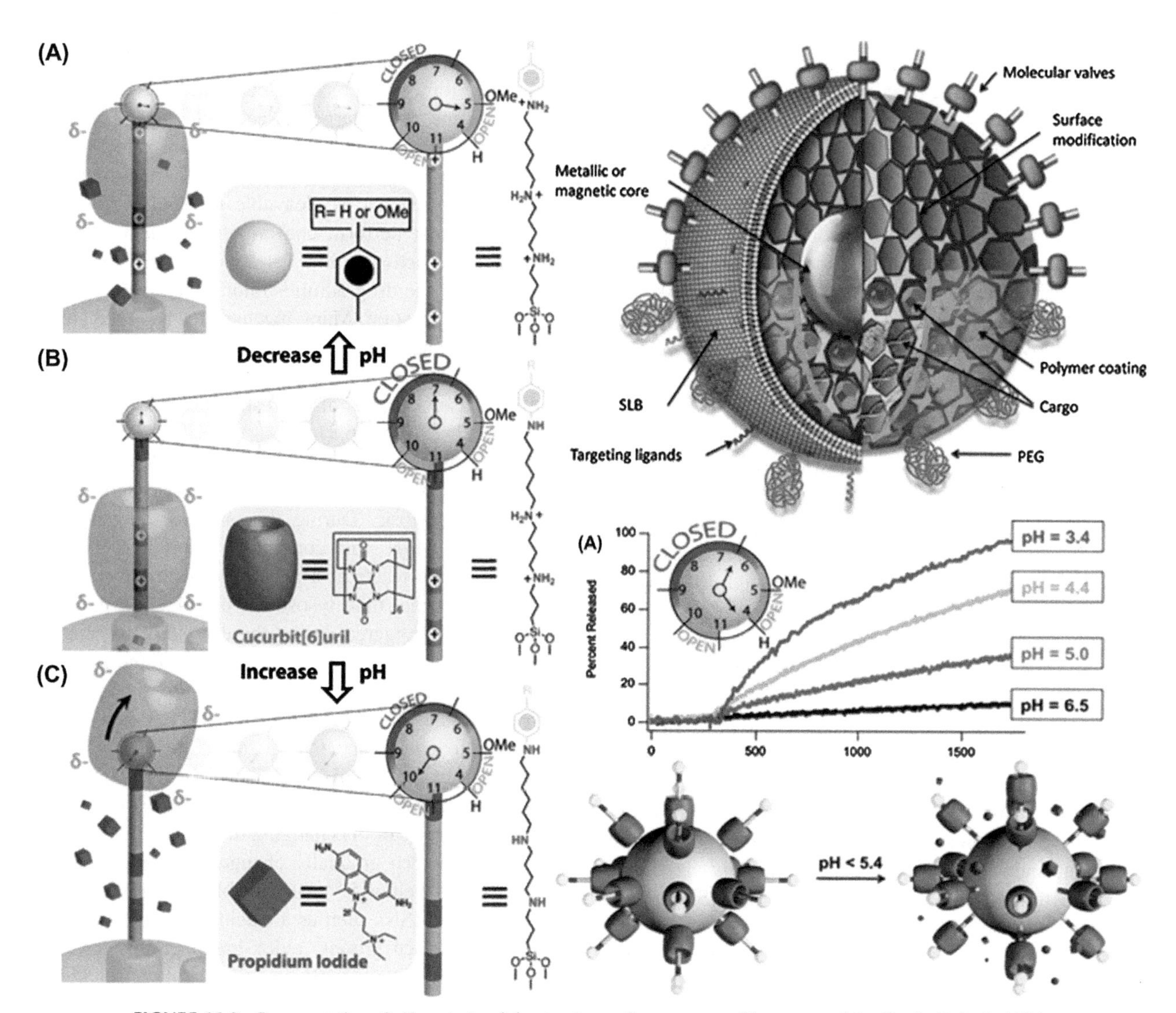

FIGURE 16.8 Representation of pH control and the structures of mesoporous silica nanoparticle. *Credit: Refs. 1, 46,80.*

used in chemotherapy-based cancer treatment can cause significant negative side effects, which can be minimized by highly specific delivery mechanisms.

Drug delivery mechanisms that are under the control of the person administering the treatment consist of light-activatable,[85] magnetically triggered,[86] and ultrasound-triggered groups.[87] For example, light-activatable nanoparticles are controlled by exposing a light to the target tissue. This treatment is limited by the attenuation of light particles through the body, which limits applicability to targets close to the skin. Light-activatable groups can be photolysis-responsive, photoisomerization-responsive, photoredox-responsive, and photothermal responsive.[85] Magnetically triggered groups can be triggered via an external magnetic field but are limited by the resolution of the applied magnetic field.[87] These are often just nanovalves with thermally decomposable bonds that are broken when the magnetic particles are exposed to an oscillating magnetic field, generating the heat required to break the bonds.[86] Ultrasound-based groups are in the early stages of research and could be a potential option for future nanoparticles.

16.5 What applications are MSNs currently used for in medicine?

MSNs currently have two main applications: imaging and drug delivery. Imaging applications have consisted of bioimaging through positron emission topography (PET) imaging, ultrasound imaging, time-gated fluorescence imaging,[88] and magnetic resonance imaging. Drug delivery has been used to deliver a variety of cargos, such as genes or proteins, gaseous molecules, and multiple drug cocktails. These various drug delivery mechanisms can be used in a variety of medical applications, such as cancer therapy, Alzheimer's disease therapy, and antibiotic treatment.

Utilizing MSNs for bioimaging takes advantage of the large storage capacity of MSNs. A key issue with in vivo bioimaging is the stability and biodistribution of imaging particles in the body. Oftentimes, delivery vectors are the solution to these issues, as they provide protection from the various enzymes and molecules present in the body. One example of this technology being used in medical applications is bioimaging through PET; PET takes advantage of radionuclides which emit a positron during their decay. The positron then reacts with electrons nearby, annihilating into two distinct gamma rays in opposite directions, which can then be detected by a scanning device. PET traditionally has strong tissue signal penetration but has issues with low spatial resolution. This makes it useful for deep tissue imaging, though it often relies on other imaging techniques to improve its resolution. However, MSNs provide an alternative way to improve the resolution of PET directly. Through loading MSNs with radionuclides such as zirconium-89,[89–92] arsenic-72,[93] copper-64,[94–102] technetium-99,[103] titanium-45,[103,104] fluorine-18,[105–107] or carbon-11,[108] it is possible to increase both the tissue selectivity and the resolution due to higher overall signals. The MSNs protect the radionucleotides from being lost during systemic circulation, which increases the quantity of molecules that make it to the target tissues. MSNs provide a novel way of improving the specificity and resolution of PET that were not previously possible.

Another imaging technique utilizing MSNs is ultrasound imaging. This technology works by using high intensity focused ultrasound (HIFU) which uses mechanical vibrations on the order of 1–20 MHz frequency.[87] This form of imaging is already an FDA-approved technology but has one key issue: poor resolution. One way to improve the resolution issue is to utilize enhancement agents (EAs),[109] which can enlarge the tissue site and improve imaging. This tissue enlargement is often done through bubble formation; MSNs provide a unique way of adding "bubbles" due to their porosity. Delivery of hollow MSNs to the tissues of interest is a way of adding "bubbles" to improve HIFU imaging resolution. This has been performed in a coupled system, where the hollow MSNs also delivered additional EAs on their surface, further improving HIFU imaging resolution.[109] The porosity of MSNs provides unique ways of carrying cargo that is useful for imaging, whether that is radionuclides, or just hollow "bubbles" for HIFU.

MSNs are synonymous with drug delivery due to their diverse cargo-carrying capacity and medical applications. Originally, MSNs were mainly used for small drug delivery because pore size limited protein loading to only the surface of MSNs, but recently as MSN engineering has improved pore sizes, larger proteins are being delivered. Large molecules such as plasmid DNA have been successfully delivered with MSNs' with pore sizes around 20 nm.[110] MSNs have also been used to deliver siRNA with a concentration of 380-μg siRNA/mg MSN.[111] Delivery of extremely small molecules such as nitric oxide (NO) and carbon monoxide (CO) via MSNs has also been shown.[112] Small molecule drug delivery of CO and NO is done through carrying releaser molecules that can be externally triggered to release CO or NO. This is important because CO and NO, at a certain dose, can cause cell apoptosis, a trait that is utilized to kill cancer cells. Because of the ability for one MSN to have different pore sizes, it is possible to create a cocktail drug therapy within one MSN particle. This delivery mixture is important for medical applications as cancer and many other diseases often show improved treatment under multiple drugs. This process is known as combination therapy and is often used through the delivery of multiple drugs alongside siRNA for cancer treatment. While independently siRNA and cancer treatment drugs work, the combination has been shown to greatly increase efficiency. In one study, codelivery of siRNA and doxorubicin was shown to cause cell apoptosis in 37% of breast cancer cells versus 14% for just doxorubicin by itself.[113] This combination therapy approach allows MSNs to be uniquely effective for complex drug delivery applications. MSNs' drug delivery can also be used as a disease marker. For example, in Alzheimer's disease, it is theorized that aggregation of amyloid-β (Aβ) proteins leads to the progression of the disease. It is also known that during this aggregation process, cytotoxic reactive oxygen species are formed, such as H_2O_2. Scientists utilized this fact to design MSNs with an H_2O_2-responsive trigger to deliver a drug known for reducing Alzheimer's progression, clioquinol, to the brain.[114] This controlled mechanism was important for reducing cytotoxicity through increased specificity. MSNs provide a great way for targeting brain-based diseases such as Alzheimer's disease because of their ability to be designed small enough (<30 nm) to pass the blood–brain barrier. MSNs can also be used to deliver antibiotics systematically through the body. Through loading MSNs with antimicrobial ionic liquids without a surface coating, passive drug delivery is possible.[115] Similarly, one group delivered antimicrobial peptides via MSNs to combat lung infections.[116,117] Another delivery mechanism is coating the surface of MSNs with antimicrobial lysosome enzymes that will become active once the MSNs are endocytosed into the bacterial cells.[118] A combination of these two methods could prove useful for future antibiotic MSNs. The challenges remaining for utilizing MSNs in the clinic consist mainly of study-design issues such as quantifying biodistribution in humans. In addition, methods for determining MSN concentration in tissues can be challenging as most methods used on animal models are invasive and not applicable to humans.

16.6 New types of silica NPs, MONs, and PMOs: what makes them different?

While MSNs have historically been the major, if not the only, area of silica nanoparticle research, two additional types, MONs and PMOs, are budding sectors in current silica nanoparticle research. Despite the already highly customizable MSNs, the more complex MONs and PMOs provide exponentially more design possibilities. This order of magnitude increase in variability has everything to do with the structure of MONs and PMOs. The only difference from MSNs to PMOs is the replacement of one of the OMethyl or OEthyl groups in the silica precursors in TMOS or TEOS with an organic R group (Fig. 16.9).

This additional organic group is only limited by the ability to allow the periodic structure of silica nanoparticles to be formed as shown in Fig. 16.10.

This allows for a wide variety of additional silica nanoparticles to be formed with a variety of new chemistries due to the organic R group. To add additional complexity, MONs, that are silica nanoparticles, have regions of MSNs and PMOs that create a hybrid. These hybrids can have different proportions of the organic and nonorganic variants, creating unique porous structures. While PMOs and MONs are quite new, they already account for at least 10% of the papers currently being published on silica nanoparticles.

MONs and PMOs have a lot of potential for making uniquely functional silica nanoparticles. This is due to the flexibility of the organic R group. The R group can have a drastic effect on what types of cargo the nanoparticle can carry, which is due to both the physical changes to the pore size and shape and the chemical changes affecting the hydrophobicity/hydrophilicity and charge of the particle. For example, creating nanoparticles with an R group that has a triggerable group such as a light-activated photocleavable group can drastically change the control of drug delivery or degradability of the structure. It will also change the possibilities for surface modifications. In traditional MSNs, the surface groups will always be silanols or siloxanes. With MONs and PMOs, the options for surface groups open up the types of chemical modifications that can be made, allowing for unique triggerable groups to be used as "pore-gates." PMOs and MONs have already been designed to do a variety of tasks such as traditional cargo delivery and release, imaging, cell adhesion, bacterial inhibition, and photodynamic therapy.

There are many challenges to utilizing MONs and PMOs for medical applications. Most of these challenges are due to not being able to fall back on studies performed on MSNs. Although MSNs only have the safety considerations of the drugs being carried and the surface modifications, MONs and PMOs also have their baseline structure to consider. Despite the FDA's consideration of silica as safe, MONs and PMOs do not receive benefit from this as they are considered a completely new compound. Furthermore, no two PMOs or MONs are the same, meaning each new R group or mix will have to be approved separately, adding additional complexity to medical use. Therefore, any clinical studies performed will require additional research on safety (toxicology, degradability, etc.) before being approved for every PMO or MON. Degradability of the PMO or MON structures is a source of concern, as the mechanism for degradation is not clearly defined and will differ from R group to R group. Understanding the effects of these changes is key for medical applications.

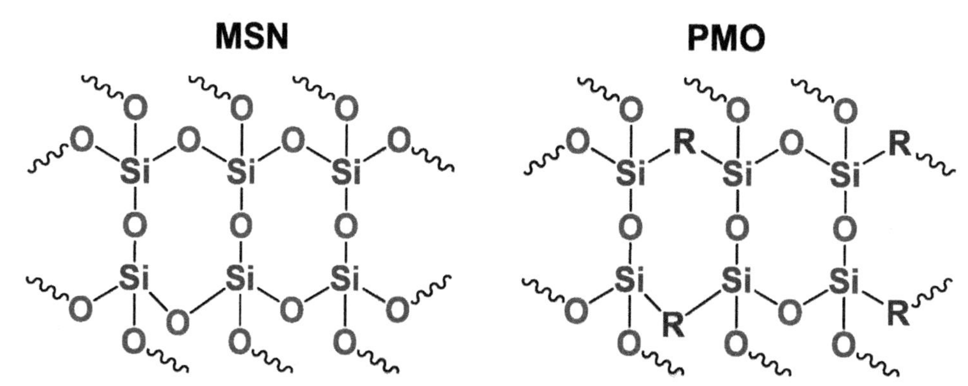

FIGURE 16.9 Mesoporous silica nanoparticle (MSN) versus periodic mesoporous organosilica (PMO) Structure. *Credit: Original Work.*

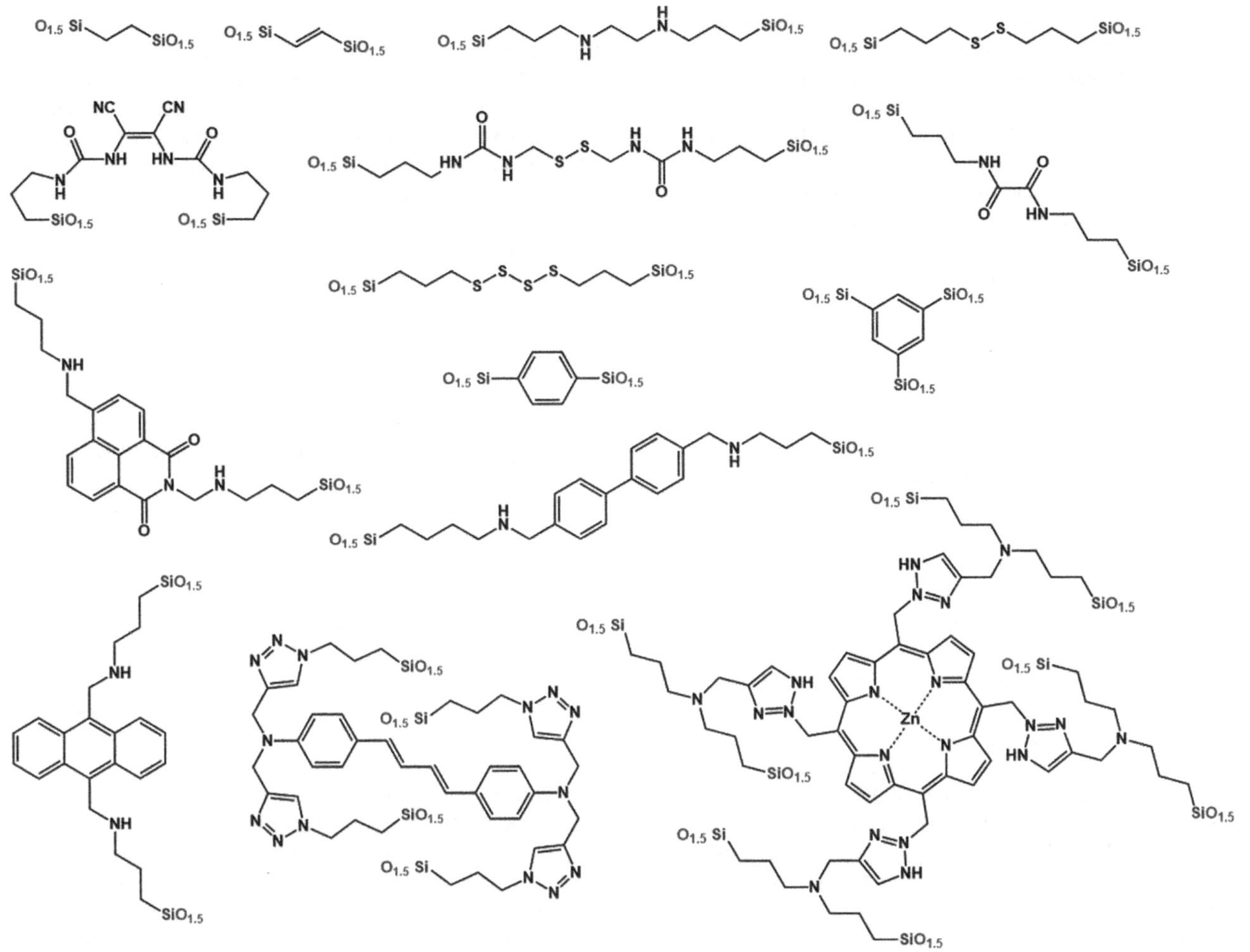

FIGURE 16.10 Published mesoporous organosilica nanoparticle and periodic mesoporous organosilica precursors. Different functional R groups are represented in orange. *Credit: Refs. 1,36,37,40,41,119–132.*

References

1. Croissant JG, Fatieiev Y, Almalik A, Khashab NM. Mesoporous silica and organosilica nanoparticles: physical chemistry, biosafety, delivery strategies, and biomedical applications. *Adv Healthc Mater* 2018;**7**. https://doi.org/10.1002/adhm.201700831. UNSP 1700831-UNSP 1700831.
2. Cotí KK, et al. Mechanised nanoparticles for drug delivery. Royal Society of Chemistry *Nanoscale* 2009:16–39.
3. Wu S-H, Hung Y, Mou C-Y. Mesoporous silica nanoparticles as nanocarriers. Royal Society of Chemistry *Chem Commun* 2011:9972–85.
4. Croissant J, Fatieiev Y, Khashab N. Degradability and clearance of silicon, organosilica, silsesquioxane, silica mixed oxide, and mesoporous silica nanoparticles. *Adv Mater* 2017;**29**:1–51.
5. Corriu R, Leclercq D. Recent developments of molecular chemistry for sol-gel processes. *Angew Chem* 1996;**35**.
6. Corriu R, Moreau J, Thepot P, Chi Man MW. New mixed organic-inorganic polymers: hydrolysis and polycondensation of bis(-trimethoxysilyl) organometallic precursors. *Chem Mater* 1992;**4**:1217–24.
7. Alauzun J, Besson E, Mehdi A, Reye C, Corriu RJP. Reversible covalent chemistry of CO2: an opportunity for nano-structured hybrid organic-inorganic materials. *Chem Mater* 2008;**20**:503–13. https://doi.org/10.1021/cm701946w.
8. Corriu R, Moreau J, Thepot P, Chi Man MW. Hybrid silica gels containing 1,3-butadiyne bridging units. Thermal and chemical reactivity of the organic fragment. *Chem Mater* 1996;**8**:100–6.
9. Andrianainarivelo M, Corriu R, Leclercq D, Mutin PH, Vioux A. Mixed oxides SiO_2–ZrO_2 and SiO_2–TiO_2 by a non-hydrolytic sol–gel route. *J Mater Chem* 1996;**6**:1665–71.
10. Boury B, Corriu R. Auto-organisation of hybrid organic–inorganic materials prepared by sol–gel chemistry. *Chem Commun* 2002:795–802.
11. Bourget L, Corriu RJP, Leclercq D, Mutin PH, Vioux A. Non-hydrolytic sol-gel routes to silica. *J Non-Cryst Solids* 1998;**242**:81–91.
12. Zhao L, Loy D, Shea K. Photodeformable spherical hybrid nanoparticles. *J Am Chem Soc* 2006;**128**:14250–1.
13. Shea KJ, Loy DA. Bridged polysilsesquioxanes. Molecular-engineered hybrid organic–inorganic materials. *Chem Mater* 2001;**13**:3306–19.

14. Qhobosheane M, Santra S, Zhang P, Tan W. Biochemically functionalized silica nanoparticles. *Analyst* 2001;**126**:1274–8.
15. Hobson S, Shea KJ. Bridged bisimide polysilsesquioxane Xerogels: new hybrid Organic–Inorganic materials. *Chem Mater* 1997;**9**:616–23.
16. Loy D, Shea KJ. Bridged polysilsesquioxanes. Highly porous hybrid organic-inorganic. *Chem Rev* 1995;**95**:1431–42.
17. Oviatt H, et al. Applications of organic bridged polysilsesquioxane xerogels to nonlinear optical materials by the sol-gel method. *Chem Mater* 1995;**7**:493–8.
18. Croissant JG, Fatieiev Y, Khashab NM. Degradability and clearance of silicon, organosilica, silsesquioxane, silica mixed oxide, and mesoporous silica nanoparticles. *Adv Mater* 2017;**29**. https://doi.org/10.1002/adma.201604634.
19. Yang P, Gai S, Lin J. Functionalized mesoporous silica materials for controlled drug delivery. *Chem Soc Rev* 2012;**41**:3679–98. https://doi.org/10.1039/c2cs15308d.
20. Liu J, Liu T, Pan J, Liu S, Lu GQM. Advances in multicompartment mesoporous silica micro/nanoparticles for theranostic applications. *Annu Rev Chem Biomol Eng* 2018;**9**:389–411. https://doi.org/10.1146/annurev-chembioeng-060817-084225.
21. Li Z, Barnes JC, Bosoy A, Stoddart JF, Zink JI. Mesoporous silica nanoparticles in biomedical applications. *Chem Soc Rev* 2012;**41**:2590–605. https://doi.org/10.1039/c1cs15246g.
22. Croissant J, Cattoën X, Wong Chi Man M, Durand J-O, Khashab N. Syntheses and applications of periodic mesoporous organosilica nanoparticles. *Nanoscale* 2015;**7**:20318–34.
23. Lu Y, et al. Aerosol-assisted self-assembly of mesostructured spherical nanoparticles. *Nature* 1999;**398**:223–6.
24. Brinker CJ, Scherer G. *Sol-gel Science*. Acedemic Press; 2013.
25. Wu S-H, Mou C-Y, Lin H-P. Synthesis of mesoporous silica nanoparticles. *Chem Soc Rev* 2013;**42**:3862–75. https://doi.org/10.1039/c3cs35405a.
26. Liu N, et al. Self-directed assembly of photoactive hybrid silicates derived from an azobenzene-bridged silsesquioxane. *J Am Chem Soc* 2002;**124**:14540–1.
27. Lu Y, et al. Evaporation-induced self-assembly of hybrid bridged silsesquioxane film and particulate mesophases with integral organic functionality. *J Am Chem Soc* 2000;**122**:5258–61.
28. Brinker CJ, Lu Y, Sellinger A, Fan H. Evaporation-induced self-assembly: nanostructures made easy. *Adv Mater* 1999;**11**.
29. Owens GJ, et al. Sol–gel based materials for biomedical applications. *Prog Mater Sci* 2016;**77**:1–79. https://doi.org/10.1016/j.pmatsci.2015.12.001.
30. Bitounis D, Fanciullino R, Iliadis A, Ciccolini J. Optimizing druggability through liposomal formulations: new approaches to an old concept. *ISRN Pharm* 2012:738432. https://doi.org/10.5402/2012/738432.
31. Beck JS, et al. A new family of mesoporous molecular sieves prepared with. *J Am Chem Soc* 1992;**114**:10834–43.
32. Zhang Q, et al. Biocompatible, uniform, and redispersible mesoporous silica nanoparticles for cancer-targeted drug delivery in vivo. *Adv Funct Mater* 2013;**24**.
33. Meng H, et al. Use of size and a copolymer design feature to improve the biodistribution and the enhanced permeability and retention effect of doxorubicin-loaded mesoporous silica nanoparticles in a Murine Xenograft tumor model. *ACS Nano* 2011;**5**:4131–44. https://doi.org/10.1021/nn200809t.
34. Yang J, et al. Spatially confined fabrication of core–shell gold Nanocages@Mesoporous silica for near-infrared controlled photothermal drug release. *Chem Mater* 2013;**25**:3030–7.
35. Li X, Xie QR, Zhang J, Xia W, Gu H. The packaging of siRNA within the mesoporous structure of silica nanoparticles. *Biomaterials* 2011;**32**:9546–56. https://doi.org/10.1016/j.biomaterials.2011.08.068.
36. Croissant J, et al. Mixed periodic mesoporous organosilica nanoparticles and core-shell systems, application to in vitro two-photon imaging, therapy, and drug delivery. *Chem Mater* 2014;**26**:7214–20. https://doi.org/10.1021/cm5040276.
37. Hu H, et al. Synthesis of Janus Au@periodic mesoporous organosilica (PMO) nanostructures with precisely controllable morphology: a seed-shape defined growth mechanism. *Nanoscale* 2017;**9**:4826–34. https://doi.org/10.1039/c7nr01047h.
38. Teng Z, et al. Facile synthesis of yolk-shell-structured triple-hybridized periodic mesoporous organosilica nanoparticles for biomedicine. *Small* 2016;**12**:3550–8. https://doi.org/10.1002/smll.201600616.
39. Wang T, et al. Mesostructured TiO2 gated periodic mesoporous organosilica-based nanotablets for multistimuli-responsive drug release. *Small* 2015;**11**:5907–11. https://doi.org/10.1002/smll.201501835.
40. Wang X, et al. A controllable asymmetrical/symmetrical coating strategy for architectural mesoporous organosilica nanostructures. *Nanoscale* 2016;**8**:13581–8. https://doi.org/10.1039/c6nr03229j.
41. Wu J, et al. Synergistic chemo-photothermal therapy of breast cancer by mesenchymal stem cell-encapsulated yolk-shell GNR@HPMO-PTX nanospheres. *Acs Applied Mater Interfaces* 2016;**8**:17927–35. https://doi.org/10.1021/acsami.6b05677.
42. Ma K, Sai H, Wiesner U. Ultrasmall sub-10 nm near-infrared fluorescent mesoporous silica nanoparticles. *J Am Chem Soc* 2012;**134**:13180–3. https://doi.org/10.1021/ja3049783.
43. Huang M, et al. Dendritic mesoporous silica nanospheres synthesized by a novel dual-templating micelle system for the preparation of functional nanomaterials. *Langmuir* 2017;**33**:519–26. https://doi.org/10.1021/acs.langmuir.6b03282.
44. Lu J, Li Z, Zink JI, Tamanoi F. In vivo tumor suppression efficacy of mesoporous silica nanoparticles-based drug-delivery system: enhanced efficacy by folate modification. *Nanomed Nanotechnol Biol Med* 2012;**8**:212–20. https://doi.org/10.1016/j.nano.2011.06.002.
45. Kim T-W, Chung P-W, Lin VSY. Facile synthesis of monodisperse spherical MCM-48 mesoporous silica nanoparticles with controlled particle size. *Chem Mater* 2010;**22**:5093–104. https://doi.org/10.1021/cm1017344.
46. Tarn D, et al. Mesoporous silica nanoparticle nanocarriers: biofunctionality and biocompatibility. *Acc Chem Res* 2013;**46**:792–801. https://doi.org/10.1021/ar3000986.
47. Moon D-S, Lee J-K. Tunable synthesis of hierarchical mesoporous silica nanoparticles with radial wrinkle structure. *Langmuir* 2012;**28**:12341–7. https://doi.org/10.1021/la302145j.
48. Kim M-H, et al. Facile synthesis of monodispersed mesoporous silica nanoparticles with ultralarge pores and their application in gene delivery. *ACS Nano* 2011;**5**:3568–76. https://doi.org/10.1021/nn103130q.
49. Argyo C, Weiss V, Braeuchle C, Bein T. Multifunctional mesoporous silica nanoparticles as a universal platform for drug delivery. *Chem Mater* 2014;**26**:435–51. https://doi.org/10.1021/cm402592t.

50. Niu D, Ma Z, Li Y, Shi J. Synthesis of core-shell structured dual-mesoporous silica spheres with tunable pore size and controllable shell thickness. *J Am Chem Soc* 2010;**132**:15144–7. https://doi.org/10.1021/ja1070653.
51. Lundqvist M, et al. Nanoparticle size and surface properties determine the protein corona with possible implications for biological impacts. *Proc Natl Acad Sci USA* 2008;**105**:14265–70. https://doi.org/10.1073/pnas.0805135105.
52. Shen D, et al. Biphase stratification approach to three-dimensional dendritic biodegradable mesoporous silica nanospheres. *Nano Lett* 2014;**14**:923–32. https://doi.org/10.1021/nl404316v.
53. Cedervall T, et al. Understanding the nanoparticle-protein corona using methods to quantify exchange rates and affinities of proteins for nanoparticles. *Proc Natl Acad Sci USA* 2007;**104**:2050–5. https://doi.org/10.1073/pnas.0608582104.
54. Monopoli MP, et al. Physical-chemical aspects of protein corona: relevance to in vitro and in vivo biological impacts of nanoparticles. *J Am Chem Soc* 2011;**133**:2525–34. https://doi.org/10.1021/ja107583h.
55. Tenzer S, et al. Rapid formation of plasma protein corona critically affects nanoparticle pathophysiology. *Nat Nanotechnol* 2013;**8**:772–U1000. https://doi.org/10.1038/nnano.2013.181.
56. Casals E, Pfaller T, Duschl A, Oostingh GJ, Puntes V. Time evolution of the nanoparticle protein corona. *ACS Nano* 2010;**4**:3623–32. https://doi.org/10.1021/nn901372t.
57. Del Pino P, et al. Protein corona formation around nanoparticles - from the past to the future. *Materials Horizons* 2014;**1**:301–13. https://doi.org/10.1039/c3mh00106g.
58. Nash T, Allison AC, Harington JS. Physico-chemical properties of silica in relation to its toxicity. *Nature* 1966;**210**. https://doi.org/10.1038/210259a0. 259-+.
59. Zhang H, et al. Processing pathway dependence of amorphous silica nanoparticle toxicity: colloidal vs pyrolytic. *J Am Chem Soc* 2012;**134**:15790–804. https://doi.org/10.1021/ja304907c.
60. Huang X, et al. The shape effect of mesoporous silica nanoparticles on biodistribution, clearance, and biocompatibility in vivo. *ACS Nano* 2011;**5**:5390–9. https://doi.org/10.1021/nn200365a.
61. Lu J, Liong M, Li Z, Zink JI, Tamanoi F. Biocompatibility, biodistribution, and drug-delivery efficiency of mesoporous silica nanoparticles for cancer therapy in animals. *Small* 2010;**6**:1794–805. https://doi.org/10.1002/smll.201000538.
62. Liu T, et al. Single and repeated dose toxicity of mesoporous hollow silica nanoparticles in intravenously exposed mice. *Biomaterials* 2011;**32**:1657–68. https://doi.org/10.1016/j.biomaterials.2010.10.035.
63. Dobrovolskaia MA, et al. Interaction of colloidal gold nanoparticles with human blood: effects on particle size and analysis of plasma protein binding profiles. *Nanomed Nanotechnol Biol Med* 2009;**5**:106–17. https://doi.org/10.1016/j.nano.2008.08.001.
64. Pisani C, et al. The timeline of corona formation around silica nanocarriers highlights the role of the protein interactome. *Nanoscale* 2017;**9**:1840–51. https://doi.org/10.1039/c6nr04765c.
65. Paula AJ, Martinez DST, Araujo Junior RT, Souza Filho AG, Alves OL. Suppression of the hemolytic effect of mesoporous silica nanoparticles after protein corona interaction: independence of the surface microchemical environment. *J Braz Chem Soc* 2012;**23**:1807–14. https://doi.org/10.1590/S0103-50532012005000048.
66. Martinez DST, et al. Monitoring the hemolytic effect of mesoporous silica nanoparticles after human blood protein corona formation. *Eur J Inorg Chem* 2015:4595–602. https://doi.org/10.1002/ejic.201500573.
67. Lesniak A, et al. Effects of the presence or absence of a protein corona on silica nanoparticle uptake and impact on cells. *ACS Nano* 2012;**6**:5845–57. https://doi.org/10.1021/nn300223w.
68. Kreuter J, et al. Apolipoprotein-mediated transport of nanoparticle-bound drugs across the blood-brain barrier. *J Drug Target* 2002;**10**:317–25. https://doi.org/10.1080/10611860290031877.
69. Monopoli MP, Bombelli FB, Dawson KA. Nanobiotechnology Nanoparticle coronas take shape. *Nat Nanotechnol* 2011;**6**:11–2. https://doi.org/10.1038/nnano.2011.267.
70. Botella P, et al. Surface-modified silica nanoparticles for tumor-targeted delivery of camptothecin and its biological evaluation. *J Control Release* 2011;**156**:246–57. https://doi.org/10.1016/j.jconrel.2011.06.039.
71. Mirshafiee V, Mahmoudi M, Lou K, Cheng J, Kraft ML. Protein corona significantly reduces active targeting yield. *Chem Commun* 2013;**49**:2557–9. https://doi.org/10.1039/c3cc37307j.
72. Liu J, Yu M, Zhou C, Zheng J. Renal clearable inorganic nanoparticles: a new frontier of bionanotechnology. *Mater Today* 2013;**16**:477–86. https://doi.org/10.1016/j.mattod.2013.11.003.
73. Giri S, Trewyn BG, Stellmaker MP, Lin VSY. Stimuli-responsive controlled-release delivery system based on mesoporous silica nanorods capped with magnetic nanoparticles. *Angew Chem Int Ed* 2005;**44**:5038–44. https://doi.org/10.1002/anie.200501819.
74. He Q, Zhang Z, Gao Y, Shi J, Li Y. Intracellular localization and cytotoxicity of spherical mesoporous silica nano- and microparticles. *Small* 2009;**5**:2722–9. https://doi.org/10.1002/smll.200900923.
75. Finnie KS, et al. Biodegradability of sol-gel silica microparticles for drug delivery. *J Sol Gel Sci Technol* 2009;**49**:12–8. https://doi.org/10.1007/s10971-008-1847-4.
76. Ehrlich H, Demadis KD, Pokrovsky OS, Koutsoukos PG. Modern views on desilicification: biosilica and abiotic silica dissolution in natural and artificial environments. *Chem Rev* 2010;**110**:4656–89. https://doi.org/10.1021/cr900334y.
77. Tzur-Balter A, Shatsberg Z, Beckerman M, Segal E, Artzi N. Mechanism of erosion of nanostructured porous silicon drug carriers in neoplastic tissues. *Nat Commun* 2015;**6**. https://doi.org/10.1038/ncomms7208. 6208-6208.
78. Lu W, et al. Photoluminescent mesoporous silicon nanoparticles with siCCR2 improve the effects of mesenchymal stromal cell transplantation after acute myocardial infarction. *Theranostics* 2015;**5**:1068–82. https://doi.org/10.7150/thno.11517.
79. Knezevic NZ, Durand J-O. Large pore mesoporous silica nanomaterials for application in delivery of biomolecules. *Nanoscale* 2015;**7**:2199–209. https://doi.org/10.1039/c4nr06114d.
80. Angelos S, et al. pH clock-operated mechanized nanoparticles. *J Am Chem Soc* 2009;**131**. https://doi.org/10.1021/ja9010157. 12912-+.
81. Lee C-H, et al. Intracellular pH-responsive mesoporous silica nanoparticles for the controlled release of anticancer chemotherapeutics. *Angew Chem Int Ed* 2010;**49**:8214–9. https://doi.org/10.1002/anie.201002639.
82. Rim HP, Min KH, Lee HJ, Jeong SY, Lee SC. pH-tunable calcium phosphate covered mesoporous silica nanocontainers for intracellular controlled release of guest drugs. *Angew Chem Int Ed* 2011;**50**:8853–7. https://doi.org/10.1002/anie.201101536.
83. Kim H, et al. Glutathione-induced intracellular release of guests from mesoporous silica nanocontainers with cyclodextrin gatekeepers. *Adv Mater* 2010;**22**:4280. https://doi.org/10.1002/adma.201001417.
84. Patel K, et al. Enzyme-responsive snap-top covered silica nanocontainers. *J Am Chem Soc* 2008;**130**:2382–3. https://doi.org/10.1021/ja0772086.

85. Ferris DP, et al. Light-operated mechanized nanoparticles. *J Am Chem Soc* 2009;**131**:1686–8. https://doi.org/10.1021/ja807798g.
86. Thomas CR, et al. Noninvasive remote-controlled release of drug molecules in vitro using magnetic actuation of mechanized nanoparticles. *J Am Chem Soc* 2010;**132**:10623–5. https://doi.org/10.1021/ja1022267.
87. Chen Y, et al. Multifunctional mesoporous composite nanocapsules for highly efficient MRI-guided high-intensity focused ultrasound cancer surgery. *Angew Chem Int Ed* 2011;**50**:12505–9. https://doi.org/10.1002/anie.201106180.
88. Gu L, et al. In vivo time-gated fluorescence imaging with biodegradable luminescent porous silicon nanoparticles. *Nat Commun* 2013;**4**:2326. https://doi.org/10.1038/ncomms3326.
89. Miller L, et al. Synthesis, characterization, and biodistribution of multiple Zr-89-labeled pore-expanded mesoporous silica nanoparticles for PET. *Nanoscale* 2014;**6**:4928–35. https://doi.org/10.1039/c3nr06800e.
90. Chen F, et al. In vivo integrity and biological fate of chelator-free zirconium-89-labeled mesoporous silica nanoparticles. *ACS Nano* 2015;**9**:7950–9. https://doi.org/10.1021/acsnano.5b00526.
91. Goel S, et al. Engineering intrinsically zirconium-89 radiolabeled self-destructing mesoporous silica nanostructures for in vivo biodistribution and tumor targeting studies. *Adv Sci* 2016;**3**. https://doi.org/10.1002/advs.201600122. 1600122-1600122.
92. Kamkaew A, et al. Cerenkov radiation induced photodynamic therapy using Chlorin e6-loaded hollow mesoporous silica nanoparticles. *Acs Appl Mater Interfaces* 2016;**8**:26630–7. https://doi.org/10.1021/acsami.6b10255.
93. Ellison PA, et al. Intrinsic and stable conjugation of thiolated mesoporous silica nanoparticles with radioarsenic. *Acs Appl Mater Interfaces* 2017;**9**:6772–81. https://doi.org/10.1021/acsami.6b14049.
94. Huang X, et al. Long-term multimodal imaging of tumor draining sentinel lymph nodes using mesoporous silica-based nanoprobes. *Biomaterials* 2012;**33**:4370–8. https://doi.org/10.1016/j.biomaterials.2012.02.060.
95. Chen F, et al. In vivo tumor targeting and image-guided drug delivery with antibody-conjugated, radio labeled mesoporous silica nanoparticles. *ACS Nano* 2013;**7**:9027–39. https://doi.org/10.1021/nn403617J.
96. Huang X, et al. Mesenchymal stem cell-based cell engineering with multifunctional mesoporous silica nanoparticles for tumor delivery. *Biomaterials* 2013;**34**:1772–80. https://doi.org/10.1016/j.biomaterials.2012.11.032.
97. Chen F, et al. Engineering of hollow mesoporous silica nanoparticles for remarkably enhanced tumor active targeting efficacy. *Sci Rep* 2014;**4**. https://doi.org/10.1038/srep05080. 5080-5080.
98. Chen F, et al. In vivo tumor vasculature targeted PET/NIRF imaging with TRC105(Fab)-conjugated, dual-labeled mesoporous silica nanoparticles. *Mol Pharm* 2014;**11**:4007–14. https://doi.org/10.1021/mp500306k.
99. Goel S, et al. VEGF(121)-Conjugated mesoporous silica nanoparticle: a tumor targeted drug delivery system. *Acs Appl Mater Interfaces* 2014;**6**:21677–85. https://doi.org/10.1021/am506849p.
100. Chakravarty R, et al. Hollow mesoporous silica nanoparticles for tumor vasculature targeting and PET image-guided drug delivery. *Nanomedicine* 2015;**10**:1233–46. https://doi.org/10.2217/nnm.14.226.
101. Chen F, et al. In vivo tumor vasculature targeting of CuS@MSN based theranostic nanomedicine. *ACS Nano* 2015;**9**:3926–34. https://doi.org/10.1021/nn507241v.
102. Cheng B, et al. Gold nanosphere gated mesoporous silica nanoparticle responsive to near-infrared light and redox potential as a theranostic platform for cancer therapy. *J Biomed Nanotechnol* 2016;**12**:435–49. https://doi.org/10.1166/jbn.2016.2195.
103. Chen F, et al. Intrinsic radiolabeling of Titanium-45 using mesoporous silica nanoparticles. *Acta Pharmacol Sin* 2017;**38**:907–13. https://doi.org/10.1038/aps.2017.1.
104. Valdovinos H, et al. Positron emission tomography imaging of intrinsically titanium-45 radiolabeled mesoporous silica nanoparticles. *J Nucl Med* 2016;**57**.
105. Lee SB, et al. Mesoporous silica nanoparticle pretargeting for PET imaging based on a rapid bioorthogonal reaction in a living body. *Angew Chem Int Ed* 2013;**52**:10549–52. https://doi.org/10.1002/anie.201304026.
106. Kim DW. Bioorthogonal click chemistry for fluorine-18 labeling protocols under physiologically friendly reaction condition. *J Fluorine Chem* 2015;**174**:142–7. https://doi.org/10.1016/j.jfluchem.2014.11.009.
107. Rojas S, et al. Novel methodology for labelling mesoporous silica nanoparticles using the F-18 isotope and their in vivo biodistribution by positron emission tomography. *J Nanoparticle Res* 2015;**17**. https://doi.org/10.1007/s11051-015-2938-0. 131-131.
108. Denk C, et al. Design, synthesis, and evaluation of a low-molecular-weight C-11-Labeled tetrazine for pretargeted PET imaging applying bioorthogonal in vivo click chemistry. *Bioconjug Chem* 2016;**27**:1707–12. https://doi.org/10.1021/acs.bioconjchem.6b00234.
109. Wang X, et al. Perfluorohexane-encapsulated mesoporous silica nanocapsules as enhancement agents for highly efficient high intensity focused ultrasound (HIFU). *Adv Mater* 2012;**24**:785–91. https://doi.org/10.1002/adma.201104033.
110. Gao F, Botella P, Corma A, Blesa J, Dong L. Monodispersed mesoporous silica nanoparticles with very large pores for enhanced adsorption and release of DNA. *J Phys Chem B* 2009;**113**:1796–804. https://doi.org/10.1021/jp807956r.
111. Moeller K, et al. Highly efficient siRNA delivery from core-shell mesoporous silica nanoparticles with multifunctional polymer caps. *Nanoscale* 2016;**8**:4007–19. https://doi.org/10.1039/c5nr06246b.
112. Chakraborty I, Mascharak PK. Mesoporous silica materials and nanoparticles as carriers for controlled and site-specific delivery of gaseous signaling molecules. *Microporous Mesoporous Mater* 2016;**234**:409–19. https://doi.org/10.1016/j.micromeso.2016.07.028.
113. Zhou X, et al. Dual-responsive mesoporous silica nanoparticles mediated codelivery of doxorubicin and Bcl-2 SiRNA for targeted treatment of breast cancer. *J Phys Chem C* 2016;**120**:22375–87. https://doi.org/10.1021/acs.jpcc.6b06759.
114. Geng J, Li M, Wu L, Chen C, Qu X. Mesoporous silica nanoparticle-based H2O2 responsive controlled-release system used for alzheimer's disease treatment. *Adv Healthc Mater* 2012;**1**:332–6. https://doi.org/10.1002/adhm.201200067.
115. Trewyn BG, Whitman CM, Lin VSY. Morphological control of room-temperature ionic liquid templated mesoporous silica nanoparticles for controlled release of antibacterial agents. *Nano Lett* 2004;**4**:2139–43. https://doi.org/10.1021/nl048774r.

116. Izquierdo-Barba I, et al. Incorporation of antimicrobial compounds in mesoporous silica film monolith. *Biomaterials* 2009;**30**:5729–36. https://doi.org/10.1016/j.biomaterials.2009.07.003.
117. Kwon EJ, et al. Porous silicon nanoparticle delivery of tandem peptide anti-infectives for the treatment of *Pseudomonas aeruginosa* lung infections. *Adv Mater* 2017;**29**. https://doi.org/10.1002/adma.201701527.
118. Li L-l, Wang H. Enzyme-coated mesoporous silica nanoparticles as efficient antibacterial agents in vivo. *Adv Healthc Mater* 2013;**2**:1351–60. https://doi.org/10.1002/adhm.201300051.
119. Lu D, Lei J, Wang L, Zhang J. Multifluorescently traceable nanoparticle by a single-wavelength excitation with color-related drug release performance. *J Am Chem Soc* 2012;**134**:8746–9. https://doi.org/10.1021/ja301691j.
120. Li X, et al. Anisotropic growth-induced synthesis of dual-compartment *Janus mesoporous* silica nanoparticles for bimodal triggered drugs delivery. *J Am Chem Soc* 2014;**136**:15086–92. https://doi.org/10.1021/ja508733r.
121. Teng Z, et al. Yolk-shell structured mesoporous nanoparticles with thioether-bridged organosilica frameworks. *Chem Mater* 2014;**26**:5980–7. https://doi.org/10.1021/cm502777e.
122. Teng Z, et al. A facile multi-interface transformation approach to monodisperse multiple-shelled periodic mesoporous organosilica hollow spheres. *J Am Chem Soc* 2015;**137**:7935–44. https://doi.org/10.1021/jacs.5b05369.
123. Yang Y, et al. Structure-dependent and glutathione-responsive biodegradable dendritic mesoporous organosilica nanoparticles for safe protein delivery. *Chem Mater* 2016;**28**:9008–16. https://doi.org/10.1021/acs.chemmater.6b03896.
124. Chen Y, et al. Hollow mesoporous organosilica nanoparticles: a generic intelligent framework-hybridization approach for biomedicine. *J Am Chem Soc* 2014;**136**:16326–34. https://doi.org/10.1021/ja508721y.
125. Guan B, et al. Highly ordered periodic mesoporous organosilica nanoparticles with controllable pore structures. *Nanoscale* 2012;**4**:6588–96. https://doi.org/10.1039/c2nr31662e.
126. Lin CX, et al. Synthesis of magnetic hollow periodic mesoporous organosilica with enhanced cellulose tissue penetration behaviour. *J Mater Chem* 2011;**21**:7565–71. https://doi.org/10.1039/c1jm10615e.
127. Jimenez CM, et al. Nanodiamond-PMO for two-photon PDT and drug delivery. *J Mater Chem B* 2016;**4**:5803–8. https://doi.org/10.1039/c6tb01915c.
128. Xiong L, Qiao S-Z. A mesoporous organosilica nano-bowl with high DNA loading capacity - a potential gene delivery carrier. *Nanoscale* 2016;**8**:17446–50. https://doi.org/10.1039/c6nr06777h.
129. Ni Q, et al. Gold nanorod embedded large-pore mesoporous organosilica nanospheres for gene and photothermal cooperative therapy of triple negative breast cancer. *Nanoscale* 2017;**9**:1466–74. https://doi.org/10.1039/c6nr07598c.
130. Dang M, et al. Mesoporous organosilica nanoparticles with large radial pores via an assembly-reconstruction process in bi-phase. *J Mater Chem B* 2017;**5**:2625–34. https://doi.org/10.1039/c6tb03327j.
131. Mauriello-Jimenez C, et al. Porphyrin-functionalized mesoporous organosilica nanoparticles for two-photon imaging of cancer cells and drug delivery. *J Mater Chem B* 2015;**3**:3681–4. https://doi.org/10.1039/c5tb00315f.
132. Croissant JG, et al. Disulfide-gated mesoporous silica nanoparticles designed for two-photon-triggered drug release and imaging. *J Mater Chem B* 2015;**3**:6456–61. https://doi.org/10.1039/c5tb00797f.

Chapter 17

Biomedical applications of cerium oxide nanoparticles: a potent redox modulator and drug delivery agent

Nicholas J. Abuid[1], Kerim M. Gattás-Asfura[1], Daniel J. LaShoto[1], Alexia M. Poulos[1] and Cherie L. Stabler[1,2]

[1]*J. Crayton Pruitt Family Department of Biomedical Engineering, University of Florida, Gainesville, FL, United States;* [2]*University of Florida Diabetes Institute, Gainesville, FL, United States*

17.1 Background

17.1.1 Reactive oxygen species and reactive nitrogen species in human physiology and pathophysiology

In biological systems, redox reactions occur in numerous processes, such as respiration and energy storage. Redox reactions include free radical reactions that generate reactive oxygen species (ROS) and reactive nitrogen species (RNS).[1] ROS are reactive molecules or radicals derived from O_2 and include hydrogen peroxide (H_2O_2), superoxide anion ($O_2{\bullet}^-$), hydroxyl radical (HO•), and hydroperoxyl radical ($HO_2\bullet$).[2–4] RNS are reactive molecules derived from nitric oxide (•NO) and include agents such as peroxynitrite ($ONOO^-$).[5] ROS and RNS are typically produced within a cell as a part of natural metabolic processes. They play various roles in cell physiology, from intracellular signaling and cell–cell communication to control of vascular diameter, a sensor for hypoxia, and regulation of the immune system.[6,7] ROS/RNS levels generated for these physiological signaling pathways are typically classified as low,[8] e.g., approximately 82 nmol/min of H_2O_2 is produced per g of rat liver.[9] Immune cells in the body generate ROS in higher concentrations that act as a defense mechanism against invading bacteria and pathogens.[10] To regulate intracellular ROS/RNS levels, cells produce antioxidants, such as glutathione, superoxide dismutase (SOD), and catalase (CAT). Synthesis of these proteins is modulated by ROS/RNS levels, where antioxidant generation increases and decreases to maintain the cell's specific acceptable concentration range.[7]

When ROS/RNS concentrations exceed the antioxidant capacity of the cell and/or the antioxidant levels are insufficient to scavenge ROS/RNS, an imbalance, collectively known as oxidative stress, arises. Elevated ROS/RNS levels are not only detrimental to the body, where they serve to oxidize macromolecules, fragment proteins, and impart DNA damage, they also typically serve as a signal of a pathological event. For example, ROS is a key player in several pathophysiological conditions including cancer, obesity, and autoimmune diseases. While oxidative stress can arise from multiple pathological factors (e.g., hyperglycemia, hypoxia, apoptosis),[11,12] the most common impetus for this imbalance is inflammation. Thus, this section will focus on the role of free radicals in inflammatory diseases.

Inflammation is a defense mechanism used by host cells to protect against foreign agents or insults/injuries that threaten organism homeostasis. This inflammatory response is a general component of the immune system and is classically identified by the hallmarks of swelling, redness, pain, and fever. These responses are due to increased permeability of blood vessels that results in increased fluidic and leukocyte infiltration into the tissue. Because of its nonspecific nature, inflammation is typically binned into the innate arm of the immune system, although inflammatory pathways, cells, and signals play key roles in instructing adaptive immune cell responses.[13] During inflammation, a redox imbalance occurs where ROS/RNS serves as a key player in destroying pathogens, signaling between cells, and dictating the phenotype of recruited cells. First responder cells, neutrophils, produce ROS to destroy foreign pathogens.[14] This oxidative environment promotes naïve resident macrophages to mature into a proinflammatory (M1) phenotype.[15] Furthermore, ROS/RNS recruits monocytes to the target site that also transition

Nanoparticles for Biomedical Applications. https://doi.org/10.1016/B978-0-12-816662-8.00017-5

into M1 macrophages. Macrophages are key players in regulating inflammation and resolving the insult, as they are responsible for removing debris from the injury site and orchestrating tissue repair via secretion of ROS, RNS, and proinflammatory cytokines, such as interferon gamma, tumor necrosis factor-alpha (TNF-α), and interleukin-1 (IL-1).[16] These macrophage-derived signals can serve to further recruit additional immune cells, as well as to signal cells within the adaptive arm, such as T and B cells.[13]

In most cases, acute inflammation is resolved by the clearance of the foreign body, insult, or pathogen. Subsequently, the recruitment of immune cells to the site is halted as vascular permeability retracts, and the remaining immune cells undergo phenotype switching to promote tissue healing/repair (e.g., macrophage transition from M1 to antiinflammatory (M2)) and/or initiate programmed cell death (apoptosis).[17,18] However, in select cases, inflammation is unresolved, which leads to a state of chronic inflammation. This prolonged state of inflammation is a key feature of several diseases including autoimmunity, neurodegeneration, type 2 diabetes, and respiratory conditions.[19]

Given that ROS and RNS are key agents in sustaining a chronic inflammatory environment, considerable research efforts are focused on deactivating or scavenging these agents. Decreasing oxidative stress not only mitigates cell damage and death but also globally alters the environment. By modulating ROS and RNS in the injury site, it is possible to control cell phenotype and cytokine expression.[20] Reducing the levels of ROS can decrease the expression of TNF-α and IL-1β in innate immune cells. These cytokines and ROS also serve as a signal between cells of the innate and the adaptive branches of the immune system.[21] These pathways linking ROS and inflammation indicate that redox modulation can have a trickle-down effect on inflammatory conditions and diseases. Thus, the identification and validation of novel antioxidant materials that are compatible with biological applications would have a profound impact on multiple medical conditions, from heart disease to cancer. Oxidative stress relief can be achieved by elevating or boosting cell-generated antioxidants or delivering exogenous agents such as flavonoids, carotenoids, magnolol, omega-3, and omega-6 fatty acids.[22,23] However, these antioxidant agents have poor bioavailability. To address many of these challenges, researchers have explored leveraging nanoparticle therapeutics for redox modulation, in particular, cerium oxide nanoparticles (CONPs).

17.1.2 Properties of cerium oxide nanoparticles

Cerium (Ce), a lanthanoid element, exhibits unique redox behavior due to its electron configuration, which starts to fill the 4f orbital in the ground state.[24] It has common oxidation numbers of +3 or +4 and can be found in selected minerals, including bastnäsite and monazite, which are important commercial sources.[25] Oxide forms of cerium include CeO_2 (dioxide or ceria) and Ce_2O_3 (dicerium trioxide or sesquioxide).[26] Cerium oxide has been broadly utilized for various applications, such as electrolyte in fuel and solar cells, detection systems, surface polishing, ultraviolet light absorbent, fertilizer, and an active component for heterogeneous catalysis.[24,27–32] This last application takes advantage of cerium cycling (autoregeneration) redox equilibrium between its two oxidation states and Lewis acid/base sites. This results in the capacity of cerium oxide to catalyze a broad spectrum of agents, including ROS and RNS.[33] The reactivity of cerium oxide is particularly effective at the nanoscale, as the high surface-to-volume ratio results in elevated surface oxygen vacancies, hence Ce^{3+}.[34] Thus, the smaller the particle, the stronger the redox activity per unit volume. This boost in activity has led to a strong interest in CONPs for biomedical applications, as shown in Fig. 17.1A.[35]

Of particular biomedical interest is the use of CONP in radical-mediated reactions, either against oxidative stress and radiation or as a selective cytotoxic prooxidation therapeutic. CONPs can mimic the catalytic property of major natural antioxidant systems including the metalloenzymes, SOD, and CAT.[36] Nanoparticle reaction with superoxide or hydrogen peroxide has been assayed, respectively, utilizing the reduction of ferricytochrome C by superoxide or oxidation of 3,3′,5,5′-tetramethylbenzidine, 10-acetyl-3,7-dihydroxyphenoxazine, and 2,2-azinobis-(3-ethylbenzothizoline-6-sulfonic acid) (AzBTS), and/or H_2O_2, as monitored spectrophotometrically.[37–40] These studies have also established that CONP can serve as an oxidizing agent, and that the oxidizing capacity of CONP depends on the pH of the particular solution and the ratio of surface cerium 3+/4+.[39] In acidic pH, CONP has oxidase-like activity (highest at pH 4) and tends to exhibit more SOD-mimetic than CAT-mimetic properties.[38,41] The mechanisms of SOD and CAT activity are summarized in Fig. 17.1B and C. Preferential reactivity has also been correlated to the number of oxygen vacancies, where CONPs are able to scavenge ROS or RNS when having a higher or lower cerium 3+/4 + ratio, respectively.[42] Thus, the smaller the particle, the stronger the ROS catalytic activity, due to its elevated surface Ce^{3+}.[43] However, in a noninternalized CONP cell model, a higher surface Ce^{3+} concentration on CONP has been linked with increased cytotoxicity as a result of ROS formation and nanoparticle cell wall attachment.[44]

CONP can be engineered to scavenge different radicals or act as an oxidant depending on particle characteristics and destination. For example, the modulation of bulk (e.g., size and shape) and chemical (e.g., composition,

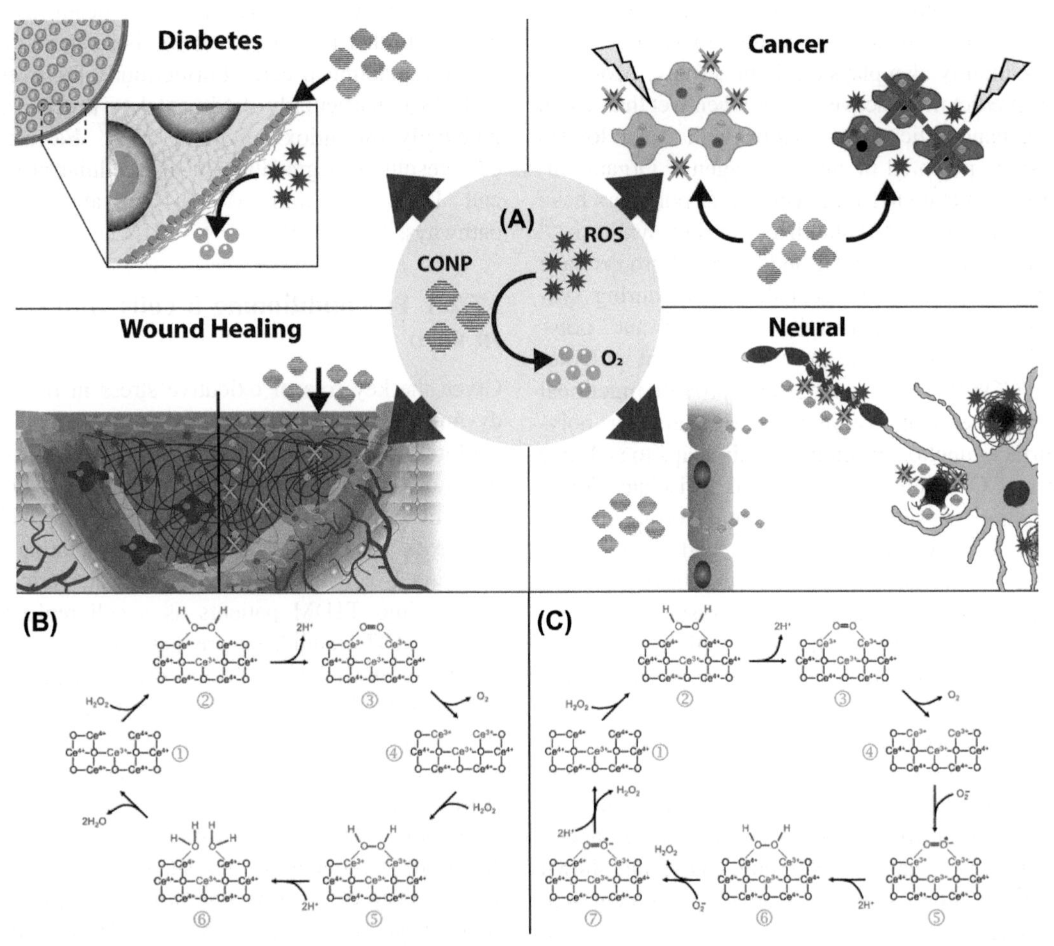

FIGURE 17.1 Cerium oxide nanoparticle (CONP) has adaptable redox properties and can modulate reactive oxygen species for multiple pathological conditions and at various stages of disease development and progression (A). Several factors can dictate the redox activity of CONP. The postulated mechanisms of catalase mimetic activity (B) and superoxide dismutase–mimetic activity (C) are depicted. The enzyme-like activity is beneficial when treating redox imbalances at different stages of disease development and progression. *Figure (B–C) adapted from Celardo I., et al., Pharmacological potential of cerium oxide nanoparticles.* Nanoscale *2011;3(4):1411–1420.*

coatings, and surfactants used during fabrication) characteristics has been shown to influence the catalytic activity of these nanostructures.[24,34] CONP fabrication methods include precipitation, coprecipitation, wet-chemical, hydrothermal process, and microwave-mediated synthesis.[45] Resulting nanoparticle properties are manipulated by the method of fabrication, as well as by parameters of the method used, such as the period of aging, temperature, and pH.[46] Manipulating these factors can yield nanoparticles with distinct shape, size, stability, and oxidative ratio of 3+/4+,[46–48] resulting in variations in cellular trafficking and activity, i.e., prooxidant or antioxidant.[46] Karakoti et al. provided a comprehensive review of the role of different factors during the synthesis process on CONP properties.[45] Briefly, CONP synthesis involves stirring a cerium precursor, such as cerium (III) nitrate,[49–51] cerium (III) sulfate,[52] or cerium (II) chloride,[53,54] with an oxidizer, such as hydrogen peroxide or ammonia.[47] Simple modifications in the concentration of these reagents, as well as the ratio of precursor to oxidizer, can also alter CONP's resulting oxidation state. The precipitation method is one of the most common methods of CONP synthesis, and it consists of adding cerium precursor to an oxidizer, followed by stirring and purification.[50–52] Alternative protocols dry and furnace the precipitant at different temperatures, again providing tailorability in the ratio of 3+/4+.[52] Another synthesis method uses the coprecipitation of cerium nitrate and potassium carbonate to yield a precursor of cerium (III) carbonate, which ages under stirring to cerium oxide particles.[49] Heat-mediated methods include hydrothermal and microwave-mediated synthesis, where heat is added to Teflon-lined autoclave containing a cerium precursor.[53,55] Flame spray pyrolysis generates CONP by the addition of a cerium precursor solution to the center of a flame in the presence of a controlled oxygen stream; this method provides fine control of nanoparticle size via manipulation of the rate of precursor addition and oxygen.[56,57] Understanding each of these fabrication techniques and the effect of the different parameters during the reaction allows for tailorability in the features of the resulting CONP.

CONP solubility also plays a role in activity. Atomistic simulations predict more active CONP when wet than when dry because nanoparticle coordination with water lowers the electrostatic potential of surface oxygen.[58] Organic alcohols, amines, metal-chelating agents, and polymers have all been utilized as CONP stabilizers during synthesis.[24] Polymers containing carboxylate and hydroxyl groups have been utilized to stabilize and coat the CONP during synthesis. Dextran,[59,60] poly (acrylic acid),[61,62] and polyethylene glycol (PEG)[63] are some examples of polymer coatings on CONP. These coatings also provide functional groups for further conjugation to other agents or polymers.[64] Surface functionalization not only helps to stabilize and disperse CONP but can be utilized to isolate CONP from environmental solutes (e.g., protein corona in biological fluids),[65] control cytotoxicity,[66,67] and direct CONP localization.[62,68] Overall, the surface-related factors such as particle characteristics, surface coating, crystal facets, and local environment can impact the redox activity of CONP and can direct either toward a prooxidant or an antioxidant route.[69]

In subsequent sections, we outline the application of CONP toward multiple biomedical applications where modulation of oxidative stress is essential to mitigate disease progression or to provide an interventional agent. While still in early stages of exploration, CONP has shown significant potential to serve as a broad and potent free radical scavenger.

17.2 Diabetes

Diabetes mellitus (DM) is a disease that involves abnormal blood glucose levels and dysfunction of the pancreatic insulin–producing β cells. There are two main types of DM, type I diabetes mellitus (T1DM) and type II diabetes mellitus (T2DM). Both types differ in etiology; however, they share common disease traits such as blood glucose instability, loss in β-cell function, and oxidative stress.[70] Redox imbalances play a key role in the pathogenesis of both diseases. In autoimmune T1DM, ROS is a critical contributor to both β-cell death and dysfunction and the propagation of the autoimmune response.[21,71] In T2DM, the combination of genetic and environmental factors, such as nutritional excess and physical inactivity, leads to peripheral insulin resistance in muscle and fat tissues.[72–74] The development of this resistance is postulated to be a protective mechanism against excessive ROS generated due to excess glucose transport into fat and muscle cells.[75] To account for this insulin resistance, β cells increase in mass and insulin production, but these overworked cells eventually succumb to metabolic burnout.[74] Both T1DM and T2DM are self-perpetuated by the hyperglycemia that results from β-cell dysfunction and death, as high blood glucose further leads to metabolic burnout and dysfunction of the remaining β cells. Furthermore, the overabundance of ROS is particularly detrimental to β cells, due to their inherently low antioxidant defenses.[76,77] Elevated ROS in β cells results in degradation of intracellular proteins, lipids, and DNA, as well as the activation of apoptotic pathways.[21,78]

17.2.1 Preconditioning β cells with CONP *In vitro*

Given the key role of oxidative stress in β-cell death and dysfunction, antioxidant supplementation has been explored as an option to preserve β-cell mass. A strong focus of this approach in diabetes has been in supporting the efficacy of clinical islet transplantation (CIT). In CIT, pancreatic islets, the cluster of cells containing the insulin-secreting β cells, are isolated from cadaveric donors and infused into T1DM patients as a cell replacement therapy.[79,80] CIT candidates are patients with poor glucose instability and repeated occurrences of unaware hypoglycemic events.[81] A challenge with CIT, however, is the significant loss of β-cell mass during culture and post-transplant due to oxidative stress. Numerous antioxidant agents, such as edaravone and gliclazide, have been incorporated into islet transplants, via systemic infusion, preculture treatment, or transgenic overexpression, with varying degrees of protective effects[82–86]; however, these approaches are limited by the need for systemic delivery, the decreased duration of effect, and the complexities of transfection, respectively. To provide more durable protection, studies have explored the impact of supplementing islet or β-cell cultures with CONP. In the first report of CONP benefits for β-cell culture, Simpson et al. described the intracellular uptake of CONP and their subsequent capacity to scavenge intracellular free radicals under an oxidant challenge.[87] In another approach, CONP was combined with sodium selenite and added to pancreatic islet cultures.[88] Sodium selenite contains antioxidant and antidiabetic properties, as it has been shown to improve glucose response, insulin secretion, and islet graft survival.[89,90]

Elevated β-cell viability and insulin secretion was observed over the culture period, indicating the capacity of these supplements to preserve these cells longer in culture. In a subsequent paper, Abdollahi's group replaced sodium selenite with yttrium oxide nanoparticle (YONP) as a complementary antioxidant strategy.[91] Yttrium behaves similar to lanthanide metals and is known for having one of the highest free energy of oxide formation of all the metal oxides.[92,93] Pretreatment of pancreatic islets with CONP/YONP resulted in cytoprotection from physiologically harmful H_2O_2 challenges. Antioxidant nanoparticles also decreased intracellular ROS levels, which reduced β-cell apoptosis and mitigated ROS-mediated impairment of insulin secretion.[91] While supplementation of β-cell cultures with CONP is highly promising, there are concerns over the cytotoxic effects of cellular internalization and accumulation of these nanoparticles, particularly for CONP larger than 100 nm or dosages greater than 1 mM for smaller particle sizes.[33,35,94–97] Finally, as many cellular processes are mediated by intracellular free radical signaling, the internalization of CONP may have unpredictable consequences on these processes and lead to pathological conditions in these cells.[98] As such, approaches that seek to control cellular internalization of these particles or modulate the surface properties of CONP would be highly beneficial.

17.2.2 CONP in β-cell transplantation

While antioxidant supplements may preserve islet survival in culture, transplanted islets are subjected to significant inflammatory reactions, immune recognition, and attack that lead to reduction in therapeutic efficacy.[80,99] This is due to both the inherent inflammation and immune attack associated with the implantation of foreign allogeneic cells, as well as the autoimmune recognition of β cells associated with T1DM. Thus, CIT recipients are subjected to a potent regimen of antiinflammatory and immunosuppressive drugs to prevent allogeneic and autogenic-associated immune attack.[80] This drug cocktail imparts broad and adverse side effects. To avoid the need for systemic immunosuppression, biomaterial encapsulation has been employed. The encapsulation of islets within a biomaterial helps to prolong graft viability by serving as a physical barrier to prevent direct interactions between islets and host cells.[100–102] While most of these materials used for cellular encapsulation (e.g., alginate, PEG, and hydroxyethyl methacrylate-co-methyl methacrylate) are branded as "biocompatible," any material implant will instigate nonspecific inflammatory host responses, which can be detrimental to the graft. This inflammatory environment initiates the foreign body response (FBR), which terminates in a thick fibrotic layer of cells and matrix encapsulating the implant. This fibrotic layer not only prevents the exchange of nutrients and the efficient diffusion of secreted insulin but the cells within this layer also secrete ROS to degrade the offending material.[103] ROS can easily diffuse through the alginate bead and cause toxicity to the encapsulated cells. In addition, ROS serves as a key signal to adaptive immune cells to provoke a more specialized immune attack.[21] The incorporation of antioxidants within immunoisolation encapsulating biomaterials would serve to not only protect the underlying cells from ROS-mediated damage but it will also dampen the activation of host responses that lead to FBR and adaptive immune activation. Several groups have explored this complementary approach by tethering or incorporating agents, such as tannic acid and curcumin, within encapsulating hydrogels.[104–107] To provide a potentially more durable and broader ROS scavenging approach, our laboratory has explored incorporating CONP into islet encapsulation platforms.[60,108] In one approach, CONP was distributed throughout the alginate to form a nanocomposite material, where their complementary charge properties facilitated CONP entrapment, depicted in Fig. 17.2A.[60] Binding of the CONP within the material not only reduced cytotoxicity associated with cellular internalization but provided enhanced safety of nanoparticle delivery by mitigating host phagocytosis. Protection of the entrapped cells from ambient ROS was further demonstrated.[60] In another approach, nanoscale layers of CONP were coated onto alginate microcapsules in a discreet layer-by-layer manner (Fig. 17.2B).[108] Layers of CONP were formed via alternating CONP with alginate, resulting in nanoscale control of layer thickness and permeability. Furthermore, surface coatings localize the ROS scavenging capacity of CONP to the periphery of the bead, where it can serve to scavenge and potentially modulate host immune cell responses, as shown in Fig. 17.2C. Results found these layers to scavenge H_2O_2 in a manner that protected β cells from ROS-mediated toxicity and preserved insulin responsiveness.[108] Future efforts will explore the capacity of these coatings to not only enhance the biocompatibility of these implants but to prevent the activation of adaptive immune responses. In future work, the reduction of this encapsulation platform from a micro- to nanoscale will promote more efficient delivery of nutrients and secretion of insulin, as well as substantially reduce the overall volume of the transplant.[104,105,107,109,110]

17.2.3 CONP for alleviation of diabetic complications

In both T1DM and T2DM, chronic hyperglycemia due to β-cell loss is the primary contributing factor to multiple micro- and macrovasculature complications associated with diabetes, such as cardiovascular diseases, chronic kidney disease, retinopathy, and limb amputation.[111,112] Oxidative stress also plays a key role in the progression of these complications.[113] Elevated glucose in the bloodstream results in increased protein–glucose interactions, as well as the influx of glucose within endothelial cells. This leads to extracellular and intracellular redox imbalances, with the generation of detrimental advanced glycation end products and glucose oxidation in the bloodstream, as well as intracellular overproduction of superoxide, nitric oxide, and hydrogen peroxide.[114,115]

Targeted antioxidant delivery has the potential to prevent, delay, or reverse these complications; however, the benefits of systemic antioxidant nutritional supplements in

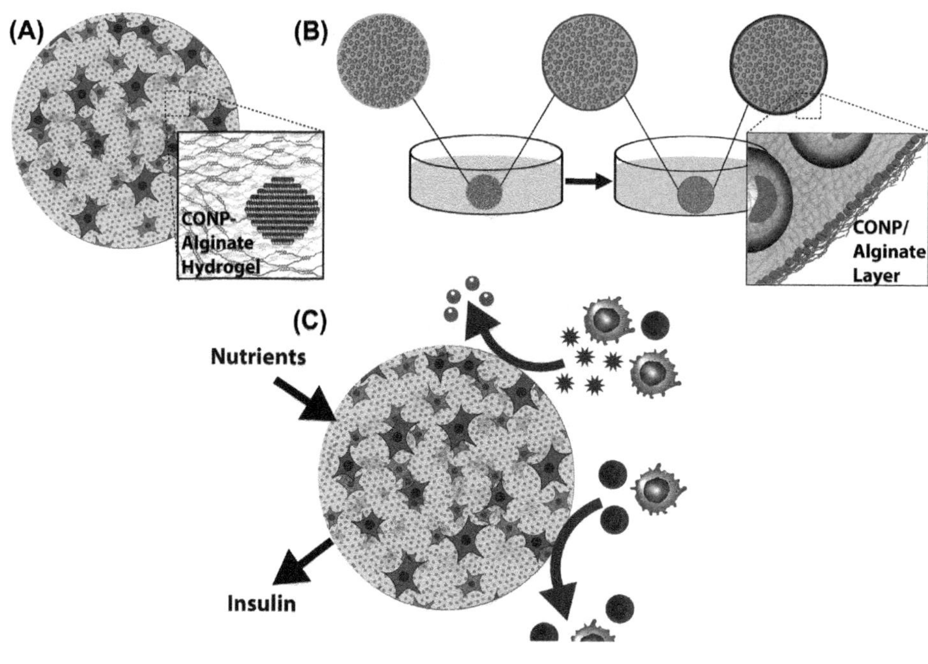

FIGURE 17.2 Implementation of cerium oxide nanoparticle (CONP) into cellular encapsulation platforms or onto its surface can serve to prevent reactive oxygen species (ROS)–induced cell death in encapsulated cells. (A) Multilayer coatings with CONP can be achieved via electrostatic interactions to form nanocomposite hydrogels or (B) layered onto the surface in a layer-by-layer manner. (C) Resulting CONP-encapsulation platforms exhibit bioactivity to scavenge ambient ROS generated during the foreign body response to the implant. In addition, permselectivity of encapsulation hydrogel is retained, permitting nutrient and insulin exchange, but blocking cellular infiltration. *Adapted from Weaver JD, Stabler CL. Antioxidant cerium oxide nanoparticle hydrogels for cellular encapsulation.* Acta Biomater *2015;**16**:136–144; Abuid NJ, et al., Layer-by-Layer cerium oxide nanoparticle coating for anti oxidant protection of encapsulated beta cells* . Adv Healthc Mater *2019;**0**(0):1801493.*

mitigating disease in clinical trials have been mixed.[116–119] The lack of clear efficacy alludes to insufficiencies of antioxidant delivery, potency, and durability. As previously outlined, antioxidant nanoparticles are superior to most antioxidant agents due to their high surface-to-volume ratio, their high antioxidant capabilities, superior bioavailability, and pharmacokinetics. Thus, CONP may serve as an antioxidant able to overcome these limitations.

17.2.3.1 Diabetes neuropathy, wound healing, and the diabetic foot

Neuropathy is a common complication of diabetes and the leading cause of nontraumatic amputations.[120] ROS generated under chronic hyperglycemia results in neuronal cell death and nerve damage, leading to weakness and desensitization of extremities.[121] Desensitization of lower extremities imparts undetected stress and wounds in the foot, which can lead to chronic, nonhealing wounds or diabetic foot ulcers (DFUs).[121] In one approach, the combination of CONP and YONP was explored as a therapy to protect nerve cells from glucose toxicity. High-glucose concentrations induce ROS overproduction in nerve cells.[122] Pretreatment of cells with CONP/YONP decreased intracellular ROS and prevented lipid peroxidation and nerve cell apoptosis. While this cytoprotection can prevent neuropathies in the early stages of diabetes, fully established DFUs require a shift in focus to regenerating the tissue in these nonhealing wounds.

Wound healing is a highly coordinated process categorized into four main overlapping stages: (1) hemostasis, (2) inflammation, (3) migration/proliferation, and (4) remodeling.[123] ROS serves as a significant signal in all of these stages. First, immune cells use ROS as a defense mechanism from foreign pathogens in the wound.[124] It is also a secondary signaling molecule between nonlymphoid and lymphoid cells, as well as signaling between different branches of the immune system.[123,125] These cells communicate to promote angiogenesis, new extracellular matrix deposition (ECM), and tissue remodeling; however, in diabetic patients, the synchrony of the wound healing process is altered by redox imbalances and chronic inflammation.[126–128] Furthermore, there is evidence to support that antioxidant defense mechanisms in the body are compromised in elder and diabetic patients.[129] As such, diabetes and age contribute to the accumulation of ROS, resulting in a chronic inflammatory environment. This impairs the highly coordinated wound healing process, with suppression of the migration and proliferation of keratinocytes, fibroblasts, and vascular endothelial cells (VECs) that work synergistically to remodel the damaged tissue, deposit ECM, and form new blood vessels.[126,130] Oxidative stress also promotes additional tissue damage at the wound site via induction of cell death that is involved in maintaining and restoring skin integrity and function.[128]

Modulation of ROS and RNS to promote healthy closure is being explored as a therapy for chronic wounds. Antioxidant therapy to the wound site includes systemic antioxidant supplementation,[131,132] localized antioxidant hydrogels,[133–135] and metal-based redox catalysts.[94,136–138] Zinc oxide, silver oxide, titanium oxide,

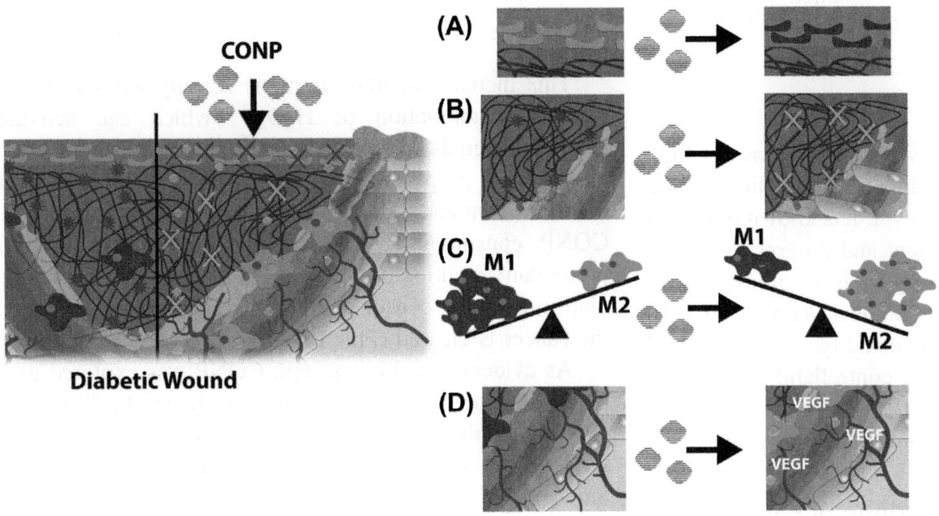

FIGURE 17.3 The versatile properties of cerium oxide nanoparticle (CONP) can be used to promote wound healing in a multifaceted manner. CONP can serve as (A) an antimicrobial agent; (B) a general reactive oxygen species scavenger to promote cell infiltration and remodeling; (C) a supporter of M2 phenotype in macrophages, and (D) a promoter of angiogenesis.

and manganese oxide nanoparticles are some of the metal-based catalysts currently being researched for wound healing; however, most antioxidants lack the self-renewing capability and controllable redox properties of CONP. In addition, CONP can scavenge broader types of ROS and RNS molecules that play a role at different stages of wound healing. In response to the wound microenvironment, it is possible for CONP to switch redox properties to scavenge or produce ROS.[94,136,137] It is also possible to engineer the particles to be prone to certain types of ROS or RNS (i.e., CAT vs. SOD mimetic activity). Therefore, the therapeutic potential of CONP to promote wound healing is high.

In addition, uptake of CONP results in the scavenging of intracellular NO within macrophages, which helps decrease the inflammatory response by these cells.[139] For example, the addition of CONP to macrophage cultures inhibits the synthesis of inducible nitric oxide synthase and proinflammatory cytokines, which also reduces ROS and RNS production.[139,140] The local dampening of the inflammatory environment allows for cells to initiate mechanisms for wound healing, e.g., proliferate and migrate to the wound site, restore blood vessels, and replace ECM (Fig. 17.3). Several studies have shown that CONP treatment can promote migration and proliferation of keratinocytes,[136,141] VECs,[142] and fibroblasts.[136] Cell internalization of CONP further reduces ROS-induced cell death via CONP scavenging of intracellular ROS and blockage of H_2O_2-activated apoptotic pathways.[136] In rodent studies of wound healing, CONP treatment resulted in enhanced skin closure and revascularization, when compared to control groups. CONP delivery also correlated with increased leukocyte infiltration, which potentially contributed to increased blood vessel formation.[136]

Promoting angiogenesis in chronic wounds is a common approach, as increased blood vessels can influence various stages of the wound healing process, such as elevating nutrient delivery to improve resident cell viability and promoting stromal and immune cell migration. The most common approach is to locally deliver a proangiogenic factor, such as vascular endothelial growth factor (VEGF); however, the local delivery of biologics is complicated by the harsh inflammatory environment of the wound, which typically leads to prompt degradation of the growth factor.[143] Promotion of native angiogenic factor expression from endothelial cells (ECs) is another option, as the cells are potent promoters of capillary formation.[144] The stimulation of angiogenic pathways in ECs is typically achieved via hypoxia-induced factor 1- α (HIF-1α) in response to low oxygen conditions[143,145] While CONP typically generates oxygen as a by-product of ROS scavenging, it has been shown that certain formulations of CONP can induce hypoxia in ECs; this feature can be achieved by controlling the ratio of Ce^{3+}/Ce^{4+}.[146] Specifically, CONP can bind to O_2 molecules without generating ROS as a side product, as shown in Eq. a:

$$CeO_{2\text{-}x} + 0.5\,x\,O_2 \rightarrow CeO_2 \quad \text{(a)}$$

Thus, CONP can induce targeted angiogenesis by promoting EC proliferation, migration, and VEGF expression.[146]

As it relates to wound healing, CONP can also promote wound resolution by mitigating infection. Modulation of CONP fabrication can generate prooxidant nanoparticles that can serve as an antimicrobial agent by generating free radicals to fight bacterial infection in the wound site.[133,147–150] Given the versatile roles of CONP in wound healing, researchers have developed and tested CONP-containing gels on human subjects with late-stage DFUs.[151] Pilot case results show encouraging potential for clinical translation, where the treatment of neuropathic

DFUs with CONP-containing gels resulted in enhanced wound closure when treated with CONP gels.[151]

17.3 Cancer

Cancer is a heterogeneous disease that often leads to high morbidity and mortality.[152,153] The etiology of this disease is yet to be fully understood; however, it is known that ROS plays a role in cancer development and progression. ROS role in cancer is multifaceted varying from promoting tumor growth and cancer cell migration to enhancing anticancer therapies, where ROS cytotoxicity is harnessed.[154] Because of its ubiquitous nature, controllability of redox properties, and pharmacokinetics, CONP is a promising candidate for augmenting traditional cancer therapies.

17.3.1 CONP for targeted killing of cancerous cells

Current treatment for cancer includes chemotherapy, radiotherapy, and surgery. However, these treatments are limited by effective delivery, cellular resistance, and peripheral and off-target toxicity.[155] The selective redox properties of CONP can be exploited to engineer alternative cancer therapies that cause toxicity to cancer cells, with minimal to no effect on the surrounding tissue.[59,156] Because of elevated metabolism, cancer cells produce high concentrations of lactic acid, which lead to acidic environments in the cytosolic and extracellular space.[59,157,158] At low pHs, CONP biases to scavenging $O_2^{\bullet-}$ rather than H_2O_2, as shown below in Eqs. (b) and (c).[40,156,159–162]

$$Ce^{4+} + O_2^{\bullet -} \rightarrow Ce^{3+} + O_2 \quad \text{(b)}$$

$$Ce^{3+} + 2H^{+} + O_2^{\bullet -} \rightarrow Ce^{4+} + H_2O_2 \quad \text{(c)}$$

This increase in SOD mimetic activity leads to intracellular accumulation of H_2O_2,[40] which can activate apoptotic signals in cancer cells.[163,164] Moreover, CONP can switch properties based on changes in the local microenvironment. For example, at physiological pH, CONP consumes ROS, switching its properties from prooxidant to antioxidant.[41,156,164] This provides a versatile platform to treat cancer while mitigating cytotoxicity once the cancer is cleared (Fig. 17.4).[41]

As evidence of this concept, CONP was explored as a potential bone cancer therapeutic. Incubating healthy bone cells (osteoblasts) or bone cancer cells (osteosarcomas) with CONP resulted in biased toxicity. Under the low intracellular pH presenting within osteosarcomas, CONP generated ROS and induced cell apoptosis, while healthy cells were minimally impacted.[164] This same trend was observed when treating malignant skin cancer, melanoma, with CONP.[59,165,166] Human melanoma cells also contain high lactase concentrations compared with noncancerous cells, making these cells more sensitive to CONP treatment.[157,158,167,168] When internalized by melanoma cells, CONP generated ROS in response to the acidic microenvironment. Elevated intracellular ROS imparted lipid peroxidation and DNA damage, which pushed the cells to activate apoptotic pathways.[59,165,169] In addition, CONP can alter the antioxidant defense mechanisms in cancer cells, pushing the overexpression of oxidative stress markers.[165,169] While research is still in the early stage, CONP illustrates the strong potential to provide targeted cytotoxicity to cancerous cells.

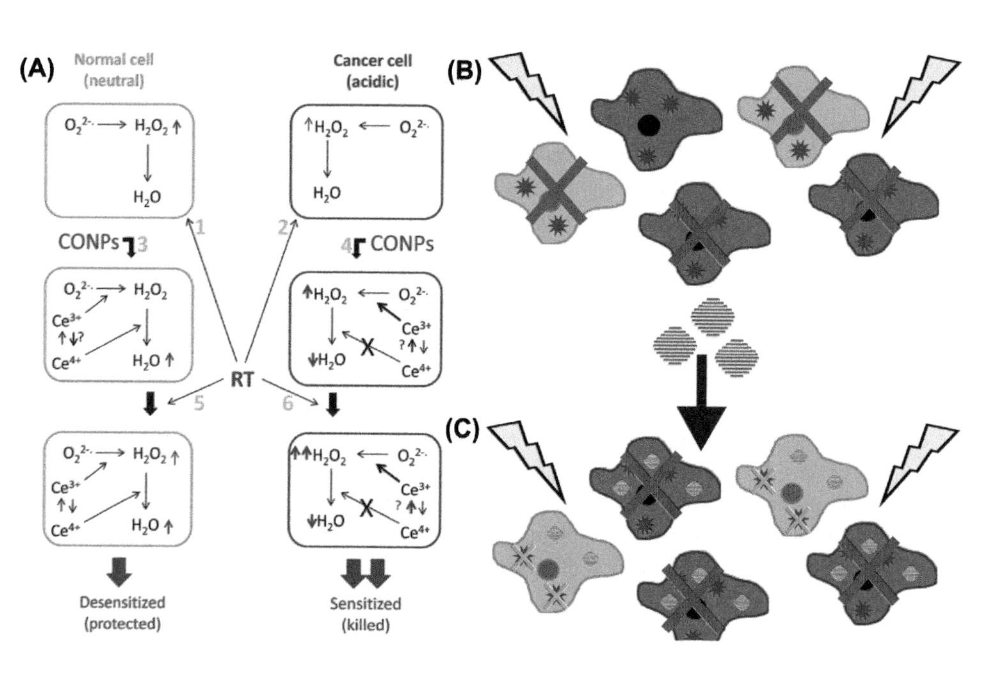

FIGURE 17.4 (A) Cerium oxide nanoparticle (CONP) can act as a prooxidant in acidic conditions and an antioxidant in a neutral environment. These properties make CONP an ideal therapeutic that is toxic to cancer cells without damaging normal cells. (B–C) This treatment has been combined with radiation therapy (RT) to protect normal cells from reactive oxygen species generated by radiation while sensitizing cancer cells to RT. *Adapted from Wason MS, et al., Sensitization of pancreatic cancer cells to radiation by cerium oxide nanoparticle-induced ROS production.* Nanomedicine *2013;9(4):558–569.*

17.3.2 CONP and radiation therapy

Cancer patients undergoing radiation therapy (RT) suffer tissue deterioration that often leads to poor quality of life. The source of cytotoxicity in RT is ROS generated via ionization reactions.[170] Thus, reducing intracellular ROS pretreatment or preventing ROS generation during treatment could serve to protect healthy tissue. Dr. Baker's group at the University of Central Florida has published extensively on the use of CONP in RT.[41,160,161,171] Collectively, their research has shown that combining CONP with RT can both reduce the negative effects of radiation on the surrounding healthy tissue of the tumor and augment the potency of the treatment in cancer cells. Specifically, the pretreatment of healthy cells in vitro with CONP protected from radiation in various cell types, e.g., lung fibroblasts, colon, breast, and pancreatic cells.[41,160,161,171] The translation of this approach to systemic CONP delivery in rodents before radiation exposure further validated its potential.[160,161]

In addition to protecting healthy cells, CONP has also been shown to reduce the resistance of certain cancer cells to RT. Generally, cancer cells that are refractory to RT are those that achieve a low intracellular pH, which prevents radiation-induced H_2O_2 production.[170] Using the same pH-dependent redox properties of CONP outlined above to impart selective toxicity to cancer cells, CONP treatment can augment the efficacy of RT. For example, the cotreatment of CONP with radiation elevated H_2O_2 accumulation and increased the efficacy of RT to kill pancreatic cancer cells, while protecting healthy peripheral cells (Fig. 17.4).[40,41] The synergistic impact of CONP and RT was further validated in pancreatic cancer rodent models.[40] With these promising reports, it would be of interest to explore the potential of CONP to enhance efficacy in radiation treatment−resistant cancers in larger animals.

17.3.3 CONP applied to combinatory radiation and chemotherapy

A common clinical approach for treating aggressive cancers is to combine surgery with radiotherapy and chemotherapy to reduce the risk of metastasis and cancer reoccurrence.[172] In an attempt to reduce adjuvant therapies and minimize side effects while retaining efficacy, CONP could be included in this approach. In one example, CONP was functionalized with the anticancer drug neogambogic acid (NGA) and combined with radiotherapy.[162] The resulting combinatory treatment induced elevated autophagy and apoptosis in breast cancer cells when compared with control or single agent groups.[162] The mechanism of action was postulated to be the prolongation of the G2/M phase of the cell cycle, which enhanced the sensitivity of the cancer cells to RT.[162,163] Of interest, the CONP-NGA agent did not modulate intracellular ROS in the breast cancer cells. Thus, the mechanism of CONP action and cancer cell death needs further study.

17.3.4 CONP role in tumor development

The roles of ROS in tumor development vary from directing proliferation and migration to modulating the stromal cell niche to promote tumor growth and expansion.[173] Within the tumor niche, elevated intracellular ROS concentrations can dictate the phenotype and fate of stromal cells in the tumor microenvironment, playing a key role in supporting tumor survival, expansion, and distal invasion. For example, fibroblasts under oxidative conditions differentiate into myofibroblasts and upregulate alpha-smooth muscle actin (αSMA) and matrix metalloproteinase 2 (MMP-2), which then serves to potentiate tumor development, growth, and invasion.[174−176] Cancer cells also promote stromal cell activity by synthesizing and expressing transforming growth factor β (TGF-β) to direct angiogenesis, immune tolerance, fibroblast recruitment, and an oxidative microenvironment.[177] Reducing ROS in the local microenvironment could inhibit these pathways.[178] For example, CONP was found to inhibit TGF-β-mediated differentiation of fibroblasts into myofibroblasts.[156] This suppression prevented the resident tumor cells from proliferating, migrating, and invading the surrounding tissue. Furthermore, CONP can also act as a prooxidant when internalized by squamous and melanoma cells.[59,156] By inhibiting pathways and stromal cell phenotypes that support the tumor microenvironment, CONP delivery resulted in reduced tumor size and decreased neovascularization in tumor-bearing mice.[59]

The antioxidant effects of CONP also play a similar role in suppressing EC-mediated tumor growth. When seeking to expand, cancer cells secrete both VEGF and MMP, factors that serve to stimulate EC proliferation and to degrade the surrounding extracellular matrix, respectively, to promote EC migration and capillary tube formation.[179,180] In one application for treatment of ovarian cancer, CONP treatment was found to selectively inhibit VEGF within ECs.[181] This resulted in a decline of tumor size and vascularization in mice treated with CONP.[181]

While CONP has shown significant impact in multiple rodent models, CONP is highly dependent on its specific microenvironment. Because CONP acts as an antioxidant in some types of cancer cells[41,59,162,182] and as a prooxidant in others,[171,181] it is possible that the redox behavior of CONP is influenced by the type of cancer cell. For example, CONP was shown to induce toxicity in breast cancer models in one approach[162,171] but was not effective in another.[181] Other factors that alter redox behavior in CONP include charge, size, and shape, as well as other not-yet-discovered features.[43,44,69,181] Thus, this provides an opportunity to control the function of these ambidextrous nanoparticles, such as modulating charge to direct CONP toward different compartments of the cell.[62] It also calls for further studies to elucidate methods to control and/or predict their behavior within a specific cancer microenvironment.

17.4 Neurodegenerative diseases

Parkinson's, Alzheimer's, and multiple sclerosis (MS) are neurodegenerative diseases involving loss of brain function over time. Several factors contribute to neural degeneration, with each of these diseases exhibiting variant mechanisms of development and progression. Despite this disparate pathology, all share the similarity that oxidative stress is involved in exacerbating their progression.[183] The physiological level of ROS generated in neural cells is higher than most other cells, due to their elevated metabolic demand.[184] While typically mitigated by intracellular antioxidants, pathological conditions and aging decreases the brain's natural antioxidant defense mechanisms, resulting in oxidative stress.[183,184] Because of the key role of oxidative stress in neurodegenerative diseases, ROS scavenging agents have been explored as potential therapeutics, including lipoic acid, vitamin C, tocopherol (vitamin E), and docosahexaenoic acid.[183] A major challenge in their efficacy, however, is efficient delivery through the blood–brain barrier (BBB).[185] With the potential of CONP to transverse the BBB in rodent models, as well as their ease of functionalization, size, and shape make CONP a promising treatment for neurodegenerative conditions, as shown in Fig. 17.5A.[186–188]

17.4.1 CONP as a therapeutic in Alzheimer's disease

Alzheimer's disease (AD) is a neurodegenerative disease characterized by a progressive decline in memory and overall mental function. Even though the exact mechanisms of disease development and progression have not yet been elucidated, patients with AD typically exhibit extracellular plaque formation, composed of amyloid-beta (Aβ) peptide aggregates, and intracellular neurofibrillary tangles, comprised of hyperphosphorylated tau proteins.[189] The formation of these plaques and tangles induces neuroinflammation and elevates ROS and RNS generation, which, in turn, promotes further plaque buildup.[189,190] This oxidative environment also promotes the binding of metal ions, such as copper, zinc, and iron to Aβ peptides, leading to additional Aβ aggregation and ROS generation.[191] All of these abnormal processes, e.g., metal-Aβ complexes, plaque buildup, and consequential ROS/RNS generation lead to neural cell death and degeneration.[192,193]

The use of CONP as a therapeutic for oxidative stress and neurodegeneration relief in AD is multifaceted. Reports have shown that CONP can prevent the formation of toxic metal–Aβ complexes by impeding metal ions (Cu^{2+}) from interacting with Aβ.,[194] while also scavenging ROS produced by preexisting Cu^{2+}-Aβ complexes.[194,195] In a combinatory approach, the drug clioquinol (CQ), a metal chelator that can bind to Cu^{2+} ions and prevent Cu^{2+}-Aβ complexes, and CONP were integrated into a dual drug delivery platform.[194] Mesoporous silica nanoparticles (MSNs) were used as the CQ delivery carrier, CONP was then conjugated to the MSN surface via phenylboronic acid moieties on the MSN and glucose on the CONP. This resulted in multiple benefits: retention of the CQ drug during delivery; a reversible H_2O_2-responsive CONP release; and localized antioxidant capacity. This yielded a system that combined the benefits of CONP, additional H_2O_2 buffering, and metal ion chelation.[194] In vitro, the resulting dual-delivery platform destabilized the formation of Cu^{2+}-Aβ complexes and Aβ fibrils and decreased intracellular ROS within adrenal gland carcinoma cells (PC12).[194] Although additional validation and animal studies are required to firmly establish delivery, targeting, and efficacy, this approach highlights the potential of CONP to serve not only as a potent bioactive component but as a modulator of controlled drug delivery.

Analogous to ROS, RNS also play a role in neurodegeneration in AD by contributing to the formation of neural aggregates and neural cytotoxicity.[196,197] An imbalance of nitric oxide in the brain can aggravate neurodegeneration by activating cell death pathways or reacting with superoxide molecules to form peroxynitrite ($ONOO^-$). Peroxynitrite can cause direct damage to neurons, accelerate Aβ plaque formation, trigger intracellular release of metal ions, and alter mitochondria respiration.[198] Soluble Aβ promotes RNS generation, especially peroxynitrite, which further induces Aβ aggregation. Both soluble and aggregated forms of Aβ are toxic to neuronal cells via RNS-dependent pathways.[196,197] With both ROS and RNS scavenging properties, CONP can thus serve as a highly potent therapeutic. Treatment of neuronal cells with CONP has been shown to not only inhibit RNS-mediated aggregation into plaque but to also scavenge peroxynitrite and halt the electrophilic nitration of tyrosine in neuronal proteins that can lead to neural cell toxicity.[198,199]

Another hallmark of neurodegenerative disease, especially AD, is neural mitochondrial dysfunction.[198] In neuronal cells, mitochondria fission and fusion regulates tasks such as mitochondrial proliferation, adaptation to changes in cell metabolism, and apoptosis. The balance of mitochondrial fission/fusion is orchestrated by GTPases such as dynamin-related protein 1 (DRP1).[200–202] An imbalance in this process induces apoptosis, either by the overactivation of fission or the inhibition of fusion, causes

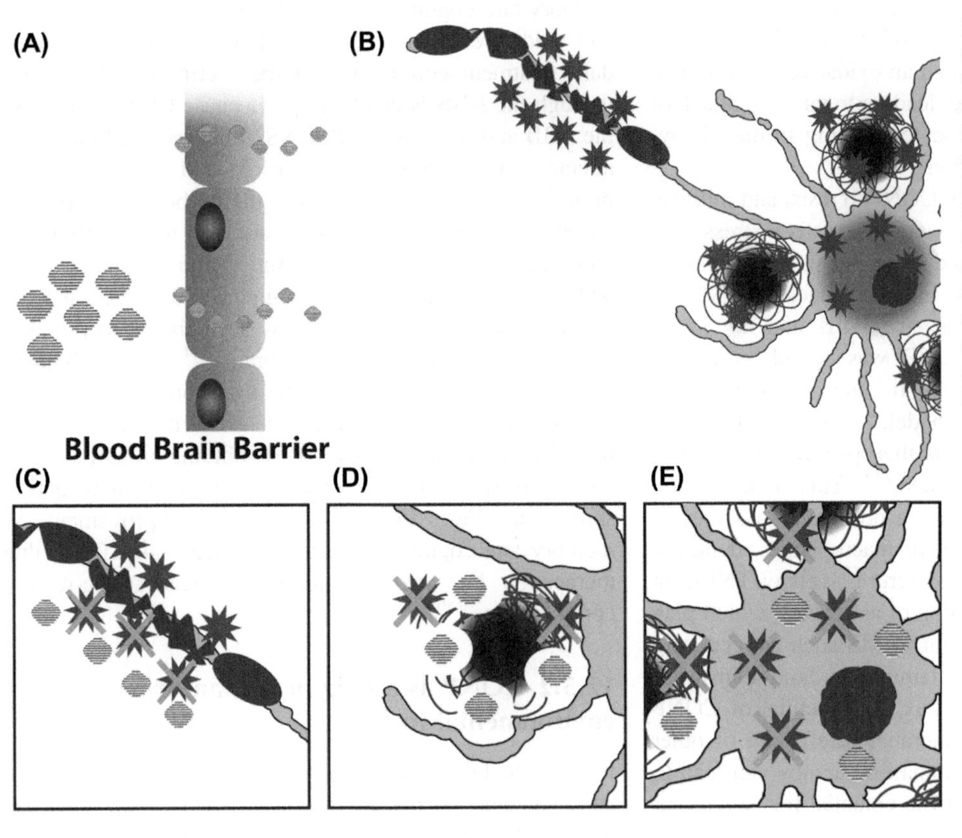

FIGURE 17.5 (A) Evidence that cerium oxide nanoparticle (CONP) can cross the blood–brain barrier makes it an ideal therapeutic for the treatment of degenerative diseases and trauma in the brain. (B) Multiple reactive oxygen species (ROS)- and reactive nitrogen species (RNS)–mediated pathways lead to neuronal dysfunction. CONP treatment can serve to (C) mitigate ROS-driven demyelination; (D) prevent and destabilize Aβ plaques, and (E) scavenge intracellular ROS and RNS to protect the neuron.

mitochondrial fragmentation.[200,202] It is known that abnormal levels of ROS/RNS and Aβ peptides can directly cause mitochondrial dysregulation by the overactivation of DRP1.[202] In addition, imbalances of glutamate and N-methyl D-aspartate receptor activity contribute to neuronal toxicity via mitochondrial fragmentation and RNS overproduction.[203] CONP treatment of stressed neural cells decreased intracellular RNS, resulting in decreased DRP1 phosphorylation and mitochondrial fragmentation, which resulted in improved mitochondrial respiration.[198]

The targeted delivery of therapeutics to the brain remains a challenge; however, CONP provides advantages over other agents due to its ease of functionalization and controllable physical/chemical properties. For example, the destination of CONP to the desired target could be promoted via functionalization of the surface with an antibody specific to the affected site. In one application, CONP was functionalized with an anti-Aβ antibody via a PEG linker to promote particle homing to Aβ plaques in the brain.[188] By targeting to the pathological plaque, the potent scavenging capacity of CONP was localized, thereby impairing additional aggregate formation and toxicity. The reduction of such aggregates can also lead to elevated healing and neural survival. For example, brain-derived neurotrophic factor (BDNF) plays an important role in both supporting neural cell viability and memory retention.[204] The precursor of BDNF, pro-BDNF, however, can cause neuronal toxicity at high concentrations.[205–207] In AD, there is an imbalance in the ratio of mature to immature BDNF.[206] Interestingly, neural cell treatment with CONP promoted a healthy ratio of mature/immature BDNF, in a redox-independent manner.[188,208] The mechanism of action of CONP needs further research; however, it is encouraging that these nanoparticles contain therapeutic properties beyond simply scavenging ROS/RNS.

17.4.2 CONP and multiple sclerosis

MS is an autoimmune disease of the central nervous system (CNS) characterized by a loss in cognition and motor function due to changes in microglia phenotype.[209] Microglia are CNS-resident cells responsible for modulating the production and remodeling of myelin, which are the protective sheaths surrounding nerve fibers.[210] Depending on the conditions of the microenvironment, microglia can be proinflammatory or antiinflammatory. Proinflammatory microglia promote the destruction of myelin, whereas antiinflammatory microglia replace old myelin.[210] Chronic inflammation overextends the demyelination process, which then causes impairment of the electrical signals that are necessary for neuronal communication. Chronic inflammation also induces microglia and astrocytes to overproduce ROS and impart myelin damage and cytotoxicity on axons, oligodendrocytes, and neurons.[210,211] An inflammatory and an oxidative environment also promote T-cell trafficking, leading to targeted attack of myelin-producing oligodendrocytes causing further demyelination and neurodegeneration.[211]

The therapeutic potential of CONP to resist and mitigate immune response and inflammation/oxidative stress was explored in mice with induced experimental autoimmune encephalomyelitis (EAE), a mouse model for MS.[212] Because of its ability to cross the BBB and act as an antioxidant in the brain, CONP was found to reduce inflammation, astrocyte activation, and improve motor function in this EAE rodent model.[212] To further elevate therapeutic efficacy, CONP was then paired with an anti-inflammatory drug, lenalidomide.[213] This combination therapy reduced levels of IL-17, a proinflammatory cytokine involved in the activation of macrophages, dendritic cells, and T cells, and decreased serum levels of TNF-α in EAE mice. In addition, activation of astrocytes, which play several roles in the development of MS such as recruiting lymphocytes, exacerbating inflammation, and demyelination, was suppressed.[213,214] Thus, the potential of CONP to synergize and elevate the therapeutic efficacy of other drugs is established. This combination therapy can lead to improved outcomes, as well as the potential for targeted or decreased drug loads.

17.5 CONP in other biomedical applications

While CONP has been primarily applied to diabetes, neurodegenerative diseases, and cancer, there are other pathological conditions that could benefit from CONP treatment. Herein, we highlight two other major areas of potential impact for CONP-based therapy.

17.5.1 CONP applied to ischemic stroke

Stroke-induced cerebral ischemia is one of the leading causes of long-term disability in the United States.[215,216] Strokes occur when a blood vessel is occluded, causing blood to stop flowing. Lack of blood flow to the brain causes acidosis and the deprivation of glucose and oxygen, which leads to ischemia and neural cell death.[217] To protect the nutritionally deprived cells, mitochondria in neural cells decrease oxygen consumption.[218] When blood supply is replenished to the brain, however, this quick shift in oxygen supply results in the cellular conversion of excess oxygen into ROS and RNS.[215] As described earlier, this oxidative/nitrosative imbalance leads to neural inflammation and brain damage.[215] This can be particularly detrimental to the hippocampus, the region of the brain responsible for memory and cognition, as it is highly sensitive to hypoxic and oxidative damage.[215] As outlined previously, antioxidant treatment could mitigate these effects, but delivery through the BBB is challenging. Because CONP can cross the BBB and scavenge ROS/RNS, it has received increased attention as a drug carrier for targeted delivery to the brain.[186,187,212,219,220] Protection of the brain, specifically the hippocampus, has been demonstrated in rodent models when treating with CONP within 4 h postischemia.[221] In addition to preventing ischemia-induced damage via ROS and RNS scavenging, CONP has been shown to promote adult neurogenesis in damaged brains.[186] The mechanism of this effect is postulated to be the promotion of AMP-activated protein kinase, which leads to the phosphorylation of protein kinase C and CREB-binding protein, both of which promote adult neurogenesis (mechanism of action shown in Fig. 17.5B).[186,222] With improvement in memory and cognition in rats pretreated with CONP, this therapeutic has strong potential to treat stroke-related complications.[186,212]

17.5.2 CONP as a lung protectant from environmental toxins

Environmental toxins, such as ionizing radiation, cigarette smoking, and chemicals in consumables in the environment, are generating significant worldwide health issues. The lungs, liver, kidney, brain, and skin are generally the organs most affected by environmental contaminants. Disease mechanisms vary depending on toxicity source; however, ROS- and RNS-induced damage is universal in environmental pathophysiology.[223]

As a critical and delicate interface with the environment, the lungs are particularly susceptible to environmental toxins. Ionizing radiation from medical imaging, UV light, and even dietary iodine can induce ROS overproduction and damage pulmonary and ECs in the lungs.[224] These environmental factors disrupt physiological homeostasis and lead to hypoxia, oxidative stress, and inflammation in the lungs and the cardiovascular system.[225,226] While initial impacts start in the lung, toxicity can propagate to the rest of the body through the vasculature.[225,227,228] Cell death in the lungs, in addition to hypoxia, instigates inflammatory conditions that signal tissue remodeling; however, this chronic inflammatory state leads to the overexpression of tissue remodeling growth factors and enzymes, such as MMPs, VEGF, and TGF-β, that results in pathological lung tissue.[226,228] Improper tissue remodeling disrupts the integrity and mechanics of vascular and lung tissue. Furthermore, pathological angiogenesis alters pulmonary and arterial pressures leading to pulmonary hypertension that progresses to chronic obstructive pulmonary disease.[225–230]

Given the various roles of ROS in the development of respiratory conditions, researchers have explored antioxidant for prevention and treatment. Targeted delivery of antioxidants to the lungs is a challenge that impedes easy delivery of potential agents.[231] Because of its controllable size, shape, and surface properties, nanoparticles are an ideal format for lung therapy. The delivery of redox-active particles such as CONP to the lung can be achieved if their properties are meticulously engineered. For example, prevention of radiation-induced damage to mouse lungs was demonstrated via the intraperitoneal administration of CONP.[160] Effective delivery of an adequate CONP concentration to the lung resulted in reduced macrophage invasion, with resulting macrophages favoring the antiinflammatory phenotype.[139,160] Controlling the macrophage phenotype also helped ameliorate the overall inflammatory response, resulting in healthy restoration of the degraded ECM and increased supportive angiogenesis.

In addition to modulating the inflammatory response, CONP can also serve as a protector of lung tissue and its supporting vasculature. *In vitro* studies show that CONP treatment provides antioxidant protection to pulmonary and ECs, with the internalization of CONP resulting in decreased intracellular ROS and oxidative stress.[232,233] Several in vivo studies have designed CONP in a manner that promotes targeting and accumulation in the lungs.[234,235] Following the instigation of lung injury in these rodent models, CONP-treated animals exhibited decreased inflammatory cytokines when compared with nanoparticle controls. These reports are encouraging as it shows the feasibility of nanoparticle treatment to reduce respiratory complications induced by environmental toxicity and hypoxia. While the most successful administration route for CONP in rodents is intraperitoneal administration, this may not translate well to larger animals. Therefore, further studies comparing administration routes (e.g., aerosol, intravenous) and size properties (e.g., size, shape, and surface charge) should be examined.

17.6 Conclusions and future directions

In this chapter, we highlighted the most widely studied biomedical applications for CONP, with an emphasis on alleviating oxidative/nitrative stress in diseases such as neurodegeneration, diabetes, and cancer. The controllable redox properties of CONP have also shown promise in other biomedical applications, such as eye-related diseases, liver toxicity from environmental factors, and cardiovascular disease.[233,236–239] Of special interest for CONP applications is for treatment of cardiovascular (CV) disease, the leading cause of death in the world. CV disease is a multifactorial family of pathologies where the main characteristic is the restriction of blood flow.[240] Lack of blood flow to the heart leads to myocardial infarction, colloquially known as heart attack. This lack of blood supply to cardiac tissues leads to ischemia, cardiomyocyte death, and tissue necrosis. Similar to stroke, inflammation and oxidative stress pathways are also activated, which further propagates cell death and global tissue damage.[241] Promising reports of the potential of antioxidant supplementation with CONP to defend cardiac cells from oxidative insults has emerged[233,238,239]; however, its full potential to treat diseases have not been fully exploited.

In addition to expanding CONP applications to various pathological conditions, it is also important to fully understand the role and downstream impacts of CONP at different stages of a disease. In addition, a detailed understanding of the particular disease etiology and the physiological conditions of each disease stage can facilitate and improve CONP efficacy via modulation of timing, dosage, and targeting. The literature reports multiple contradictions on the properties and behavior of CONP particles under different conditions, specifically in cancer. Separate studies use different formulations of CONP to treat similar disease models; however, the synthesis method, the ratio of Ce^{3+}/Ce^{4+}, and even surface coating can affect the behavior of these particles.[47,48,237] Therefore, various CONP configurations can yield contradictory results when applied to the same disease condition. Because these particles can be engineered to generate or scavenge ROS/RNS under certain conditions, the specific formulations of CONP should be tailored to treat different redox imbalances. Another caveat that should be identified is that researchers commonly generalize different types of cell lines; however, different types of cancers cells (i.e., pancreatic, breast, and melanoma) have variable phenotypes that may induce changes in CONP activity.

Furthermore, other factors such as cell media composition and passage number may affect the conditions of the studies. Finally, cell lines should be used only as a first screening method to establish feasibility, while primary cell sources provide a more robust validation of observed trends. Therefore, CONP research should focus more on primary cell lines and the specific phenotype of those cells to ensure reproducibility and appropriate tailoring of CONP formulations to ensure optimal impact. Finally, because the properties of CONP can change under altered conditions, it is important to fully characterize the particles, using typical nanoparticle characterization methods, and the conditions of the study when reporting protection and toxicity.

References

1. Ray PD, Huang B-W, Tsuji Y. Reactive oxygen species (ROS) homeostasis and redox regulation in cellular signaling. *Cell Signal* 2012;**24**(5):981–90.
2. Bayr H. Reactive oxygen species. *Crit Care Med* 2005;**33**(12):S498–501.

3. Halliwell B. Reactive oxygen species and the central nervous system. *J Neurochem* 1992;**59**(5):1609–23.
4. Simon HU, Haj-Yehia A, Levi-Schaffer F. Role of reactive oxygen species (ROS) in apoptosis induction. *Apoptosis* 2000;**5**(5):415–8.
5. Patel RP, et al. Biological aspects of reactive nitrogen species. *Biochim Biophys Acta* 1999;**1411**(2):385–400.
6. Alfadda AA, Sallam RM. Reactive oxygen species in health and disease. *J Biomed Biotechnol* 2012;**2012**.
7. Hensley K, et al. Reactive oxygen species, cell signaling, and cell injury. *Free Radic Biol Med* 2000;**28**(10):1456–62.
8. Murphy MP. How mitochondria produce reactive oxygen species. *Biochem J* 2009;**417**(1):1–13.
9. Oshino N, Jamieson D, Chance B. The properties of hydrogen peroxide production under hyperoxic and hypoxic conditions of perfused rat liver. *Biochem J* 1975;**146**(1):53–65.
10. Fang FC. Antimicrobial reactive oxygen and nitrogen species: concepts and controversies. *Nat Rev Microbiol* 2004;**2**:820.
11. Evans JL, et al. Oxidative stress and stress-activated signaling pathways: a unifying hypothesis of type 2 diabetes. *Endocr Rev* 2002;**23**(5):599–622.
12. Papaharalambus CA, Griendling KK. Basic mechanisms of oxidative stress and reactive oxygen species in cardiovascular injury. *Trends Cardiovasc Med* 2007;**17**(2):48–54.
13. Iwasaki A, Medzhitov R. Control of adaptive immunity by the innate immune system. *Nat Immunol* 2015;**16**:343.
14. Chen GY, Nuñez G. Sterile inflammation: sensing and reacting to damage. *Nat Rev Immunol* 2010;**10**:826.
15. Tan HY, et al. The reactive oxygen species in macrophage polarization: reflecting its dual role in progression and treatment of human diseases. *Oxid Med Cell Longev* 2016;**2016**.
16. Martin P, Leibovich SJ. Inflammatory cells during wound repair: the good, the bad and the ugly. *Trends Cell Biol* 2005;**15**(11):599–607.
17. Wynn TA, Vannella KM. Macrophages in tissue repair, regeneration, and fibrosis. *Immunity* 2016;**44**(3):450–62.
18. Serhan CN, Savill J. Resolution of inflammation: the beginning programs the end. *Nat Immunol* 2005;**6**:1191.
19. Mittal M, et al. Reactive oxygen species in inflammation and tissue injury. *Antioxid Redox Signal* 2014;**20**(7):1126–67.
20. Naik E, Dixit VM. Mitochondrial reactive oxygen species drive proinflammatory cytokine production. *J Exp Med* 2011;**208**(3):417.
21. Padgett LE, et al. The role of reactive oxygen species and proinflammatory cytokines in type 1 diabetes pathogenesis. *Ann N Y Acad Sci* 2013;**1281**:16–35.
22. Pham-Huy LA, He H, Pham-Huy C. Free radicals, antioxidants in disease and health. *Int J Biomed Sci* 2008;**4**(2):89–96.
23. Álvarez-Mejía AL, et al. Effect of natural exogenous antioxidants on aging and on neurodegenerative diseases AU - Guerra-Araiza, Christian. *Free Radic Res* 2013;**47**(6–7):451–62.
24. Reed K, et al. Exploring the properties and applications of nanoceria: is there still plenty of room at the bottom? *Environ Sci Nano* 2014;**1**(5):390–405.
25. Dahle JT, Arai Y. Environmental geochemistry of cerium: applications and toxicology of cerium oxide nanoparticles. *Int J Environ Res Public Health* 2015;**12**(2):1253–78.
26. Gangopadhyay S, et al. Structure and properties of cerium oxides in bulk and nanoparticulate forms. *J Alloy Compd* 2014;**584**:199–208.
27. Chockalingam R, Amarakoon V, Giesche H. Alumina/cerium oxide nano-composite electrolyte for solid oxide fuel cell applications. *J Eur Ceram Soc* 2008;**28**(5):959–63.
28. Subbiah D, et al. Nano ceria as xylene sensor – role of cerium precursor. *J Alloy Compd* 2018;**753**:771–80.
29. Olgun F, et al. A novel cerium oxide nanoparticles-based colorimetric sensor using tetramethyl benzidine reagent for antioxidant activity assay. *Talanta* 2018;**182**:55–61.
30. Bulbul G, et al. DNA assay based on nanoceria as fluorescence quenchers (NanoCeracQ DNA assay). *Sci Rep* 2018;**8**.
31. Pang X, Li D, Peng A. Application of rare-earth elements in the agriculture of China and its environmental behavior in soil. *Environ Sci Pollut R* 2002;**9**(2):143–8.
32. Saadat-Monfared A, Mohseni M. Polyurethane nanocomposite films containing nano-cerium oxide as UV absorber; Part 2: structural and mechanical studies upon UV exposure. *Colloids Surf, A* 2014;**441**:752–7.
33. Pirmohamed T, et al. Nanoceria exhibit redox state-dependent catalase mimetic activity. *Chem Commun* 2010;**46**(16):2736–8.
34. Ma Y, et al. Regulating the surface of nanoceria and its applications in heterogeneous catalysis. *Surf Sci Rep* 2018;**73**(1):1–36.
35. Celardo I, et al. Pharmacological potential of cerium oxide nanoparticles. *Nanoscale* 2011;**3**(4):1411–20.
36. Singh S, et al. A phosphate-dependent shift in redox state of cerium oxide nanoparticles and its effects on catalytic properties. *Biomaterials* 2011;**32**(28):6745–53.
37. Soh M, et al. Ceria-zirconia nanoparticles as an enhanced multi-antioxidant for sepsis treatment. *Angew Chem* 2017;**56**(38):11399–403.
38. Asati A, et al. Oxidase-like activity of polymer-coated cerium oxide nanoparticles. *Angew Chem* 2009;**48**(13):2308–12.
39. Ni P, et al. On the origin of the oxidizing ability of ceria nanoparticles. *RSC Adv* 2015;**5**(118):97512–9.
40. Korsvik C, et al. Superoxide dismutase mimetic properties exhibited by vacancy engineered ceria nanoparticles. *ChemComm* 2007;(10):1056–8.
41. Wason MS, et al. Sensitization of pancreatic cancer cells to radiation by cerium oxide nanoparticle-induced ROS production. Sensitization of pancreatic cancer cells to radiation by cerium oxide nanoparticle-induced ROS production *Nanomedicine* 2013;**9**(4):558–69.
42. Dowding JM, et al. Cerium oxide nanoparticles scavenge nitric oxide radical (NO). *Chem Commun (Camb)* 2012;**48**(40):4896–8.
43. Lu M, et al. Insight into several factors that affect the conversion between antioxidant and oxidant activities of nanoceria. *ACS Appl Mater Interfaces* 2016;**8**(36):23580–90.
44. Pulido-Reyes G, et al. Untangling the biological effects of cerium oxide nanoparticles: the role of surface valence states. *Sci Rep* 2015;**5**:15613.
45. Rajeshkumar S, Naik P. Synthesis and biomedical applications of Cerium oxide nanoparticles – a review. *Biotechnol Rep (Amst)* 2018;**17**:1–5.
46. Karakoti AS, et al. Preparation and characterization challenges to understanding environmental and biological impacts of ceria nanoparticles. *Surf Interface Anal* 2012;**44**(8):882–9.
47. Karakoti AS, et al. Nanoceria as antioxidant: synthesis and biomedical applications. *JOM* 2008;**60**(3):33–7.
48. Das S, et al. Cerium oxide nanoparticles: applications and prospects in nanomedicine. *Nanomedicine* 2013;**8**(9):1483–508.
49. Farahmandjou M, Zarinkamar M, Firoozabadi TP. Synthesis of Cerium Oxide (CeO_2) nanoparticles using simple CO-precipitation method. *Rev Mex Fis* 2016;**62**(5):496–9.

50. Ketzial JJ, Nesaraj AS. Synthesis of CeO_2 nanoparticles by chemical precipitation and the effect of a surfactant on the distribution of particle sizes. *J Ceram Process Res* 2011;**12**(1):74–9.
51. Babitha KK, et al. Structural characterization and optical studies of CeO_2 nanoparticles synthesized by chemical precipitation. *Indian J Pure Appl Phys* 2015;**53**(9):596–603.
52. Liu YH, et al. Synthesis and character of cerium oxide (CeO_2) nanoparticles by the precipitation method. *Metalurgija* 2014;**53**(4):463–5.
53. Masui T, et al. Synthesis of cerium oxide nanoparticles by hydrothermal crystallization with citric acid. *J Mater Sci Lett* 2002;**21**(6):489–91.
54. Wang W, et al. A surfactant and template-free route for synthesizing ceria nanocrystals with tunable morphologies. *J Mater Chem* 2010;**20**(36):7776–81.
55. Soren S, et al. Antioxidant potential and toxicity study of the cerium oxide nanoparticles synthesized by microwave-mediated synthesis. *Appl Biochem Biotechnol* 2015;**177**(1):148–61.
56. Mädler L, Stark WJ, Pratsinis SE. Flame-made ceria nanoparticles. *J Mater Res* 2002;**17**(6):1356–62.
57. Lord MS, et al. Cellular uptake and reactive oxygen species modulation of cerium oxide nanoparticles in human monocyte cell line U937. *Biomaterials* 2012;**33**(31):7915–24.
58. Sayle T, et al. Environment-mediated structure, surface redox activity and reactivity of ceria nanoparticles. *Nanoscale* 2013;**5**(13):6063–73.
59. Alili L, et al. Downregulation of tumor growth and invasion by redox-active nanoparticles. *Antioxid Redox Signal* 2013;**19**(8):765–78.
60. Weaver JD, Stabler CL. Antioxidant cerium oxide nanoparticle hydrogels for cellular encapsulation. *Acta Biomater* 2015;**16**:136–44.
61. Safi M, et al. Interactions between sub-10-nm iron and cerium oxide nanoparticles and 3T3 fibroblasts: the role of the coating and aggregation state. *Nanotechnology* 2010;**21**(14):145103.
62. Asati A, et al. Surface-charge-dependent cell localization and cytotoxicity of cerium oxide nanoparticles. *ACS Nano* 2010;**4**(9):5321–31.
63. Karakoti AS, et al. PEGylated nanoceria as radical scavenger with tunable redox chemistry. *J Am Chem Soc* 2009;**131**(40):14144–5.
64. Asati A, Kaittanis C, Santra S, Perez JM. pH-Tunable oxidase-like activity of cerium oxide nanoparticles achieving sensitive fluorigenic detection of cancer biomarkers at neutral pH. *Anal Chem* 2011;**83**(7):2547–53.
65. Konduru N, et al. Silica coating influences the corona and biokinetics of cerium oxide nanoparticles. *Part Fibre Toxicol* 2015;**12**.
66. Ould-Moussa N, et al. In vitro toxicity of nanoceria: effect of coating and stability in biofluids. *Nanotoxicology* 2014;**8**(7):799–811.
67. Yazici H, Alpaslan E, Webster T. The role of dextran coatings on the cytotoxicity properties of ceria nanoparticles toward bone cancer cells. *JOM* 2015;**67**(4):804–10.
68. Lord M, et al. Hyaluronan coated cerium oxide nanoparticles modulate CD44 and reactive oxygen species expression in human fibroblasts. *J Biomed Mater Res A* 2016;**104**(7):1736–46.
69. Grulke E, Reed K, Beck M, Huang X, Cormack A, Seal S. Nanoceria: factors affecting its pro- and anti-oxidant properties. *Environ Sci Nano* 2014;**1**(5):429–44.
70. Leahy JL. Pathogenesis of type 2 diabetes mellitus. *Arch Med Res* 2005;**36**(3):197–209.
71. Thayer TC, et al. Superoxide production by macrophages and T cells is critical for the induction of autoreactivity and type 1 diabetes. *Diabetes* 2011:DB_101222.
72. Chang YC, Chuang LM. The role of oxidative stress in the pathogenesis of type 2 diabetes: from molecular mechanism to clinical implication. *Am J Transl Res* 2010;**2**(3):316–31.
73. Akash MSH, Rehman K, Chen S. Role of inflammatory mechanisms in pathogenesis of type 2 diabetes mellitus. *J Cell Biochem* 2013;**114**(3):525–31.
74. Kahn SE. The relative contributions of insulin resistance and beta-cell dysfunction to the pathophysiology of Type 2 diabetes. *Diabetologia* 2003;**46**(1):3–19.
75. Ceriello A, Motz E. Is oxidative stress the pathogenic mechanism underlying insulin resistance, diabetes, and cardiovascular disease? The common soil hypothesis revisited. *Arter Thromb Vasc Biol* 2004;**24**(5):816–23.
76. Drews G, Krippeit-Drews P, Düfer M. Oxidative stress and beta-cell dysfunction. *Pflugers Arch* 2010;**460**(4):703–18.
77. Gusdon AM, Corbett JA, Mathews CE. Type 1 diabetes: islet inflammation – the contribution of cytokines and beta cells. *Drug Discov Today* 2006;**3**(3):367–72.
78. Nakamura U, et al. Rapid intracellular acidification and cell death by H2O2 and alloxan in pancreatic beta cells. *Free Radic Biol Med* 2006;**40**(11):2047–55.
79. Shapiro AMJ, et al. Islet transplantation in seven patients with type 1 diabetes mellitus using a glucocorticoid-free immunosuppressive regimen. *N Engl J Med* 2000;**343**(4):230–8.
80. Shapiro AMJ, Pokrywczynska M, Ricordi C. Clinical pancreatic islet transplantation. *Nat Rev Endocrinol* 2016;**13**(5):268.
81. Ryan EA, Bigam D, Shapiro AM. Current indications for pancreas or islet transplant. *Diabetes Obes Metab* 2006;**8**(1):1–7.
82. Mancarella R, et al. Beneficial effect of the nonpeptidyl low molecular weight radical scavenger IAC on cultured human islet function. *Cell Transplant* 2008;**17**(10–11):1271–6.
83. Fukudome D, et al. The radical scavenger edaravone counteracts diabetes in multiple low-dose streptozotocin-treated mice. *Eur J Pharmacol* 2008;**583**(1):164–9.
84. Kimoto K, et al. Gliclazide protects pancreatic beta-cells from damage by hydrogen peroxide. *Biochem Biophys Res Commun* 2003;**303**(1):112–9.
85. Li X, Chen H, Epstein PN. Metallothionein protects islets from hypoxia and extends islet graft survival by scavenging most kinds of reactive oxygen species. *J Biol Chem* 2004;**279**(1):765–71.
86. Padmasekar M, et al. Exendin-4 protects hypoxic islets from oxidative stress and improves islet transplantation outcome. *Endocrinology* 2013;**154**(4):1424–33.
87. Tsai Y-Y, et al. Novel synthesis of cerium oxide nanoparticles for free radical scavenging. *Nanomedicine* 2007;**2**(3):325–32.
88. Hosseini A, et al. Improvement of isolated rat pancreatic islets function by combination of cerium oxide nanoparticles/sodium selenite through reduction of oxidative stress AU - Pourkhalili, Nazila. *Toxicol Mech Methods* 2012;**22**(6):476–82.
89. Campbell SC, et al. Selenium stimulates pancreatic beta-cell gene expression and enhances islet function. *FEBS (Fed Eur Biochem Soc) Lett* 2008;**582**(15):2333–7.
90. Monfared SSMS, Larijani B, Abdollahi M. Islet transplantation and antioxidant management: a comprehensive review. *World J Gastroenterol* 2009;**15**(10):1153.
91. Hosseini A, et al. Antiapoptotic effects of cerium oxide and yttrium oxide nanoparticles in isolated rat pancreatic islets. *Hum Exp Toxicol* 2013;**32**(5):544–53.

92. Hosseini A, et al. Cerium and yttrium oxide nanoparticles against lead-induced oxidative stress and apoptosis in rat hippocampus. *Biol Trace Elem Res* 2015;**164**(1):80–9.
93. Schubert D, et al. Cerium and yttrium oxide nanoparticles are neuroprotective. *Biochem Biophys Res Commun* 2006;**342**(1):86–91.
94. Das M, et al. Auto-catalytic ceria nanoparticles offer neuroprotection to adult rat spinal cord neurons. *Biomaterials* 2007;**28**(10):1918–25.
95. Hussain S, et al. Cerium dioxide nanoparticles induce apoptosis and autophagy in human peripheral blood monocytes. *ACS Nano* 2012;**6**(7):5820–9.
96. Stern ST, et al. Induction of autophagy in porcine kidney cells by quantum dots: a common cellular response to nanomaterials? *Toxicol Sci* 2008;**106**(1):140–52.
97. Patil S, et al. Protein adsorption and cellular uptake of cerium oxide nanoparticles as a function of zeta potential. *Biomaterials* 2007;**28**(31):4600–7.
98. Dröge W. Free radicals in the physiological control of cell function. *Physiol Rev* 2002;**82**(1):47–95.
99. Cantarelli E, Piemonti L. Alternative transplantation sites for pancreatic islet grafts. *Curr Diab Rep* 2011;**11**(5):364–74.
100. Sakata N, et al. Encapsulated islets transplantation: past, present and future. *World J Gastrointest Pathophysiol* 2012;**3**(1):19–26.
101. De Vos P, Hamel A, Tatarkiewicz K. Considerations for successful transplantation of encapsulated pancreatic islets. *Diabetologia* 2002;**45**(2):159–73.
102. Desai T, Shea LD. Advances in islet encapsulation technologies. *Nat Rev Drug Discov* 2016;**16**:338.
103. Anderson JM, Rodriguez A, Chang DT. Foreign body reaction to biomaterials. *Semin Immunol* 2008;**20**(2):86–100.
104. Kozlovskaya V, et al. Hydrogen-bonded multilayers of tannic acid as mediators of T-cell immunity. *Adv Healthc Mater* 2015;**4**(5):686–94.
105. Kozlovskaya V, et al. Ultrathin polymeric coatings based on hydrogen-bonded polyphenol for protection of pancreatic islet cells. *Adv Funct Mater* 2012;**22**(16):3389–98.
106. Zhang Y, et al. Drug-eluting conformal coatings on individual cells. *Cell Mol Bioeng* 2016;**9**(3):382–97.
107. Pham-Hua D, et al. Islet encapsulation with polyphenol coatings decreases pro-inflammatory chemokine synthesis and T cell trafficking. *Biomaterials* 2017;**128**:19–32.
108. Abuid NJ, et al. Layer-by-Layer cerium oxide nanoparticle coating for antioxidant protection of encapsulated beta cells. *Adv Healthc Mater* 2019;**0**(0):1801493.
109. Gattás-Asfura KM, Stabler CL. Bioorthogonal layer-by-layer encapsulation of pancreatic islets via hyperbranched polymers. *ACS Appl Mater Interfaces* 2013;**5**(20):9964–74.
110. Gattas-Asfura K, et al. Covalent layer-by-layer assembly of hyperbranched polymers on alginate microcapsules to impart stability and permselectivity. *J Mater Chem* 2014;**2**(46):8208–19.
111. Domingueti CP, et al. Diabetes mellitus: the linkage between oxidative stress, inflammation, hypercoagulability and vascular complications. *J Diabetes Complications* 2016;**30**(4):738–45.
112. Kowluru RA, Mishra M. Oxidative stress, mitochondrial damage and diabetic retinopathy. *Biochim Biophys Acta* 2015;**1852**(11):2474–83.
113. Kawahito S, Kitahata H, Oshita S. Problems associated with glucose toxicity: role of hyperglycemia-induced oxidative stress. *World J Gastroenterol* 2009;**15**(33):4137–42.
114. Newsholme P, et al. Molecular mechanisms of ROS production and oxidative stress in diabetes. *Biochem J* 2016;**473**(24):4527–50.
115. Francesca Bonomini LFR, Rezzani R. Metabolic syndrome, aging and involvement of oxidative stress. *Aging Dis* 2015;**6**(2):109–20.
116. Montonen J, et al. Dietary antioxidant intake and risk of type 2 diabetes. *Diabetes Care* 2004;**27**(2):362–6.
117. Sheikh-Ali M, Chehade JM, Mooradian AD. The antioxidant paradox in diabetes mellitus. *Am J Ther* 2011;**18**(3):266–78.
118. Cardiovascular and other outcomes postintervention with insulin glargine and omega-3 fatty acids (ORIGINALE). *Diabetes Care* 2016;**39**(5):709–16.
119. Ziegler D, et al. Treatment of symptomatic diabetic polyneuropathy with the antioxidant alpha-lipoic acid: a meta-analysis. *Diabet Med* 2004;**21**(2):114–21.
120. Ojalvo AG, et al. Healing enhancement of diabetic wounds by locally infiltrated epidermal growth factor is associated with systemic oxidative stress reduction. *Int Wound J* 2017;**14**(1):214–25.
121. Gary Sibbald R, Woo KY. The biology of chronic foot ulcers in persons with diabetes. *Diabetes Metab Res Rev* 2008;**24**(S1):S25–30.
122. Ghaznavi H, et al. Neuro-protective effects of cerium and yttrium oxide nanoparticles on high glucose-induced oxidative stress and apoptosis in undifferentiated PC12 cells. *Neurol Res* 2015;**37**(7):624–32.
123. Dunnill C, et al. Reactive oxygen species (ROS) and wound healing: the functional role of ROS and emerging ROS-modulating technologies for augmentation of the healing process. *Int Wound J* 2017;**14**(1):89–96.
124. Spooner R, Yilmaz Ö. The role of reactive-oxygen-species in microbial persistence and inflammation. *Int J Mol Sci* 2011:334–52.
125. Bryan N, et al. Reactive oxygen species (ROS)–a family of fate deciding molecules pivotal in constructive inflammation and wound healing. *Eur Cell Mater* 2012;**24**:249–65.
126. Falanga V. Wound healing and its impairment in the diabetic foot. *Lancet* 2005;**366**(9498):1736–43.
127. Kunkemoeller B, Kyriakides TR. Redox signaling in diabetic wound healing regulates extracellular matrix deposition. *Antioxid Redox Signal* 2017;**27**(12):823–38.
128. Zhao R, Liang H, Clarke E, Jackson C, Xue M. Inflammation in chronic wounds. *Int J Mol Sci* 2016;**17**(12):2085.
129. Kupczyk D, et al. Age-related changes in an antioxidant defense system in elderly patients with essential hypertension compared with healthy controls. AU - Rybka, Joanna *Redox Rep* 2011;**16**(2):71–7.
130. Kunkemoeller B, Kyriakides TR. Redox signaling in diabetic wound healing regulates extracellular matrix deposition. *Antioxidants Redox Signal* 2017;**27**(12):823–38.
131. Kant V, et al. Antioxidant and anti-inflammatory potential of curcumin accelerated the cutaneous wound healing in streptozotocin-induced diabetic rats. *Int Immunopharmacol* 2014;**20**(2):322–30.
132. MacKay D, Miller AL. Nutritional support for wound healing. *Altern Med Rev* 2003;**8**(4):359–77.
133. Zhao X, et al. Antibacterial anti-oxidant electroactive injectable hydrogel as self-healing wound dressing with hemostasis and adhesiveness for cutaneous wound healing. *Biomaterials* 2017;**122**:34–47.
134. Gong C, et al. A biodegradable hydrogel system containing curcumin encapsulated in micelles for cutaneous wound healing. *Biomaterials* 2013;**34**(27):6377–87.
135. Altiok D, Altiok E, Tihminlioglu F. Physical, antibacterial and antioxidant properties of chitosan films incorporated with thyme oil for potential wound healing applications. *J Mater Sci Mater Med* 2010;**21**(7):2227–36.

136. Chigurupati S, et al. Effects of cerium oxide nanoparticles on the growth of keratinocytes, fibroblasts and vascular endothelial cells in cutaneous wound healing. *Biomaterials* 2013;**34**(9):2194–201.
137. Marzorati S, et al. Culture medium modulates proinflammatory conditions of human pancreatic islets before transplantation. *Am J Transplant* 2006;**6**(11):2791–5.
138. Xia T, et al. Comparison of the mechanism of toxicity of zinc oxide and cerium oxide nanoparticles based on dissolution and oxidative stress properties. *ACS Nano* 2008;**2**(10):2121–34.
139. Hirst SM, et al. Anti-inflammatory properties of cerium oxide nanoparticles. *Small* 2009;**5**(24):2848–56.
140. Selvaraj V, et al. Effect of cerium oxide nanoparticles on sepsis induced mortality and NF-kappaB signaling in cultured macrophages. *Nanomedicine* 2015;**10**(8):1275–88.
141. Singh R, Karakoti AS, Self W, Seal S, Singh S. Redox-sensitive cerium oxide nanoparticles protect human keratinocytes from oxidative stress induced by glutathione depletion. *Langmuir* 2016;**32**(46):12202–11.
142. Chen S, et al. Cerium oxide nanoparticles protect endothelial cells from apoptosis induced by oxidative stress. *Biol Trace Elem Res* 2013;**154**(1):156–66.
143. Saghazadeh S, et al. Drug delivery systems and materials for wound healing applications. *Adv Drug Deliv Rev* 2018;**127**:138–66.
144. Okonkwo UA, DiPietro LA. Diabetes and wound angiogenesis. *Int J Mol Sci* 2017;**18**(7):1419.
145. Kim YW, Byzova TV. Oxidative stress in angiogenesis and vascular disease. *Blood* 2014;**123**(5):625–31.
146. Das S, et al. The induction of angiogenesis by cerium oxide nanoparticles through the modulation of oxygen in intracellular environments. *Biomaterials* 2012;**33**(31):7746–55.
147. Farias IAP, Santos CC Ld, Sampaio FC. Antimicrobial activity of cerium oxide nanoparticles on opportunistic microorganisms: a systematic review. *BioMed Res Int* 2018;**2018**:14.
148. Mohanta YK, et al. Antimicrobial, antioxidant and cytotoxic activity of silver nanoparticles synthesized by leaf extract of Erythrina suberosa (Roxb.). *Front Mol Biosci* 2017;**4**.
149. Pelletier DA, et al. Effects of engineered cerium oxide nanoparticles on bacterial growth and viability. *Appl Environ Microbiol* 2010;**76**(24):7981–9.
150. Kamika I, Tekere M. Impacts of cerium oxide nanoparticles on bacterial community in activated sludge. *Amb Express* 2017;**7**(1):63.
151. Kobyliak N, et al. Neuropathic diabetic foot ulcers treated with cerium dioxide nanoparticles: a case report. *Diabetes Metab Syndr* 2019;**13**(1):228–34.
152. Kumari S, et al. Reactive oxygen species: a key constituent in cancer survival. *Biomark Insights* 2018;**13**. pp. 1177271918755391–1177271918755391.
153. Panieri E, Santoro MM. ROS homeostasis and metabolism: a dangerous liaison in cancer cells. *Cell Death Dis* 2016;**7**(6).
154. Galadari S, et al. Reactive oxygen species and cancer paradox: to promote or to suppress? *Free Radic Biol Med* 2017;**104**:144–64.
155. Rosenblum D, et al. Progress and challenges towards targeted delivery of cancer therapeutics. *Nat Commun* 2018;**9**(1):1410.
156. Alili L, et al. Combined cytotoxic and anti-invasive properties of redox-active nanoparticles in tumor-stroma interactions. *Biomaterials* 2011;**32**(11):2918–29.
157. De Milito A, Fais S. Tumor acidity, chemoresistance and proton pump inhibitors. *Future Oncol* 2005;**1**(6):779–86.
158. Kato Y, et al. Acidic extracellular microenvironment and cancer. *Cancer Cell Int* 2013:89.
159. Alpaslan E, et al. pH-dependent activity of dextran-coated cerium oxide nanoparticles on Prohibiting osteosarcoma cell proliferation. *ACS Biomater Sci Eng* 2015;**1**(11):1096–103.
160. Colon J, et al. Protection from radiation-induced pneumonitis using cerium oxide nanoparticles. *Nanomedicine* 2009;**5**(2):225–31.
161. Colon J, et al. Cerium oxide nanoparticles protect gastrointestinal epithelium from radiation-induced damage by reduction of reactive oxygen species and upregulation of superoxide dismutase 2. *Nanomedicine* 2010;**6**(5):698–705.
162. Chen F, et al. Enhancement of radiotherapy by ceria nanoparticles modified with neogambogic acid in breast cancer cells. *Int J Nanomedicine* 2015:4957–69.
163. Roa W, et al. Gold nanoparticle sensitize radiotherapy of prostate cancer cells by regulation of the cell cycle. *Nanotechnology* 2009;**20**(37):375101.
164. Alpaslan E, et al. pH-dependent activity of dextran-coated cerium oxide nanoparticles on Prohibiting osteosarcoma cell proliferation. *ACS Biomater Sci Eng* 2015.
165. Pešić M, et al. Anti-cancer effects of cerium oxide nanoparticles and its intracellular redox activity. *Chem Biol Interact* 2015;**232**:85–93.
166. Wittgen HG, van Kempen LC. Reactive oxygen species in melanoma and its therapeutic implications. *Melanoma Res* 2007;**17**(6):400–9.
167. Kumari M, et al. Toxicity study of cerium oxide nanoparticles in human neuroblastoma cells. *Int J Toxicol* 2014;**33**(2):86–97.
168. Semenza GL. Tumor metabolism: cancer cells give and take lactate. *J Clin Invest* 2008:3835–7.
169. Ali D, et al. Cerium oxide nanoparticles induce oxidative stress and genotoxicity in human skin melanoma cells. *Cell Biochem Biophys* 2015;**71**(3):1643–51.
170. Trachootham D, Alexandre J, Huang P. Targeting cancer cells by ROS-mediated mechanisms: a radical therapeutic approach? *Nat Rev Drug Discov* 2009;**8**:579.
171. Tarnuzzer RW, et al. Vacancy engineered ceria nanostructures for protection from radiation-induced cellular damage. *Nano Lett* 2005;**5**(12):2573–7.
172. Ebctcg. Effect of radiotherapy after mastectomy and axillary surgery on 10-year recurrence and 20-year breast cancer mortality: meta-analysis of individual patient data for 8135 women in 22 randomised trials. *Lancet* 2014;**383**(9935):2127–35.
173. Liotta LA, Kohn EC. The microenvironment of the tumour–host interface. *Nature* 2001;**411**:375.
174. Reuter S, et al. Oxidative stress, inflammation, and cancer: how are they linked? *Free Radic Biol Med* 2010;**49**(11):1603–16.
175. Martinez-Outschoorn UE, et al. Understanding the "lethal" drivers of tumor-stroma co-evolution AU - Lisanti, Michael P. *Cancer Biol Ther* 2010;**10**(6):537–42.
176. Otranto M, et al. The role of the myofibroblast in tumor stroma remodeling. *Cell Adh Migr* 2012:203–19.
177. De Wever O, Mareel M. Role of tissue stroma in cancer cell invasion. *J Pathol* 2003;**200**(4):429–47.
178. Costa A, Scholer-Dahirel A, Mechta-Grigoriou F. The role of reactive oxygen species and metabolism on cancer cells and their microenvironment. *Semin Cancer Biol* 2014;**25**:23–32.
179. Panieri E, Santoro MM. ROS homeostasis and metabolism: a dangerous liaison in cancer cells. *Cell Death Dis* 2016;**7**:e2253.

180. Paley PJ, et al. Vascular endothelial growth factor expression in early stage ovarian carcinoma. *Cancer* 1997;**80**(1):98–106.
181. Giri S, et al. Nanoceria: a rare-earth nanoparticle as a novel anti-angiogenic therapeutic agent in ovarian cancer. *PLoS One* 2013;**8**(1):e54578.
182. Luetke A, et al. Osteosarcoma treatment – where do we stand? A state of the art review. *Cancer Treat Rev* 2014;**40**(4):523–32.
183. Kim GH, et al. The role of oxidative stress in neurodegenerative diseases. *Exp Neurobiol* 2015;**24**(4):325–40.
184. Haddadi M, et al. Brain aging, memory impairment and oxidative stress: a study in Drosophila melanogaster. *Behav Brain Res* 2014;**259**:60–9.
185. Liu Z, et al. Oxidative stress in neurodegenerative diseases: from molecular mechanisms to clinical applications. *Oxid Med Cell Longev* 2017;**2017**.
186. Arya A, et al. Cerium oxide nanoparticles promote neurogenesis and abrogate hypoxia-induced memory impairment through AMPK-PKC-CBP signaling cascade. *Int J Nanomedicine* 2016;**11**:1159–73.
187. Yokel RA, et al. Biodistribution and biopersistence of ceria engineered nanomaterials: size dependence. *Nanomedicine* 2013;**9**(3):398–407.
188. Cimini A, et al. Antibody-conjugated PEGylated cerium oxide nanoparticles for specific targeting of Abeta aggregates modulate neuronal survival pathways. *Acta Biomater* 2012;**8**(6):2056–67.
189. Cheignon C, et al. Oxidative stress and the amyloid beta peptide in Alzheimer's disease. *Redox Biol* 2018;**14**:450–64.
190. Ittner LM, Götz J. Amyloid-β and tau — a toxic. *Nat Rev Neurosci* 2010;**12**(2):67.
191. Sastre M, Ritchie C, Hajji N. Metal ions in Alzheimer's disease brain. *JSM Alzheimer's Dis Related Dementia* 2015.
192. Chen X, Guo C, Kong J. Oxidative stress in neurodegenerative diseases☆. *Neural Regen Res* 2012:376–85.
193. Faller P, Hureau C. Bioinorganic chemistry of copper and zinc ions coordinated to amyloid-β peptide. *Dalton Trans* 2009;(7):1080–94.
194. Li M, et al. Cerium oxide caged metal chelator: anti-aggregation and anti-oxidation integrated H2O2-responsive controlled drug release for potential Alzheimer's disease treatment. *Chem Sci* 2013;**4**(6):2536–42.
195. Zhao Y, et al. Probing the molecular mechanism of cerium oxide nanoparticles in protecting against the neuronal cytotoxicity of Abeta1-42 with copper ions. *Metallomics* 2016;**8**(7):644–7.
196. Knott AB, Bossy-Wetzel E. Nitric oxide in health and disease of the nervous system. *Antioxid Redox Signal* 2009;**11**(3):541–54.
197. Guix FX, et al. Amyloid-dependent triosephosphate isomerase nitrotyrosination induces glycation and tau fibrillation. *Brain* 2018;**132**(5):1335–45.
198. Dowding JM, et al. Cerium oxide nanoparticles protect against Aβ-induced mitochondrial fragmentation and neuronal cell death. *Cell Death Differ* 2014;**21**(10):1622.
199. Smith MA, et al. Widespread peroxynitrite-mediated damage in Alzheimer's disease. *J Neurosci* 1997;**17**(8):2653.
200. Wang X, et al. Amyloid-β overproduction causes abnormal mitochondrial dynamics via differential modulation of mitochondrial fission/fusion proteins. *Proc Natl Acad Sci U S A* 2008;**105**(49):19318–23.
201. Knott AB, et al. Mitochondrial fragmentation in neurodegeneration. *Nat Rev Neurosci* 2008;**9**(7):505.
202. Reddy PH, et al. Dynamin-related protein 1 and mitochondrial fragmentation in neurodegenerative diseases. *Brain Res Brain Res Rev* 2011;**67**(1):103–18.
203. Danysz W, Parsons CG. Alzheimer's disease, β-amyloid, glutamate, NMDA receptors and memantine – searching for the connections. *Br J Pharmacol* 2012;**167**(2):324–52.
204. Binder DK, Scharfman HE. Brain-derived neurotrophic factor. *Growth Factors* 2004;**22**(3):123–31.
205. Connor B, et al. Brain-derived neurotrophic factor is reduced in Alzheimer's disease. *Brain Res Mol Brain Res* 1997;**49**(1–2):71–81.
206. Lim JY, Reighard CP, Crowther DC. The pro-domains of neurotrophins, including BDNF, are linked to Alzheimer's disease through a toxic synergy with Aβ. *Hum Mol Genet* 2015:3929–38.
207. Teng HK, et al. ProBDNF induces neuronal apoptosis via activation of a receptor complex of p75NTR and sortilin. *J Neurosci* 2005;**25**(22):5455–63.
208. Barbara D'Angelo SS, Benedetti E, Silvia Di Loreto, Phani RA, Falone Stefano, Amicarelli Fernanda, Ceru Maria Paola, Cimini Annamaria. Cerium oxide nanoparticles trigger neuronal survival in a human alzheimer disease model by modulating BDNF pathway. *Curr Nanosci* 2018;**5**(2):167–76.
209. Compston A, Coles A. Multiple sclerosis. *Lancet* 2008;**372**(9648):1502–17.
210. Luo C, et al. The role of microglia in multiple sclerosis. *Neuropsychiatr Dis Treat* 2017:1661–7.
211. Gilgun-Sherki Y, Melamed E, Offen D. The role of oxidative stress in the pathogenesis of multiple sclerosis: the need for effective antioxidant therapy. *J Neurol* 2004;**251**(3):261–8.
212. Heckman KL, et al. Custom cerium oxide nanoparticles protect against a free radical mediated autoimmune degenerative disease in the brain. *ACS Nano* 2013;**7**(12):10582–96.
213. Eitan E, et al. Combination therapy with lenalidomide and nanoceria ameliorates CNS autoimmunity. *Exp Neurol* 2015;**273**:151–60.
214. Ponath G, Park C, Pitt D. The role of astrocytes in multiple sclerosis. *Front Immunol* 2018;**9**. pp. 217–217.
215. Chen H, et al. Oxidative stress in ischemic brain damage: mechanisms of cell death and potential molecular targets for neuroprotection. *Antioxid Redox Signal* 2011:1505–17.
216. Progress AWM. Neuroprotection in ischemic stroke. *Circulation* 2014;**130**:2002–4.
217. Maiti P, et al. Hypobaric hypoxia induces oxidative stress in rat brain. *Neurochem Int* 2006;**49**(8):709–16.
218. Papandreou I, et al. HIF-1 mediates adaptation to hypoxia by actively downregulating mitochondrial oxygen consumption. *Cell Metab* 2006;**3**(3):187–97.
219. Hardas SS, et al. Brain distribution and toxicological evaluation of a systemically delivered engineered nanoscale ceria. *Toxicol Sci* 2010;**116**(2):562–76.
220. Hardas SS, et al. Rat brain pro-oxidant effects of peripherally administered 5nm ceria 30 days after exposure. *Neurotoxicology (Little Rock)* 2012;**33**(5):1147–55.
221. Estevez AY, et al. Neuroprotective mechanisms of cerium oxide nanoparticles in a mouse hippocampal brain slice model of ischemia. *Free Radic Biol Med* 2011;**51**(6):1155–63.
222. Ramamurthy S, et al. AMPK activation regulates neuronal structure in developing hippocampal neurons. *Neuroscience* 2014;**259**:13–24.
223. Ryter SW, et al. Mechanisms of cell death in oxidative stress. *Antioxid Redox Signal* 2007;**9**(1):49–89.
224. Wartofsky L. Increasing world incidence of thyroid cancer: increased detection or higher radiation exposure? *Hormones (Basel)* 2010;**9**(2):103–8.

225. Talukder MA, et al. Chronic cigarette smoking causes hypertension, increased oxidative stress, impaired NO bioavailability, endothelial dysfunction, and cardiac remodeling in mice. *Am J Physiol Heart Circ Physiol* 2011;**300**(1):H388−96.
226. Churg A, Cosio M, Wright JL. Mechanisms of cigarette smoke-induced COPD: insights from animal models. *Am J Physiol Lung Cell Mol Physiol* 2008;**294**(4):L612−31.
227. Pittilo MR. Cigarette smoking, endothelial injury and cardiovascular disease. *Int J Exp Pathol* 2000;**81**(4):219−30.
228. Zuo L, et al. Interrelated role of cigarette smoking, oxidative stress, and immune response in COPD and corresponding treatments. *Am J Physiol Lung Cell Mol Physiol* 2014;**307**(3):L205−18.
229. Ferrer E, et al. Effects of cigarette smoke and hypoxia on pulmonary circulation in the Guinea pig. *Eur Respir J* 2011;**38**(3):617−27.
230. Wright JL, Levy RD, Churg A. Pulmonary hypertension in chronic obstructive pulmonary disease: current theories of pathogenesis and their implications for treatment. *Thorax* 2005;**60**(7):605−9.
231. Foronjy R, Wallace A, D'Armiento J. The pharmokinetic limitations of antioxidant treatment for COPD. *Pulm Pharmacol Ther* 2008;**21**(2):370−9.
232. Rubio L, et al. Antioxidant and anti-genotoxic properties of cerium oxide nanoparticles in a pulmonary-like cell system. *Arch Toxicol* 2016;**90**(2):269−78.
233. Niu J, Wang K, Kolattukudy PE. Cerium oxide nanoparticles inhibits oxidative stress and nuclear factor-κB activation in H9c2 cardiomyocytes exposed to cigarette smoke extract. *J Pharmacol Exp Ther* 2011:53−61.
234. Xu P-T, et al. Cerium oxide nanoparticles: a potential medical counter measure to mitigate radiation-induced lung injury in CBA/J mice. *Radiat Res* 2016;**185**(5):11.
235. Arya A, et al. Cerium oxide nanoparticles protect rodent lungs from hypobaric hypoxia-induced oxidative stress and inflammation. *Int J Nanomedicine* 2013:4507−20.
236. Amin KA, et al. The protective effects of cerium oxide nanoparticles against hepatic oxidative damage induced by monocrotaline. *Int J Nanomedicine* 2011;**6**:143−9.
237. Walkey C, et al. Catalytic properties and biomedical applications of cerium oxide nanoparticles. *Environ Sci Nano* 2015;**2**(1):33−53.
238. Rim KT, et al. Effect of cerium oxide nanoparticles to inflammation and oxidative DNA damages in H9c2 cells. *Mol Cell Toxicol* 2012;**8**(3):271−80.
239. Pagliari F, et al. Cerium oxide nanoparticles protect cardiac progenitor cells from oxidative stress. *ACS Nano* 2012;**6**(5):3767−75.
240. Cervantes Gracia K, Llanas-Cornejo D, Husi H. CVD and Oxidative Stress. *J Clin Med* 2017;**6**(2):22.
241. Sun Y. Myocardial repair/remodelling following infarction: roles of local factors. *Cardiovasc Res* 2009;**81**(3):482−90.

Chapter 18

Polymeric Nanoparticles

Bader M. Jarai, Emily L. Kolewe, Zachary S. Stillman, Nisha Raman and Catherine A. Fromen
Department of Chemical and Biomolecular Engineering, University of Delaware, Newark, DE, United States

18.1 Introduction

"I just want to say one word to you. Just one word... Are you listening?... Plastics .... There's a great future in plastics." Discuss as you will the cultural implications of Mr. McGuire's comments to Dustin Hoffman's character in the 1967 movie, The Graduate, but the underlying reality of this statement has persisted; "plastics" or polymers are everywhere. In drug delivery, "plastics" have transformed the pharmaceutical landscape and offer tremendous benefits toward controlling and tuning drug release profiles. Polymers are macromolecular structures that are built from a large number of repeating units called monomers. The diverse nature of these building units gives rise to a spectrum of chemical and physical properties, enabling designer materials that are tunable for a given application. The field of polymer chemistry has exploded as Mr. McGuire predicted, with novel synthesis methods giving rise to a host of new and precisely controlled polymer materials; so too has the use of polymers exploded in the fields of drug delivery and nanomedicine.

The introduction of polymers to pharmaceutical applications has revolutionized the drug delivery field in a few staggering ways. Polymers have been used to alter the pharmacokinetic (PK) profile of active pharmaceutical ingredients (APIs), capable of providing both sustained release and altered clearance profiles. The use of polymers to sustain API release dates back to the mid-1960s, with independent pioneering research from Harvard researcher Judah Folkman, MD, and Alza Corporation founder Alejandro Zaffaroni, PhD, establishing first-order kinetic release of APIs from polymer matrices.[1] The sustained release field was further transformed by the work of Robert Langer, a former postdoctoral fellow for Folkman, who demonstrated the sustained release of sensitive protein molecules from a hydrophobic polymer, poly (ethylene-vinyl acetate) (PEVA), with protein release lasting over 100 days.[2] These advances led to a wide variety of sustained release pharmaceutical devices, implants, and depots that all use polymers to control and sustain drug release, including ocular, oral, vaginal, and topical products.[1] Also, stemming back to the mid-1960s, polymers have been used to alter the PK of APIs, with Rutgers professor Frank Davis introducing the concept of conjugating poly(ethylene glycol) (PEG) to protein APIs to increase circulation times.[3] This concept of adding PEG to an API, called "PEGylation," has resulted in countless clinically approved protein, antibody, and nanoparticle (NP) formulations with low immunogenicity, increased half-lives, and improved PK profiles.[4]

These examples demonstrate the deep history of polymers in drug delivery and highlight the distinct utility of polymers in pharmaceutical applications. Perhaps unsurprisingly, the observed benefits of using polymers for controlled release and altered PK profiles of small molecules have found similar benefits within the field of nanomedicine. Polymeric NPs offer the same benefits of all NP formulations, including protecting delivered therapeutic agents from degradation and limiting off-target API-related cytotoxicity upon administration. Uniquely, polymeric NPs can offer additional advantages of tailor-made material considerations, stemming from the inherent properties of the molecules beginning at the monomeric level. Thus, polymer NPs can be generated with control over size, shape, and surface chemistry, customizable API release profiles, inherent biocompatibility, and stimuli-responsiveness.

As mentioned earlier, polymers are built from monomer building blocks. Natural polymers, those formed in nature, are often composed of monomers with vastly different chemistries, whereas synthetic polymers are typically composed of a much smaller number of well-defined monomer units. These blocks can be arranged in a number of configurations, yielding long single chains or highly branched structures, which can result in a wide range of chain conformations and microstructures. Polymers are often described by their chain length, the number of monomer units in the polymer backbone, and their molecular weight (MW). Polymers can also demonstrate regions of ordering, resulting in crystalline domains. The degree of crystallinity within the polymer material will dramatically influence its phase behavior. The phase behavior is of particular importance for nanomedicine applications, as it will control the formulation behavior needed for processing as well

Nanoparticles for Biomedical Applications. https://doi.org/10.1016/B978-0-12-816662-8.00018-7

as the interactions with the API. This is described by the polymer's melting temperature (T_m), which describes the transition from a crystalline or semicrystalline phase to a completely amorphous phase, and the polymer's glass transition temperature (T_g), which describes a phase transition from a glassy to a rubbery state.[5] Because polymers can have varying degrees of crystallinity, some polymers can have either one or both of these characteristic phase transitions. Other relevant polymeric properties include their hydrophobicity, as measured by water contact angle, and their mechanical properties, defined by their Young's elastic modulus and tensile strength. Varied analytical techniques are used by polymer scientists to fully characterize their polymer material, including gel permeation chromatography,[6] dynamic scanning calorimetry,[7] thermal gravimetric analysis,[8] and rheometry.[9]

Depending on the specific polymer properties and synthetic conditions, a wide range of polymer NP structures can be formed.[10] Nanoshells, nanospheres, polyplexes, polymersomes, and dendrimers are among the most commonly reported morphologies of polymeric NPs (Fig. 18.1).[11–13] These various structures facilitate unique API incorporation and release properties that can be precisely controlled by tuning the physiochemical properties such as size, molecular weight, degradation rate, and shape. Nanoshells or nanocapsules have a vesicle-like morphology and are utilized to encapsulate APIs in the liquid core of the particle, which is surrounded by the particle's polymeric shell. The liquid core may be oil or water based, depending on the setup of the fabrication process used to generate the nanoshells. The structure of nanospheres consists of a continuous polymer matrix with the API distributed within the matrix through encapsulation or covalent bonding, though the drug can also be adsorbed to the surface of the nanosphere. While solid polymer morphologies are usually spherical, nonspherical structures have been widely reported.[14,15] Polyplexes are polyelectrolyte complexes formed by electrostatic attractions between polycations and polyanions.[16] Polyplexes have been extensively used in gene delivery applications by conjugating different polycations to negatively charged oligonucleotides.[17] They have a strong advantage over other polymeric nanoassemblies due to their ease of fabrication via self-assembly.[18] Dendrimers are repeating large structures that "hyperbranch" in controllable, reproducible designs.[19] The size, reaction kinetics, and surface reaction groups are precisely controllable through the dendrimer framework, which can have advantages in therapeutic applications.[19,20] APIs can be conjugated to the surface or encapsulated in the highly structured network of the dendrimers.[19,20] However, synthesis of dendrimer NPs is often complex and involves multiple steps and post-modifications.[21] Polymersomes are vesicular structures of amphiphilic block copolymers, which are two distinct polymers that have been covalently joined together.[22,23] Polymersomes have significant advantage over liposomes (lipid-based vesicles) in their chemical versatility and *in vivo* circulation stability, making them an attractive choice to encapsulate and deliver cargo.[24,25] Overall, these morphologically diverse polymer-based assemblies highlight the design flexibility of polymers, which is instrumental for specializing drug delivery for various applications.

The topic of polymeric NPs for nanomedicine alone is a vast subject worthy of an entire textbook. Within this chapter, our goal is to provide the reader with an overview of the most common polymeric materials and fabrication methods used in nanomedicine, as well as some key examples of applications of polymeric NPs that capitalize on the unique attributes of the polymer material. We note that this chapter is by no means exhaustive and highly recommend the reader to consult with many excellent reviews in the literature to complement this chapter, including in-depth reviews of common nanomedicine polymer materials of PEG,[4,26–28] poly(lactic-co-glycolic acid) (PLGA),[29,30] hydrogels,[31] pluronics,[32] dendrimers,[33] proteins,[34] responsive polymeric NP systems,[35–37] and applications,[38,39] as well as others noted throughout the chapter.

18.2 Common polymers in nanomedicine

Polymeric materials used to prepare NPs are commonly categorized into natural and synthetic polymers. Natural polymers are naturally occurring polymers derived from a wide range of plant- or animal-based sources. Synthetic polymers are often created from petroleum-derived raw materials through precision growth methods; because of

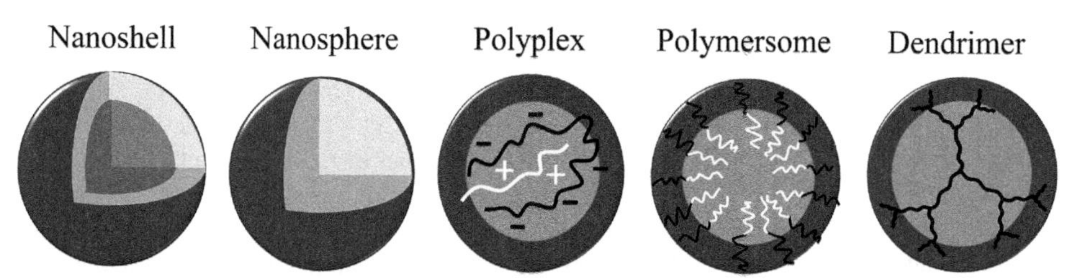

FIGURE 18.1 Nanoparticle types: nanoshells or nanocapsules (A), solid polymer particles or nanospheres (B), charge-induced complexes between cationic and ionic polymers or polyplexes (C), immiscible phase-induced liposome-like structures or polymersomes (D), and repeated, highly ordered structures or dendrimer nanoparticles (E).

their defined chemical structure, their physical and chemical properties can be more easily tuned than natural polymers, though the narrow MW distribution of natural polymers allows for very well-defined properties. In this section, we give an overview of some of the commonly used natural and synthetic polymeric materials in designing NP systems for biomedical applications, with a focus on biodegradable polymers.

18.2.1 Natural polymers

Natural polymers offer key advantages for use in biomedical applications. Derived from plant- or animal-based sources, natural polymers are often highly biocompatible, nontoxic at a wide range of concentrations, and generally inexpensive.[40–42] Natural polymers are derived from a diverse pool of sources and can have significant batch-to-batch variability in NP formulations. These may be extracted from raw materials through complicated separation processes or reproduced synthetically through often complicated multistep pathways. As a result, natural polymer NP formulations can have a range of physical and chemical properties, which may lead to poor control over synthesis and fabrication. Poor mechanical performance is also a concern for using natural polymers; however, their ubiquity can often provide worthwhile benefits. Natural polymers often found in nanomedicine can be categorized into two major subfamilies: polysaccharides and proteins. Examples of structures of natural polymers are included in Table 18.1.

18.2.1.1 Natural polysaccharides

Polysaccharides are carbohydrate-based polymers consisting of different sugar molecules joined together by glycosidic bonds. Polysaccharides can have linear or branched structures, which gives rise to a range of physical properties that influence their choice as a material for drug delivery and tissue engineering applications. Polysaccharide-based NPs have been reviewed extensively.[43] Chitosan, cellulose, and hyaluronic acid (HA) are among the most common polysaccharide-based polymers used in biomedical applications.

18.2.1.1.1 Hyaluronic acid

HA is a linear chain polysaccharide consisting of repeating D-glucuronic acid and N-acetyl-D-glucosamine units. HA is a biocompatible and biodegradable polymer and is naturally found within the extracellular matrix of many human tissues. Due to its ubiquity in the human body, HA has been extensively used for controlling API release and also for improving targeted drug delivery.[44] Interestingly, the human receptor CD44, which is specific for HA, is often overexpressed on tumor cells, which has prompted many researchers to incorporate HA in NP-based formulations to enhance delivery to tumors.[45]

18.2.1.1.2 Cellulose

Cellulose is a linear chain polysaccharide built from glucose units connected through $\beta(1 \rightarrow 4)$ glycosidic bonds. Cellulose is the most abundant polysaccharide in nature and is inherently biocompatible with human tissue.[46] Nanosized cellulose-based particles can be categorized into two groups: cellulose nanocrystals and nanofibrillated cellulose.[47] Cellulose nanocrystals have a very high surface area and a net negative charge, both of which are advantageous for conjugating APIs to the surface of the crystals. For example, doxorubicin (DOX) has been successfully bound to the surface of cellulose nanocrystals, indicating the ability of cellulose-based NPs to be used for anticancer drug delivery.[48] In addition, nanofibrillated cellulose has been used for the controlled release of beclomethasone dipropionate, a steroidal small molecule.[49]

18.2.1.1.3 Chitosan

Chitosan is a polysaccharide consisting of $\beta(1 \rightarrow 4)$ joined D-glucosamine and *N*-acetyl-D-glucosamine that are randomly distributed throughout the polymer. Chitosan is synthesized through the deacetylation of chitin derived from shells of crustaceans.[50] The linear chain polysaccharide has a structure similar to that of cellulose, which gives chitosan the potential to form both nanocrystals and nanofibers. Chitosan has shown potential as a biocompatible and biodegradable API nanocarrier. Chitosan degradation *in vivo* occurs through an enzymatic degradation, with a degradation rate proportional to the degree of deacetylation.[51] Therefore, the rate of API release from chitosan NPs may be modulated by tuning the degree of deacetylation in the polymer matrix. Chitosan has also been shown to be a mucoadhesive, with interesting applications for NP delivery at mucosal surfaces,[52] as well as gene delivery because of its cationic charge.[53,54]

18.2.1.2 Natural proteins

Proteins are macromolecules composed of one or more amino acid chains and can loosely be considered natural polymers, with complex self-assembly of the amino acid chains capable of macromolecular structures. Proteins are used for NP preparation because of their biodegradability and ease of modification. In addition, the ability of proteins to recognize molecules can be utilized to improve targeted drug delivery when incorporated into an NP. Protein polymers used in biomedical applications are most commonly derived from albumin,[55] elastin,[56] collagen,[57] and silk.[58] Notably, a number of protein-based NP therapeutics are FDA approved, including Abraxane, an injectable NP albumin-bound chemotherapeutic used for treating different cancers.[59] Protein NP design and material selection have been reviewed elsewhere.[60]

TABLE 18.1 Common natural polymeric materials used for fabricating nanoparticles and the structures of each material.

Polymer	Structure
Hyaluronic acid (HA)	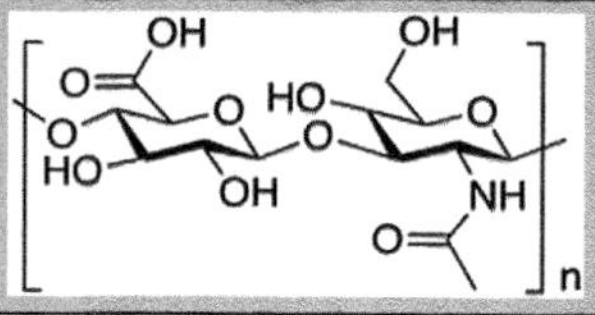
Cellulose	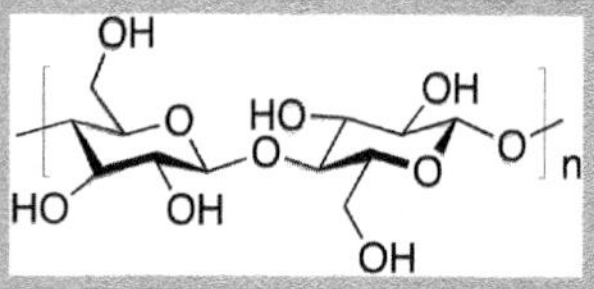
Chitosan	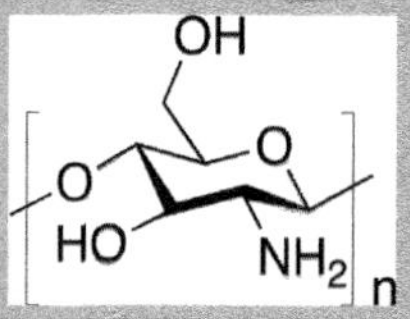
Silk	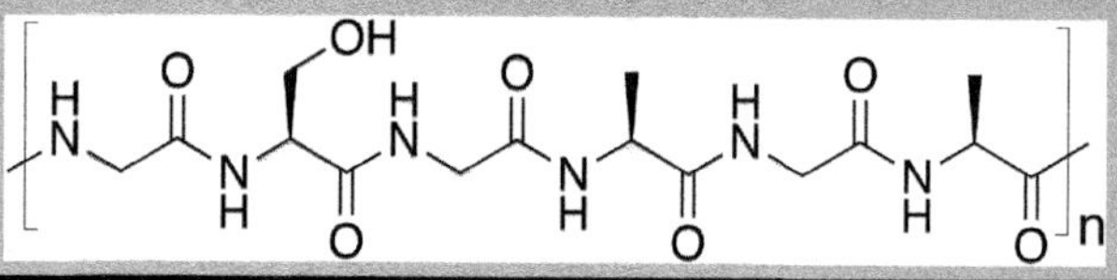

18.2.2 Synthetic polymers

Synthetic polymers are polymers not generally found in nature and are synthesized through polymerization reactions beginning from a wide range of monomeric units. Synthetic polymers are highly tunable, easily controllable materials that offer advantages over natural polymers. Synthetic polymers can be designed to possess mechanical properties similar to those of biological tissue, which highlights the ability of synthetic polymers to be used as tissue or cell mimics.[61,62] In addition, the tunability of synthetic polymers allows the precise control of API release, a key requirement in drug delivery applications. However, without careful consideration, many synthetic polymers may not show sufficient biocompatibility as compared with natural polymers, and therefore, the choice of material is a key parameter in designing an effective drug delivery vehicle. Synthetic polymers span an extremely wide library of materials, including polyesters, the most commonly explored polymers for drug delivery. Other biodegradable materials have also been used due to their range of chemical and physical properties, including polyamides and polyanhydrides. Active research in stimuli-responsive synthetic polymers has also provided further control of API release from NP carriers, highlighting the benefit of rationally designed synthetic polymers in nanomedicine.

Polymer synthesis generally falls under one of three categories: step-growth, radical, or ionic polymerization. Each of these methods has its own advantages and disadvantages, as well as an associated set of polymers which can be synthesized with the method.[63,64] Step-growth polymerization involves sequential reaction of bifunctional monomers either with themselves or with another bifunctional monomer, which allows for continuous reaction. Radical polymerizations utilize the generation of radical species to promote the continuous reaction of the monomer species. Radical polymerizations, unlike step-growth polymerizations, typically utilize an initiator to begin the polymerization process, generating radicals after exposure to UV light, redox reactions, induced decomposition, or thermolysis.[63] The radical initiator will then begin the chain of reactions for the polymerization, referred to as propagation steps.[63] Radical polymerization reactions are difficult to control; thus, techniques have been developed to control the length of polymers and rates of polymerization.[63] Some of these techniques include atom-transfer radical polymerization (ATRP), reversible addition fragmentation chain-transfer (RAFT) radical polymerization, and ring-opening metathesis polymerization (ROMP).[64] Ionic polymerizations, much like radical polymerizations, often utilize an initiator to generate the ion to begin the propagation. Generally, these initiators include nucleophiles such as ionic metal

TABLE 18.2 Common synthetic polymeric materials used for nanoparticle fabrication and the structures of each material.

Polymer	Structure
Poly(lactic acid)(PLA)	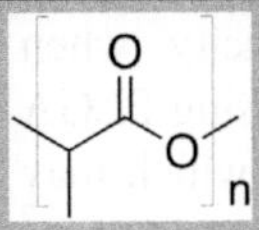
Poly(lactic-co-glycolic acid)(PLGA)	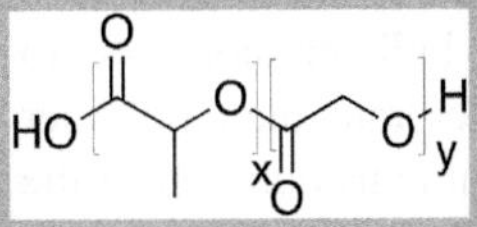
Poly(ε-caprolactone)(PCL)	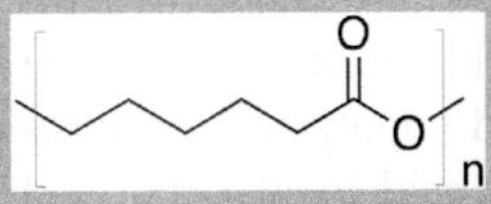
Poly(ethylenimine)(PEI)	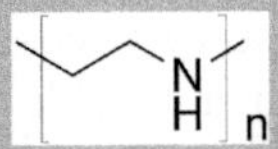
Poly(*N*-isopropyl acrylamide)(PNIPAM)	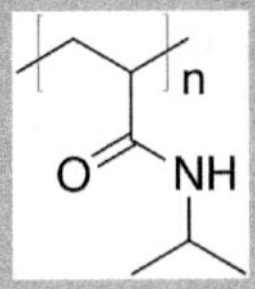

amides, cyanides, and amines in addition to certain organometallic compounds such as Grignard reagents and alkyllithium compounds. Unlike radical polymerizations, most ionic polymerizations lack a termination step.[65] Collectively, these methods can be used to create a wide range of synthetic polymers, with a few major classes described briefly in the following section. Examples of structures of synthetic polymers are included in Table 18.2.

18.2.2.1 Polyesters

Biodegradability and low immunogenicity are key requirements of polymeric materials in drug delivery applications. Polyesters have shown outstanding biocompatibility and biodegradability, and degradation products are usually metabolites that are consumed by natural pathways.[66] As a result, polyesters, especially PLGA, have been used extensively in biomedical applications.

18.2.2.1.1 Poly(glycolic acid)

Poly(glycolic acid) (PGA) is one of the first biodegradable synthetic polymers to be used for biomedical applications. PGA is most commonly synthesized via ring-opening polymerization or polycondensation of glycolic acid.[67,68] PGA was used in the first US Food and Drug Administration (FDA)–approved biodegradable suture in the 1960s.[69] PGA has high crystallinity, which contributes to its rigidity and low solubility in most organic solvents.[70] The main drawback of using PGA as a drug delivery vehicle is its rapid degradation rate, which results in loss of mechanical strength upon administration. As a result, PGA is incorporated with other polymers such as poly(ε-caprolactone) (PCL) and poly(lactic acid) (PLA) to improve mechanical properties and degradability.[71,72]

18.2.2.1.2 Poly(lactic acid)

PLA is a polymer consisting of repeating units of lactic acid. Similar to PGA, PLA is synthesized by ring-opening polymerization or direct polycondensation of lactic acid.[73] Unlike glycolic acid, lactic acid is a chiral molecule that has two enantiomers, L-lactic acid and D-lactic acid. L-lactic acid is the naturally occurring isomer and is crystalline following polymerization, whereas D-lactic acid results in an amorphous polymer.[74] Monomeric units of lactic acid are released upon PLA hydrolysis. PLA's biocompatibility stems from the fact that lactic acid is a metabolite and an intermediate for many metabolic pathways. The rate of PLA degradation is relatively slow, which makes it disadvantageous to solely use PLA in applications requiring rapid degradation or API release. The degradation rate of PLA can be altered by incorporating amounts of structurally similar monomers that degrade at different rates. For example, glycolic acid is one of the most commonly incorporated materials to increase the degradation of PLA while maintaining its biocompatibility and low toxicity.[75]

18.2.2.1.3 Poly(lactic-co-glycolic acid)

PLGA, a copolymer of lactic acid and glycolic acid, is one of the most widely used polymers in the biomedical field.[29,76] PLGA hydrolyzes into lactic acid and glycolic acid, two metabolites that are present in the body. As a result, PLGA shows very minimal cytotoxicity when administered *in vivo*. A potential drawback to using PLGA is the acidic nature of its degradation products, which may make it inapplicable in pH-sensitive environments.[77] PLGA degrades uniformly through bulk erosion due to water penetrating the NP at a higher rate than polymer degradation.[78] Erosion is an important consideration in the design of NP drug carriers to control the release of API. The degradation rate of PLGA is highly tunable and can be manipulated by tuning the MW and copolymer composition.[30] For example, a 50:50 lactic acid to glycolic acid molar ratio has been shown to exhibit the highest susceptibility to hydrolysis.[79] Polymer MW is also a tunable parameter to control API incorporation and release.[77] PLGA NPs have been used for a variety of medical purposes including vaccines,[80] cancer treatments,[81] and gene delivery[82] as described later in this chapter.

18.2.2.1.4 Poly(ε-caprolactone)

PCL is synthesized through the ring-opening polymerization of ε-caprolactonc.[83] It is notcworthy to mcntion PCL for its slow degradation rate as compared with PLGA and other commonly used polyesters. PCL's slow degradation rate in addition to its biocompatibility makes it an attractive choice for a slow API release polymeric matrix over periods of several months to over a year.[84] PCL NPs have been used to deliver and study the release and distribution of numerous therapeutic agents including hormone modulators,[85] antifungals,[86] and nonsteroidal anti-inflammatory APIs[87] over prolonged periods of time.

18.2.2.2 Polyanhydrides

Polyanhydrides are a class of biodegradable synthetic polymers that have widely been used in biomedical applications and especially in drug delivery due to their biocompatibility.[88] Polyanhydride-based materials are surface eroding, which allows for more control of sustained API release as compared with bulk-eroding polyesters.[89] Degradation of polyanhydrides through the cleavage of the anhydride bond results in dicarboxylic acid units.[90] Examples of polyanhydrides used in NP fabrication include poly(sebacic acid)[91] and poly(1,6-bis(*p*-carboxyphenoxy)hexane).[92]

18.2.2.3 Polyamines

Poly(ethylenimine) (PEI) is one of the most commonly used polymers for gene delivery. PEI is a cationic polyamine, and its positive charge allows for the formation of complexes with negatively charged DNA, referred to as polyplexes.[93] PEI comes in both linear and branched forms, and the extent of polyplex formation depends on the degree of branching as well as the ratio of DNA to PEI.[94] While PEI/DNA complexes have shown promise in gene delivery applications, they cause severe *in vivo* cytotoxicity due to PEI impairing cell function.[95] As a result, there have been many attempts to improve the biocompatibility of PEI-based complexes by shielding with biocompatible materials, especially PEG.[96,97]

18.2.3 Stimuli-responsive polymers

Stimuli-responsive polymers have been especially considered for their use as potential "smart" drug delivery devices.[98] Drug delivery vehicles that are based on stimuli-responsive materials are viewed as a major improvement to finely tune the control of API release. The most commonly studied and physiologically relevant stimuli in the field of drug delivery are temperature and pH, although stimuli-responsive polymers have been also engineered to respond to external stimuli such as light and magnetic fields.[99,100] In this section, we give an overview of the commonly used stimuli-responsive polymeric systems for control of API dosage and delivery.

18.2.3.1 Temperature-responsive polymers

Temperature-responsive polymers are materials that experience a sharp change in solubility following a small temperature difference. The presence of hydrophobic groups is a common feature of temperature-responsive polymers. Thermosensitive polymers used in drug delivery have a lower critical solution temperature, the temperature below which the polymers are soluble.[101] As a result, an increase in temperature (e.g., increase from body temperature to overheated tumor location) causes polymer insolubility, which ultimately leads to the collapse of the polymeric vehicle and release of the delivered API.[102] The most prominent example of a thermosensitive polymer is poly(*N*-isopropylacrylamide) (PNIPAM).[103] PNIPAM-based NPs have been used in drug and gene delivery applications, especially in cases of hyperthermia and in tumor microenvironments.[104,105]

18.2.3.2 pH-responsive polymers

While temperature-responsive polymers often require an externally applied heat source, pH-responsive polymers can harness physiological changes that occur naturally in many disease states, making pH the most commonly utilized stimulus for drug delivery applications. Variations of pH in the body can result in localized API release at a controlled location. For example, healthy tissue and blood have a pH of about 7.4, whereas extracellular tumor and intracellular microenvironments are slightly acidic (pH ~ 6.5 and 5, respectively).[106] Some pH-labile materials include acetals,[107] hydrazones,[108] and diorthoesters.[109] These pH-labile linkages degrade at low pH and enable the rapid release of API when incorporated with NP formulations. Other materials using pH-responsive behavior contain ionizable groups that experience solubility changes or cleavage upon exposure to a change in pH. For example, poly(acrylic acid) and poly(methacrylic acid) reversibly swell in response to pH change and have been studied for drug delivery purposes.[110,111] As a result, these polymers may be used as swelling-controlled release systems tuned to pH-sensitive physiological environments.[112]

18.3 Common methods of fabrication

Once the polymer material has been selected, taking the application, cost, phase behavior, and synthesis approach into consideration, polymers must then be formed into the desired NP structure. There are two main classifications for the methods of fabrication of polymeric NPs: top-down (TD) and bottom-up (BU). The key distinction between the two classes is that TD methods remove material away from the bulk to define NPs, whereas BU techniques develop NP assemblies through a growth process. Polymer NP assembly methods have been extensively reviewed in the literature.[113–115] In this section, we review some of the commonly used nanofabrication techniques used for biomedical applications.

18.3.1 Top-down methods

TD approaches are usually based on bulk material processing to generate NPs. Here, we review some of the more precise TD methods for NP fabrication, including emulsification, soft lithography, and electrohydrodynamic cojetting. A pictorial list of TD nanofabrication is included in Table 18.3.

18.3.1.1 Emulsification–solvent evaporation

Emulsification–solvent evaporation relies on dissolving an already-synthesized polymer into a volatile solvent such as dichloromethane and then forming an emulsion between the polymer solution and an aqueous phase.[114] The organic solvent is then removed, and as a result, a colloidal suspension of polymeric nanospheres is formed. Solvent removal is usually achieved by continuous agitation at room temperature or by using a vacuum system to reduce the pressure and extract the solvent.[116] Different emulsification techniques may be utilized, including homogenization and ultrasound sonication. The main advantage for this method is the ability to encapsulate APIs with a range of hydrophobicity. Furthermore, particle size control may be achieved by tuning process parameters such as temperature and pressure during solvent removal and speed of emulsification. However, the emulsification–solvent evaporation method has several disadvantages. The main disadvantage is the coalescence and the collapse of polymer droplets during the evaporation step. In addition, solvent evaporation is a time-consuming process, which hinders the scale-up of the emulsification–solvent evaporation method.[117]

18.3.1.2 Emulsification–solvent diffusion

Similar to the emulsification–solvent evaporation method, emulsification–solvent diffusion requires the formation of an emulsion as the first step in the preparation process. A key consideration in this process is the choice of solvent. The emulsification–solvent diffusion method requires the usage of a dispersed phase solvent that is partially miscible with the continuous phase.[118] A required condition for this process is the initial saturation of the organic and aqueous solvents such that the thermodynamic liquid–liquid equilibrium is satisfied.[119] Following emulsion formation, excess aqueous solvent is added to prime the diffusion of the partially miscible organic solvent into the aqueous phase, leaving behind polymeric nanospheres or nanocapsules. The solvent is then removed by filtration or evaporation. The emulsification–solvent diffusion method has several advantages, making it an attractive method for drug delivery applications. This method has shown high reproducibility and low batch-to-batch variability. In addition, emulsification–solvent diffusion has high NP throughput, easy scalability, and high API encapsulation efficiency, making it advantageous for delivery of cargo.[120] However, the emulsification–solvent diffusion method suffers from a few disadvantages. The main disadvantage is the need for large volumes of aqueous solvent to initialize the polymer solvent diffusion process.[121] Another disadvantage is the possible leakage of partially soluble APIs and encapsulated agents. Therefore, to avoid these drawbacks, it is encouraged to select an inexpensive aqueous solvent that does not easily dissolve the encapsulated API.[122] Emulsification–solvent diffusion may be performed via double emulsification of the primary emulsion before the solvent diffusion step. Two types of double emulsions are possible: water-oil-water (w/o/w) and oil-water-oil (o/w/o).[113]

18.3.1.3 Soft lithography–based methods

Building from precision approaches developed in the microelectronics industry including lithography and thin film processing, NPs fabricated using soft lithography utilize elastomeric templates generated from a mask to mold polymeric NPs.[123] The general approach is to first form a patterned array on a silicon wafer using traditional lithographic techniques, then transfer the inverted array to a soft template, resulting in an elastic mold with cavities or pillars of a precise designed shape. This soft template can then be

TABLE 18.3 Schematic summary of the commonly used top-down polymeric nanoparticle (NP) methods with examples of their advantages and disadvantages.

Method	Schematic	Advantages	Disadvantages
Solvent Evaporation Emulsification	Organic Solvent Evaporation	• Flexibility with loaded material	• Possible coalescence • Time-consuming
Solvent Diffusion Emulsification	Aqueous Solvent Dilution	• High NP throughput • Highly scalable	• Drug leakage • Large solvent volumes required
Soft Lithography		• High reproducibility • Precise control over shape and size	• Low NP throughput • High cost
Electrohydrodynamic Co-jetting	Polymer A Polymer B A B	• Precise control over shape, size, and chemistry	• Complex setup • Proprietary process

used as a mold, generating particles within the cavities, or as a stamp, with particles formed using coating processes of the pillars. With the control afforded from lithography, the shapes and sizes of the template can be readily varied and the polymers can easily take the shape of the stamp[124]; combined, these characteristics of lithography result in polymer NPs having improved size and shape dispersion as compared with other NPs, with capacity to generate truly monodisperse NPs. Soft lithography techniques are most often used to generate polymeric particles of controlled geometry, with capacities to mold both synthetic and natural NPs, as well as proteins, pure API, and other biopharmaceuticals. Due to the inherent nature of the process requiring definition from a 2D array, most lithography-based methods suffer from high costs and low throughput, which hinders the manufacturing scalability as compared with BU approaches.

The most commercially successful soft lithography–based NP templating approach was developed by DeSimone and colleagues in 2005.[125] The technology has since been commercialized by Liquidia Technologies, which announced its initial public offering in fall of 2018 and uses one of the first TD processes to achieve a good manufacturing practices rating. The particle replication in nonwetting templates (PRINT) technique uses an elastomeric perfluoropolyether mold and a continuous roll-to-roll manufacturing process to generate monodisperse particles.[15,38,126] The PRINT method has been used to generate polymeric and pure API NPs for a wide range of nanomedical applications, including cancer treatments,[127–130] siRNA delivery,[131] pulmonary delivery,[132–135] immune modulation,[136] and vaccines.[137,138] Liquidia Technologies has also demonstrated clinical safety of NPs fabricated with the PRINT process with at least two polymers: API NP formulations in current phase 1 and phase 2 clinical trials at the time of publication. The precision control afforded by PRINT has also led to impactful evaluation of isolated physical NP variables, including size,[139,140] shape,[134,141] charge,[142,143] modulus,[62] PEGylation,[144] and drug loading[81,129] as well as generation of biomimetic particles that can mimic aspects of red blood cells.[62,145,146] These studies have greatly added to the fundamental understanding of polymer NPs for drug delivery applications.

18.3.1.4 Electrohydrodynamic cojetting

Electrohydrodynamic (EHD) cojetting is a micro- and nanofabrication method developed to generate compartmentalized particles with more than one distinct composition.[147] Two miscible polymeric solutions are injected from different capillary needles under laminar flow regimes. An electric field is applied at the needle outlet, resulting in a high-speed jet, which causes rapid solvent evaporation and formation of anisotropic solid particles with defined compartmentalization.[148] Modification of the EHD cojetting process conditions enables the precise control of properties of the formed particles. For example, changes in the conductivity gradient across the polymeric solutions can result in particles of varying morphologies.[149] The ability to incorporate different chemistries within a single anisotropic polymeric NP has significant implications in drug delivery applications, mainly to widen the NP design space to incorporate heterogeneous APIs and, ultimately, enhance NP therapeutic efficacy. EHD cojetting is, among other fabrication methods, able to compartmentalize particles and is extensively reviewed elsewhere.[150,151]

18.3.2 Bottom-up methods

In contrast to TD approaches, BU nanofabrication methods usually start at the molecular level and, through a growth process, form nanostructured assemblies. BU methods benefit from relatively facile approaches but can suffer some batch-to-batch variability and broad NP size distributions. Here, we discuss some of the BU nanofabrication approaches, including nanoprecipitation, emulsion polymerization, and layer-by-layer (LbL) assemblies. Self-assembled polymer NPs are also formed through BU methods and are discussed later in this book. BU nanofabrication methods are summarized in Table 18.4.

18.3.2.1 Nanoprecipitation

Nanoprecipitation is often referred to as interfacial deposition or solvent displacement. In this method, the polymer is usually dissolved in the organic phase and is slowly injected into a continuously stirred aqueous phase, but the opposite order of addition may be used. Nanoprecipitation results in the formation of polymeric NPs, usually nanocapsules, as the organic solvent is removed from the droplets. Acetone is one of the most commonly used organic solvents in this process due to its ease of removal and its miscibility in common aqueous solvents such as water.[113] Nanoprecipitation does not require the presence of a surfactant, though they can be utilized to stabilize the droplet suspension and aid in achieving monodispersity. Several process parameters such as polymer concentration, mixing speed, and organic phase injection rate may be optimized to tune the characteristics of the resulting polymer NPs.[152] For example, increasing the concentration of polymer will increase the size of NPs formed, whereas increasing the agitation will lead to smaller-sized particles.[153] However, nanoprecipitation can suffer from low loading efficiency of hydrophilic APIs.[154] Since the discovery of nanoprecipitation, many different designs have been implemented to enhance its outcome,[155] the most notable being microfluidics[156] and flash nanoprecipitation.[157] Flash nanoprecipitation was first developed by Johnson and Prud'homme and is based on particle nucleation of a small molecular weight compound with a block copolymer through rapid mixing.[158,159] This process results in a more controlled NP size as compared with simple nanoprecipitation.[160]

18.3.2.2 Emulsion polymerization

Emulsion polymerization is one of the most widely used techniques for the preparation of polymeric NPs. In emulsion polymerization, the monomer is emulsified in a continuous phase of an immiscible liquid. A polymerization reaction is then initiated *in situ*, resulting in nanospheres.[161] Depending on the hydrophobicity of the desired monomer, emulsion systems can be oil-in-water (o/w) or water-in-oil (w/o). Surfactants are commonly used to stabilize emulsions and control particle size.[162] The process is usually carried out using high speed mixing, homogenization, or ultrasound sonication. Therefore, emulsification can lead to various particle size distributions and must be optimized to obtain narrower particle size populations. Depending on the chemical composition of the desired polymeric system, post-polymerization processing steps may be required to eliminate unpolymerized monomers, initiators, and remaining surfactants from the formed particles.[121]

18.3.2.3 Interfacial polymerization

In interfacial polymerization, two monomers are dissolved separately in two immiscible phases that are then emulsified. The polymerization reaction occurs at the organic–aqueous interface, resulting in a polymeric shell.[163] This system may be utilized to encapsulate APIs in the core of the formed nanocapsule. The polymerization reactions take place very rapidly, minimizing polymer preparation time and resulting in high loading efficiencies.[164] However, interfacial polymerization requires the elimination of organic solvents, monomers, and initiators, which increases the process complexity and the risk for potential cytotoxicity due to residual toxic materials.[165]

18.3.2.4 Layer-by-layer

LbL is an assembly process that relies on the sequential and irreversible assembly of polymers most commonly through electrostatic attractions.[166,167] An array of charged polymers, commonly referred to as polyelectrolytes, can be incorporated to build the NP, spanning both natural and synthetic polyelectrolytes.[168] LbL requires the use of a colloidal system as a template for the adsorption of the first polyelectrolyte layer.[169] Subsequent layers of polyelectrolytes can then be added following the initial adsorption onto the colloidal template, alternating between anionic and cationic polymer groups. The template may consist of a variety of materials, including carboxylated latex NPs, metals, or other solid polymer NPs.[170–172] One

TABLE 18.4 Schematic summary of the commonly used bottom-up methods with examples of their advantages and disadvantages.

Method	Schematic	Advantages	Disadvantages
Nano-precipitation	Organic Phase; Aqueous Phase	• Highly scalable • Low energy costs	• Ineffective for hydrophilic drugs
Layer-by-layer	(+) NP; (−) Polymer; (+) Polymer	• Precise control over chemistry and surface charge	• Possible particle collapse if electrostatic interactions are weak
Self-assembly	(-) Polymer; (+) Polymer	• Simple setup • High yield	• Ineffective for weak electrostatic attractions
Emulsion polymerization	Phase I; Phase II	• High loading efficiency • Rapid formation	• Purification and post-fabrication steps required • Residual toxic materials
Interfacial polymerization	Mono A; Mono B	• Highly scalable • Rapid formation	• Purification and postfabrication steps required • Residual toxic materials

potential issue in using LbL methods is the surface recharging at each layer addition step;[173] to maintain the stability of the adsorbed polyelectrolyte layers, molecules should adequately possess charged groups.

18.4 Applications of polymeric nanoparticles

As described earlier in this chapter, polymeric NPs possess key features that make them extremely valuable in biomedical applications. Biocompatibility, flexibility of design, sustained API release, stimuli-responsiveness, and control over shape and size are among these features inspiring the wide use of polymeric NPs in biomedical applications. In this section, we discuss some applications that have been revolutionized through the use of polymeric NPs, including cancer therapy, immune engineering, infectious diseases, and pulmonary and cardiovascular diseases. We also highlight a few of the landmark discoveries and breakthroughs in each of these applications.

18.4.1 Polymer nanoparticles for cancer therapy

Undoubtedly, the most widely studied and most advanced drug delivery application for polymer NPs to date is in cancer therapy. Between the 1980s and 2010s, countless polymeric NP formulations have been created and explored to improve cancer outcomes, establishing the overall framework of NP utility in medicine.[174] However, despite these overwhelming efforts, only a handful of polymeric NP formulations have made it to clinical trials.[175–177] To date, the most advanced polymeric cancer NP formulations in the clinic are from Bind Therapeutics, which had advanced through phase II clinical trials before the company declared bankruptcy in 2016 and was subsequently bought out by Pfizer.[175] As the fleeting successes of Bind Therapeutics may indicate, these efforts have yet to deliver on the original "magic bullet" promise of polymeric nanomedicine as cancer therapeutics.[1,175] However, the nanomedical field would not be in existence without the persistence of NP oncology efforts, particularly using polymeric NPs.

The general concept of all nanomedicine for cancer applications, but most notably for polymeric formulations, is the incorporation of an otherwise toxic API, which can be encapsulated within an NP and delivered directly to the tumor, thus mitigating side effects and enhancing therapeutic efficacy. Research energies in this area can be summarized into two major efforts: (1) enhancing specific tumor accumulation[178] and (2) efficient API incorporation and release, summarized in the following sections.

18.4.1.1 Polymer nanoparticles to enhance tumor accumulation

NP delivery to tumors has been widely proposed to occur through the enhanced permeation and retention (EPR) effect, resulting in passive NP accumulation directly in the tumor due to the "leaky vasculature" that forms following rapid tumor angiogenesis.[179] The applicability of the EPR effect in cancer has recently come under question, as solid tumors in humans have varied degrees of vascularization, different organization than artificially generated xenografts, and pressure gradients opposing diffusion.[180,181] The EPR effect alone is likely not significant enough to completely shift the biodistribution; the median passive NP tumor accumulation from formulations made between 2006 and 2016 has been estimated to be less than 1%.[182] Despite this increasing knowledge of the EPR effect, the concept has shaped the nanomedical field for the past few decades. Many landmark studies attempting to harness the EPR effect have utilized polymeric NPs to determine the optimal NP size and shape to promote passive tumor accumulation.[183,184]

Inherently coupled to the concept of EPR effect is the concept that an NP formulation must be long circulating to increase the likelihood of passing the tumor and allowing the EPR effect to occur.[178] This has prompted many significant fundamental advancements in development of long circulating NPs, led again by landmark studies using polymeric NPs. Numerous research groups have established the optimal particle size for long circulation and avoidance of the mononuclear phagocyte system.[185,186] Rod- and disk-shaped particles have been found to extend the circulation times over spherical counterparts,[187] with shape being a major factor in particle internalization.[188] In general, an inverse relationship between particle aspect ratio and internalization efficiency has been reported.[186,189–191] The effect of shape has been hypothesized to be due to actin-dependent processes that dictate phagocytosis and, thus, is dependent on the overall NP size and the local curvature at the angle of attachment.[189,192] Particle modulus has also been explored, establishing that soft NPs, often made through low cross-linking densities of PEG hydrogels, can increase circulation times.[62,193,194]

Beyond the EPR effect, a large body of research has been pursued to further enhance tumor accumulation of polymeric NPs.[178] Active targeting approaches involve decorating polymeric NPs with ligands specific to overexpressed receptors found on tumor cells, including a wide range of ligands.[178,195–198] Here, the design control of polymeric NPs allows for precision surface chemistry needed for specific ligand accumulation.[199] One major limitation of such active targeting approaches is that the ligand must be in close proximity to its cognate receptor; thus, if the overall NP transport into the tumor is not achieved, the active targeting will not be effective.[178,200,201] Research understanding polymer transport within blood flow has subsequently received attention, with particle size, shape, and modulus all contributing to a particle's distribution and margination to a vessel wall.[187,193,200,202,203] Overall, these studies with polymeric NPs for cancer applications have paved the way to current understanding of how intravenously administered NPs behave in the body, providing a solid fundamental foundation for NPs in medical applications.

18.4.1.2 Polymer nanoparticles for efficient active pharmaceutical ingredient incorporation

API incorporation and subsequent controlled release of the cargo has been widely studied for cancer applications, encompassing natural and synthetic polymer NPs of every morphology shown in Fig. 18.1. Polymer NP formulations have been developed to deliver an enormous host of chemotherapeutic drugs, including DOX,[23,58,127,170,204,205] docetaxel,[48,59,129,141] cisplatin,[205–207] fluorouracil,[74,208,209] and gemcitabine,[210,211] as a few representative examples. In general, tuning the polymer properties to the nature of the cargo has resulted in successful encapsulation strategies. For example, PLGA has been a common choice for encapsulation of hydrophobic chemotherapeutic drugs such as DOX, with loading as high as 40% wt/wt reported for some fabrication methods.[81] Other API incorporation strategies rely on covalent attachment of the molecule to the polymer matrix,[206] with largely successful prodrug polymeric NP approaches capable of controlling both API loading and release.[55,207,212] Other stimuli-responsive polymer NPs have been designed to respond to the slightly acidic tumor microenvironment or regions of hypoxia to trigger release.[98,103,213] Excellent reviews expanding on these concepts of polymer NP formulations for cancer therapeutics can be found in the literature.[39,178,214–216]

18.4.2 Polymer nanoparticles for immune engineering

The immune system is designed to fight infection, but improper responses can result in a host of detrimental effects. A growing area of research in polymer NPs involves controlling immune responses by tailoring interactions between immune cells and NPs. Due to their inherent size, NPs are naturally internalized by phagocytic antigen-presenting cells (APCs), the frontline defense of the innate immune system. APCs are responsible for internalizing foreign particulates and driving adaptive immune responses to combat infections, leveraging precise cellular signaling pathways to recognize protein fragments from both external and internal sources.[217,218] These protein fragments, called antigens, can be incorporated into NPs to mimic the surface chemistry, size, and shape of a pathogen or apoptotic cell, providing the correct stimulation to direct the APC and subsequent responses. Such NP pathogen mimicry can drive APCs to have antigen-specific responses without the presence, and potentially detrimental effects, of the pathogen itself, whereas NP self-mimicry in the presence of other molecular cues can repurpose APCs to fight various autoimmune diseases. Here, we discuss some of the areas of immune engineering using this concept, including promotion of immune tolerance and vaccine development, highlighting the potential for polymeric NPs in the immune engineering realm.

18.4.2.1 Polymer nanoparticles for vaccines

While there are multiple early historical mentions of disease prevention through inoculation,[219] one of the first purposeful attempts to develop vaccines is attributed to Louis Pasteur in the early 1880s after inoculating chickens with attenuated *Pasteurella multocida* and ultimately causing their immunity.[220] Following many similar discoveries, the vaccine journey responsible for eradicating many of the deadliest diseases is considered to be the greatest breakthrough in modern medicine.[221] Vaccines are formulations geared toward priming cells of the adaptive immune system (B cells and T cells) with APCs to elicit a response to specific antigens upon future recognition. Vaccines can accomplish different medical purposes and can be prophylactic or therapeutic. In both forms, precision cues must be delivered to the innate immune system to promote an adaptive memory response. Here, we highlight the benefits of polymeric NPs toward that aim as well as progress in utilizing polymeric NPs for novel vaccine platforms.

18.4.2.1.1 Polymer nanoparticles for prophylactic vaccines

Prophylactic vaccines are preventative vaccines administered to promote antigen-specific immunologic memory that can be rapidly recalled upon future exposure to disease-causing pathogens. One approach relies on the conjugation of antigenic peptides to the surface of polymeric NPs.[137,222] Surface conjugation approaches enable proper antigen delivery to specific APCs and may also improve vaccine targeting.[222] Antigen delivery via NP approaches has also been achieved based on the encapsulation of antigens in polymeric matrices made from biodegradable materials such as PLGA.[223] However, using encapsulation methods poses the risk of antigen damage during the fabrication process. As a result, there has been strong consideration of developing alternative approaches, notably through LbL assembly for antigen delivery to overcome limitations associated with traditional NP systems.[224] In addition to antigen delivery, codelivery with an appropriate adjuvant can be readily achieved with a polymeric NP. For example, Demento *et al.* developed antigen-loaded PLGA NPs that are surface-modified to display CpG oligodeoxynucleotide as an adjuvant.[80] The antigen/adjuvant NP system showed improved immunization results in a mouse model of West Nile virus encephalitis,[80] demonstrating the benefit of codelivery afforded by the polymer NP.

18.4.2.1.2 Polymer nanoparticles for therapeutic vaccines

Therapeutic vaccines aim to elicit an immune response to treat already occurring diseases, such as cancer. Therapeutic cancer vaccines require delivery of an overexpressed cancer peptide with the NP that must escape the endosome to promote proper antigen presentation on the APC. They also require an appropriate adjuvant to activate the APC and promote antigen-specific cytotoxic T cell proliferation. Therapeutic vaccines face many obstacles that may compromise their efficacy *in vivo*, especially pathogen-induced immune dysfunctions (e.g., cancer immunosuppression).[225] Therefore, new therapeutic vaccines must be able to overcome these challenges to have promise for treating target diseases. Saluja *et al.* designed melanoma antigen-associated PLGA NPs with a dendritic cell targeting ligand displayed on the NP surface as a dendritic cell–based antitumor vaccine.[226] Another strategy relied on CpG conjugation to the surface of NPs to enhance antigen-specific cancer immunity.[227] In addition to high therapeutic antigen loading capacity, the physiochemical properties of polymeric NPs can be tuned to promote therapeutic vaccine efficacy. For example, Fifis *et al.* demonstrated NP size-dependent tumor growth protection following *in vivo* immunization with antigen-conjugated polystyrene NPs.[228]

18.4.2.2 Polymer nanoparticles for promoting immune tolerance

APCs play a critical role in the onset and progression of autoimmune diseases, where immune cells mistake self-antigens for foreign objects and, as a result, attack and inflame healthy tissue.[229] APCs activate self-reactive T cells, which contribute to the pathogenesis of many autoimmune diseases such as multiple sclerosis (MS), type 1 diabetes mellitus, and rheumatoid arthritis.[230] Regulatory T cells are suppressive populations present in a balance with self-reactive T cells and are responsible for the natural control of self-reactive T cell response among other adaptive immune responses. Aberrant immune reactions and regulatory T cell imbalances are reflected in many autoimmune diseases.[231,232] Most tolerance-promoting therapies rely on systemic immunosuppression, which has been shown to have poor efficacy and cause vulnerability to infections.[233,234]

NP-based therapeutics have offered a potential solution to off-target side effects of broad immunosuppression therapies due to their ability to target APCs and elicit a precise immune response. The tunability of polymeric NPs is a key advantage for promoting controlled immune tolerance, which can be achieved by engineering the physiochemical properties of the administrated NPs.[235] For example, Roberts *et al.* delivered phosphatidylserine, known to promote anti-inflammatory effects following internalization by phagocytes,[236,237] using differently shaped PRINT particles. Delivery via particles enabled controlled phosphatidylserine release and subsequent activation of regulatory T cells while downregulating effector T cell activity.[238] Polymeric NPs have also been engineered to deliver autoantigenic peptides to provide a "marker of self" or a host protein signal to APCs.[239] Hunter *et al.* demonstrated the ability to induce antigen-specific T cell tolerance in experimental autoimmune encephalitis (EAE), an animal model of human MS.[240] PLGA NPs coupled with autoantigenic peptides were able to prevent as well as treat EAE symptoms following administration at the onset or peak of the disease. Hess *et al.* developed polyplexes of self-peptides and tolerogenic immune signals to drive T cells away from inflammatory phenotypes in EAE models as well.[241] Therefore, incorporating antigenic peptides with biocompatible NPs may have a promising potential for ameliorating and preventing autoimmune and inflammatory diseases. Other NP-based tolerance-promoting strategies are extensively reviewed elsewhere.[229,242,243]

Interestingly, recent reports have shown that inert polymeric NPs with no added tolerizing moieties possess the intrinsic ability to turn APCs away from their proinflammatory form in models of West Nile virus encephalitis, EAE, inflammatory bowel disease,[244] and acute lung injury.[245] Other recent work has demonstrated the role of inert PLGA particles in shifting dendritic cells toward an anti-inflammatory phenotype.[66] Unlike the previous examples of tolerance promotion through antigen recognition or known molecular pattern, these reports highlight the promise of inert polymeric NPs for immune skewing in many disease applications, as well as the role of specific polymer compositions in directing APC immune responses.

18.4.3 Polymer nanoparticles for infectious diseases

Both bacteria and viruses invade body tissue and cells, proliferate, and secrete proteins and cell signaling molecules to create an infection site. Infections are treated with antibiotics or virulence-suppressing APIs, which usually target proliferation mechanisms, cell wall integrity, or mitochondrial mechanisms.[246] In certain infections, there are quiescent pathogens capable of avoiding APIs that can ultimately lead to resistance.[246] Many antibiotic APIs suffer from poor aqueous solubility and stability, which further lowers their bioavailability and biodistribution.[247,248] Thus, polymer NPs have been considered as possibly advantageous carriers to improve pharmaceutical formulations.

In the 1990s, Patrick Couvreur was a leading researcher in loading polymer NPs with antibiotics and observed sustained API release and stability, design flexibility, and stimuli-responsiveness.[248,249] Polymer NPs are more versatile than liposomes or metallic NPs due to design flexibility, such as the ability to create copolymers for varied functionality. For example, by creating a polymeric NP with a copolymer of PEG for bioinert interactions and poly(L-histidine) for protonation in an acidic environment, the release of antibiotics was localized to the infection site.[247] This also demonstrates a stimulus-responsive behavior in a polymer NP. The versatility in design allows for a wide range of APIs to be used with polymer NP systems, improving the solubility and stability of the API *in vivo*. For example, poly(hexyl cyanoacrylate) particles loaded with azidothymidine, a poorly water-soluble antiviral nucleoside analog, showed potential as a preventative treatment of human immunodeficiency virus.[250] Some natural polymers, such as chitosan, can interact with bacteria to cause cell death, which, in NPs formulation, has natural antibiotic properties.[251] Control over release kinetics, stability, retention, and stimuli response in polymer NPs has demonstrated improved efficacy of encapsulated antibiotics by 120-fold as compared to free antibiotics.[248,252]

Extensive literature on the polymers used to create NPs as well as the lack of postmodification steps in creating polymer NPs to fight infections has been attractive to researchers from a manufacturing perspective.[248,253–255] For example, *N*-thiolated β-lactam antibiotic was covalently linked to polyacrylate and formed NPs in a one-pot system.[253] Polymer NPs are also often able to be dehydrated and rehydrated with little effect on the particle size or API content. Research on polymer NP carriers to overcome the limitation facing infection treatments has been reviewed extensively previously.[246] While there has yet to be an FDA-approved polymer NP carrier for the treatment of infections, there are patents in place and trials of clinically isolated bacteria that have been performed,[254,256] which has made polymer NPs a promising investigational therapeutic carrier to treat infections.[176]

18.4.4 Polymer nanoparticles for pulmonary diseases

Respiratory diseases remain a significant cause of morbidity and mortality worldwide, with combined pulmonary conditions contributing to more than 7.8 million annual deaths globally and estimated over $88 billion in annual health care costs in the United States alone.[257,258] Direct aerosol administration to the lung can result in as much as 100 times higher local drug concentrations when compared with systemic or oral delivery of the same molecule, dramatically increasing efficacy. As with intravenously administered NPs, inhaled formulations limit off-target side effects, avoid first-pass metabolism, and can provide superior patient compliance by avoiding needles and cold chain storage.[259–262] Despite these advantages, lung administration is not an option for most lung diseases, with commercial inhaled therapies limited to a few small molecule drugs.[259,260]

Polymer NPs are being increasingly investigated for pulmonary drug delivery.[262–264] Historically, "large" porous polymer particles (LPPs) have been successful in pulmonary API delivery, providing unique attributes of controlled API release, avoidance of macrophage clearance, and deep lung penetration stemming from their low density and large geometric size of greater than 20 μm.[265] Using biodegradable polymers such as PLGA, these LPPs led to the advent of inhalable insulin with sustained release in the lungs.[266] The concept of LPPs has also been translated to the delivery of polymer NPs through a Trojan Horse strategy, with the LPP providing efficient aerosol properties and the NPs providing superior drug release and tissue penetration.[267] While particle aerodynamic sizes between 1 and 5 μm are traditionally thought to be optimal for pulmonary deposition,[259,268] growing research suggests that NPs less than 100 nm are also efficient at deep lung deposition.[262,263,269] Furthermore, NPs smaller than approximately 6 nm in size are able to diffuse across the epithelium into circulation, whereas anionic NPs around 30 nm in size can diffuse to the lymphatics.[270] By tuning the size, NPs can be vehicles for sustained and controlled release of a therapeutic payload for both local and systemic action.[262] Thus, polymer NPs have been developed to deliver a wide range of payloads for pulmonary applications, including inhaled vaccines, insulin, antibiotics, and chemotherapeutics.[262–264]

18.4.5 Polymer nanoparticles for cardiovascular diseases

Atherosclerosis is one of the most prominent causes of cardiovascular disease, which is the leading cause of death across all developed countries. As a chronic inflammatory cardiovascular disease, atherosclerosis upregulates immune response at infected sites and is characterized by restricted blood flow from narrowed arteries caused by the formation of fatty plaque deposits along vessel walls.[271] Aggravation of inflected endothelium due to macrophage recruitment in atherosclerotic vasculature can lead to destabilization of plaque and potential thrombosis.[272] During thrombosis, these deposits can rupture and cause fatal blockages in the vasculature typical of myocardial infarction or stroke.[271]

Outside of surgical intervention to physically remove plaque deposits, current treatments for atherosclerosis generally aim to reduce lipid levels with statins or reduce immune response with anticoagulants.[272] However, statin therapy for atherosclerosis may be obscured with muscle-related myopathy and other undesirable side effects,[273] whereas both statin and anticoagulant therapy have limited bioavailability, with administration of higher dosages approaching toxicity.[274] Polymeric NPs can be utilized for sustained delivery over time for long-term treatment of a high-potency API due to the flexibility in setting size and surface charge parameters for increased bioavailability. For example, PLGA NPs have been synthesized to mimic the size, shape, and surface charge of high-density lipoprotein to target atherosclerotic tissue.[275] Lewis *et al.* have extensively reviewed these properties and particle formulations.[272]

Additionally, the dysfunctional endothelium in atherosclerosis can promote a similar EPR effect that allows for passive, controlled NP accumulation in atherosclerotic buildup and lesions.[276] Taking advantage of this concept, Katsuki *et al.* developed pitavastatin-incorporated PLGA NPs that were shown to have sustained uptake in plaque macrophages, leading to stabilization of remaining plaque and reduction of plaque area.[277] Other characteristics of atherosclerosis, such as clotting factors and upregulated cellular adhesive molecules (CAMs) on endothelial cells, can also be utilized to deliver polymer-encapsulated APIs that may otherwise be toxic in the high dosages required for effective treatment to affected tissue. For example, Peters *et al.* demonstrated that PEG-incorporated multifunctional lipid micelles functionalized with targeting clot-binding factors and synthesized with anticoagulants localize to the shoulders of vascular plaque deposits and deliver anticoagulants directly to the affected site for thrombin inhibition.[278] Polymer NPs decorated with CAM-specific ligands have been demonstrated to enhance NP localization to the plaque for API release, which is highly dependent on the NP properties, including modulus and ligand density.[193,279]

Other novel polymer therapeutics developed by Korin *et al.* exploit the shear modulation of the vasculature to disperse therapeutic PLGA NP aggregates that disassemble under high shear conditions that are typical of blood flow through atherosclerotic vasculature.[280] Shear-activated nanotherapeutics (SA-NTs) composed of aggregates of spray-dried PLGA NPs containing a thrombolytic API (tissue plasminogen activator, tPA) successfully eroded clots from murine vasculature by continuously binding to and degrading the embolism until full clearance was achieved.[280] Results show that tPA-SA-NTs allow for administration of a lower dosage of thrombolytic therapeutics to achieve the same level of efficiency as freely delivered APIs.

18.5 Concluding remarks

The use of polymers in NP-based formulations has been extremely advantageous in biomedical applications. With a wide range of materials to choose from, polymer NPs offer a significant advantage in fine-tuning NP physiochemical properties for a range of drug delivery applications. In addition, several characteristics of polymeric NPs including tunability of design, flexibility of fabrication, biocompatibility, high API loading capacity, sustained API release, stimuli-responsiveness, and control over shape and size have advanced the use of polymeric NPs in countless fields. Polymer NP therapeutics have shown impressive potential in a variety of applications especially in cancer, immune engineering, infectious diseases, and cardiovascular disease. Some of the studies highlighted earlier in this chapter represent a stepping stone toward clinical translations in hopes of eradicating these diseases. Future progress and success in the drug delivery field relies heavily on the development of novel systems as well as precise fabrication techniques to improve the development of the next-generation of therapeutics. With polymeric NPs gaining momentum in the field of drug delivery, we expect many more polymer NP-based therapeutics to make their way into the clinic in the near future. Taking advantage of the boom of novel engineered materials, polymeric NPs are poised to lead the field in developing new therapeutics from vaccines to cancer immunotherapies.

References

1. Hoffman AS. The origins and evolution of "controlled" drug delivery systems. *J Control Release* 2008;**132**(3):153–63.
2. Langer R, Folkman J. Polymers for the sustained release of proteins and other macromolecules. *Nature* 1976;**263**:797.
3. Davis FF, Abuchowski A, van Es T, et al. Enzyme-Polyethylene glycol adducts: modified enzymes with unique properties BT. In: Broun GB, Manecke G, Wingard LB, editors. *Enzyme engineering*, vol. 4. Boston, MA: Springer US; 1978. p. 169–73.
4. Harris JM, Chess RB. Effect of pegylation on pharmaceuticals. *Nat Rev Drug Discov* 2003;**2**:214.
5. Liechty WB, Kryscio DR, Slaughter BV, Peppas NA. Polymers for drug delivery systems. *Annu Rev Chem Biomol Eng* 2010;**1**(1):149–73.
6. Cho EJ, Holback H, Liu KC, Abouelmagd SA, Park J, Yeo Y. Nanoparticle characterization: state of the art, challenges, and emerging technologies. *Mol Pharm* 2013.
7. Lin PC, Lin S, Wang PC, Sridhar R. Techniques for physicochemical characterization of nanomaterials. *Biotechnol Adv* 2014.
8. Fornaguera C, Solans C. Analytical methods to characterize and purify polymeric nanoparticles. *Int J Polym Sci* 2018;**2018**:1–10.
9. Kloxin AM, Kloxin CJ, Bowman CN, Anseth KS. Mechanical properties of cellularly responsive hydrogels and their experimental determination. *Adv Mater* 2010;**22**(31):3484–94.
10. Alexis F, Pridgen E, Molnar LK, Farokhzad OC. Factors affecting the clearance and biodistribution of polymeric nanoparticles. *Mol Pharm* 2008;**5**(4):505–15.
11. Vauthier C. Polymer nanoparticles for in vivo applications: progress on preparation methods and future challenges. In: *Polymer nanoparticles for nanomedicines*. Cham: Springer International Publishing; 2016. p. 3–16.
12. Zhang S, Sun H-J, Hughes AD, et al. Self-assembly of amphiphilic Janus dendrimers into uniform onion-like dendrimersomes with predictable size and number of bilayers. *Proc Natl Acad Sci* 2014.
13. Parelkar SS, Letteri R, Chan-Seng D, et al. Polymer-peptide delivery platforms: effect of oligopeptide orientation on polymer-based DNA delivery. *Biomacromolecules* 2014.
14. Champion JA, Katare YK, Mitragotri S. Making polymeric micro- and nanoparticles of complex shapes. *Proc Natl Acad Sci* 2007.
15. Canelas DA, Herlihy KP, DeSimone JM. Top-down particle fabrication: control of size and shape for diagnostic imaging and drug delivery. *Wiley Interdiscip Rev Nanomedicine Nanobiotechnology* 2009.
16. Duncan R. The dawning era of polymer therapeutics. *Nat Rev Drug Discov* 2003.
17. Boussif O, Lezoualc'h F, Zanta MA, et al. A versatile vector for gene and oligonucleotide transfer into cells in culture and in vivo: polyethylenimine. *Proc Natl Acad Sci* 1995.
18. Lynn DM, Langer R. Degradable poly(??-amino esters): synthesis, characterization, and self-assembly with plasmid DNA. *J Am Chem Soc* 2000.
19. Scott RWJ, Wilson OM, Crooks* RM. Synthesis, characterization, and applications of dendrimer-encapsulated nanoparticles. *J Phys Chem B* 2004.
20. Zhang L, Gu FX, Chan JM, Wang AZ, Langer RS, Farokhzad OC. Nanoparticles in medicine: therapeutic applications and developments. *Clin Pharmacol Ther* 2008.
21. Pearson RM, Sunoqrot S, Hsu HJ, Bae JW, Hong S. Dendritic nanoparticles: the next generation of nanocarriers? *Ther Deliv* 2012.
22. Discher BM, Won YY, Ege DS, et al. Polymersomes: tough vesicles made from diblock copolymers. *Science* 1999.
23. Quadir MA, Morton SW, Deng ZJ, et al. PEG-polypeptide block copolymers as pH-responsive endosome-solubilizing drug nanocarriers. *Mol Pharm* 2014.
24. Meng F, Zhong Z. Polymersomes spanning from nano- to microscales: advanced vehicles for controlled drug delivery and robust vesicles for virus and cell mimicking. *J Phys Chem Lett* 2011.

25. Photos PJ, Bacakova L, Discher B, Bates FS, Discher DE. Polymer vesicles in vivo: correlations with PEG molecular weight. *J Control Release* 2003.
26. Suk JS, Xu Q, Kim N, Hanes J, Ensign LM. PEGylation as a strategy for improving nanoparticle-based drug and gene delivery. *Adv Drug Deliv Rev* 2016;**99**:28–51.
27. Duncan R, Vicent MJ. Polymer therapeutics-prospects for 21st century: the end of the beginning. *Adv Drug Deliv Rev* 2013;**65**(1):60–70.
28. KnopK, HoogenboomR, FischerD, SchubertUS. Poly(ethylene glycol) in drug delivery: pros and cons as well as potential alternatives. Angew Chemie Int Ed. 49(36):6288-6308. doi:10.1002/anie.200902672.
29. Danhier F, Ansorena E, Silva JM, Coco R, Le Breton A, Préat V. PLGA-based nanoparticles: an overview of biomedical applications. *J Control Release* 2012;**161**(2):505–22.
30. Makadia HK, Siegel SJ. Poly lactic-co-glycolic acid (PLGA) as biodegradable controlled drug delivery carrier. *Polymers (Basel)* 2011;**3**(3):1377–97.
31. Hoare TR, Kohane DS. Hydrogels in drug delivery: progress and challenges. *Polymer (Guildf)* 2008;**49**(8):1993–2007.
32. Batrakova EV, Kabanov AV. Pluronic block copolymers: evolution of drug delivery concept from inert nanocarriers to biological response modifiers. *J Control Release* 2008;**130**(2):98–106.
33. Calderón M, Quadir MA, Sharma SK, Haag R. Dendritic polyglycerols for biomedical applications. *Adv Mater* 2009;**22**(2):190–218.
34. MaHam A, Tang Z, Wu H, Wang J, Lin Y. Protein-based nanomedicine platforms for drug delivery. *Small* 2009;**5**(15):1706–21.
35. Jochum FD, Theato P. Temperature- and light-responsive smart polymer materials. *Chem Soc Rev* 2013;**42**(17):7468–83.
36. Karimi M, Ghasemi A, Sahandi Zangabad P, et al. Smart micro/nanoparticles in stimulus-responsive drug/gene delivery systems. *Chem Soc Rev* 2016;**45**(5):1457–501.
37. de la Rica R, Aili D, Stevens MM. Enzyme-responsive nanoparticles for drug release and diagnostics. *Adv Drug Deliv Rev* 2012;**64**(11):967–78.
38. Petros RA, DeSimone JM. Strategies in the design of nanoparticles for therapeutic applications. *Nat Rev DRUG Discov* 2010;**9**(8):615–27.
39. Park JH, Lee S, Kim J-H, Park K, Kim K, Kwon IC. Polymeric nanomedicine for cancer therapy. *Prog Polym Sci* 2008;**33**(1):113–37.
40. Fedel M, Endogan T, Hasirci N, et al. Blood compatibility of polymers derived from natural materials. *J Bioact Compat Polym* 2012.
41. Malafaya PB, Silva GA, Reis RL. Natural-origin polymers as carriers and scaffolds for biomolecules and cell delivery in tissue engineering applications. *Adv Drug Deliv Rev* 2007.
42. Dang JM, Leong KW. Natural polymers for gene delivery and tissue engineering. *Adv Drug Deliv Rev* 2006.
43. Liu Z, Jiao Y, Wang Y, Zhou C, Zhang Z. Polysaccharides-based nanoparticles as drug delivery systems. *Adv Drug Deliv Rev* 2008.
44. UleryBD, NairLS, LaurencinCT. Biomedical applications of biodegradable polymers. J Polym Sci Part B Polym Phys. 49(12):832-864.
45. Alaniz L, Cabrera PV, Blanco G, et al. Interaction of CD44 with different forms of hyaluronic acid. Its role in adhesion and migration of tumor cells. *Cell Commun Adhes* 2002;**9**(3):117–30.
46. Klemm PDD, Schmauder, Hans-Peter Heinze PDT. Cellulose. In: *Biopolym Vol 6 polysaccharides II polysaccharides from Eukaryotes*; 2002.
47. Siqueira G, Bras J, Dufresne A. Cellulosic bionanocomposites: a review of preparation, properties and applications. *Polymers (Basel)* 2010.
48. Jackson JK, Letchford K, Wasserman BZ, Ye L, Hamad WY, Burt HM. The use of nanocrystalline cellulose for the binding and controlled release of drugs. *Int J Nanomedicine* 2011.
49. Valo H, Arola S, Laaksonen P, et al. Drug release from nanoparticles embedded in four different nanofibrillar cellulose aerogels. *Eur J Pharm Sci* 2013.
50. Zargar V, Asghari M, Dashti A. A review on chitin and chitosan polymers: structure, chemistry, solubility, derivatives, and applications. *ChemBioEng Rev* 2015.
51. Kean T, Thanou M. Biodegradation, biodistribution and toxicity of chitosan. *Adv Drug Deliv Rev* 2010.
52. Sogias IA, Williams AC, Khutoryanskiy VV. Why is chitosan mucoadhesive? *Biomacromolecules* 2008;**9**(7):1837–42.
53. Roy K, Mao HQ, Huang SK, Leong KW. Oral gene delivery with chitosan-DNA nanoparticles generates immunologic protection in a murine model of peanut allergy. *Nat Med* 1999.
54. Mao HQ, Roy K, Troung-Le VL, et al. Chitosan-DNA nanoparticles as gene carriers: synthesis, characterization and transfection efficiency. *J Control Release* 2001.
55. Kratz F. Albumin as a drug carrier: design of prodrugs, drug conjugates and nanoparticles. *J Control Release* 2008.
56. Wu Y, Mackay JA, Mcdaniel JR, Chilkoti A, Clark RL. Fabrication of elastin-like polypeptide nanoparticles for drug delivery by electrospraying. *Biomacromolecules* 2009.
57. Rössler B, Kreuter J, Scherer D. Collagen microparticles: preparation and properties. *J Microencapsul* 1995.
58. Seib FP, Jones GT, Rnjak-Kovacina J, Lin Y, Kaplan DL. pH-dependentanticancer drug release from silk nanoparticles. *Adv Healthc Mater* 2013.
59. Hawkins MJ, Soon-Shiong P, Desai N. Protein nanoparticles as drug carriers in clinical medicine. *Adv Drug Deliv Rev* 2008;**60**(8):876–85.
60. Hurtado-López P, Murdan S, Regier MC, et al. Protein nanoparticles as drug delivery carriers for cancer therapy. *Chem Pharm Bull* 2012.
61. Cascone MG, Sim B, Sandra D. Blends of synthetic and natural polymers as drug delivery systems for growth hormone. *Biomaterials* 1995.
62. Merkel TJ, Jones SW, Herlihy KP, et al. Using mechanobiological mimicry of red blood cells to extend circulation times of hydrogel microparticles. *Proc Natl Acad Sci* 2011;**108**(2):586–91.
63. Moad G, Soloman DH. *The chemistry of radical polymerization*. 2nded. Oxford, U.K.: Elsevier; 2006.
64. Young RJ, Lovell PA. *Introduction to polymers*. 3rded. Boca Raton, FL: CRC Press; 2011.
65. Stevens MP. *Polymer chemistry: an introduction*. 3rded. New York, NY: Oxford University Press; 1998.
66. Allen RP, Bolandparvaz A, Ma JA, Manickam VA, Lewis JS. Latent, immunosuppressive nature of poly(lactic-co-glycolic acid) microparticles. *ACS Biomater Sci Eng* 2018;**4**(3):900–18.
67. Báez JE, Marcos-Fernández Á. A simple and rapid preparation of poly(Glycolide) (Pga) oligomers catalyzed by decamolybdate anion in the presence of aliphatic alcohols. *Int J Polym Anal Charact* 2011.

68. Schwarz K, Epple M. A detailed characterization of polyglycolide prepared by solid-state polycondensation reaction. *Macromol Chem Phys* 1999.
69. Pillai CKS, Sharma CP. Review paper: absorbable polymeric surgical sutures: chemistry, production, properties, biodegradability, and performance. *J Biomater Appl* 2010.
70. Amass W, Amass A, Tighe B. A review of biodegradable polymers: uses, current developments in the synthesis and characterization of biodegradable polyesters, blends of biodegradable polymers and recent advances in biodegradation studies. *Polym Int* 1998.
71. Lee SH, Kim BS, Kim SH, et al. Elastic biodegradable poly(-glycolide-co-caprolactone) scaffold for tissue engineering. *J Biomed Mater Res - Part A* 2003.
72. Cha Y, Pitt CG. The biodegradability of polyester blends. *Biomaterials* 1990.
73. Avérous L. Polylactic acid: synthesis, properties and applications. *Monomers Polym Compos Renew Resour* January 2008:433–50.
74. Nair LS, Laurencin CT. Biodegradable polymers as biomaterials. *Prog Polym Sci* 2007.
75. Gilding DK, Reed AM. Biodegradable polymers for use in surgery-polyglycolic/poly(actic acid) homo- and copolymers: 1. *Polymer (Guildf)* 1979.
76. Mundargi RC, Babu VR, Rangaswamy V, Patel P, Aminabhavi TM. Nano/micro technologies for delivering macromolecular therapeutics using poly(d,l-lactide-co-glycolide) and its derivatives. *J Control Release* 2008.
77. Kapoor DN, Bhatia A, Kaur R, Sharma R, Kaur G, Dhawan S. PLGA: a unique polymer for drug delivery. *Ther Deliv* 2015;**6**(1):41–58.
78. Faisant N, Siepmann J, Benoit JP. PLGA-based microparticles: elucidation of mechanisms and a new, simple mathematical model quantifying drug release. *Eur J Pharm Sci* 2002.
79. Miller RA, Brady JM, Cutright DE. Degradation rates of oral resorbable implants (polylactates and polyglycolates): rate modification with changes in PLA/PGA copolymer ratios. *J Biomed Mater Res* 1977.
80. Demento SL, Bonafe N, Cui W, et al. TLR9-Targeted biodegradable nanoparticles as immunization vectors protect against West Nile encephalitis. *J Immunol* 2010;**185**(5):2989–97.
81. Enlow EM, Luft JC, Napier ME, DeSimone JM. Potent engineered PLGA nanoparticles by virtue of exceptionally high chemotherapeutic loadings. *Nano Lett* 2011;**11**(2):808–13.
82. Kumar R, Mohapatra SS, Kong X, Jena PK, Bakowsky U, Lehr CM. Cationic poly(lactide-co-glycolide) nanoparticles as efficient in vivo gene transfection agents. *J Nanosci Nanotechnol* 2004.
83. Labet M, Thielemans W. Synthesis of polycaprolactone: a review. *Chem Soc Rev* 2009.
84. Sinha VR, Bansal K, Kaushik R, Kumria R, Trehan A. Poly-ε-caprolactone microspheres and nanospheres: an overview. *Int J Pharm* 2004.
85. Chawla JS, Amiji MM. Biodegradable poly(ε-caprolactone) nanoparticles for tumor-targeted delivery of tamoxifen. *Int J Pharm* 2002.
86. Espuelas MS, Legrand P, Loiseau PM, Bories C, Barratt G, Irache JM. In vitro antileishmanial activity of amphotericin B loaded in poly(ε-caprolactone) nanospheres. *J Drug Target* 2002.
87. Gamisans F, Lacoulonche F, Chauvet A, Espina M, Garcıa M, Egea M. Flurbiprofen-loaded nanospheres: analysis of the matrix structure by thermal methods. *Int J Pharm* 1999.
88. Petersen LK, Sackett CK, Narasimhan B. High-throughput analysis of protein stability in polyanhydride nanoparticles. *Acta Biomater* 2010.
89. Göpferich A. Mechanisms of polymer degradation and erosion1. In: *The biomaterials: silver jubilee compendium*; 2006.
90. Binnebose AM, Haughney SL, Martin R, Imerman PM, Narasimhan B, Bellaire BH. Polyanhydride nanoparticle delivery platform dramatically enhances killing of filarial worms. *PLoS Negl Trop Dis* 2015.
91. Mathiowitz E, Langer R. Polyanhydride microspheres as drug carriers I. Hot-melt microencapsulation. *J Control Release* 1987.
92. Kipper MJ, Shen E, Determan A, Narasimhan B. Design of an injectable system based on bioerodible polyanhydride microspheres for sustained drug delivery. *Biomaterials* 2002.
93. Lungwitz U, Breunig M, Blunk T, Göpferich A. Polyethylenimine-based non-viral gene delivery systems. *European Journal of Pharmaceutics and Biopharmaceutics* 2005.
94. Godbey WT, Wu KK, Mikos AG. Poly(ethylenimine) and its role in gene delivery. *J Control Release* 1999;**60**(2):149–60.
95. Lv H, Zhang S, Wang B, Cui S, Yan J. Toxicity of cationic lipids and cationic polymers in gene delivery. *J Control Release* 2006.
96. Tang GP, Zeng JM, Gao SJ, et al. Polyethylene glycol modified polyethylenimine for improved CNS gene transfer: effects of PEGylation extent. *Biomaterials* 2003.
97. Kursa M, Walker GF, Roessler V, et al. Novel shielded transferrin-polyethylene glycol-polyethylenimine/DNA complexes for systemic tumor-targeted gene transfer. *Bioconjug Chem* 2003.
98. Kelley EG, Albert JNL, Sullivan MO, Thomas H, Epps III . Stimuli-responsive copolymer solution and surface assemblies for biomedical applications. *Chem Soc Rev* 2013;**42**(17):7057–71.
99. Torchilin V. Multifunctional and stimuli-sensitive pharmaceutical nanocarriers. *Eur J Pharm Biopharm* 2009.
100. Jhaveri A, Deshpande P, Torchilin V. Stimuli-sensitive nanopreparations for combination cancer therapy. *J Control Release* 2014.
101. Priya James H, John R, Alex A, Anoop KR. Smart polymers for the controlled delivery of drugs – a concise overview. *Acta Pharm Sin B* 2014.
102. Fleige E, Quadir MA, Haag R. Stimuli-responsive polymeric nanocarriers for the controlled transport of active compounds: concepts and applications. *Adv Drug Deliv Rev* 2012.
103. Mura S, Nicolas J, Couvreur P. Stimuli-responsive nanocarriers for drug delivery. *Nat Mater* 2013;**12**(11):991–1003.
104. Huang G, Gao J, Hu Z, StJohn JV, Ponder BC, Moro D. Controlled drug release from hydrogel nanoparticle networks. *J Control Release* 2004.
105. Türk M, Dinçer S, Yuluğ IG, Pişkin E. In vitro transfection of HeLa cells with temperature sensitive polycationic copolymers. *J Control Release* 2004.
106. Lee ES, Gao Z, Bae YH. Recent progress in tumor pH targeting nanotechnology. *J Control Release* 2008.
107. Gu Y, Zhong Y, Meng F, Cheng R, Deng C, Zhong Z. Acetal-linked paclitaxel prodrug micellar nanoparticles as a versatile and potent platform for cancer therapy. *Biomacromolecules* 2013.
108. Biswas S, Dodwadkar NS, Sawant RR, Torchilin VP. Development of the novel PEG-PE-based polymer for the reversible attachment of specific ligands to liposomes: synthesis and in vitro characterization. *Bioconjug Chem* 2011.

109. Huang Z, Guo X, Li W, MacKay JA, Szoka FC. Acid-triggered transformation of diortho ester phosphocholine liposome. *J Am Chem Soc* 2006.
110. Donini C, Robinson DN, Colombo P, Giordano F, Peppas NA. Preparation of poly(methacrylic acid-g-poly(ethylene glycol)) nanospheres from methacrylic monomers for pharmaceutical applications. *Int J Pharm* 2002.
111. Kyriakides TR, Cheung CY, Murthy N, Bornstein P, Stayton PS, Hoffman AS. pH-Sensitive polymers that enhance intracellular drug delivery in vivo. *Journal of Controlled Release* 2002.
112. Brannon-Peppas L, Peppas NA. Solute and penetrant diffusion in swellable polymers. IX. The mechanisms of drug release from ph-sensitive swelling-controlled systems. *J Control Release* 1989.
113. Mora-Huertas CE, Fessi H, Elaissari A. Polymer-based nanocapsules for drug delivery. *Int J Pharm* 2010;**385**(1−2):113−42.
114. Crucho CIC, Barros MT. Polymeric nanoparticles: a study on the preparation variables and characterization methods. *Mater Sci Eng C* 2017;**80**:771−84.
115. Rao JP, Geckeler KE. Polymer nanoparticles: preparation techniques and size-control parameters. *Prog Polym Sci* 2011.
116. Gurny R, Peppas NA, Harrington DD, Banker GS. Development of biodegradable and injectable latices for controlled release of potent drugs. *Drug Dev Ind Pharm* 1981.
117. Soppimath KS, Aminabhavi TM, Kulkarni AR, Rudzinski WE. Biodegradable polymeric nanoparticles as drug delivery devices. *J Control Release* 2001.
118. Quintanar-Guerrero D, Allémann E, Doelker E, Fessi H. Preparation and characterization of nanocapsnles from preformed polymers by a new process based on emulsification-diffusion technique. *Pharm Res* 1998.
119. Moinard-Chécot D, Chevalier Y, Briançon S, Beney L, Fessi H. Mechanism of nanocapsules formation by the emulsion-diffusion process. *J Colloid Interface Sci* 2008.
120. Quintanar-Guerrero D, Allémann E, Doelker E, Fessi H. A mechanistic study of the formation of polymer nanoparticles by the emulsification-diffusion technique. *Colloid Polym Sci* 1997.
121. Pinto Reis C, Neufeld RJ, Ribeiro AJ, Veiga F, Nanoencapsulation I. Methods for preparation of drug-loaded polymeric nanoparticles. *Nanomedicine Nanotechnology, Biol Med* 2006.
122. Galindo-Rodríguez SA, Puel F, Briançon S, Allémann E, Doelker E, Fessi H. Comparative scale-up of three methods for producing ibuprofen-loaded nanoparticles. *Eur J Pharm Sci* 2005.
123. Xia Y, Whitesides GM. SOFT LITHOGRAPHY. *Annu Rev Mater Sci* 1998.
124. Whitesides GM, Ostuni E, Takayama S, Jiang X, Ingber DE. Soft lithography in biology and biochemistry. *Annu Rev Biomed Eng* 2001.
125. Rolland JP, Maynor BW, Euliss LE, Exner AE, Denison GM, DeSimone JM. Direct fabrication and harvesting of monodisperse, shape-specific nanobiomaterials. *J Am Chem Soc* 2005;**127**(28).
126. Merkel TJ, Herlihy KP, Nunes J, Orgel RM, Rolland JP, DeSimone JM. Scalable, shape-specific, top-down fabrication methods for the synthesis of engineered colloidal particles. *Langmuir* 2010;**26**(16):13086−96.
127. Petras RA, Ropp PA, DeSimone JM. Reductively labile PRINT particles for the delivery of doxorubicin to HeLa cells. *J Am Chem Soc* 2008.
128. Kai MP, Brighton HE, Fromen CA, et al. Tumor presence induces global immune changes and enhances nanoparticle clearance. *ACS Nano* 2016;**10**(1):861−70.
129. Chu KS, Schorzman AN, Finniss MC, et al. Nanoparticle drug loading as a design parameter to improve docetaxel pharmacokinetics and efficacy. *Biomaterials* 2013;**34**(33):8424−9.
130. Chu KS, Finniss MC, Schorzman AN, et al. Particle replication in nonwetting templates nanoparticles with tumor selective alkyl silyl ether docetaxel prodrug reduces toxicity. *Nano Lett* 2014;**14**(3):1472−6.
131. Dunn SS, Tian S, Blake S, et al. Reductively-responsive siRNA-conjugated hydrogel nanoparticles for gene silencing. *J Am Chem Soc* 2012;**11**:300174.
132. Garcia A, Mack P, Williams S, et al. Microfabricated engineered particle systems for respiratory drug delivery and other pharmaceutical applications. *J Drug Deliv* 2012;**2012**:1−10.
133. Shen TW, Fromen CA, Kai MP, et al. Distribution and cellular uptake of PEGylated polymeric particles in the lung towards cell-specific targeted delivery. *Pharm Res* 2015;**32**(10):3248−60.
134. Fromen CA, Shen TW, Larus AE, et al. Synthesis and characterization of monodisperse uniformly shaped respirable aerosols. *AIChE J* 2013;**59**(9):3184−94.
135. Rahhal TB, Fromen CA, Wilson EM, et al. Pulmonary delivery of butyrylcholinesterase as a model protein to the lung. *Mol Pharm* 2016;**13**(5):1626−35.
136. Roberts RA, Shen T, Allen IC, Hasan W, DeSimone JM, Ting JPY. Analysis of the murine immune response to pulmonary delivery of precisely fabricated nano- and microscale particles. *PLoS One* 2013,**8**(4).
137. Fromen CA, Robbins GR, Shen TW, Kai MP, Ting JPY, DeSimone JM. Controlled analysis of nanoparticle charge on mucosal and systemic antibody responses following pulmonary immunization. *Proc Natl Acad Sci* 2015;**112**(2):488−93.
138. Galloway AL, Murphy A, DeSimone JM, et al. Development of a nanoparticle-based influenza vaccine using the PRINT technology. *Nanomedicine* 2013;**9**(4):523−31.
139. Gratton SEA, Pohlhaus PD, Lee J, Guo J, Cho MJ, DeSimone JM. Nanofabricated particles for engineered drug therapies: a preliminary biodistribution study of PRINT™ nanoparticles. *J Control Release* 2007;**121**(1−2):10−8.
140. Merkel TJ, Chen K, Jones SW, et al. The effect of particle size on the biodistribution of low-modulus hydrogel PRINT particles. *J Control Release* 2012;**162**(1):37−44.
141. Chu KS, Hasan W, Rawal S, et al. Plasma, tumor and tissue pharmacokinetics of Docetaxel delivered via nanoparticles of different sizes and shapes in mice bearing SKOV-3 human ovarian carcinoma xenograft. *Nanomedicine* 2013;**9**(5):686−93.
142. Fromen CA, Rahhal TB, Robbins GR, et al. Nanoparticle surface charge impacts distribution, uptake and lymph node trafficking by pulmonary antigen-presenting cells. *Nanomedicine Nanotechnol Biol Med* 2016;**12**(3):677−87.
143. Mueller SN, Tian S, DeSimone JM. Rapid and persistent delivery of antigen by lymph node targeting PRINT nanoparticle vaccine carrier to promote humoral immunity. *Mol Pharm* 2015;**12**(5).
144. Perry JL, Reuter KG, Kai MP, et al. PEGylated PRINT nanoparticles: the impact of PEG density on protein binding, macrophage association, biodistribution, and pharmacokinetics. *Nano Lett* 2012;**12**(10):5304−10.

145. Chen K, Xu J, Luft JC, Tian S, Raval JS, DeSimone JM. Design of asymmetric particles containing a charged interior and a neutral surface charge: comparative study on in vivo circulation of polyelectrolyte microgels. *J Am Chem Soc* 2014;**136**(28):9947–52.
146. Chen K, Merkel TJ, Pandya A, et al. Low modulus biomimetic microgel particles with high loading of hemoglobin. *Biomacromolecules* 2012;**13**(9):2748–59.
147. Bhaskar S, Pollock KM, Yoshida M, Lahann J. Towards designer microparticles: simultaneous control of anisotropv, shape and size. *Small* 2010.
148. Lahann J. Recent progress in nano-biotechnology: compartmentalized micro- and nanoparticles via electrohydrodynamic Co-jetting. *Small* 2011;**7**(9):1149–56.
149. Kazemi A, Lahann J. Environmentally responsive core/shell particles via electrohydrodynamic co-jetting of fully miscible polymer solutions. *Small* 2008.
150. Yoon J, Lee KJ, Lahann J. Multifunctional polymer particles with distinct compartments. *J Mater Chem* 2011.
151. Walther A, Müller AHE. Janus particles: synthesis, self-assembly, physical properties, and applications. *Chem Rev* 2013.
152. Plasari E, Grisoni PH, Villermaux J. Influence of process parameters on the precipitation of organic nanoparticles by drowning-out. *Chem Eng Res Des* 1997.
153. Chorny M, Fishbein I, Danenberg HD, Golomb G. Lipophilic drug loaded nanospheres prepared by nanoprecipitation: effect of formulation variables on size, drug recovery and release kinetics. *J Control Release* 2002.
154. Govender T, Stolnik S, Garnett MC, Illum L, Davis SS. PLGA nanoparticles prepared by nanoprecipitation: drug loading and release studies of a water soluble drug. *J Control Release* 1999.
155. Miladi K, Sfar S, Fessi H, Elaissari A. Nanoprecipitation process: from particle preparation to in vivo applications. In: *Polymer nanoparticles for nanomedicines*; 2016.
156. Bally F, Garg DK, Serra CA, et al. Improved size-tunable preparation of polymeric nanoparticles by microfluidic nanoprecipitation. *Polymer (Guildf)* 2012.
157. D'Addio SM, Prud'homme RK. Controlling drug nanoparticle formation by rapid precipitation. *Adv Drug Deliv Rev* 2011;**63**(6):417–26.
158. Johnson BK, Prud'homme RK. Chemical processing and micromixing in confined impinging jets. *AIChE J* 2003.
159. Saad WS, Prud'homme RK. Principles of nanoparticle formation by flash nanoprecipitation. *Nano Today* 2016;**11**(2):212–27.
160. Pustulka KM, Wohl AR, Lee HS, et al. Flash nanoprecipitation: particle structure and stability. *Mol Pharm* 2013;**10**(11):4367–77.
161. Craparo EF, Cavallaro G, Bondi ML, Mandracchia D, Giammona G. PEGylated nanoparticles based on a polyaspartamide. Preparation, physico-chemical characterization, and intracellular uptake. *Biomacromolecules* 2006.
162. Antonietti M, Landfester K. Polyreactions in miniemulsions. *Prog Polym Sci* 2002.
163. Weiss CK, Ziener U, Landfester K. A route to nonfunctionalized and functionalized poly (n-butylcyanoacrylate) nanoparticles: preparation in miniemulsion. *Macromolecules* 2007.
164. Al Khouri Fallouh N, Roblot-Treupel L, Fessi H, Devissaguet JP, Puisieux F. Development of a new process for the manufacture of polyisobutylcyanoacrylate nanocapsules. *Int J Pharm* 1986.
165. Vauthier C, Bouchemal K. Methods for the preparation and manufacture of polymeric nanoparticles. *Pharm Res* 2009.
166. Poon Z. Layer-by-Layer nanoparticles with a pH sheddable layer for in vivo targeting of tumor hypoxia. *ACS Nano* 2011.
167. Sukhorukov GB, Donath E, Lichtenfeld H, et al. Layer-by-layer self assembly of polyelectrolytes on colloidal particles. *Colloids Surfaces A Physicochem Eng Asp* 1998.
168. Preetz C, Rübe A, Reiche I, Hause G, Mäder K. Preparation and characterization of biocompatible oil-loaded polyelectrolyte nanocapsules. *Nanomedicine Nanotechnology, Biol Med* 2008.
169. Radtchenko IL, Sukhorukov GB, Möhwald H. Incorporation of macromolecules into polyelectrolyte micro- and nanocapsules via surface controlled precipitation on colloidal particles. *Colloids Surfaces A Physicochem Eng Asp* 2002.
170. Deng ZJ, Morton SW, Ben-Akiva E, Dreaden EC, Shopsowitz KE, Hammond PT. Layer-by-layer nanoparticles for systemic codelivery of an anticancer drug and siRNA for potential triple-negative breast cancer treatment. *ACS Nano* 2013.
171. Rachel R, Elbakry A, Liebl R, Breunig M, Goepferich A, Zaky A. Layer-by-Layer assembled gold nanoparticles for siRNA delivery. *Nano Lett* 2009.
172. Morton SW, Herlihy KP, Shopsowitz KE, et al. Scalable manufacture of built-to-order nanomedicine: spray-assisted layer-by-layer functionalization of PRINT nanoparticles (Adv. Mater. 34/2013). *Adv Mater* 2013;**25**(34):4706.
173. Radtchenko IL, Sukhorukov GB, Leporatti S, Khomutov GB, Donath E, Möhwald H. Assembly of alternated multivalent ion/polyelectrolyte layers on colloidal particles. Stability of the multilayers and encapsulation of macromolecules into polyelectrolyte capsules. *J Colloid Interface Sci* 2000.
174. Park K. Controlled drug delivery systems: past forward and future back. *J Control Release* 2014;**190**:3–8.
175. Anselmo AC, Mitragotri S. Nanoparticles in the clinic. *Bioeng Transl Med* 2016;**1**(1):10–29.
176. Ventola CL. Progress in nanomedicine: approved and investigational nanodrugs. *P T* 2017;**42**(12):742–55.
177. Min Y, Caster JM, Eblan MJ, Wang AZ. Clinical translation of nanomedicine. *Chem Rev* 2015;**115**(19):11147–90.
178. Bertrand N, Wu J, Xu X, Kamaly N, Farokhzad OC. Cancer nanotechnology: the impact of passive and active targeting in the era of modern cancer biology. *Adv Drug Deliv Rev* 2014;**66**:2–25.
179. Fang J, Nakamura H, Maeda H. The EPR effect: unique features of tumor blood vessels for drug delivery, factors involved, and limitations and augmentation of the effect. *Adv Drug Deliv Rev* 2011;**63**(3):136–51.
180. Nakamura Y, Mochida A, Choyke PL, Kobayashi H. Nanodrug delivery: is the enhanced permeability and retention effect sufficient for curing cancer? *Bioconjug Chem* 2016;**27**(10):2225–38.
181. Danhier F. To exploit the tumor microenvironment: since the EPR effect fails in the clinic, what is the future of nanomedicine? *J Control Release* 2016;**244**:108–21.
182. Wilhelm S, Tavares AJ, Dai Q, et al. Analysis of nanoparticle delivery to tumours. *Nat Rev Mater* 2016;**1**:16014.
183. Albanese A, Tang PS, Chan WCW. The effect of nanoparticle size, shape, and surface chemistry on biological systems. *Annu Rev Biomed Eng* 2012;**14**(1):1–16.
184. Perry JL, Reuter KG, Luft JC, Pecot CV, Zamboni W, DeSimone JM. Mediating passive tumor accumulation through particle size, tumor type, and location. *Nano Lett* 2017;**17**(5):2879–86.

185. Yoo J-W, Chambers E, Mitragotri S. Factors that control the circulation time of nanoparticles in blood: challenges, solutions and future prospects. *Curr Pharm Des* 2010;**16**(21):2298–307.
186. Sharma G, Valenta DT, Altman Y, et al. Polymer particle shape independently influences binding and internalization by macrophages. *J Control Release* 2010;**147**(3):408–12.
187. Fish MB, Thompson AJ, Fromen CA, Eniola-Adefeso O. Emergence and utility of nonspherical particles in biomedicine. *Ind Eng Chem Res* 2015;**54**(16):4043–59.
188. Champion JA, Katare YK, Mitragotri S. Particle shape: a new design parameter for micro- and nanoscale drug delivery carriers. *J Control Release* 2007;**121**(1–2):3–9.
189. Champion JA, Mitragotri S. Role of target geometry in phagocytosis. *Proc Natl Acad Sci* 2006;**103**(13):4930–4.
190. Chithrani BD, Ghazani AA, Chan WCW. Determining the size and shape dependence of gold nanoparticle uptake into mammalian cells. *Nano Lett* 2006.
191. Gratton SEA, Ropp PA, Pohlhaus PD, et al. The effect of particle design on cellular internalization pathways. *Proc Natl Acad Sci* 2008;**105**(33):11613–8.
192. Champion JA, Mitragotri S. Shape induced inhibition of phagocytosis of polymer particles. *Pharm Res* 2009.
193. Fish MB, Fromen CA, Lopez-Cazares G, et al. Exploring deformable particles in vascular-targeted drug delivery: softer is only sometimes better. *Biomaterials* 2017;**124**:169–79.
194. Anselmo AC, Zhang M, Kumar S, et al. Elasticity of nanoparticles influences their blood circulation, phagocytosis, endocytosis, and targeting. *ACS Nano* 2015;**9**(3):3169–77.
195. Yang X, Chen Q, Yang J, et al. Tumor-targeted accumulation of ligand-installed polymeric micelles influenced by surface PEGylation crowdedness. *ACS Appl Mater Interfaces* 2017;**9**(50):44045–52.
196. Choi KY, Chung H, Min KH, et al. Self-assembled hyaluronic acid nanoparticles for active tumor targeting. *Biomaterials* 2010;**31**(1):106–14.
197. Sykes EA, Chen J, Zheng G. Investigating the impact of nanoparticle size on active and passive tumor targeting E fficiency. *ACS Nano* 2014;**8**(6):5696–706.
198. Wang J, Tian S, Petros RA, Napier ME, Desimone JM. The complex role of multivalency in nanoparticles targeting the transferrin receptor for cancer therapies. *J Am Chem Soc* 2010;**132**(32):11306–13.
199. Reuter KG, Perry JL, Kim D, Luft JC, Liu R, DeSimone JM. Targeted PRINT hydrogels: the role of nanoparticle size and ligand density on cell association, biodistribution, and tumor accumulation. *Nano Lett* 2015;**15**(10):6371–8.
200. Carboni E, Tschudi K, Nam J, Lu X, Ma AWK. Particle margination and its implications on intravenous anticancer drug delivery. *AAPS PharmSciTech* 2014;**15**(3):762–71.
201. Gentile F, Curcio A, Indolfi C, Ferrari M, Decuzzi P. The margination propensity of spherical particles for vascular targeting in the microcirculation. *J Nanobiotechnology* 2008;**6**:9.
202. Toy R, Hayden E, Shoup C, Baskaran H, Karathanasis E. The effects of particle size, density and shape on margination of nanoparticles in microcirculation. *Nanotechnology* 2011;**22**(11):115101.
203. Coclite A, Pascazio G, de Tullio MD, Decuzzi P. Predicting the vascular adhesion of deformable drug carriers in narrow capillaries traversed by blood cells. *J Fluids Struct* 2018;**82**:638–50.
204. Xu S, Wang W, Li X, Liu J, Dong A, Deng L. Sustained release of PTX-incorporated nanoparticles synergized by burst release of DOX•HCl from thermosensitive modified PEG/PCL hydrogel to improve anti-tumor efficiency. *Eur J Pharm Sci* 2014;**62**:267–73.
205. Gagnadoux F, Hureaux J, Vecellio L, et al. Aerosolized chemotherapy. *J Aerosol Med Pulm Drug Deliv* 2008;**21**(1):61–70.
206. Kai MP, Keeler AW, Perry JL, et al. Evaluation of drug loading, pharmacokinetic behavior, and toxicity of a cisplatin-containing hydrogel nanoparticle. *J Control Release* 2015;**204**:70–7.
207. Dhar S, Kolishetti N, Lippard SJ, Farokhzad OC, Mirkin CA. Targeted delivery of a cisplatin prodrug for safer and more effective prostate cancer therapy in vivo. *Proc Natl Acad Sci U S A* 2011;**108**(5):1850–5.
208. Huang X, Shen S, Zhang Z, Zhuang J. Cross-linked polyethylenimine–tripolyphosphate nanoparticles for gene delivery. *Int J Nanomedicine* 2014;**9**:4785–94.
209. Cheng M, He B, Wan T, et al. 5-Fluorouracil nanoparticles inhibit hepatocellular carcinoma via activation of the p53 pathway in the orthotopic transplant mouse model. *PLoS One* 2012;**7**(10):e47115.
210. Oliveira C, Neves NM, Reis RL, Martins A, Silva TH. Gemcitabine delivered by fucoidan/chitosan nanoparticles presents increased toxicity over human breast cancer cells. *Nanomedicine* 2018;**13**(16):2037–50.
211. Joubert F, Martin L, Perrier S, Pasparakis G. Development of a gemcitabine-polymer conjugate with prolonged cytotoxicity against a pancreaticcancer cell line. *ACS Macro Lett* 2017;**6**(5):535–40.
212. Parrott MC, Luft JC, Byrne JD, Fain JH, Napier ME, Desimone JM. Tunable bifunctional silyl ether cross-linkers for the design of acid-sensitive biomaterials. *J Am Chem Soc* 2010;**132**(50):17928–32.
213. Meng F, Zhong Z, Feijen J. Stimuli-responsive polymersomes for programmed drug delivery. *Biomacromolecules* 2009;**10**(2):197–209.
214. Azarmi S, Roa WH, Löbenberg R. Targeted delivery of nanoparticles for the treatment of lung diseases. *Adv Drug Deliv Rev* 2008;**60**(8):863–75.
215. Mitchell MJ, Jain RK, Langer R. Engineering and physical sciences in oncology: challenges and opportunities. *Nat Rev Cancer* 2017;**17**(11):659–75.
216. Nel AE, Mädler L, Velegol D, et al. Understanding biophysicochemical interactions at the nano–bio interface. *Nat Mater* 2009;**8**:543.
217. Pulendran B, Ahmed R. Translating innate immunity into immunological memory: implications for vaccine development. *Cell* 2006;**124**(4):849–63.
218. Iwasaki A, Medzhitov R. Regulation of adaptive immunity by the innate immune system. *Science* 2010;**327**(5963):291–5.
219. Plotkin SA. Vaccines: past, present and future. *Nat Med* 2005;**10**(4s):S5–11.
220. Translation of an address on the germ theory. *Lancet* 1881;**118**(3024):271–2.
221. Pulendran B, Li S, Nakaya HI. Systems vaccinology. *Immunity* 2010.
222. Nembrini C, Stano A, Dane KY, et al. Nanoparticle conjugation of antigen enhances cytotoxic T-cell responses in pulmonary vaccination. *Proc Natl Acad Sci* 2011;**108**(44):E989–97.
223. Shen H, Ackerman AL, Cody V, et al. Enhanced and prolonged cross-presentation following endosomal escape of exogenous antigens encapsulated in biodegradable nanoparticles. *Immunology* 2006;**117**(1):78–88.

224. De Geest BG, Willart MA, Lambrecht BN, et al. Surface-engineered polyelectrolyte multilayer capsules: synthetic vaccines mimicking microbial structure and function. *Angew Chemie - Int Ed* 2012.
225. Irvine DJ, Swartz MA, Szeto GL. Engineering synthetic vaccines using cues from natural immunity. *Nat Mater* 2013;**12**:978.
226. Saluja SS, Hanlon DJ, Sharp FA, et al. Targeting human dendritic cells via DEC-205 using PLGA nanoparticles leads to enhanced cross-presentation of a melanoma-associated antigen. *Int J Nanomedicine* 2014.
227. de Titta A, Ballester M, Julier Z, et al. Nanoparticle conjugation of CpG enhances adjuvancy for cellular immunity and memory recall at low dose. *Proc Natl Acad Sci* 2013.
228. Fifis T, Gamvrellis A, Crimeen-Irwin B, et al. Size-dependent immunogenicity: therapeutic and protective properties of nano-vaccines against tumors. *J Immunol* 2004.
229. Serra P, Santamaria P. Nanoparticle-based approaches to immune tolerance for the treatment of autoimmune diseases. *Eur J Immunol* 2018.
230. Riedhammer C, Weissert R. Antigen presentation, autoantigens, and immune regulation in multiple sclerosis and other autoimmune diseases. *Front Immunol* 2015.
231. Sakaguchi S. Naturally arising Foxp3-expressing CD25+ CD4+ regulatory T cells in immunological tolerance to self and non-self. *Nat Immunol* 2005.
232. Izcue A, Coombes JL, Powrie F. Regulatory lymphocytes and intestinal inflammation. *Annu Rev Immunol* 2009.
233. Van Der Kooij SM, De Vries-Bouwstra JK, Goekoop-Ruiterman YPM, et al. Limited efficacy of conventional DMARDs after initial methotrexate failure in patients with recent onset rheumatoid arthritis treated according to the disease activity score. *Ann Rheum Dis* 2007.
234. Feldmann M, Steinman L. Design of effective immunotherapy for human autoimmunity. *Nature* 2005.
235. Maldonado RA, LaMothe RA, Ferrari JD, et al. Polymeric synthetic nanoparticles for the induction of antigen-specific immunological tolerance. *Proc Natl Acad Sci* 2015.
236. Henson PM, Bratton DL. Antiinflammatory effects of apoptotic cells. *J Clin Invest* 2013.
237. Huynh MLN, Fadok VA, Henson PM. Phosphatidylserine-dependent ingestion of apoptotic cells promotes TGF-β1 secretion and the resolution of inflammation. *J Clin Invest* 2002.
238. Roberts RA, Eitas TK, Byrne JD, et al. Towards programming immune tolerance through geometric manipulation of phosphatidylserine. *Biomaterials* 2015.
239. Gharagozloo M, Majewski S, Foldvari M. Therapeutic applications of nanomedicine in autoimmune diseases: from immunosuppression to tolerance induction. *Nanomedicine Nanotechnology, Biol Med* 2015;**11**(4):1003–18.
240. Hunter Z, McCarthy DP, Yap WT, et al. A biodegradable nanoparticle platform for the induction of antigen-specific immune tolerance for treatment of autoimmune disease. *ACS Nano* 2014.
241. Hess KL, Andorko JI, Tostanoski LH, Jewell CM. Polyplexes assembled from self-peptides and regulatory nucleic acids blunt toll-like receptor signaling to combat autoimmunity. *Biomaterials* 2017.
242. Serra P, Santamaria P. Nanoparticle-based autoimmune disease therapy. *Clin Immunol* 2015.
243. Mccarthy DP, Hunter ZN, Chackerian B, Shea LD, Miller SD. Targeted immunomodulation using antigen-conjugated nanoparticles. *Wiley Interdiscip Rev Nanomed Nanobiotechnol* 2014.
244. Getts DR, Terry RL, Getts MT, et al. Therapeutic inflammatory monocyte modulation using immune-modifying microparticles. *Sci Transl Med* 2014;**6**(219).
245. Fromen CA, Kelley WJ, Fish MB, et al. Neutrophil-particle interactions in blood circulation driveparticle clearance and alter neutrophil responses in acute inflammation. *ACS Nano* 2017;**11**(11):10797–807.
246. Zhu X, Radovic-Moreno A, Wu J, Langer R, Shi J. Nanomedicine in the management of microbial infection – overview and perspectives. *Nano Today* 2014;**20**:41–5.
247. Radovic-Moreno AF, Lu TK, Puscasu VA, Yoon CJ, Langer R, Farokhzad OC. Surface charge-switching polymeric nanoparticles for bacterial cell wall-targeted delivery of antibiotics. *ACS Nano* 2012;**6**(5):4279–87.
248. Pinto-Alphandary H, Andremont A, Couvreur P. Targeted delivery of antibiotics using liposomes and nanoparticles: research and applications. *Int J Antimicrob Agents* 2000;**13**:155–68.
249. Seijo B, Fattal E, Roblot-Treupel L, Couvreur P. Design of nanoparticles of less than 50 nm diameter - preparation, characterization and drug loading. *International Journal of Pharmaceutics* 1990:1–7.
250. Bender A, Schäfer V, Steffan AM, et al. Inhibition of HIV in vitro by antiviral drug-targeting using nanoparticles. *Res Virol* 1994;**145**(C):215–20.
251. Birch NP, Schiffman JD. Characterization of self-Assembled polyelectrolyte complex nanoparticles formed from chitosan and pectin. *Langmuir* 2014;**30**(12):3441–7.
252. Turos E, Reddy GSK, Greenhalgh K, et al. Penicillin-bound polyacrylate nanoparticles: restoring the activity of β-lactam antibiotics against MRSA. *Bioorganic Med Chem Lett* 2007;**17**(12):3468–72.
253. Turos E, Shim JY, Wang Y, et al. Antibiotic-conjugated polyacrylate nanoparticles: new opportunities for development of anti-MRSA agents. *Bioorganic Med Chem Lett* 2007;**17**(1):53–6.
254. Nam-Cha SH, Pérez-Tanoira R, Pérez-Martínez J, et al. Antimicrobial evaluation of quaternary ammonium polyethyleneimine nanoparticles against clinical isolates of pathogenic bacteria. *IET Nanobiotechnology* 2015;**9**(6):342–8.
255. Yin Y, Papavasiliou G, Zaborina OY, Alverdy JC, Teymour F. De novo synthesis and functional analysis of polyphosphate-loaded poly(ethylene) glycol hydrogel nanoparticles targeting pyocyanin and pyoverdin production in *Pseudomonas aeruginosa* as a model intestinal pathogen. *Ann Biomed Eng* 2017;**45**(4):1058–68.
256. Gref R, Minamitake Y, Langer R. *Biodegradable injectable nanoparticles*. 1996.
257. *The top 10 causes of death, fact sheet 310*. 2012.
258. Morbidity & Mortality. *Chart book on cardiovascular, lung, and blood diseases*, vol. 2012; 2012.
259. Patton JS, Byron PR. Inhaling medicines: delivering drugs to the body through the lungs. *Nat Rev Drug Discov* 2007;**6**:67.
260. Weers JG, Bell J, Chan H-K, et al. Pulmonary formulations: what remains to be done? *J Aerosol Med Pulm Drug Deliv* 2010;**23**(Suppl. 2):S5–23.
261. Muralidharan P, Malapit M, Mallory E, Hayes DJ, Mansour HM. Inhalable nanoparticulate powders for respiratory delivery. *Nanomedicine* 2015;**11**(5):1189–99.

262. Mansour HM, Rhee YS, Wu X. Nanomedicine in pulmonary delivery. *Int J Nanomedicine* 2009;**4**:299–319.
263. Yang W, Peters JI, Williams RO. Inhaled nanoparticles—a current review. *Int J Pharm* 2008;**356**(1):239–47.
264. Ungaro F, d'Angelo I, Miro A, La Rotonda MI, Quaglia F. Engineered PLGA nano- and micro-carriers for pulmonary delivery: challenges and promises. *J Pharm Pharmacol* 2012;**64**(9):1217–35.
265. Edwards DA, Hanes J, Caponetti G, et al. Large porous particles for pulmonary drug delivery. *Science* 1997;**276**(5320):1868 LP–1872.
266. Patton B, Nagarajan. Inhaled insulin. *Adv Drug Deliv Rev* 1999;**35**(2–3):235–47.
267. Tsapis N, Bennett D, Jackson B, Weitz DA, Edwards DA. Trojan particles: large porous carriers of nanoparticles for drug delivery. *Proc Natl Acad Sci* 2002;**99**(19):12001 LP–12005.
268. Newman SP. Drug delivery to the lungs: challenges and opportunities. *Ther Deliv* 2017;**8**(8):647–61.
269. Sung JC, Pulliam BL, Edwards DA. Nanoparticles for drug delivery to the lungs. *Trends Biotechnol* 2007;**25**(12):563–70.
270. Choi HS, Ashitate Y, Lee JH, et al. Rapid translocation of nanoparticles from the lung airspaces to the body. *Nat Biotechnol* 2010;**28**(12):1300–3.
271. Falk E. Pathogenesis of atherosclerosis. *J Am Coll Cardiol* 2006;**47**(8):C7–12.
272. Lewis DR, Kamisoglu K, York AW, Moghe PV. Polymer-based therapeutics: nanoassemblies and nanoparticles for management of atherosclerosis. *Wiley Interdiscip Rev Nanomedicine Nanobiotechnology* 2011.
273. Sewright KA, Clarkson PM, Thompson PD. Statin myopathy: incidence, risk factors, and pathophysiology. *Curr Atheroscler Rep* 2007.
274. Nguyen LTH, Muktabar A, Tang J, et al. Engineered nanoparticles for the detection, treatment and prevention of atherosclerosis: how close are we? *Drug Discov Today* 2017.
275. Sanchez-Gaytan BL, Fay F, Lobatto ME, et al. HDL-mimetic PLGA nanoparticle to target atherosclerosis plaque macrophages. *Bioconjug Chem* 2015.
276. Aizik G, Grad E, Golomb G. Monocyte-mediated drug delivery systems for the treatment of cardiovascular diseases. *Drug Deliv Transl Res* 2018;**8**(4):868–82.
277. Katsuki S, Matoba T, Nakashiro S, et al. Nanoparticle-mediated delivery of pitavastatin inhibits atherosclerotic plaque destabilization/rupture in mice by regulating the recruitment of inflammatory monocytes. *Circulation* 2014.
278. Peters D, Kastantin M, Kotamraju VR, et al. Targeting atherosclerosis by using modular, multifunctional micelles. *Proc Natl Acad Sci* 2009.
279. Fromen CA, Fish MB, Zimmerman A, Adili R, Holinstat M, Eniola-Adefeso O. Evaluation of receptor-ligand mechanisms of dual-targeted particles to an inflamed endothelium. *Bioeng Transl Med* 2016;**1**(1):103–15.
280. Korin N, Kanapathipillai M, Matthews BD, et al. Shear-activated nanotherapeutics for drug targeting to obstructed blood vessels. *Science* 2012.

Chapter 19

Hydrophobically assembled nanoparticles

Self-assembled nanoparticles

Jonathan Wang[1], Michael Mellas[2], Matthew Tirrell[3] and Eun Ji Chung[1,4,5,6,7,8]

[1]Biomedical Engineering, University of Southern California, Los Angeles, CA, United States; [2]Institute for Molecular Engineering, University of Chicago, Chicago, IL, United States; [3]Pritzker School of Molecular Engineering, University of Chicago, Chicago, IL, United States; [4]Department of Chemical Engineering and Materials Science, University of Southern California, Los Angeles, CA, United States; [5]Eli and Edythe Broad Center for Regenerative Medicine and Stem Cell Research, Keck School of Medicine, University of Southern California, Los Angeles, CA, United States; [6]Norris Comprehensive Cancer Center, Keck School of Medicine, University of Southern California, Los Angeles, CA, United States; [7]Department of Surgery, Division of Vascular Surgery and Endovascular Therapy, Keck School of Medicine, University of Southern California, Los Angeles, CA, United States; [8]Department of Medicine, Division of Nephrology and Hypertension, Keck School of Medicine, University of Southern California, Los Angeles, CA, United States

19.1 Introduction

Intermolecular forces, or forces experienced between different molecules, drive a wide range of organic nanoparticle assemblies and can include van der Waals forces, hydrophobic effects, hydrogen bonds, and electrostatic interactions.[1] These forces fall under the class of "supramolecular" interactions, which is a term coined by the 1987 Nobel Laureate in Chemistry, Jean-Marie Lehn.[2] Currently, supramolecular chemistry is an interdisciplinary field with a broad array of applications including molecular imaging, metal extraction, drug delivery, etc.[3,4]

The macroscale determination of hydrophobicity, or the lack of attraction to water, is often measured by the static contact angle, defined as the tangential angle at the liquid–solid–air interface of a droplet on a flat surface.[5] A surface is generally termed hydrophobic when a static droplet of water has a contact angle >90 degrees and is hydrophilic when the opposite is true. However, this extrinsic property may manifest differently depending on the length scale.[6] On the nanoscale, techniques such as molecular dynamics simulations,[7–9] surface adsorption,[10] measurement of the affinity (partitioning) coefficient,[11] hydrophobic interaction chromatography,[12] and contact angle via the sessile drop Young–Laplace method[13] are used instead to quantify hydrophobic force.

These hydrophobic forces can be utilized in the field of biomedical engineering to create structures for applications such as drug delivery or imaging. Generalized equations for idealized systems can provide a tool for predicting the magnitude of the hydrophobic force driving self-assembly of particles. J.N. Israelachvili was the first to utilize the surface force apparatus (Fig. 19.1)[14] and two lipid bilayers[15] to measure the attractive force between two hydrophobic surfaces (Eq. 19.1) when they were brought together in close proximity.

$$\boldsymbol{E_{hydro}} = -\boldsymbol{\gamma}(\boldsymbol{a}-\boldsymbol{a}_0)\boldsymbol{e}^{-d/D_{hydro}} \quad [19.1]$$

where γ is the interfacial tension and
D_{hydro} is the hydrophobic decay length.

Derjaguin–Landau–Verwey–Overbeek (DLVO) theory is another model which originates from the mathematical description of colloids in suspension (Fig. 19.2). The force acting between two colloidal particles, F(h), acting at a distance h can be captured in Eq. (19.2). Researchers have successfully utilized this theory to give baseline approximations of stability of colloidal suspensions.[16]

$$\boldsymbol{F}(\boldsymbol{h}) = 2\pi \boldsymbol{R_{eff}} \boldsymbol{W}(\boldsymbol{h}) \quad [19.2]$$

where

F(h) = force acting between two colloidal particles by surface separation h,
W(h) = free energy of two plates per unit area,
R_{eff} = effective radius.

Nanoparticles for Biomedical Applications. https://doi.org/10.1016/B978-0-12-816662-8.00019-9

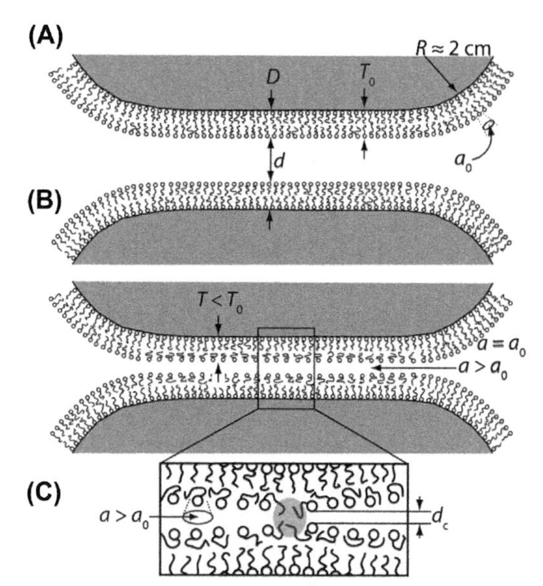

FIGURE 19.1 Schematic diagrams depicting the process by which two supported surfactant or lipid bilayers fuse. (A) Initially, two bilayers are separated by 30 nm and begin to interact due to long-range electrostatic double-layer forces. (B) As the bilayers approach, they are forced together (2–3 nm), and the strong normal stresses associated with steric and electrostatic repulsions cause the outer layers to thin normally and spread laterally, exposing the hydrophobic interior of the bilayer. (C) A close-up of the instability that occurs near $d_c \approx 1$ nm: Stress opens a hydrophobic pore, causing the hydrophobic interiors to strongly attract each other, while the highly stressed outer monolayers begin to be pushed out of the contact area. *Adapted and reprinted from S.H. Donaldson, C.T. Lee, B.F. Chmelka, and J.N. Israelachvili, General hydrophobic interaction potential for surfactant/lipid bilayers from direct force measurements between light-modulated bilayers. Proc Natl Acad Sci, 2011. 108(38): p. 15699 with permission from PNAS.*

Despite historical development of mathematical models, researchers sometimes find the predictions are inadequate to describe real-world phenomena or colloids in an in vivo biomedical engineering application.[18] Regardless of mathematical model used, the overarching motif for nanoparticle synthesis in biomedical engineering is to create molecules with both hydrophilic and hydrophobic portions, which will behave in a predictable fashion in an aqueous environment. Hydrophobic portions will cluster together usually in the core of a nanoparticle in solution to minimize contact with water, while the hydrophilic portions form a "corona" around the core to allow for solubility in aqueous media such as blood. Four main classes of molecules have seen significant progress in biomedical engineering applications in the past two decades: (1) peptide amphiphiles, (2) nucleic acid constructs, (3) block copolymers, and (4) dendrimers. We will focus on an introduction to the principles behind their hydrophobic self-assembly and highlight key studies demonstrating the advantages conferred by their supramolecular architecture.

19.2 Peptide amphiphiles

Peptide amphiphiles are a class of amphiphilic molecule defined by the presence of a hydrophilic peptide in the headgroup. The hydrophobic tail is typically an oil (i.e., alkyl chain or fatty acid) or a hydrophobic peptide. The head and tail may be linked directly or with a spacer moiety. The breadth of the peptide amphiphile class provides many potential applications as well as important fundamental questions about their assembly.

The assembly thermodynamics of peptide amphiphiles are driven primarily by the hydrophobic effect.[19] In general, a hydrophobic solute in aqueous solution will be surrounded by a layer of water molecules with high surface tension, which increases the free energy of solution, G_{soln},

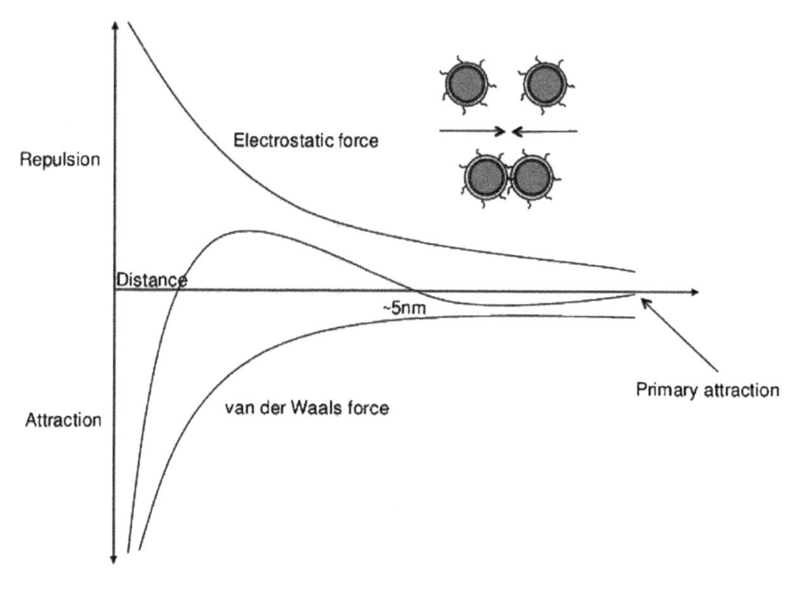

FIGURE 19.2 Schematic of the Derjaguin–Landau–Verwey–Overbeek theory. The tendency of colloids to agglomerate or separate can be derived by combining two curves of electrostatic repulsion and van der Waals attraction. *Adapted and reprinted from Peter Kaali, E.S.a.S.K., Prevention of biofilm associated infections and degradation of polymeric materials used in biomedical applications, in Biomedical engineering, trends in materials science. 2011. with permission from IntechOpen.*

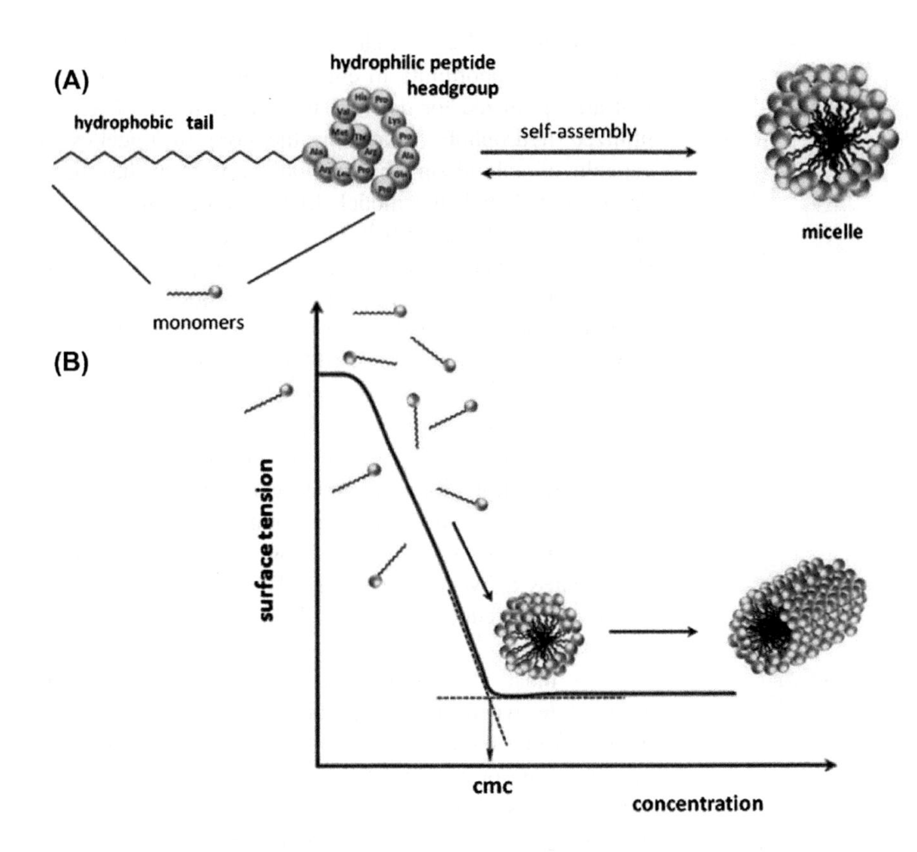

FIGURE 19.3 Characteristic curve of the surface tension for aqueous surfactants solution. (A) Schematic presentation of the peptide amphiphile with the hydrophobic C16 alkyl chain and the hydrophilic peptide headgroup forming micelles by self-assembly above the critical micelle concentration (CMC). (B) Idealized curve of surface tension as a function of surfactant concentration with the CMC representing the point, where surfactant molecules start to form aggregates known as spherical micelles, with further increasing concentration, the micelles may change the shape to cylindric forms. *Adapted and reprinted from C. Hüttl, C. Hettrich, R. Miller, B.-R. Paulke, P. Henklein, H. Rawel, and F.F. Bier, Self-assembled peptide amphiphiles function as multivalent binder with increased hemagglutinin affinity. BMC Biotechnol, 2013. 13(1): p. 51 with permission from BioMed Central Ltd.*

due to the reduced entropy of the surrounding water layer. G_{soln}, namely, is the free energy of the assembled nanoparticle, relative to that of the dispersed monomers. Since the enthalpy of the solution depends primarily on the volume of solute, which remains constant regardless of solute–solute interaction, but the entropy depends on surface area of the solute–water interface, G_{soln} decreases as more solute molecules associate together into a separate phase to minimize the surface area exposed to aqueous solution per solute molecule.

Amphiphiles are driven to assemble by the same kinetics, but the presence of the hydrophilic moiety in the solute molecules provides a force favoring solution with the water. The result is a micelle wherein the hydrophobic moiety acts as an oil phase while the hydrophilic moiety maximizes contact with water and simultaneously minimizes the oil–water contact, providing a cap on micelle size.

The presence of the hydrophilic moiety also reduces G_{soln} for individual amphiphile molecules, creating a minimum concentration of amphiphiles below which micelle formation is disfavored, known as the critical micelle concentration (CMC) (Fig. 19.3). For derivation of CMC from the law of mass action, refer to the work by Maibaum et al.[19] Generally, forces that strengthen the hydrophobic effect also lower the CMC. Because of this correlation, the CMC is often taken as a proxy for the stability of the micelles in solution.[20]

Micelle shape is determined by the packing parameter[22,23] of the amphiphile molecule. The packing parameter P is given by equation $P = v/al$, where v is the volume the molecule occupies in solution, a is the area of the hydrophilic headgroup when solvated, and l is the length of the hydrophobic tail in the oil phase. The critical packing parameter (C_{pp}) can be thought of as a measurement of the shape an individual amphiphile preferentially takes in solution: for $C_{pp} < 1/3$, the monomer shape is conical, and the resulting micelles are generally spheroids, while for $C_{pp} > 1/2$, the monomer shape is more cylindrical, driving formation of long wormlike micelles (Fig. 19.4). Kinetic observations by Tirrell et al. suggest that most micelle formation begins with sphere formation, even for higher packing parameters, but that the spheres then subsequently merge to form the wormlike structures observed in the case of high C_{pp}.[24] According to these observations, spherical micelle formation is relatively fast, and the packing parameter correlates with the thermodynamic favorability of merging these micelles to form worms.

The fundamental relationship between peptide secondary structure and packing parameter is an integral component of peptide amphiphile micelle formation in particular and cannot be overlooked when designing peptide amphiphiles for specific applications.[23,26,27] However, this relationship provides a relatively simple means by which to tune the shape of the micelle. The formation of β-sheets in the peptide headgroup tends to greatly reduce the area of headgroup solvation in water, increasing the packing parameter and driving the formation of wormlike micelles,

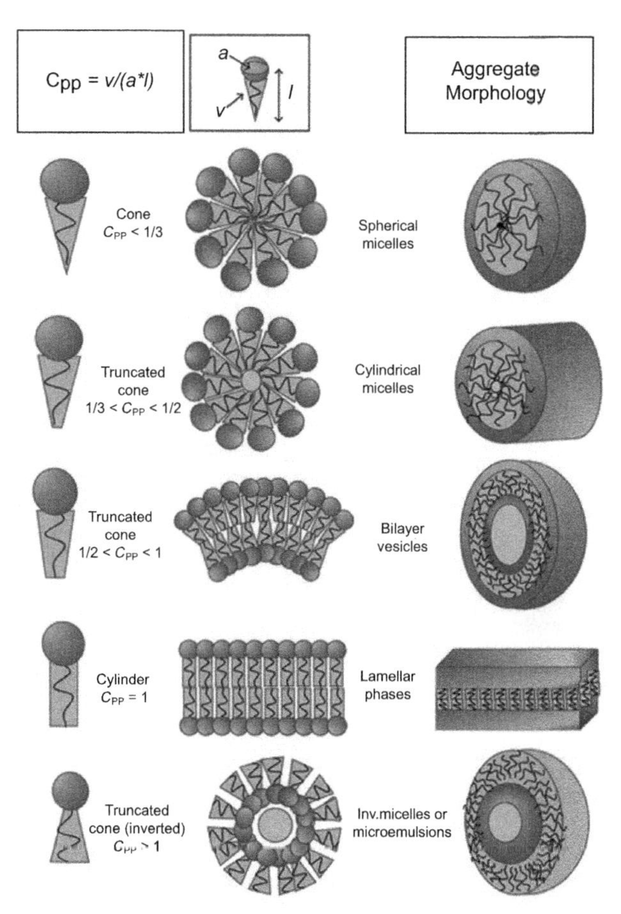

FIGURE 19.4 Amphiphile morphology and summary of the aggregate structures that can be predicted from the critical packing parameter. *Adapted and reprinted from Lombardo, D., M.A. Kiselev, Magazu, S. , and P. Calandra, Amphiphiles self-assembly: basic concepts and future perspectives of supramolecular approaches. Adv Condens Matter Phys, 2015. 2015: p. 22. with permission from Hindawi.*

while a lack of secondary structure tends to correlate to a lower packing parameter. It has been suggested that if the degree of secondary structure formation can be tuned, so can the shape of the micelles and the viscoelastic properties of the solution.[28] This tunability makes peptide amphiphiles suitable for a wide array of applications from drug delivery to tissue and regenerative medicine. In this text, we focus mostly on spherical nanoparticles, while Cui et al. provide an interesting review of amphiphiles forming cylindrical micelles, which are used for biomedical applications in a hydrogel format.[29]

19.2.1 Biomedical application of peptide amphiphiles

19.2.1.1 Drug delivery

Peptide amphiphile micelles have been explored as drug carriers in a wide variety of pharmaceutical applications.[30–34] The modularity of amphiphile synthesis presents the opportunity to engineer designer amphiphiles that are optimized for delivery to a target tissue. The solubilized hydrophobic phase in the core of micelles is capable of solubilizing hydrophobic drugs, as has been demonstrated with the model drugs doxorubicin,[30] paclitaxel,[31] and cabozantinib.[32] Furthermore, the hydrophilic shell can be functionalized with bioactive peptide ligands to promote tissue-specific delivery of micelles.[30,31,34] Most peptides produced in the laboratory today take advantage of solid-phase peptide synthesis (SPPS), invented in the 1960s by Merrifield.[35] Amino acids are added sequentially to a solid support via a series of addition reactions, and finally cleaved from the support once chain elongation is completed. These custom peptide ligands permit a suitably engineered drug-loaded peptide amphiphile micelle to provide higher efficacy and fewer off-target effects, due to the targeted delivery of the drug. The method has shown promise in reducing tumor load[31] as well as in atherosclerosis.[34]

One must also consider the safety of the peptide amphiphile when designing the delivery system. It is important that the amphiphile or micelle does not damage healthy tissue or accumulate in areas that can cause detrimental effects. While the lack of comprehensive theory of micelle safety necessitates individual testing of any engineered amphiphile design, some findings do provide useful guidelines. Since the peptide amphiphiles in question are constructed with biomimetic amino acids and phospholipid components, they are largely biodegradable, biocompatible, and nontoxic.[34,36,37] In general, smaller particles (<10 nm) tend to be cleared via glomerular filtration in the kidneys, while larger particles are more likely to bind to macrophages and be cleared by the reticuloendothelial system (RES).[34,38–40] Protein adsorption onto the nanoparticle surface, or opsonization, is another key factor which can lead to heightened RES clearance in circulation or in tissues such as the liver and spleen.[41] PEGylation, or the addition of polyethylene glycol (PEG) to the surface of a peptide amphiphile micelle can screen surface charge and help prevent uptake by the RES.[34] Placing a bulky PEG as a spacer in between a peptide and the hydrophobic lipid tail has been experimentally shown to drive PAs to assemble into spherical micelles.[23] Other strategies, such as incorporating the drug into the amphiphile itself via biodegradable linkers for in situ release, can also assist with clearance of micelles. Zhao et al. demonstrated that this method was viable for codelivery of naproxen and curcumin, by using naproxen dendrimers as the hydrophobic core of the micelle, which then solubilized the curcumin for simultaneous delivery.[33] Analyzing the release of the drugs in vitro revealed that the naproxen was separated and activated after cell uptake.

19.2.1.2 Immunomodulation

The immune system plays a central role in preventing and fighting infection as well as in promoting healing of wounded or damaged tissue. Proper function of the immune system requires a fine balance in the expression of a wide array of receptors and ligands to maintain feedback communication between innate and adaptive immune responses.[42]

To briefly summarize the complex system, the immune system comprises two fundamental parts: the innate immune system and the adaptive immune system. The innate immune system can be thought of as the nonspecific first response to injury or infection. Macrophages, dendritic cells, natural killer (NK) cells, and antigen-presenting cells all play roles in the innate immune response, and they respond first to proinflammatory signals and mediate the inflammatory response. The adaptive immune system acts more slowly, but will target a specific antigen with little collateral damage. B cells and T cells mediate the innate immune response; T cells are further specialized into helper T cells, cytotoxic T cells, and regulatory T cells (T_H, T_C, and T_{reg} respectively).[43] Communication between innate and adaptive immune cells triggers adaptive immune response. Upon clearing of an infection, the adaptive immune system will retain memory cells, which can recognize a previously fought threat and mount a secondary immune response to it quickly.

Because the immune response is mediated by peptide–receptor binding, it is possible to engineer peptide amphiphile micelles which express an immunomodulatory receptor-binding peptide, functioning as adjuvants, which modify immune response in a targeted fashion. Hudalla et al. show peptide nanofiber assemblies that contain a high density of adjuvants in both folded protein native epitope conformations, allowing for immune responses not achievable with unmodified vaccines.[44] For example, work by Ulery et al. has demonstrated the effectiveness of micelles composed of vasoactive intestinal peptide directly conjugated to palmitic acid (pVIPA) (Fig. 19.5).[45–47] Because vasoactive intestinal peptide suppresses tumor necrosis factor-alpha (TNF-α) expression, there has been interest in its application as a therapeutic agent against autoimmune disorders.[48–50] The zwitterion linker had a significant effect on the CMC and shape of the micelles conjugated to palmitic acid via a glutamate-lysine zwitterion linker (pzVIPA).[51] The vasoactive intestinal peptide had been previously shown to reduce inflammation by inhibiting the inflammatory marker TNF-α, which is ordinarily produced by antigen presenting cells to activate macrophages and dendritic cells. This activation plays a role in innate immunity, but can exacerbate dysfunctional immune response in many disease states. The synthesized pVIPA formed cylindrical micelles, while the pzVIPA formed braided wormlike micelles instead. While the pzVIPA had a much higher CMC, it was found to reduce TNF-α expression and suppress pro-inflammatory behavior in innate immune cells more effectively compared to the pVIPA. However, pVIPA did promote chemokine receptor–mediated regulatory T-cell recruitment, which can also play a role in immune tolerance.[45–47]

Because of the specific immune responses achievable by conjugating immunomodulatory peptides into amphiphiles, other immune applications such as wound healing and vaccination have been of interest. Hyaluronan-polycaprolactone (HA-PCL) amphiphiles with incorporated fibroblast growth factor 1 (FGF1) were demonstrated to promote healing of wounds in rat models.[52] FGF1 is not only much safer than other angiogenic growth factors, having demonstrated no adverse effects, but it is also much less soluble and more prone to aggregation. Micellization was found to reduce FGF1 aggregation and permitted sustained release of FGF1 in wounded tissue. Finally, peptide amphiphiles have proven useful in vaccination, where either aggregation into micelles[30] or adjuvants incorporated into the core[53] strengthened the resulting immune response significantly. Significant research done by Collier et al. using self-assembled fibrillar peptide vaccines have improved vaccine thermal stability,[54] associated CD4+ helper T cell responses,[55] and activated B cell responses in hosts without causing inflammation.[56] It is likely that micellization will be a useful strategy to pursue when designing future vaccines.

19.2.1.3 Site-specific targeting and imaging

Because a site-specific peptide ligand can be directly incorporated into the design of the amphiphile according to its water solubility, it is possible to target specific sites with the micelles themselves. Peptide amphiphiles can therefore act as both active agent and carrier in medical applications such as regenerative medicine or imaging. Depending on the binding motif in the hydrophilic layer, some micelles may have a wide variety of applications.

As a case study, we will consider the fibrin-binding REKA motif employed by Tirrell et al.[57] Using cysteine–maleimide conjugation, REKA peptide was bound to amphiphilic 1,2-distearoyl-sn-glycero-3-phosphoethanolamine-PEG (DSPE-PEG) to generate DSPE-PEG-CREKA amphiphile, which formed ellipsoid micelles. Testing micelle affinity for fibrin residue in glioblastoma[57] and atherosclerosis[58] indicated that the micelles bound the residual fibrin in each of these diseases in a progression-dependent fashion. Furthermore, it was demonstrated that REKA micelles could be conjugated with diethylenetriaminepentaacetic acid (DTPA), a gadolinium chelator, and employed in MRI contrast imaging, whereupon MRI contrast signal was found to quantitate the

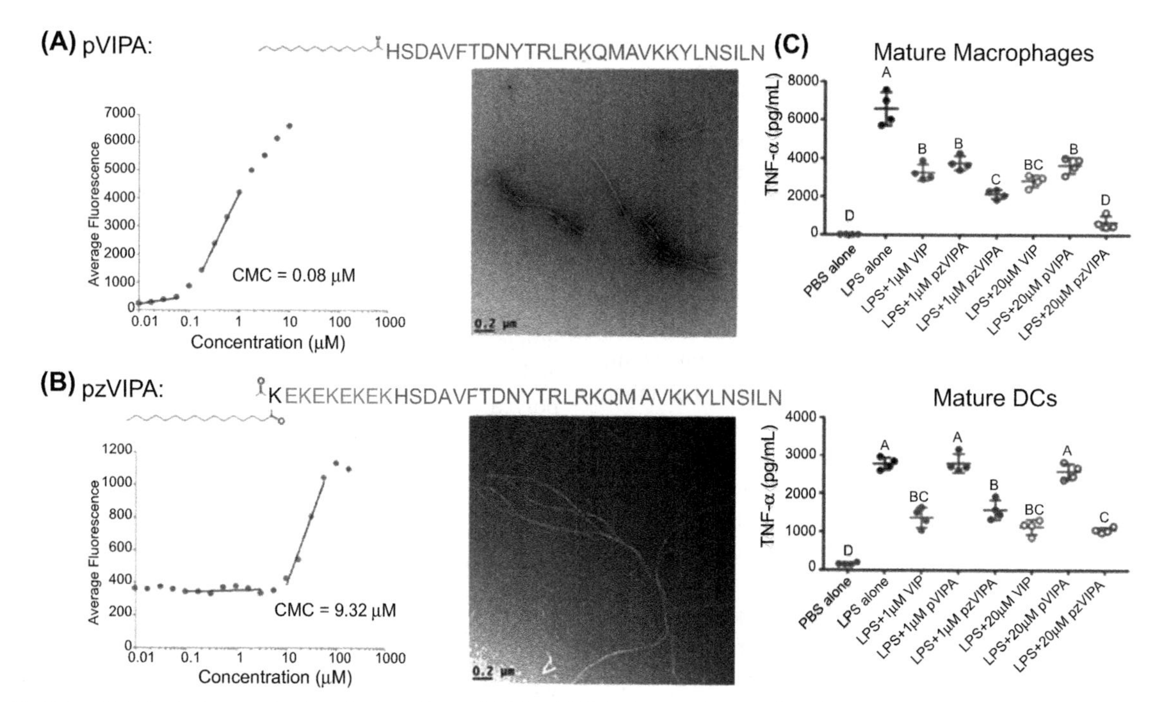

FIGURE 19.5 (A) Palmitoyl-vasoactive intestinal peptide amphiphiles (pVIPA) form stable wormlike micelles above their critical micelle concentration (CMC). (B) Palmitoyl-zwitterionic(glutamate-lysine)-VIP amphiphiles (pzVIPA) require higher concentrations to assemble and form braided assemblies of wormlike micelles above their CMC. Despite the decreased CMC, the pzVIPA remains of interest due to its efficacy reducing TNF-α levels in macrophages and dendritic cells activated with lipopolysaccharides (LPS) (C). *Adapted and reprinted from Zhang, R., C.N. Leeper, X. Wang, T.A. White, and B.D. Ulery, Immunomodulatory vasoactive intestinal peptide amphiphile micelles. Biomaterials Science, 2018. with permission from Royal Society of Chemistry.*

presence of fibrin in atherosclerotic lesions.[58] Follow-up work on atherosclerosis demonstrated that while REKA was effective at binding the fibrin present in micelles, fibrin accumulation was indicative of late-stage lesions.[59] An earlier plaque detection system was subsequently developed to bind vascular cell adhesion molecule 1 (DSPE-PEG-VCAM-1) (Fig. 19.6),[60] which is expressed at atherosclerotic plaque sites at an early stage in humans.[61,62] Tirrell et al. were able to demonstrate that VCAM-1-binding micelles localized at atherosclerotic plaque sites before lesions formed, and that VCAM-1 expression (and micelle binding) correlated with sites of later lesion formation.[60] Further work utilizing a CCR2 binding motif of monocyte chemoattractant protein 1 (DSPE-PEG-MCP-1) found the micelles to be latently capable of binding monocytes at atherosclerotic lesions. Because monocyte accumulation at lesions is correlated to progression of atherosclerosis,[63] the presence of micelles bound to monocytes could be used as a proxy for disease progression.[64] The MCP1 micelles were further found to interfere with CCR2 signaling in prostate cancer cells, increasing cytotoxicity of the cells, which suggests possible antitumor function as well.[65] This series of work, utilizing DSPE-PEG conjugated with a few peptides or mixed functionalities for diagnostic detection or treatment of a diverse set of disease states, demonstrates the breadth and versatility of applications a peptide amphiphile micelle may have, with relatively minor modifications.

Site-specific targeting permits a peptide amphiphile micelle to perform the double duty of carrying therapeutic molecules in their core while also functionalized with a diagnostic marker. The class of "theranostic" micelles has demonstrated utility for most types of medical imaging, for which follow a few examples. Cho et al. used[45] functional positron emission tomography (F PET) to establish the efficacity of a PEG-PCL system for delivering paclitaxel, cyclopamine, and gossypol simultaneously to ovarian cancer.[66,67] Steinbach et al. have demonstrated the potential of ultrasound imaging to trigger image-guided delivery of micelle-bound drugs to a site of interest before using the ultrasound to pulse burst the micelle, releasing its internal cargo.[67] A variety of strategies have been employed to achieve in vivo fluorescence imaging, including nanofibers with attached quantum dots,[68] micelles with incorporated near-infrared Cy5[65,66] or Cy7[60] dye, micelles with a gemcitabine or camptothecin prodrug core and quenched fluorescent linker that fluoresce upon in situ cleavage,[69,70] and a quenched fluorescent core attached to a degradable linker to measure endosomal degradation.[71] Finally, MRI has been established as a particularly useful method for its potential to achieve high contrast with minimal invasiveness, though the accumulation and cytotoxicity of

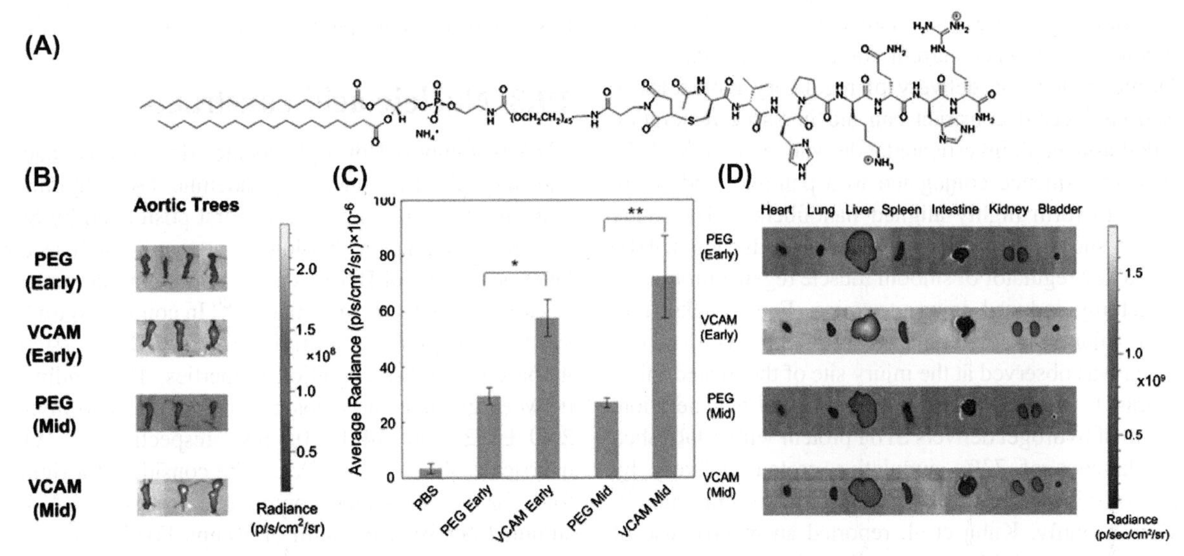

FIGURE 19.6 (A) Structure of DSPE-PEG(2000)-VCAM (seq: VHPKQHR). (B) Ex vivo imaging of mouse aortas show both increased localization of Cy7-labeled micelles by DSPE-PEG(2000)-VCAM and increased association of micelles to aortas with later-stage atherosclerosis, suggesting that the VCAM micelles could be used to track disease progression. Fluorescence is quantified in (C). (D) Biodistribution of micelles shows minimal accumulation, with the exception of the clearance organs. *Adapted and reprinted from Chung, E.J., Y. Cheng, R. Morshed, K. Nord, Y. Han, M.L. Wegscheid, B. Auffinger, D.A. Wainwright, M.S. Lesniak, and M.V. Tirrell, Fibrin-binding, peptide amphiphile micelles for targeting glioblastoma(☆). Biomaterials, 2014. 35(4): p. 1249–1256 and Mlinar, L.B., E.J. Chung, E.A. Wonder, and M. Tirrell, Active targeting of early and mid-stage atherosclerotic plaques using self-assembled peptide amphiphile micelles. Biomaterials, 2014. 35(30): p. 8678–8686 with permission from Elsevier.*

gadolinium-based micelle imaging has led to safety concerns. Some methods designed to minimize the risk of Gd toxicity include Gd-chelating tetracarboxylic acid (DOTA) or DPTA-attached micelles[58,72] and Gd-free imaging.[73] The latter method, termed chemical exchange saturation transfer (CEST) MRI, is especially interesting because it takes advantage of the exchangeability of protons between the micelle-encapsulated drug and the water in vivo to produce high-contrast MRI imaging without gadolinium, circumventing the risks of Gd toxicity entirely. Through these imaging methods, it is possible to examine the in situ behavior of site-specific micelles with high fidelity.

The ability to tune the biodistribution and improve imaging modalities demonstrates the usefulness of PAs. The final cellular fate of the nanoparticle depends highly on micelle internalization and intracellular trafficking, which may utilize pathways such as pinocytosis and nonspecific or receptor-mediated endocytosis. A comprehensive review on the physiochemical properties affecting cellular internalization of micelles can be explored in the work of Duan and Li.[39]

19.2.1.4 Tissue engineering

These nanostructures designed through self-assembly strategies have the potential to enhance bioactivity for tissue regeneration and wound repair. Investigations by the pioneering Stupp group have created self-assembling peptide amphiphiles toward applications in the regeneration of the central nervous system, vasculature, and hard tissue.[74] The assemblies used for cell scaffolds ideally incorporate both the necessary mechanical support and elasticity, as well as the ability to trigger cell signaling pathways, mimicking the native extracellular matrix. Furthermore, molecular design can be used to create structures that biodegrade over an appropriate time scale. To achieve a minimally invasive solution, these amphiphiles can be introduced into the site of interest as an injectable liquid, but self-assemble in situ into solid scaffolds or nanostructures.

Although possessing different form factors compared to spherical peptide amphiphile micelles is previously mentioned, the ordered supramolecular structure conveys cellular benefits not seen in traditional random covalent polymers. For example, Richter et al. utilized an aligned peptide amphiphile nanofiber neurograft for facial nerve repair. This neurograft was constructed with amphiphile molecules of palmitoyl and the amino acid sequence VVVAAAEE, which was previously shown to display a high degree of nanoscale alignment for lengths of several centimeters. Its self-assembly into nanofibers is triggered by gelation of ions present in the synthesis buffering solution which screen the charged amino acid residues.[75] A maximum neurograft length of 7.5 and 2.5 mm in diameter was tested in a rat model of nerve injury, which showed no statistical difference compared to the autograft repair group.[76] Similar degrees of neural regeneration and recovery were seen between these two repair techniques, which are attributed to the enhanced recruitment of

Schwann cells producing myelinated regeneration.[37] These results show promise that nanoengineered tissue replacements may replace current autograft standards.

As mentioned, the delivery of regulatory molecules in a tissue engineered construct can aid in tissue restoration time. Podlasek et al. investigated a derivative of the $V_nA_nE_n$ amino acid sequence conjugated to a palmitic acid (C16) alkyl tail to form highly aligned nanofibers.[77] The study showed a successful delivery of Sonic Hedgehog (SHH) protein, a key regulator of smooth muscle regeneration, after prostatectomy induced injury to mice. Four weeks after induced injury, nerve regeneration along with axonal sprouting was observed at the injury site of the treated mice, in contrast to controls which showed axonal degeneration. This type of hydrogel delivers SHH protein with established release kinetics of 73% cumulative protein delivery by 6 days, showing optimal muscle regeneration properties.[78]

More recently, Kuhn et al. reported an in vivo use of self-assembling peptide amphiphile micelles carrying a migratory bioactive Tenascin-C (Ten-C) derived peptide sequence, for the redirection of endogenous neuroblasts in the rodent brain. Ten-C is an oligomeric extracellular glycoprotein linked to neural precursor cell migration. Due to the highly aligned supramolecular structure, nanofibers were able to stimulate the migration of neuroblasts to the cortex of the brain 24-fold higher than control, with minimum inflammation normally associated with the pro-inflammatory properties of free Ten-C.[79] Such exciting results can open new avenues for utilizing an adult patient's own neuroblasts and stem cells for regenerating damaged tissue and replacing parenchyma lost to injury.

19.3 Nucleic acid constructs

DNA is composed of a phosphate−deoxyribose backbone and natural bases including adenine (A), thymine (T), cytosine (C), and guanine (G). First postulated by Seeman in 1982, DNA nanotechnology is now a research sector that takes advantage of DNA as a structural material, rather than as carrier for genetic information.[80] In contrast to traditional synthetic polymers, the driving force of DNA assembly is its base pair self-recognition properties. The binding force between guanine and cytosine, and adenine and thymine is 20.0 ± 0.2 and 14.0 ± 0.3 pN, respectively.[81] On the nanoscale, therefore, DNA can be considered a rigid scaffold for length scales comparable to the DNA double stranded persistence length of 50 nm. For length scales on larger magnitudes, it can conveniently be modeled as an elastic rod with an equivalent Young's modulus and tethered boundary conditions.[81,82]

In 2006, Ruthemund adopted a simple "scaffolded DNA origami" method to fold DNA into arbitrary 2D shapes, allowing a myriad of complex geometries to be formed (Fig. 19.7).[83] Short oligonucleotide "staple strands" were used to fold long DNA strands with spatial resolution of about 6 nm.

Investigators have conjugated short-sequence DNA, which are generally hydrophilic, to hydrophobic molecules.

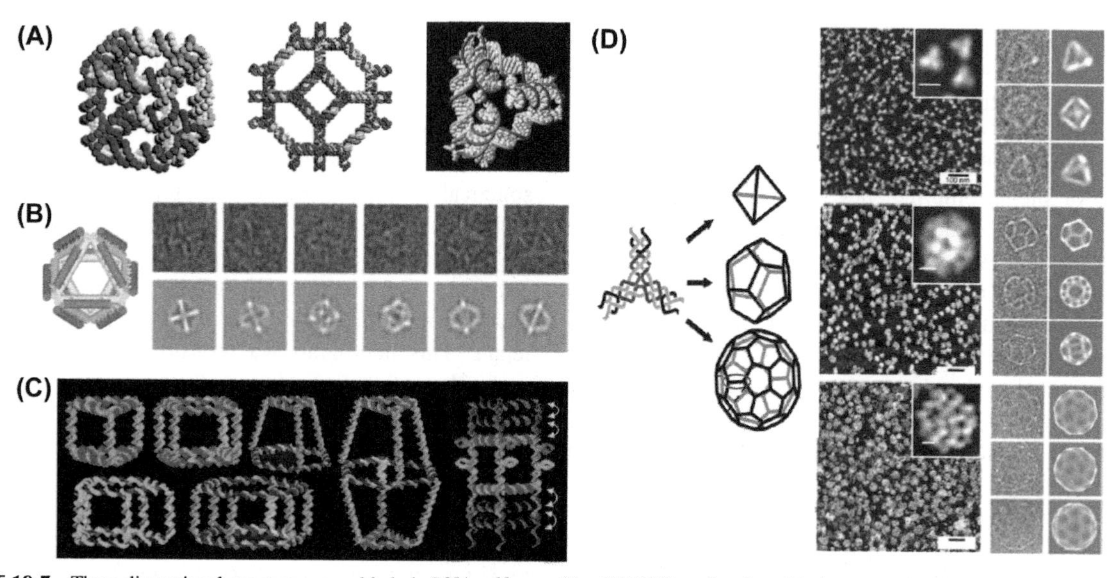

FIGURE 19.7 Three-dimensional structures assembled via DNA self-assembly. (A) DNA molecules with the connectivity of a cube, an octahedron and a tetrahedron. (B) Design of DNA octahedron from 1669-nucleotide DNA and cryo-electron micrograph images of individual octahedron particles corresponding projections of their 3D map. (C) Three-dimensional triangular prism, cube, pentameric and hexameric prisms, heteroprism and biprism generated from single-stranded and cyclic DNA triangles, squares, pentagons, and hexagons with organic vertices (D) DNA tetrahedra, dodecahedra and "buckyballs" assembled from three-point-star motifs. *Adapted and reprinted from Li, H., J.D. Carter, and T.H. LaBean, Nanofabrication by DNA self-assembly. Mater Today, 2009. 12(5): p. 24−32 with permission from Elsevier.*

These are termed amphiphilic oligonucleotides (AONs), and behave much like the peptide amphiphiles previously discussed; AONs generally self-assemble into structures with simple geometries such as spherical or cylindrical micelles in aqueous solutions.[85] Uniquely, the molecular recognition properties of DNA are intact, and thus DNA micelles can hybridize with complimentary sequences while maintaining supramolecular integrity. Importantly, when interacting with cell membranes, the highly charged nature of DNA is able to insert into the cell membrane, driving endocytosis pathways of cell uptake.

Solid-phase synthesis (SPS) and solution coupling are two main methodologies for the construction of DNA modified with functional groups. In SPS, fragments of DNA up to approximately 200 nucleotides are built up by iterative chemical synthesis on solid supports using activated phosphoramidite building blocks. The four-step procedure includes deprotection, coupling, capping, and oxidation, which is followed by cleaving DNA off the solid support. The SPS technique makes it possible not only to prepare precise oligonucleotides with near perfect sequences, but introduce functional groups into the DNA sequence.[86] Solution coupling is a more straightforward method to make covalent bonds between reaction-ready DNAs supplied from industry. Amine, thiol functionalization onto DNA, for example, is conjugated to biomolecules containing the complementary carboxylic acid or maleimide reactive group.

More complex architectures can be achieved by insertion of nongenetic blocks into hydrophilic DNA. Wang et al. linked hydrophobic perylene chromophore units within a hydrophilic DNA chain, which underwent folding processes induced by noncovalent interactions (Fig. 19.8). Unique properties emerged such as structural stability during thermal cycling between 20 and 90°C, an advantage conferred over traditional nanoparticle assemblies.[87] These perylene DNA nanoparticles could be disassembled when presented with the complementary DNA strand in solution, creating potential applications as colorimetric DNA biosensors.

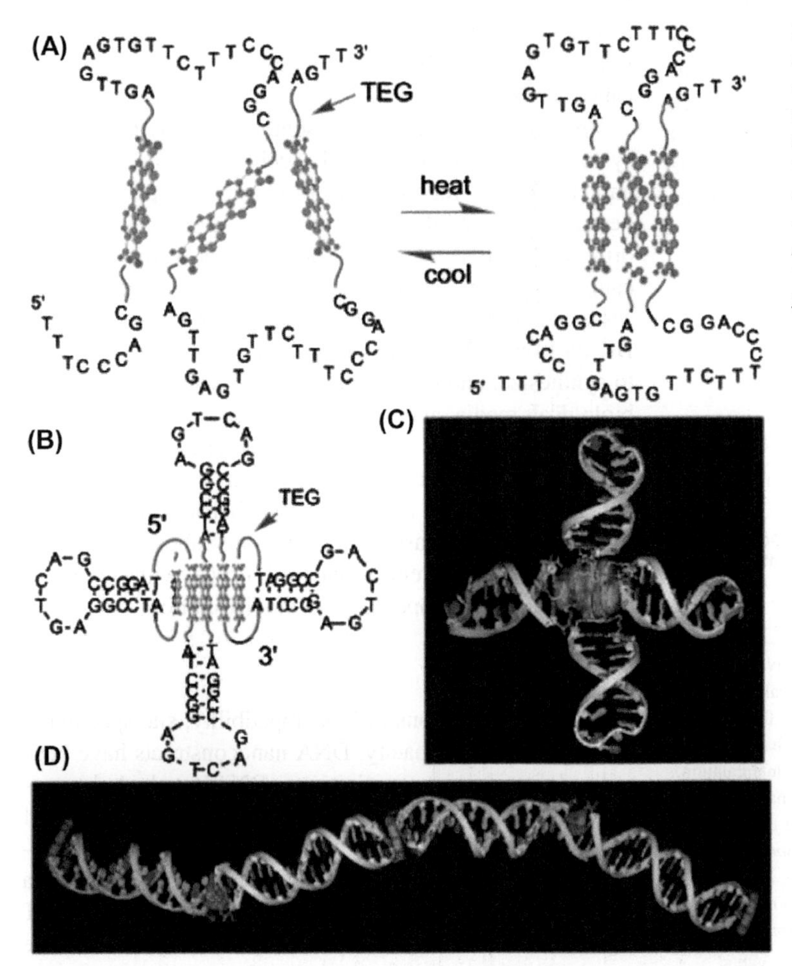

FIGURE 19.8 Schematic of self-assembled DNA phenylene nanostructure. (A) Thermophilic property of the chromophoric trimer linked nanoparticle schematic and nucleotide sequence. (B, C) A chromophoric pentamer surrounded by DNA hairpin structures (D) that can be unfolded through binding to the complementary DNA. *Adapted and reprinted from Wang, W., W. Wan, H.-H. Zhou, S. Niu, and A.D.Q. Li, Alternating DNA and π-conjugated sequences. Thermophilic foldable polymers. J Am Chem Soc, 2003. 125(18): p. 5248–5249. with permission from American Chemical Society.*

19.3.1 Biomedical applications of nucleic acid constructs

19.3.1.1 Drug/gene delivery

Supramolecular DNA nanostructures have a high potential to be universal vehicles for targeted drug or genetic payload delivery.[88] DNA is inherently biocompatible, but naked DNA molecules are usually impermeable to mammalian cell membranes unless accompanied by transfection agents. However, with mechanisms still under investigation, studies revealed that many pure DNA nanostructures have high uptake efficiency compared to free small molecules in solution.[89]

Doxorubicin, a potent anticancer drug used to treat a wide variety of cancers, is known to have side effects that are difficult to tolerate, such as cardiac, renal, pulmonary, testicular toxicity.[90] Additionally, it is prone to significant tumor resistance as chemotherapy duration increases. Therefore, a highly selective nanocarrier for doxorubicin is a desired research outcome, for which DNA nanocarriers have been extensively researched. Ding and coworkers created a DNA origami structure with triangular supramolecular self-assembly results (Fig. 19.9). When intercalated with doxorubicin, the nanocarrier system significantly enhanced cytotoxicity to both regular human breast adenocarcinoma (MCF-7) cells, as well as a doxorubicin-resistant MCF-7 cell line. This is attributed to the avoidance of lysosome acidification of doxorubicin, as different uptake mechanisms are proposed to govern nanoparticle uptake.[91] The expression of associated drug efflux pumps are consequently expressed to a lesser degree in nanoparticle formulations compared to free drug.

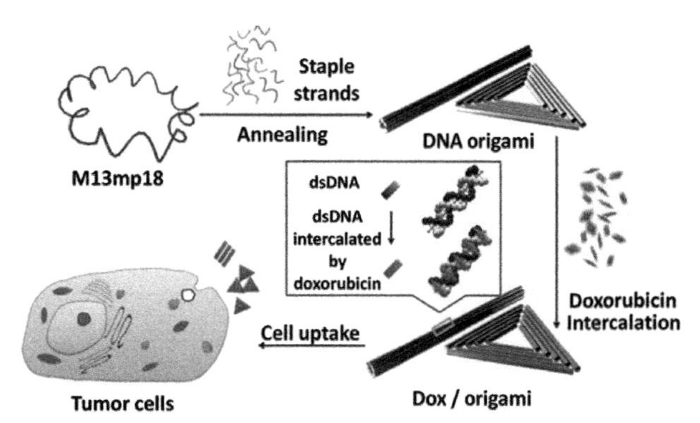

FIGURE 19.9 DNA origami and doxorubicin origami delivery system assembly. The long single-strand M13mp18 genomic DNA scaffold strand (blue) is folded into the triangle and tube structures through the hybridization of rationally designed staple strands. Watson–Crick base pairs in the double helices serve as docking sites for doxorubicin intercalation. After incubation with doxorubicin, the drug-loaded DNA nanostructure delivery vessels were administered to MCF-7 cells, and the effects were investigated. *Adapted and reprinted from Jiang, Q., C. Song, J. Nangreave, X. Liu, L. Lin, D. Qiu, Z.-G. Wang, G. Zou, X. Liang, H. Yan, and B. Ding, DNA origami as a carrier for circumvention of drug resistance. J Am Chem Soc, 2012. 134(32): p. 13396–13403 with permission from American Chemical Society Publications.*

Similarly, Mok et al. report a successful combination therapy of small interfering ribonucleic acids (siRNAs) and chemical drugs for effective drug resistant cancer treatment.[92] In this study, PEG-siRNA-polycaprolactone (PEG-siRNA-PCL) micelles that encapsulate the hydrophobic drug paclitaxel enabled efficient codelivery of siRNA and drugs to cancer cells. PEG-siRNA-PCL micelles containing anti-apoptotic Bcl-2-specific siRNA were shown to have superior anticancer effects, assessed by caspase-3 activity analysis, apoptotic cell staining, and a cytotoxicity test, to those of paclitaxel-free micelles and unmodified siRNAs. This synergistic effect of Bcl-2 siRNA and paclitaxel is attributed to the high loading capacity achieved when incorporating siRNA into the nanoparticle structure, leaving larger hydrophobic drug loading capacity. This work provides an efficient codelivery platform for combination anticancer therapy with siRNA and chemotherapy. Hong et al. achieved a similar cancer cell–specific targeting in vitro using a cationic lipid-nucleic acid nanoparticle which were homogenously sized spheres between 70 and 100 nm (Genospheres). Insertion of an antibody–lipopolymer reactive to human epidermal growth factor receptor 2 (HER2) allowed for selective targeting and transfection of HER2 overexpressing SK-BR-3 breast cancer cells.[93]

In vivo, a spherical, self-assembled nucleic acid (SNA) system was developed for the delivery of BKM120, an anticancer drug for treatment of chronic lymphocytic leukemia (CLL). While promising for cancer treatment, this drug leaks across the blood–brain barrier, causing significant side effects in patients. The DNA nanoparticle possesses the ideal properties of a drug carrier: (1) encapsulates BKM120 with high efficiency, (2) monodisperse and easy to synthesize, and (3) biocompatible and stable in different biological media and in serum. Evaluation of this drug delivery system in vivo shows long circulation half-life times up to 12 h, accumulation at tumor sites, and minimal passage through the blood–brain barrier (Fig. 19.10).[94] This and other self-assembled structures allow researchers to modify the current arsenal of drugs with favorable pharmacokinetic properties and biodistribution.[95]

19.3.1.2 Imaging

For the similar reasons of biocompatibility, site specificity, and high loading capacity, DNA nanoconstructs have been utilized for imaging applications. DNA tetrahedral nanostructures with an anti-ATP sequence embedded in one of the edges were developed as an intracellular energy reporter. This nanostructure would interact with ATP via a conformational change upon binding and generates a FRET signal with a pair of fluorophores (Cy3 and Cy5) within the

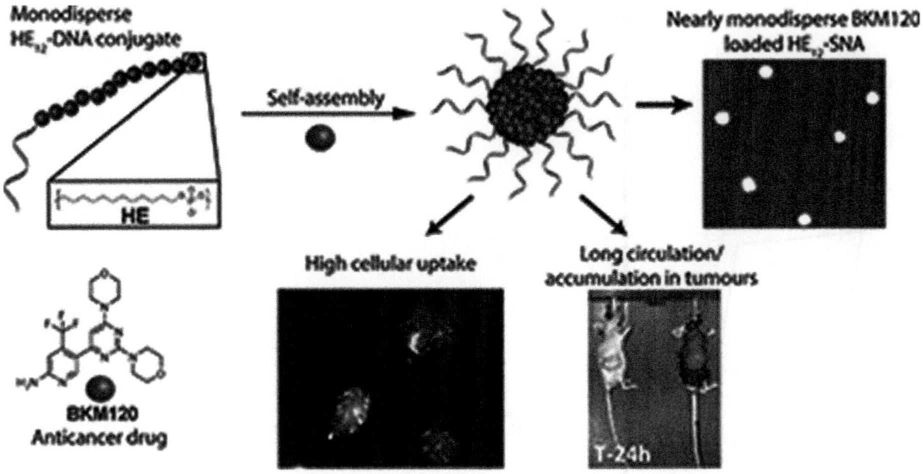

FIGURE 19.10 Schematic of spherical nucleic acid (SNA) system for the delivery of BKM120 in vivo, which uses the typical amphiphilic self-assembly scheme for monodisperse nanoparticle formation. *Adapted and reprinted from Bousmail, D., L. Amrein, J.J. Fakhoury, H.H. Fakih, J.C.C. Hsu, L. Panasci, and H.F. Sleiman, Precision spherical nucleic acids for delivery of anticancer drugs. Chem Sci, 2017. 8(9): p. 6218–6229 with permission from American Chemical Society Publications.*

structure.[96] Subnanomolar detection of the target was achieved due to the high binding affinity measured and an ability to alter supramolecular structure upon union with the target ATP molecule.[97]

Krishnan and colleagues encapsulated a fluorescent biopolymer that functions as a pH reporter within a synthetic icosahedral DNA cage, assembled via hydrophobic partitioning.[98] Used here without molecular recognition between host and cargo, only cells bearing receptors for the DNA casing of the capsule complex could engulf it. They show that the encapsulated cargo is therefore received specifically by the coelomocytes, a scavenger cell type, in *Caenorhabditis elegans*. The cell-specific uptake of highly controlled nanostructures is useful in distinguishing physiological detail and is key in achieving high spatial resolution in future clinical engineering applications.

19.4 Block copolymer nanoparticles

Interest in synthetic polymers as materials for biomedical applications has led to rising interest in the use of block copolymer micelles.[99–101] Block copolymers are named for their structure, which consists of at least two polymer "blocks" joined together. The advantages of block copolymers for engineering nanoscale materials includes their ease and reproducibility of polymerization, the tunability of their constituent block sizes, and the ability to easily functionalize the blocks to allow for modular synthesis and covalent drug or ligand loading. Block copolymer micelles are typically assembled via a diblock or triblock strategy wherein one block or the center block, respectively, is neutral and hydrophilic to solvate the micelle, while the other blocks drive the micellization or gelation at higher concentrations (Fig. 19.11). The other block is typically one of the three types, which determines the core force driving the assembly. A hydrophobic block creates amphiphilic micelles which assemble via the hydrophobic force and behave according to packing parameter dynamics. A polyionic block allows for polyion complex micelles (PICMs), also known as polyelectrolyte complex micelles (PECMs), by electrostatic complexation with an oppositely charged polyion. Additional electrostatically driven nanoparticles are described in more detail in Chapter 20. A metal-complexed block generates metal-complexed micelles which will form around the metal in the core.[101–103] Typically, while micelle shape depends on a number of factors such as packing parameter as previously described, the length of the blocks also plays a major role in determining shape: a longer hydrophilic block will favor spheres, while a longer core block will favor rods or lamellar structures.[104]

Most commonly, the hydrophilic block of the copolymer will be PEG, also called polyethylene oxide (PEO). PEG is widely known and used for its inertness in vivo and is considered the gold standard for the hydrophilic block.[101] While this property can be a disadvantage for tissue engineering applications where binding to the injury site is desirable, PEG can be readily functionalized with a peptide or ligand to permit adhesion.[106] Another hydrophilic polymer explored is polyvinylpyrrolidone (PVP), which is also biocompatible and better suited to freeze-drying than PEG. However, its synthesis remains a major challenge to its use.[101]

A wide variety of core block polymers exist, depending upon the application and desired properties. The core is generally a biodegradable hydrophobic polyester, charged polyamine, or polycarboxylate.[100] For amphiphiles, the core is most often polylactic acid (PLA), polyglycolic acid (PGA), poly(lactic-co-glycolic acid) (PLGA), polycaprolactone (PCL), and polybutylene terephthalate (PBT) (Fig. 19.12). In some cases, the structural properties can be varied by varying the enantiopurity, such as the use of

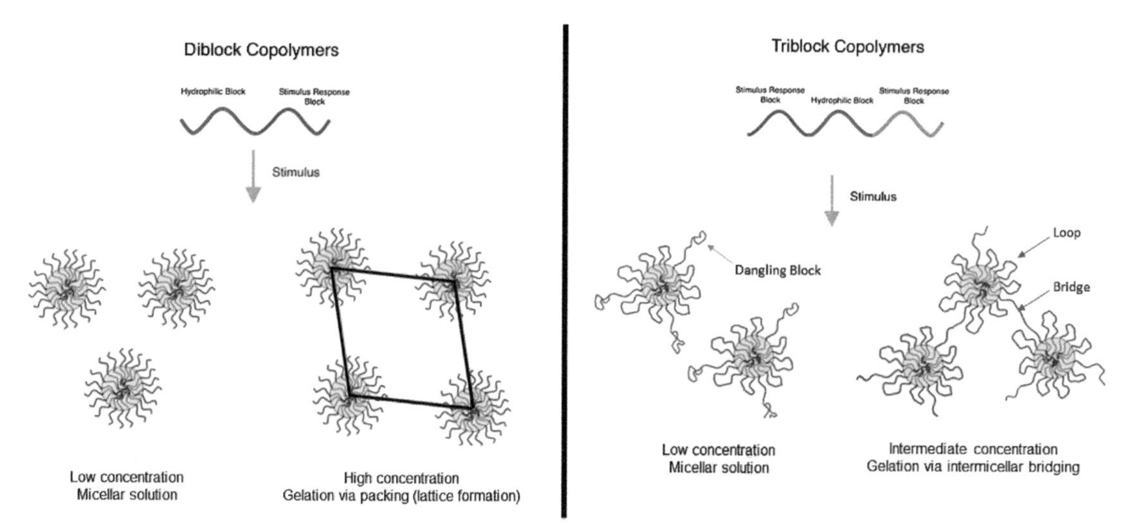

FIGURE 19.11 Micellization and gelation mechanisms of diblock (left) and triblock (right) copolymers. It is possible for hydrophobic portions to exist outside the core in "dangling blocks" when deformation of the hydrophilic block is energetically unfavorable. *Adapted from Madsen, J. and S.P. Armes, (Meth)acrylic stimulus-responsive block copolymer hydrogels. Soft Matter, 2012. 8(3): p. 592–605.*

poly(L-lactic acid) (PLLA) or racemic PLA (PDLLA) to obtain a semicrystalline or amorphous core, respectively.[100] PLA generates dense but flexible nanostructures, but it degrades slowly, and there have been concerns with the immunogenicity of lactic acid accumulation during degradation.[107] PGA degrades more quickly but its stiffness and melting point (225°C) are too high for practical use. PLGA has properties between those of PLA and PGA, and its properties are tunable by varying the lactic/glycolic acid ratio in synthesis. This allows for fine control of the properties of PLGA toward the particular areas of interest.[100] PCL is used for its low (60°C) melting point and ease of processing, with slow degradation. PBT-PEG has been shown to have properties and degradation tunable by the length ratio of PEG to PBT block, but PBT itself is not fully biodegradable.[100] Generally, amphiphiles will need to be optimized for properties desirable for the specific application.

For PECMs, the most common core blocks are polyethyleneimine (PEI), poly(dimethylamino)ethyl methacrylate (PDMAEMA), polymethacrylate (PMA) and the polyamino acids polyaspartate (PLD), polyglutamate

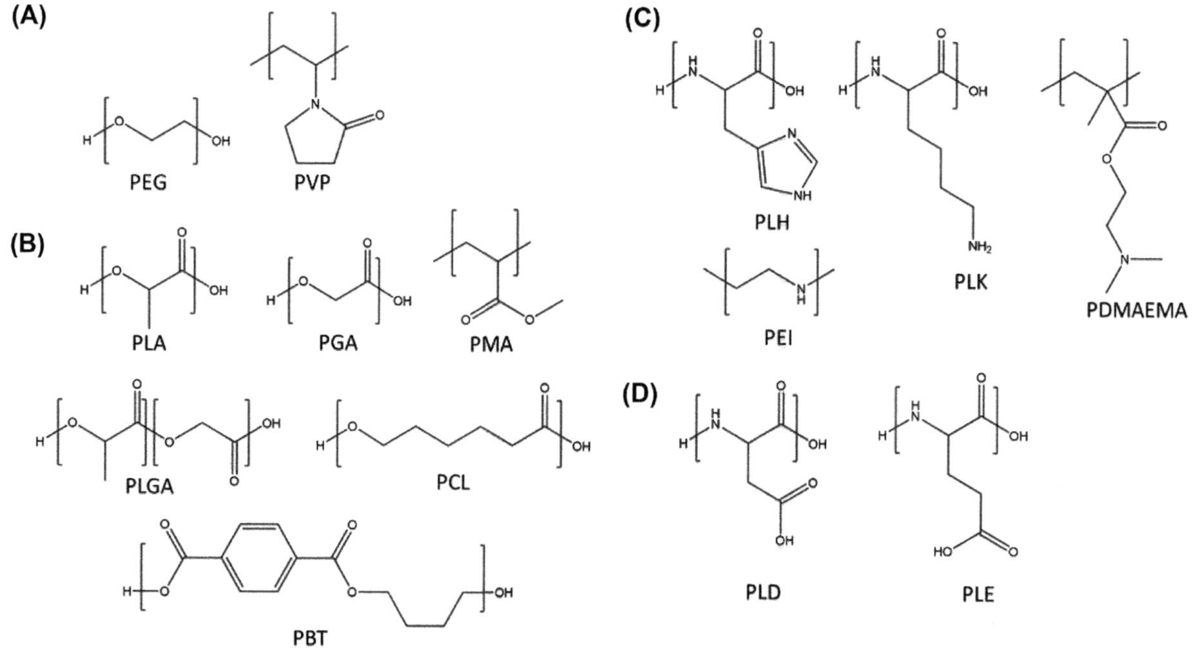

FIGURE 19.12 Structures of commonly used (A) hydrophilic, (B) hydrophobic, (C) cationic, and (D) anionic polymers.

(PLE), polyhistidine (PLH), and polylysine (PLK). The choice of charge depends on the charge of the desired cargo: for polyanionic oligonucleotides and plasmids, a polycation (PEI, PDMAEMA, PLK) is desired; for polycations, a polyanion (PMA, PLD, PLE) will be more suitable.[100,108,109] The properties and stability of PECMs tend to vary by the relative length of the polyion block to the PEG block, as well as the pKa of the polyion block. For example, at sufficiently high pH, polycations will neutralize and the micelle will degrade, but PLH-based micelles (pKa ~6.7) will be much less stable in general than PLK- or PEI-based micelles (pKa ~10).[101]

19.4.1 Biomedical applications of block copolymer nanoparticles

19.4.1.1 Drug delivery

Similar to peptide amphiphiles, block copolymer amphiphiles can solubilize hydrophobic molecules in their core for delivery. In general, the presence of the hydrophobic polymer will lead to incorporation of small hydrophobic molecules into the core of the micelle,[110,111] but the critical properties of drug solubility, micelle stability, and drug release kinetics will be influenced by the choice of hydrophobic polymer.[101] For example, Shuai et al. determined that the crystallinity of PCL in doxorubicin-encapsulated PEG-PCL micelles influenced the intermolecular interactions between drug and PCL, which ultimately reflected in the solubility of the doxorubicin in the micelle.[112] Lin et al. similarly demonstrated that the differential hydrophobicity of PLLA, PCL, and polyvalerolactone influenced the partitioning of indomethacin into the micelles' cores.[113,114] Further research suggests a general relationship between the calculated solubility of drug and polymer derived from group contribution theory and the empirical parameters of actual micelles.[114] Seta et al. demonstrated the utility of a hybrid polyion-hydrophobic core micelle for delivering siRNA to the brain, bypassing the blood–brain barrier.[115] Taking advantage of HIV Tat peptide as a polycation, they synthesized a self-assembling triphasic micelle upon incorporation of siRNA and was subsequently delivered intranasally to mice. The work demonstrated the utility of intranasal delivery of RNA as well as the ability of the micelle structure to facilitate uptake through the blood–brain barrier.

Like with peptide amphiphile micelles, active surface-targeting ligands are used in block copolymer systems to achieve enhanced drug delivery. In addition to peptide-targeting agents as previously discussed, antibodies have also been used on the surface of nanoparticles, such as Trastuzumab, a clinically approved, humanized antibody used to bind HER2. Investigators in the Shoichet group have coupled maleimide-modified Trastuzumab to the polymer poly(D,L-lactide-co-2-methyl-2-carboxytrimethylene carbonate)-graft-poly(ethylene glycol)-X (P(LA-co-TMCC)-g-PEG-X), with X representing furan.[116] Confocal imaging studies showed internalization of the particle in a human ovary cancer cell line, SKOV-3luc, while nonfunctionalized micelles showed no uptake. The targeting of HER2-overexpressing cells to promote receptor-mediated endocytosis demonstrates the feasibility of active ligands in vitro.

Another rising strategy for sustained drug delivery and tissue engineering is controlled degradation. Normally, the hydrophobic block will slowly degrade in vivo, but ideal degradation rates allow for a steady dosage of an encapsulated drug or coordinated replacement of a polymer scaffold with healing tissue.[100] The presence of the hydrophilic PEG block also speeds degradation by attracting water molecules to the vicinity of the hydrophobic block and thus facilitating hydrolytic degradation of the copolymer. Furthermore, the degradation rate has been found to be dependent upon PEG–polyester ratio.[117] Linker blocks such as polydioxanone (DX) can provide further control of degradation by providing different functionalities available for enzymatic reaction.[118] Miyamoto et al. demonstrated that when loaded with osteoinductive growth factor bone morphogenetic protein-2 (BMP-2), PLA-DX-PEG gels sustained steady growth of ectopic bone. For drug delivery, Moroni et al. demonstrated as a proof-of-concept a PEGT-PBT scaffold loaded with two different dyes.[119] The dyes were partially released in a large initial burst followed by sustained release for over a month. They were able to obtain similar results when tested with the drug dexamethasone.[120] Finally, PLA-PEG-PLA triblock copolymer was found to be effective for encapsulating and releasing angiogenic sphingosine 1-phosphate for wound healing, diabetic, and ischemic injury.[121–123] The tunability of block copolymers will likely permit further advances into sustained drug delivery.

19.4.1.2 Imaging

The properties of polymer micelles that make them suitable for drug delivery, such as tunable degradation and flexible incorporation of drug molecules into the structure, also make block copolymers suitable for imaging. As a case study, Gong et al. synthesized a branched amphiphilic block copolymer with doxorubicin incorporated covalently into the core of the micelle using an acid labile hydrazone linker, designated Boltorn H40-poly(L-glutamate-hydrazone-doxorubicin)-b-poly(ethylene glycol) (H40–P(LE-Hyd-DOX)-PEG) (Fig. 19.13).[124] The branches were variably functionalized with RGD peptide for tumor targeting or NOTA, a macrocyclic Cu-chelator, for[119] Cu PET imaging. The so-named H40-DOX-cRGD micelles were

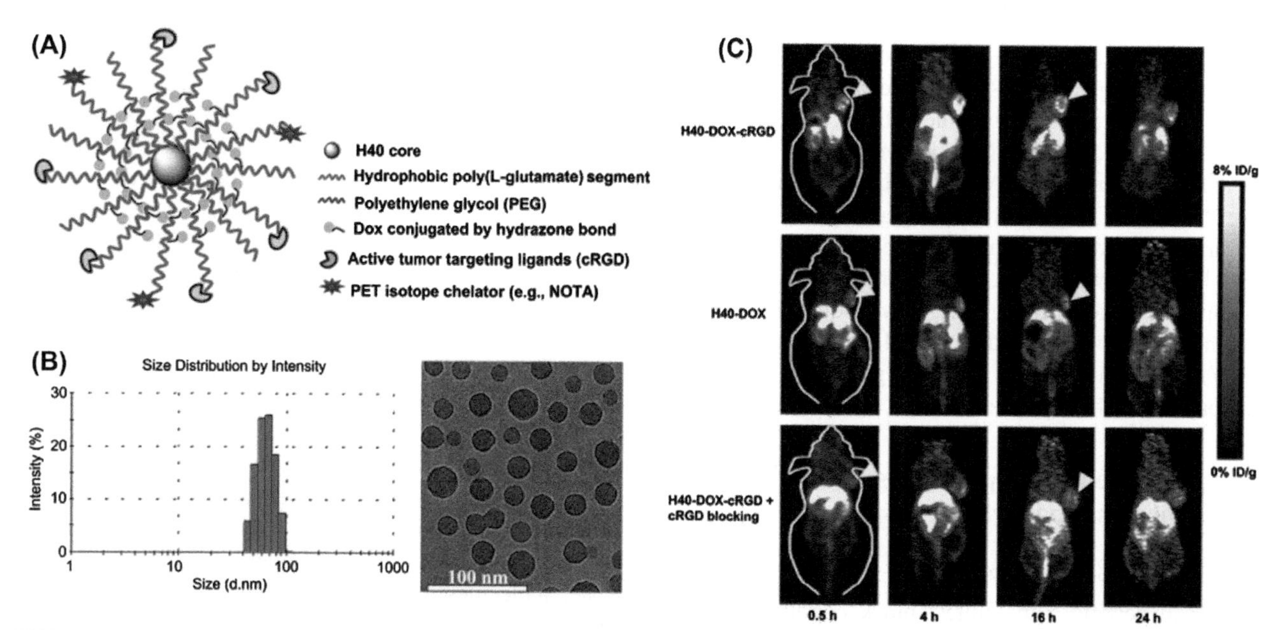

FIGURE 19.13 (A) Schematic of theranostic particles of Xiao et al. combining internally incorporated doxorubicin with copper-chelating NOTA moiety and tumor-targeting cRGD moiety. (B) H40-DOX-cRGD assemblies form spherical particles of approximately 60–70 nm diameter. (C) 64Cu-PET images of tumor-bearing mice demonstrate localization of H40-DOX-cRGD particles at the tumor site. *Adapted and reprinted from Xiao, Y., H. Hong, A. Javadi, J.W. Engle, W. Xu, Y. Yang, Y. Zhang, T.E. Barnhart, W. Cai, and S. Gong, Multifunctional unimolecular micelles for cancer-targeted drug delivery and positron emission tomography imaging. Biomaterials, 2012. 33(11): p. 3071–3082 with permission from Elsevier.*

found, using PET imaging, to accumulate in human glioblastoma cells via $\alpha_v\beta_3$-mediated endocytosis, whereas micelles without the RGD peptide were found not to accumulate nearly as well. The drug-loaded micelles were found to exhibit increased cytotoxicity in vivo as compared to a free doxorubicin control, which is likely due to the increased local concentration of doxorubicin due to the active targeting of the micelle construct. By incorporating engineering functionalities such as covalent labile linkage, hydrophobic assembly, and hydrophilic block functionalization for active targeting and imaging, the H40-DOX-cRGD system demonstrates the versatility afforded to engineering theranostic and diagnostic block copolymer micelles.

19.5 Dendrimers

The word "dendrimer" is derived from the Greek words "dendros," meaning trees, and "meros," meaning part. They are macromolecules, and their molecular weight is controlled by the repeated addition of functional sites, also known as focal points, to branching subunits. Each additional layer generates an increasing number of focal points, giving the dendrimer its characteristic exponential branching.[125] Traditionally, the total number of repeated focal point layers is defined as the dendrimer's generation number. Various chemistries have been used to generate these focal point linkages; the three most commonly used are "Lego," click, and ligation chemistries.[126] Commonly used dendrimer platforms include polyamidoamine (PAMAM), poly (propylene imine) (PPI), poly-L-lysine, melamine, poly (etherhydroxylamine) (PEHAM), poly (esteramine) (PEA), and polyglycerol.[127]

Dendrimers differ from classical polymers as they are not synthesized by uncontrolled polymerization reactions, but by stepwise protection and deprotection of functional sites.[128] The iterative strategy of linking monomers has been categorized into two main modalities. In divergent assembly, initially introduced by Vogtle et al.,[129] molecular growth proceeds from the central core outwards. In convergent assembly developed by Frechet et al.[130] in 1990, smaller constituents referred to as dendrons are synthesized, then combined to form the final dendrimer product (Fig. 19.14). While each technique offers distinct advantages and disadvantages, divergent synthesis methods are more prone to cumulative deletion errors and steric hindrance as generation number increases. Convergent methods generally require more individual reactions compared to a divergent counterpart of comparable generation. A comprehensive analysis of the considerations between divergent and convergent methods has been made by Meeijer et al.[131] Regardless of synthesis method, various interior layers composed of repeating units emanate from the core in the final product, while the spaces between branches can be quantified as "void space." One particular interest to biomedical engineering is the encapsulation of various small molecules within these void spaces. Furthermore, the multivalent surface of a dendrimer defines

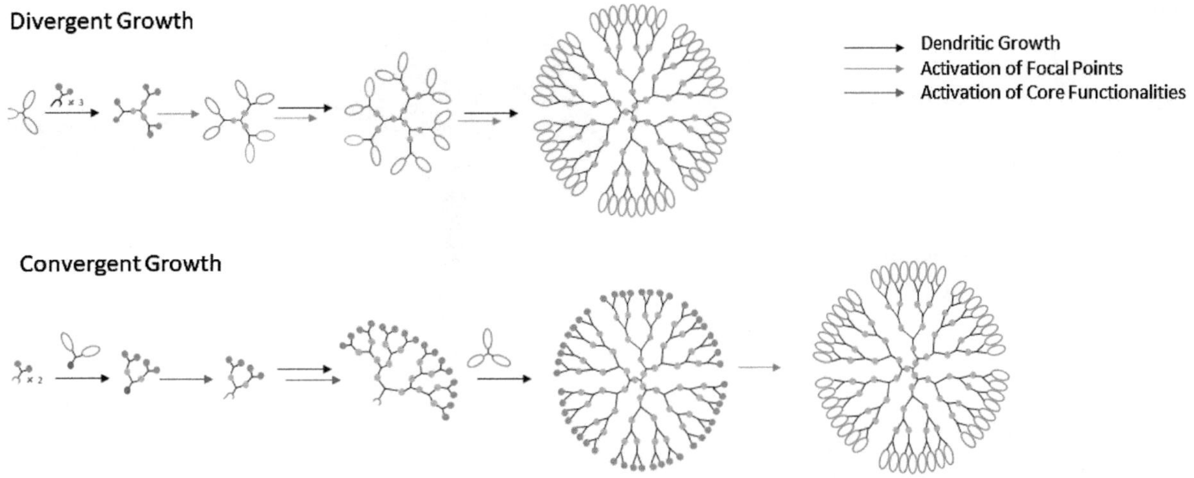

Divergent Growth

Convergent Growth

Dendritic Growth
Activation of Focal Points
Activation of Core Functionalities

FIGURE 19.14 Schematic overview of divergent and convergent dendrimer synthesis strategies, including growth and activation steps. *Adapted from Walter, M.V. and M. Malkoch, Simplifying the synthesis of dendrimers: accelerated approaches. Chem Soc Rev, 2012. 41(13): p. 4593–4609.*

the dendrimer's macroscopic properties and can be functionalized to display various moieties to the surrounding environment.[132]

PAMAM dendrimers are the most commonly studied and commercialized family of dendrimers and were firstly synthesized by coupling N-(2-aminoethyl) acryl amide monomers to an ammonia core.[127] However, one barrier to commercialization is the difficulty of carrying out a large-scale synthesis that reproducibly yields a uniform composition of the dendrimer product. Often touted for the ability to form the "perfect molecule" due to precise control of material layer by layer, the divergent and convergent synthesis methods are prone to populations of product that are only near-perfect. For example, in 2010, J R. Baker Jr. et al. revisited a previously published G5 dendrimer composed of four folic acid and five methotrexate molecules. This supposedly pure single molecule was instead found to be 182 different species when subjected to analytical high-performance liquid chromatography and ^{1}H nuclear magnetic resonance characterization; only about 4% of the dendrimer sample is composed of the nominal target molecule.[134] Therefore, efforts to boost reaction efficiency and reaction specificity are crucial for the widespread adoption of dendrimers.

Self-assembled dendrimers were explored as early as 1995 by Van Hest, utilizing amphiphilic dendrimers composed of a combination of polystyrene (PS) and poly(propylene imine). Based on generation number, spherical micelles, micellar rods, or vesicular structures were observed, while inverted micelles were observed at low generation numbers.[135] One common architecture is to utilize alkyl tails and other hydrophobic lipids conjugated to hydrophilic dendrimers to allow self-assembly in aqueous conditions. More complex, multilamellar self-assembled structures have been investigated, and take advantage of Janus dendrimers (Fig. 19.15), which are defined as dendrimers composed of different functional groups emanating from the core, often with differing hydrophobicity.[136,137] Interestingly, many researchers have used dendrimers as template scaffolds to direct the assembly of peptide amphiphiles as well, which is highlighted by the Tirrell group.[138] Precise control of supramolecular shape and size can be achievable with dendrimers to form the nanoparticle system, as physiochemical properties will dictate performance in eventual clinical applications. In this text, we will limit our scope to hydrophobically self-assembled dendrimers applied to biomedical engineering applications.

19.5.1 Biomedical applications of dendrimers

19.5.1.1 Drug delivery

The targeted delivery of drugs such as chemotherapeutics has seen quite an increase in research interest in the past decade. Reduction of the negative off-target organ side effects of traditional therapies is the main impetus, while decreasing tumor load and metastatic potential. Like many other nanocarriers previously discussed in this text, targeting is achieved by either passive size-based accumulation via EPR, or the utilization of targeting moieties presented on the outer layer of the dendrimer, which can be peptides, antibodies, antibody fragments, etc.

Self-assembled dendrimers composed of the ubiquitous PAMAM dendron and two hydrophobic C18 alkyl chains were used to encapsulate the anticancer drug doxorubicin.[139] Able to achieve 40% drug loading efficiency, these amphiphilic dendrimer (AmDM) nanocarriers showed a propensity to avoid drug efflux, a characteristic response of cells to many traditional small molecule chemotherapies.

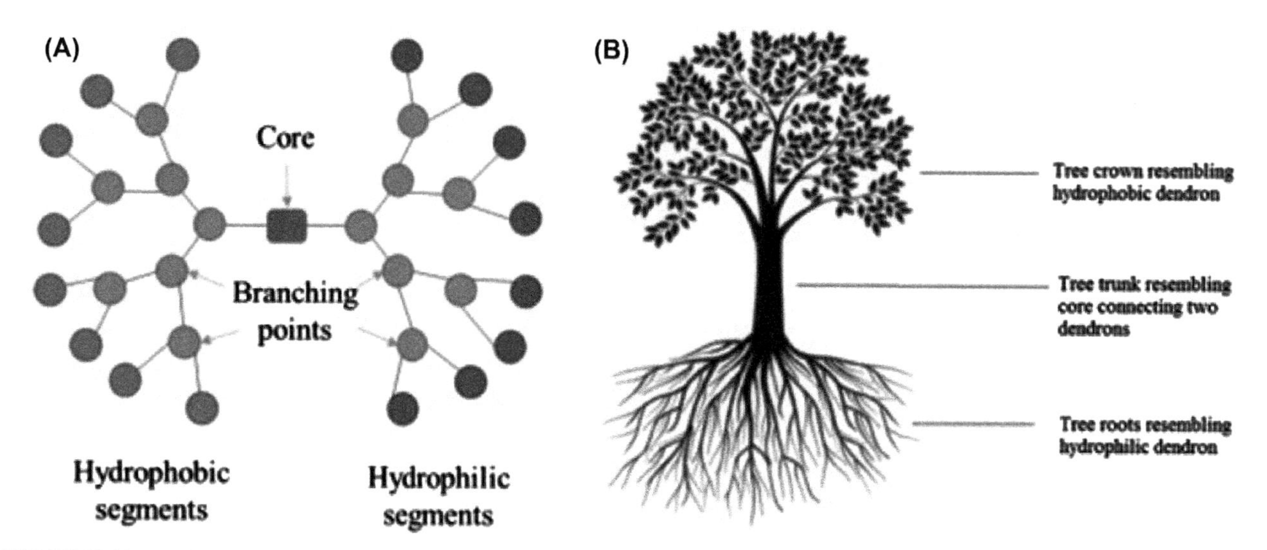

FIGURE 19.15 (A) Schematic representation of Janus dendrimers (JDs). (B) Structural homology of JDs to a tree. *Adapted and reprinted from Sikwal, D.R., R.S. Kalhapure, and T. Govender, An emerging class of amphiphilic dendrimers for pharmaceutical and biomedical applications: janus amphiphilic dendrimers. Eur J Pharm Sci, 2017. 97: p. 113–134 with permission from Elsevier.*

When administered to NOD scid gamma (NSG)-immunodeficient mice bearing subcutaneous tumors derived from drug resistant breast cancer MCF-7R cells, tumor volume was seen to be reduced by approximately 25% compared to free doxorubicin. Weight loss of the AmDM-treated mice was comparable to control mice, while considerable weight loss was observed for mice treated with free doxorubicin. This can be attributed to the preferential accumulation of the 10 nm diameter AmDMs at the tumor site, which is achieved with passive targeting via the EPR effect. Upon histological analysis of off-target organs, a reduction in cardiotoxicity and hepatotoxicity was seen.

In addition to the EPR effect, Janus dendrimers have been shown to differentiate healthy and diseased cells in vitro to preferentially deliver therapeutics. Polyester dendrimers based on 2,2-bis(hydroxymethyl)propionic acid (bis-MPA) monomers were used to administer the antimalarial drugs chloroquine (CQ) and primaquine (PQ) to *Plasmodium*-infected red blood cells (pRBCs), while leaving healthy RBCs unaffected.[140] This specificity can be attributed to the permeation pathways *Plasmodium* generates in its host cell, not present in healthy RBCs.[141] Interestingly, all the diameters for the Janus dendrimers were above 70 nm, which is the upper limit described for entry of simple macromolecules into malaria-infected erythrocytes. While specific a mechanism has yet to be elucidated in this study, the interplay of dendrimer supramolecular structure and diseased cell-specific uptake can be a powerful tool for targeted delivery.

One of the first reports to successfully utilize self-assembling dendrimers to deliver a genetic payload was published in 2012, with successful gene silencing in vivo. Yu et al. created PAMAM dendrimers conjugated to an alkyl chain, which self-assemble into complexes with siRNA.[142] SiRNA against heat shock protein 27 (Hsp27), a potent regulator of prostate cancer metastasis, was successfully delivered to nude mice bearing PC-3 xenograft tumors. Downregulation of Hsp27 at the mRNA and protein levels was 50% greater than scrambled siRNA. Advantages of dendrimer-based delivery vehicle over traditional viral delivery include a reduction in inflammatory, immunogenic, and mutagenic effects in the host, as shown by biocompatible results in MTT and LDH assays. Traditionally, PAMAM and similarly structured dendrimers are presumed to escape the late endosome due to the proton sponge effect, where the protonation of their interior primary amines causes the endosome to burst and release contents into the cytoplasm.[143,144] Similar amphiphilic dendrimers presented by Yu. et al. with either shorter alkyl chains or lower-generation dendrons failed to elicit significant gene silencing, validating the unique performance of the supramolecular nanostructures.

In addition to diffusive drug release, triggered release from physiochemical stimulus, such as light or pH, has also been investigated (Fig. 19.16).[145] Wang et al. demonstrated this using biocompatible crosslinkers such as coumarin, which has additional anticoagulant and anticancer properties. Coumarin undergoes cyclodimerization upon irradiation with 300 nm light, and upon irradiation with shorter wavelength UV light, displays the reversible dissociation into monomers. Coumarin was linked to a low-generation PAMAM dendrimer, which formed nanoclusters capable of light-sensitive payload release. Delivery of an enhanced green fluorescent protein (EGFP) plasmid into human breast adenocarcinoma cells increased transfection efficiency by 119-fold compared to commercial transfection

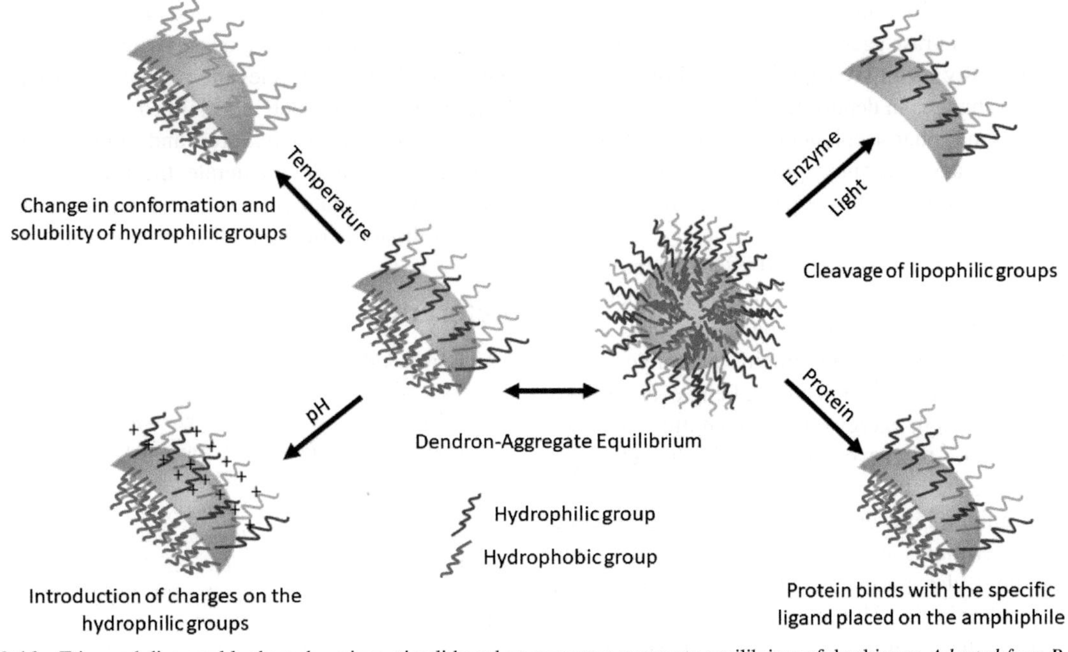

FIGURE 19.16 Triggered disassembly through various stimuli based on monomer-aggregate equilibrium of dendrimers. *Adapted from R. Ramireddy, R., K.R. Raghupathi, D.A. Torres, and S. Thayumanavan, Stimuli sensitive amphiphilic dendrimers. New J Chem, 2012. 36(2): p. 340–349.*

reagents such as Lipofectamine 2000.[146] The precise mechanisms of dendrimer genetic transfection are actively being investigated, but may be due to the hydrophobic coumarin allowing polyplexing with the nuclear membrane.

Most of the polymeric gene vectors are associated with negative correlation between transfection efficacy and cytotoxicity, especially PAMAMs. Dendrimer supramolecular structures, however, can achieve a balance between both. Genetic delivery with triggered release has been investigated in a study using hydrophobic, reactive oxygen species (ROS)-responsive poly-(propylenesulfide) (PPS) conjugated with low-generation PAMAMs. The thioether cores of the nanomicelles dissociated upon contact with intracellular ROS and released DNA payloads for transfection. While achieving similar transfection efficiency compared to Lipofectamine 2000 controls, these nonviral supramolecular dendrimers showed >90% cell viability due to ROS scavenging, while controls displayed <40% viability.[147]

19.5.1.2 Imaging

The ideal molecular imaging probe would be biocompatible, contain a high density of imaging payload, and selectively target the areas of interest in vivo. As focal point numbers increase exponentially with generation number, terminal focal points can have a fluorophore or imaging agent conjugated. Conventional imaging agents for magnetic resonance (MR) and computer tomography (CT) are small molecules, which exhibit rapid renal clearance. This

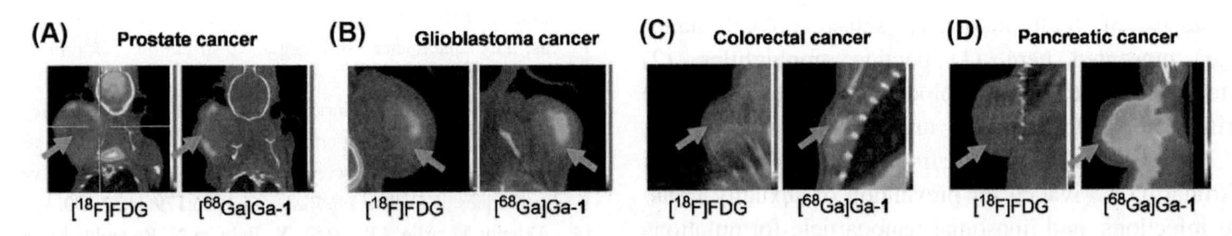

FIGURE 19.17 Radiolabeled dendrimer [68Ga]Ga-1 for Positron emission tomography (PET) imaging of various tumors. Tumor targeting and uptake assessment of [68Ga]Ga-1 in mouse ectopic xenograft models of (A) prostate adenocarcinoma (22Rv1 cell line), (B) glioma (U87 cell line), (C) colorectal adenocarcinoma (HT-29 cell line), and (C) pancreatic adenocarcinoma (SOJ-6 cell line) in comparison with [18F] FDG, the clinical gold reference for PET imaging in oncology. Up to a 14-fold increase in PET signal ratios are seen compared to [18F] FDG. *Adapted and reprinted from P. Garrigue, J. Tang, L. Ding, A. Bouhlel, A. Tintaru, E. Laurini, Y. Huang, Z. Lyu, M. Zhang, S. Fernandez, L. Balasse, W. Lan, E. Mas, D. Marson, Y. Weng, X. Liu, S. Giorgio, J. Iovanna, S. Pricl, B. Guillet, and L. Peng, Self-assembling supramolecular dendrimer nanosystem for PET imaging of tumors. Proc Natl Acad Sci, 2018 with permission from PNAS.*

limits their applicability to short-term imaging sessions on the order of hours. Unlike small molecules, supramolecular dendrimer-based contrast agents offer much greater flexibility and tuneability for in vivo applications. For example, even nanoscale changes in dendrimer size result in changes in biodistribution, pharmacokinetics, imaging payload loading capacity, and clearance properties, allowing the most optimal conditions to be selected for specific purposes.

Positron emission tomography (PET) imaging is a commonly used nuclear imaging modality which has femtomolar sensitivity and high tissue penetration. Combined with X-ray computed tomography, anatomic localization of PET targets can be colocalized. Peng et al. utilized gallium-68 as the high-energy positron emitter radioisotope. Dendritic 1,4,7-triazacyclononane-1,4,7-triacetic acid (NOTA) was used as the gallium chelator, forming the characteristic amphiphilic dendrimer construct composed of four NOTA terminals and one hydrophobic alkyl chain. These supramolecular micelles increased the radiotracer half-life from 68 min to 171 ± 42 min. PET imaging was carried out using the dendrimer nanomicelles, designated as [68Ga]Ga-1, to quantify their tumor targeting and uptake in various xenograft mouse models of cancer, including human prostate carcinoma, human glioblastoma, human colorectal adenocarcinoma, and human pancreatic adenocarcinoma (Fig. 19.17). In almost all cases, the observed effective tumor uptake and tumor-to-background ratios with [68Ga] Ga-1 were superior to those obtained with fludeoxyglucose F 18 ([18F]FDG), the clinical gold standard for PET imaging in oncology.[148] Interestingly, the supramolecular assemblies avoided off-tumor accumulation in the metabolically active tissues such as muscle and heart, a known drawback of current [18F]FDG formulations.

19.5.1.3 Conclusion

Control over the nanoscale in medicine, and more specifically in drug delivery and imaging applications, is set to increase at a hastened pace. A conceptual understanding of biological responses to nanomaterials is needed to develop and apply nanomaterials in biomedical engineering. The four classes of hydrophobically self-assembled nanoparticles presented here, (1) peptide amphiphiles, (2) nucleic acid constructs, (3) block copolymers, and (4) dendrimers, provide their own unique benefits and drawbacks. With the emergence of commercial dendrimers such as Starpharma's VivaGel for prevention of sexually transmitted infections, and liposomal nanoparticle formulations of Dox in Janssen's Doxil, we are witnessing the steady translation of nanomedicine from the lab bench to the clinic. This is especially evident in the pipeline of nanosized solutions in clinical trials, such as Paclitaxel-loaded micelles, and Auroshell nanoparticles by Nanospectra for MRI imaging. The challenges that lie ahead include the optimization of synthesis methods to generate homogenous nanoparticle products in a cost-efficient manner, as well as the identification of relevant patient subgroups that will benefit from any such specialized targeted therapies.[149] After two decades of research and clinical trial work, opportunities lie ahead to iterate these designs in the next generation, ultimately to improve clinical outcomes and sharpen the tools of biomedical engineering.

References

1. Ferreira LMB, Kiill CP, Pedreiro LN, Santos AM, Gremião MPD. Chapter 5 – supramolecular design of hydrophobic and hydrophilic polymeric nanoparticles A2 – grumezescu, Alexandru Mihai. In: *Design and development of new nanocarriers*. William Andrew Publishing; 2018. p. 181–221.
2. Lehn JM. Cryptates: the chemistry of macropolycyclic inclusion complexes. *Accounts of Chemical Research* 1978;**11**(2):49–57.
3. Kolesnichenko IV, Anslyn EV. Practical applications of supramolecular chemistry. *Chem Soc Rev* 2017;**46**(9):2385–90.
4. Lehn J-M. Toward complex matter: supramolecular chemistry and self-organization. *Proc Natl Acad Sci* 2002;**99**(8):4763.
5. Law K-Y, Zhao H. Contact angle measurements and surface characterization techniques. In: *Surface Wetting: characterization, contact angle, and fundamentals*. Cham: Springer International Publishing; 2016. p. 7–34.
6. Dan G, Guoxin X, Jianbin L. Mechanical properties of nanoparticles: basics and applications. *J Phys D Appl Phys* 2014;**47**(1):013001.
7. Zhu C, Gao Y, Li H, Meng S, Li L, Francisco JS, Zeng XC. Characterizing hydrophobicity of amino acid side chains in a protein environment via measuring contact angle of a water nanodroplet on planar peptide network. *Proc Natl Acad Sci* 2016;**113**(46):12946.
8. Bandyopadhyay D, Choudhury N. Characterizing hydrophobicity at the nanoscale: a molecular dynamics simulation study. *J Chem Phys* 2012;**136**(22):224505.
9. Fu IW, Markegard CB, Chu BK, Nguyen HD. Role of hydrophobicity on self-assembly by peptide amphiphiles via molecular dynamics simulations. *Langmuir* 2014;**30**(26):7745–54.
10. Xiao Y, Wiesner MR. Characterization of surface hydrophobicity of engineered nanoparticles. *J Hazard Mater* 2012;**215–216**:146–51.
11. Sangster J. Octanol-water partition coefficients of simple organic compounds. *J Phys Chem Ref Data* 1989;**18**(3):1111–229.
12. Sven S, Keck CM, Muller RH. The "real environment" quantification of surface hydrophobicity of differently stabilized nanocrystals as key parameter for organ distribution. *Macromol Symp* 2014;**345**(1):32–41.
13. Drelich J, Miller JD, Good RJ. The effect of drop (bubble) size on advancing and receding contact angles for heterogeneous and rough solid surfaces as observed with sessile-drop and captive-bubble techniques. *J Colloid Interface Sci* 1996;**179**(1):37–50.
14. Akbulut M, Alig ARG, Min Y, Belman N, Reynolds M, Golan Y, Israelachvili J. Forces between surfaces across nanoparticle Solutions: role of size, shape, and concentration. *Langmuir* 2007;**23**(7):3961–9.
15. Donaldson SH, Lee CT, Chmelka BF, Israelachvili JN. General hydrophobic interaction potential for surfactant/lipid bilayers from

direct force measurements between light-modulated bilayers. *Proc Natl Acad Sci* 2011;**108**(38):15699.

16. Ruiz-Cabello FJM, Maroni P, Borkovec M. Direct measurements of forces between different charged colloidal particles and their prediction by the theory of Derjaguin, Landau, Verwey, and Overbeek (DLVO). *J Chem Phys* 2013;**138**(23):234705.
17. Kaali Peter, Stromberg Emma, Karlsson Sigbritt. Prevention of biofilm associated infections and degradation of polymeric materials used in biomedical applications. In: *Biomedical engineering, trends in materials science*; 2011.
18. Rennie R. *DLVO theory*. Oxford University Press; 2016.
19. Maibaum L, Dinner AR, Chandler D. Micelle formation and the hydrophobic effect. *J Phys Chem B* 2004;**108**(21):6778−81.
20. Patist A, Bhagwat SS, Penfield KW, Aikens P, Shah DO. On the measurement of critical micelle concentrations of pure and technical-grade nonionic surfactants. *J Surfactants Deterg* 2000;**3**(1):53−8.
21. Hüttl C, Hettrich C, Miller R, Paulke B-R, Henklein P, Rawel H, Bier FF. Self-assembled peptide amphiphiles function as multivalent binder with increased hemagglutinin affinity. *BMC Biotechnol* 2013;**13**(1):51.
22. Israelachvili JN. 10 - unifying concepts in intermolecular and interparticle forces. In: Israelachvili JN, editor. *Intermolecular and surface forces*. 3rd ed. Boston: Academic Press; 2011. p. 191−204.
23. Trent A, Marullo R, Lin B, Black M, Tirrell M. Structural properties of soluble peptide amphiphile micelles. *Soft Matter* 2011;**7**(20):9572−82.
24. Shimada T, Sakamoto N, Motokawa R, Koizumi S, Tirrell M. Self-assembly process of peptide amphiphile worm-like micelles. *J Phys Chem B* 2012;**116**(1):240−3.
25. Lombardo D, Kiselev MA, Magazu S, Calandra P. Amphiphiles self-assembly: basic concepts and future perspectives of supramolecular approaches. *Adv Condens Matter Phys* 2015;**2015**:22.
26. Missirlis D, Chworos A, Fu CJ, Khant HA, Krogstad DV, Tirrell M. Effect of the peptide secondary structure on the peptide amphiphile supramolecular structure and interactions. *Langmuir* 2011;**27**(10):6163−70.
27. Shrestha RG, Nomura K, Yamamoto M, Yamawaki Y, Tamura Y, Sakai K, Sakamoto K, Sakai H, Abe M. Peptide-based gemini amphiphiles: phase behavior and rheology of wormlike micelles. *Langmuir* 2012;**28**(44):15472−81.
28. Shimada T, Megley K, Tirrell M, Hotta A. Fluid mechanical shear induces structural transitions in assembly of a peptide−lipid conjugate. *Soft Matter* 2011;**7**(19):8856−61.
29. Cui H, Webber MJ, Stupp SI. Self-assembly of peptide amphiphiles: from molecules to nanostructures to biomaterials. *Peptide Science* 2010;**94**(1):1−18.
30. Accardo A, Vitiello M, Tesauro D, Galdiero M, Finamore E, Martora F, Mansi R, Ringhieri P, Morelli G. Self-assembled or mixed peptide amphiphile micelles from Herpes simplex virus glycoproteins as potential immunomodulatory treatment. *Int J Nanomed* 2014;**9**:2137−48.
31. Javali NM, Raj A, Saraf P, Li X, Jasti B. Fatty acid−RGD peptide amphiphile micelles as potential paclitaxel delivery carriers to αvβ3Integrin overexpressing tumors. *Pharm Res* 2012;**29**(12):3347−61.
32. Yang Q, Moulder k R, Cohen MS, Cai S, Forrest LM. Cabozantinib loaded DSPE-PEG(2000) micelles as delivery system: formulation, characterization and cytotoxicity evaluation. *BAOJ Pharma Sci* 2015;**1**:001.
33. Zhao Y, Zeng Q, Wu F, Li J, Pan Z, Shen P, Yang L, Xu T, Cai L, Guo L. Novel naproxen-peptide-conjugated amphiphilic dendrimer self-assembly micelles for targeting drug delivery to osteosarcoma cells. *RSC Adv* 2016;**6**(65):60327−35.
34. Chung EJ, Mlinar LB, Sugimoto MJ, Nord K, Roman BB, Tirrell M. In vivo biodistribution and clearance of peptide amphiphile micelles. *Nanomed Nanotechnol Biol Med* 2015;**11**(2):479−87.
35. Fields GB. Introduction to peptide synthesis. In: *Current protocols in protein science*; 2002 [Chapter 18]: p. Unit-18.1.
36. Samad MB, Chhonker YS, Contreras JI, McCarthy A, McClanahan MM, Murry DJ, Conda-Sheridan M. Developing polyamine-based peptide amphiphiles with tunable morphology and physicochemical properties. *Macromol Biosci* 2017;**17**(8):1700096.
37. Black KA, Lin BF, Wonder EA, Desai SS, Chung EJ, Ulery BD, Katari RS, Tirrell MV. Biocompatibility and characterization of a peptide amphiphile hydrogel for applications in peripheral nerve regeneration. *Tissue Eng A* 2015;**21**(7−8):1333−42.
38. Choi HS, Liu W, Misra P, Tanaka E, Zimmer JP, Ipe BI, Bawendi MG, Frangioni JV. Renal clearance of nanoparticles. *Nat Biotechnol* 2007;**25**(10):1165−70.
39. Duan X, Li Y. Physicochemical characteristics of nanoparticles affect circulation, biodistribution, cellular internalization, and trafficking. *Small* 2013;**9**(9-10):1521−32.
40. Burns AA, Vider J, Ow H, Herz E, Penate-Medina O, Baumgart M, Larson SM, Wiesner U, Bradbury M. Fluorescent silica nanoparticles with efficient urinary excretion for nanomedicine. *Nano Lett* 2009;**9**(1):442−8.
41. Lu J, Owen SC, Shoichet MS. Stability of self-assembled polymeric micelles in serum. *Macromolecules* 2011;**44**(15):6002−8.
42. Iwasaki A, Medzhitov R. Control of adaptive immunity by the innate immune system. *Nat Immunol* 2015;**16**(4):343−53.
43. Janeway Jr CA, Travers P, Walport M, et al. *Immunobiology: the immune system in health and disease*. 5th ed. New York: Garland Science; 2001.
44. Hudalla GA, Modica JA, Tian YF, Rudra JS, Chong AS, Sun T, Mrksich M, Collier JH. A self-adjuvanting supramolecular vaccine carrying a folded protein antigen. *Adv Healthc Mater* 2013;**2**(8):1114−9.
45. Tan Y-V, Abad C, Wang Y, Lopez R, Waschek J. VPAC2 (vasoactive intestinal peptide receptor type 2) receptor deficient mice develop exacerbated experimental autoimmune encephalomyelitis with increased Thl/Th17 and reduced Th2/Treg responses. *Brain Behav Immun* 2015;**44**:167−75.
46. Delgado M, Ganea D. Vasoactive intestinal peptide: a neuropeptide with pleiotropic immune functions. *Amino Acids* 2013;**45**(1). https://doi.org/10.1007/s00726-011-1184-8.
47. Delgado M, Munoz-Elias EJ, Gomariz RP, Ganea D. Vasoactive intestinal peptide and pituitary adenylate cyclase-activating polypeptide enhance IL-10 production by Murine macrophages: in vitro and in vivo studies. *J Immunol* 1999;**162**(3):1707.
48. Delgado M, Abad C, Martinez C, Leceta J, Gomariz RP. Vasoactive intestinal peptide prevents experimental arthritis by downregulating both autoimmune and inflammatory components of the disease. *Nat Med* 2001;**7**:563.
49. Gonzalez-Rey E, Fernandez-Martin A, Chorny A, Martin J, Pozo D, Ganea D, Delgado M. Therapeutic effect of vasoactive intestinal peptide on experimental autoimmune encephalomyelitis : down-regulation of inflammatory and autoimmune responses. *Am J Pathol* 2006;**168**(4):1179−88.
50. Villanueva-Romero R, Gutiérrez-Cañas I, Carrión M, Pérez-García S, Seoane IV, Martínez C, Gomariz RP, Juarranz Y. The

anti-inflammatory mediator, vasoactive intestinal peptide, Modulates the differentiation and function of Th subsets in rheumatoid arthritis. *J Immunol Res* 2018:6043710. 2018.

51. Zhang R, Leeper CN, Wang X, White TA, Ulery BD. Immunomodulatory vasoactive intestinal peptide amphiphile micelles. *Biomater Sci* 2018.
52. Lin T-C, Chen J-H, Chen Y-H, Teng T-m, Su C-H, Hsu S-h. Biodegradable micelles from a hyaluronan-poly(ε-caprolactone) graft copolymer as nanocarriers for fibroblast growth factor 1. *J Mater Chem B* 2013;**1**(43):5977–87.
53. Zhang R, Kramer JS, Smith JD, Allen BN, Leeper CN, Li X, Morton LD, Gallazzi F, Ulery BD. Vaccine adjuvant incorporation strategy dictates peptide amphiphile micelle immunostimulatory capacity. *AAPS J* 2018;**20**(4):73.
54. Sun T, Han H, Hudalla GA, Wen Y, Pompano RR, Collier JH. Thermal stability of self-assembled peptide vaccine materials. *Acta Biomater* 2016;**30**:62–71.
55. Pompano RR, Chen J, Verbus EA, Han H, Fridman A, McNeely T, Collier JH, Chong AS. Titrating T-cell epitopes within self-assembled vaccines optimizes CD^{4+} helper T cell and antibody outputs. *Adv Healthc Mater* 2014;**3**(11):1898–908.
56. Chen J, Pompano RR, Santiago FW, Maillat L, Sciammas R, Sun T, Han H, Topham DJ, Chong AS, Collier JH. The use of self-adjuvanting nanofiber vaccines to elicit high-affinity B cell responses to peptide antigens without inflammation. *Biomaterials* 2013;**34**(34):8776–85.
57. Chung EJ, Cheng Y, Morshed R, Nord K, Han Y, Wegscheid ML, Auffinger B, Wainwright DA, Lesniak MS, Tirrell MV. Fibrin-binding, peptide amphiphile micelles for targeting glioblastoma(☆). *Biomaterials* 2014;**35**(4):1249–56.
58. Yoo SP, Pineda F, Barrett JC, Poon C, Tirrell M, Chung EJ. Gadolinium-functionalized peptide amphiphile micelles for Multimodal imaging of atherosclerotic lesions. *ACS Omega* 2016;**1**(5):996–1003.
59. Finn AV, Nakano M, Narula J, Kolodgie FD, Virmani R. Concept of vulnerable/unstable plaque. *Arterioscler Thromb Vasc Biol* 2010;**30**:1282–92.
60. Mlinar LB, Chung EJ, Wonder EA, Tirrell M. Active targeting of early and mid-stage atherosclerotic plaques using self-assembled peptide amphiphile micelles. *Biomaterials* 2014;**35**(30):8678–86.
61. Libby P. History of discovery: inflammation in atherosclerosis. *Arterioscler Thromb Vasc Biol* 2012;**32**(9):2045–51.
62. Ley K, Huo Y. VCAM-1 is critical in atherosclerosis. *J Clin Investig* 2001;**107**(10):1209–10.
63. Swirski FK, Pittet MJ, Kircher MF, Aikawa E, Jaffer FA, Libby P, Weissleder R. Monocyte accumulation in mouse atherogenesis is progressive and proportional to extent of disease. *Proc Natl Acad Sci USA* 2006;**103**(27):10340–5.
64. Chung EJ, Nord K, Sugimoto MJ, Wonder E, Tirrell M, Mlinar LB, Alenghat FJ, Fang Y. Monocyte-targeting supramolecular micellar assemblies: a molecular diagnostic tool for atherosclerosis. *Adv Healthc Mater* 2015;**4**(3):367–76.
65. Poon C, Chowdhuri S, Kuo C-H, Fang Y, Alenghat FJ, Hyatt D, Kani K, Gross ME, Chung EJ. Protein Mimetic and anticancer properties of monocyte-targeting peptide amphiphile micelles. *ACS Biomater Sci Eng* 2017;**3**(12):3273–82.
66. Chakravarty R, Hong H, Cai W. Positron emission tomography image-guided drug delivery: current status and future perspectives. *Mol Pharm* 2014;**11**(11):3777–97.
67. Cho H, Lai TC, Kwon GS. Poly(ethylene glycol)-block-poly(ε-caprolactone) micelles for combination drug delivery: evaluation of paclitaxel, cyclopamine and gossypol in intraperitoneal xenograft models of ovarian cancer. *J Control Release* 2013;**166**(1):1–9.
68. Su Z, Shen H, Wang H, Wang J, Li J, Nienhaus GU, Shang L, Wei G. Motif-designed peptide nanofibers decorated with graphene quantum dots for simultaneous targeting and imaging of tumor cells. *Adv Funct Mater* 2015;**25**(34):5472–8.
69. Yang Z, Lee JH, Jeon HM, Han JH, Park N, He Y, Lee H, Hong KS, Kang C, Kim JS. Folate-based near-infrared fluorescent theranostic gemcitabine delivery. *J Am Chem Soc* 2013;**135**(31):11657–62.
70. Wu X, Sun X, Guo Z, Tang J, Shen Y, James TD, Tian H, Zhu W. In vivo and in situ tracking cancer chemotherapy by highly photostable NIR fluorescent theranostic prodrug. *J Am Chem Soc* 2014;**136**(9):3579–88.
71. Lock LL, Cheetham AG, Zhang P, Cui H. Design and construction of supramolecular nanobeacons for enzyme detection. *ACS Nano* 2013;**7**(6):4924–32.
72. Langereis S, Geelen T, Grüll H, Strijkers GJ, Nicolay K. Paramagnetic liposomes for molecular MRI and MRI-guided drug delivery. *NMR Biomed* 2013;**26**(7):728–44.
73. Lock LL, Li Y, Mao X, Chen H, Staedtke V, Bai R, Ma W, Lin R, Li Y, Liu G, Cui H. One-component supramolecular filament hydrogels as theranostic label-free magnetic resonance imaging agents. *ACS Nano* 2017;**11**(1):797–805.
74. Webber MJ, Kessler JA, Stupp SI. Emerging peptide nanomedicine to regenerate tissues and organs. *J Intern Med* 2010;**267**(1):71–88.
75. Zhang S, Greenfield MA, Mata A, Palmer LC, Bitton R, Mantei JR, Aparicio C, de la Cruz MO, Stupp SI. A self-assembly pathway to aligned monodomain gels. *Nat Mater* 2010;**9**:594.
76. Greene JJ, McClendon MT, Stephanopoulos N, Álvarez Z, Stupp SI, Richter C-P. Electrophysiological assessment of a peptide amphiphile nanofiber nerve graft for facial nerve repair. *J Tissue Eng Regenerat Med* 2018;**12**(6):1389–401.
77. Angeloni NL, Bond CW, Tang Y, Harrington DA, Zhang S, Stupp SI, McKenna KE, Podlasek CA. Regeneration of the cavernous nerve by Sonic hedgehog using aligned peptide amphiphile nanofibers. *Biomaterials* 2011;**32**(4):1091–101.
78. Hehemann M, Kalmanek E, Choe S, Dynda D, Hu W-Y, Quek ML, Harrington DA, Stupp SI, McVary KT, Podlasek CA. Sonic hedgehog regulation of human rhabdosphincter muscle:Potential implications for treatment of stress urinary incontinence. *Neurourol Urodyn* 2018;**37**(8):2551–9.
79. Motalleb R, Berns EJ, Patel P, Gold J, Stupp SI, Kuhn HG. In vivo migration of endogenous brain progenitor cells guided by an injectable peptide amphiphile biomaterial. *J Tissue Eng Regenerat Med* 2018;**12**(4):e2123–33.
80. Seeman NC. Nucleic acid junctions and lattices. *J Theor Biol* 1982;**99**(2):237–47.
81. Zhang T-b, Zhang C-l, Dong Z-l, Guan Y-f. Determination of base binding strength and base stacking interaction of DNA duplex using atomic force microscope. *Sci Rep* 2015;**5**. pp. 9143–9143.
82. Schiffels D, Liedl T, Fygenson DK. Nanoscale structure and Microscale stiffness of DNA nanotubes. *ACS Nano* 2013;**7**(8):6700–10.
83. Rothemund PWK. Folding DNA to create nanoscale shapes and patterns. *Nature* 2006;**440**:297.

84. Li H, Carter JD, LaBean TH. Nanofabrication by DNA self-assembly. *Mater Today* 2009;**12**(5):24–32.
85. Haipeng L, Zhi Z, Huaizhi K, Yanrong W, Kwame S, Weihong T. DNA-Based micelles: synthesis, micellar properties and size-dependent cell permeability. *Chem Eur J* 2010;**16**(12):3791–7.
86. Kwak M, Herrmann A. Nucleic acid amphiphiles: synthesis and self-assembled nanostructures. *Chem Soc Rev* 2011;**40**(12):5745–55.
87. Wang W, Wan W, Zhou H-H, Niu S, Li ADQ. Alternating DNA and π-conjugated sequences. Thermophilic foldable polymers. *J Am Chem Soc* 2003;**125**(18):5248–9.
88. Jeong JH, Park TG. Novel Polymer–DNA hybrid polymeric micelles composed of hydrophobic poly(d,l-lactic-co-glycolic acid) and hydrophilic oligonucleotides. *Bioconjug Chem* 2001;**12**(6):917–23.
89. Li J, Fan C, Pei H, Shi J, Huang Q. Smart drug delivery nanocarriers with self-assembled DNA nanostructures. *Adv Mater* 2013;**25**(32):4386–96.
90. Tang J, Zhang R, Guo M, Shao L, Liu Y, Zhao Y, Zhang S, Wu Y, Chen C. Nucleosome-inspired nanocarrier obtains encapsulation efficiency enhancement and side effects reduction in chemotherapy by using fullerenol assembled with doxorubicin. *Biomaterials* 2018;**167**:205–15.
91. Jiang Q, Song C, Nangreave J, Liu X, Lin L, Qiu D, Wang Z-G, Zou G, Liang X, Yan H, Ding B. DNA origami as a carrier for circumvention of drug resistance. *J Am Chem Soc* 2012;**134**(32):13396–403.
92. Lee SH, Lee JY, Kim JS, Park TG, Mok H. Amphiphilic siRNA conjugates for Co-delivery of nucleic acids and hydrophobic drugs. *Bioconjug Chem* 2017;**28**(8):2051–61.
93. Hayes ME, Drummond DC, Kirpotin DB, Zheng WW, Noble Iv CO, Park JW, Marks JD, Benz CC, Hong K. Genospheres: self-assembling nucleic acid-lipid nanoparticles suitable for targeted gene delivery. *Gene Ther* 2005;**13**:646.
94. Bousmail D, Amrein L, Fakhoury JJ, Fakih HH, Hsu JCC, Panasci L, Sleiman HF. Precision spherical nucleic acids for delivery of anticancer drugs. *Chem Sci* 2017;**8**(9):6218–29.
95. Yuliia V, Mykhailo V, Rudnev AV, Robert H. DNA-grafted supramolecular polymers: helical ribbon structures formed by self-assembly of pyrene–DNA chimeric oligomers. *Angew Chem Int Ed* 2015;**54**(27):7934–8.
96. Lin C, Katilius E, Liu Y, Zhang J, Yan H. Self-assembled signaling aptamer DNA arrays for protein detection. *Angew Chem Int Ed* 2006;**45**(32):5296–301.
97. Jhaveri SD, Kirby R, Conrad R, Maglott EJ, Bowser M, Kennedy RT, Glick G, Ellington AD. Designed signaling aptamers that transduce molecular recognition to changes in fluorescence intensity. *J Am Chem Soc* 2000;**122**(11):2469–73.
98. Bhatia D, Surana S, Chakraborty S, Koushika SP, Krishnan Y. A synthetic icosahedral DNA-based host–cargo complex for functional in vivo imaging. *Nat Commun* 2011;**2**:339.
99. Kim MP, Yi G-R. Nanostructured colloidal particles by confined self-assembly of block copolymers in evaporative droplets. *Frontiers in Materials* 2015;**2**(45).
100. Kutikov AB, Song J. Biodegradable PEG-based amphiphilic block copolymers for tissue engineering applications. *ACS Biomater Sci Eng* 2015;**1**(7):463–80.
101. Gaucher G, Dufresne M-H, Sant VP, Kang N, Maysinger D, Leroux J-C. Block copolymer micelles: preparation, characterization and application in drug delivery. *J Control Release* 2005;**109**(1):169–88.
102. Wu J, Akaike T, Maeda H. Modulation of enhanced vascular permeability in tumors by a bradykinin antagonist, a cyclooxygenase inhibitor, and a nitric oxide scavenger. *Cancer Res* 1998;**58**(1):159–65.
103. Nishiyama N, Kato Y, Sugiyama Y, et al. Cisplatin-loaded polymer-metal complex micelle with time-modulated decaying property as a novel drug delivery system. *Pharm Res* 2001;**18**:1035.
104. Zhang L, Eisenberg A. Multiple Morphologies and characteristics of "Crew-Cut" micelle-like aggregates of polystyrene-b-poly(acrylic acid) diblock copolymers in aqueous solutions. *J Am Chem Soc* 1996;**118**(13):3168–81.
105. Madsen J, Armes SP. (Meth)acrylic stimulus-responsive block copolymer hydrogels. *Soft Matter* 2012;**8**(3):592–605.
106. Yamamoto Y, Nagasaki Y, Kato Y, Sugiyama Y, Kataoka K. Long-circulating poly(ethylene glycol)–poly(d,l-lactide) block copolymer micelles with modulated surface charge. *J Control Release* 2001;**77**(1):27–38.
107. Miller RA, Brady JM, Cutright DE. Degradation rates of oral resorbable implants (polylactates and polyglycolates): rate modification with changes in PLA/PGA copolymer ratios. *J Biomed Mater Res* 1977;**11**(5):711–9.
108. Oishi M, Sasaki S, Nagasaki Y, Kataoka K. pH-responsive oligodeoxynucleotide (ODN)–Poly(Ethylene glycol) conjugate through acid-labile β-thiopropionate linkage: preparation and polyion complex micelle formation. *Biomacromolecules* 2003;**4**(5):1426–32.
109. Wakebayashi D, Nishiyama N, Yamasaki Y, Itaka K, Kanayama N, Harada A, Nagasaki Y, Kataoka K. Lactose-conjugated polyion complex micelles incorporating plasmid DNA as a targetable gene vector system: their preparation and gene transfecting efficiency against cultured HepG2 cells. *J Control Release* 2004;**95**(3):653–64.
110. Fournier E, Dufresne M-H, Smith DC, Ranger M, Leroux J-C. A novel one-step drug loading procedure for water-soluble amphiphilic nanocarriers. *Pharm Res* 2006;**23**(8). pp. 1948–1948.
111. Allen C, Han J, Yu Y, Maysinger D, Eisenberg A. Polycaprolactone–b-poly(ethylene oxide) copolymer micelles as a delivery vehicle for dihydrotestosterone. *J Control Release* 2000;**63**(3):275–86.
112. Shuai X, Ai H, Nasongkla N, Kim S, Gao J. Micellar carriers based on block copolymers of poly(ε-caprolactone) and poly(ethylene glycol) for doxorubicin delivery. *J Control Release* 2004;**98**(3):415–26.
113. Lin W-J, Juang L-W, Lin C-C. Stability and release performance of a series of pegylated copolymeric micelles. *Pharm Res* 2003;**20**(4):668–73.
114. Liu J, Xiao Y, Allen C. Polymer–drug compatibility: a guide to the development of delivery systems for the anticancer agent, ellipticine. *J Pharm Sci* 2004;**93**(1):132–43.
115. Kanazawa T, Akiyama F, Kakizaki S, Takashima Y, Seta Y. Delivery of siRNA to the brain using a combination of nose-to-brain delivery and cell-penetrating peptide-modified nano-micelles. *Biomaterials* 2013;**34**(36):9220–6.
116. Chan DPY, Owen SC, Shoichet MS. Double click: dual functionalized polymeric micelles with antibodies and peptides. *Bioconjug Chem* 2013;**24**(1):105–13.

117. Saito N, Okada T, Toba S, Miyamoto S, Takaoka K. New synthetic absorbable polymers as BMP carriers: plastic properties of poly-D,L-lactic acid-polyethylene glycol block copolymers. *J Biomed Mater Res* 1999;**47**(1):104–10.
118. Saito N, Okada T, Horiuchi H, Murakami N, Takahashi J, Nawata M, Ota H, Nozaki K, Takaoka K. A biodegradable polymer as a cytokine delivery system for inducing bone formation. *Nat Biotechnol* 2001;**19**:332.
119. Moroni L, Licht R, de Boer J, de Wijn JR, van Blitterswijk CA. Fiber diameter and texture of electrospun PEOT/PBT scaffolds influence human mesenchymal stem cell proliferation and morphology, and the release of incorporated compounds. *Biomaterials* 2006;**27**(28):4911–22.
120. Gaharwar AK, Mihaila SM, Kulkarni AA, Patel A, Di Luca A, Reis RL, Gomes ME, van Blitterswijk C, Moroni L, Khademhosseini A. Amphiphilic beads as depots for sustained drug release integrated into fibrillar scaffolds. *J Control Release* 2014;**187**:66–73.
121. Kawanabe T, Kawakami T, Yatomi Y, Shimada S, Soma Y. Sphingosine 1-phosphate accelerates wound healing in diabetic mice. *J Dermatol Sci* 2007;**48**(1):53–60.
122. Zhang J, Song J. Amphiphilic degradable polymers for immobilization and sustained delivery of sphingosine 1-phosphate. *Acta Biomaterialia* 2014;**10**(7):3079–90.
123. Qi X, Okamoto Y, Murakawa T, Wang F, Oyama O, Ohkawa R, Yoshioka K, Du W, Sugimoto N, Yatomi Y, Takuwa N, Takuwa Y. Sustained delivery of sphingosine-1-phosphate using poly(lactic-co-glycolic acid)-based microparticles stimulates Akt/ERK-eNOS mediated angiogenesis and vascular maturation restoring blood flow in ischemic limbs of mice. *Eur J Pharmacol* 2010;**634**(1):121–31.
124. Xiao Y, Hong H, Javadi A, Engle JW, Xu W, Yang Y, Zhang Y, Barnhart TE, Cai W, Gong S. Multifunctional unimolecular micelles for cancer-targeted drug delivery and positron emission tomography imaging. *Biomaterials* 2012;**33**(11):3071–82.
125. Cheng Y. Dendrimer-based drug delivery systems from theory to practice. In: Cheng Y, editor. *Wiley series in drug discovery and development*. Hoboken, N.J.: John Wiley & Sons; 2012.
126. Šebestík J, Reiniš M, Ježek J. Synthesis of dendrimers: convergent and divergent approaches. In: Sebestik J, Reinis M, Jezek J, editors. *Biomedical applications of peptide-, Glyco- and Glycopeptide dendrimers, and Analogous dendrimeric structures*. Vienna: Springer Vienna; 2012. p. 55–81.
127. Madaan K, Kumar S, Poonia N, Lather V, Pandita D. Dendrimers in drug delivery and targeting: drug-dendrimer interactions and toxicity issues. *J Pharm BioAllied Sci* 2014;**6**(3):139–50.
128. Caminade A-M, Turrin C-O. Dendrimers for drug delivery. *J Mater Chem B* 2014;**2**(26):4055–66.
129. Buhleier E, Wehner W, Vögtle F. Cascade and nonskid chain like syntheses of molecular cavity topologies. *Synthesis* 1978;**1978**(02):155–8.
130. Hawker CJ, Frechet JMJ. Preparation of polymers with controlled molecular architecture. A new convergent approach to dendritic macromolecules. *J Am Chem Soc* 1990;**112**(21):7638–47.
131. Hummelen JC, Van Dongen JLJ, Meijer EW. Electrospray mass spectrometry of poly(propylene imine) dendrimers—the issue of dendritic purity or polydispersity. *Chem Eur J* 1997;**3**(9):1489–93.
132. Tomalia DA. Birth of a new macromolecular architecture: dendrimers as quantized building blocks for nanoscale synthetic polymer chemistry. *Prog Polym Sci* 2005;**30**(3):294–324.
133. Walter MV, Malkoch M. Simplifying the synthesis of dendrimers: accelerated approaches. *Chem Soc Rev* 2012;**41**(13):4593–609.
134. Mullen DG, Borgmeier EL, Desai AM, van Dongen MA, Barash M, Cheng X-m, Baker JR, Banaszak Holl MM. Isolation and characterization of dendrimers with precise numbers of functional groups. *Chem Eur J* 2010;**16**(35):10675–8.
135. van Hest JCM, Delnoye DAP, Baars MWPL, van Genderen MHP, Meijer EW. Polystyrene-dendrimer amphiphilic block copolymers with a generation-dependent aggregation. *Science* 1995;**268**(5217):1592–5.
136. Zhang S, Sun H-J, Hughes AD, Moussodia R-O, Bertin A, Chen Y, Pochan DJ, Heiney PA, Klein ML, Percec V. Self-assembly of amphiphilic Janus dendrimers into uniform onion-like dendrimersomes with predictable size and number of bilayers. *Proc Natl Acad Sci USA* 2014;**111**(25):9058–63.
137. Sikwal DR, Kalhapure RS, Govender T. An emerging class of amphiphilic dendrimers for pharmaceutical and biomedical applications: janus amphiphilic dendrimers. *Eur J Pharm Sci* 2017;**97**:113–34.
138. Lin BF, Marullo RS, Robb MJ, Krogstad DV, Antoni P, Hawker CJ, Campos LM, Tirrell MV. De novo design of bioactive protein-resembling nanospheres via dendrimer-templated peptide amphiphile assembly. *Nano Lett* 2011;**11**(9):3946–50.
139. Wei T, Chen C, Liu J, Liu C, Posocco P, Liu X, Cheng Q, Huo S, Liang Z, Fermeglia M, Pricl S, Liang X-J, Rocchi P, Peng L. Anticancer drug nanomicelles formed by self-assembling amphiphilic dendrimer to combat cancer drug resistance. *Proc Natl Acad Sci* 2015;**112**(10):2978.
140. Movellan J, Urbán P, Moles E, de la Fuente JM, Sierra T, Serrano JL, Fernàndez-Busquets X. Amphiphilic dendritic derivatives as nanocarriers for the targeted delivery of antimalarial drugs. *Biomaterials* 2014;**35**(27):7940–50.
141. Goodyer ID, Pouvelle B, Schneider TG, Trelka DP, Taraschi TF. Characterization of macromolecular transport pathways in malaria-infected erythrocytes. *Mol Biochem Parasitol* 1997;**87**(1):13–28.
142. Yu T, Liu X, Bolcato-Bellemin A-L, Wang Y, Liu C, Erbacher P, Qu F, Rocchi P, Behr J-P, Peng L. An amphiphilic dendrimer for effective delivery of small interfering RNA and gene silencing In Vitro and In Vivo. *Angew Chem Int Ed* 2012;**51**(34):8478–84.
143. Sonawane ND, Szoka FC, Verkman AS. Chloride accumulation and swelling in endosomes enhances DNA transfer by polyamine-DNA polyplexes. *J Biol Chem* 2003.
144. Liu X, Zhou J, Yu T, Chen C, Cheng Q, Sengupta K, Huang Y, Li H, Liu C, Wang Y, Posocco P, Wang M, Cui Q, Giorgio S, Fermeglia M, Qu F, Pricl S, Shi Y, Liang Z, Rocchi P, Rossi JJ, Peng L. Adaptive amphiphilic dendrimer-based nanoassemblies as robust and versatile siRNA delivery systems. *Angew Chem Int Ed* 2014;**53**(44):11822–7.
145. Rajasekhar Reddy R, Raghupathi KR, Torres DA, Thayumanavan S. Stimuli sensitive amphiphilic dendrimers. *New J Chem* 2012;**36**(2):340–9.
146. Wang H, Miao W, Wang F, Cheng Y. A self-assembled coumarin-anchored dendrimer for efficient gene delivery and light-responsive drug delivery. *Biomacromolecules* 2018;**19**(6):2194–201.

147. Xu C-T, Chen G, Nie X, Wang L-H, Ding S-G, You Y-Z. Low generation PAMAM-based nanomicelles as ROS-responsive gene vectors with enhanced transfection efficacy and reduced cytotoxicity in vitro. *New J Chem* 2017;**41**(9):3273–9.
148. Garrigue P, Tang J, Ding L, Bouhlel A, Tintaru A, Laurini E, Huang Y, Lyu Z, Zhang M, Fernandez S, Balasse L, Lan W, Mas E, Marson D, Weng Y, Liu X, Giorgio S, Iovanna J, Pricl S, Guillet B, Peng L. Self-assembling supramolecular dendrimer nanosystem for PET imaging of tumors. *Proc Natl Acad Sci* 2018.
149. Hare JI, Lammers T, Ashford MB, Puri S, Storm G, Barry ST. Challenges and strategies in anti-cancer nanomedicine development: an industry perspective. *Adv Drug Deliv Rev* 2017;**108**:25–38.

Chapter 20

Electrostatically driven self-assembled nanoparticles and coatings

Sachit Shah[1], Allen Eyler[1], Sara Tabandeh[1] and Lorraine Leon[1,2]

[1]*Department of Materials Science and Engineering, University of Central Florida, Orlando, FL, United States;* [2]*NanoScience and Technology Center, University of Central Florida, Orlando, FL, United States*

20.1 Introduction

Over the past several decades, electrostatically self-assembled nanoparticles have emerged as a promising new technology for biomedical applications such as drug and gene delivery, biosensing, and nanoreactors. Self-assembly at the nanoscale enables the facile fabrication of intricately structured particles, which can be small enough to be internalized by human cells and can possess tailored surfaces promoting biocompatibility as well as the targeting of specific cell types. Electrostatically driven self-assembly is particularly promising because the interactions can be tuned, or reversed, depending on environmental conditions such as solvent, ionic strength, and pH; this environmental responsiveness leads to truly "smart" nanomedicine.

This chapter reviews several types of electrostatically self-assembled nanoparticles, as well as nanoparticle coatings, and their applications in the biomedical field. Polyplexes, which consist of nucleic acids bound electrostatically to a cationic polymer (CP), have the potential to replace viral vectors for gene therapy applications, delivering nucleic acids safely and effectively. A similar approach is used to encapsulate charged proteins that can be used as therapeutics. Block copolymer polyelectrolyte complex micelles, consisting of charged and hydrophilic polymer segments assembled into core and corona structures, have applications in gene delivery, where the outer corona serves to protect the cargo and facilitate cellular entry. Layer-by-layer nanoparticle coatings are formed when oppositely charged polyelectrolytes are alternately deposited onto a nanoparticle core, producing a precisely controlled layered structure; these structures, which have functionalities imparted by the shell layers as well as the core, have applications in drug delivery, in biosensing, and as nanoreactors. Each of these technologies is described in detail in the following sections, with a focus on fabrication and structural control, as well as behavior and efficacy in application studies.

20.2 Nanoscale Homopolymer Polyelectrolyte Complexes

Homopolymer polyelectrolyte complexes, generally called polyelectrolyte complexes (PECs) are formed as a result of interactions between oppositely charged polyelectrolytes in solution.[1,2] This interaction can lead to phase separation in the form of precipitates (solids)[3–6] or coacervates (liquids).[3,6–10] The driving force for PEC formation is largely entropic in nature. The entropy gain is due to counterion release that occurs when the double layers of the two oppositely charged macroions are disrupted after mixing.[2] The structure of charged polyelectrolyte assemblies includes intrinsic (polycation and polyanion) and extrinsic (polyelectrolyte and counterion) ion pairing, and the strength of intrinsic ion pairing is a key determinant in the formation of solid or liquid complexes.[6,11] The stronger the electrostatic interactions, the greater the tendency of the complexes to be in the form of a solid. Weak pairs of oppositely charged polyelectrolytes contain more water and are more likely to form coacervates, which allow for more mobility of small molecules or ions.[12] Besides electrostatic interactions, short-range forces, combined with steric packing and hydration, can influence the physical state of PECs.[6] While precipitates have limited utility in the absence of special processing,[13] complex coacervates, due to their low interfacial tension with water, can be used in a variety of applications such as encapsulation of drugs[14,15] and flavors,[16,17] compartmentalization,[18,19] adhesives,[20–22] and nano-/bioreactors.[23,24]

Nanoparticles for Biomedical Applications. https://doi.org/10.1016/B978-0-12-816662-8.00020-5

Here, we limit our discussions to nanoscale PECs, as bulk and micron-sized PECs are covered elsewhere.[3–10,25] The focus is on PECs comprising polycations/nucleic acids (polyplexes), and protein-polyelectrolytes due to their relevance in biomedical applications.

Polyplexes are formed by a combination of CPs and nucleic acids in aqueous solution.[26,27] They have attracted a lot of attention in gene therapy applications as an alternative for viral carriers due to their ability to overcome hurdles like immune and toxic reactions, low nucleic acid carrying capacity, and high cost.[26–28] The electrostatically driven interaction between the positive charges of the polycation and negative charges of the nucleic acid in polyplexes leads to the spontaneous formation of complexes as a result of nucleic acid condensation via charge compensation and hydrophobic interactions.[28–30] Light scattering,[31] circular dichroism,[32,33] and optical microscopy[34] have been used to study the compaction of DNA upon interaction with polycations. Besides the electrostatic interactions, secondary interactions such as hydrogen bonding and hydrophobic interactions can also contribute to polyplex formation.[29] Nonstoichiometric polyplexes which have excess negative (nucleic acid) or excess positive (polycation) charges form soluble nanometer-sized polyplexes, in contrast to charge-balanced complexes that phase separate from solution into larger aggregates.[35,36] Negatively charged complexes, with an excess of DNA, repel the negatively charged cell membrane, limiting their ability for cellular uptake. Cationic particles, however, can interact with the negatively charged plasma membrane of the cell resulting in DNA endocytosis,[37] though their pharmacokinetic and biodistribution properties depend on biological interactions.[36] Nonstoichiometric complexes of chitosan and DNA/siRNA can form nanosized complexes that enter endocytic vessels because their diameter does not exceed 100 nm.[29,38] The size-limiting cellular uptake explains the need for DNA compaction.[30] Different optimal sizes have been suggested for targeting versus nontargeting polyplexes,[39] as well as different types of nucleic acids.[40]

Polyplexes have been investigated as nonviral carriers for both DNA[30,36,41] and RNA.[38,42–45] However, due to the small size of certain RNA molecules, like siRNA, electrostatic complexes with CPs are less stable compared to DNA/polycation complexes and intracellular delivery of lower efficacy has been reported.[46] The stability of PECs has been studied using a variety of different polymer systems, and it is well understood that polymers with higher molecular weight have higher stabilities.[47] As an attempt to increase polyplex stability, Heissig et al.[46] have connected siRNA to a 181-nucleotide adaptor DNA extension. The electrostatic interactions between polymers and DNA/siRNA must not only condense and protect the nucleic acids from degradation but also allow them to be released at the target site. Thus very strong interactions with nucleic acids can impair their delivery efficiency.[29]

PEC nanoparticles containing proteins also have great potential to be used in drug delivery applications and for microencapsulation in the cosmetic and food industries.[29,48–50] Using isothermal titration calorimetry, it has been determined that complex formation between polyelectrolytes and proteins is mainly due to the coulombic forces, although hydrophobic interactions can also be involved.[51,52] Besides delivery, protein-PECs can be used to immobilize proteins via incorporation into layer-by-layer (LbL) assemblies, which will be discussed in Section 20.4.[49] Related to protein-PECs, charged peptides can also form complexes capable of delivering enzymes.[53]

20.2.1 Physiochemical parameters affecting complexation

Parameters such as the polymer structure, molecular weight, charge density, polymer mixing ratios, ionic strength, and pH of the solution influence PEC formation, stability, and the efficiency of delivery or transfection of the proteins and nucleic acids which will be discussed in the following sections.

20.2.1.1 Polymer structure and strength of polyelectrolyte

CPs have the ability to condense and neutralize the charges of nucleic acids, which is necessary for successful gene transfection.[27] The structure of CPs (linear vs. branched) can affect gene transfer efficiency of the polyplex.[37,54,55] Branched structures can be further divided into symmetric and nonsymmetric structures such as dendrimers which have radial symmetry, and polyethyleneimine (PEI), a branched polyelectrolyte which lacks a symmetry center.[55] Tang et al.[55] studied the role of CP structure by comparing linear, branched, and dendritic polymer's interactions with DNA and concluded that all formed a toroidal structure with a diameter of about 55 nm. However, linear and intact dendrimer (perfect radial branched) CPs formed aggregated clusters, while branched and fractured dendrimer (defective radial branched) CPs remained discrete entities in solution. This difference in behavior was attributed to differences in CP rigidity causing more rigid chains to aggregate, possibly as a result of bridging.[37,55] Evaluation of physiochemical properties of polyplexes has indicated that the presence of nonionic hydrophilic groups such as hydroxyl or amide groups can improve transfection efficiency of linear polypeptides (e.g., polylysine derivatives). In the case of branched structures (e.g., polyamidoamine (PAMAM) dendrimers), increasing surface charge density can enhance transfection efficiency.[54]

Polysaccharides, which are biomedically relevant polyelectrolytes, can have different branching structures and behave as both strong and weak polyelectrolytes. Examples of these are heparin, hyaluronic acid (HA), and chitosan which have the ability to form nanostructures with demonstrated use in tissue engineering applications.[56] Heparin, a strong polyanion, can be highly variable in its saccharide sequence and sulfation pattern, which can influence its ability to bind proteins including enzymes and growth factors.[56,57] Chitosan is a cationic nontoxic biopolymer, and due to its high charge density it is antimicrobial and can be used in wound healing applications.[58] Hyaluronic acid, a weak polyanion, is a nonimmunogenic and biodegradable polymer and many of its biological functions are based on the specific interactions it has with cell-surface HA receptors such as CD44.[59]

Cationic block and graft copolymers have also been developed to improve polyplexes stability and prevent their interaction with serum proteins.[37] For example, poly (ethylene glycol) (PEG) has been grafted to PEI to decrease cytotoxicity and increase solubility of polyplexes[60] and also improve transfection efficiency.[61] PEG can prevent complex precipitation even when stoichiometric ratios of DNA and polycation are used. However, due to its nonbiodegradable nature, it can cause antibody formation and hypersensitivity reactions. Carbohydrate-based cationic block copolymers have been explored as an alternative to PEG and demonstrated low toxicity, high luciferase expression, and cellular uptake.[62] Block copolymer (BCP) complexes will be discussed in detail later in this chapter (Section 20.3).

20.2.1.2 Stoichiometry of mixing (charge ratio)

When mixing oppositely charged polymers, one can control the ratio of positively charged monomers to negatively charged monomers. For polyplexes, this ratio is expressed as the ratio of positively charged amino groups (N) to negatively charged phosphate groups (P), N/P ratio. The charge ratio can determine the size of the complex and therefore cellular interactions, biodistribution, and finally gene transfection efficiency,[26,28,63,64] and is more broadly expressed as the f^+ value, given by

$$f^+ = \frac{[+]}{[+] + [-]}$$

Here, $[+]$ is the molar concentration of all positive charges of the polycation and $[-]$ is the molar concentration of all negative charges of the polyanion, and an f^+ value of 0.50 is equimolar charge. Importantly, manipulation of the charge ratio keeps PECs within the nanoparticle size domain, while neutral complexes, with a charge ratio of 1, can aggregate together and form larger particles.[65,66] For polyplexes, high N:P ratios lead to more nucleic acid condensation and improved cellular uptake due to the affinity of the positively charged complex with the negatively charged cell surface.[26] For DNA/transferrin−PEI complexes under physiological salt conditions, N/P ratios of 6 or higher prevented the formation of large aggregates.[63] However, larger DNA/PEI complexes (300−600 nm) had more luciferase gene expression efficiency than the smaller particles (30−60 nm), due to enhanced uptake and endosome destabilizing activity. In another study by Gebhart and Kabanov,[28] transfection efficiency as well as cellular toxicity showed a dependence on the charge ratio, where optimal charge ratios corresponded to the maximum luciferase expression with tolerable levels of cytotoxicity. A unique example is chitosan/siRNA complexes which demonstrated an increase in particle size with excess siRNA, possibly due to greater bridge formation between chitosan chains via siRNA causing interparticle aggregation.[64] A different study using polysaccharide-based PECs, illustrated that the particle size and distribution increased close to charge neutrality. Interestingly, this only occurred when a relatively high-molecular-weight weak polycation (chitosan) was paired with a relatively low-molecular-weight strong polyanion (heparin). The opposite situation (low-molecular-weight weak polycation (chitosan)/high-molecular-weight weak polyanion (hyaluronan)) did not show the same trend of particle aggregation.[56]

20.2.1.3 Polyelectrolyte molecular weight

Molecular weight (Mw) of the polymers affects complex size and stability, cellular uptake, dissociation, and transfection efficiency of the carriers.[29] Longer polymer chains, as well as higher degree of branching, increases condensation of DNA resulting in better stability against degradation in extracellular environments.[26] At low charge ratios (N/P < 4), high Mw PEI can reportedly condense plasmid DNA more efficiently than low Mw PEI.[67] However, for shorter nucleic acids such as mRNA, peptide-modified low Mw CPs showed efficient transfection.[68] The difference in stability in the cytosol might account for this, as high Mw PEI can provide pDNA stability until nuclear entry, though this stability is too high for mRNA which must be released in the cytosol to be biologically active.[65] To understand the condensation mechanism of polyplexes, Mann et al.[69] utilized atomic force microscopy (AFM) to describe the molecular morphologies formed during condensation of DNA with polylysine of different chain lengths at increasing charge ratios. The smallest length polylysine (average 19 residues) showed the best condensation ability at low DNA concentrations. One possible explanation is that shorter polymers could better compensate the loss in conformational entropy in the complexed state with the gained entropy due to the counterion release, compared to longer polymers.[69] For natural biopolymers, like chitosan, the charge density can be increased via the degree of deacetylation (DD) or the percentage of deacetylated primary amine groups along the molecular chain which can result in a greater DNA/siRNA binding capacity.[29] Chitosan with adequately high DD and Mw was reported to retain condensed DNA and show high transfection efficiency.[70] For siRNA/chitosan nanoparticles the highest gene silencing was achieved by using high Mw chitosan (114 and 110 kDa) and DD (84%) due to the formation of stable nanoparticles using longer, more flexible molecules with increased charge density.[71] However, when designing a PEC-based carrier system, optimum molecular weight should be considered for the polycation with regards to the cytotoxicity (generally, the higher Mw of the polycation, the higher the cytotoxicity), so that the final complex has both high delivery efficiency and tolerable cytotoxicity.

20.2.1.4 Ionic strength

Ionic strength and counterions can affect the interactions in PECs.[72] The addition of salt decreases the number of intrinsic pairs, by forming extrinsic pairs more readily, thereby reducing the degree of electrostatic interaction between the polyelectrolytes.[11,73] An alternate explanation is that increasing salt concentration reduces the Debye length, which represents the distance over which two opposite charges interact. The reduction in Debye length decreases the strength of interaction between the polyelectrolytes in the PEC, causing more polyelectrolytes to be suspended in the non-PEC phase. The addition of salt also reduces the overall entropic gain from counterion release, increasing the water content in the PEC, thereby reducing the interfacial energy. This results in a decrease in the amount of PEC that is formed.[74] Also, the addition of salt to solid PECs can facilitate liquid coacervate formation.[8] The addition of an excessive amount of salt prevents any complexation and hence no PEC formation occurs; this is known as the critical salt concentration.

It has been shown that at charge ratios that normally cause particle aggregation, complexation of plasmid DNA with PEI or transferrin-PEI formed nonaggregated particles in the 30–50 nm range only in low ionic strength solutions, below physiological ranges.[63] Other systems show that the average size of polyplexes increases in the presence of NaCl solution (0.15 M), likely due to swelling of the polyplexes.[75] Charge ratio is also important when considering the effect of salt on PECs. For instance the hydrodynamic radii of siRNA/chitosan nanoparticles were not substantially affected by the addition of salt over 24 h, due to their significant positive charge, illustrated using zeta potential.[64] Unlike, synthetic polyelectrolytes or nucleic acids that have regular charge spacing, for proteins the anisotropy of electrostatic domains plays an important role in the ionic strength dependency of protein–polyelectrolyte binding.[72] Complex formation between catalase and chitosan as well as Eudragit E100 (a cationic copolymer based on dimethylaminoethyl methacrylate esters) in the presence of electrolytes was evaluated by measuring turbidity.[76] Catalase–chitosan complexation diminished at any concentration of NaCl but catalase–Eudragit E100 showed gradual dissolving as the ionic strength increased. Boeris et al.[76] also tried other salt halides (NaBr and NaF) and observed no difference in the turbidity versus ionic strength plots for the catalase–chitosan complex. However, the catalase–Eudragit E100 complex diminished in turbidity as the Hofmeister series increased ($F^- < Cl^- < Br^-$). This suggests that catalase–Eudragit E100 complexes may also involve hydrophobic interactions since the decreased ability of F- to disrupt the structure of water influenced complexation, and hydrophobic effects are driven by decreases in water entropy.[77] Under physiological conditions, polyplexes can undergo exchange reactions between DNA and other anionic biological macromolecules, leading to the release of DNA. The rate and position of equilibrium in the exchange reaction is highly dependent on ionic strength and the chemical nature of the salt present in solution.[30]

20.2.1.5 pH

In general, the pH of aqueous solutions affects complexation behavior due to modulation of the ionization extent of the polyelectrolytes, and it is important to consider the possibility of significant changes in the pH environment with different routes of administration when evaluating a gene delivery system.[36,66] For example, PEC nanoparticles made using chitosan (polycation) and pectin (polyanion), decrease in average size to a significant extent above pH 3.5, which is the pKa of pectin.[58] As the pH increases toward 6, the dissociation of chitosan (pKa ~6.5) is expected and a negative value of zeta potential was measured.[58] CPs such as PEI and polyamidoamine (PAMAM) dendrimers that contain amine groups with pKa values near physiological pH have been reported to show good transgene expression due to the "proton sponge" effect leading to endosomal escape.[36,67,78,79] CPs can absorb protons during endocytic trafficking, preventing the acidification of endocytic vesicles necessary for the maturation from endosome to lysosome. Consequently, more protons, as well as chloride ions (to maintain charge neutrality) will be pumped into the endosome. This increase in ion concentration causes osmotic swelling and subsequent rupture of the endosomes which leads to polyplex release into the cytosol and prevents nucleic acids from lysosomal degradation.[65,80,81] Sonawane et al.[82] tested and provided support for the proton sponge hypothesis by measuring the chloride ion concentration, pH, and volume of endosomes after internalization of polyplexes composed of plasmid DNA and polylysine or polyamines like PEI and PAMAM. Chloride ion accumulation was found to be remarkably greater in endosomes-containing PEI and PAMAM polyamines, versus polylysine complexes. Their results confirmed that PEI and PAMAM buffer endosomal pH, increase chloride content, and produce endosomes which are more sensitive to osmotic stress. However, the proton sponge hypothesis alone does not fully explain the remarkable ability of these CPs as transfection reagents providing endosomal escape.[26]

20.2.2 Endocytosis and nuclear entering of polyplexes

To have effective gene transfection, carrier systems should overcome several cellular barriers to deliver their cargo.[83] Besides using positively charged polyplexes to interact with cell-surface proteoglycans,[26,27] soluble, charge-neutralized polyplexes also interact with the cell surface using ligands.[27] Polyplexes made with hydrophobized polycations (containing a side-chain cetyl group) have been shown to adsorb onto a liposome surface providing a mechanism for cell membrane penetration.[84] Different cellular internalization mechanisms have been proposed such as phagocytosis, (macro) pinocytosis, clathrin-dependent and independent endocytosis, and caveolae-mediated endocytosis.[81,83,85] Rejman et al.[83] concluded that polyplexes taken up by clathrin-mediated endocytosis will encounter degradation due to lysosomal compartment targeting and those internalized via caveolae tend to have more efficient transfection by escaping this compartment. Particle size can strongly affect the internalization mechanism and subsequent route of complexes as larger particles (at least 200 nm, but less than 1 μm in diameter) have been reported to be preferentially internalized with caveolae-mediated endocytosis, whereas smaller particles (<200 nm) undergo clathrin-mediated endocytosis.[86] Chemical structure and surface of polyplex particles can also influence the endocytic pathway.[87,88] Cationic glycopolymers which were treated with low concentrations of heparin, endocytosed primarily through micropinocytosis and clathrin-mediated pathways while in the absence of heparin, caveolae, and micropinocytosis were indicated to be the main endocytosis routes.[88] Barriers to successful in vivo delivery of nucleic acids has been schematically showed by Yin et al.[89] in Fig. 20.1. For DNA, after cell entry, trafficking of DNA through the cytoplasm is followed by the entry into the nucleus and transcription.[37,65] siRNA and miRNA must be loaded into RNA-induced silencing complex (RISC), while mRNA has to bind to the translational machinery.[81,90] However, the process of entry and further pathways through the intracellular environment are not well understood and require further detailed investigation.

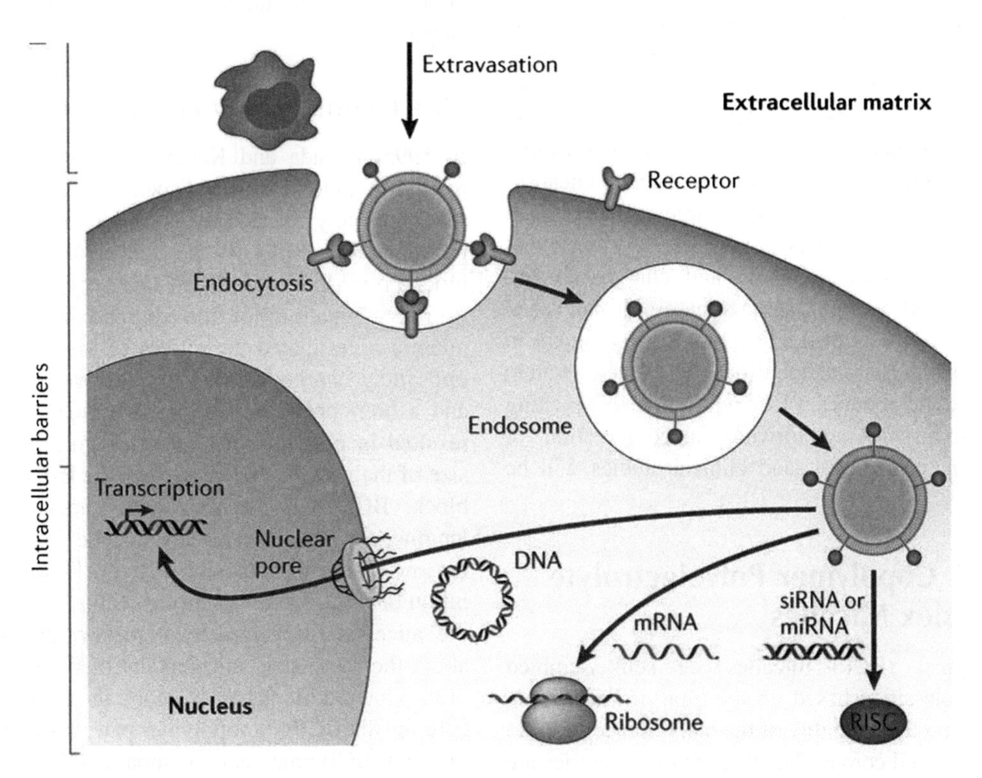

FIGURE 20.1 Barriers to successful in vivo delivery of nucleic acids using nonviral vectors. RISC, RNA-induced silencing complex. *Adapted with permission from Yin et al.*[89].

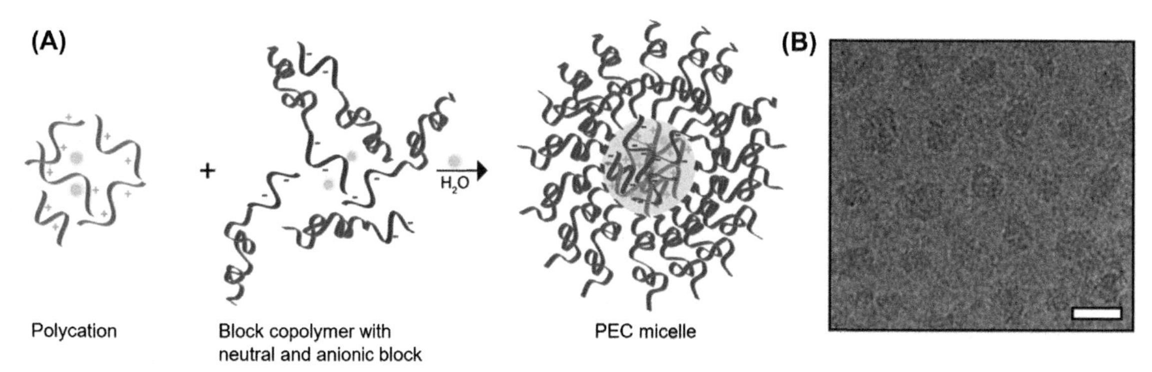

FIGURE 20.2 (A) Schematic representation of polyelectrolyte complex (PEC) micelle formation of block copolymer/homopolymer pair. (B) Cryo-TEM image of PEC micelles. Scale bar represents 40 nm. *Reprinted with permission from Ting et al.*[101] *Copyright © 2018 American Chemical Society.*

20.2.3 Outlook on nanoscale homopolymer PECs

Protein and nucleic acid polyelectrolyte nanocomplexes have been the focus of much ongoing fundamental and biomedical research. In order to properly design a nanoscale PEC for delivery applications, structural parameters and physicochemical properties should be considered to give an appropriate balance between protection of cargo and subsequent release at the target point. Despite the analysis of many different systems, nanoscale PECs for gene delivery have not yet achieved efficient uptake and sustained gene expression in vivo.[91] Issues arise with achieving high efficiency combined with low cytotoxicity, as these properties are inversely proportional for polycations. One promising strategy to overcome this trade-off between efficacy and toxicity is the use of zinc-dipicolylamine-based ligands to functionalize inefficient low Mw CPs. The zinc ligand has a large binding affinity for phosphate groups, leading to increased DNA encapsulation and endosomal escape.[92] For larger, micron-sized PECs, new synthetic polymers have been developed that combine the benefits of lipophilic and charged assemblies,[93] which could be a promising strategy for nanosized vehicles for future use. Considering rapid development in both polymer synthesis and identification of new protein and nucleic acid therapeutics, PECs will remain an exciting area of research. Moving forward, a combination of fundamental, pharmaceutical, and clinical studies will be required.

20.3 Block Copolymer Polyelectrolyte Complex Micelles

Block Copolymer (BCP) micelles are self-assembled nanostructures classified based on the type of intermolecular forces driving the assembly of the macromolecules into a segregated core and corona. The three main categories are amphiphilic micelles formed due to solvophobic interactions, PEC micelles due to electrostatic interactions, and micelle formation due to metal complexation.[94] Here we focus on PEC micelles, also referred to as polyion complex micelles,[95,96] interpolyelectrolyte complex micelles,[36,97] block ionomer complex micelles,[36,98] or complex coacervate core micelles.[97,99,100] PEC micelles contain a neutral hydrophilic corona and a PEC core (Fig. 20.2A). They have potential use in targeted delivery of charged molecules such as nucleic acids and proteins. These nanometric particles emulate certain features of viruses, where the protective corona of the micelle is analogous to the capsid layer of a virus. Additionally, stimulus responsive functionalities and selective targeting features can be engineered to provide target-specific control over release of cargo.

20.3.1 Formation of PEC micelles

In 1995, Harada and Kataoka[102] first illustrated the formation of spherical monodisperse PEC micelles by mixing two oppositely charged BCPs (poly(ethylene glycol)-block-poly(L-lysine) (PEG-PLK) and poly(ethylene glycol)-block-poly(aspartic acid) (PEG-PAsp)) with equal degrees of polymerization for the charged blocks. They subsequently investigated the effects of mixing two BCPs with oppositely charged blocks together versus mixing a BCP and a homopolymer. Mixing two BCPs of equal lengths resulted in monodisperse spherical micelles, in which the size of the micelle increased with the length of the charged block. BCP/BCP mixtures with unequal charged block lengths, did not result in any micelle formation, indicated by low scattering intensity of light. However, when a solution of PEG-PAsp was mixed with a homopolymer, PLK, the micelles formed were of narrow distribution and of about the same size, independent of the length or equality of the charged blocks.[103] Notably, the radius of the micellar core for the BCP/homopolymer pair was larger than that of the BCP/BCP pair, using comparable lengths. This difference in size was explained by an increased ability for molecular rearrangement in the BCP/homopolymer system, leading to an increased aggregation number and larger radius.[103,104] The ability to rearrange is related to the core–corona interface. A smooth interface due to complete demixing occurs when BCP/BCP pairs of equal charged lengths are used. However, BCP/homopolymer samples and BCP/BCP samples with unequal charged lengths showed intermixing between the core and the corona.[104] Interestingly, BCP electrolytes selectively form micelles with oppositely charged BCPs of equal length in a mixture containing multiple block lengths, a phenomenon termed chain length recognition. Chain length recognition is driven by complete phase separation of the core and corona which allows for the junction connecting the charged and neutral blocks to be aligned at the core–corona interface.[104,105] This phenomenon is unique to electrostatically driven micelles and is not featured in amphiphilic micelle formation.[105]

As mentioned earlier in this chapter, oppositely charged polyelectrolytes tend to aggregate at charge neutral conditions but the presence of the hydrophilic block in the BCPs helps restrict this phase separation to the nanoscale regime. Therefore, PEC micelle formation is heavily influenced by the ratio of charged block length to neutral block length. For example, BCPs with equal neutral and charged blocks result in macroscopic phase separation (precipitation/sedimentation observed by the naked eye), but a charged-to-neutral block length ratio of 1:3 results in monodisperse micelles.[106,107] When a charged-to-neutral block length ratio of 1:9 was used, there was almost no scattering, suggesting that the length of the charged block was too small to cause phase separation, since the authors reported that at least 12 repeat units are needed for complexation.[106,108]

As discussed for mixtures of homopolymers in Section 20.2.1, PEC micelle formation is also largely dependent on the molar ratio of positive and negative charges, or f^+ value. Titration of two oppositely charged species (either BCP/BCP pairs or BCP/homopolymer pairs) with varying f^+ values can be observed using light scattering. As the concentration of the positive species is increased, more PEC micelles are formed, increasing the intensity of scattered light. Typically, a sharp intensity peak is observed around $f^+ = 0.50$, when maximum micelle formation would occur, with relatively lower levels of scattering for $f^+ \neq 0.50$.[100] The order of addition is also a delicate experimental parameter. When mixing polyelectrolytes in stoichiometric ratios, in the absence of salt, addition of polycation to polyanion or vice versa is inconsequential when equilibrium structures are formed. However, dynamic light scattering studies have revealed that the scattering intensities differ for the addition of polyanion to polycation versus the addition of polycation to polyanion.[109]

Secondary structure of polymers, predominantly polypeptides, plays a role in PEC micelle formation as well.[110] For example, when homochiral PEG-PLK was mixed with poly(L-glutamic acid) (PGlu), β-sheet formation in the core was observed, but when racemic PGlu was used, a random coil structure was formed.[2,6] The solid core micelles (β-sheet structure) had slower formation kinetics and were more polydisperse than their liquid core (random coil) counterparts due to their inability to rearrange into equilibrium structures because of interchain hydrogen bonding. The discovery of PEC micelles with solid and liquid cores is fairly recent, and the understanding of the differences between them is currently being explored.

20.3.2 Structural properties of micelles

The morphology of PEC micelles is dictated by numerous factors including block lengths of charged and neutral blocks, block rigidity, pH, and salt concentration. Relatively longer neutral blocks generally lead to spherical micelle formation, while shorter neutral blocks can lead to the formation of cylindrical or wormlike micelles.[111,112] This is similar to amphiphilic BCPs, where shape is dictated by a critical packing parameter which is the ratio of the volume of the solvophobic chain divided by the head group area multiplied by the length of the solvophobic chain (v/a_0L).[113] For PEC micelles, wormlike micelles can also be obtained when the charged blocks are rigid because of the excess energy required to cause chain deformation.[100,114] At equilibrium, the structure of PEC micelles is fundamentally determined by the relative free energies of the structural contributions of the core, corona, and the interface between the two.

Kataoka and coworkers have related micelle morphology to the neutral block or PEG corona density, defined as the ratio of the association number of the PEG chains to the surface area of the inner core of the PEC micelle (Fig. 20.3).[103,104] Shorter charged blocks form cores of smaller radii and increased curvature, causing the crowded corona chains to relax in an outward direction, allowing for higher PEG density.[95] The converse is also true. It can be seen that an increase in association number (and subsequently size) of the micelle increases the PEG density, forcing the corona segments to take a stretched conformation. The stretching of the core and corona segments with a higher association number causes a decrease in conformational entropy, which compensates for the decrease in interfacial energy when the micelle is formed.[104] This balance between interfacial energy and conformational entropy determines the thermodynamically favorable morphology of the micelles. A higher PEG density, therefore, forces the formation of spherical

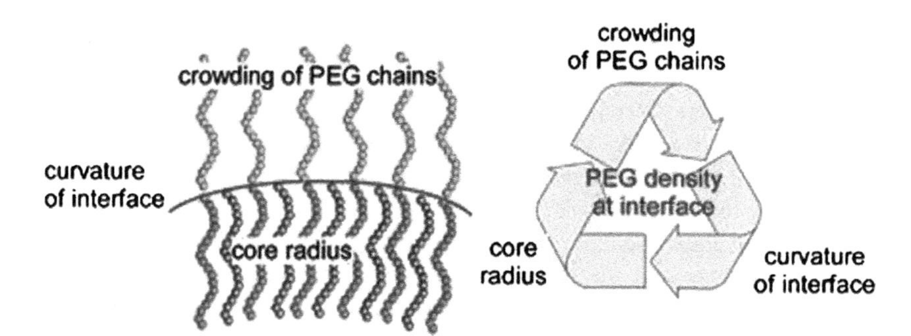

FIGURE 20.3 Illustration of poly (ethylene glycol) (PEG) corona density and the parameters that influence it, such as block lengths and association numbers. PEG corona density determines micelle shape. *Reprinted with permission from Harada et al.*[103] *Copyright © 2017 The Society of Polymer Science.*

micelles as the PEG chains repel each other under osmotic pressure,[114] by increasing the core curvature. Additionally, if the fraction of neutral hydrophilic segments is reduced (as in the case of BCP/homopolymer pairs) beyond a threshold level, lamellar structures of the PEC are favored, inducing a transition from spherical to wormlike micelles.[99]

Unique alterations to the BCP components have been shown to yield interesting multimolecular structures. "Polymersomes" are polymer-based vesicles that enclose some volume and have a thin membrane; these are called PICsomes (polyion complex-somes) when made with a PEC membrane and a neutral, hydrophilic block such as PEG.[111,115] The formation of these architectures is driven by the segregation of the PEG and PEC phases, and there is a strong dependence on the weight fraction, and hence the density of PEG, to determine whether micelles or PICsomes are formed. It has been reported that a 10% weight fraction of PEG leads to micelle formation, and a lower fraction of PEG leads to PICsome formation.[116] The transition from spherical micelles to PICsomes with decreasing PEG weight fraction is attributed to the lowered number of PEG chains at the core–corona interface, despite an increased PEC volume.[115] The PEC volume would increase if the method to reduce PEG weight fraction was the addition of polyion homopolymer. The observed transition phases were spherical micelle, cylinder, connected cylinder, connected plane, and lamella.[115] Related polymersome structures have been formed by mixing oppositely charged hydrophobic block copolymers.[117] Clearly, the structure of the polyions is a determinant in the morphology of PEC micelles and can be used to engineer desired properties. For instance, a trehalose-based cationic BCP complexed with plasmid deoxyribonucleic acid (pDNA) was shown to form nanoscale polyplexes instead of micelles, which were colloidally stable during in vivo circulation.[62] Another mode of improving the colloidal stability of these self-assembled structures is by using an ABC-type triblock copolymer with pDNA to form core–shell–corona micelles.[118]

Similar to solvophobic systems, PEC micelles form different structures with increasing total polymer concentration. As the concentration increases, micelle coronas begin to entangle and form hydrogels. Initially, disordered micelle cores form the hydrogel network, but as the concentration continues to increase the micelle cores organize into a body-centered cubic lattice, which transitions to hexagonally packed cylinders at even higher concentrations. This has been demonstrated using both diblock and triblock systems using small-angle X-ray scattering (SAXS), where microphase separation and ordering was observed.[74,119]

20.3.3 Effect of salt on PEC micelles

Since PEC micelles are electrostatically driven assemblies, a small amount of added salt forms larger PEC cores.[120] An excess amount of salt hinders PEC formation, and hence no micelles are formed. The reduction in electrostatic interaction between the polyelectrolytes caused by salt addition can be harnessed to induce spherical to wormlike transitions.[112] Salt can also be used as a controlled trigger for release of cargo by causing complete micelle dissolution.[120] Work done by Lindhoud presents one possible benefit from the alteration of PEC micelle behavior in the presence of salt.[121] PEC micelles were formed using a low charge density molecule (lipase) and two high charge density polyelectrolytes. The addition of salt screened the polyelectrolyte and lipase interactions, and since the lipase protein was large and of low charge density, it was ejected from the micelle.[121] This specific micellar system would not be very useful for biomedical applications because lipase release was triggered at a salt concentration lower than physiological concentrations. However, with proper engineering of the system, salt-triggered micelles have the potential to be used in controlled release drug delivery.

Similar to solvophobic systems, PEC micelles also have a critical micelle concentration (CMC), which is defined as the concentration at which polymer chains begin to assemble into micelles; below the CMC, only single chains exist.[122,123] Compared to amphiphilic micelles, whose CMC can be measured by surface tension measurements or hydrophobic dyes, the CMC of PEC micelles has been measured with light scattering techniques, resulting in less precise measurements. Theoretical predictions indicate that an increase in charged block length results in an increase in CMC up to a maximum, after which the CMC decreases with an increase in charged block length. The addition of salt presented a linear relationship between $\log_{10}$CMC and $\sqrt{C_s}$, where C_s is the salt concentration.[122]

20.3.4 Characterization methods and imaging

PEC micelles are difficult to characterize because micelles are small and dynamic nanoparticles and both the core and corona are highly solvated.[100] The high solvent content in the core and corona domains makes imaging with electron microscopy difficult due to low phase contrast. With TEM, the two conventional methods of imaging PEC micelles are using negatively stained samples[124,125] and using cryogenic-TEM (cryo-TEM).[126,127] Static and dynamic light scattering are frequently used tools in investigation of PEC micelle systems. Dynamic light scattering is informative of particle size, size distribution, and sphericity.[102] Static light scattering can be used to find Mw and aggregation numbers, as well as the CMC. Since PEC micelles are two-component systems, titration with varying f^+ can be done to establish the preferred micelle composition, which is the point with maximum light scattering intensity and complexation between oppositely charged polymers.[106] X-ray and neutron scattering are used to identify micellar domains, radii of gyration, shape, structure, and architectures over a range of length scales.[74] UV-vis absorption is another way that micelle formation can be observed, when a fluorescent anionic derivative, such as polyfluorene (PF_{22}) is used.[100] Upon micelle formation, a strong decay in the intensity of the fluorescence curve is observed (superquenching). By varying f^+ the ratio of intensities of the primary and secondary bands remained constant, and only the magnitude of intensities changed indicating that the PF_{22} chains did not stretch or twist inside the micelle. Fourier transform infrared spectroscopy, like the previously described UV-vis experiment, can be used to observe complexation, by looking at the deformation peaks of the ligands participating in complexation.[128]

20.3.5 Nucleic acid and protein delivery

Despite the potential of nucleic acid therapeutics, delivery has been difficult due to the negative charge of the molecule, enzymatic degradation, accumulation in nontarget organs/tissues, and insufficient cellular uptake.[96,129] PEC micelles can overcome these barriers.[129–131] Compared to polyplexes formed using homopolymers discussed in Section 20.2, nucleic acids complexed with BCPs show higher stability and higher resistance toward nuclease attack.[61] Different nucleic acid PEC micelles exist, in which the nucleic acid may be used as a homopolymer and mixed with an oppositely charged BCP, or a neutral polymer is conjugated to the nucleic acid which is subsequently mixed with a cationic homopolymer or BCP. These systems have been studied for the purpose of delivering a large variety of nucleic acids differing in size, hybridization, and function such as pDNA,[114,132] antisense oligonucleotides (AON),[133,134] oligodeoxynucleotides (ODN),[129,135] small interfering ribonucleic acid (siRNA),[130,136] microRNA (miRNA),[125] and mRNA.[137] Nucleic acid delivery can be confirmed by measuring the expression of downstream targets. For example, the use of plasmid containing PEC micelles allowed delivery to be confirmed via luciferase expression, demonstrating that increased expression was achieved with excess polycation.[138]

Targeting capabilities of nucleic acid delivering PEC micelles are significant to their efficacy as a therapeutic. For example, a lactosylated-PEG/siRNA conjugate complexed with PLK was developed to target asialoglycoprotein receptors of human hepatoma cells.[130] Similarly, a PEC micelle system with a folate ligand (used to target malignant tumors) has been shown to produce high targeting capabilities in vitro.[129] Another system has used cyclic RGD (arginine–glycine–aspartic acid) conjugated to PEG, siRNA, and cholesterol.[139] This multifunctional molecule was complexed with lysine to form tumor-targeting PEC micelles. Another example of creating multifunctional BCP electrolytes was aimed at treating atherosclerosis.[125] Two multifunctional peptide-PEG-polycation molecules were synthesized containing different targeting peptides, one that targets fibrin deposits found in atherosclerotic plaque and the other that targets inflamed endothelial cells via vascular cell adhesion molecule (VCAM-1), located on the cell surface. Micelles were formed using the two peptide-PEG-polycation molecules and miRNA inhibitors. This study was the first demonstration of targeting dysregulated miRNAs in atherosclerosis using targeted PEC micelles.

Proteins and enzymes can also be delivered using PEC micelles, although much fewer examples exist compared to nucleic acids. Work by Kataoka showed the formation of micelles between PEG-PAsp and lysozyme.[140,141] This system provided evidence that enzymatic activity can be controlled by modifying the corona thickness of the micelles, by increasing the block length of the neutral, hydrophilic block.

Despite considerable progress, there remains a need for higher efficiency of cellular uptake to improve efficacy of PEC micelles, and hence stimulus–responsive systems are rapidly gaining momentum. For instance, pH-sensitive peptides and polymers can undergo conformational changes that disrupt cell membranes[142] and have been developed for improved pDNA or siRNA delivery.[143] Thermoresponsive systems using poly(N-isopropylacrylamide) (PNIPAM), a neutral, hydrophilic polymer that undergoes a hydrophilic to hydrophobic transition above its lower critical solubility temperature (LCST), have also produced promising results.[144–146] This transition occurs between about 32 and 40°C, depending on molecular weight and solution conditions such as salt concentration. PNIPAM is one of the most common thermoresponsive polymers used in the biomedical field due to its acceptable biocompatibility.[147,148] A PEI-PNIPAM system to condense pDNA has been shown to improve accumulation and transfection in hyperthermia-treated tumor sites.[149,150] In addition to using pH and temperature as triggers, other avenues are also being explored, such as optical and magnetic triggers.[142]

20.3.6 Cell internalization

As previously mentioned, cellular uptake or cell internalization and targeting are the biggest challenges in *in vivo* efficacy of PEC micelle drug delivery systems. One proposed mechanism for this is via the enhanced permeability and retention (EPR) effect, which describes the tendency for macromolecules to selectively accumulate in regions of higher vascular permeability such as tumor tissue.[151,152] This has been demonstrated using PEC micelles loaded with mitoxantrone and doxorubicin which are complexed with poly(ethylene oxide)-poly(acrylic acid) and experience greater ease of transvascular transport via the EPR effect.[151]

PEG-stabilized micelles are readily taken up by cells via endocytosis, as the shell shields the charges within the core.[136] This can be enhanced using cell-penetrating peptides such as the HIV1-Tat peptide (Tat) which has been functionalized with PEGylated poly(ε-caprolactone) and complexed with vascular endothelial growth factor (VEGF) siRNA to form PEC micelles. The Tat peptide contains a high concentration of arginine which interacts with carbonate, sulfate, and phosphate of the proteoglycans at the surface of cells leading to enhanced intracellular transport with increasing N/P ratio (amine of the Tat peptide to the phosphate of the proteoglycan).[153,154]

Cellular uptake is often confirmed using fluorescently labeled polymers and imaging of cells, but more quantitative measurements can be achieved using flow cytometry.[136,142,155,156] Although PEC micelles are clearly entering cells, the exact mechanism of transport within the cell and the different pathways involved remain unclear.

20.3.7 In vivo studies

For PEC micelles to progress toward clinical applications, their biodistribution as well as systemic and local toxicity need to be evaluated. Although not fully established for PEC micelles, the biodistribution is likely governed by the particle's size and surface charge as it is for other nanoparticle systems.[157] PEC micelles have shown high circulation times, and low surface charge.[158] For instance, using PEG-PLK and plasmid DNA, PEC micelles improved the circulation time of supercoiled DNA in the blood to 30 min, and linear DNA to 3 h, compared to naked DNA which was degraded within 5 min.[138] The size (typically a function of molecular weight) of particles is an important factor for passing through vascular tissue to reach blood vessels. Given that micelles occur at the nanoscale, the size is sufficient for intercellular transport, which has a cutoff size of about 600 nm.[159]

Toxicity of the cationic components forming the particles is an important aspect to consider in nucleic acid delivery, owing to their propensity for interacting with negatively charged molecules.[160] As mentioned in Section 20.2, polycations tend to bind to the negatively charged plasma membrane and disrupt it, which can be quantified by the degree of lactose dehydrogenase leakage.[161,162] Higher molecular weight polycations display higher membrane disruption, but become less efficient for cellular uptake. This is the reason for employing neutral hydrophilic blocks, that are biocompatible (like PEG), in conjunction with polycations to reduce the effects of toxicity. Some PEC micelle systems have suffered from poor stability when tested in vivo, leading to the development of disulfide cross-linked micelles that showed increased circulation time.[139,163,164] For example, a PEG-siRNA disulfide-linked conjugate with PEI silenced VEGF in prostate cancer cells, with up to 96.5% efficacy.[165,166] Additionally, cholesterol has been conjugated to the charged block, such as siRNA, because the hydrophobized group reduces micelle disruption and prevents the leakage of cargo.[139] Although most PEC micelles have been delivered via intravenous administration, ocular delivery of PEC micelles has also been successfully demonstrated.[167]

20.3.8 Outlook

Pioneering work by Kataoka[95,102,104,105] and Stuart[98,99,106,107,127] have demonstrated the role of polymer block lengths and neutral block density on the size and morphology of PEC micelles. These dynamic assemblies are responsive to different charge ratios, salt concentration, polymer concentration, pH, and temperature when using a thermoresponsive corona forming segment. PEC micelles have the ability to overcome challenges associated with nucleic acid delivery (charge, enzymatic degradation) leading to delivery vehicles that can provide protection for the cargo, aid in longer circulation times, and be used for specific targeting of cells and tissues. These benefits have allowed PEC micelles to proceed to clinical trials. For instance, CALAA-01 by Calando Pharmaceuticals is a PEG-stabilized micelle, where a cyclodextrin polymer is complexed with siRNA used to reduce the expression of the M2 subunit of ribonucleotide reductase, which is a known anticancer target.[168] It was one of the first targeted polymer-based nanoparticles carrying siRNA that was administered to humans (clinical trials beginning in 2008).[169] Despite the trial ending due to toxic events, the efficacy of the particles was demonstrated in humans leaving room for new, less toxic, PEC micelles to be developed. Due to the versatility of this platform and new advances in polymer synthesis, it is possible that PEC micelles will play a role in the treatment of various diseases that are currently incurable.

20.4 Layer-by-layer self-assembled nanoparticles for biomedical applications

20.4.1 Introduction

Over the past few decades, the LbL technique has emerged as a promising technique for the fabrication of films and particles with precisely controlled structure and composition. LbL assembly was first described by Iler, who demonstrated the deposition of alternating layers of charged particles onto a solid surface.[170] In the 1990s, Decher and Hong[171] extended this technique to the deposition of layers of alternately charged polyelectrolytes onto solid surfaces. Since then, the technique has expanded to the deposition of a variety of charged components onto different types of substrates, including colloids, which this section focuses on.

The LbL technique has numerous advantages that make it ideal for a broad range of applications. It is a simple and inexpensive procedure, requiring equipment no more specialized or costly than beakers, solvent, and a substrate. Furthermore, LbL allows for the precise control of the composition and thickness of the deposited layers, simply by controlling the order in which the substrate is exposed to the various charged species. LbL assembly is especially well suited for biomedical applications, since it can be used with biocompatible and biodegradable materials; additionally, the tunable porosity of the polyelectrolyte layers has clear advantages for drug delivery systems.

LbL assembly has an additional advantage of scalability, which can be accomplished through multiple routes. In one example, the particle replication in nonwetting templates (PRINT) technique was used to create particles with specific size and geometry by growing them within a cross-linked polyvinyl alcohol (PVA) mold.[172] Subsequently, the mold was sprayed with alternating polyelectrolyte solutions, which could penetrate the mold and deposit the polyanions and polycations onto the particle surfaces. Another potential avenue for scaling up the LbL deposition onto nanoparticles is electrophoretic polymer assembly. Richardson et al. demonstrated this technique with the deposition of poly(allylamine hydrochloride) (PAH) and poly(styrene sulfonate) (PSS) onto silica particles.[173] The silica cores were suspended in a porous hydrogel. PSS and PAH were alternately passed through the gel by an electric field applied by an anode and cathode, coating the silica cores. 85% of particles were recovered, showing the high efficiency of this method.

Due to the broad range of techniques and applications of LbL, it is worth mentioning some studies that fall outside the scope of this section. Many researchers have studied the use of hollow capsules of micron size or larger for the delivery of drugs, vaccines, or other therapeutic cargo.[174–179] In addition to LbL-produced colloids, there has been much interest in LbL films for biomedical applications, such as drug delivery, biosensing, adhesion of proteins and cells, mediation of cellular functions, and implantable materials.[180] Moreover, while this section focuses on electrostatically driven self-assembly, LbL films can be assembled through other forces; for example, hydrogen-bonded LbL films have the potential to be more sensitive to pH or temperature, enabling the controlled release of cargo from drug delivery materials[181]; these materials may also have improved biocompatibility relative to electrostatically assembled materials.[182] LbL assembly driven by hydrophobic interactions[183] and DNA complementarity[184] has also been demonstrated.

20.4.2 Procedures

The general procedure for assembly of nanoparticles through LbL is very simple, although additional steps can be added to induce further structural modifications. The process begins with a suspension of charged particles that serve as nanoparticle cores. The cores are exposed to solutions or suspensions of charged species (such as polyelectrolytes or charged nanoparticles) with alternating charge, which bind electrostatically to the growing nanoparticle. Between adsorption steps, centrifugation and washing are performed to remove unadsorbed charged species from suspension. Each step results in the deposition of a single charged layer.[185] The general procedure is shown in Fig. 20.4.

Once a layered structure has been assembled onto the core, the nanoparticle can be modified in various ways. Drugs or other therapeutic cargo can be introduced into the

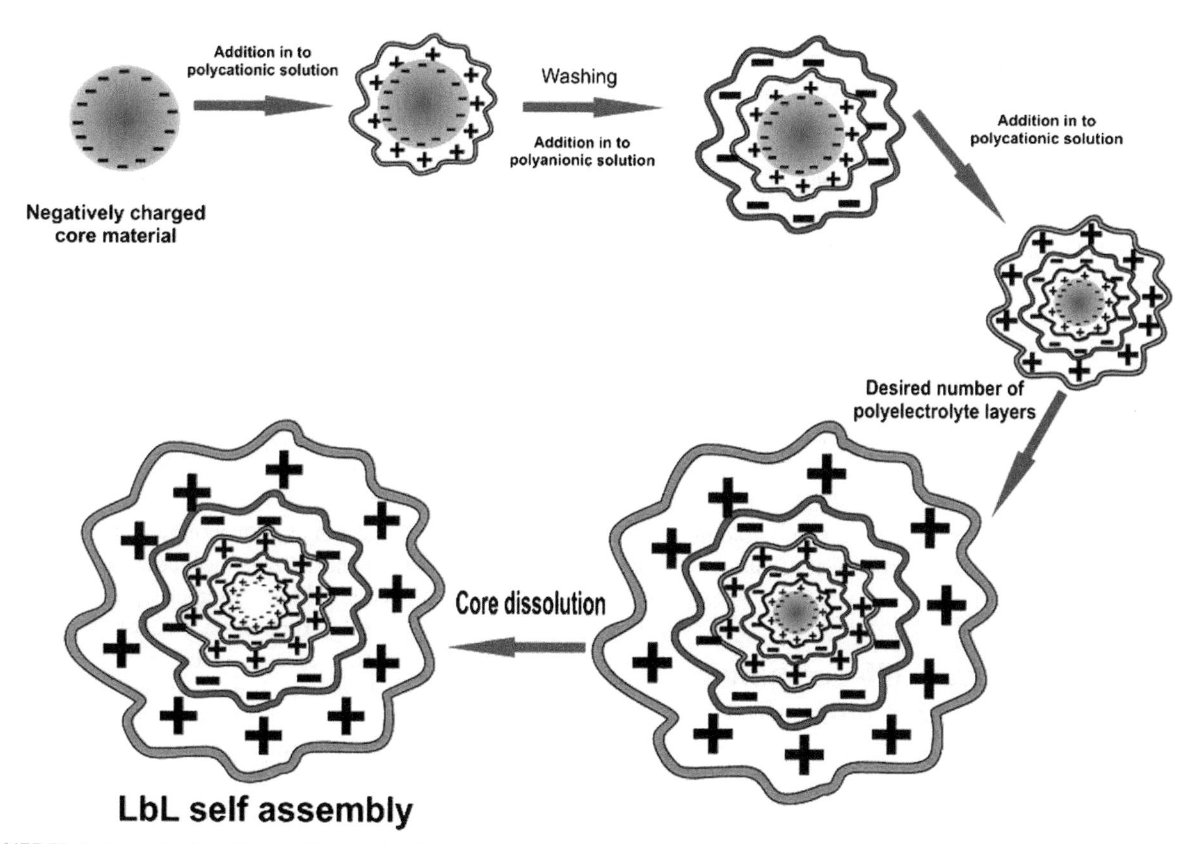

FIGURE 20.4 Layer-by-layer (LbL) self-assembly of core–shell nanoparticle followed by core dissolution. *Reprinted with permission from Deshmukh et al.*[186]

polyelectrolyte layers for later delivery. Alternatively, the core can be removed through various means to produce a hollow shell, into which other components can later be introduced. Examples of such sacrificial cores include melamine formamide, which decomposes in aqueous solutions of pH less than 1.6[174]; silica, which is similarly dissolved under acidic conditions[187]; and polystyrene, which is dissolved by tetrahydrofuran.[188] Furthermore, hollow inorganic capsules can be prepared by first introducing inorganic nanoparticles or precursors into the deposited layers, followed by calcination to sinter the inorganic components and destroy the core; some examples of inorganic capsules produced by this method include hollow TiO_2 spheres and Au/SiO_2 nanospheres.[189]

20.4.3 Applications

20.4.3.1 Combined approaches: LbL assemblies with polyplexes

In some cases, the benefits of polyplexes and LbL assembly can be combined to create gene or vaccine delivery systems with controlled release and longer circulation times. Blacklock et al.[190] demonstrated a gene delivery system consisting of LbL films in which the anionic layer consisted of bare DNA, while the cationic layer was a positively charged polyplex of DNA and hyperbranched poly (amido amine), a bioreducible polymer. The combination of bare DNA and polyplexes served to modulate the DNA release, as the polyplexes were released rapidly and the bare DNA slowly. Furthermore, the DNA release rate could be modulated by salt concentration, with higher concentration resulting in faster release.

Kim et al.[191] combined LbL assembly with polyplexes to create more effective DNA vaccines deliverable by microneedles. Alternating layers of heparin and albumin were deposited onto the polydopamine-coated surface of the polycarbonate microneedles. Polyplexes consisting of plasmid DNA encoding the beta-amyloid peptide (the vaccine target, which is implicated in Alzheimer's disease) and a CP were deposited onto the surface heparin layer and served as the DNA delivery vehicle. The vaccine is administered simply by applying a patch containing these polyplex-loaded microneedles to the skin, releasing the DNA-loaded polyplexes into the cutaneous tissue. In addition to being facile and painless, this approach was found to induce more antibodies in mice than conventional subcutaneously injected vaccines.

In addition to the incorporation of polyplexes into LbL layers, it is possible to deposit polyelectrolyte layers onto the surface of polyplexes to improve their performance. As the transfection efficiency and cytotoxicity of gene delivery vehicles are largely determined by surface properties, Ke et al.[192] sought to improve these properties by depositing layers of PAA and poly(N-(8-aminooctyl)-acrylamide) (P8Am) onto the surface of pDNA/PEI polyplexes, demonstrating greater transfection and reduced cytotoxicity when applied to HeLa and HepG2 cells (immortal cell lines derived from human cervical cancer and hepatocellular carcinoma cells, respectively).

Boyle et al.[88] demonstrated improved gene transfection efficiency by coating a polyplex consisting of pDNA and a trehalose-based polycation by coating the polyplex with anionic heparin. When heparin was added to the polyplexes, their zeta potential changed from around 4 mV to −1.2 mV, indicating adsorption of heparin onto the polyplex surface. As a result of this surface coating, the transfection efficiency of green fluorescent protein was increased in three different cell types (HepG2, primary fibroblasts, and U87 cells); the magnitude of this increase in efficiency ranged from 20% (in HepG2) to 60% (in U87 cells). Although a negative charge is typically detrimental to transfection, as discussed in Section 20.2, it was found that the heparin coating improved transfection by invoking different endocytotic pathways (clathrin-coated pits and micropinocytosis, rather than caveolae and micropinocytosis). As with the other studies mentioned here, this example shows the promise and versatility of combining polyplexes with LbL assembly.

20.4.3.2 Drug delivery

LbL-assembled nanoparticles are particularly well suited for drug delivery applications due to their ability to encapsulate various therapeutic materials, as well as the tunable nature of the shell, whose surface properties and porosity enable the targeting of specific cells as well as the controlled release of the cargo. Several approaches are used for the delivery of therapeutics via LbL nanoparticles.

The first of these approaches is the encapsulation of drugs into a hollow capsule. This method has the advantage of protecting the drug from being prematurely degraded in the body, as well as protecting the body from the side effects of the drug.[193] Loading of drugs into the capsules can be accomplished by controlling the porosity of the shell layers through the addition of salt, or by loading the capsules with a low molecular weight sequestering agent with high affinity for the drug of interest. The release characteristics of the drugs are also critically important and are generally categorized as burst or sustained release. Burst release may be desirable when cellular uptake of the capsule occurs and the drug is released within the cell, while sustained release is preferred when the drug component is released extracellularly to prevent excessive localized drug concentration.[193] Burst release can be triggered by an external stimulus such as laser light, or by the cellular uptake process; sustained release tends to occur via diffusion of the drug through the capsule wall.

Another approach to drug encapsulation via LbL is to adsorb the polyelectrolyte layers directly onto a drug nanocrystal, resulting in a very high concentration of the drug within the core as compared to approaches with drug-loaded porous or hollow cores. Zahr et al.[194] demonstrated this technique using nanocrystals of dexamethasone, a steroid used to treat inflammation and ameliorate the side effects of chemotherapy. PAH and PSS were alternately deposited onto the nanocrystal, and the PAH/PSS shell was then modified with PEG to improve biocompatibility. The resulting encapsulated drug nanocrystals were around 130 nm in diameter; the small size of these particles would allow them to penetrate through the smallest human capillary pores and into tumors.

A third approach is to absorb the drug molecules into the polyelectrolyte shell layers, while leaving the nanoparticle core intact. This technique is commonly used with magnetic cores, which provide multifold advantages: through the application of an external magnetic field, it is possible to target the nanoparticles to specific regions; furthermore, an applied magnetic field can induce heating of the nanoparticles, which is useful both for hyperthermia treatment of tumors and for localized, thermally controlled drug delivery. These applications of LbL nanoparticles with magnetic cores are comprehensively reviewed by Kumar and Mohommad.[195] In one example of this technique, Huang et al. demonstrated the delivery of the anticancer drug doxorubicin via oral administration of LbL nanoparticles. Iron oxide nanoparticles were coated with polyelectrolyte layers via LbL, followed by loading of the polyelectrolytes with doxorubicin, and finally capping of the shell layers with casein to prevent precipitation of the particles in the acidic stomach environment. The magnetic nanoparticles provided MRI contrast to map the distribution of particles in mouse models, which confirmed effective delivery of the drug to the small intestine.[196]

In addition to the use of inorganic cores, a porous organic core may be used, allowing for the loading of drug molecules into the core itself as well as into the shell layers. In one example, Shutava et al. created LbL particles with cross-linked gelatin cores, which were encased in different types of polyelectrolyte layers with thicknesses of 5−20 nm. The gel-like cores, with sizes of 200−300 nm, were loaded with several polyphenol drugs including epigallocatechin gallate (EGCG), which is found in green tea and possessing anticancer properties. The deposited polyelectrolyte layers served to modulate the cell uptake behavior of the particles and to control the release characteristics of the drug. A sustained release over a period of 8 h was achieved, and the EGCG-loaded nanoparticles remained as effective as free EGCG in blocking intracellular signaling via hepatocyte growth factor in breast cancer cells.[197]

When the therapeutic cargo to be delivered is itself a charged polymer such as DNA or RNA, it can simply be deposited onto the nanoparticle core in an LbL fashion without the need for an additional drug-loading step. Elbakry et al.[198] demonstrated this technique as a viable platform for gene silencing applications. Anionic small interfering RNA (siRNA) and cationic PEI were alternately adsorbed onto 15-nm gold nanoparticles. The siRNA sequence blocked the expression of enhanced green fluorescent protein (EGFP), which provided an indicator of the knockdown in gene expression when the nanoparticles were introduced into EGFP-expressing CHO−K1 cells. It was found that the siRNA-coated gold nanoparticles reduced the production of EGFP by 28%. Guo et al.[199] applied a similar approach, but incorporated a charge-reversal polymer PAH-Cit (which reverses from negatively to positively charged in acidic environments) as one of the polyelectrolyte layers. This charge reversal facilitated the release of the siRNA resulting in a greater concentration of siRNA in the cell cytoplasm, leading to an 80% knockdown efficiency of lamin A/C protein expression in HeLa cells.

In addition to the individual approaches described in previous paragraphs, combinations of these methods can be versatile and powerful. Such a combined approach was developed by Deng at al. for the treatment of aggressive triple-negative breast cancer (TNBC). In addition to a carboxyl-modified polystyrene latex nanoparticle core loaded with doxorubicin to attack cancer cells, siRNA in the LbL-applied polyelectrolyte coating served to knockdown drug-resistance pathways, making the cells more vulnerable to the doxubicin.[200] Specifically, the siRNA was selected to target the gene for multidrug resistance protein 1 (MRP1), a membrane pump that reduces drug concentrations in the cancer cell and whose presence is correlated with more severe TNBC. An outer shell was applied over the siRNA/HA layers to facilitate the targeting of tumor cells. From in vivo experiments in mice, it was found that the siRNA/doxorubicin nanoparticles were four times more effective at reducing tumor size than a control particle containing doxorubicin with a random RNA sequence, demonstrating the effectiveness of gene silencing combined with the anticancer drug.

One of the signature advantages of the use of LbL-assembled nanoparticles for drug delivery is the ability to functionalize the outer shell of the nanoparticles to effectively target-specific cell types, which can maximize the effectiveness of the treatment and reduce side effects. Cortez et al. achieved this specificity using antibody-functionalized LbL nanoparticles to target colorectal cancer cells via an antigen commonly expressed by these cells, A33.[188] Polystyrene nanoparticles with a diameter of 488 nm were coated with PAH/PSS layers, followed by the adsorption of the humanized A33 monoclonal antibody (huA33) to the outer PSS layer. In binding experiments, the huA33-functionalized nanoparticles showed a fourfold binding increase to LIM1215 colorectal cells compared to control nanoparticles (which were functionalized with a different antibody, mouse IgG). Furthermore, confocal microscopy confirmed the improved internalization of these particles by LIM1215 compared to the control particles.

Poon et al. demonstrated another targeting strategy for LbL nanoparticles, taking advantage of the lower pH found in tumor microenvironments. Unlike the previous approach which requires functionalization by specific ligands, this method is broadly applicable to different types of tumors. In this study, three layers were deposited onto the nanoparticle core: a PLK layer, a neutravidin layer, and finally a PEG layer. The PLK layer contributes to cellular uptake due to its charge. The neutravidin behaves as a pH-sensitive linker between PLK and PEG; at low pH (as found in tumor microenvironments), these links are broken, releasing the outer PEG layer. In healthy tissues, however, the PEG layer inhibits cellular uptake. Fluorescence imaging confirmed the absorption and retention of the nanoparticles by tumors in mice.[201]

20.4.3.3 Biosensing

LbL-fabricated nanoparticles have attracted much interest for biosensing applications, due to their high surface area and controllable surface properties. In one example, Trau et al. sought to improve on conventional immunoassays by encapsulating fluorescent crystals of fluorescein diacetate (FDA) in PAH/PSS polyelectrolyte layers.[202] The LbL-applied polyelectrolyte layers served dual functions: to improve the colloidal stability of the nanoparticles and to allow for the functionalization of the particle surface with antibodies. After the immunoreaction took place, FDA crystals were dissolved, releasing a strong fluorescent signal. The advantage of this approach relative to conventional immunoassays is that the ratio between fluorescent dye to biomolecules (F/P ratio), an important factor in the sensitivity of immunoassays, is greatly increased; the sensitivity of the immunoassay was increased 2000-fold compared to conventional immunoassays. In another study with potential biosensing applications, Schneider and Decher[203] created LbL-coated gold nanoparticles with LbL-deposited layers containing fluorophores; the number of layers (and therefore the distance between the fluorophores and the core) controlled the fluorescence intensity.

20.4.3.4 Biomimetic reactors

Due to their customizable structure and composition, and ability to encapsulate smaller components, LbL particles have drawn interest as nanoreactors, artificial organelles, and even as artificial cells. Most of these studies have focused on micron-sized or larger particles and have been reviewed by Shchukin and Sukhorukov,[204] as well as Städler.[205] In one example of a nanoscale LbL biomimetic reactor, He et al. synthesized calcium carbonate within the interior of LbL-assembled polymer nanotubes loaded with urease.[206] The nanotubes consisted of inner alternating layers of PSS and PAH, with PSS replaced by magnetic Fe_3O_4 nanoparticles in the outer layers (which allowed for separation of the final product). The urease loaded into the nanotubes catalyzed the reaction of aqueous urea and $CaCl_2$ into $CaCO_3$; depending on the diameter of the tubes, different polymorphs of $CaCO_3$ were obtained (vaterite or calcite). The process developed in this study mimics the biomineralization process that forms bones or shells in nature.

20.4.3.5 Layer-by-layer composite films containing nanoparticles

In addition to nanoparticles formed via LbL assembly on colloidal templates, there are numerous examples of LbL films containing nanoparticles that have biomedical applications.[207–216] These applications, which are too broad to discuss in depth here, include biosensors,[207,208,216] antibacterial films,[209,212,214] and drug delivery systems.[215] In another example, Kommireddy et al. created LbL films consisting of PSS, PDDA, and TiO_2 nanoparticles for the attachment of stem cells.[210] It was found that increasing the number of TiO_2 layers increased the surface roughness, which promoted spreading of cells on the surface. This type of film has potential applications in biomedical devices to support stem cell attachment for tissue repair. Xi et al. created nanoporous LbL films by depositing alternating layers of gold nanoparticles and graphene films onto a substrate.[211] The resulting films were effective as electrochemical sensors for H_2O_2, which may have applications in biosensing.

20.4.4 Outlook

LbL assembly of nanoparticles represents a powerful new technique for biomedical applications due to its facile procedures, low cost, and ability to control structures with nanoscale precision. While many promising laboratory studies have been reported, much fewer animal studies have been performed, and there have been no known clinical trials in humans. Städler et al. identify the main issues with LbL capsules in particular as poor colloidal stability, a labor-intensive and low-yield fabrication process, poor control over drug loading and release, and poor control over cell targeting and internalization.[205] For capsules and other in vivo applications, it is critical that the materials used are biocompatible; however, some of the polyelectrolytes most commonly used in these studies, such as PAH, do not meet this requirement.[175] Furthermore, additional study of nonspherical particles is needed since the particle geometry is known to affect biological interactions.[217] Although significant challenges remain before LbL nanoparticle assembly is widely adopted in biomedical technology, it remains the subject of ongoing and intensive research to overcome these challenges.

20.5 Conclusion

Studies on homopolymer PECs, BCP PEC micelles, and LbL-assembled nanoparticles demonstrate the great potential of electrostatically assembled nanoparticles for biomedical applications. The stabilization of PECs on the nanoscale is achieved either by manipulating the charge ratio of complexes (Section 20.2.1), by using block copolymers (Section 20.3), or through the number and sequence of polyelectrolyte layers deposited in an LbL process. Electrostatically driven self-assembly is a powerful technique for obtaining precisely controlled nanostructures, since these structures can be controlled simply by altering a few factors during the fabrication process, such as composition, polyelectrolyte molecular weight, or ionic strength. These designed structures, in turn, lead to specific interactions with cells or biological materials, making the nanoparticles multifunctional and intelligent materials. Although these materials have shown impressive results in the laboratory, it is not clearly understood how they perform in the human body as relatively few studies have advanced to the stage of clinical trials. For the potential of these materials to be fully realized, further work must be undertaken to transfer this area of research from the laboratory to the clinic.

References

1. Müller M. *Polyelectrolyte complexes in the dispersed and solid state I–principles and theory*. Springer; 2014.
2. Marciel AB, Chung EJ, Brettmann BK, Leon L. Bulk and nanoscale polypeptide based polyelectrolyte complexes. *Adv Colloid Interface Sci* 2017;**239**:187–98.
3. Vieregg JR, Lueckheide M, Marciel AB, Leon L, Bologna AJ, Rivera JR, Tirrell MV. Oligonucleotide-peptide complexes: phase control by hybridization. *J Am Chem Soc* 2018;**140**:1632–8.
4. Galazka VB, Smith D, Ledward DA, Dickinson E. Complexes of bovine serum albumin with sulphated polysaccharides: effects of pH, ionic strength and high pressure treatment. *Food Chem* 1999;**64**:303–10.

5. Chollakup R, Beck JB, Dirnberger K, Tirrell M, Eisenbach CD. Polyelectrolyte molecular weight and salt effects on the phase behavior and coacervation of aqueous solutions of poly(acrylic acid) sodium salt and poly(allylamine) hydrochloride. *Macromolecules* 2013;**46**:2376–90.
6. Perry SL, Leon L, Hoffmann KQ, Kade MJ, Priftis D, Black KA, Wong D, Klein RA, Pierce CF, Margossian KO, Whitmer JK, Qin J, de Pablo JJ, Tirrell M. Chirality-selected phase behaviour in ionic polypeptide complexes. *Nat Commun* 2015;**6**:6052.
7. Priftis D, Leon L, Song Z, Perry SL, Margossian KO, Tropnikova A, Cheng J, Tirrell M. Self-assembly of α-helical polypeptides driven by complex coacervation. *Angew Chem Int Ed Engl* 2015;**54**:11128–32.
8. Wang Q, Schlenoff JB. The polyelectrolyte complex/coacervate continuum. *Macromolecules* 2014;**47**:3108–16.
9. Weinbreck F, de Vries R, Schrooyen P, de Kruif CG. Complex coacervation of whey proteins and gum Arabic. *Biomacromolecules* 2003;**4**:293–303.
10. Girod S, Boissière M, Longchambon K, Begu S, Tourne-Pétheil C, Devoisselle JM. Polyelectrolyte complex formation between iota-carrageenan and poly(L-lysine) in dilute aqueous solutions: a spectroscopic and conformational study. *Carbohydr Polym* 2004;**55**:37–45.
11. Zhang Y, Batys P, O'Neal JT, Li F, Sammalkorpi M, Lutkenhaus JL. Molecular origin of the glass transition in polyelectrolyte assemblies. *ACS Cent Sci* 2018;**4**:638–44.
12. Fu J, Fares HM, Schlenoff JB. Ion-pairing strength in polyelectrolyte complexes. *Macromolecules* 2017;**50**:1066–74.
13. Shamoun RF, Hariri HH, Ghostine RA, Schlenoff JB. Thermal transformations in extruded saloplastic polyelectrolyte complexes. *Macromolecules* 2012;**45**:9759–67.
14. Black KA, Priftis D, Perry SL, Yip J, Byun WY, Tirrell M. Protein encapsulation via polypeptide complex coacervation. *ACS Macro Lett* 2014;**3**:1088–91.
15. Kataoka K, Harada A, Nagasaki Y. Block copolymer micelles for drug delivery: design, characterization and biological significance. *Adv Drug Deliv Rev* 2001;**47**:113–31.
16. Madene A, Jacquot M, Scher J, Desobry S. Flavour encapsulation and controlled release - a review. *Int J Food Sci Technol* 2006;**41**:1–21.
17. Augustin MA, Hemar Y. Nano- and micro-structured assemblies for encapsulation of food ingredients. *Chem Soc Rev* 2009;**38**:902–12.
18. Keating CD. Aqueous phase separation as a possible route to compartmentalization of biological molecules. *Acc Chem Res* 2012;**45**:2114–24.
19. Frankel EA, Bevilacqua PC, Keating CD. Polyamine/nucleotide coacervates provide strong compartmentalization of Mg^{2+}, nucleotides, and RNA. *Langmuir* 2016;**32**:2041–9.
20. Lim S, Choi YS, Kang DG, Song YH, Cha HJ. The adhesive properties of coacervated recombinant hybrid mussel adhesive proteins. *Biomaterials* 2010;**31**:3715–22.
21. Winslow BD, Shao H, Stewart RJ, Tresco PA. Biocompatibility of adhesive complex coacervates modeled after the sandcastle glue of Phragmatopoma californica for craniofacial reconstruction. *Biomaterials* 2010;**31**:9373–81.
22. Wang W, Xu Y, Li A, Li T, Liu M, Von Klitzing R, Ober CK, Kayitmazer AB, Li L, Guo X. Zinc induced polyelectrolyte coacervate bioadhesive and its transition to a self-healing hydrogel. *RSC Adv* 2015;**5**:66871–8.
23. Kawamura A, Harada A, Kono K, Kataoka K. Self-assembled nano-bioreactor from block ionomers with elevated and stabilized enzymatic function. *Bioconjug Chem* 2007;**18**:1555–9.
24. Anraku Y, Kishimura A, Kamiya M, Tanaka S, Nomoto T, Toh K, Matsumoto Y, Fukushima S, Sueyoshi D, Kano MR, Urano Y, Nishiyama N, Kataoka K. Systemically injectable enzyme-loaded polyion complex vesicles as in vivo nanoreactors functioning in tumors. *Angew Chem Int Ed* 2016;**55**:560–5.
25. Hammond PT. Recent explorations in electrostatic multilayer thin film assembly. *Curr Opin Colloid Interface Sci* 2000;**4**:430–42.
26. Tros de Ilarduya C, Sun Y, Düzgüneş N. Gene delivery by lipoplexes and polyplexes. *Eur J Pharm Sci* 2010;**40**:159–70.
27. De Smedt SC, Demeester J, Hennink WE. Cationic polymer based gene delivery systems. *Pharm Res* 2000;**17**:113–26.
28. Gebhart CL, Kabanov AV. Evaluation of polyplexes as gene transfer agents. *J Control Release* 2001;**73**:401–16.
29. Mao S, Sun W, Kissel T. Chitosan-based formulations for delivery of DNA and siRNA. *Adv Drug Deliv Rev* 2010;**62**:12–27.
30. Kabanov AV, Kabanov VA. DNA complexes with polycations for the delivery of genetic material into cells. *Bioconjug Chem* 1995;**6**:7–20.
31. Shapiro JT, Leng M, Felsenfeld G. Deoxyribonucleic acid-polylysine complexes. Structure and nucleotide specificity. *Biochemistry* 1969;**8**:3219–32.
32. Zama M, Ichimura S. Difference between polylysine and polyarginine in changing DNA structure upon complex formation. *Biochem Biophys Res Commun* 1971;**44**:936–42.
33. Zama M. Structure and circular dichroism of DNA-polylysine-polyarginine complex. *Biochim Biophys Acta* 1974;**366**:124–34.
34. Wagner E, Cotten M, Foisner R, Birnstiel ML. Transferrin-polycation-DNA complexes: the effect of polycations on the structure of the complex and DNA delivery to cells. *Proc Natl Acad Sci USA* 1991;**88**:4255–9.
35. Kabanov VA, Zezin AB. A new class of water soluble polyelectrolytes. *Makromol. Chem. Suppl.* 1984;**6**:259–76.
36. Kabanov AV, Kabanov VA. Interpolyelectrolyte and block ionomer complexes for gene delivery: physico-chemical aspects. *Adv Drug Deliv Rev* 1998;**30**:49–60.
37. Kabanov AV. Taking polycation gene delivery systems from in vitro to in vivo. *Pharm Sci Technol Today* 1999;**2**:365–72.
38. Ragelle H, Vandermeulen G, Préat V. Chitosan-based siRNA delivery systems. *J Control Release* 2013;**172**:207–18.
39. Mintzer MA, Simanek EE. Nonviral vectors for gene delivery. *Chem Rev* 2009;**109**:259–302.
40. Dohmen C, Edinger D, Fröhlich T, Schreiner L, Lächelt U, Troiber C, Rädler J, Hadwiger P, Vornlocher H-P, Wagner E. Nanosized multifunctional polyplexes for receptor-mediated SiRNA delivery. *ACS Nano* 2012;**6**:5198–208.
41. Luo D, Saltzman WM. Synthetic DNA delivery systems. *Nat Biotechnol* 2000;**18**:33–7.
42. Derouchey J, Schmidt C, Walker GF, Koch C, Plank C, Wagner E, Rädler JO. Monomolecular assembly of siRNA and poly (ethylene glycol)-peptide copolymers. *Biomacromolecules* 2008;**9**:724–32.
43. Zintchenko A, Philipp A, Dehshahri A, Wagner E. Simple modifications of branched PEI lead to highly efficient siRNA carriers with low toxicity. *Bioconjug Chem* 2008;**19**:1448–55.
44. Creusat G, Thomann JS, Maglott A, Pons B, Dontenwill M, Guérin E, Frisch B, Zuber G. Pyridylthiourea-grafted

polyethylenimine offers an effective assistance to siRNA-mediated gene silencing in vitro and in vivo. *J Control Release* 2012;**157**:418–26.
45. Martirosyan A, Olesen MJ, Howard KA. Chitosan-based nanoparticles for mucosal delivery of RNAi therapeutics. *Adv Genet* 2014;**88**:325–52.
46. Heissig P, Klein PM, Hadwiger P, Wagner E. DNA as tunable adaptor for siRNA polyplex stabilization and functionalization. *Mol Ther – Nucleic Acids* 2016;**5**:e288.
47. Priftis D, Tirrell M. Phase behaviour and complex coacervation of aqueous polypeptide solutions. *Soft Matter* 2012;**8**:9396–405.
48. Schmitt C, Sanchez C, Desobry-Banon S, Hardy J. Structure and technofunctional properties of protein-polysaccharide complexes: a review. *Crit Rev Food Sci Nutr* 1998;**38**:689–753.
49. Vander Straeten A, Bratek-Skicki A, Germain L, D'Haese C, Eloy P, Fustin CA, Dupont-Gillain C. Protein-polyelectrolyte complexes to improve the biological activity of proteins in layer-by-layer assemblies. *Nanoscale* 2017;**9**:17186–92.
50. Schmitt C, Turgeon SL. Protein/polysaccharide complexes and coacervates in food systems. *Adv Colloid Interface Sci* 2011;**167**:63–70.
51. Picó GA, Woitovich Valetti N. Complexes formation between proteins and polyelectrolytes and their application in the downstream processes of enzyme purification. In: Visakh PM, Bayraktar O, Picó GA, editors. *Polyelectrolytes: Thermodynamics and Rheology*. Springer; 2014. p. 245–73.
52. Ball V, Winterhalter M, Schwinte P, Lavalle P, Voegel JC, Schaaf P. Complexation mechanism of bovine serum albumin and poly(allylamine hydrochloride). *J Phys Chem B* 2002;**106**:2357–64.
53. Hu B, Wang SS, Li J, Zeng XX, Huang QR. Assembly of bioactive peptide-chitosan nanocomplexes. *J Phys Chem B* 2011;**115**:7515–23.
54. Kimura T, Yamaoka T, Iwase R, Murakami A. Structure/function relationship in the polyplexes containing cationic polypeptides for gene delivery. *Nucleic Acids Symp Ser* 2001;**1**:203–4.
55. Tang MX, Szoka FC. The influence of polymer structure on the interactions of cationic polymers with DNA and morphology of the resulting complexes. *Gene Ther* 1997;**4**:823–32.
56. Boddohi S, Moore N, Johnson PA, Kipper MJ. Polysaccharide-based polyelectrolyte complex nanoparticles from chitosan, heparin, and hyaluronan. *Biomacromolecules* 2009;**10**:1402–9.
57. Guimond S, Maccarana M, Olwin BB, Lindahl U, Rapraeger AC. Activating and inhibitory heparin sequences for FGF-2 (basic FGF): distinct requirements for FGF-1, FGF-2, and FGF-4. *J Biol Chem* 1993;**268**:23906–14.
58. Birch NP, Schiffman JD. Characterization of self-assembled polyelectrolyte complex nanoparticles formed from chitosan and pectin. *Langmuir* 2014;**30**:3441–7.
59. de la Fuente M, Seijo B, Alonso MJ. Novel hyaluronan-based nanocarriers for transmucosal delivery of macromolecules. *Macromol Biosci* 2008;**8**:441–50.
60. Petersen H, Fechner PM, Martin AL, Kunath K, Stolnik S, Roberts CJ, Fischer D, Davies MC, Kissel T. Polyethylenimine-graft-poly(ethylene glycol) copolymers: influence of copolymer block structure on DNA complexation and biological activities as gene delivery system. *Bioconjug Chem* 2002;**13**:845–54.
61. Katayose S, Kataoka K. Water-soluble polyion complex associates of DNA and poly(ethylene glycol)-poly(L-lysine) block copolymer. *Bioconjug Chem* 1997;**8**:702–7.
62. Tolstyka ZP, Phillips H, Cortez M, Wu Y, Ingle N, Bell JB, Hackett PB, Reineke TM. Trehalose-based block copolycations promote polyplex stabilization for lyophilization and in vivo pDNA delivery. *ACS Biomater Sci Eng* 2016;**2**:43–55.
63. Ogris M, Steinlein P, Kursa M, Mechtler K, Kircheis R, Wagner E. The size of DNA/transferrin-PEI complexes is an important factor for gene expression in cultured cells. *Gene Ther* 1998;**10**:1425–33.
64. Howard KA, Rahbek UL, Liu X, Damgaard CK, Glud SZ, Andersen MØ, Hovgaard MB, Schmitz A, Nyengaard JR, Besenbacher F, Kjems J. RNA interference in vitro and in vivo using a novel chitosan/siRNA nanoparticle system. *Mol Ther* 2006;**14**:476–84.
65. Lee Y, Kataoka K. Delivery of nucleic acid drugs. In: Murakami A, editor. *Nucleic acid drugs*, **249**. Berlin, Heidelberg: Springer; 2011. p. 95–134.
66. Liu W, Sun S, Cao Z, Zhang X, Yao K, Lu WW, Luk KDK. An investigation on the physicochemical properties of chitosan/DNA polyelectrolyte complexes. *Biomaterials* 2005;**26**:2705–11.
67. Kunath K, von Harpe A, Fischer D, Petersen H, Bickel U, Voigt K, Kissel T. Low-molecular-weight polyethylenimine as a non-viral vector for DNA delivery: comparison of physicochemical properties, transfection efficiency and in vivo distribution with high-molecular-weight polyethylenimine. *J Control Release* 2003;**89**:113–25.
68. Bettinger T, Carlisle RC, Read ML, Ogris M, Seymour LW. Peptide-mediated RNA delivery: a novel approach for enhanced transfection of primary and post-mitotic cells. *Nucleic Acids Res* 2001;**29**:3882–91.
69. Mann A, Richa R, Ganguli M. DNA condensation by poly-l-lysine at the single molecule level: role of DNA concentration and polymer length. *J Control Release* 2008;**125**:252–62.
70. Huang M, Fong CW, Khor E, Lim LY. Transfection efficiency of chitosan vectors: effect of polymer molecular weight and degree of deacetylation. *J Control Release* 2005;**106**:391–406.
71. Liu X, Howard KA, Dong M, Andersen MØ, Rahbek UL, Johnsen MG, Hansen OC, Besenbacher F, Kjems J. The influence of polymeric properties on chitosan/siRNA nanoparticle formulation and gene silencing. *Biomaterials* 2007;**28**:1280–8.
72. Seyrek E, Dubin PL, Tribet C, Gamble EA. Ionic strength dependence of protein-polyelectrolyte interactions. *Biomacromolecules* 2003;**4**:273–82.
73. Perry SL, Li Y, Priftis D, Leon L, Tirrell M. The effect of salt on the complex coacervation of vinyl polyelectrolytes. *Polymers* 2014;**6**:1756–72.
74. Krogstad DV, Choi S-H, Lynd NA, Audus DJ, Perry SL, Gopez JD, Hawker CJ, Kramer EJ, Tirrell MV. Small angle neutron scattering study of complex coacervate micelles and hydrogels formed from ionic diblock and triblock copolymers. *J Phys Chem B* 2014;**118**:13011–8.
75. Ren Y, Jiang X, Pan D, Mao HQ. Charge density and molecular weight of polyphosphoramidate gene carrier are key parameters influencing its DNA compaction ability and transfection efficiency. *Biomacromolecules* 2010;**11**:3432–9.
76. Boeris V, Romanini D, Farruggia B, Picó G. Interaction and complex formation between catalase and cationic polyelectrolytes: chitosan and Eudragit E100. *Int J Biol Macromol* 2009;**45**:103–8.
77. Boeris V, Spelzini D, Salgado JP, Picó G, Romanini D, Farruggia B. Chymotrypsin-poly vinyl sulfonate interaction studied by

dynamic light scattering and turbidimetric approaches. *Biochim Biophys Acta — Gen Subj* 2008;**1780**:1032—7.

78. Behr J-P. The proton sponge: a trick to enter cells the viruses did not exploit. *Chim Int J Chem* 1997;**51**:34—6.
79. Lächelt U, Wagner E. Nucleic acid therapeutics using polyplexes: a journey of 50 years (and beyond). *Chem Rev* 2015;**115**:11043—78.
80. Pack DW, Hoffman AS, Pun S, Stayton PS. Design and development of polymers for gene delivery. *Nat Rev Drug Discov* 2005;**4**:581—93.
81. Santos-Carballal B, Fernández EF, Goycoolea FM. Chitosan in non-viral gene delivery: role of structure, characterization methods, and insights in cancer and rare diseases therapies. *Polymers* 2018;**10**:444.
82. Sonawane ND, Szoka FC, Verkman AS. Chloride accumulation and swelling in endosomes enhances DNA transfer by polyamine-DNA polyplexes. *J Biol Chem* 2003;**278**:44826—31.
83. Rejman J, Bragonzi A, Conese M. Role of clathrin- and caveolae-mediated endocytosis in gene transfer mediated by lipo- and polyplexes. *Mol Ther* 2005;**12**:468—74.
84. Yaroslavov AA, Sukhishvili SA, Obolsky OL, Yaroslavova EG, Kabanov AV, Kabanov VA. DNA affinity to biological membranes is enhanced due to complexation with hydrophobized polycation. *FEBS Lett* 1996;**384**:177—80.
85. Rejman J, Conese M, Hoekstra D. Gene transfer by means of lipo- and polyplexes: role of clathrin and caveolae-mediated endocytosis. *J Liposome Res* 2006;**16**:237—47.
86. Rejman J, Oberle V, Zuhorn IS, Hoekstra D. Size-dependent internalization of particles via the pathways of clathrin- and caveolae-mediated endocytosis. *Biochem J* 2004;**377**:159—69.
87. McLendon PM, Fichter KM, Reineke TM. Poly(glycoamidoamine) vehicles promote pDNA uptake through multiple routes and efficient gene expression via caveolae-mediated endocytosis. *Mol Pharm* 2010;**7**:738—50.
88. Boyle WS, Senger K, Tolar J, Reineke TM. Heparin enhances transfection in concert with a trehalose-based polycation with challenging cell types. *Biomacromolecules* 2017;**18**:56—67.
89. Yin H, Kanasty RL, Eltoukhy AA, Vegas AJ, Dorkin JR, Anderson DG. Non-viral vectors for gene-based therapy. *Nat Rev Genet* 2014;**15**:541—55.
90. Ha M, Kim VN. Regulation of microRNA biogenesis. *Nat Rev Mol Cell Biol* 2014;**15**:509—24.
91. Collins M, Thrasher A. Gene therapy: progress and predictions. *Proc R Soc B Biol Sci* 2015;**282**:20143003.
92. Liu S, Jia H, Yang J, Pan J, Liang H, Zeng L, Zhou H, Chen J, Guo T. Zinc coordinated cationic polymers break up the paradox between low molecular weight and high transfection efficacy. *Biomacromolecules* 2018;**19**(11):4270—6.
93. Wu Y, Smith AE, Reineke TM. Lipophilic polycation vehicles display high plasmid DNA delivery to multiple cell types. *Bioconjug Chem* 2017;**28**:2035—40.
94. Sant VP, Kang N, Maysinger D, Leroux J. Block copolymer micelles: preparation, characterization and application in drug delivery. *J Control Release* 2005;**109**:169—88.
95. Harada A, Kataoka K. Polyion complex micelle formation from double- hydrophilic block copolymers composed of charged and non-charged segments in aqueous media. *Polym J* 2018;**50**:95—100.
96. Oishi M, Nagatsugi F, Sasaki S, Nagasaki Y, Kataoka K. Smart polyion complex micelles for targeted intracellular delivery of PEGylated antisense oligonucleotides containing acid-labile linkages. *Chembiochem* 2005;**6**:718—25.
97. Pergushov DV, Müller AHE, Schacher FH. Micellar interpolyelectrolyte complexes. *Chem Soc Rev* 2012;**41**:6888—901.
98. Voets IK, de Keizer A, Cohen Stuart MA. Complex coacervate core micelles. *Adv Colloid Interface Sci* 2009;**147—148**:300—18.
99. Van Der Kooij HM, Spruijt E, Voets IK, Fokkink R, Cohen Stuart MA, Van Der Gucht J. On the stability and morphology of complex coacervate core micelles: from spherical to wormlike micelles. *Langmuir* 2012;**28**:14180—91.
100. Aloi A, Guibert C, Olijve LLC, Voets IK. Morphological evolution of complex coacervate core micelles revealed by iPAINT microscopy. *Polymer* 2016;**107**:450—5.
101. Ting JM, Wu H, Herzog-Arbeitman A, Srivastava S, Tirrell MV. Synthesis and assembly of designer styrenic diblock polyelectrolytes. *ACS Macro Lett* 2018;**7**:726—33.
102. Harada A, Kataoka K. formation of polyion complex micelles in an aqueous milieu from a pair of oppositely-charged block copolymers with poly(ethylene glycol) segments. *Macromolecules* 1995;**28**:5294—9.
103. Harada A, Kataoka K. Polyion complex micelle formation from double- hydrophilic block copolymers composed of charged and non-charged segments in aqueous media. *Polymer Journal* 2017;**50**:95—100.
104. Harada A, Kataoka K. Effect of charged segment length on physicochemical properties of core-shell type polyion complex micelles from block ionomers. *Macromolecules* 2003;**36**:4995—5001.
105. Harada A, Kataoka K. Chain length recognition: core-shell supramolecular assembly from oppositely charged block copolymers. *Science* 1999;**283**:65—7.
106. Stuart MAC, Besseling NAM, Fokkink RG, Cohen Stuart MA, Besseling NAM, Fokkink RG. Formation of micelles with complex coacervate cores. *Langmuir* 1998;**14**:6846—9.
107. van Der Burgh S, de Keizer A, Cohen Stuart MA. Complex coacervation core micelles. colloidal stability and aggregation mechanism. *Langmuir* 2004;**20**:1073—84.
108. Tsuchida E, Abe K. Interactions between macromolecules in solution and intermacromolecular complexes. *Adv Polym Sci* 1982;**45**.
109. Lueckheide M, Vieregg JR, Bologna AJ, Leon L, Tirrell MV. Structure-property relationships of oligonucleotide polyelectrolyte complex micelles. *Nano Lett* 2018;**18**(11):7111—7.
110. Mutaf OF, Kishimura A, Mochida Y, Kim A, Kataoka K. Induction of secondary structure through micellization of an oppositely charged pair of homochiral block- and homopolypeptides in an aqueous medium. *Macromol Rapid Commun* 2015;**36**:1958—64.
111. Koide A, Kishimura A, Osada K, Jang W-D, Yamasaki Y. Semipermeable polymer vesicle (PICsome) self-assembled in aqueous medium from a pair of oppositely charged block Copolymers: physiologically stable micro-/nanocontainers of water-soluble macromolecules. *J Am Chem Soc* 2006;**128**:5988—9.
112. Štěpánek M, Škvarla J, Uchman M, Procházka K, Angelov B, Kováčik L, Garamus VM, Mantzaridis C, Pispas S. Wormlike core-shell nanoparticles formed by co-assembly of double hydrophilic block polyelectrolyte with oppositely charged fluorosurfactant. *Soft Matter* 2012;**8**:9412—7.
113. Israelachvili JN. *Intermolecular and surface forces*. 3rd ed. Elsevier Science; 2011.

114. Tockary TA, Osada K, Motoda Y, Hiki S, Chen Q, Takeda KM, Dirisala A, Osawa S, Kataoka K. Rod-to-Globule transition of pDNA/PEG-Poly(l-Lysine) polyplex micelles induced by a collapsed balance between DNA rigidity and PEG crowdedness. *Small* 2016;**12**:1193–200.
115. Wibowo A, Osada K, Matsuda H, Anraku Y, Hirose H, Kishimura A, Kataoka K. Morphology control in water of polyion complex nanoarchitectures of double-hydrophilic charged block copolymers through composition tuning and thermal treatment. *Macromolecules* 2014;**47**:3086–92.
116. Dong WF, Kishimura A, Anraku Y, Chuanoi S, Kataoka K. Monodispersed polymeric nanocapsules: spontaneous evolution and morphology transition from reducible hetero-PEG PICmicelles by controlled degradation. *J Am Chem Soc* 2009;**131**:3804–5.
117. Schrage S, Sigel R, Schlaad H. Formation of amphiphilic polyion complex vesicles from mixtures of oppositely charged block ionomers. *Macromolecules* 2003;**36**:2–5.
118. Jiang Y, Lodge TP, Reineke TM. Packaging pDNA by polymeric ABC micelles simultaneously achieves colloidal stability and structural control. *J Am Chem Soc* 2018;**140**:11101–11.
119. Hunt JN, Feldman KE, Lynd NA, Deek J, Campos LM, Spruell JM, Hernandez BM, Kramer EJ, Hawker CJ. Tunable, high modulus hydrogels driven by ionic coacervation. *Adv Mater* 2011;**23**:2327–31.
120. Förster S, Abetz V, Müller AHE. Polyelectrolyte block copolymer micelles. In: *Polyelectrolytes with defined molecular architecture II*; 2004. p. 173–210.
121. Lindhoud S, de Vries R, Schweins R, Cohen Stuart MA, Norde W. Salt-induced release of lipase from polyelectrolyte complex micelles. *Soft Matter* 2009;**5**:242–50.
122. Astafieva I, Khougaz K, Eisenberg A. Micellization in block polyelectrolyte solutions. 2. Fluorescence study of the critical micelle concentration as a function of soluble block length and salt concentration. *Macromolecules* 1995;**28**:7127–34.
123. Astafieva I, Zhong XF, Eisenberg A. Critical micellization phenomena in block polyelectrolyte solutions. *Macromolecules* 1993;**26**:7339–52.
124. Zhang Q, Vakili MR, Li XF, Lavasanifar A, Le XC. Terpolymer micelles for the delivery of arsenic to breast cancer cells: the effect of chain sequence on polymeric micellar characteristics and cancer cell uptake. *Mol Pharm* 2016;**13**:4021–33.
125. Kuo C-H, Leon L, Chung EJ, Huang R-T, Sontag TJ, Reardon CA, Getz GS, Tirrell M, Fang Y. Inhibition of atherosclerosis-promoting microRNAs via targeted polyelectrolyte complex micelles. *J Mater Chem B* 2014;**2**:8142–53.
126. ten Hove JB, Wang J, van Oosterom MN, van Leeuwen FWB, Velders AH. Size-sorting and pattern formation of nanoparticle-loaded micellar superstructures in biconcave thin films. *ACS Nano* 2017;**11**:11225–31.
127. Voets IK, de Keizer A, Cohen Stuart MA. Irreversible structural transitions in mixed micelles of oppositely charged diblock copolymers in aqueous solution. *Macromolecules* 2007;**40**:2158–64.
128. Dai Z, Yin J, Yan S, Cao T, Ma J, Chen X. Polyelectrolyte complexes based on chitosan and poly(L-glutamic acid). *Polym Int* 2007;**56**:1122–7.
129. Kim SH, Jeong JH, Mok H, Lee SH, Kim SW, Park TG. Folate receptor targeted delivery of polyelectrolyte complex micelles prepared from ODN-PEG-folate conjugate and cationic lipids. *Biotechnol Prog* 2007;**23**:232–7.
130. Oishi M, Nagasaki Y, Itaka K, Nishiyama N, Kataoka K. Lactosylated poly(ethylene glycol)-siRNA conjugate through acid-labile β-thiopropionate linkage to construct pH-sensitive polyion complex micelles achieving enhanced gene silencing in hepatoma cells. *J Am Chem Soc* 2005;**127**:1624–5.
131. Höbel S, Aigner A. Polyethylenimines for siRNA and miRNA delivery in vivo. *WIREs Nanomed Nanobiotechnol* 2013;**5**:484–501.
132. Tockary TA, Osada K, Chen Q, MacHitani K, Dirisala A, Uchida S, Nomoto T, Toh K, Matsumoto Y, Itaka K, Nitta K, Nagayama K, Kataoka K. Tethered PEG crowdedness determining shape and blood circulation profile of polyplex micelle gene carriers. *Macromolecules* 2013;**46**:6585–92.
133. Jeong JH, Kim SH, Kim SW, Park TG. Polyelectrolyte complex micelles composed of c-raf antisense oligodeoxynucleotide-poly(ethylene glycol) conjugate and poly(ethylenimine): effect of systemic administration on tumor growth. *Bioconjug Chem* 2005;**16**:1034–7.
134. Jeong JH, Kim SH, Kim SW, Park TG. Intracellular delivery of poly(ethylene glycol) conjugated antisense oligonucleotide using cationic lipids by formation of self-assembled polyelectrolyte complex micelles. *J Nanosci Nanotechnol* 2006;**6**:2790–5.
135. Jeong JH, Kim SW, Park TG. A new antisense oligonucleotide delivery system based on self-assembled ODN-PEG hybrid conjugate micelles. *J Control Release* 2003;**93**:183–91.
136. Kanazawa T, Sugawara K, Tanaka K, Horiuchi S, Takashima Y, Okada H. Suppression of tumor growth by systemic delivery of anti-VEGF siRNA with cell-penetrating peptide-modified MPEG-PCL nanomicelles. *Eur J Pharm Biopharm* 2012;**81**:470–7.
137. Baba M, Itaka K, Kondo K, Yamasoba T, Kataoka K. Treatment of neurological disorders by introducing mRNA in vivo using polyplex nanomicelles. *J Control Release* 2015;**201**:41–8.
138. Harada-Shiba M, Yamauchi K, Harada A, Takamisawa I, Shimokado K, Kataoka K. Polyion complex micelles as vectors in gene therapy – pharmacokinetics and in vivo gene transfer. *Gene Ther* 2002;**9**:407–14.
139. Oe Y, Christie RJ, Naito M, Low SA, Fukushima S, Toh K, Miura Y, Matsumoto Y, Nishiyama N, Miyata K, Kataoka K. Actively-targeted polyion complex micelles stabilized by cholesterol and disulfide cross-linking for systemic delivery of siRNA to solid tumors. *Biomaterials* 2014;**35**:7887–95.
140. Harada A, Kataoka K. Pronounced activity of enzymes through the incorporation into the core of polyion complex micelles made from charged block copolymers. *J Control Release* 2001;**72**:85–91.
141. Harada A, Kataoka K. Novel polyion complex micelles entrapping enzyme molecules in the core: preparation of narrowly-distributed micelles from lysozyme and poly(ethylene glycol)-poly(aspartic acid) block copolymer in aqueous medium. *Macromolecules* 1998;**31**:288–94.
142. Du F-S, Wang Y, Zhang R, Li Z-C. Intelligent nucleic acid delivery systems based on stimuli-responsive polymers. *Soft Matter* 2010;**6**:835–48.
143. Convertine AJ, Benoit DSW, Duvall CL, Hoffman AS, Stayton PS. Development of a novel endosomolytic diblock copolymer for siRNA delivery. *J Control Release* 2009;**133**:1263–72.
144. Xu J, Liu S. Polymeric nanocarriers possessing thermoresponsive coronas. *Soft Matter* 2008;**4**:1745.
145. Dähling C, Lotze G, Drechsler M, Mori H, Pergushov DV, Plamper FA. Temperature-induced structure switch in thermo-responsive micellar interpolyelectrolyte complexes: toward core–

shell−corona and worm-like morphologies. *Soft Matter* 2016;**12**:5127−37.
146. Bastakoti BP, Guragain S, Nakashima K, Yamauchi Y. Stimuli-induced core-corona inversion of micelle of poly (acrylic acid)-block-Poly (N-isopropylacrylamide) and its application in drug delivery. *Macromol Chem Phys* 2015;**216**:287−91.
147. Lima LH, Morales Y, Cabral T. Ocular biocompatibility of poly-N-isopropylacrylamide (pNIPAM). *J. Ophthalmol* 2016;**2016**:6.
148. Cooperstein MA, Canavan HE. Assessment of cytotoxicity of (N-isopropyl acrylamide) and poly(N-isopropyl acrylamide)-coated surfaces. *Biointerphases* 2013;**8**(1).
149. Schwerdt A, Zintchenko A, Concia M, Roesen N, Fisher K, Lindner LH, Issels R, Wagner E, Ogris M. Hyperthermia-induced targeting of thermosensitive gene carriers to tumors. *Hum Gene Ther* 2008;**19**:1283−92.
150. Zintchenko A, Ogris M, Wagner E. Temperature dependent gene expression induced by PNIPAM-based copolymers: potential of hyperthermia in gene transfer. *Bioconjug Chem* 2006;**17**:766−72.
151. Ramasamy T, Kim H, Choi Y, Tran H. pH sensitive polyelectrolyte complex micelles for highly effective combination chemotherapy. *J Mateirals Chem B* 2014;**2**:6324−33.
152. Azzopardi EA, Ferguson EL, Thomas DW. The enhanced permeability retention effect: a new paradigm for drug targeting in infection. *J Antimicrob Chemother* 2013;**68**:257−74.
153. Futaki S, Ohashi W, Suzuki T, Niwa M, Tanaka S, Ueda K, Harashima H, Sugiura Y. Stearylated arginine-rich peptides: a new class of transfection systems. *Bioconjug Chem* 2001;**12**:1005−11.
154. Wender PA, Mitchell DJ, Pattabiraman K, Pelkey ET, Steinman L, Rothbard JB. The design, synthesis, and evaluation of molecules that enable or enhance cellular uptake: peptoid molecular transporters. *Proc Natl Acad Sci USA* 2000;**97**:13003−8.
155. Suma T, Miyata K, Ishii T, Uchida S, Uchida H, Itaka K, Nishiyama N, Kataoka K. Enhanced stability and gene silencing ability of siRNA-loaded polyion complexes formulated from polyaspartamide derivatives with a repetitive array of amino groups in the side chain. *Biomaterials* 2012;**33**:2770−9.
156. Müller M. Sizing, shaping and pharmaceutical applications of polyelectrolyte complex nanoparticles. *Adv Polym Sci* 2014;**256**:197−260.
157. Shang L, Nienhaus K, Nienhaus GU. Engineered nanoparticles interacting with cells : size matters. *J Nanobiotechnol* 2014;**12**:1−11.
158. Yamamoto Y, Nagasaki Y, Kato Y, Sugiyama Y, Kataoka K. Long-circulating poly(ethylene glycol)-poly(D,L-lactide) block copolymer micelles with modulated surface charge. *J Control Release* 2001;**77**:27−38.
159. Yuan F, Dellian M, Fukumura D, Leunig M, Berk DA, Jain RK, Torchilin VP. Vascular permeability in a human tumor xenograft: molecular size dependence and cutoff size. *Cancer Res* 1995;**55**:3752−6.
160. Kakizawa Y, Kataoka K. Block copolymer micelles for delivery of gene and related compounds. *Adv Drug Deliv Rev* 2002;**54**:203−22.
161. Fischer D, Bieber T, Li Y, Elsässer HP, Kissel T. A novel non-viral vector for DNA delivery based on low molecular weight, branched polyethylenimine: effect of molecular weight on transfection efficiency and cytotoxicity. *Pharm Res* 1999;**16**:1273−9.
162. Choksakulnimitr S, Masuda S, Tokuda H, Takakura Y, Hashida M. In vitro cytotoxicity of macromolecules in different cell culture systems. *J Control Release* 1995;**34**:233−41.
163. Kakizawa Y, Harada A, Kataoka K. Environment-sensitive stabilization of core-shell structured polyion complex micelle by reversible cross-linking of the core through disulfide bond. *J Am Chem Soc* 1999;**121**:11247−8.
164. Christie RJ, Miyata K, Matsumoto Y, Nomoto T, Menasco D, Lai TC, Pennisi M, Osada K, Fukushima S, Nishiyama N, Yamasaki Y, Kataoka K. Effect of polymer structure on micelles formed between siRNA and cationic block copolymer comprising thiols and amidines. *Biomacromolecules* 2011;**12**:3174−85.
165. Kim SH, Jeong JH, Lee SH, Kim SW, Park TG. PEG conjugated VEGF siRNA for anti-angiogenic gene therapy. *J Control Release* 2006;**116**:123−9.
166. Hwa S, Hoon J, Hyeon S, Wan S, Gwan T. Local and systemic delivery of VEGF siRNA using polyelectrolyte complex micelles for effective treatment of cancer. *J Control Release* 2008;**129**:107−16.
167. Bachu RD, Chowdhury P, Al-saedi ZHF, Karla PK, Boddu SHS. Ocular drug delivery barriers — role of nanocarriers in the treatment of anterior segment ocular diseases. *Pharmaceutics* 2018;**10**:28.
168. Zuckerman JE, Gritli I, Tolcher A, Heidel JD, Lim D, Morgan R, Chmielowski B, Ribas A, Davis ME, Yen Y. Correlating animal and human phase Ia/Ib clinical data with CALAA-01, a targeted, polymer-based nanoparticle containing siRNA. *Proc Natl Acad Sci USA* 2014;**111**:11449−54.
169. Anselmo AC, Mitragotri S. An overview of clinical and commercial impact of drug delivery systems. *J Control Release* 2014;**190**:15−28.
170. Iler RK. Multilayers of colloidal particles. *J Colloid Interface Sci* 1966;**21**:569−94.
171. Decher G, Hong J-D. Buildup of ultrathin multilayer films by a self-assembly process: i. Consecutive adsorption of anionic and cationic bipolar amphiphiles on charged surfaces. *Makromol Chem Macromol Symp* 1991;**46**:321−7.
172. Morton SW, Herlihy KP, Shopsowitz KE, Deng ZJ, Chu KS, Bowerman CJ, Desimone JM, Hammond PT. Scalable manufacture of built-to-order nanomedicine: spray-assisted layer-by-layer functionalization of PRINT nanoparticles. *Adv Mater* 2013;**25**:4707−13.
173. Richardson JJ, Ejima H, Lörcher SL, Liang K, Senn P, Cui J, Caruso F. Preparation of nano- and microcapsules by electrophoretic polymer assembly. *Angew Chem Int Ed* 2013;**52**:6455−8.
174. Donath E, Sukhorukov GB, Caruso F, Davis SA, Möhwald H. Novel hollow polymer shells by colloid-templated assembly of polyelectrolytes. *Angew Chem Int Ed* 1998;**37**:2201−5.
175. Shenoy DB, Antipov AA, Sukhorukov GB, Möhwald H. Layer-by-layer engineering of biocompatible, decomposable core-shell structures. *Biomacromolecules* 2003;**4**:265−72.
176. Szarpak A, Cui D, Dubreuil F, De Geest BG, De Cock LJ, Picart C, Auzély-Velty R. Designing hyaluronic acid-based layer-by-layer capsules as a carrier for intracellular drug delivery. *Biomacromolecules* 2010;**11**:713−20.
177. Yan S, Zhu J, Wang Z, Yin J, Zheng Y, Chen X. Layer-by-layer assembly of poly(l-glutamic acid)/chitosan microcapsules for high loading and sustained release of 5-fluorouracil. *Eur J Pharm Biopharm* 2011;**78**:336−45.
178. Xie YL, Wang MJ, Yao SJ. Preparation and characterization of biocompatible microcapsules of sodium cellulose sulfate/chitosan by means of layer-by-layer self-assembly. *Langmuir* 2009;**25**:8999−9005.

179. Anandhakumar S, Nagaraja V, Raichur AM. Reversible polyelectrolyte capsules as carriers for protein delivery. *Colloids Surfaces B Biointerfaces* 2010;**78**:266–74.
180. Taori VP, Liu Y, Reineke TM. DNA delivery in vitro via surface release from multilayer assemblies with poly(glycoamidoamine)s. *Acta Biomater* 2009;**5**:925–33.
181. Kharlampieva E, Koziovskaya V, Sukhishvili SA. Layer-by-layer hydrogen-bonded polymer films: from fundamentals to applications. *Adv Mater* 2009;**21**:3053–65.
182. Kozlovskaya V, Harbaugh S, Drachuk I, Shchepelina O, Kelley-Loughnane N, Stone M, Tsukruk VV. Hydrogen-bonded LbL shells for living cell surface engineering. *Soft Matter* 2011;**7**:2364–72.
183. Zhao J, Pan F, Li P, Zhao C, Jiang Z, Zhang P, Cao X. Fabrication of ultrathin membrane via layer-by-layer self-assembly driven by hydrophobic interaction towards high separation performance. *ACS Appl Mater Interfaces* 2013;**5**:13275–83.
184. Johnston APR, Mitomo H, Read ES, Caruso F. Compositional and structural engineering of DNA multilayer films. *Langmuir* 2006;**22**:3251–8.
185. Sukhorukov GB, Donath E, Lichtenfeld H, Knippel E, Knippel M, Budde A, Möhwald H. Layer-by-layer self assembly of polyelectrolytes on colloidal particles. *Colloids Surfaces A Physicochem Eng Asp* 1998;**137**:253–66.
186. Deshmukh PK, Ramani KP, Singh SS, Tekade AR, Chatap VK, Patil GB, Bari SB. Stimuli-sensitive layer-by-layer (LbL) self-assembly systems: targeting and biosensory applications. *J Control Release* 2013;**166**:294–306.
187. Wang Y, Yu A, Caruso F. Nanoporous polyelectrolyte spheres prepared by sequentially coating sacrificial mesoporous silica spheres. *Angew Chem Int Ed* 2005;**44**:2888–92.
188. Cortez C, Tomaskovic-Crook E, Johnston APR, Radt B, Cody SH, Scott AM, Nice EC, Heath JK, Caruso F. Targeting and uptake of multilayered particles to colorectal cancer cells. *Adv Mater* 2006;**18**:1998–2003.
189. Caruso F. Hollow inorganic capsules via colloid-templated layer-by-layer electrostatic assembly. *Colloid Chem* 2003;**227**:145–68.
190. Blacklock J, Mao G, Oupický D, Möhwald H. DNA release dynamics from bioreducible layer-by-layer films. *Langmuir* 2010;**26**:8597–605.
191. Kim NW, Lee MS, Kim KR, Lee JE, Lee K, Park JS, Matsumoto Y, Jo D-G, Lee H, Lee DS, Jeong JH. Polyplex-releasing microneedles for enhanced cutaneous delivery of DNA vaccine. *J Control Release* 2014;**179**:11–7.
192. Ke J-H, Young T-H. Multilayered polyplexes with the endosomal buffering polycation in the core and the cell uptake-favorable polycation in the outer layer for enhanced gene delivery. *Biomaterials* 2010;**31**:9366–72.
193. Johnston APR, Cortez C, Angelatos AS, Caruso F. Layer-by-layer engineered capsules and their applications. *Curr Opin Colloid Interface Sci* 2006;**11**:203–9.
194. Zahr AS, De Villiers M, Pishko MV. Encapsulation of drug nanoparticles in self-assembled macromolecular nanoshells. *Langmuir* 2005;**21**:403–10.
195. Kumar CSSR, Mohammad F. Magnetic nanomaterials for hyperthermia-based therapy and controlled drug delivery. *Adv Drug Deliv Rev* 2011;**63**:789–808.
196. Huang J, Shu Q, Wang L, Wu H, Wang AY, Mao H. Layer-by-layer assembled milk protein coated magnetic nanoparticle enabled oral drug delivery with high stability in stomach and enzyme-responsive release in small intestine. *Biomaterials* 2015;**39**:105–13.
197. Shutava TG, Balkundi SS, Vangala P, Steffan JJ, Bigelow RL, Cardelli JA, O'Neal DP, Lvov YM. Layer-by-layer-coated gelatin nanoparticles as a vehicle for delivery of natural polyphenols. *ACS Nano* 2009;**3**:1877–85.
198. Elbakry A, Zaky A, Liebl R, Rachel R, Goepferich A, Breunig M. Layer-by-layer assembled gold nanoparticles for siRNA delivery. *Nano Lett* 2009;**9**:2059–64.
199. Guo S, Huang Y, Jiang Q, Sun Y, Deng L, Liang Z, Du Q, Xing J, Zhao Y, Wang PC, Dong A, Liang X. Enhanced gene delivery and siRNA silencing by gold nanoparticles coated with charge-reversal polyelectrolyte. *ACS Nano* 2010;**4**:5505–11.
200. Deng ZJ, Morton SW, Ben-Akiva E, Dreaden EC, Shopsowitz KE, Hammond PT. Layer-by-layer nanoparticles for systemic codelivery of an anticancer drug and siRNA for potential triple-negative breast cancer treatment. *ACS Nano* 2013;**7**:9571–84.
201. Poon Z, Chang D, Zhao X, Hammond PT. Layer-by-layer nanoparticles with a pH-sheddable layer for in vivo targeting of tumor hypoxia. *ACS Nano* 2011;**5**:4284–92.
202. Trau D, Yang W, Seydack M, Caruso F, Yu NT, Renneberg R. Nanoencapsulated microcrystalline particles for superamplified biochemical assays. *Anal Chem* 2002;**74**:5480–6.
203. Schneider G, Decher G, Nerambourg N, Praho R, Werts MHV, Blanchard-Desce M. Distance-dependent fluorescence quenching on gold nanoparticles ensheathed with layer-by-layer assembled polyelectrolytes. *Nano Lett* 2006;**6**:530–6.
204. Shchukin DG, Sukhorukov GB. Nanoparticle synthesis in engineered organic nanoscale reactors. *Adv Mater* 2004;**16**:671–82.
205. Städler B, Price AD, Zelikin AN. A critical look at multilayered polymer capsules in biomedicine: drug carriers, artificial organelles, and cell mimics. *Adv Funct Mater* 2011;**21**:14–28.
206. He Q, Möhwald H, Li J. Layer-by-layer assembled nanotubes as biomimetic nanoreactors for calcium carbonate deposition. *Macromol Rapid Commun* 2009;**30**:1538–42.
207. Zhao W, Xu JJ, Shi CG, Chen HY. Multilayer membranes via layer-by-layer deposition of organic polymer protected prussian blue nanoparticles and glucose oxidase for glucose biosensing. *Langmuir* 2005;**21**:9630–4.
208. Wu BY, Hou SH, Yin F, Zhao ZX, Wang YY, Wang XS, Chen Q. Amperometric glucose biosensor based on multilayer films via layer-by-layer self-assembly of multi-wall carbon nanotubes, gold nanoparticles and glucose oxidase on the Pt electrode. *Biosens Bioelectron* 2007;**22**:2854–60.
209. Fu J, Ji J, Fan D, Shen J. Construction of antibacterial multilayer films containing nanosilver via layer-by-layer assembly of heparin and chitosan-silver ions complex. *Wiley Intersci* 2006;**33**:97–103.
210. Kommireddy DS, Sriram SM, Lvov YM, Mills DK. Stem cell attachment to layer-by-layer assembled TiO2 nanoparticle thin films. *Biomaterials* 2006;**27**:4296–303.
211. Xi Q, Chen X, Evans DG, Yang W. Gold nanoparticle-embedded porous graphene thin films fabricated via layer-by-layer self-assembly and subsequent thermal annealing for electrochemical sensing. *Langmuir* 2012;**28**:9885–92.
212. Shen L, Wang B, Wang J, Fu J, Picart C, Ji J. Asymmetric free-standing film with multifunctional anti-bacterial and self-cleaning properties. *ACS Appl Mater Interfaces* 2012;**4**:4476–83.

213. Orozco VH, Kozlovskaya V, Kharlampieva E, López BL, Tsukruk VV. Biodegradable self-reporting nanocomposite films of poly(lactic acid) nanoparticles engineered by layer-by-layer assembly. *Polymer* 2010;**51**:4127–39.
214. Nie C, Yang Y, Cheng C, Ma L, Deng J, Wang L, Zhao C. Bioinspired and biocompatible carbon nanotube-Ag nanohybrid coatings for robust antibacterial applications. *Acta Biomater* 2017;**51**:479–94.
215. Vrana NE, Erdemli O, Francius G, Fahs A, Rabineau M, Debry C, Tezcaner A, Keskin D, Lavalle P. Double entrapment of growth factors by nanoparticles loaded into polyelectrolyte multilayer films. *J Mater Chem B* 2014;**2**:999–1008.
216. Liu S, Yan J, He G, Zhong D, Chen J, Shi L, Zhou X, Jiang H. Layer-by-layer assembled multilayer films of reduced graphene oxide/gold nanoparticles for the electrochemical detection of dopamine. *J Electroanal Chem* 2012;**672**:40–4.
217. Cui J, Van Koeverden MP, Müllner M, Kempe K, Caruso F. Emerging methods for the fabrication of polymer capsules. *Adv Colloid Interface Sci* 2014;**207**:14–31.

Chapter 21

Nanoemulsions

Ankur Gupta[1,2]
[1]*Department of Mechanical and Aerospace Engineering;* [2]*Princeton University, Princeton, NJ, United States*

21.1 Introduction

Emulsions consist of two immiscible liquids where droplets of one liquid are suspended in the other liquid. Emulsions are broadly classified into two categories: oil-in-water (O/W) emulsions where oil droplets are suspended in water and water-in-oil (W/O) emulsions where water droplets are suspended in oil. An example of O/W emulsion is milk. In milk, droplets of fat are dispersed in water. In contrast, butter is an example of W/O emulsion where water droplets are suspended in fat. Since emulsions consist of two immiscible liquids, they are kinetically stable, i.e., they separate into oil and water phases over a period of time. Therefore, surfactants and emulsifiers are typically required to stabilize emulsions and prolong their shelf life. Surfactants and emulsifiers are molecules that sit at the interface of oil and water and stabilize emulsions through different mechanisms such as steric stabilization and electrostatic repulsion. For instance, casein protein acts as a surfactant to stabilize the fat droplets in milk.

Typically, emulsions possess an average droplet size ranging from a few microns to hundreds of microns. However, nanoemulsions are a subset of emulsions with droplet sizes in the range of 20–500 nm.[1–4] Nanoemulsions are sometimes also referred to as miniemulsions. They are an attractive candidate to deliver hydrophobic drugs/nutrients[5–7] as they exhibit enhanced pharmacological activity.[8] Nanoemulsions also possess interesting rheological properties (i.e., response to mechanical deformation) that can be readily tuned. For instance, they can be transformed from viscous (liquid-like) to elastic (solid-like) just by decreasing the droplet size.[9,10] Lastly, nanoemulsions display robust stability that allows them to have a long shelf life.[11]

Broadly speaking, there are three different approaches to utilize nanoemulsions for biomedical applications. The first and most common approach employs nanoemulsions to create formulations for different hydrophobic drugs.[12–21] In these formulations, the hydrophobic drug is dissolved in the oil phase of O/W nanoemulsions. To achieve appreciable level of drug loading, studies optimize nanoemulsion formulations with respect to choice of oil phases, surfactant(s), and formulation composition. These formulations are then exploited for different modes of drug delivery including topical, ocular, intravenous, and intranasal. Though the first approach presents a number of advantages, it also suffers from concerns related to toxicity, mainly due to the presence of oil and surfactant in the final formulation.[22] The second approach attempts to circumvent these concerns. Much like the first approach, the second approach also includes hydrophobic drug laden O/W nanoemulsions. However, in this approach, the oil phase is chosen to be volatile. Additionally, a cross-linking agent is added in the water phase. Upon evaporation of the oil phase, this technique enables generation of hydrogel beads with embedded crystals (or amorphous particles) of hydrophobic drug.[5,6,23–25] Since the surfactant is no longer required to stabilize the oil phase, it is washed away from the final product. Furthermore, as the hydrophobic drug crystal is confined by the size of the patent nanoemulsion drop, the crystal size can be tuned by changing the nanoemulsion drop size (hence the nanoemulsion serves as a template), which in turn enables controlled delivery of the drug.[5]

The last approach where nanoemulsions are utilized in biomedical applications is synthesis of advanced materials.[26–28] Since nanoemulsions are quite flexible with respect to composition, they serve as an ideal candidate to template variety of advance materials with tunable properties. For instance, W/O nanoemulsions can be transformed into hydrogel nanoparticles with different elasticity that can influence the biological fate of hydrogel nanoparticles being used as drug carriers.[26]

In this chapter, we first review the different methods to make nanoemulsions. We emphasize the advantages and disadvantages of different methods and describe the preferred routes to make nanoemulsions depending on the desired application. We also briefly discuss the stability and rheological properties of nanoemulsions. Next, we detail

Nanoparticles for Biomedical Applications. https://doi.org/10.1016/B978-0-12-816662-8.00021-7

the three different approaches to biomedical applications outlined above, i.e., (i) nanoemulsions formulations for hydrophobic drugs, (ii) nanoemulsions as a template to create hydrophobic drug nanocrystals, and (iii) nanoemulsions for advanced material synthesis in biomedical applications. We conclude by providing a summary of nanoemulsions in biomedical applications and potential directions for future research.

21.2 Nanoemulsion preparation

Nanoemulsions consist of two immiscible liquids where 20–500 nm sized droplets of one liquid phase (dispersed phase) are suspended in the other liquid phase (continuous phase). If the oil droplets are suspended in water, i.e., O/W nanoemulsions, oil is defined as the dispersed phase and water is defined as the continuous phase, and vice-verse for W/O nanoemulsions. To stabilize nanoemulsion droplets, a surfactant (or emulsifier) is almost always required. Surfactants could be ionic as well as nonionic. Some common ionic surfactants are sodium dodecyl sulfate (SDS, anionic) and cetyltrimethylammonium bromide (CTAB, cationic), and some typical nonionic surfactants are Tween, Span, and Brij. Though the majority of nanoemulsions have been prepared using synthetic surfactants, some studies have also made nanoemulsions using natural biopolymers.[29–32]

Nanoemulsion preparation can be divided into two groups of methods: high-energy methods and low-energy methods. High-energy methods are energy intensive methods and typically require power density input of 10^7–10^9 W/kg[1]. In contrast, low-energy methods only require power density input of 10^3–10^5 W/kg.[1] We first describe some examples of each kind of method and then discuss the advantages and disadvantages of both types of methods.

High-energy methods typically include high-pressure homogenization and ultrasonication. In high-pressure homogenizers (Fig. 21.1), a mixture of oil, water, and surfactant(s) is pushed through a small gap of 5–10 μm.[11,33–38] Due to the relatively small gap size, pressure drops rise up to a few thousands of bars and the droplets are deformed by extremely large values of shear forces that break the drop into small sizes.[39,40] Typically, the mixture is processed through the homogenizer 15–20 times before the droplet size becomes constant.[2,33,34] The mechanism of ultrasonication is similar to high-pressure homogenization. In an ultrasonicator, electrical input is converted into pressure fluctuations that then generate cavitation bubbles (Fig. 21.1). When the cavitation bubbles break, shear forces are generated that ultimately break the bigger drops into smaller ones.[33] Like the high-pressure homogenize, the ultrasonicator is run for about 15–20 min before the droplet size becomes roughly constant.[11,33,37,41]

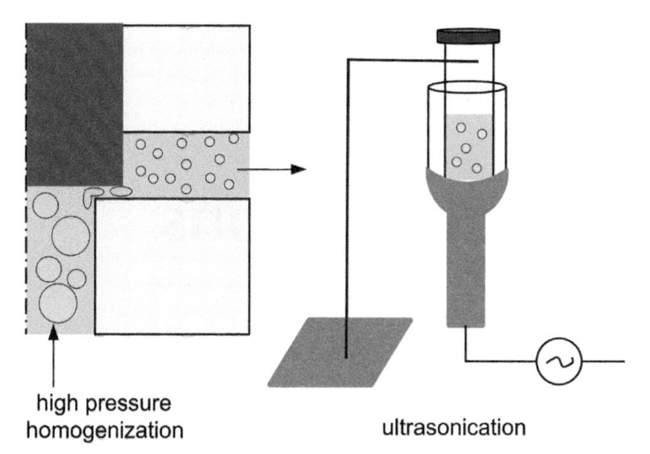

FIGURE 21.1 Schematic of high-energy methods used to prepare nanoemulsions. The two most widely used high-energy methods are high-pressure homogenization and ultrasonication.

In high-energy methods, it has been well established that average droplet size (d) follows an exponential decay with the number of homogenization passes[33,36] (N) and ultrasonication time[11,33,37,41]; see Fig. 21.2A for an example. The kinetics of nanoemulsion formation is dictated by the efficiency of droplet breakup.[34] We note that droplet size also decreases with an increase in the pressure drop of homogenization (Fig. 21.2A). This is expected since an increase in pressure drop increases the shear force that then breaks droplets into even smaller sized droplets. A useful parameter to control the droplet size of nanoemulsions is the droplet phase viscosity; an increase in dispersed phase viscosity leads to an increase in droplet size.[33,36,42] To quantitatively predict the droplet size for high-energy methods, Gupta et al.[33] derived and experimentally validated a dimensionless relationship

$$\mathrm{We} = C\,\mathrm{Oh}^{2/5}, \tag{21.1}$$

where Weber number is defined as $\mathrm{We} = \frac{\sqrt{\mu_c \varepsilon \rho_c}}{\sigma/d}$, Ohnesorge number is defined as $\mathrm{Oh} = \frac{\mu_d}{\sqrt{\rho_d \sigma d}}$, μ_c and ρ_c are continuous phase viscosity and density, μ_d and ρ_d are dispersed phase viscosity and density, σ is the interfacial tension between dispersed and continuous phases, ε is the power density (i.e., input energy per unit mass per unit time) of homogenization, d is the average droplet diameter of nanoemulsions, and C is a constant. Weber number is the ratio of applied stress (i.e., the stress trying to break the drop) to the interfacial stress (i.e., the stress trying to hold the droplet together), and Ohnesorge number quantifies the effect of droplet viscosity. For nanoemulsions, since the droplet size d is small, $Oh \gg 1$. The importance of surfactant in Eq. (21.1) comes through interfacial tension σ. One of the interesting features of the relation in Eq. (21.1) is that $d \propto \left(\frac{\mu_d}{\mu_c}\right)^{\frac{1}{3}}$ is approximately followed.

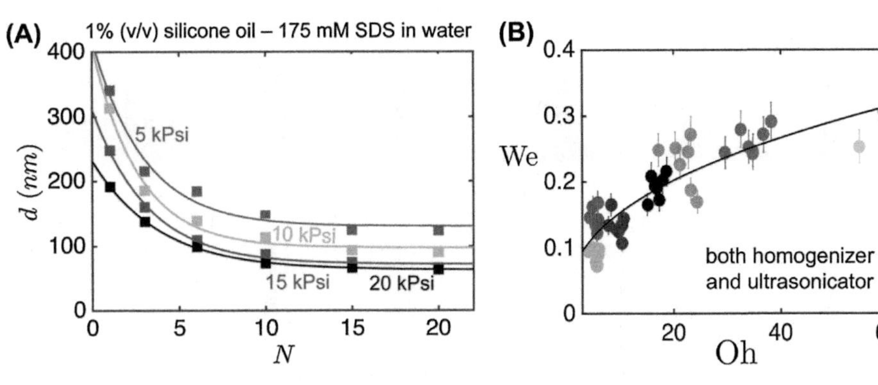

FIGURE 21.2 Overview of experimental measurements using high-energy methods. (A) The average droplet size (***d***) exponentially decreases with number of passes (***N***) in a homogenizer. Here, ***d*** versus ***N*** data for O/W nanoemulsions with silicone oil as the dispersed phase and SDS as the surfactant are shown. The data show that size also decreases with increase in pressure drop. (B) The experimentally measured droplet size validates the theoretically derived scaling relationship $\mathbf{We} = \mathbf{C\,Oh}^{2/5}$. Here, the data include several different nanoemulsion formulations prepared with both the homogenizer and ultrasonicator. *The figure is adapted with permission from Gupta, A., Eral, H. B., Hatton, T. A. & Doyle, P. S. Controlling and predicting droplet size of nanoemulsions: scaling relations with experimental validation. Soft Matter 12, 1452–1458 (2016).*

Therefore, different parameters can be utilized to tune the nanoemulsion droplet size. Eq. (21.1) was experimentally validated; see Fig. 21.2B. The experimental data include several different types of nanoemulsions prepared using both the homogenizer and ultrasonicator.

In contrast to high-energy methods, low-energy methods simply require to mix the components, i.e., oil, water, and surfactant(s), using a stirrer.[43–52] Low-energy methods are energy efficient because of two reasons. First, the quantity of surfactant is significantly higher than high-energy methods. Second, the surfactant is specifically chosen to bring down the interfacial tension by a factor of $10^3 - 10^4$ relative to the interfacial tension used in high-energy methods. Specifically, $\sigma = O(10)$ mN/m in high-energy methods[33] and $\sigma = O(10^{-2})$ mN/m in low-energy methods.[48]

Two types of low-energy methods are the emulsion inversion point and phase inversion temperature (Fig. 21.3). In the former method, nanoemulsions are prepared via change in composition (Fig. 21.3), and in the latter method, nanoemulsions are prepared through change in temperature (Fig. 21.3). First, we focus on emulsion inversion point. There are broadly two ways to mix components: (i) mix water and surfactant, and then add oil (labeled as method A in Fig. 21.3) or (ii) mix oil and surfactant, and then add water (labeled as method B in Fig. 21.3). Previously, several studies argued that only method B is the correct order of mixing components to make nanoemulsions.[3,4,47,48] However, more recently, Gupta et al.[6] demonstrated that the mixing order is dictated by the choice of surfactant and liquid phases (Fig. 21.4). The researchers prepared O/W nanoemulsions with decane as the oil phase. They used a mixture of Tween 80 and Span 80 to change the hydrophilic–lipophilic number (HLB) of the system. A higher HLB number represents a more hydrophilic surfactant. Gupta et al.[6] showed that method B works for higher HLB, whereas method A works for lower HLB (Fig. 21.4). The authors argued that for nanoemulsion formation to be effective using emulsion inversion point, *the surfactant should dislike the initial mixing phase*. Thus when the second liquid phase is introduced, the surfactant migrates toward the interface and generates nanoemulsions. Simply put, when a surfactant is mixed with water (method A), it should be less hydrophilic or should have a lower HLB. In contrast, when surfactant is mixed with oil (method B), it should be more hydrophilic or should possess a higher

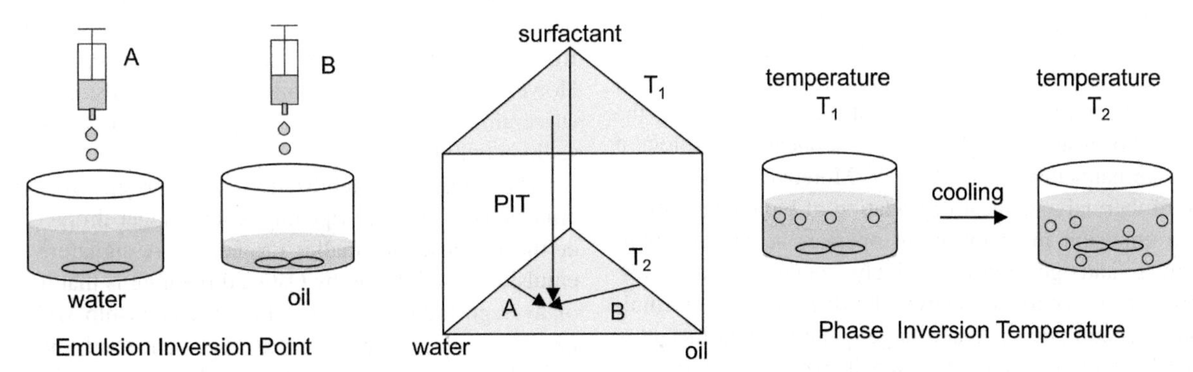

FIGURE 21.3 Schematic of low-energy methods to prepare nanoemulsions. Emulsion inversion point method utilizes two different orders to mix components (A or B) to create nanoemulsions. In phase inversion temperature, mixture of oil, water, and surfactant is cooled from a higher temperature (T_1) to a lower temperature (T_2) to make nanoemulsions.

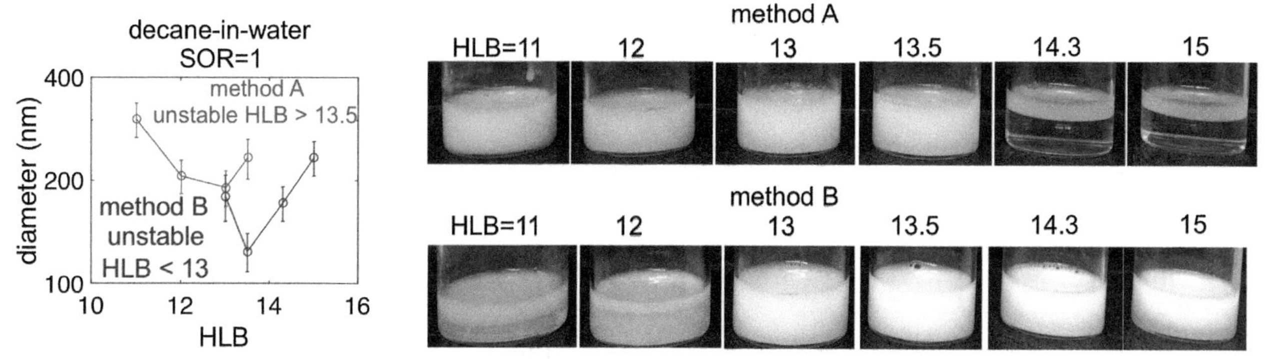

FIGURE 21.4 An example of the effect of order of mixing for O/W nanoemulsions prepared using emulsion inversion point method. Decane in water nanoemulsions remains stable when prepared using method A for lower HLB. In contrast, nanoemulsions form using method B for higher HLB. *The figure is reproduced with permission from Gupta, A., Badruddoza, A. Z. M. & Doyle, P. S. A general route for nanoemulsion synthesis using low-energy methods at constant temperature. Langmuir 33, 7118–7123 (2017).*

HLB. This is consistent with experimental observations (Fig. 21.4). In phase inversion temperature, the components are mixed at higher temperature and then the mixture is brought to a lower temperature.[43–45]

There are advantages and disadvantages of both high- and low-energy methods. High-energy methods are more robust since they are less restrictive about surfactant choice. Furthermore, they also require less amount of surfactant to make nanoemulsions. Since the surfactant amount is flexible, it has been shown that high-energy methods can prepare nanoemulsions with dispersed phase volume fraction as high as 40%.[9,10] However, as noted previously, high-energy methods require significantly more energy input than low-energy methods. Also, since high-energy methods are energetically inefficient, they tend to heat up the sample that can cause matter degradation, especially if biological entities utilized in making the nanoemulsions are temperature sensitive.

On the other hand, though low-energy methods are energy efficient, they are restrictive about surfactant choice and quite often require two surfactants to be effective. Moreover, the quantity of surfactant required is significantly higher as compared to high-energy methods. Therefore, typically, dispersed volume fraction is lower than 25%. Lastly, low-energy nanoemulsions are less stable than high-energy methods (see Fig. 21.5 for details).

Since emulsion inversion point requires simple unit operations and typically operates at room temperature, the majority of research for biomedical applications exploits it to make nanoemulsions.[14,17,53–55] Moreover, there is less risk of thermal and shear degradation of biological entities since emulsion inversion point operates at constant temperature and generates relatively modest shear rates. However, as mentioned above, the disadvantage of emulsion inversion point is that a large quantity of surfactant is typically required that can make it expensive to prepare nanoemulsion-based formulations. In addition, larger amount of surfactant can also lead to toxicity concerns in formulations.[22] Therefore, some formulations employ high-pressure homogenization to make nanoemulsions.[12,13,56] We summarize the advantages and disadvantages for both categories of methods in Table 21.1.

21.3 Nanoemulsion stability and rheology

As mentioned earlier, nanoemulsions are a kinetically stable system and over a period of time, they tend to separate into their native phases of oil and water. To control the stability of nanoemulsions, it is important to understand the destabilization mechanism. There are different mechanisms through which emulsions destabilize. Here, we briefly discuss a few of these mechanisms and detail the most relevant mechanism for nanoemulsions.

The most common mechanism through which emulsions destabilize is coalescence. In coalescence, two or more droplets combine to become a larger drop. Typically, creaming or sedimentation succeeds coalescence. In creaming or sedimentation, density difference between oil and water phases results in a net gravitational force which in turn creates a vertically upward/downward motion of droplets. Hence, at the end, the dispersed phase separates from the continuous phase and collects as a separate layer. However, due to their small size, nanoemulsions are not susceptible to either coalescence or creaming/sedimentation.[1]

The major destabilization mechanism for nanoemulsions is Ostwald ripening where bigger droplets grow at the expense of smaller droplets.[57] A signature of an emulsion destabilizing by Ostwald ripening is that the cube of average radius follows a linear relationship with time, i.e., $r^3 = \omega t$, where r is the average nanoemulsion radius, ω is the ripening rate constant, and t is time. This relationship between r and t has been reported in several

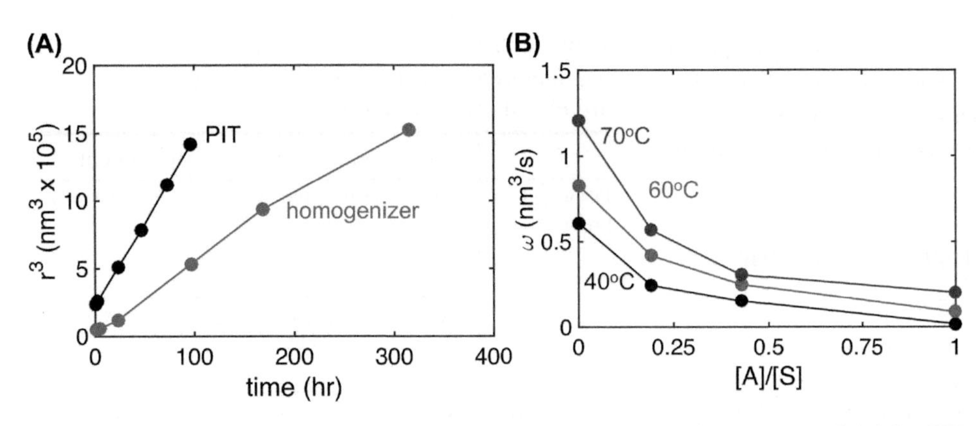

FIGURE 21.5 Destabilization mechanism of nanoemulsions. (A) Nanoemulsions destabilize through the process of Ostwald ripening. In Ostwald ripening, smaller droplets become smaller and larger droplets become larger. A signature of Ostwald ripening mechanism is that cube of average radius of nanoemulsions r^3 is a linear function of time t, or $r^3 = \omega t$, where ω is the ripening rate. The data show that nanoemulsion droplet size indeed follows the expected trend. Here, destabilization rates for two different methods are shown. It is clear that nanoemulsions prepared using phase inversion temperature (labeled as PIT) destabilize faster than nanoemulsions prepared using a homogenizer. The data have been taken from *Tadros, T., Izquierdo, P., Esquena, J., & Solans, C. Formation and stability of nanoemulsion, Adv. Colloid. Interface Sci. 108–109, 303–318 (2004).* (B) The ripening rate ω increases with increase in temperature. However, ω can be reduced through trapped species method. Here [A]/[S] is the concentration ratio of trapped species (Lipoid s75) to the surfactant (Myrj s40). The higher the amount of additional species, smaller is the ripening rate. *The data has been taken from Delmas, T. et al. How to prepare and stabilize very small nanoemulsions. Langmuir 27, 1683–1692 (2011). The figure has been adapted with permission from Gupta, A., Burak, H. E., & Hatton T. A. Nanoemulsions: formation, properties and applications. Soft Matter 12, 2826–2841 (2016).*

TABLE 21.1 Summary of advantages and disadvantages of high- and low-energy methods to prepare nanoemulsions for biomedical applications.

	High-energy methods	Low-energy methods
Composition	Dispersed phase volume fraction as high as 40%, more flexibility in composition, less amount of surfactant required	Dispersed volume fraction typically lower than 25%; composition is not flexible, larger amount of surfactant required
Energy	Requires input of 10^7–10^9 W/kg; needs specialized unit operations	Requires input of 10^3–10^5 W/kg; needs simple unit operations
Stability	Stability is relatively robust and can be tuned depending on needs	Stability is highly dependent on components and composition
Heat and shear	Nanoemulsion preparation includes high shear and thermal changes	Emulsion inversion point operates at constant temperature and modest shear

nanoemulsions studies that confirm Ostwald ripening is the dominant destabilization mechanism for nanoemulsions[11,28,42,43]; see Fig. 21.5A. As shown in the figure, the ω of high-energy methods is typically lower than ω of low-energy methods.

In Ostwald ripening, the dispersed phase molecules from the smaller drop diffuse through the continuous phase and merge into the bigger drop. Hence, the ripening rate depends significantly on the solubility of the dispersed phase in the continuous phase.[1,11,57] A lower solubility of the dispersed phase implies a lower ripening rate. This property is exploited to improve the stability of nanoemulsions in *trapped species method*[11,28]. In this method, a species insoluble in the continuous phase is mixed with the dispersed phase (such as wax in O/W nanoemulsions). This effectively creates an additional chemical potential penalty and lowers the driving force for the dispersed phase molecule to diffuse through the continuous phase, and hence the Ostwald ripening rate decreases. This is demonstrated in Fig. 21.5B. Here, the oil phase is composed of Labrafac and the surfactant is chosen as Myrj s40; see Delmas et al. for details.[11] The trapped species is Lipoid s75. The concentration of the trapped species is denoted as [A] and the concentration of surfactant is denoted as [S]. Therefore, when [A] is increased with respect to [S], a decrease in ω is observed.

Since dispersed phase molecules diffuse more slowly in the continuous phase at a lower temperature, ω also decreases with decrease in temperature.[11] Another variation to control stability is to introduce a species in the continuous phase instead of the dispersed phase. However, this method was found to be less effective, especially at longer times.[11]

Other than robust stability, nanoemulsions also possess interesting rheological properties. Literature reports show that the viscosity and elasticity of nanoemulsions can be tuned by simply changing the nanoemulsion size without changing the composition.[9,10] For instance, Helgeson et al.[9] showed that when nanoemulsion droplet size decreases from 100 to 30 nm, the storage modulus (a measure of elasticity) increases from 10^3 to 10^4 Pa. Thus tuning droplet size provides a convenient way to tune the rheological property of nanoemulsions. In Sections 2 and 3, we discussed the preparation methods and properties of nanoemulsions. Next, we will focus on nanoemulsions in biomedical applications.

21.4 Nanoemulsion formulations for hydrophobic drugs

The most common approach of exploiting nanoemulsions for biomedical applications is creating O/W nanoemulsion formulations where one or more hydrophobic drugs are dissolved in the oil phase.[12–21] The basic idea behind these formulations is that nanodroplets serve as a medium to transport hydrophobic drugs. The advantage of nanoemulsions when compared to the larger droplet–sized emulsions is the enhanced stability[1,4] and improved pharmacological activity.[8] For instance, Schwarz et al.[8] systematically showed that smaller droplet size enhances the drug activity during topical mediation. Furthermore, Benita and Levy[58] argue that oil droplet size should be smaller than the smallest vein inside the body to avoid embolism. In summary, nanoemulsions are preferred due to improved stability, improved pharmacological activity, and safer mode of administration.

The most common method to create nanoemulsion formulations is emulsion inversion point method.[14,17,53–55] However, as reviewed in Table 21.1, this method requires a relatively large amount of surfactant to stabilize nanoemulsions. Moreover, emulsion inversion point formulations require a very laborious effort to optimize components and composition. Therefore, some studies also employ high-pressure homogenization and ultrasonication.[8,12,13,56,58]

The objective of this section is to focus on reviewing some of the nanoemulsion formulations for different modes of delivery: topical, ocular, intravenous, and others.

21.4.1 Topical formulations that are applied directly to the skin

The objective of these nanoemulsion formulations is to enable improved drug permeation through the skin while also providing an ease of application. These O/W nanoemulsions are prepared either using emulsion inversion point or through high-pressure homogenization. A summary of typical composition of this class of nanoemulsions is provided in Table 21.2. The oil phases are always organic such as medium chain triglycerides, propylene glycol (or a close derivative), benzyl alcohol, olive oil, soybean oil, triacetin, and others. Some studies also exploit cosmetic grade oils such as Eutanol G.[56] The content of the oil is typically about 15–20 wt% in the overall formulation.

TABLE 21.2 Overview of composition for nanoemulsions used in topical formulations that are directly applied to skin.

	Component	Amount
Dispersed phase	Oil such as medium chain triglycerides, propylene glycol, benzyl alcohol, olive oil, triacetin	15–20 wt%
	Hydrophobic active material like celecoxib, ketoprofen, progesterone, etc.	1–1.5 wt%
Continuous phase	Surfactant such as Tween 20, Tween 80, poloxamers, polyvinyl alcohol.	15–20 wt% (low energy) 3–5 wt% (high energy)
	Cross-linking agent such as carbopol 940 to convert the formulation into a gel	0.5–1 wt%
	Water	Remaining

In the oil phase, a hydrophobic drug or nutrient (sometimes also referred as an active pharmaceutical ingredient, API) is dissolved, generally to the maximum capacity in order to achieve the largest API loading. Typical solubility levels of these API in the oil phase are 80–100 mg/g. Since the oil phase is typically about 15–20 wt% of the entire formulation, the overall loading of the drug is about 10–15 mg/g. Some examples of API include celecoxib[14] (for arthritis and osteoarthritis), ketoprofen[59] (for rheumatoid arthritis), progesterone[12] (for hormone replacement therapy), and ceramide III[56] (for skin hydration and smoothness). The surfactant phase is typically nonionic such as Tween 20, Tween 80, polyvinyl alcohol, solutol HS 15, and poloxamers. However, to utilize more natural products due to toxicity concerns, sucrose esters and cyclodextrins[12] have also been utilized.

The relative composition of oil and surfactant phases is determined by the preparation method. When emulsion inversion point is exercised, the amount of surfactant weight fraction is similar to the oil phase weight fraction, i.e., 15–20 wt%.[14,17,53–55] Simply put, surfactant-to-oil (SOR) ratio is about unity. In fact, even when the amount of oil phase is small, amount of surfactant is adjusted to keep SOR = 1. For instance, Kim et al. prepared nanoemulsion formulation by emulsion inversion point method with 2 wt % oil phase and 2 wt% surfactant phase.[59] In contrast, when nanoemulsion formulation is created using high-pressure homogenization, values of SOR can be kept as low as 0.2.[12,13,56] As an example, Yilmaz et al. employed a high-pressure homogenizer to formulate nanoemulsions with 20 wt% oil-phase nanoemulsion and only 5 wt% surfactant, or SOR = 0.25. Thus, as mentioned previously in Table 21.1, low-energy methods are energy efficient but need a significantly larger quantity of surfactant when compared to high-energy methods. Next, we discuss the aqueous phase composition.

Since one of the primary objectives of these formulations is the ease of application on the skin, it is desired to increase the viscosity of the aqueous phase. The most common modification is to add a cross-linking agent, such as carbopol 940, that converts the continuous phase (water) into a gel.[14,18,53] Therefore, the addition of a cross-linking agent enables the formulation to be applied to the skin as a gel. Instead of adding a cross-linking agent, it is also possible to induce gelation by simultaneously increasing the viscosity of aqueous through additives such as glycerol and polyethylene glycol (PEG) and also increasing the oil-phase fraction. For instance, Sonneville-Aubrun et al.[60] reported that with the same continuous phase, nanoemulsion turned from liquid to a gel when oil weight fraction was increased from 15 wt% to 25 wt% (Fig. 21.6A).

To address the influence of addition of a cross-linking agent on performance of a nanoemulsion formulation, Baboota et al.[14] prepared three different samples with celecoxib as API: (i) control gel loaded with celecoxib, (ii) O/W nanoemulsion with celecoxib as API but no cross-linking agent, and (iii) O/W nanoemulsion with celecoxib as API as well as a cross-linking agent. The authors reported that both nanoemulsions with/without cross-linking result in a significantly larger skin permeation of the API as compared to the control group (Fig. 21.6B). The inclusion of a cross-linking agent in the nanoemulsion formulation only leads to minor decrease in cumulative API permeation. In addition to the cross-linking agent, the effective charge on nanoemulsion droplets can modify the permeation levels. For instance, Yilmaz et al.[13] reported that a positively charged nanoemulsion cream hydrates the skin better than a negative charged nanoemulsion cream (Fig. 21.6C). This phenomenon occurs since the skin is negatively charged. We discuss the details of similar charged interactions in the next subsection.

21.4.2 Ocular formulations

These formulations involve administering the drugs through eye drops. The delivery of an active ingredient through eye drops poses several challenges. First, the standard aqueous eye drops cannot administer hydrophobic drugs. Second, and more importantly, the tear duct clears 80% of the drug within a couple of minutes. Hence, it is common to see multiple dosages of eye drops. To resolve these challenges simultaneously, nanoemulsions have been utilized. In fact, they have already been commercially exploited in the Novasorb product series. Interested readers are referred to the review article by Lallemand et al.[21] that

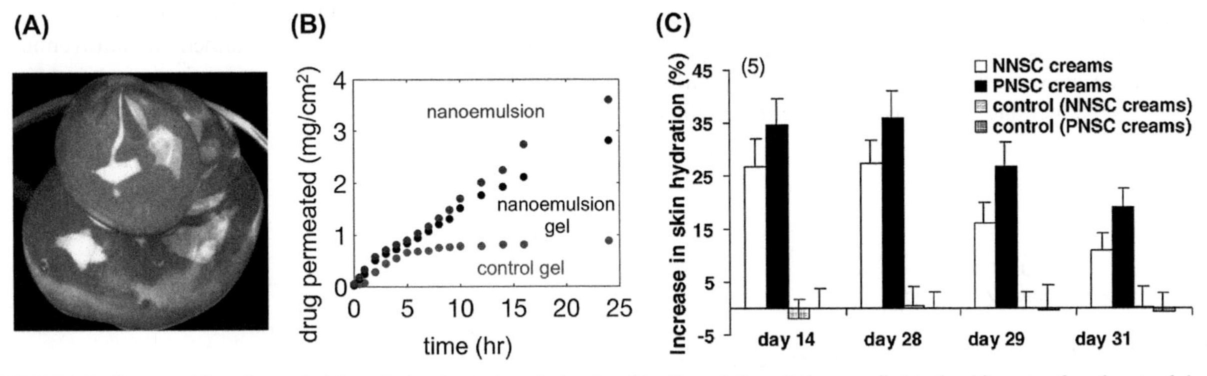

FIGURE 21.6 Nanoemulsions for topical formulation that are applied to the skin. Formulations that are applied to the skin are preferred as a gel due to improved ease of application. Nanoemulsions provide a convenient way to create gels. O/W nanoemulsions can be converted into a gel simply by addition of a cross-linking agent in the aqueous phase. (A) It is also possible to induce gelation by simply increasing the oil fraction. *The figure has been reproduced with permission from Sonneville-Aubrun, O., Simonnet, J.-T., & L'Alloret, F. Nanoemulsions: a new vehicle for skincare products, Adv. Colloid. Interface Sci. 108–109, 145–149 (2004).* (B) O/W nanoemulsions with celecoxib as API in the oil phase and with/without a cross-linking agent in the aqueous phase were prepared. The data here show the cumulative in-vitro skim permeation of celecoxib. The data show that nanoemulsion and nanoemulsion gel outperform the control gel significantly. The inclusion of a cross-linking agent has a minor negative influence on the API permeation. *The data have been taken from Baboota, S., Shakeel, F., Ahuja, A., Ali, J., & Shafiq, S. Design, development and evaluation of novel nanoemulsion formulations for transdermal potential of celecoxib, Acta Pharm 57, 315–332 (2007).* (C) Nanoemulsions have also been utilized to improve skin hydration. Here, a comparison of increase in skin hydration with time for different nanoemulsion creams is demonstrated. Since the human skin is negatively charged, positively charged nanoemulsion creams (labeled as PNSC) perform better than negatively charged nanoemulsion creams (labeled as NNSC). *The figure has been reproduced with permission Yilmaz, E. & Borchert, H. H. Effect of lipid-containing, positively charged nanoemulsions on skin hydration, elasticity and erythema - an in vivo study. Int. J. Pharm. 307, 232–238 (2006).*

details the milestones and rationale of Novasorb. Here, we briefly describe the main developments.

The human eye consists of a tear film that is protected against evaporation by the lipid layer (Fig. 21.7A). The tear film is also in touch with the mucin layer that is negatively charged. As mentioned previously, the tear film is constantly cleared through the tear duct. Therefore, when an eye drop is introduced in the tear film, it is preferred that the active component stays longer in the tear film. To prolong the retention time of active components, the Novasorb technology develops positively charged nanodroplets (also referred to as cationic nanoemulsions) and exploits the property that mucin layer is negatively charged. The electrostatic attraction between the negatively charged mucin layer and positively charged nanodroplets results in improved bioavailability (Fig. 21.7B). Lallemand et al.[21] show that the drug bioavailability from a cationic nanoemulsion formulations of cyclosporine A, a drug used in treatment of severe dry eyes, outperforms a commercially available anionic emulsion. To impart a positive charge to the oil droplet, in addition to the surfactant, a cationic agent is also required. Since the cationic agents tend to be toxic, they are used in a relatively low concentration. For instance, cetalkonium chloride (CKC) is utilized in Novasorb. CKC gets its positive charge from the ammonium ions.

A summary of composition of nanoemulsion formulations for ocular delivery is provided in Table 21.3. The oil phase is typically based on oil such as medium chain triglycerides, mineral oil, and vegetable oil, among others. The hydrophobic drugs such as cyclosporine (for dry eye) and dorzolamide[61,62] (for treating glaucoma) are dissolved in the oil phase. The oil phase also consists of cationic agents such as CKC and a surfactant such as tylopaxol. In contrast, the aqueous phase consists of another surfactant such as poloxamer and also consists of NaOH to adjust the pH. Some glycerol is also added since it serves as an osmotic agent. Since one of the considerations is to minimize the amount of the cationic agent and surfactants (to avoid toxicity concerns), high-pressure homogenizer is employed to create nanoemulsions.[21]

TABLE 21.3 Overview of composition for nanoemulsions used in ocular formulations.

	Component	Amount
Dispersed phase	Medium chain triglyceride, mineral oil, vegetable oil	1−2 wt%
	Cetalkonium chloride (cationic agent), tylopaxol (surfactant)	0.005 wt%, 0.2 wt%
Continuous phase	Poloxamer (surfactant), NaOH (adjust pH), glycerol (viscosity adjustment)	0.01 wt%, as required
	Water	

21.4.3 Others

There are other modes of delivery that have also been investigated using nanoemulsions. For instance, O/W nanoemulsion formulations for intravenous applications have been developed for drugs such as rifampicin[63] (for tuberculosis treatment), aminoalkanethiosulfuric acids[64] (for treatment of schistosomiasis, an infectious disease), carbamazepine[22] (for therapy of seizures), ramipril[16,17] (an antihypertensive drug), and saquinavir[65] (an HIV-protease inhibitor), among others. Here, majority of studies utilize emulsion inversion point method to make nanoemulsions. Since these formulations were aimed for intravenous applications, no cross-linking agent is introduced in the continuous phase.

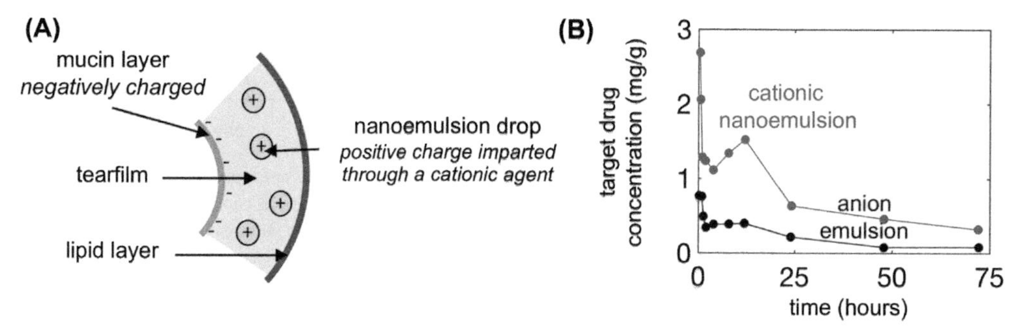

FIGURE 21.7 Nanoemulsions for ocular delivery. (A) Since the objective of ocular delivery is to increase the retention time of the drug in the tear film, cationic nanoemulsions, i.e., nanoemulsions that have an effective positive charge, are preferred since the mucin layer of the eye is negatively charged. (B) Target drug concentration in rabbit eye for two different modes of delivery: cationic nanoemulsion and a commercially available anionic emulsion. The target drug here is cyclosporine A that is used to treat dry eyes. The results clearly demonstrate that cationic nanoemulsion significantly improves the bioavailability of the target drug. *The data have been taken from Lallemand, F., Daull, P., Benita, S., Buggage, R. & Garrigue, J. Successfully improving ocular drug delivery using the cationic nanoemulsion , Novasorb* J Drug Deliv *(2012). https://doi.org/10.1155/2012/604204.*

In their articles, Kumar et al. created O/W nanoemulsion formulation for intranasal delivery[19,20] and incorporated antipsychotic drug risperidone in the oil phase. The authors incorporated chitosan as a cross-linking agent in the aqueous phase and tested two modes of delivery in Swiss albino rats: intranasal and intravenous. The authors found that intranasal delivery with chitosan in the aqueous phase performed best followed by intranasal delivery without chitosan in the aqueous phase. The intravenous delivery performed the worst among the three modes.

Researchers have also created nanoemulsion formulations (i) without any synthetic surfactants,[66] (ii) for cancer treatment including mouse models,[67,68] (iii) for treatment for malaria,[69] (iv) stabilized by magnetic surfactants,[70] and (v) designed for intestinal absorption.[71] Lastly, there have also been attempts to exploit W/O nanoemulsions for transport of hydrophilic compounds.[72]

21.5 Nanoemulsions as a template for hydrophobic drug nanocrystals

In Section 4, we discussed various formulations of O/W nanoemulsions where an API is dissolved in the oil phase. As evident from Tables 21.2 and 21.3, diverse range of oil and surfaces choices is available for nanoemulsion-based formulations. However, since oil and surfactants can be toxic, every new formulation requires an extensive study that characterizes the toxicity and pharmacokinetics of the formulation before it is suitable for human use. Therefore, it is preferred to avoid using the oil phase and surfactant in formulations. In this section, we discuss how nanoemulsions are exploited as templates to create nanocrystals of a hydrophobic drug.

An overview of steps followed in utilizing nanoemulsions to template hydrophobic drug nanocrystals is

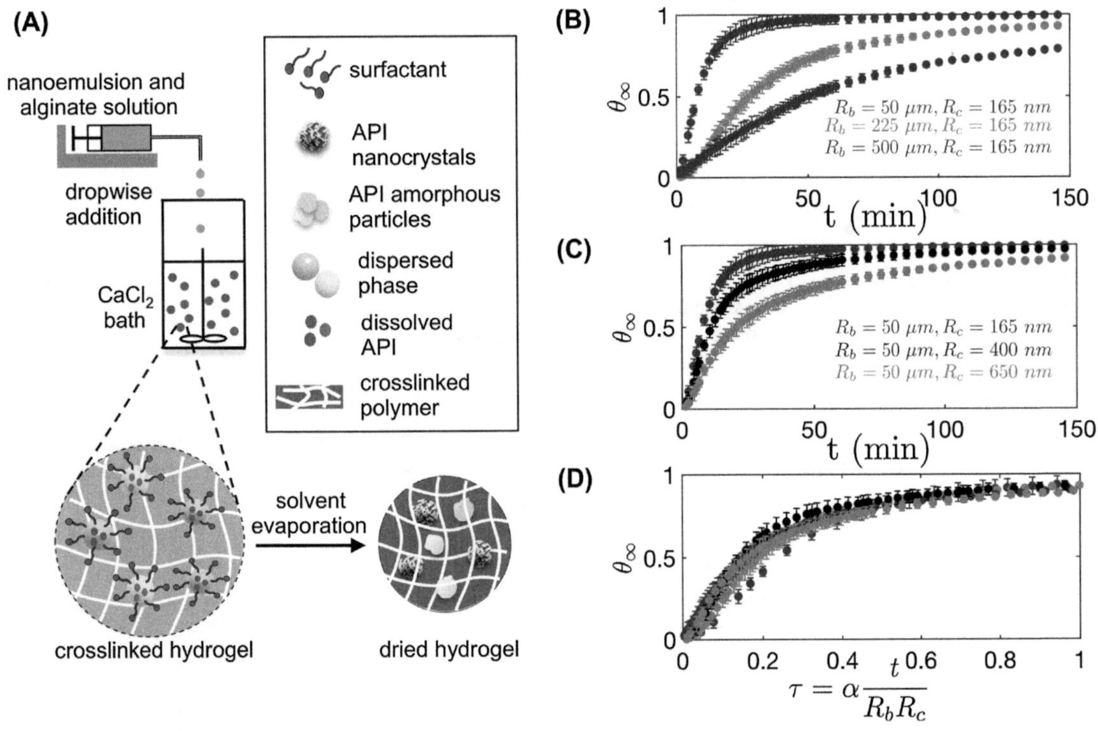

FIGURE 21.8 Nanoemulsions as templates for hydrophobic drug nanocrystals. (A) O/W nanoemulsions are prepared using either high-energy or low-energy methods. In the oil phase, hydrophobic drug(s), i.e., APIs, are dissolved. In the aqueous phase, sodium alginate is added. The nanoemulsion solution is dropped from a syringe into a calcium chloride bath. When nanoemulsion solution comes in contact with calcium chloride, cross-linking of the aqueous phase occurs. Therefore, hydrogel beads of radius R_b are created. These microbeads contain the nanodrops of oil that contain the API. The beads are then washed and dried, and thus the oil and moisture evaporate. The evaporation process induces crystallization of the API. The crytsal size is denoted by R_c. (B) In-vitro dissolution profiles of alginate microbeads containing fenofibrate drug crystals. The dimensionless concentration of dissolved alginate (θ_∞) as a function of time (t) for $R_c = 165$ nm and different values of R_b. It is observed that a larger R_b leads to a slower dissolution. (C) θ_∞ versus t for different values of R_c but same value of R_b. It can be seen that a larger R_c results in slower dissolution. (D) To collapse the data from (B) and (C), the x-axis is rescaled as $\tau = \alpha \frac{t}{R_b R_c}$, where α is a constant. *The figure is adapted with permission Badruddoza, A. Z. M., Gupta, A., Myerson, A. S., Trout, B. L. & Doyle, P. S. Low energy nanoemulsions as templates for the formulation of hydrophobic drugs. Adv Ther 1, 1700020 (2018).*

provided in Fig. 21.8A.[5,6,23–25] First, O/W nanoemulsions are created using either high-energy[23–25] or low-energy methods.[5,6] Here, the oil phase is chosen to be biocompatible and volatile (such as anisole). The API is dissolved in the oil phase. The aqueous phase contains the surfactant as well as sodium alginate. Once the nanoemulsions have been prepared, macrodrops of nanoemulsions, i.e., macrodrops of aqueous phase that contain nanodrops of the oil phase, are created using a syringe. The macrodrops are then dropped in a bath of calcium chloride that triggers an instantaneous polymerization reaction to transform aqueous drops containing sodium alginate into alginate microbeads. The alginate microbeads contain nanodrops of oil where the API is dissolved. These microbeads are thoroughly washed with water to remove any excess surfactant. Next, the beads are dried to evaporate oil and excess moisture. The drying process induces crystallization of the dissolved hydrophobic API. Therefore, the end product is microbeads with radius R_b with embedded drug nanocrystals of radius R_c. Due to the drying step and multiple washing steps, surfactant and oil phases are removed from the final product.

There are two length scales present in the microbeads embedded with nanocrystals, i.e., R_b and R_c. These length scales are readily tunable as the bead size is tuned by changing the syringe size and the crystal size can be modified by controlling the nanoemulsion drop size.[5] There is also possibility to utilize centrifugal force to achieve smaller R_b values.[73]

To measure the drug release profiles, in-vitro studies were conducted with different values of R_b and R_c. Badruddoza et al.[5] systematically studied two model drugs: fenofibrate and ibuprofen. They showed that a larger bead size results in a slower drug delivery since a larger bead size leads to a longer diffusion time (Fig. 21.8B). Similarly, a larger crystal also leads to a slower drug release since a larger crystal size decreases the surface area and hence the dissolution rate slows down (Fig. 21.8C). To quantitatively capture the effect of both bead size and crystal size, it is possible to rescale the time $\tau = \alpha \frac{t}{R_b R_c}$, where α is a constant, and collapse the dissolution rates for different R_b and R_c on a master plot (Fig. 21.8D).

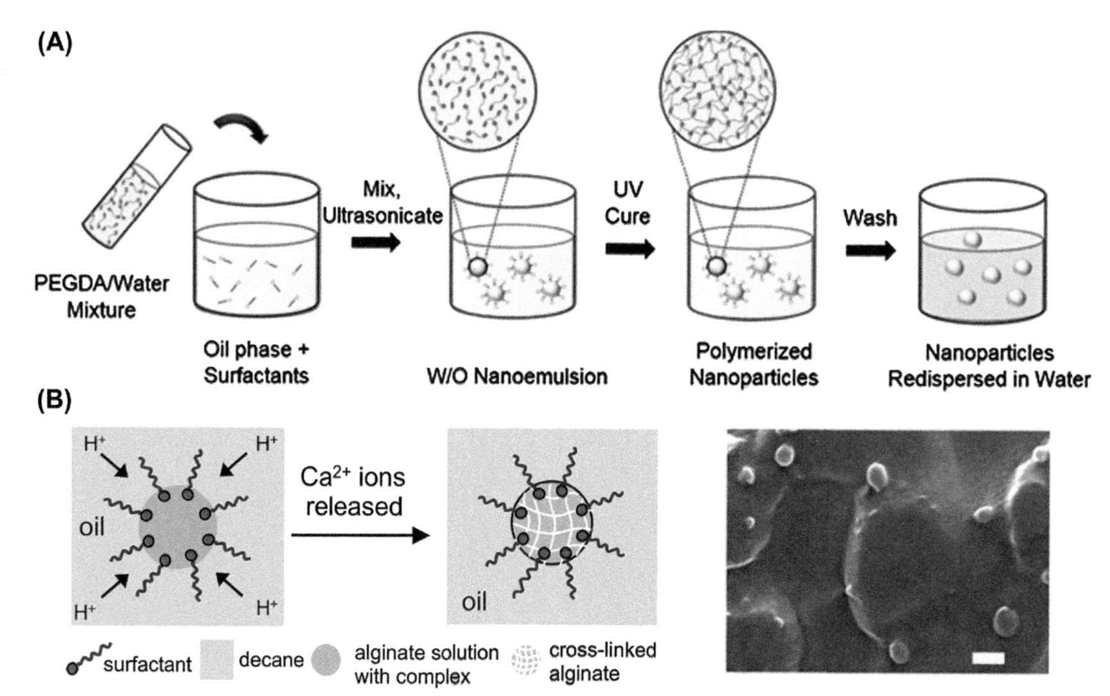

FIGURE 21.9 Summary of the processes to convert W/O nanoemulsions into hydrogel nanoparticles. These hydrogel nanoparticles can then be used for different modes of drug delivery. (A) W/O nanoemulsions are prepared with PEGDA in the water phase using ultrasonication. Next, the nanoemulsions are UV cured where aqueous drops cross-link to form hydrogel nanoparticles. The cross-linked nanoparticles are then separated and dispersed in water through washing and solvent exchange. The figure is adapted with permission from *Anselmo, A.C., Elasticity of nanoparticles influences their blood circulation, phagocytosis, endocytosis, and targeting, ACS Nano 9, 3169–3177 (2015).* (B) Instead of using a high-energy method, it is also possible to utilize a low-energy method to create hydrogel nanoparticles. Here, W/O nanoemulsions are prepared using emulsion inversion point. The aqueous phase consists of calcium–EDTA complex, sodium alginate, and sodium chloride. When acetic acid is introduced in the oil phase, the hydrogen ions from the acetic acid react with calcium–EDTA complex and release the calcium ions that trigger the cross-linking reaction. This technique enables preparation of 200-300 nm hydrogel nanoparticles. Scale bar is 200 nm. *The figure is adapted with permission from Gupta et al.Gupta, A., Badruddoza, A. Z. M. & Doyle, P. S. A general route for nanoemulsion synthesis using low-energy methods at constant temperature. Langmuir 33, 7118–7123 (2017).*

There are many advantages of this approach: (i) it avoids the use of oil and surfactant in the final product thus reducing concerns of toxicity, (ii) it provides a route to tune the release rates of hydrophobic drugs by tuning the R_b and R_c, and (iii) it provides the possibility to embed multiple drugs within the same microbead, thus improving dosing and patient compliance.[5]

21.6 Nanoemulsions for advanced material synthesis in biomedical applications

In sections 4 and 5, we discussed the application of nanoemulsions in delivering hydrophobic drugs. In this section, we discuss the application of nanoemulsions in advanced material synthesis that are then utilized in biomedical applications.

An interesting approach to utilize W/O nanoemulsions is to convert the dispersed phase into a hydrogel. To achieve this, a cross-linking agent is introduced into the aqueous phase. Anselmo et al.[26] created W/O nanoemulsions using ultrasonication with varying amounts of polyethylene (glycol) diacrylate (PEGDA) in the dispersed phase. The authors then cross-linked the dispersed phase using UV and separated out the nanohydrogel particles (Fig. 21.9A). The authors reported that they are able to vary the elasticity of the particles from 10 to 3000 kPa. It was observed that blood circulation and targeting depended significantly on the elasticity of the particles. Another approach to create hydrogel particles using nanoemulsions is through low-energy method. Gupta et al.[6] prepared W/O nanoemulsions using low-energy methods. Here, they added sodium alginate, sodium chloride, and calcium–EDTA in the aqueous phase. To trigger the cross-linking of alginate, acetic acid is introduced in the oil phase

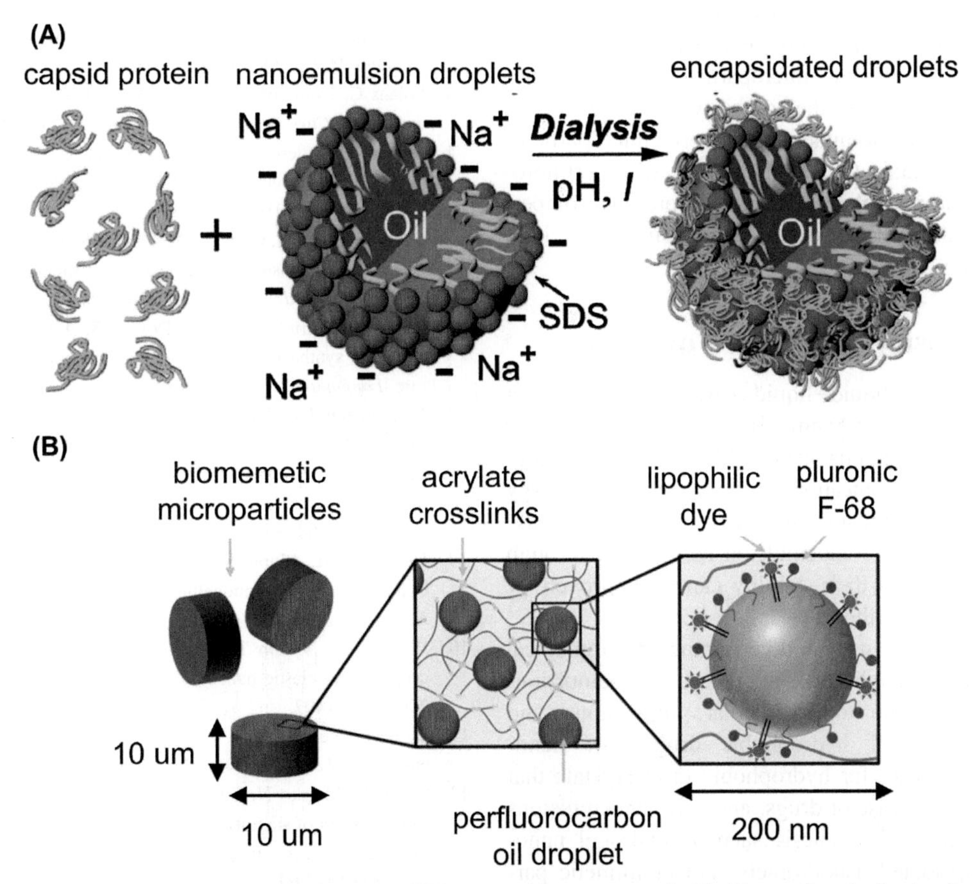

FIGURE 21.10 Nanoemulsions for biomaterial synthesis. (A) O/W nanoemulsions are created with silicone oil as the droplet phase and SDS as the surfactant. Since SDS is an anionic surfactant, positively charged protein from cowpea chlorotic mottle virus was utilized to encapsidate the nanodroplet. By varying the pH and ionic strength, the encapsidation process was tuned. *(B) O/W nanoemulsions are utilized in biomimetic microparticles. The polymeric microparticles contain the nanoemulsions with perfluorocarbon as the droplet phase. Due to the presence of perfluorocarbon, the microparticles demonstrate a high oxygen-carrying capacity. (A). The figure is adapted with permission from Chang et al.Chang, C. B., Knobler, C. M., Gelbart, W. M. & Mason, T. G. Curvature dependence of viral protein structures on encapsidated nanoemulsion droplets. ACS Nano 2, 281–286 (2008). (B) The figure is adapted with permission from An et al.An, H. Z., Safai, E. R., Burak Eral, H. & Doyle, P. S. Synthesis of biomimetic oxygen-carrying compartmentalized microparticles using flow lithography. Lab Chip 13, 4765 (2013).*

(Fig. 21.9B). When acetic acid comes in contact with calcium–EDTA present in the aqueous droplets, calcium ions are released that initiate cross-linking. Through this approach, the authors utilized low-energy nanoemulsions to create hydrogel particles. There have also been more recent efforts to prepare polymeric nanoparticles using double nanoemulsions.[74,75]

Nanoemulsions have also been utilized to encapsidate droplets using virus proteins. The overview of this process is provided in Fig. 21.10A. Here, Chang et al.[27] created nanoemulsion droplets stabilized with an anionic surfactant, i.e., SDS. Since this imparted a negative charge to the droplets, authors used capsid protein that is positively charged to encapsidate the droplets using electrostatic attraction. The protein is extracted from cowpea chlorotic mottle virus. The authors showed that by changing the pH and concentration of salt in the solution, they are able to tune the encapsidation behavior of proteins. Lastly, functional nanoemulsions can also be used in 3-D printing as printable ink. Hsiao et al.[76] created 3-D printed structure with temperature-responsive nanoemulsions that enable tissue deformation studies. Similarly, nanoemulsions are also used in biomimetic microparticles where nanoemulsions drops improved the solubility of oxygen inside the particles.[28] The biomimetic polymeric microparticles are designed to contain the nanoemulsions with perfluorocarbon as the droplet phase. Due to the presence of perfluorocarbon, the microparticles demonstrated a high oxygen-carrying capacity Fig. 21.10B.

21.7 Conclusion and future outlook

Nanoemulsions are liquid–liquid systems with droplet sizes between 20 and 500 nm. They are prepared either using high-energy methods such as high-pressure homogenization and ultrasonication, or through low-energy methods such as emulsion inversion point and phase inversion temperature. Nanoemulsion destabilizes through Ostwald ripening, and their stability can be improved by the trapped species method.

Nanoemulsions are used in diverse range of biomedical applications. These applications include (i) nanoemulsion-based formulations for topical, ocular, intravenous, and intranasal delivery of hydrophobic drugs, (ii) nanoemulsions as template for hydrophobic drug crystals that enable controlled release of drugs, and (iii) nanoemulsions for advanced material synthesis such as hydrogel nanoparticles, encapsidated nanodroplets, and biomimetic particles with improved solubility of oxygen.

Though nanoemulsions are promising for biomedical applications, to enable rapid commercialization of nanoemulsion technologies, several scientific questions need to be addressed. For instance, development of nanoemulsion formulations is mostly driven through a trial and error approach. Therefore, future research should focus on answering the following questions: can we design more systematic routes to develop these formulations? Can we find specific compositions that might serve as a good starting point for the optimization process in order to reduce the number of iterations to arrive at optimal formulation composition? Similarly, though it is recognized that nanoemulsion droplet size is the key property that differentiates nanoemulsions, most studies focusing on biomedical applications do not vary this parameter. Future studies could systematically study the effect of droplet size and droplet size distribution on in-vitro dissolution profiles, skin permeation, and other relevant parameters. Lastly, nanoemulsions should also be explored as candidates for targeted drug delivery.

References

1. Gupta A, Burak HE, Hatton TA, Doyle PS. Nanoemulsions: formation, properties and applications. *Soft Matter* 2016;**12**:2826–41.
2. Mason TG, Wilking JN, Meleson K, Chang CB, Graves SM. Nanoemulsions: formation, structure, and physical properties. *J Phys Condens Matter* 2006;**18**:R635–66.
3. Solans C, Izquierdo P, Nolla J, Azemar N, Garciacelma M. Nanoemulsions. *Curr Opin Colloid Interface Sci* 2005;**10**:102–10.
4. Tadros T, Izquierdo P, Esquena J, Solans C. Formation and stability of nano-emulsions. *Adv Colloid Interface Sci* 2004;**108–109**:303–18.
5. Badruddoza AZM, Gupta A, Myerson AS, Trout BL, Doyle PS. Low energy nanoemulsions as templates for the formulation of hydrophobic drugs. *Adv Ther* 2018;**1**:1700020.
6. Gupta A, Badruddoza AZM, Doyle PS. A general route for nanoemulsion synthesis using low-energy methods at constant temperature. *Langmuir* 2017;**33**:7118–23.
7. McClements DJ. Edible nanoemulsions: fabrication, properties, and functional performance. *Soft Matter* 2011;**7**:2297–316.
8. Schwarz JS, Weisspapir MR, Friedman DI. Enhanced transdermal delivery of diazepam by submicron emulsion (sme) creams. *Pharm Res* 1995;**12**:687–92.
9. Helgeson ME, Moran SE, An HZ, Doyle PS. Mesoporous organohydrogels from thermogelling photocrosslinkable nanoemulsions. *Nat Mater* 2012;**11**:344–52.
10. Wilking JN, Mason TG. Irreversible shear-induced vitrification of droplets into elastic nanoemulsions by extreme rupturing. *Phys Rev* 2007;**75**:041407.
11. Delmas T, et al. How to prepare and stabilize very small nanoemulsions. *Langmuir* 2011;**27**:1683–92.
12. Klang V, Matsko N, Zimmermann AM, Vojnikovic E, Valenta C. Enhancement of stability and skin permeation by sucrose stearate and cyclodextrins in progesterone nanoemulsions. *Int J Pharm* 2010;**393**:152–60.
13. Yilmaz E, Borchert HH. Effect of lipid-containing, positively charged nanoemulsions on skin hydration, elasticity and erythema - an in vivo study. *Int J Pharm* 2006;**307**:232–8.
14. Baboota S, Shakeel F, Ahuja A, Ali J, Shafiq S. Design, development and evaluation of novel nanoemulsion formulations for transdermal potential of celecoxib. *Acta Pharm* 2007;**57**:315–32.

15. Shakeel F, et al. Nanoemulsions as vehicles for transdermal delivery of aceclofenac. *AAPS PharmSciTech* 2007;**8**:E104.
16. Shafiq S, et al. Development and bioavailability assessment of ramipril nanoemulsion formulation. *Eur J Pharm Biopharm* 2007;**66**:227–43.
17. Shafiq-un-nabi S, et al. Formulation development and optimization using nanoemulsion technique: a technical note. *AAPS PharmSciTech* 2007;**8**:1–6.
18. Alves PM, Pohlmann AR, Guterres SS. Semisolid topical formulations containing nimesulide-loaded nanocapsules, nanospheres or nanoemulsion: development and rheological characterization. *Die Pharmazie* 2005;**60**:900–4.
19. Kumar M, et al. Intranasal nanoemulsion based brain targeting drug delivery system of risperidone. *Int J Pharm* 2008;**358**:285–91.
20. Kumar M, Misra A, Mishra AK, Mishra P, Kamla P. Mucoadhesive nanoemulsion-based intranasal drug delivery system of olanzapine for brain targeting. *J Drug Target* 2008;**16**:806–14.
21. Lallemand F, Daull P, Benita S, Buggage R, Garrigue J. Successfully improving ocular drug delivery using the cationic nanoemulsion. *Novasorb J Drug Deliv* 2012. https://doi.org/10.1155/2012/604204.
22. Kelmann RG, Kuminek G, Teixeira HF, Koester S. Carbamazepine parenteral nanoemulsions prepared by spontaneous emulsification process. *Int J Pharm* 2007;**342**:231–9.
23. Eral HB, et al. Composite hydrogels laden with crystalline active pharmaceutical ingredients of controlled size and loading. *Chem Mater* 2014;**26**:6213–20.
24. Eral HB, et al. Biocompatible alginate microgel particles as heteronucleants and encapsulating vehicles for hydrophilic and hydrophobic drugs. *Cryst Growth Des* 2014;**14**:2073–82.
25. Badruddoza AZM, Godfrin PD, Myerson AS, Trout BL, Doyle PS. Core-shell composite hydrogels for controlled nanocrystal formation and release of hydrophobic active pharmaceutical ingredients. *Adv Healthc Mater* 2016;**5**:1960–8.
26. Anselmo AC, et al. Elasticity of nanoparticles influences their blood circulation, phagocytosis, endocytosis, and targeting. *ACS Nano* 2015;**9**:3169–77.
27. Chang CB, Knobler CM, Gelbart WM, Mason TG. Curvature dependence of viral protein structures on encapsidated nanoemulsion droplets. *ACS Nano* 2008;**2**:281–6.
28. An HZ, Safai ER, Burak Eral H, Doyle PS. Synthesis of biomimetic oxygen-carrying compartmentalized microparticles using flow lithography. *Lab Chip* 2013;**13**:4765.
29. Lee SJ, McClements DJ. Fabrication of protein-stabilized nanoemulsions using a combined homogenization and amphiphilic solvent dissolution/evaporation approach. *Food Hydrocolloids* 2010;**24**:560–9.
30. Li M, Ma Y, Cui J. Whey-protein-stabilized nanoemulsions as a potential delivery system for water-insoluble curcumin. *LWT – Food Sci Technol* 2014;**59**:49–58.
31. Ozturk B, Argin S, Ozilgen M, McClements DJ. Formation and stabilization of nanoemulsion-based vitamin e delivery systems using natural biopolymers: whey protein isolate and gum Arabic. *Food Chem* 2015;**188**:256–63.
32. Qian C, Decker EA, Xiao H, McClements DJ. Physical and chemical stability of β-carotene-enriched nanoemulsions: influence of ph, ionic strength, temperature, and emulsifier type. *Food Chem* 2012;**132**:1221–9.
33. Gupta A, Eral HB, Hatton TA, Doyle PS. Controlling and predicting droplet size of nanoemulsions: scaling relations with experimental validation. *Soft Matter* 2016;**12**:1452–8.
34. Gupta A, Narsimhan V, Hatton TA, Doyle PS. Kinetics of the change in droplet size during nanoemulsion formation. *Langmuir* 2016;**32**:11551–9.
35. Mason TG, Graves SM, Wilking JN, Lin MY. Extreme emulsification: formation and structure of nanoemulsions. *Condens Matter Phys* 2006;**9**:193–9.
36. Meleson K, Graves S, Mason TG. Formation of concentrated nanoemulsions by extreme shear. *Soft Mater* 2004;**2**:109–23.
37. Leong TSH, Wooster TJ, Kentish SE, Ashokkumar M. Minimising oil droplet size using ultrasonic emulsification. *Ultrason Sonochem* 2009;**16**:721–7.
38. Donsì F, Sessa M, Ferrari G. Effect of emulsifier type and disruption chamber geometry on the fabrication of food nanoemulsions by high pressure homogenization. *Ind Eng Chem Res* 2012;**51**:7606–18.
39. Håkansson A, Innings F, Trägårdh C, Bergenståhl B. A high-pressure homogenization emulsification model—improved emulsifier transport and hydrodynamic coupling. *Chem Eng Sci* 2013;**91**:44–53.
40. Håkansson A, Trägårdh C, Bergenståhl B. Dynamic simulation of emulsion formation in a high pressure homogenizer. *Chem Eng Sci* 2009;**64**:2915–25.
41. Kentish S, et al. The use of ultrasonics for nanoemulsion preparation. *Innov Food Sci Emerg Technol* 2008;**9**:170–5.
42. Wooster TJ, Golding M, Sanguansri P. Impact of oil type on nanoemulsion formation and ostwald ripening stability. *Langmuir* 2008;**24**:12758–65.
43. Izquierdo P, et al. Formation and stability of nano-emulsions prepared using the phase inversion temperature method. *Langmuir* 2002;**18**:26–30.
44. Izquierdo P, et al. The influence of surfactant mixing ratio on nanoemulsion formation by the pit method. *J Colloid Interface Sci* 2005;**285**:388–94.
45. Izquierdo P, et al. Phase behavior and nano-emulsion formation by the phase inversion temperature method. *Langmuir* 2004;**20**:6594–8.
46. Esquena J, Forgiarini A. Studies of the relation between phase behavior and emulsification methods with nanoemulsion formation. In: *Trends in colloid and interface science XIV*, vol. 115; 2000. p. 36–9.
47. Esquena J, Forgiarini A. Formation and stability of nano-emulsions in mixed nonionic surfactant systems. *Trends in Colloid and Interface Science* 2001;**XV**:184–9.
48. Forgiarini A, Esquena J, González C, Solans C, Gonza C. Formation of nano-emulsions by low-energy emulsification methods at constant temperature. *Langmuir* 2001;**17**:2076–83.
49. Porras M, et al. Studies of formation of w/o nano-emulsions. *Colloids Surfaces A Physicochem Eng Asp* 2004;**249**:115–8.
50. Porras M, Solans C, Gonzalez C, Gutierrez JM. Properties of water-in-oil (w/o) nano-emulsions prepared by a low-energy emulsification method. *Colloids Surfaces A Physicochem Eng Asp* 2008;**324**:181–8.
51. Solè I, Maestro A, Gonzalez C, Solans C, Gutiérrez JM. Optimization of nano-emulsion preparation by low-energy methods in an ionic surfactant system. *Langmuir* 2006;**22**:8326–32.
52. Perazzo A, Preziosi V, Guido S. Phase inversion emulsification: current understanding and applications. *Adv Colloid Interface Sci* 2015;**222**:581–99.

53. Mou D, et al. Hydrogel-thickened nanoemulsion system for topical delivery of lipophilic drugs. *Int J Pharm* 2008;**353**:270–6.
54. Kong M, Chen XG, Kweon DK, Park HJ. Investigations on skin permeation of hyaluronic acid based nanoemulsion as transdermal carrier. *Carbohydr Polym* 2011;**86**:837–43.
55. Shakeel F, Shafiq S, Haq N, Alanazi FK, Alsarra IA. Nanoemulsions as potential vehicles for transdermal and dermal delivery of hydrophobic compounds: an overview. *Expert Opin Drug Deliv* 2012;**9**:953–74.
56. Yilmaz E, Borchert HH. Design of a phytosphingosine-containing, positively-charged nanoemulsion as a colloidal carrier system for dermal application of ceramides. *Eur J Pharm Biopharm* 2005;**60**:91–8.
57. Lifshitz IM, Slyozov VV. The kinetics of precipitation from supersaturated solid solutions. *J Phys Chem Solids* 1961;**19**:35–50.
58. Benita S, Levy MY. Submicron emulsions as colloidal drug carriers for intravenous administration: comprehensive physicochemical characterization. *J Pharm Sci* 1993;**82**:1069–79.
59. Kim BS, Won M, Lee KM, Kim CS. In vitro permeation studies of nanoemulsions containing ketoprofen as a model drug. *Drug Deliv* 2008;**15**:465–9.
60. Sonneville-Aubrun O, Simonnet J-T, L'Alloret F. Nanoemulsions: a new vehicle for skincare products. *Adv Colloid Interface Sci* 2004;**108–109**:145–9.
61. Ammar HO, Salama HA, Ghorab M, Mahmoud AA. Nanoemulsion as a potential ophthalmic delivery system for dorzolamide hydrochloride. *AAPS PharmSciTech* 2009;**10**:808–19.
62. Ammar HO, Salama HA, Ghorab M, Mahmoud AA. Development of dorzolamide hydrochloride in situ gel nanoemulsion for ocular delivery development of dorzolamide hydrochloride in situ gel nanoemulsion for ocular delivery. *Drug Dev Ind Pharm* 2010;**36**:1330–9.
63. Ahmed M, Ramadan W, Rambhu D, Shakeel F. Potential of nanoemulsions for intravenous delivery of rifampicin. *Die Pharmazie* 2008;**63**:806–11.
64. Ara C De, et al. Improvement of in vitro efficacy of a novel schistosomicidal drug by incorporation into nanoemulsions. *Int J Pharm* 2007;**337**:307–15.
65. Vyas TK, Shahiwala A, Amiji MM. Improved oral bioavailability and brain transport of saquinavir upon administration in novel nanoemulsion formulations. *Int J Pharm* 2008;**347**:93–101.
66. Zhou H, et al. Preparation and characterization of a lecithin nanoemulsion as a topical delivery system. *Nanoscale Res. Lett.* 2010;**5**:224–30.
67. Tagne J, Kakumanu S, Ortiz D, Shea T, Nicolosi RJ. Articles a nanoemulsion formulation of tamoxifen increases its efficacy in a breast cancer cell line. *Mol Pharm* 2008;**31**:129–30.
68. Tagne J, Kakumanu S, Nicolosi RJ. Articles nanoemulsion preparations of the anticancer drug dacarbazine significantly increase its efficacy in a xenograft mouse melanoma model. *Mol Pharm* 2008;**54**:61–6.
69. Singh KK, Vingkar SK. Formulation , antimalarial activity and biodistribution of oral lipid nanoemulsion of primaquine. *Int J Pharm* 2008;**347**:136–43.
70. Primo FL, et al. Magnetic nanoemulsions as drug delivery system for foscan s: skin permeation and retention in vitro assays for topical application in photodynamic therapy (pdt) of skin cancer. *J Magn Magn Mater* 2007;**311**:354–7.
71. Brusewitz C, Schendler A, Funke A, Wagner T, Lipp R. Novel poloxamer-based nanoemulsions to enhance the intestinal absorption of active compounds. *Int J Pharm* 2007;**329**:173–81.
72. Wu H, Ramachandran C, Weiner ND, Roessler BJ. Topical transport of hydrophilic compounds using water-in-oil nanoemulsions. *Int J Pharm* 2001;**220**:63–75.
73. Eral HB, et al. Governing principles of alginate microparticle synthesis with centrifugal forces. *Langmuir* 2016;**32**:7198–209.
74. Zhang M, et al. Synthesis of oil-laden poly(ethylene glycol) diacrylate hydrogel nanocapsules from double nanoemulsions. *Langmuir* 2017;**33**:6116–26.
75. Malo de Molina P, Zhang M, Bayles AV, Helgeson ME. Oil-in-water-in-oil multinanoemulsions for templating complex nanoparticles. *Nano Lett* 2016;**16**:7325–32.
76. Hsiao LC, Badruddoza AZM, Cheng L-C, Doyle PS. 3D printing of self-assembling thermoresponsive nanoemulsions into hierarchical mesostructured hydrogels. *Soft Matter* 2017;**13**:921–9.

Chapter 22

The role of artificial intelligence in scaling nanomedicine toward broad clinical impact

Jeffrey Khong[1,2,a], Peter Wang[1,2,a], Tiffany RX. Gan[1,2,4], Jiansheng Ng[1,2], Truong Thanh Lan Anh[1,2], Agata Blasiak[1,2], Theodore Kee[1,2] and Dean Ho[1,2,3]

[1]N.1 Institute for Health (N.1), National University of Singapore, Singapore; [2]Department of Biomedical Engineering, NUS Engineering, National University of Singapore, Singapore; [3]Department of Pharmacology, Yong Loo Lin School of Medicine, National University of Singapore, Singapore; [4]Department of Surgery, National University Health System, Singapore

22.1 Introduction

Nanotechnology has been broadly explored to improve everything ranging from drug exposure to reducing drug toxicity.[1–70] Particles based on a broad spectrum of polymers, metals, carbon, and other materials have been used for various preclinical studies to address a range of disease indications including solid and hematologic cancers, infectious diseases, cardiovascular disorders, obesity, ophthalmology, diabetes, and many other clinical challenges.[71–120] The field of nanomedicine has also seen multiple classes of nanoparticles move toward clinical validation studies as well as FDA (Food and Drug Administration) approvals. Notably, in 1995, Doxil (doxorubicin HCl liposome injection) became the first nanoparticle-based drug carrier approved by the FDA. Though originally approved for AIDS-related Kaposi's sarcoma, its use later expanded to the treatment of other disease indications, including ovarian cancer, multiple myeloma, and metastatic breast cancer. As with other nanoparticles seeking FDA approval, Doxil underwent preclinical, clinical, and postmarketing phases in order to validate its efficacy. Preclinical studies applying Doxil to in vivo and human-derived xenograft models were conducted prior to clinical testing. Subsequently, in 1999, a series of Phase II clinical trials were conducted among women with relapsed ovarian cancer and the treatment response rate was later validated in a Phase III trial, which accelerated full FDA approval. Currently, clinical trials using liposomal-based therapy are being widely studied for clinical applications. For example, a clinical study investigated the use of Doxil in combination with Velcade to enhance treatment response rate of 646 multiple myeloma patients (National Clinical Trial (NCT) 00103506). Additionally, an ongoing clinical trial is examining the treatment response of patients with ovarian, fallopian tube, or primary peritoneal cancer when administered Doxil in combination with Atezolizumab and/or Bevacizumab (NCT02839707).

The FDA approval of Doxil has paved the way for the use of other nanoparticles against a variety of other indications. A number of clinical studies are currently cleared for start or underway. For example, a clinical study pertaining to a nanoparticle formulation of amphotericin B is being conducted to examine its efficacy toward mucocutaneous candidiasis (NCT02629419). In the area of pain management, an interventional clinical trial to assess the efficacy of a nanoformulation of lidocaine and prilocaine was recently completed (NCT03441841). A first-in-human study of photothermal therapy to address atherosclerosis was also recently completed (NCT01270139). In the area of orthopedics, periarticular injection of liposomal bupivacaine and unmodified bupivacaine were recently assessed for total knee arthroplasty (NCT02349542). A number of trials are assessing the use of liposomal doxorubicin in combination with other therapies (e.g., paclitaxel, fludarabine) for various oncologic indications (e.g., breast cancer, ovarian cancer, etc., NCT03221881, NCT03335241). Nanocarbons such as diamond nanoparticles have also been explored for oral health applications, where nanodiamond-

a These authors contributed equally to this work.

Nanoparticles for Biomedical Applications. https://doi.org/10.1016/B978-0-12-816662-8.00022-9

embedded gutta percha was used as a postroot canal filler material (NCT02698163).[118] Aside from these studies, nanomedicine-based drug formulations such as Abraxane and Caelyx have also been approved by the FDA for nonsmall cell lung cancer, breast cancer, and pancreatic cancer (Abraxane), as well as advanced breast cancer and ovarian cancer (Caelyx).

Through these trials as well as other studies, nanomedicine has clearly made an impact in the clinic and it is likely to improve treatment outcomes for a number of additional indications.[121–170] Apart from monotherapy, nanotechnology-modified drugs are also expected to impact the design of combination therapy regimens, as demonstrated by some of the aforementioned trials.[171–200] However, as combination therapies with at least one nanoparticle drug continue to be explored, novel methods for regimen design should be considered in order to enhance the chances of trial success while optimizing patient outcomes. Conventional combination therapy, whether nano or nonnano, involves the selection of drugs that address aberrant disease pathways, drug targets of interest, followed by dose finding. Unfortunately, a large pool of drugs is often not interrogated when designing combination regimens, since target/pathway-based drug selection often results in a narrow pool to begin with. High dosages of these drugs are often used and these can lead to substantial patient side effects. If larger pools of drugs could be considered when developing a combination, it is highly likely that better outcomes can be achieved for patients. However, when considering both large pools of drugs and their possible respective dosages, the parameter space can easily become insurmountable to assess based on conventional brute force screening. This critical need can be successfully addressed using emerging artificial intelligence (AI)-based approaches, where both optimal drug and optimal dose identification can be simultaneously solved using platforms that combine experimental validation with analytics. Once these combinations are identified, a patient's evolving response to treatment will often necessitate the need to dynamically dose combination therapy regimens as opposed to fixed-dose drug administration. This is another area that can be uniquely addressed by AI-based platforms.[201–233]

To provide a roadmap toward AI-optimized nanomedicine, this chapter will highlight some recent advances in AI-based combination therapy development coupled with AI-guided dynamic combination therapy dosing. As the field of nanomedicine continues to advance, these AI strategies are expected to play a critical role in realizing patient outcomes that exceed those currently being observed with conventionally designed combination therapy and nanotherapy.

22.2 The role of digital therapeutics

Within the emerging field of integrating AI and therapeutics, digital therapeutics is being explored as an alternate treatment modality, involving digital therapy alone or in combination with drug-based treatments. These digital interventions are already being explored in greater depth for indications such as diabetes, obesity, and cognitive decline, among others.[234–236]

22.2.1 Feedback System Control (FSC)-optimized nanodiamond combination

The primary objective of drug discovery/development mostly revolves around target and combination therapy. Currently, combination therapy, which consists of multidrug regimens, serves as the standard-of-care for cancer treatment. However, the development of combinatorial drugs is usually additively determined, and combinatorial chemotherapy regimens are often determined and administered using maximum tolerated doses. Although the current administration of combination therapy ensures efficiency in cancer killing, it has yet to achieve selectivity in killing cancer cells over healthy cells for durable treatment response. As such, modifying drugs, such as adsorbing them to delivery vehicles, to reduce toxicity and drug resistance has been a primary objective in the field of nanomedicine.

Wang et al. paired nanodiamond (ND) drug delivery platform with Feedback System Control (FSC), an AI-driven platform that systemically optimizes combinatorial drug design.[237] To address the aforementioned challenges, FSC was used to optimize combination nanomedicine drug delivery, and the framework for this process was divided into three stages (Fig. 22.1). Stage 1 began with separately synthesizing doxorubicin (DOX), mitoxantrone (MTX), and bleomycin (BLEO) onto the surface of the NDs to form three distinct ND-drug complexes. Subsequently, Latin hypercube sampling method was used to generate 57 combinations with varying concentrations of ND-DOX, ND-MTX, ND-BLEO, and Paclitaxel (PAC) with varying concentrations. Stage 2 then applied all 57 combinations to three types of breast cancer cell lines (MDA-MB-231, BT20, MCF7) and three other control cell lines (MCF10A, IMR-90, H9C2) in order to determine the safety and efficacy using viability assays. Stage 3 utilized the FSC platform to create phenotypic response surfaces using the correlation between the drugs and their corresponding therapeutic windows, a measure derived from the difference in the viability assays of the cancer and control cell lines indicative of both efficacy and toxicity. FSC was able to determine a global combinatorial regimen for each cancer cell line using the FSC calibrated phenotypic response

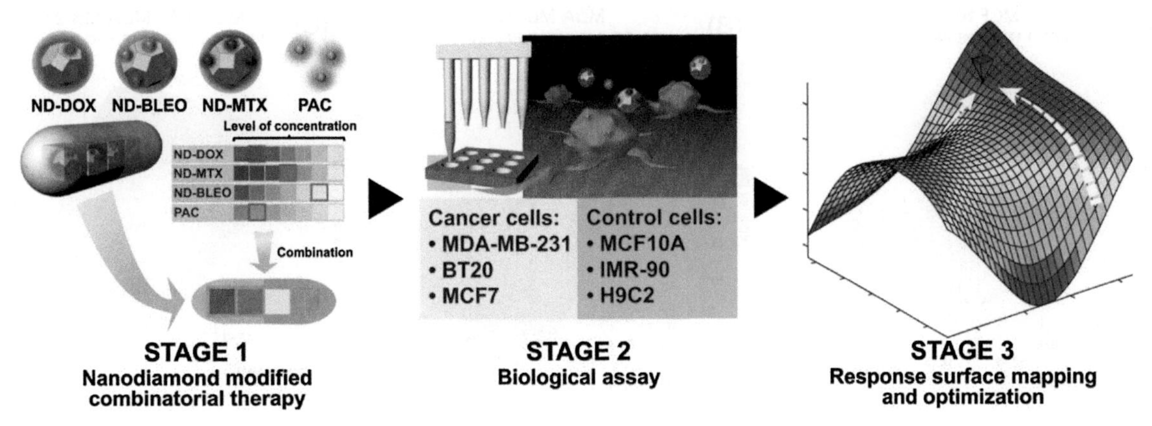

FIGURE 22.1 Schematic of Feedback System Control (FSC) Platform as used in optimizing ND combinations. Stage 1: Doxorubicin (DOX), Mitoxantrone (MTX), and Bleomycin (BLEO) were loaded onto nanodiamonds (NDs), forming ND-DOX, ND-MTX, and MD-BLEO complexes. Latin Hypercube Sampling was used to create 57 diverse combinations of these complexes and Paclitaxel (PAC). Stage 2: 57 combinations of the complexes were applied to three cancer cell lines and three control cell lines in order to determine the cell viabilities via assays. Stage 3: FSC platform correlated the drugs with therapeutic windows, a measure of difference derived from the viability assays of the cancer and control cell lines, to create a response surface that determined the globally optimized combination of the complexes. *Credit: Wang H, Lee D-K, Chen K-Y, et al. Mechanism-independent optimization of combinatorial nanodiamond and unmodified drug delivery using a phenotypically driven platform technology.* ACS Nano *2015;**9**(3):3332–44.*

surfaces (Fig. 22.2). Most importantly, each optimized regimen was verified experimentally ensuring the optimum was accurate.

To determine the effectiveness of FSC-optimized ND combinations, a series of comparisons consisting of unmodified and modified single drugs, optimal unmodified combinations, and a randomly sampled ND-drug combination were analyzed. The therapeutic window for the FSC-optimized ND combination was compared with the therapeutic windows of each single drug and the ND-conjugated single drug complexes. As observed, the FSC-optimized ND combination outperformed all single drugs, both ND-modified and unmodified. Notably, the therapeutic window of the optimal ND combination was 51.50%, which was 21.28% higher than the highest single drug ND-BLEO complex (Fig. 22.3). In addition to comparing the optimized ND combination and the single drugs, the FSC-optimized ND combination was further studied with an unmodified FSC-optimized combination of DOX, MTX, BLEO, and PAC in MDA-MB-231 cancer cell lines using all three control cell lines. The therapeutic window of the FSC-optimized ND combination outperformed that of the unmodified FSC-optimized combination (Fig. 22.4A–C). In order to perform a comparison of the FSC-optimized ND combination and current clinical standards, the average therapeutic window of 57 randomly sampled ND-drug combinations obtained from Latin hypercube sampling was determined. The FSC-optimized ND combination similarly demonstrated a greater average therapeutic index than the randomly sampled ND-drug combinations across all cell lines (Fig. 22.4D). In fact, most of the randomly sampled combinations resulted in negative therapeutic indexes, which would be representative of toxic outcomes if scaled into in vivo and in-human studies.

FSC was able to systematically determine a globally optimized ND combination that achieved high efficacy and low toxicity. In sum, this study highlights the potential of AI-optimized nanomedicine to enhance current standards of combination therapy. FSC may serve as an actionable AI-driven platform that can promptly identify patient-specific combinations for nanotherapy regimens.

22.2.2 Optimizing drug combinations against multiple myeloma using quadratic phenotypic optimization platform

Traditional combinatorial drug treatment can be highly effective in treating a wide variety of indications. However, combination treatment development encounters difficulties when finding effective drug combinations from large drug libraries. Furthermore, on top of finding working drug combinations, doses for each particular drug must be optimized in order for the treatment to be efficacious. To put this into perspective, testing all possible combinations of nine drugs at three possible concentrations each would result in 3^9 or 19,683 possible combinations. Thus, traditional high-throughput screening methods can be time-consuming, expensive, and impractical to find drug combinations for therapy.

The introduction of AI-based combination methods like FSC aims to overcome the challenges encountered by traditional methods like high-throughput screening. Rashid et al. developed the quadratic phenotypic optimization platform (QPOP), an AI computational platform that efficiently and iteratively identifies effective drug combinations and optimizes drug doses and ratios in said combinations.[238] The core technology of QPOP lies in fitting the relationship between inputs (e.g., drugs) and

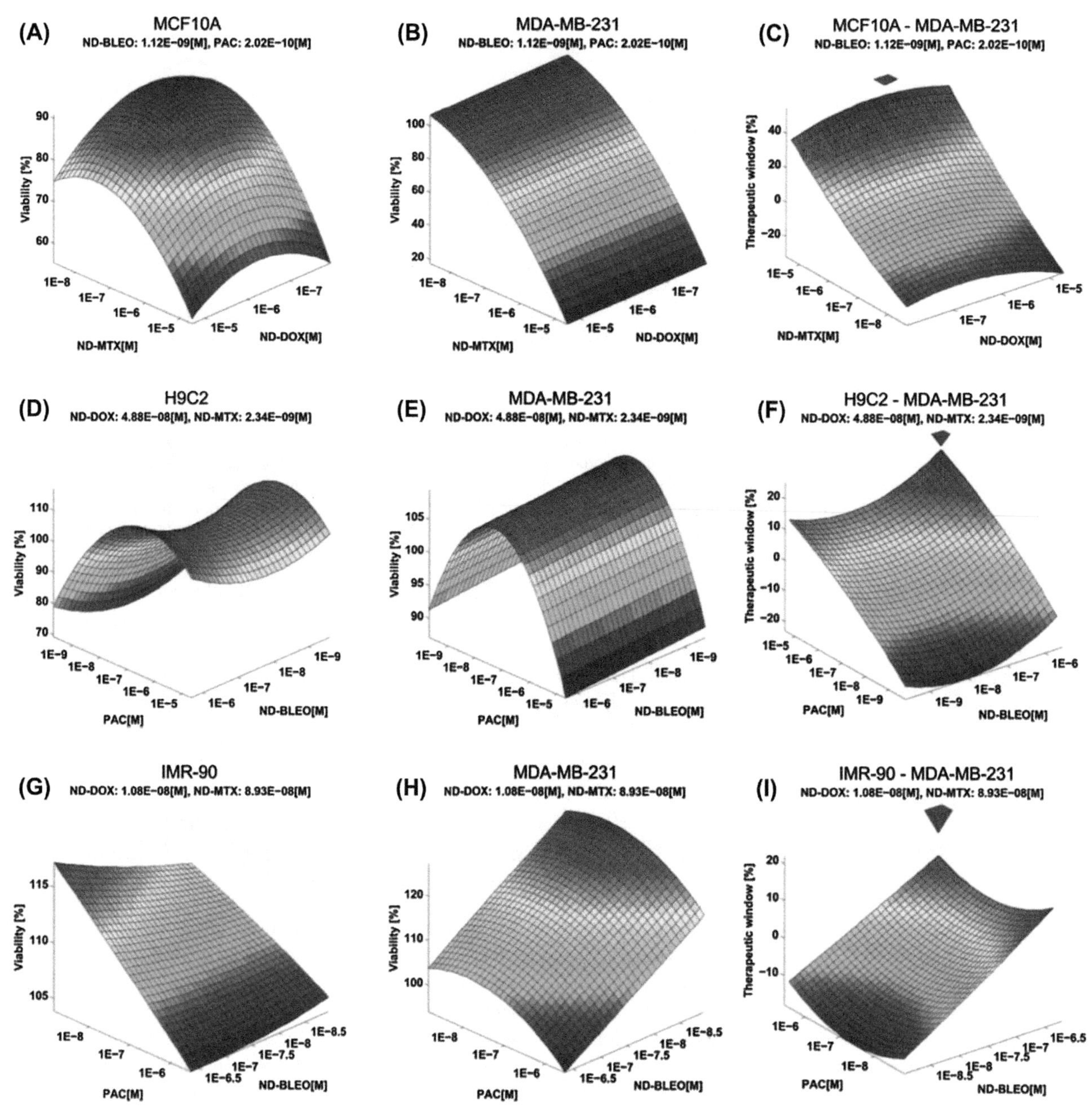

FIGURE 22.2 Using cellular response surfaces of all control cell lines and the MDA-MB-231 cancer cell lines to determine the therapeutic window response surfaces. Cellular response surfaces of (A) control cell lines MCF10A and (B) cancer cell lines MDA-MB-231 with varying combinations of ND-DOX and ND-MTX, while ND-BLEO and PAC were fixed at optimal dosage. (C) Therapeutic window response surface between the control cell lines MCF-10A and cancer cell lines MDA-MB-231 is shown. FSC determined that the optimal therapeutic window (*blue pyramid*) was 47.01%, and it was experimentally verified to be 51.50%. Cellular response surfaces of (D) H9C2 and (E) MDA-MB-231 with varying combinations of ND-BLEO and PAC, while ND-DOX and ND-MTX were fixed at optimal dosage. (F) Therapeutic window response surface between the control cell lines H9C2 and cancer cell lines MDA-MB-231 is shown. FSC determined that the optimal therapeutic window (*blue pyramid*) was 20.71%, and it was experimentally verified to be 21.46%. Cellular response surfaces of (G) IMR-90 and (H) MDA-MB-231 with varying combinations of ND-BLEO and PAC, while ND-DOX and ND-MTX were fixed at optimal dosage. (I) Therapeutic window response surface between the control cell lines IMR-90 and cancer cell lines MDA-MB-231 is shown. FSC determined that the optimal therapeutic window (*blue pyramid*) was 9.53%, and it was experimentally verified to be 15.80%. *Credit: Wang H, Lee D-K, Chen K-Y, et al. Mechanism-independent optimization of combinatorial nanodiamond and unmodified drug delivery using a phenotypically driven platform technology.* ACS Nano *2015;9(3):3332–44.*

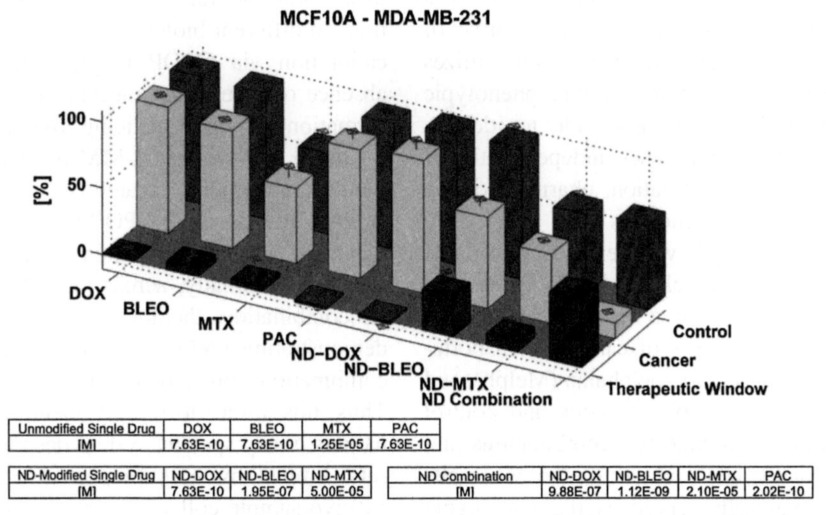

FIGURE 22.3 Comparison of optimal dosing of single drugs, ND-drug complexes, and ND-combination. This comparative study illustrates the therapeutic windows calculated from the difference between the cell viabilities of MCF10A (control) and MDA-MB-231 (cancer) for the drug doses listed in a table under the graph. *Credit: Wang H, Lee D-K, Chen K-Y, et al. Mechanism-independent optimization of combinatorial nanodiamond and unmodified drug delivery using a phenotypically driven platform technology.* ACS Nano *2015;**9**(3):3332–44.*

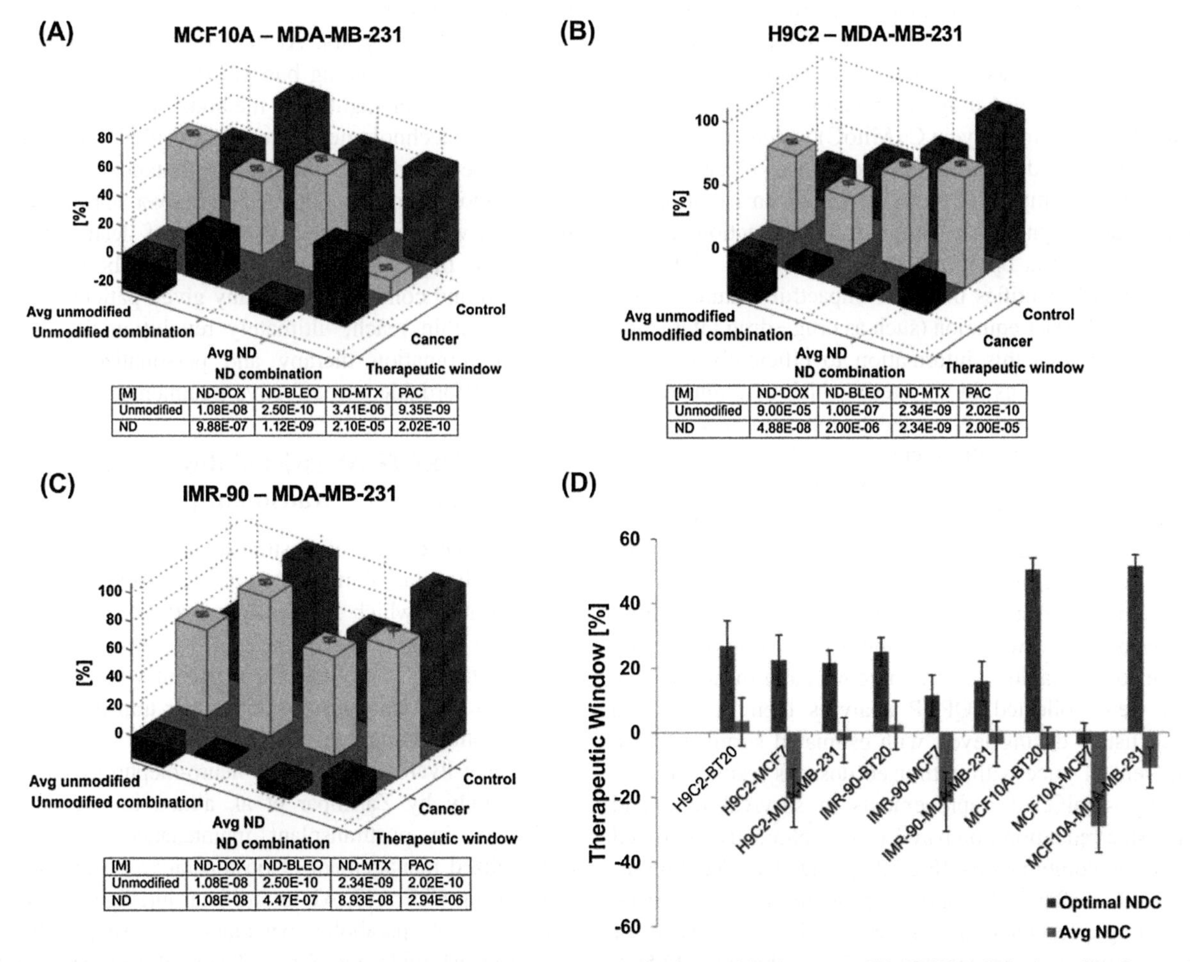

FIGURE 22.4 The comparison of therapeutic windows among FSC-optimized ND combination, unmodified FSC-optimized combination, and the average of randomly sampled ND-drug combinations. Therapeutic windows of optimal ND combination were compared with optimal unmodified combination in cancer cell lines MDA-MB-231 and control cell lines (A) MCF10A, (B) H9C2, and (C) IMR-90. (D) The optimal ND combination was compared with the average of 57 randomly sampled ND-drug combinations obtained via Latin hypercube sampling in three breast cancer cell lines (MDA-MB-231, BT20, and MCF7) and the aforementioned three control cell lines. *Credit: Wang H, Lee D-K, Chen K-Y, et al. Mechanism-independent optimization of combinatorial nanodiamond and unmodified drug delivery using a phenotypically driven platform technology.* ACS Nano *2015;**9**(3):3332–44.*

desired phenotypic outputs (e.g., cell viabilities) to a smooth, second-order quadratic surface representative of the biological system of interest. Because QPOP utilizes only the controllable inputs and measurable phenotypic outputs of the biological system, it is able to identify optimal drug combinations and doses independently of predetermined drug synergy information, pharmacokinetic properties, and patient-specific genomics.

In a recent study, QPOP was employed against bortezomib-resistant multiple myeloma (MM) to identify effective drug combinations from a variety of candidate drugs, including clinical standards of care such as bortezomib (Bort), lenalidomide (Lena), melphalan (Melph), and dexamethasone (Dex).[238] In vitro MM cells and control cells were treated with 128 unique test combinations and the difference between the cell viability of the MM cells compared to the normal cells served as the phenotypic output in QPOP analyses (to find combinations that maximized killing of cancer cells while minimized killing of normal cells). QPOP then fit cell viability differences and their corresponding drug combinations to a second-order quadratic surface, and the nine best drugs were selected based on their number of appearances in top combinations. A second analysis was performed using the nine best drugs, and optimal 2- and 4-drug combinations containing decitabine (Dec) and mitomycin C (MitoC) which are oncology drugs nonstandard for MM were identified. Notably, decitabine and mitomycin C were ineffective in isolation but demonstrated synergistic drug–drug interaction effects when combined at optimized drug–dose ratios.[238] Importantly, QPOP identifies the most impactful features of the fitted second-order equation (such as drug–drug interaction terms), then uses this information to efficiently pinpoint optimal combinations. In vitro tests which determined IC_{50} (concentration of a drug needed to inhibit a specific biological function by 50%) curves of these drugs, both independently and as combinations, further confirmed the performance of QPOP-optimized drug combinations.[238]

QPOP analyses were further performed in an in vivo P100v xenograft model and in ex vivo patient samples to validate in vitro results.[238] In the in vivo test, tumor-bearing mice were treated with combinations consisting of varying dosages of decitabine and mitomycin C, and mean survival times were collected. QPOP analyses then generated a ranked list of dosing levels with estimated survival times. Treatment of mice with optimized dosages resulted in statistically significant improvements in survival time and tumor size reduction compared to two clinically approved three-drug combinations (Fig. 22.5A,D–F). The QPOP-generated surface plot indicated increasing synergistic drug–drug effects and greater survival times as dosages of the two drugs were brought toward 1.5 mg/kg (Fig. 22.5C). Importantly, the surface plots between in vitro and in vivo tests differed, indicating the importance of reoptimization to account for translating previously optimized combinations to different biological systems (Fig. 22.5C).[238] Rapid calibration via QPOP reoptimized combinations in the absence of preexisting mechanism- and synergy-based information, all while reducing toxic effects.

In the ex vivo test, 4 MM patient samples were treated with combinations created from a six-drug library.[238] Across all samples, QPOP-generated quadratic surfaces identified similar synergistic interactions between candidate drugs. Additionally, across the patient samples, responses to combination therapies were distinctly personalized, demonstrating QPOP's ability to identify unique optimal combinations on a patient-by-patient basis (Table 22.1). Thus, this ability to rapidly identify optimal drug combinations in any specific system despite especially small data sets, limited by both pragmatic constraints like cost or ex vivo sample collection, proves the capabilities of AI in drug development. In the context of personalized medicine, where every patient's metadata vastly differs from one another, AI technology can inexpensively identify combinations within days of patient treatment, critical for interventional timelines.

In the coming years, AI developments such as QPOP will assist in overcoming barriers for combination therapy development that traditional methods encounter.[239] Using AI-driven technologies such as QPOP to identify patient-specific drug combinations in tandem with using nanodiamonds and nanotherapy to deliver optimized combinations will further push the limits of desirable patient outcomes. Implementing AI to optimize both drug and nanodiamond combinations in any given patient or system is now within reach; ultimately revolutionizing conventional combination therapy and personalized medicine, creating affordable and effective treatments.

22.2.3 CURATE.AI-assisted dosing for postoperative liver transplant patients

Conventional dosing of posttransplant immunosuppressive drugs, such as tacrolimus, often uses physician-titrated drug administration, which frequently results in deviations from the target trough level ranges.[240] The trough level—the concentration of tacrolimus in a patient's blood draw—is critical to managing postoperative liver transplant patients, as fluctuating trough levels may result in severe adverse events like liver rejections and neuro-/nephrotoxicity.[241] A recent study by Zarrinpar et al. aimed to overcome the challenges in posttransplant maintenance by providing personalized management of postoperative dosing of tacrolimus using CURATE.AI, an artificial intelligence platform comprised of parabolic personalized dosing (PPD).[242] CURATE.AI guides tacrolimus dosing of postoperative liver transplant patients using the measured trough levels of the patient, the primary efficacy measurement for liver

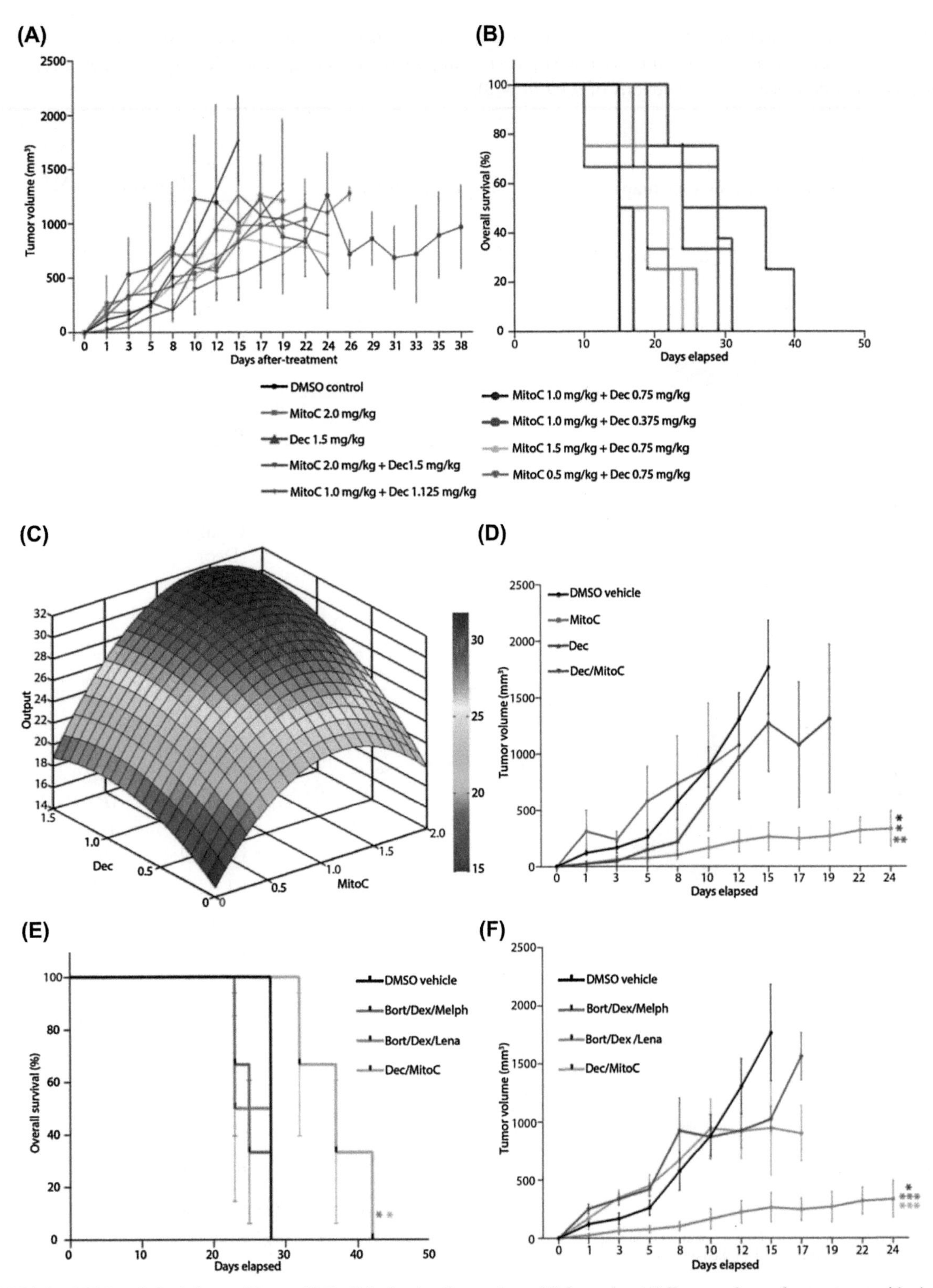

FIGURE 22.5 QPOP-optimized doses of Dec and MitoC for in vivo Bort-resistant MM samples. (A) Tumor volume after treatment with nine unique drug combinations containing varying concentrations of Dec and MitoC ($n = 4$ per group). (B) Drug treatments analyzed using Kaplan–Meier method. (C) QPOP parabolic response surface where efficacy (mean survival time of mice) subtracted by toxicity (mean change in body weight) serves as the phenotypic output. (D) Tumor volume after treatment with optimized concentrations of Dec and MitoC, independently and in combination. (E) Analysis of Dec/MitoC combination treatment versus Bort/Dex/Melph and Bort/Dex/Lena combination treatment using Kaplan–Meier method. (F) Tumor volume after treatment with Dec/MitoC, Bort/Dex/Melph, and Bort/Dex/Lena. *Credit: Rashid MBMA, Toh TB, Hooi L, et al. Optimizing drug combinations against multiple myeloma using a quadratic phenotypic optimization platform (QPOP).* Sci Transl Med *2018;**10**(453):eaan0941.*

TABLE 22.1 Ex vivo parabolic response surfaces of Dec/MitoC. Parabolic response surfaces indicate responsiveness to Dec and MitoC in ex vivo MM patient samples with varying dosing levels. R^2 values, IC_{50} values, and CIs data are shown as means of ±SD ($n = 3$).

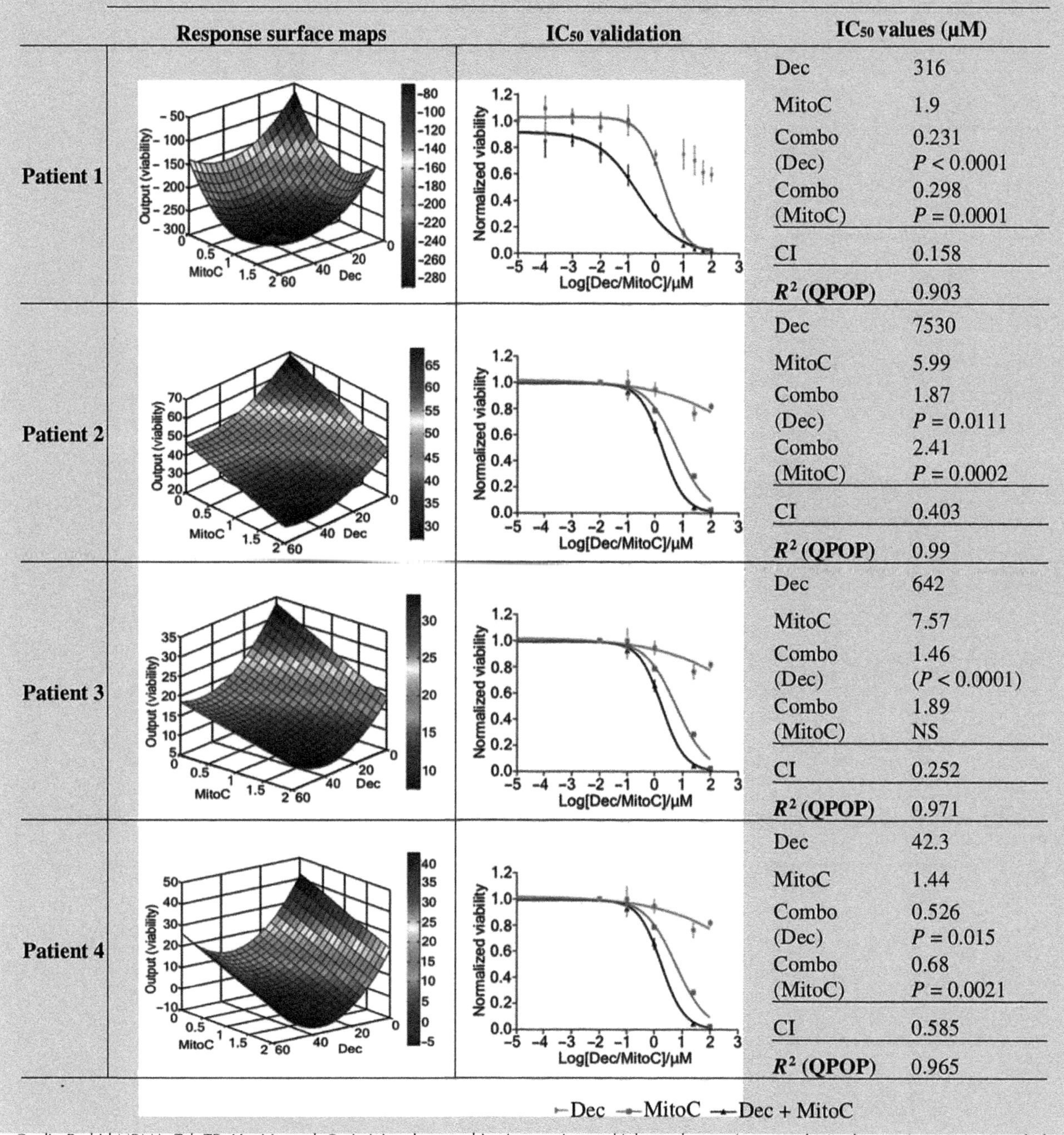

	Response surface maps	IC_{50} validation	IC_{50} values (μM)	
Patient 1			Dec	316
			MitoC	1.9
			Combo (Dec)	0.231 $P < 0.0001$
			Combo (MitoC)	0.298 $P = 0.0001$
			CI	0.158
			R^2 (QPOP)	0.903
Patient 2			Dec	7530
			MitoC	5.99
			Combo (Dec)	1.87 $P = 0.0111$
			Combo (MitoC)	2.41 $P = 0.0002$
			CI	0.403
			R^2 (QPOP)	0.99
Patient 3			Dec	642
			MitoC	7.57
			Combo (Dec)	1.46 ($P < 0.0001$)
			Combo (MitoC)	1.89 NS
			CI	0.252
			R^2 (QPOP)	0.971
Patient 4			Dec	42.3
			MitoC	1.44
			Combo (Dec)	0.526 $P = 0.015$
			Combo (MitoC)	0.68 $P = 0.0021$
			CI	0.585
			R^2 (QPOP)	0.965

Credit: Rashid MBMA, Toh TB, Hooi L, et al. Optimizing drug combinations against multiple myeloma using a quadratic phenotypic optimization platform (QPOP). *Sci Transl Med* 2018;**10**(453):eaan0941.

transplants, to calibrate and determine optimal doses that manage trough levels within target range.

Eight participants of this study were managed using physician-guided dosing for the initial 10 days after transplantation. After this initial period, four patients (PPD1, PPD2, PPD3, PPD4) were managed using CURATE.AI for personalized dynamic dosing management. The remaining four patients (C1, C2, C3, C4) served as control patients and continued physician-guided dosing after the first 10 days. Using clinical data from the physician-guided treatment period, CURATE.AI retrospectively calibrated and personalized the dosing of control patient C1.[242] Retrospectively, CURATE.AI was able to determine tacrolimus doses that corresponded to target trough levels determined by the clinical team and was able to dynamically identify drug doses to bring and maintain patient trough levels within target range, as compared to the conventional physician-guided titrated method of drug dosing.[242]

CURATE.AI-guided patients (PPD1-4) started dynamic personalized dosing after the first 10 days of physician-guided dosing. Using the initial 10 data points, CURATE.AI was able to construct a patient-specific profile for each PPD patient based on a quadratic correlation relationship between varied drug dose and efficacy termed the phenotypic response surface (PRS). Generated patient-specific profiles enabled the identification of tacrolimus doses with corresponding trough levels within the target therapeutic range (Fig. 22.6A,C–E). CURATE.AI constantly recalibrates the treatment inputs as the subject's response evolves during the course of treatment or as regimen changes occur, resulting in robust and sustainable interventional optimization. For example, PPD1 underwent hemodialysis multiple times throughout the treatment, which affected the trough levels and resulted in deviations between measured and CURATE.AI-projected trough levels. To resolve this, the time between hemodialysis sessions and measured blood trough levels were correlated with the deviations between measured and CURATE.AI-projected trough levels (Fig. 22.6B). This correlation allowed CURATE.AI to preemptively adjust tacrolimus dosing to account for deviations resulting from hemodialysis. Another example of CURATE.AI recalibration capability is demonstrated from the correlation of regimen changes and trough level deviations for patients given antibiotic and antifungal drugs (Fig. 22.7). Postoperative transplant patients are commonly administered multiple drugs including antibiotic and antifungal drugs, which are usually tapered during the postoperative maintenance phase. These other medications given prophylactically or as a result of infections often result in trough level deviations.[243] Similar to the hemodialysis-caused deviations, correlation of regimen changes and trough level deviations for patients given antibiotic and antifungal drugs allowed CURATE.AI to identify appropriate tacrolimus doses following a recalibration.

The tapering of prednisone, another critical drug in postoperative drug dosing, was found to similarly cause deviations in trough levels in patients. Despite this, CURATE.AI was able to create patient-specific profiles illustrating the interactions between tacrolimus and prednisone dosing correlated with the respective trough levels (Fig. 22.8). The surfaces indicate the nature of the drug–drug interactions for each patient with a convex surface representing a synergistic effect and concave surface representing an antagonistic effect. These correlations further illustrate the interpatient variability, as each patient responded to tacrolimus and prednisone differently. CURATE.AI recalibration resulted in corrections of tacrolimus doses that better managed patient trough levels. This ability to dynamically recalibrate during times of unstable treatment according to patient-specific responses signifies the power of AI-enabled technologies like CURATE.AI to prospectively guide treatments in real-time.

CURATE.AI-guided dosing of tacrolimus demonstrated a notable improvement in bringing trough levels within target range when compared with physician-guided dosing. Notably, C1 trough levels deviated from target range for 90% of the duration of physician-guided dosing.[242] Physician-guided dosing for control patients resulted in 72.6% of trough levels deviating from target range, and 30.7% of trough levels deviating at least 2 ng/mL. In contrast, CURATE.AI-guided patient trough levels deviated from target range for 54.2% of the entire treatment, with 10.8% of the trough levels deviating at least 2 ng/mL away from the target range. CURATE.AI-dosed patients outperformed physician-dosed patients in various metrics like the number of days that trough levels deviated more than 2 ng/mL away from the target range, and these patients were discharged, on average, nearly a month earlier than the control patients.

In sum, CURATE.AI effectively improved the management of tacrolimus dosing, while causing no adverse events/complications that would require prolonged hospitalization. This study demonstrates the potential of AI technologies like CURATE.AI to effectively improve treatment response rates and patient outcomes, while reducing the cost of care (e.g., hospitalization). Importantly, because each patient received individualized optimized doses and responded differently to certain drug concentrations, the study also evidences the need to address patients on an individualized level. Therefore, with the application of nanoparticles to further improve patient outcomes, AI-based technologies like FSC can be used to optimize nanoparticle combinations on a personalized level. In addition, within treatment regimens, nanodiomond concentrations need to fine-tuned with technologies like CURATE.AI. Overall, CURATE.AI serves as a critical complementary and scalable AI-driven platform when translating and scaling nanomedicine into the clinic, as novel nanomedicine like traditional therapies must be personalized and managed at the patient-specific level.

22.2.4 CURATE.AI-guided dosing of a metastatic prostate cancer patient

CURATE.AI serves as a universal optimization platform that optimizes patient outcomes despite varying contexts and indications. In combination therapy for oncology,

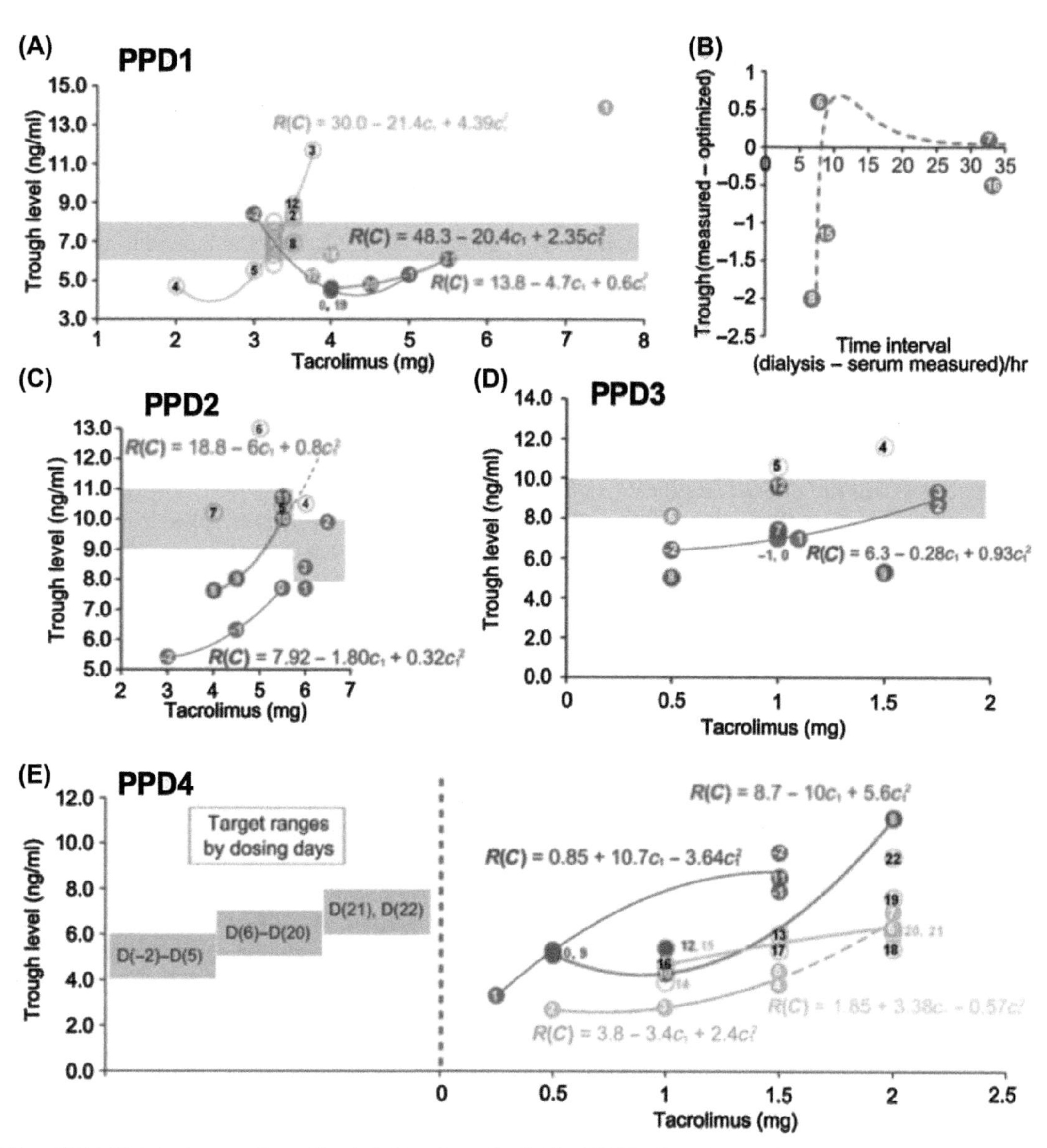

FIGURE 22.6 CURATE.AI patient-specific profiles for PPD patients. (A, C–E) CURATE.AI patient-specific profiles were calibrated based on the first 10 days of physician-guided dosing, and they were used to prospectively dose each PPD patient on the subsequent days. CURATE.AI profiles were recalibrated using trough levels from at least three successive days (dosing days denoted by numbers in circles) if the patient's regimen changed. The target ranges for each PPD patient are highlighted in gray, and the patient-specific CURATE.AI equations are shown. (B) PPD1 had multiple hemodialysis sessions throughout the treatment, and the hemodialysis caused noticeable deviations in CURATE.AI-projected trough levels. A function of trough level deviations and time between hemodialysis and blood draw was created to account for hemodialysis when dosing the patient. *Credit: Zarrinpar A, Lee D-K, Silva A, et al. Individualizing liver transplant immunosuppression using a phenotypic personalized medicine platform.* Sci Transl Med *2016;8(333):333ra49–33ra49.*

finding the optimal dose combination is challenging due to the fact that drug synergy is dose- and time-dependent with intra- and interpatient variability. Furthermore, conventional chemotherapy typically uses dose escalation to reach a maximum tolerated dose (MTD) to find an appropriate combination drug regimen. This approach often results in high toxicity experienced by the patient with various reported adverse events. Nanomedicine has made drastic improvements in treatment outcomes by reducing drug efflux, enhancing sustained drug release, and lowering experienced drug toxicity. Yet, a need for the personalization of nanoparticle-based combination therapy remains. CURATE.AI can address these obstacles via AI-assisted analysis of patient data for each specific patient. In a recent case report, CURATE.AI demonstrated the capability to optimize drug regimen by guiding the dose modulation of a combination therapy in a metastatic castration-resistant prostate cancer (mCRPC) patient.[244]

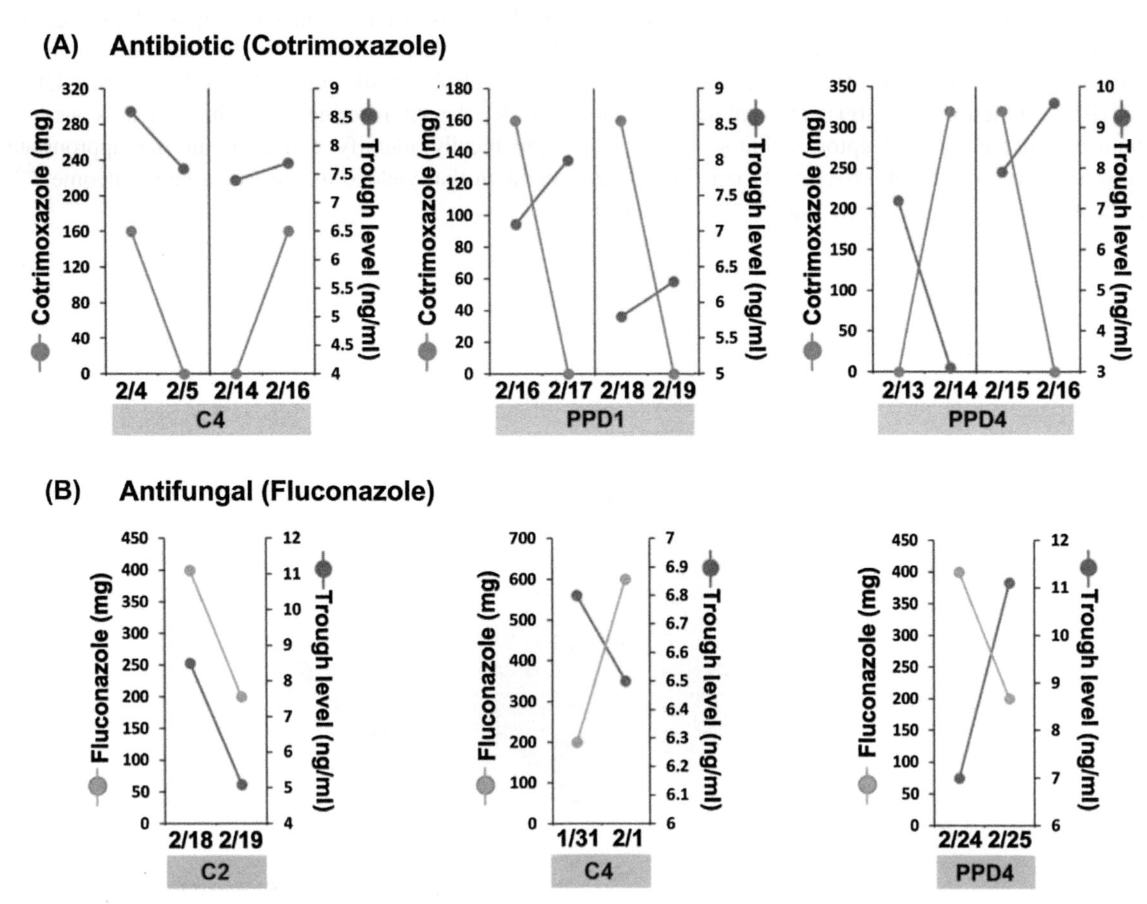

FIGURE 22.7 The correlations between cotrimoxazole/fluconazole doses and patients' trough levels. These patients were given cotrimoxazole and fluconazole during their treatments, and they each posed unique responses to the drugs. CURATE.AI used these correlations to preemptively dose (A) C4, PPD1, and PPD4 who were administered cotrimoxazole and (B) C2, C4, and PPD4 who were administered fluconazole. *Credit: Zarrinpar A, Lee D-K, Silva A, et al. Individualizing liver transplant immunosuppression using a phenotypic personalized medicine platform.* Sci Transl Med *2016;8(333):333ra49–33ra49.*

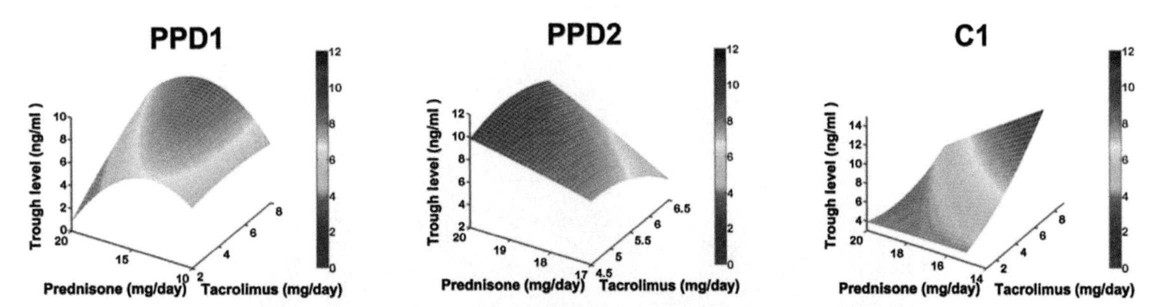

FIGURE 22.8 Tacrolimus-Prednisone interaction plots for PPD1, PPD2, and C1. These interaction plots illustrate the correlation between the drug–drug interactions and trough levels. The behavior of the interaction plots indicates the synergistic or antagonistic (convex or concave) drug–drug interactions. *Credit: Zarrinpar A, Lee D-K, Silva A, et al. Individualizing liver transplant immunosuppression using a phenotypic personalized medicine platform.* Sci Transl Med *2016;8(333):333ra49–33ra49.*

Specifically, CURATE.AI guided the treatment of an 82-year-old male patient participating in a Phase 1B/2A safety and tolerability study of a bromodomain and extra-terminal (BET) inhibitor ZEN-3694, in combination with enzalutamide, an androgen receptor inhibitor, to reduce serum prostate-specific antigen (PSA) levels, corresponding to the treatment of the resistant cancer.[244] The dose modulations from the first 6 months of physician-guided treatment were used to create an individualized CURATE.AI profile (Fig. 22.9A). Using the CURATE.AI profile, the engineering and clinical teams were able to dynamically identify and pinpoint the appropriate drug regimen that yielded the best treatment outcome.[244]

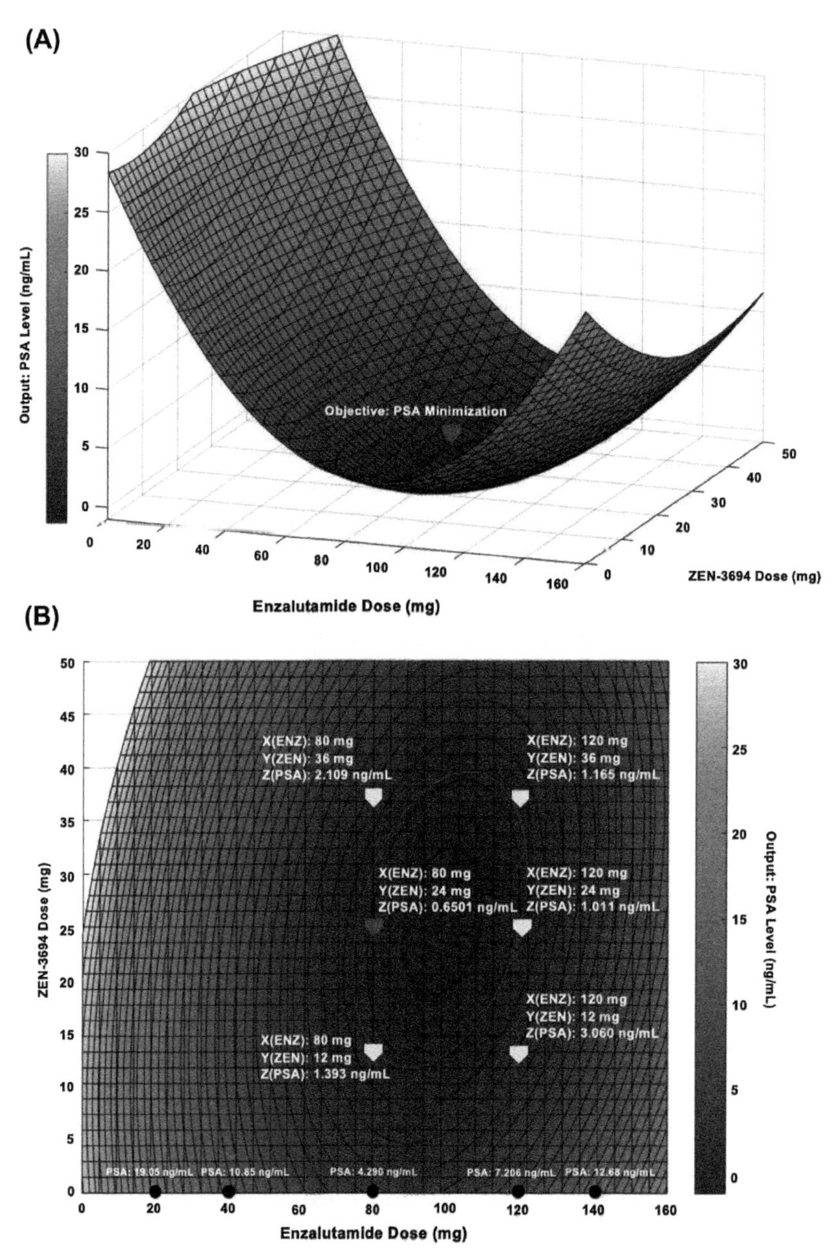

FIGURE 22.9 Patient-specific CURATE.AI profiles. (A) The inputs (Enzalutamide and ZEN-3694 doses) and output (PSA levels) were used to construct the individualized CURATE.AI profile. (B) Using the profile, CURATE.AI recommended 80 mg Enzalutamide and 24 mg ZEN-394 (*red arrow*). The regimens within the red ellipse corresponded to PSA levels <1 ng/mL as predicted by the CURATE.AI profile. *Credit: Pantuck AJ, Lee DK, Kee T, et al. Modulating BET Bromodomain Inhibitor ZEN-3694 and Enzalutamide Combination Dosing in a Metastatic Prostate Cancer Patient Using CURATE. AI, an Artificial Intelligence Platform.* Adv Ther *2018;**1**(6):1800104.*

CURATE.AI immediately identified an optimal dose combination of 80 mg Enzalutamide and 24 mg ZEN-3694 (Fig. 22.9B), which was 50% lower than the patient's originally assigned dose regimen prior to CURATE.-AI-guided dosing. Though decreasing the dosing levels challenged conventional chemotherapy dose escalation, the subsequent PSA for the patient decreased to a desirable 0.86 ng/mL—the first PSA measurement throughout treatment to be below 1.0 ng/mL. The clinical team maintained the regimen at the same doses for 10 weeks as recommended by CURATE.AI. During the period, the patient's PSA levels continuously decreased to 0.68 ng/mL, which was the lowest observed throughout the study. As the patient's reported tolerance and symptoms improved, the clinical team decided to reduce the ZEN-3694 dose from 24 to 12 mg. Prior to the reduction, CURATE.AI determined the reduction would moderately increase the PSA levels to 1.52 ng/mL. The patient was administered 80 mg Enzalutamide and 12 mg ZEN-3694 for 12 weeks, and the PSA level substantially increased to 1.6 ng/mL. After updating the CURATE.AI platform with the patient's new clinical data, CURATE.AI recommended increasing the ZEN-3694 dose to 24 mg. Subsequently, the patient's PSA level decreased to 0.99 ng/mL.

CURATE.AI successfully identified substantial dose reductions, increasing both treatment efficacy and tolerance. The reduction in PSA levels during CURATE.AI-guided treatment was validated by computed tomography (CT) imaging and nuclear medicine bone scan, which showed a sustained decrease in tumor lesion size,

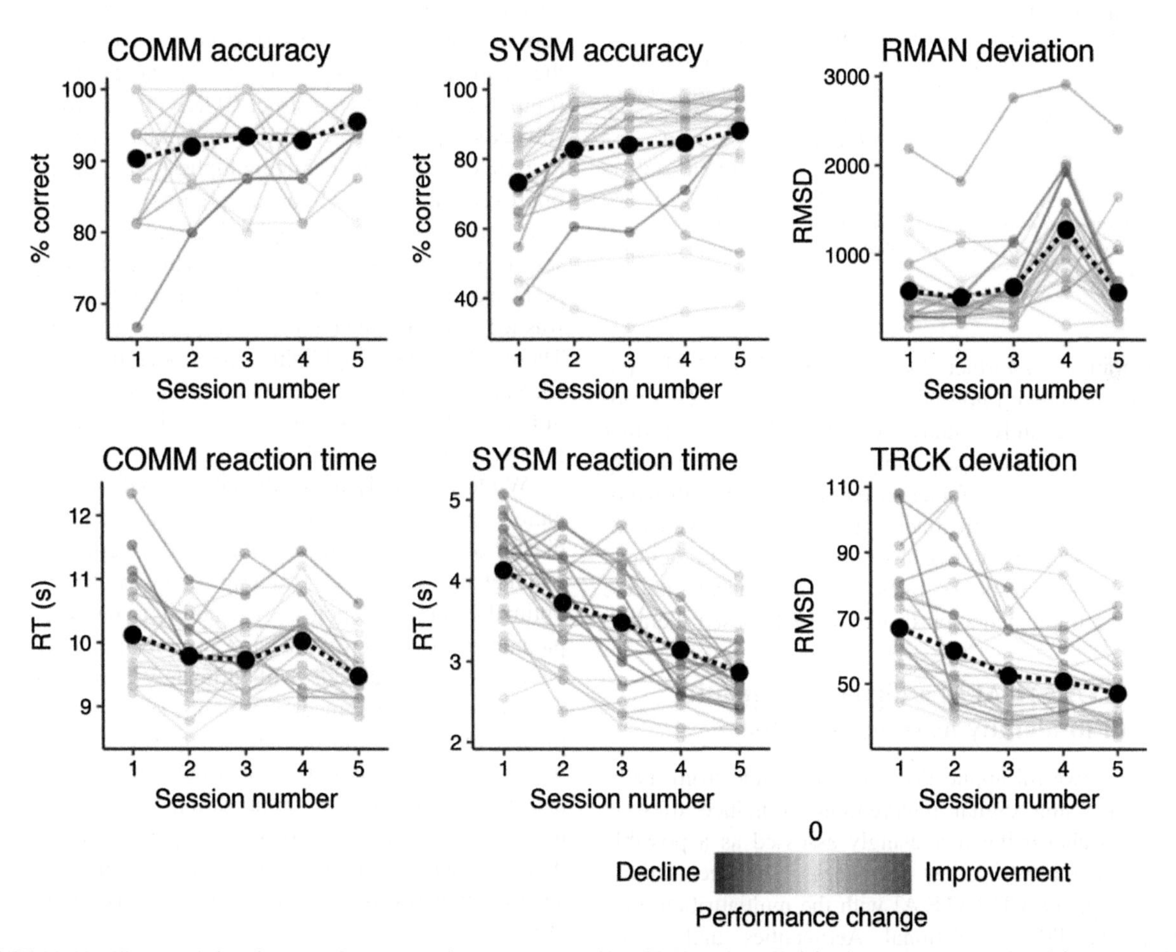

FIGURE 22.10 The recorded performance for each metric across 5 days of MATB-II sessions. Training improvements are plotted for each participant ($n = 28$) and the trend of the lines indicate the rate of change: improvement (*red*), no change (*yellow*), and decline (*blue*). The average performance for each metric is plotted in black. *COMM*, communications task; *RMAN*, resource management task; *SYSM*, system monitoring task; *TRCK*, tracking task. *Credit: Kee T, Weiyan C, Blasiak A, et al. Harnessing CURATE. AI as a Digital Therapeutics Platform by Identifying N-of-1 Learning Trajectory Profiles.* Adv Ther, *1900023.*

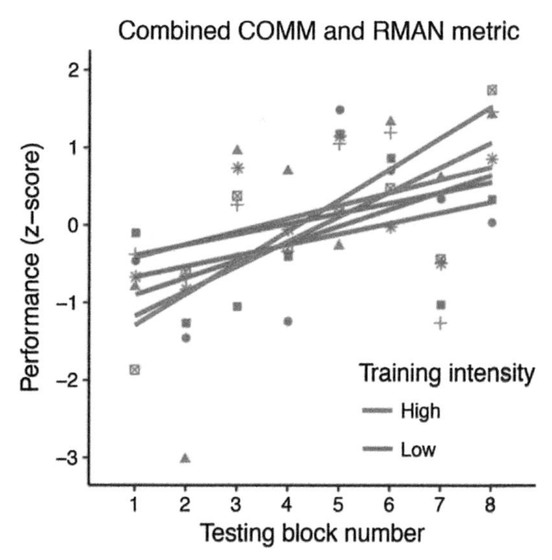

FIGURE 22.11 The effects of single-session alternating testing and training blocks experiment ($n = 6$). All subjects underwent testing blocks of medium intensity alternating with training blocks of low ($n = 3$) or high intensity ($n = 3$). Performance was worse for TRCK task and SYSM reaction time, while all subjects showed significant improvements during a single session for COMM and RMAN tasks. Thus, the performance z-scores were derived from combining COMM and RMAN tasks. The positive trendlines showed this improvement. Intersubject variability was observed despite all subjects undergoing the same event sequence. *Credit: Kee T, Weiyan C, Blasiak A, et al. Harnessing CURATE. AI as a Digital Therapeutics Platform by Identifying N-of-1 Learning Trajectory Profiles.* Adv Ther, *1900023.*

demonstrating no further disease progression.[244] The patient then resumed a normal and active lifestyle. This prospective case-study study of CURATE.AI further demonstrates the success of applying AI to real-time dosing and further supports a future of employing AI with nanomedicine to improve treatment outcomes. AI-driven platforms can scalably personalize nanotherapy to achieve better treatment response rates, and thus accelerate the widespread implementation of nanoparticle-based therapy.

22.2.5 CURATE.AI as a digital therapeutic platform to identify learning trajectory

AI poses powerful applications in fields aside from medicine, and, using digital intervention to induce lifestyle changes is also being increasingly assessed as a possible strategy to improve patient outcomes. In a recent study, Kee et al. paired CURATE.AI with the multiattribute task battery (MATB), a National Aeronautics and Space Administration (NASA) and United States Air Force-developed flight deck operations training software to assess the individualized multitasking capabilities of healthy test subjects in a prospective setting.[245] These tasks included managing fuel tank levels, tracking a target via joystick, adjusting a radio in response to verbal commands, and responding to indicator lights and gauges.

The initial studies showed that individuals performed differently on the MATB even with the same sequences and control settings and some of these interindividual differences have been associated with variation in cognitive abilities or personality traits (Fig. 22.10). Importantly, these differences emerged even though each participant experienced exactly the same event sequence. With regards to training intensity, it was shown that training intensity affects performance with subjects improving even during a single session of training (Fig. 22.11).

When CURATE.AI was implemented, subjects' intensities were varied systematically. Their intensity and current performance levels (inputs) were used to identify the corresponding rate of performance improvement (output) and used to construct CURATE.AI profiles. Each subject's profile revealed important characteristics (e.g., intensity levels mediating highest rate of performance improvement, etc.). Major differences between subjects were observed. For example, high-intensity training in select participants corresponded with greatest gains in performance improvement, while low-intensity training was identified for mediating similar gains in other subjects. These findings highlight the potential utility of CURATE.AI as a tool to guide training intensity at the individual level in order to obtain the highest performance improvement (Fig. 22.12).

While this study is not directly related to drug combination optimization with AI, it serves as an important indicator of the ability for AI to accurately capture the input parameters (e.g., dose, training intensity) that mediate optimal treatment responses. The ability to interrogate large parameter spaces across in vitro and preclinical models as well as clinical subjects will ultimately contribute to the identification of nanomedicine inputs, such as which drugs to add to which type of particles at specific doses, that mediate globally optimum patient outcomes. In addition to broader nanomedicine optimization, AI-driven digital therapy may even be a possible companion treatment modality for nanomedicine regimens for existing indications such as diabetes, obesity, and cognitive disorders, among others.

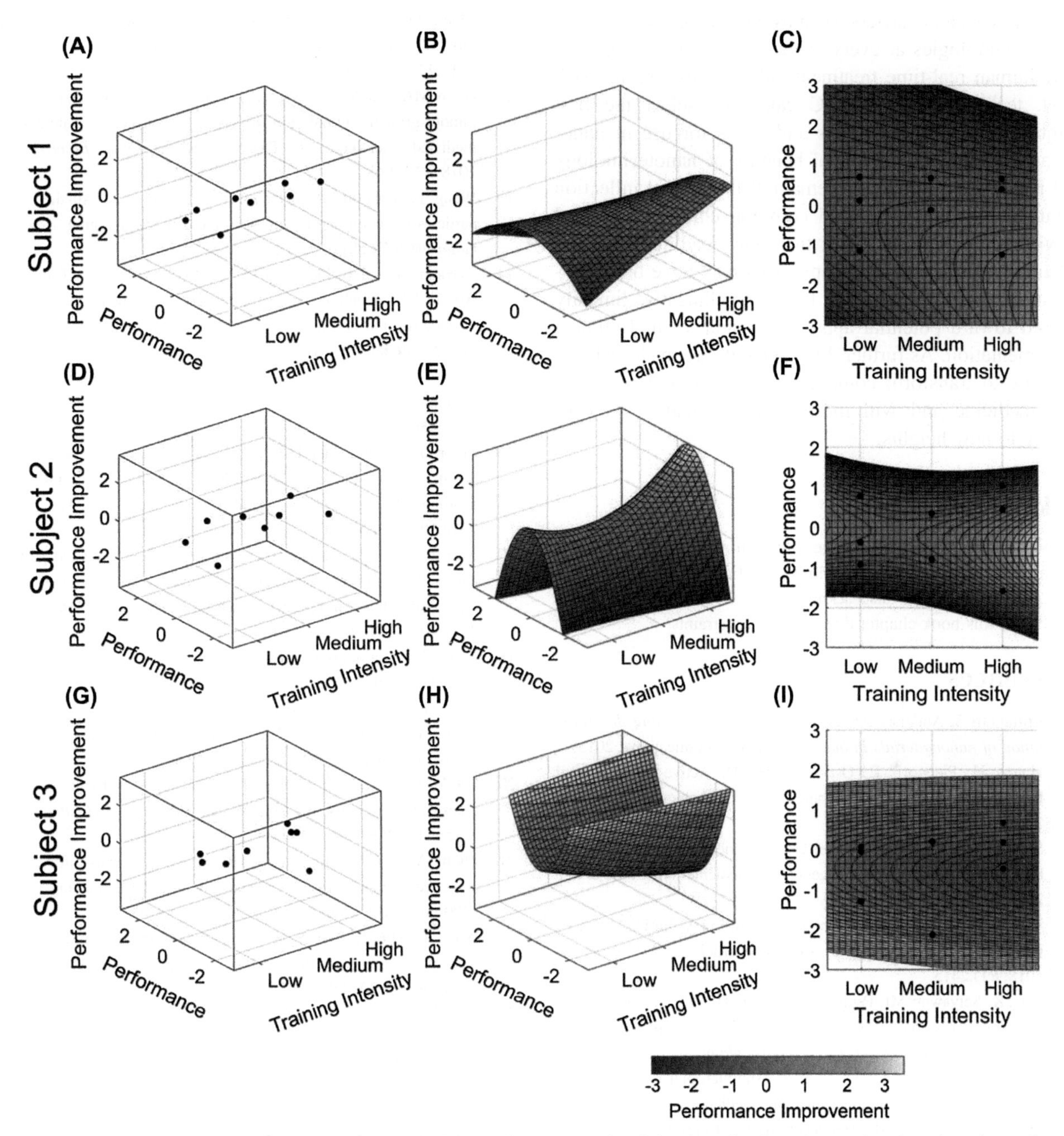

FIGURE 22.12 CURATE.AI profiles for subject 1–3. Prior performance and training intensity (inputs) are plotted against the performance improvement (output) in order to create subject-specific CURATE.AI profiles in 2D and 3D for (A–C) Subject 1, (D–F) Subject 2, and (G–I) Subject 3. Performance improvement is shown in black dots on the 2D CURATE.AI profiles. *Credit: Kee T, Weiyan C, Blasiak A, et al. Harnessing CURATE. AI as a Digital Therapeutics Platform by Identifying N-of-1 Learning Trajectory Profiles.* Adv Ther, *1900023.*

22.3 Conclusions

This chapter serves as a survey of the applications of AI in medicine to optimize patient outcomes. And while these clinically validated technologies are not directly involved with nanotherapy, one can see how these technologies provide a strong foundation for the adaptation of nanomedicine, such as nanodiamonds, into the clinic. Combining nanotherapy and AI is a field to be further explored and yielding promising improvements to personalized medicine. QPOP has demonstrated that AI-assisted identification of the best combination of drugs is necessary to treat any indication. CURATE.AI assists in selecting optimal doses to be given to patients during treatment and provides a pathway of less risky clinical implementation by avoiding the traditional clinical trial design and translation of novel nanotherapies and combinations.

Nanoparticles and carriers, such as NDs, enhance these AI-based technologies at every stage from drug development to in-human real-time treatment; additionally, within each level, technologies like FSC can even select the best combination of nanoparticles and drugs for use in nanotherapy. Despite the potential benefits of nanotechnology and nanotherapy, they still remain at the critical inflection point before widespread and common clinical usage. AI provides unique capabilities that may lead to markedly enhanced ND-mediated therapy. This may have broad implications as NDs continue to be preclinically/clinically studied toward potential approvals/clearances and clinical implementation. As further developments are made, AI will continue to transform combination therapy and personalized medicine and will most definitely scale nanotechnology to new heights.

Acknowledgments

The authors gratefully acknowledge support from National University of Singapore start-up funds, and Ministry of Education (MOE) Tier 1 FRC grant. The authors also acknowledge all studies that were not included in this book chapter due to space constraints.

References

1. Mitragotri S, Anderson DG, Chen X, et al. *Accelerating the translation of nanomaterials in biomedicine*. ACS Publications; 2015.
2. Huang H, Pierstorff E, Osawa E, Ho D. Active nanodiamond hydrogels for chemotherapeutic delivery. *Nano Lett* 2007;**7**(11):3305–14.
3. Serrano MC, Chung EJ, Ameer GA. Advances and applications of biodegradable elastomers in regenerative medicine. *Adv Funct Mater* 2010;**20**(2):192–208.
4. Wen S, Zhou J, Zheng K, Bednarkiewicz A, Liu X, Jin D. Advances in highly doped upconversion nanoparticles. *Nat Commun* 2018;**9**(1):2415.
5. Tee JK, Setyawati MI, Peng F, Leong DT, Ho HK. Angiopoietin-1 accelerates restoration of endothelial cell barrier integrity from nanoparticle-induced leakiness. *Nanotoxicology* 2019:1–19.
6. Karahan HE, Wiraja C, Xu C, et al. Antimicrobial nanomedicine: graphene materials in antimicrobial nanomedicine: current status and future perspectives (Adv. Healthcare Mater. 13/2018). *Adv Healthc Mater* 2018;7(13):1870050.
7. Ho DN. *Applications in biology and nanoscale medicine*, vol. 10. US: Springer; 2010. 978-1.
8. Ho D, Wang P, Kee T. Artificial intelligence in nanomedicine. *Nanoscale Horiz* 2019;**4**(2):365–77.
9. Heo GS, Zhao Y, Sultan D, et al. Assessment of copper nanoclusters for accurate in vivo tumor imaging and potential for translation. *ACS Appl Mater Interfaces* 2019;**11**(22):19669–78.
10. Peters EB, Tsihlis ND, Karver MR, et al. Atheroma niche-responsive nanocarriers for immunotherapeutic delivery. *Adv Healthc Mater* 2019;**8**(3):1801545.
11. Chang SL, Dwyer C, March K, et al. Atomic and electronic structures of functionalized nanodiamond particles. *Microsc Microanal* 2017;**23**(S1):2270–1.
12. Islam MA, Xu Y, Tao W, et al. Author correction: restoration of tumour-growth suppression in vivo via systemic nanoparticle-mediated delivery of PTEN mRNA. *Nat Biomed Eng* 2018;**2**(12):968.
13. Wang Y, Barhoumi A, Tong R, et al. $BaTiO_3$-core Au-shell nanoparticles for photothermal therapy and bimodal imaging. *Acta Biomater* 2018;**72**:287–94.
14. Garraud N, Dhavalikar R, Unni M, Savliwala S, Rinaldi C, Arnold DP. Benchtop magnetic particle relaxometer for detection, characterization and analysis of magnetic nanoparticles. *Phys Med Biol* 2018;**63**(17):175016.
15. Zhou S, Hokugo A, McClendon M, et al. Bioactive peptide amphiphile nanofiber gels enhance burn wound healing. *Burns* 2019;**45**(5):1112–21.
16. Moore L, Yang J, Lan TTH, et al. Biocompatibility assessment of detonation nanodiamond in non-human primates and rats using histological, hematologic, and urine analysis. *ACS Nano* 2016;**10**(8):7385–400.
17. Guo B, Sheng Z, Hu D, et al. Biocompatible conjugated polymer nanoparticles for highly efficient photoacoustic imaging of orthotopic brain tumors in the second near-infrared window. *Mater Horiz* 2017;**4**(6):1151–6.
18. Chung EJ, Sugimoto MJ, Koh JL, Ameer GA. A biodegradable tri-component graft for anterior cruciate ligament reconstruction. *J Tissue Eng Regenerat Med* 2017;**11**(3):704–12.
19. Smith AM, Mancini MC, Nie S. Bioimaging: second window for in vivo imaging. *Nat Nanotechnol* 2009,**4**(11):710.
20. Lee Y, Xu C, Sebastin M, et al. Bioinspired nanoparticulate medical glues for minimally invasive tissue repair. *Adv Healthc Mater* 2015;**4**(16):2587–96.
21. Zhong Y, Ma Z, Zhu S, et al. Boosting the down-shifting luminescence of rare-earth nanocrystals for biological imaging beyond 1500 nm. *Nat Commun* 2017;**8**(1):737.
22. Wan H, Yue J, Zhu S, et al. A bright organic NIR-II nanofluorophore for three-dimensional imaging into biological tissues. *Nat Commun* 2018;**9**(1):1171.
23. Marciel AB, Chung EJ, Brettmann BK, Leon L. Bulk and nanoscale polypeptide based polyelectrolyte complexes. *Adv Colloid Interface Sci* 2017;**239**:187–98.
24. Chow EK-H, Ho D. Cancer nanomedicine: from drug delivery to imaging. *Sci Transl Med* 2013;**5**(216). 216rv4-16rv4.
25. Rejeeth C, Vivek R, NipunBabu V, Sharma A, Ding X, Qian K. Cancer nanomedicine: from PDGF targeted drug delivery. *Med Chem Commun* 2017;**8**(11):2055–9.
26. Bu LL, Rao L, Yu GT, et al. Cancer stem cell-platelet hybrid membrane-coated magnetic nanoparticles for enhanced photothermal therapy of head and neck squamous cell carcinoma. *Adv Funct Mater* 2019;**29**(10):1807733.
27. Geiger BC, Wang S, Padera RF, Grodzinsky AJ, Hammond PT. Cartilage-penetrating nanocarriers improve delivery and efficacy of growth factor treatment of osteoarthritis. *Sci Transl Med* 2018;**10**(469):eaat8800.

28. Nguyen DN, Roth TL, Li J, et al. A Cas9 nanoparticle system with truncated Cas9 target sequences on DNA repair templates enhances genome targeting in diverse human immune cell types. *bioRxiv* 2019:591719.
29. Yen A, Zhang K, Daneshgaran G, Kim H, Ho D. A chemopreventive nanodiamond platform for oral cancer treatment. *J Calif Dent Assoc* 2016;**44**(2):121–7.
30. Loh KP, Ho D, Chiu GNC, Leong DT, Pastorin G, Chow EKH. Clinical applications of carbon nanomaterials in diagnostics and therapy. *Adv Mater* 2018;**30**(47):1802368.
31. Lee D-K, Hsiou D, Kee T, et al. *Combining nanotechnology with personalized and precision MedicineNanodiamonds as therapeutic and imaging agents. Nanomaterials handbook*. CRC Press; 2017. p. 379–90.
32. Ōsawa E, Ho D, Huang H, Korobov MV, Rozhkova NN. Consequences of strong and diverse electrostatic potential fields on the surface of detonation nanodiamond particles. *Diam Relat Mater* 2009;**18**(5–8):904–9.
33. Osumi S, Felder SE, Wang H, Lin YN, Dong M, Wooley KL. Construction of nanostructures in aqueous solution from amphiphilic glucose-derived polycarbonates. *J Polym Sci A Polym Chem* 2019;**57**(3):432–40.
34. Wang P, Su W, Ding X. Control of nanodiamond-doxorubicin drug loading and elution through optimized compositions and release environments. *Diam Relat Mater* 2018;**88**:43–50.
35. Li Q, Barrett DG, Messersmith PB, Holten-Andersen N. Controlling hydrogel mechanics via bio-inspired polymer–nanoparticle bond dynamics. *ACS Nano* 2016;**10**(1):1317–24.
36. Chow EK-H, Pierstorff E, Cheng G, Ho D. Copolymeric nanofilm platform for controlled and localized therapeutic delivery. *ACS Nano* 2007;**2**(1):33–40.
37. Fenton OS, Kauffman KJ, McClellan RL, et al. Customizable lipid nanoparticle materials for the delivery of siRNAs and mRNAs. *Angew Chem* 2018;**130**(41):13770–4.
38. Vaidya B, Parvathaneni V, Kulkarni NS, et al. Cyclodextrin modified erlotinib loaded PLGA nanoparticles for improved therapeutic efficacy against non-small cell lung cancer. *Int J Biol Macromol* 2019;**122**:338–47.
39. Liechty WB, Scheuerle RL, Ramirez JEV, Peppas NA. Cytoplasmic delivery of functional siRNA using pH-responsive nanoscale hydrogels. *Int J Pharm* 2019;**562**:249–57.
40. Wang J, Poon C, Chin D, et al. Design and in vivo characterization of kidney-targeting multimodal micelles for renal drug delivery. *Nano Res* 2018;**11**(10):5584–95.
41. Liu WK, Adnan A, Kopacz AM, et al. Design of nanodiamond based drug delivery patch for cancer therapeutics and imaging applications. In: *Nanodiamonds: applications in biology and nanoscale medicine*. Springer; 2010. p. 249–84.
42. Man HB, Ho D. Diamond as a nanomedical agent for versatile applications in drug delivery, imaging, and sensing. *Physica Status Solidi (a)* 2012;**209**(9):1609–18.
43. Ho D, Zarrinpar A, Chow EK-H. *Diamonds, digital health, and drug development: optimizing combinatorial nanomedicine*. ACS Publications; 2016.
44. Johnson NJ, He S, Diao S, Chan EM, Dai H, Almutairi A. Direct evidence for coupled surface and concentration quenching dynamics in lanthanide-doped nanocrystals. *J Am Chem Soc* 2017;**139**(8):3275–82.
45. Mirkin CA, Letsinger RL, Mucic RC, Storhoff JJ. A DNA-based method for rationally assembling nanoparticles into macroscopic materials. *Nature* 1996;**382**(6592):607.
46. Zeng X, Tao W, Wang Z, et al. Docetaxel-loaded nanoparticles of dendritic amphiphilic block copolymer H40-PLA-b-TPGS for cancer treatment. *Part Part Syst Charact* 2015;**32**(1):112–22.
47. Xu C, Xu K, Gu H, et al. Dopamine as a robust anchor to immobilize functional molecules on the iron oxide shell of magnetic nanoparticles. *J Am Chem Soc* 2004;**126**(32):9938–9.
48. Shi S, Kong N, Feng C, et al. Drug delivery strategies for the treatment of metabolic diseases. *Adv Healthc Mater* 2019:1801655.
49. Lim J-M, Cai T, Mandaric S, et al. Drug loading augmentation in polymeric nanoparticles using a coaxial turbulent jet mixer: yong investigator perspective. *J Colloid Interface Sci* 2019;**538**:45–50.
50. Bahmani B, Uehara M, Ordikhani F, et al. Ectopic high endothelial venules in pancreatic ductal adenocarcinoma: a unique site for targeted delivery. *EBioMedicine* 2018;**38**:79–88.
51. Hoshyar N, Gray S, Han H, Bao G. The effect of nanoparticle size on in vivo pharmacokinetics and cellular interaction. *Nanomedicine* 2016;**11**(6):673–92.
52. Gratton SE, Ropp PA, Pohlhaus PD, et al. The effect of particle design on cellular internalization pathways. *Proc Natl Acad Sci* 2008;**105**(33):11613–8.
53. Ma L, Liu T-W, Wallig MA, et al. Efficient targeting of adipose tissue macrophages in obesity with polysaccharide nanocarriers. *ACS Nano* 2016;**10**(7):6952–62.
54. Creixell M, Bohorquez AC, Torres-Lugo M, Rinaldi C. EGFR-targeted magnetic nanoparticle heaters kill cancer cells without a perceptible temperature rise. *ACS Nano* 2011;**5**(9):7124–9.
55. Ashtari K, Nazari H, Ko H, et al. Electrically conductive nanomaterials for cardiac tissue engineering. *Adv Drug Deliv Rev* 2019;**144**:162–79.
56. Mi Y, Hagan IVCT, Vincent BG, Wang AZ. Emerging nano-/microapproaches for cancer immunotherapy. *Adv Sci* 2019:1801847.
57. Alvarez MM, Aizenberg J, Analoui M, et al. *Emerging trends in micro-and nanoscale technologies in medicine: from basic discoveries to translation*. ACS Publications; 2017.
58. Khan OF, Kowalski PS, Doloff JC, et al. Endothelial siRNA delivery in nonhuman primates using ionizable low–molecular weight polymeric nanoparticles. *Sci Adv* 2018;**4**(6):eaar8409.
59. Mayle KM, Dern KR, Wong VK, et al. Engineering A11 minibody-conjugated, polypeptide-based gold nanoshells for prostate stem cell antigen (PSCA)–Targeted photothermal therapy. *SLAS Technol: Trans Life Sci Innovation* 2017;**22**(1):26–35.
60. Masehi-Lano JJ, Chung EJ. Engineering citric acid-based porous scaffolds for bone regeneration. In: *Biomaterials for tissue engineering*. Springer; 2018. p. 1–10.
61. Man HB, Zhang K, Robinson E, Chow EK, Ho D. Engineering nanoparticulate diamond for applications in nanomedicine and biology. In: *Ultananocrystalline diamond*. Elsevier; 2012. p. 493–518.
62. Tabandeh S, Leon L. Engineering peptide-based polyelectrolyte complexes with increased hydrophobicity. *Molecules* 2019;**24**(5):868.
63. Padmakumar S, Parayath NN, Nair SV, Menon D, Amiji MM. Enhanced anti-tumor efficacy and safety with metronomic

intraperitoneal chemotherapy for metastatic ovarian cancer using biodegradable nanotextile implants. *J Controlled Release* 2019;**305**:29–40.

64. Goh WJ, Zou S, Lee CK, et al. EXOPLEXs: chimeric drug delivery platform from the fusion of cell-derived nanovesicles and liposomes. *Biomacromolecules* 2017;**19**(1):22–30.
65. Dong M, Wessels MG, Lee JY, et al. Experiments and simulations of complex sugar-based Coil–brush block polymer nanoassemblies in aqueous solution. *ACS Nano* 2019;**13**(5):5147–62.
66. Yamankurt G, Berns EJ, Xue A, et al. Exploration of the nanomedicine-design space with high-throughput screening and machine learning. *Nat Biomed Eng* 2019;**1**.
67. Fuller EG, Sun H, Dhavalikar RD, et al. Externally triggered heat and drug release from magnetically controlled nanocarriers. *ACS Appl Polym Mater* 2019;**1**(2):211–20.
68. Karp JM, Peer D. Focus on RNA interference: from nanoformulations to in vivo delivery. *Nanotechnology* 2018;**29**(1): 010201.
69. Yoo SP, Pineda F, Barrett JC, Poon C, Tirrell M, Chung EJ. Gadolinium-functionalized peptide amphiphile micelles for multimodal imaging of atherosclerotic lesions. *ACS Omega* 2016;**1**(5):996–1003.
70. Patel AK, Kaczmarek JC, Bose S, et al. Gene delivery: inhaled nanoformulated mRNA polyplexes for protein production in lung epithelium (Adv. Mater. 8/2019). *Adv Mater* 2019;**31**(8):1970053.
71. Han S, Samanta A, Xie X, et al. Gold and hairpin DNA functionalization of upconversion nanocrystals for imaging and in vivo drug delivery. *Adv Mater* 2017;**29**(18):1700244.
72. Setyawati MI, Tay CY, Bay BH, Leong DT. Gold nanoparticles induced endothelial leakiness depends on particle size and endothelial cell origin. *ACS Nano* 2017;**11**(5):5020–30.
73. Wang M, Wiraja C, Wee M, Yeo D, Hu L, Xu C. Hairpin-structured probe conjugated nano-graphene oxide for the cellular detection of connective tissue growth factor mRNA. *Anal Chim Acta* 2018;**1038**:140–7.
74. Bahou C, Richards DA, Maruani A, et al. Highly homogeneous antibody modification through optimisation of the synthesis and conjugation of functionalised dibromopyridazinediones. *Org Biomol Chem* 2018;**16**(8):1359–66.
75. Au KM, Balhorn R, Balhorn MC, Park SI, Wang AZ. High-performance concurrent chemo-immuno-radiotherapy for the treatment of hematologic cancer through selective high-affinity ligand antibody mimic-functionalized doxorubicin-encapsulated nanoparticles. *ACS Cent Sci* 2018;**5**(1):122–44.
76. Poon C, Gallo J, Joo J, Chang T, Bañobre-López M, Chung EJ. Hybrid, metal oxide-peptide amphiphile micelles for molecular magnetic resonance imaging of atherosclerosis. *J Nanobiotechnol* 2018;**16**(1):92.
77. Liu J, Wang S, Cai X, Zhou S, Liu B. Hydrogen peroxide degradable conjugated polymer nanoparticles for fluorescence and photoacoustic bimodal imaging. *Chem Commun* 2018;**54**(20):2518–21.
78. Kokubun K, Matsumura S, Yudasaka M, Iijima S, Shiba K. Immobilization of a carbon nanomaterial-based localized drug-release system using a bispecific material-binding peptide. *Int J Nanomed* 2018;**13**:1643.
79. Pusuluri A, Wu D, Mitragotri S. Immunological consequences of chemotherapy: single drugs, combination therapies and nanoparticle-based treatments. *J Controlled Release* 2019;**305**:130–54.
80. Pentecost A, Kim MJ, Jeon S, et al. Immunomodulatory nanodiamond aggregate-based platform for the treatment of rheumatoid arthritis. *Regener Biomater* 2019;**6**(3):163–74.
81. Chew SW, Zeng Y, Cui M, et al. In situ generation of zinc oxide nanobushes on microneedles as antibacterial coating. *SLAS Technol: Trans Life Sci Innovation* 2018;**24**(2). 2472630318812350.
82. Lance KD, Bernards DA, Ciaccio NA, et al. In vivo and in vitro sustained release of ranibizumab from a nanoporous thin-film device. *Drug Deliv Transl Res* 2016;**6**(6):771–80.
83. Urbano L, Clifton L, Ku HK, et al. Influence of the surfactant structure on photoluminescent π-conjugated polymer nanoparticles: interfacial properties and protein binding. *Langmuir* 2018;**34**(21):6125–37.
84. Patel AK, Kaczmarek JC, Bose S, et al. Inhaled nanoformulated mRNA polyplexes for protein production in lung epithelium. *Adv Mater* 2019;**31**(8):1805116.
85. Neburkova J, Sedlak F, Zackova Suchanova J, et al. Inhibitor–gcpii interaction: selective and robust system for targeting cancer cells with structurally diverse nanoparticles. *Mol Pharm* 2018;**15**(8):2932–45.
86. Ramos DM, Abdulmalik S, Arul MR, et al. Insulin immobilized PCL-cellulose acetate micro-nanostructured fibrous scaffolds for tendon tissue engineering. *Polym Adv Technol* 2019;**30**(5):1205–15.
87. Wang Y, Liu C-H, Ji T, et al. Intravenous treatment of choroidal neovascularization by photo-targeted nanoparticles. *Nat Commun* 2019;**10**(1):804.
88. Culver HR, Wechsler ME, Peppas NA. Label-free detection of tear biomarkers using hydrogel-coated gold nanoshells in a localized surface plasmon resonance-based biosensor. *ACS Nano* 2018;**12**(9):9342–54.
89. Mensah LB, Morton SW, Li J, et al. Layer-by-layer nanoparticles for novel delivery of cisplatin and PARP inhibitors for platinum-based drug resistance therapy in ovarian cancer. *Bioeng Transl Med* 2019;**4**(2): e10131.
90. Li W, Szoka FC. Lipid-based nanoparticles for nucleic acid delivery. *Pharm Res* 2007;**24**(3):438–49.
91. Chiu GN, Wong M-Y, Ling L-U, et al. Lipid-based nanoparticulate systems for the delivery of anti-cancer drug cocktails: implications on pharmacokinetics and drug toxicities. *Curr Drug Metabol* 2009;**10**(8):861–74.
92. Liu Y, Ng Y, Toh MR, Chiu GN. Lipid-dendrimer hybrid nanosystem as a novel delivery system for paclitaxel to treat ovarian cancer. *J Controlled Release* 2015;**220**:438–46.
93. Vavra J, Rehor I, Rendler T, et al. Long-term imaging: supported lipid bilayers on fluorescent nanodiamonds: a structurally defined and versatile coating for bioapplications (Adv. Funct. Mater. 45/ 2018. *Adv Funct Mater* 2018;**28**(45):1870319.
94. Say JM, van Vreden C, Reilly DJ, Brown LJ, Rabeau JR, King NJ. Luminescent nanodiamonds for biomedical applications. *Biophys Rev* 2011;**3**(4):171–84.
95. Luo Y-L, Xu C-F, Li H-J, et al. Macrophage-specific in vivo gene editing using cationic lipid-assisted polymeric nanoparticles. *ACS Nano* 2018;**12**(2):994–1005.
96. Tong S, Zhu H, Bao G. Magnetic iron oxide nanoparticles for disease detection and therapy. *Mater Today* 2019.
97. Pallares RM, Choo P, Cole LE, Mirkin CA, Lee A, Odom TW. Manipulating immune activation of macrophages by tuning the

oligonucleotide composition of gold nanoparticles. *Bioconjug Chem* 2019;**30**(7):2032–7.
98. Kadakia E, Bottino D, Amiji M. Mathematical modeling and simulation to investigate the CNS transport characteristics of nanoemulsion-based drug delivery following intranasal administration. *Pharm Res* 2019;**36**(5):75.
99. Costa DF, Torchilin VP. Micelle-like nanoparticles as siRNA and miRNA carriers for cancer therapy. *Biomed Microdevices* 2018;**20**(3):59.
100. Jarvis M, Arnold M, Ott J, Pant K, Prabhakarpandian B, Mitragotri S. Microfluidic co-culture devices to assess penetration of nanoparticles into cancer cell mass. *Bioeng Transl Med* 2017;**2**(3):268–77.
101. Wang Z, Guo B, Middha E, et al. Microfluidics prepared uniform conjugated polymer nanoparticles for photo-triggered immune microenvironment modulation and cancer therapy. *ACS Appl Mater Interfaces* 2019;**11**(12):11167–76.
102. Bari S, Chu PPY, Lim A, et al. Mitochondrial superoxide reduction and cytokine secretion skewing by carbon nanotube scaffolds enhance ex vivo expansion of human cord blood hematopoietic progenitors. *Nanomed Nanotechnol Biol Med* 2015;**11**(7):1643–56.
103. DiStasio N, Lehoux S, Khademhosseini A, Tabrizian M. The multifaceted uses and therapeutic advantages of nanoparticles for atherosclerosis research. *Materials* 2018;**11**(5):754.
104. Adjei IM, Yang H, Plumton G, et al. Multifunctional nanoparticles for intracellular drug delivery and photoacoustic imaging of mesenchymal stem cells. *Drug Deliv Transl Res* 2019;**9**:1–15.
105. Zhang XQ, Lam R, Xu X, Chow EK, Kim HJ, Ho D. Multimodal nanodiamond drug delivery carriers for selective targeting, imaging, and enhanced chemotherapeutic efficacy. *Adv Mater* 2011;**23**(41):4770–5.
106. Low WC, Rujitanaroj PO, Lee DK, et al. Mussel-Inspired modification of nanofibers for REST siRNA delivery: understanding the effects of gene-silencing and substrate topography on human mesenchymal stem cell neuronal commitment. *Macromol Biosci* 2015;**15**(10):1457–68.
107. Lee H, Dellatore SM, Miller WM, Messersmith PB. Mussel-inspired surface chemistry for multifunctional coatings. *Science* 2007;**318**(5849):426–30.
108. Tao W, Wang J, Parak WJ, Farokhzad OC, Shi J. Nanobuffering of pH-responsive polymers: a known but sometimes overlooked phenomenon and its biological applications. *ACS Nano* 2019;**13**(5):4876–82.
109. Peer D, Karp JM, Hong S, Farokhzad OC, Margalit R, Langer R. Nanocarriers as an emerging platform for cancer therapy. *Nat Nanotechnol* 2007;**2**(12):751.
110. Brown KA, Hedrick JL, Eichelsdoerfer DJ, Mirkin CA. Nanocombinatorics with cantilever-free scanning probe arrays. *ACS Nano* 2018;**13**(1):8–17.
111. Osawa E, Ho D. Nanodiamond and its application to drug delivery. *J Med Allied Sci* 2012;**2**(2):31.
112. Houshyar S, Padhye R, Shanks R, Nayak R. Nanodiamond fabrication of superhydrophilic wool fabrics. *Langmuir,* 2019;**35**(22):7105–11.
113. Chow EK, Zhang X-Q, Chen M, et al. Nanodiamond therapeutic delivery agents mediate enhanced chemoresistant tumor treatment. *Sci Transl Med* 2011;**3**(73). 73ra21–73ra21.
114. Ho D. Nanodiamond-based chemotherapy and imaging. In: *Nanotechnology-based precision tools for the detection and treatment of cancer*. Springer; 2015. p. 85–102.
115. Gu M, Wang X, Toh TB, Hooi L, Tenen DG, Chow EKH. Nanodiamond-based platform for intracellular-specific delivery of therapeutic peptides against hepatocellular carcinoma. *Adv Therap* 2018;**1**(8):1800110.
116. Lam R, Chen M, Pierstorff E, Huang H, Osawa E, Ho D. Nanodiamond-embedded microfilm devices for localized chemotherapeutic elution. *ACS Nano* 2008;**2**(10):2095–102.
117. Waddington DE, Sarracanie M, Zhang H, et al. Nanodiamond-enhanced MRI via in situ hyperpolarization. *Nat Commun* 2017;**8**:15118.
118. Lee D-K, Kim SV, Limansubroto AN, et al. Nanodiamond–gutta percha composite biomaterials for root canal therapy. *ACS Nano* 2015;**9**(11):11490–501.
119. Hou W, Toh TB, Abdullah LN, et al. Nanodiamond–Manganese dual mode MRI contrast agents for enhanced liver tumor detection. *Nanomed Nanotechnol Biol Med* 2017;**13**(3):783–93.
120. Huang H, Pierstorff E, Liu K, Ōsawa E, Ho D. Nanodiamond-mediated delivery of therapeutics via particle and thin film architectures. In: *Nanodiamonds: applications in biology and nanoscale medicine*. Springer; 2010. p. 151–74.
121. Chen M, Pierstorff ED, Lam R, et al. Nanodiamond-mediated delivery of water-insoluble therapeutics. *ACS Nano* 2009;**3**(7):2016–22.
122. Toh T-B, Lee D-K, Hou W, et al. Nanodiamond–mitoxantrone complexes enhance drug retention in chemoresistant breast cancer cells. *Mol Pharm* 2014;**11**(8):2683–91.
123. Man HB, Ho D. Nanodiamonds as platforms for biology and medicine. *J Lab Autom* 2013;**18**(1):12–8.
124. HO D. Nanodiamonds for drug delivery and diagnostics. *Nanodiamond* 2014:151.
125. Ho D, Wang C-HK, Chow EK-H. Nanodiamonds: the intersection of nanotechnology, drug development, and personalized medicine. *Sci Adv* 2015;**1**(7):e1500439.
126. Nuhn H, Blanco CE, Desai TA. Nanoengineered stent surface to reduce in-stent restenosis in vivo. *ACS Appl Mater Interfaces* 2017;**9**(23):19677–86.
127. Saveh-Shemshaki N, Nair LS, Laurencin CT. Nanofiber-based matrices for rotator cuff regenerative engineering. *Acta Biomater,* 2019;**94**:64–81.
128. Bisso PW, Gaglione S, Guimarães PP, Mitchell MJ, Langer R. Nanomaterial interactions with human neutrophils. *ACS Biomater Sci Eng* 2018;**4**(12):4255–65.
129. Ong V, Mei V, Cao L, Lee K, Chung EJ. Nanomedicine for cystic fibrosis. *SLAS Technol: Trans Life Sci Innovation* 2019;**24**(2):169–80.
130. Tsai N, Lee B, Kim A, et al. Nanomedicine for global health. *J Lab Autom* 2014;**19**(6):511–6.
131. Gao J, Li W, Guo Y, Feng S-S. Nanomedicine strategies for sustained, controlled and targeted treatment of cancer stem cells. *Nanomedicine* 2016;**11**(24):3261–82.
132. Leong DT, Bay BH. Nanomedicine's multi-pronged approach in tackling cancer. *Curr Med Chem* 2018;**25**(12):1377.
133. Metz SW, Thomas A, Brackbill A, et al. Nanoparticle delivery of ad subunit vaccine induces balanced, type-specific neutralizing

antibodies to each dengue virus serotype. *PLoS Negl Trop Dis* 2018;**12**(9). e0006793–e93.

134. Chung EJ. Nanoparticle strategies for biomedical applications: reviews from the University of Southern California Viterbi School of Engineering, 2019.
135. Nam J-M, Thaxton CS, Mirkin CA. Nanoparticle-based bio-bar codes for the ultrasensitive detection of proteins. *Science* 2003;**301**(5641):1884–6.
136. Wu C, Leon L, Chung EJ, Tirrell M, Fang Y. Nanoparticle-mediated targeting of endothelial mir92a-PPAP2B signaling Axis in atherosclerosis. *Circulation* 2015;**132**(Suppl. 1_3). A16526–A26.
137. Ma L, Kohli M, Smith A. Nanoparticles for combination drug therapy. *ACS Nano* 2013;**7**(11):9518–25.
138. Simon-Yarza T, Mielcarek A, Couvreur P, Serre C. Nanoparticles of metal-organic frameworks: on the road to in vivo efficacy in biomedicine. *Adv Mater* 2018;**30**(37):1707365.
139. Wang X, Wang J, Feng S, et al. Nano-porous silica aerogels as promising biomaterials for oral drug delivery of paclitaxel. *J Biomed Nanotechnol* 2019;**15**(7):1532–45.
140. Weldon C, Ji T, Nguyen M-T, et al. Nanoscale bupivacaine formulations to enhance the duration and safety of intravenous regional anesthesia. *ACS Nano* 2018;**13**(1):18–25.
141. Rosi NL, Mirkin CA. Nanostructures in biodiagnostics. *Chem Rev* 2005;**105**(4):1547–62.
142. Muthu MS, Mei L, Feng S-S. Nanotheranostics: advanced nanomedicine for the integration of diagnosis and therapy. *Nanomedicine* 2014;**9**(9):1277–80.
143. Chen S, Weitemier AZ, Zeng X, et al. Near-infrared deep brain stimulation via upconversion nanoparticle–mediated optogenetics. *Science* 2018;**359**(6376):679–84.
144. Reineck P, Trindade LF, Havlik J, et al. Not all fluorescent nanodiamonds are created equal: a comparative study. *Part Part Syst Charact* 2019;**36**(3):1900009.
145. Wu W, Mao D, Cai X, et al. ONOO–and ClO–responsive organic nanoparticles for specific in vivo image-guided photodynamic bacterial ablation. *Chem Mater* 2018;**30**(11):3867–73.
146. Pichot V, Muller O, Seve A, Yvon A, Merlat L, Spitzer D. Optical properties of functionalized nanodiamonds. *Sci Rep* 2017;**7**(1):14086.
147. Choe S, Kalmanek E, Bond C, et al. Optimization of sonic hedgehog delivery to the penis from self-assembling nanofiber hydrogels to preserve penile morphology after cavernous nerve injury. *Nanomed Nanotechnol Biol Med* 2019:102033.
148. Coffman JE, Metz SW, Brackbill A, et al. Optimization of surface display of DENV2 E protein on a nanoparticle to induce virus specific neutralizing antibody responses. *Bioconjug Chem* 2018;**29**(5):1544–52.
149. Kurtanich T, Roos N, Wang G, Yang J, Wang A, Chung EJ. Pancreatic cancer gene therapy delivered by nanoparticles. *SLAS Technol: Trans Life Sci Innovation* 2019;**24**(2):151–60.
150. Girard M, Wang S, Du JS, et al. Particle analogs of electrons in colloidal crystals. *Science* 2019;**364**(6446):1174–8.
151. Champion JA, Katare YK, Mitragotri S. Particle shape: a new design parameter for micro-and nanoscale drug delivery carriers. *J Controlled Release* 2007;**121**(1–2):3–9.
152. Perry JL, Reuter KG, Kai MP, et al. PEGylated PRINT nanoparticles: the impact of PEG density on protein binding, macrophage association, biodistribution, and pharmacokinetics. *Nano Lett* 2012;**12**(10):5304–10.
153. Hartgerink JD, Beniash E, Stupp SI. Peptide-amphiphile nanofibers: a versatile scaffold for the preparation of self-assembling materials. *Proc Natl Acad Sci* 2002;**99**(8):5133–8.
154. Zhang X-Q, Chen M, Lam R, Xu X, Osawa E, Ho D. Polymer-functionalized nanodiamond platforms as vehicles for gene delivery. *ACS Nano* 2009;**3**(9):2609–16.
155. Mayle KM, Dern KR, Wong VK, et al. Polypeptide-based gold nanoshells for photothermal therapy. *SLAS Technol: Trans Life Sci Innovation* 2017;**22**(1):18–25.
156. Barnard AS. Predicting the impact of structural diversity on the performance of nanodiamond drug carriers. *Nanoscale* 2018;**10**(19):8893–910.
157. Hu J, Dong Y, Ng WK, Pastorin G. Preparation of drug nanocrystals embedded in mannitol microcrystals via liquid antisolvent precipitation followed by immediate (on-line) spray drying. *Adv Powder Technol* 2018;**29**(4):957–63.
158. Nie S, Emory SR. Probing single molecules and single nanoparticles by surface-enhanced Raman scattering. *Science* 1997;**275**(5303):1102–6.
159. Mochalin VN, Shenderova O, Ho D, Gogotsi Y. The properties and applications of nanodiamonds. *Nat Nanotechnol* 2012;**7**(1):11.
160. Bari S, Chu PPY, Lim A, et al. Protective role of functionalized single walled carbon nanotubes enhance ex vivo expansion of hematopoietic stem and progenitor cells in human umbilical cord blood. *Nanomed Nanotechnol Biol Med* 2013;**9**(8):1304–16.
161. Huang H, Pierstorff E, Osawa E, Ho D. Protein-mediated assembly of nanodiamond hydrogels into a biocompatible and biofunctional multilayer nanofilm. *ACS Nano* 2008;**2**(2):203–12.
162. Partain B, Unni M, Dobson J, Rinaldi C, Allen K. Quantifying particle distribution in healthy and osteoarthritic rat knee joints using fluorescent imaging and electron paramagnetic resonance spectroscopy. *Osteoarthr Cartil* 2019;**27**:S478–9.
163. Sheikhi A, Hayashi J, Eichenbaum J, et al. Recent advances in nanoengineering cellulose for cargo delivery. *J Controlled Release* 2019;**294**:53–76.
164. Chung EJ, Tirrell M. Recent advances in targeted, self-assembling nanoparticles to address vascular damage due to atherosclerosis. *Adv Healthc Mater* 2015;**4**(16):2408–22.
165. Torchilin VP. Recent advances with liposomes as pharmaceutical carriers. *Nat Rev Drug Discov* 2005;**4**(2):145.
166. Ganta S, Devalapally H, Shahiwala A, Amiji M. A review of stimuli-responsive nanocarriers for drug and gene delivery. *J Controlled Release* 2008;**126**(3):187–204.
167. Akbarzadeh A, Khalilov R, Mostafavi E, et al. Role of dendrimers in advanced drug delivery and biomedical applications: a review. *Exp Oncol,* 2018;**40**(3):178–83.
168. Kapadia CH, Tian S, Perry JL, Luft JC, DeSimone JM. Role of linker length and antigen density in nanoparticle peptide vaccine. *ACS Omega* 2019;**4**(3):5547–55.
169. Chen D, Ganesh S, Wang W, Amiji M. The role of surface chemistry in serum protein corona-mediated cellular delivery and gene silencing with lipid nanoparticles. *Nanoscale* 2019;**11**:8760–75.
170. Hu Y-S, Do J, Edamakanti CR, et al. Self-assembling vascular endothelial growth factor nanoparticles improve function in spinocerebellar ataxia type 1. *Brain* 2019;**142**(2):312–21.

171. Bao Y, Boissenot T, Guegain E, et al. Simple synthesis of cladribine-based anticancer polymer prodrug nanoparticles with tunable drug delivery properties. *Chem Mater* 2016;**28**(17):6266–75.
172. Halbur C, Choudhury N, Chen M, Kim JH, Chung EJ. siRNA-conjugated nanoparticles to treat ovarian cancer. *SLAS Technol: Trans Life Sci Innovation* 2019;**24**(2):137–50.
173. Zhu H, Zhang L, Tong S, Lee CM, Deshmukh H, Bao G. Spatial control of in vivo CRISPR–Cas9 genome editing via nanomagnets. *Nat Biomed Eng* 2019;**3**(2):126.
174. Caudill CL, Perry JL, Tian S, Luft JC, DeSimone JM. Spatially controlled coating of continuous liquid Interface production microneedles for transdermal protein delivery. *J Controlled Release* 2018;**284**:122–32.
175. El-Sawy HS, Al-Abd AM, Ahmed TA, El-Say KM, Torchilin VP. Stimuli-responsive nano-architecture drug-delivery systems to solid tumor micromilieu: past, present, and future perspectives. *ACS Nano* 2018;**12**(11):10636–64.
176. Wang X, Gu M, Toh TB, Abdullah NLB, Chow EK-H. Stimuli-responsive nanodiamond-based biosensor for enhanced metastatic tumor site detection. *SLAS Technol: Trans Life Sci Innovation* 2018;**23**(1):44–56.
177. Petros RA, DeSimone JM. Strategies in the design of nanoparticles for therapeutic applications. *Nat Rev Drug Discov* 2010;**9**(8):615.
178. Zhang X-Q, Xu X, Lam R, Giljohann D, Ho D, Mirkin CA. Strategy for increasing drug solubility and efficacy through covalent attachment to polyvalent DNA–nanoparticle conjugates. *ACS Nano* 2011;**5**(9):6962–70.
179. Lueckheide M, Vieregg JR, Bologna AJ, Leon L, Tirrell MV. Structure–property relationships of oligonucleotide polyelectrolyte complex micelles. *Nano Lett* 2018;**18**(11):7111–7.
180. Lee SS, Fyrner T, Chen F, et al. Sulfated glycopeptide nanostructures for multipotent protein activation. *Nat Nanotechnol* 2017;**12**(8):821.
181. Cheng H, Chabok R, Guan X, et al. Synergistic interplay between the two major bone minerals, hydroxyapatite and whitlockite nanoparticles, for osteogenic differentiation of mesenchymal stem cells. *Acta Biomater* 2018;**69**:342–51.
182. Messersmith PB, Giannelis EP. Synthesis and characterization of layered silicate-epoxy nanocomposites. *Chem Mater* 1994;**6**(10):1719–25.
183. Bang JYR, Ting C, Wang P, et al. Synthesis and characterization of nanodiamond–growth factor complexes toward applications in oral implantation and regenerative medicine. *J Oral Implantol* 2018;**44**(3):207–11.
184. Poon C, Sarkar M, Chung EJ. Synthesis of monocyte-targeting peptide amphiphile micelles for imaging of atherosclerosis. *JoVE (J Vis Exp)* 2017;**129**:e56625.
185. Man HB, Kim H, Kim H-J, et al. Synthesis of nanodiamond–daunorubicin conjugates to overcome multidrug chemoresistance in leukemia. *Nanomed Nanotechnol Biol Med* 2014;**10**(2):359–69.
186. Asadi N, Annabi N, Mostafavi E, et al. Synthesis, characterization and in vitro evaluation of magnetic nanoparticles modified with PCL–PEG–PCL for controlled delivery of 5FU. *Artif Cells Nanomed Biotechnol* 2018;**46**(Suppl. 1):938–45.
187. Satpathy M, Wang L, Zielinski RJ, et al. Targeted drug delivery and image-guided therapy of heterogeneous ovarian cancer using HER2-targeted theranostic nanoparticles. *Theranostics* 2019;**9**(3):778.
188. Fang Y, Huang R-T, Wu D, et al. Targeting dys-regulated mechanotransduction mechanisms in treating arterial and pulmonary vascular diseases by nanomedicine. *FASEB J* 2017;**31**(1_Supplment). 1015.13–15.13.
189. Yang G, Chen Q, Wen D, et al. A therapeutic microneedle patch made from hair-derived keratin for promoting hair regrowth. *ACS Nano* 2019;**13**(4):4354–60.
190. Gloag L, Benedetti TM, Cheong S, et al. Three-dimensional branched and faceted gold–ruthenium nanoparticles: using nanostructure to improve stability in oxygen evolution electrocatalysis. *Angew Chem* 2018;**130**(32):10398–402.
191. Yang M, Zhang M, Nakajima H, Yudasaka M, Iijima S, Okazaki T. Time-dependent degradation of carbon nanotubes correlates with decreased reactive oxygen species generation in macrophages. *Int J Nanomed* 2019;**14**:2797.
192. Ye Y, Wang J, Sun W, Bomba HN, Gu Z. Topical and transdermal nanomedicines for cancer therapy. In: *Nanotheranostics for cancer applications*. Springer; 2019. p. 231–51.
193. Schroeder A, Heller DA, Winslow MM, et al. Treating metastatic cancer with nanotechnology. *Nat Rev Cancer* 2012;**12**(1):39.
194. Smith AH, Robinson EM, Zhang X-Q, et al. Triggered release of therapeutic antibodies from nanodiamond complexes. *Nanoscale* 2011;**3**(7):2844–8.
195. Smith AM, Mohs AM, Nie S. Tuning the optical and electronic properties of colloidal nanocrystals by lattice strain. *Nat Nanotechnol* 2009;**4**(1):56.
196. Huang H, Chen M, Bruno P, et al. Ultrananocrystalline diamond thin films functionalized with therapeutically active collagen networks. *J Phys Chem B* 2009;**113**(10):2966–71.
197. Zha RH, Delparastan P, Fink TD, Bauer J, Scheibel T, Messersmith PB. Universal nanothin silk coatings via controlled spidroin self-assembly. *Biomat Sci* 2019;**7**(2):683–95.
198. Amin DR, Higginson CJ, Korpusik AB, Gonthier AR, Messersmith PB. Untemplated resveratrol-mediated polydopamine nanocapsule formation. *ACS Appl Mater Interfaces* 2018;**10**(40):34792–801.
199. Culver HR, Steichen SD, Herrera-Alonso M, Peppas NA. Versatile route to colloidal stability and surface functionalization of hydrophobic nanomaterials. *Langmuir* 2016;**32**(22):5629–36.
200. Merz V, Lenhart J, Vonhausen Y, Ortiz-Soto ME, Seibel J, Krueger A. Zwitterion-Functionalized detonation nanodiamond with superior protein repulsion and colloidal stability in physiological media. *Small* 2019:1901551.
201. Clemens DL, Lee B-Y, Silva A, et al. Artificial intelligence enabled parabolic response surface platform identifies ultra-rapid near-universal TB drug treatment regimens comprising approved drugs. *PLoS One* 2019;**14**(5):e0215607.
202. Ronen M, Rosenberg R, Shraiman BI, Alon U. Assigning numbers to the arrows: parameterizing a gene regulation network by using accurate expression kinetics. *Proc Natl Acad Sci* 2002;**99**(16):10555–60.
203. Ding X, Liu W, Weiss A, et al. Discovery of a low order drug-cell response surface for applications in personalized medicine. *Phys Biol* 2014;**11**(6):065003.
204. Kaplan S, Bren A, Zaslaver A, Dekel E, Alon U. Diverse two-dimensional input functions control bacterial sugar genes. *Mol Cell* 2008;**29**(6):786–92.

205. Lee B-Y, Clemens DL, Silva A, et al. Drug regimens identified and optimized by output-driven platform markedly reduce tuberculosis treatment time. *Nat Commun* 2017;**8**:14183.
206. Ding X, Njus Z, Kong T, Su W, Ho C-M, Pandey S. Effective drug combination for Caenorhabditis elegans nematodes discovered by output-driven feedback system control technique. *Sci Adv* 2017;**3**(10):eaao1254.
207. Jorgensen WL. Efficient drug lead discovery and optimization. *Acc Chem Res* 2009;**42**(6):724–33.
208. Janes KA, Chandran PL, Ford RM, et al. An engineering design approach to systems biology. *Integr Biol* 2017;**9**(7):574–83.
209. Shoval O, Sheftel H, Shinar G, et al. Evolutionary trade-offs, Pareto optimality, and the geometry of phenotype space. *Science* 2012;**336**(6085):1157–60.
210. Weiss A, Ding X, Van Beijnum JR, et al. A feedback loop optimized vascular targeted drug combination for the treatment of cancer. *Angiogenesis* 2014;**17**(CONF). 725–25.
211. Ma Y, Sun CP, Haake DA, Churchill BM, Ho CM. A high-order alternating direction implicit method for the unsteady convection-dominated diffusion problem. *Int J Numer Methods Fluids* 2012;**70**(6):703–12.
212. Fleury M, Belkina AC, Proctor EA, et al. Increased expression and modulated regulatory activity of coinhibitory receptors PD-1, TIGIT, and TIM-3 in lymphocytes from patients with systemic sclerosis. *Arthritis Rheumatol* 2018;**70**(4):566–77.
213. Edington CD, Chen WLK, Geishecker E, et al. Interconnected microphysiological systems for quantitative biology and pharmacology studies. *Sci Rep* 2018;**8**(1):4530.
214. Clark AM, Wheeler SE, Taylor DP, et al. A microphysiological system model of therapy for liver micrometastases. *Exp Biol Med* 2014;**239**(9):1170–9.
215. Nicolaou CA, Brown N. Multi-objective optimization methods in drug design. *Drug Discov Today Technol* 2013;**10**(3):e427–35.
216. Dekel E, Alon U. Optimality and evolutionary tuning of the expression level of a protein. *Nature* 2005;**436**(7050):588.
217. Nowak-Sliwinska P, Weiss A, Ding X, et al. Optimization of drug combinations using feedback system control. *Nat Protoc* 2016;**11**(2):302.
218. Lee D-K, Chang VY, Kee T, Ho C-M, Ho D. Optimizing combination therapy for acute lymphoblastic leukemia using a phenotypic personalized medicine digital health platform: retrospective optimization individualizes patient regimens to maximize efficacy and safety. *SLAS Technol: Trans Life Sci Innovation* 2017;**22**(3):276–88.
219. Yu H, Zhang WL, Ding X, et al. Optimizing combinations of flavonoids deriving from astragali radix in activating the regulatory element of erythropoietin by a feedback system control scheme. *Evid Based Complement Altern Med* 2013;**2013**.
220. Iliadis A, Barbolosi D. Optimizing drug regimens in cancer chemotherapy by an efficacy–toxicity mathematical model. *Comput Biomed Res* 2000;**33**(3):211–26.
221. Silva A, Lee B-Y, Clemens DL, et al. Output-driven feedback system control platform optimizes combinatorial therapy of tuberculosis using a macrophage cell culture model. *Proc Natl Acad Sci* 2016;**113**(15):E2172–9.
222. Liu Q, Zhang C, Ding X, et al. Preclinical optimization of a broad-spectrum anti-bladder cancer tri-drug regimen via the Feedback System Control (FSC) platform. *Sci Rep* 2015;**5**:11464. https://doi.org/10.1038/srep11464.
223. Weiss A, Ding X, Van Beijnum JR, et al. Rapid optimization of drug combinations for the optimal angiostatic treatment of cancer. *Angiogenesis* 2015;**18**(3):233–44.
224. Wei F, Bai B, Ho C-M. Rapidly optimizing an aptamer based BoNT sensor by feedback system control (FSC) scheme. *Biosens Bioelectron* 2011;**30**(1):174–9.
225. Chen Y, Ho C-M. *Real-time feedback system control technology platform with dynamically changing stimulations*. Google Patents; 2016.
226. Wu S, Lan L, Jiang J, et al. Simultaneous determination of the potent anti-tuberculosis regimen—pyrazinamide, ethambutol, protionamide, clofazimine in beagle dog plasma using LC–MS/MS method coupled with 96-well format plate. *J Pharm Biomed Anal* 2019;**168**:44–54.
227. Weiss A, Berndsen RH, Ding X, et al. A streamlined search technology for identification of synergistic drug combinations. *Sci Rep* 2015;**5**:14508.
228. Al-Shyoukh I, Yu F, Feng J, et al. Systematic quantitative characterization of cellular responses induced by multiple signals. *BMC Syst Biol* 2011;**5**(1):88.
229. Cattaneo D, Merlini S, Pellegrino M, et al. Therapeutic drug monitoring of sirolimus: effect of concomitant immunosuppressive therapy and optimization of drug dosing. *Am J Transplant* 2004;**4**(8):1345–51.
230. Freire E. A thermodynamic approach to the affinity optimization of drug candidates. *Chem Biol Drug Des* 2009;**74**(5):468–72.
231. Lee B-Y, Clemens DL, Silva A, et al. Ultra-rapid near universal TB drug regimen identified via parabolic response surface platform cures mice of both conventional and high susceptibility. *PLoS One* 2018;**13**(11):e0207469.
232. Jaynes J, Zhao Y, Xu H, Ho CM. Use of orthogonal array composite designs to study lipid accumulation in a cell-free system. *Qual Reliab Eng Int* 2016;**32**(5):1965–74.
233. Khemtong C, Kessinger CW, Gao J. Polymeric nanomedicine for cancer MR imaging and drug delivery. *Chem Commun* 2009;(24):3497–510.
234. Berman MA, Guthrie NL, Edwards KL, et al. Change in glycemic control with use of a digital therapeutic in adults with type 2 diabetes: cohort study. *JMIR Diabetes* 2018;**3**(1):e4.
235. Cho C-H, Lee H-J. Could digital therapeutics be a game changer in psychiatry? *Psychiatry Investig* 2019;**16**(2):97.
236. Cho C-H, Lee T, Kim M-G, In HP, Kim L, Lee H-J. Mood prediction of patients with mood disorders by machine learning using passive digital phenotypes based on the circadian rhythm: prospective observational cohort study. *J Med Internet Res* 2019;**21**(4):e11029.
237. Wang H, Lee D-K, Chen K-Y, et al. Mechanism-independent optimization of combinatorial nanodiamond and unmodified drug delivery using a phenotypically driven platform technology. *ACS Nano* 2015;**9**(3):3332–44. https://doi.org/10.1021/acsnano.5b00638.
238. Rashid MBMA, Toh TB, Hooi L, et al. Optimizing drug combinations against multiple myeloma using a quadratic phenotypic optimization platform (QPOP). *Sci Transl Med* 2018;**10**(453). eaan0941.

239. Rashid MBMA, Chow EK-H. Artificial intelligence-driven designer drug combinations: from drug development to personalized medicine. *SLAS Technol: Trans Life Sci Innovation* 2019;**24**(1):124–5.
240. Størset E, Åsberg A, Skauby M, et al. Improved tacrolimus target concentration achievement using computerized dosing in renal transplant recipients—a prospective, randomized study. *Transplantation* 2015;**99**(10):2158.
241. Tolou-Ghamari Z. Nephro and neurotoxicity of calcineurin inhibitors and mechanisms of rejections: a review on tacrolimus and cyclosporin in organ transplantation. *J Nephropathol* 2012;**1**(1):23.
242. Zarrinpar A, Lee D-K, Silva A, et al. Individualizing liver transplant immunosuppression using a phenotypic personalized medicine platform. *Sci Transl Med* 2016;**8**(333). https://doi.org/10.1126/scitranslmed.aac5954. 333ra49–33ra49.
243. Trofe-Clark J, Lemonovich T, Practice AIDCo. Interactions between anti-infective agents and immunosuppressants in solid organ transplantation. *Am J Transplant* 2013;**13**(s4):318–26.
244. Pantuck AJ, Lee DK, Kee T, et al. Modulating BET bromodomain inhibitor ZEN-3694 and enzalutamide combination dosing in a metastatic prostate cancer patient using CURATE. AI, an artificial intelligence platform. *Adv Ther* 2018;**1**(6):1800104.
245. Kee T, Weiyan C, Blasiak A, et al. Harnessing CURATE. AI as a digital therapeutics platform by identifying N-of-1 learning trajectory profiles. *Adv Ther* 2019;**2**:1900023.

Index

'*Note*: Page numbers followed by f indicate figures and t indicate tables.'

F

G

H

I

N

O

P

Q

R

9780128166628